W9-BSZ-270

FIFTH EDITION

Tresch and Aronow's
Cardiovascular Disease
in the Elderly

FIFTH EDITION

Tresch and Aronow's
Cardiovascular Disease
in the Elderly

Edited by

Wilbert S. Aronow, MD

Jerome L. Fleg, MD

Michael W. Rich, MD

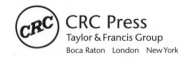

CRC Press
Taylor & Francis Group
Boca Raton   London   New York

CRC Press is an imprint of the
Taylor & Francis Group, an **informa** business

CRC Press
Taylor & Francis Group
6000 Broken Sound Parkway NW, Suite 300
Boca Raton, FL 33487-2742

© 2014 by Taylor & Francis Group, LLC
CRC Press is an imprint of Taylor & Francis Group, an Informa business

No claim to original U.S. Government works

Printed and bound in India by Replika Press Pvt. Ltd.

Printed on acid-free paper
Version Date: 20130503

International Standard Book Number-13: 978-1-84214-543-2 (Hardback)

Visit the Taylor & Francis Web site at
http://www.taylorandfrancis.com

and the CRC Press Web site at
http://www.crcpress.com

Contents

CONTENTS vii

About the editors

Wilbert S. Aronow, MD, FACC, FAHA   Professor of Medicine, Attending Physician, Divisions of Cardiology, Geriatrics, and Pulmonary/Critical Care Medicine, and Director, Cardiology Clinic, Westchester Medical Center/New York Medical College, Valhalla; Senior Associate Program Director, Cardiology Fellowship Program, Westchester Medical Center/New York Medical College; Senior Associate Program Director, and Research Mentor for the Residency and Fellowship Programs, Department of Medicine, Westchester Medical Center/New York Medical College; and Senior Associate Director, Center for Educational Innovations Project Quality Research, Westchester Medical Center/New York Medical College. Dr. Aronow received his MD from Harvard Medical School. He has edited or co-edited 11 books and authored or co-authored 1290 papers and 199 commentaries or Letters to the Editor. Dr. Aronow is a Fellow of the American College of Cardiology, the American Heart Association, the American College of Physicians, the American College of Chest Physicians, the American Geriatrics Society (Founding Fellow of Western Section), the Gerontological Society of America, and the New York Cardiological Society. He has been a member of 78 editorial boards of medical journals, an associate editor for 11 medical journals, and a guest editor for 6 other medical journals. Each year from 2001 to 2012, he has received an outstanding teacher and researcher award from the medical residents and also from the cardiology fellows at Westchester Medical Center/New York Medical College. He has received awards from the Society of Geriatric Cardiology, the Gerontological Society of America, New York Medical College, the Walter Bleifeld Memorial Award for distinguished contributions to clinical research from the International Academy of Cardiology at the 15th World Congress on Heart Disease in July, 2010, and a Distinguished Fellowship Award from the International Academy of Cardiology at the 17th World Congress on Heart Disease in July, 2012.

Jerome L. Fleg, MD, FACC, FAHA   Medical Officer, Division of Cardiovascular Sciences, National Heart, Lung, and Blood Institute, Bethesda, Maryland and Guest Researcher, Laboratory of Cardiovascular Science, Gerontology Research Center, National Institute on Aging, Baltimore, Maryland. Dr. Fleg received his MD from the University of Cincinnati College of Medicine, and has authored over 200 peer-reviewed articles and more than 100 book chapters and reviews related to cardiovascular aging and disease. He serves on multiple journal editorial boards and is an associate editor for the *Journal of Cardiopulmonary Rehabilitation and Prevention*.

Michael W. Rich, MD, FACC, AGSF   Professor of Medicine, Washington University School of Medicine, and Director, Cardiac Rapid Evaluation Unit, Barnes-Jewish Hospital, St. Louis, Missouri. Dr. Rich received his MD from the University of Illinois College of Medicine, Chicago, and he has published over 250 journal articles (11 in 2012) and more than 50 books and book chapters. Dr. Rich is an associate editor for the *American Journal of Medicine* and the *Journal of the American Geriatrics Society*.

Contributors

Philip A. Ades, MD, FACC Fletcher-Allen Health Care, University of Vermont College of Medicine, Burlington, Vermont

Ali Ahmed, MD, MPH, FGSA, FACC, FAHA, FESC University of Alabama at Birmingham and VA Medical Center, Birmingham, Alabama

Melissa M. Anastacio, MD Cardiothoracic Surgery Resident, Department of Cardiothoracic Surgery, University of Pittsburgh Medical Center, Pittsburgh, Pennsylvania

Wilbert S. Aronow, MD, FACC, FAHA Department of Medicine, Divisions of Cardiology, Geriatrics and Pulmonary Critical Care Medicine, New York Medical College, Westchester Medical Center, Valhalla, New York

Hendren Bajillan, MD, MBBS Department of Internal Medicine/Section on Infectious Diseases, Wake Forest School of Medicine, Winston-Salem, North Carolina

Maciej Banach, MD, FAHA, FESC Department of Hypertension, Medical University of Lodz, Poland

Henny H. Billett, MD Division of Hematology, Montefiore Medical Center and Albert Einstein College of Medicine, Bronx, New York

Roger S. Blumenthal, MD The Johns Hopkins Ciccarone Center for the Prevention of Heart Disease, Baltimore, Maryland

Andrew Cassar, MD, MRCP Division of Cardiovascular Diseases, Mayo Clinic College of Medicine, Mayo Clinic, Rochester, Minnesota

Melvin D. Cheitlin, MD Cardiology Division, University of California, San Francisco, California

Angela Cheng-Lai, PharmD, BCPS Department of Pharmacy, Montefiore Medical Center, Bronx, New York

Lovely Chhabra, MD Department of Internal Medicine, Saint Vincent Hospital, University of Massachusetts Medical School, Worcester, Massachusetts

Rose S. Cohen, MD, MSc, FACC Department of Cardiology, Contra Costa Regional Medical Center, Martinez, California

Mark D. Corriere, MD Division of Endocrinology and Metabolism, Johns Hopkins University School of Medicine, Baltimore, Maryland

Samuel C. Durso, MD, MBA Division of Geriatrics and Gerontology, Johns Hopkins University School of Medicine, Baltimore, Maryland

Gregory A. Fishbein, MD   Department of Pathology and Laboratory Medicine, David Geffen School of Medicine at UCLA, Los Angeles, California

Michael C. Fishbein, MD, FACC   Department of Pathology and Laboratory Medicine, David Geffen School of Medicine at UCLA, Los Angeles, California

Jerome L. Fleg, MD, FACC, FAHA   Division of Cardiovascular Sciences, National Heart, Lung, and Blood Institute, National Institutes of Health, Maryland

Lee A. Fleisher, MD, FACC   Department of Anesthesiology and Critical Care, University of Pennsylvania School of Medicine, Philadelphia, Pennsylvania

Stanley S. Franklin, MD, FACC   Heart Disease Prevention Program, Division of Cardiology, University of California, Irvine, California

William H. Frishman, MD, FACC, MACP   Department of Medicine, Division of Cardiology, New York Medical College, Westchester Medical Center, Valhalla, New York

Steven R. Gambert, MD, AGSF, MACP   Department of Medicine, University of Maryland School of Medicine; and UMMC and R Adams Cowley Shock Trauma Center, Baltimore, Maryland

Sarah Goodlin, MD, FACC, FAAHPM   Department of Medicine, Division of General Internal Medicine and Geriatrics, Oregon Health and Science University and Portland Veterans Affairs Medical Center, Portland, Oregon

Kevin P. High, MD, MS, FIDSA   Department of Internal Medicine/Section on Infectious Diseases, Wake Forest School of Medicine, Winston-Salem, North Carolina

David R. Holmes Jr., MD, MACC   Division of Cardiovascular Diseases, Mayo Clinic College of Medicine, Mayo Clinic, Rochester, Minnesota

Laurie G. Jacobs, MD, FACP, AGSF   Division of Geriatrics, Department of Medicine, Montefiore Medical Center and Albert Einstein College of Medicine, Bronx, New York

Rita Rastogi Kalyani, MD, MHS   Division of Endocrinology and Metabolism, Johns Hopkins University School of Medicine, Baltimore, Maryland

Jennifer S. Lawton, MD, FACS   Division of Cardiothoracic Surgery, Department of Surgery, Washington University School of Medicine, St. Louis, Missouri

Andrew J. Litwack, MD   Department of Medicine, Division of Cardiology, University of Pennsylvania, Philadelphia, Pennsylvania

Seth S. Martin, MD   The Johns Hopkins Ciccarone Center for the Prevention of Heart Disease, Baltimore, Maryland

Mathew S. Maurer, MD   Department of Medicine, Division of Cardiology, Columbia University Medical Center; and Clinical Cardiovascular Research Laboratory for the Elderly, Allen Hospital of New York Presbyterian Hospital, New York, New York

John Arthur McClung, MD, FACC   Department of Medicine, Division of Cardiology, New York Medical College, Westchester Medical Center, Valhalla, New York

Myron Miller, MD Department of Medicine, Johns Hopkins University School of Medicine; and Division of Geriatric Medicine, Department of Medicine, Sinai Hospital of Baltimore, Baltimore, Maryland

John E. Morley, MD, BCh Division of Geriatric Medicine, Saint Louis University School of Medicine, St. Louis, Missouri

Vikram Prasanna, MD Department of Medicine, Division of Cardiology, University of Pennsylvania, Philadelphia, Pennsylvania

Michael W. Rich, MD, FACC, AGSF Division of Cardiology, Department of Internal Medicine, Washington University School of Medicine, St. Louis, Missouri

Atsuko Seki, MD The Pathology Division, Clinical Laboratories, National Hospital Organization, Tokyo Medical Center, Tokyo, Japan

Marina Shcherba, MD Division of Hematology, Montefiore Medical Center and Albert Einstein College of Medicine, Bronx, New York

Win-Kuang Shen, MD Mayo Clinic Arizona, Scottsdale, Arizona

David H. Spodick, MD, DSc Department of Cardiovascular Medicine, Saint Vincent Hospital, University of Massachusetts Medical School, Worcester, Massachusetts

Craig Tanner, MD Department of Medicine, Division of General Internal Medicine and Geriatrics, Oregon Health and Science University and Portland Veterans Affairs Medical Center, Portland, Oregon

David M. Tehrani, BS Heart Disease Prevention Program, Division of Cardiology, University of California, Irvine, California

Fernando Tondato, MD Mayo Clinic Arizona, Scottsdale, Arizona

Jesse Weinberger, MD Department of Neurology, Mount Sinai School of Medicine, New York, New York

Nathan D. Wong, MD, PhD, FACC, FAHA Heart Disease Prevention Program, Division of Cardiology, University of California, Irvine, California

Foreword

It is indeed a pleasure to write this foreword for the new 5th edition of *Tresch and Aronow's Cardiovascular Disease in the Elderly*. I wrote the foreword to the 4th edition of this excellent text and was happy to see that the new edition expands and improves on what was already a classic work.

This edition contains much new material: for example, extensive discussion has been added concerning the new antithrombotic agents that became available to US practitioners during the last two years, and a number of chapters have been comprehensively revised with new authors and/or co-authors. Also, a summary has been added at the outset of each chapter in order to facilitate easy reading; important references in the bibliography are highlighted for simplified access, and evidence-based recommendations are suggested as much as possible with strong emphasis on new research findings.

This is truly a lovely book that should be studied by cardiologists throughout the world, given the remarkable increase in the number of elderly patients seeking care in recent years. The editors and authors are to be congratulated for this outstanding contribution to the clinical care and science of elderly patients with cardiovascular disease.

Joseph S. Alpert, MD
University of Arizona College of Medicine
Tucson, Arizona, USA
Editor in Chief
The American Journal of Medicine

Preface

In 2010, the first of the "baby boomers" turned 65 years old. We have now entered a period of explosive growth in the older adult population in the USA, from just over 40 million in 2010 to approximately 73 million by 2030, an increase of over 80%.[1] Concomitantly, the proportion of the populace over age 65 will increase from about 1 in 8 to about 1 in 5. Similar demographic shifts are occurring in many countries around the world. Accompanying this "graying" of the population, there will be a dramatic rise in the number of older persons with clinically manifest—or at risk for developing—cardiovascular disorders, including hypertension, coronary artery disease, valvular heart disease, heart failure, and cardiac rhythm disturbances. Since persons over age 65 already account for more than 80% of all deaths attributable to cardiovascular disease, it will become imperative in the years ahead for all clinicians involved in the care of older adults—not just primary care physicians, geriatricians, and cardiologists, but also surgeons, anesthesiologists, other medical subspecialists, and nurse practitioners—to have a basic understanding of the effects of aging on cardiovascular structure and function, as well as of the impact of aging and prevalent comorbid conditions on the clinical presentation, diagnosis, and response to therapy in older adults with cardiovascular disease.

As with prior editions, the primary objective of the present volume is to provide an up-to-date and in-depth, yet clinically relevant and "readable" overview of the epidemiology, pathophysiology, evaluation, and treatment of cardiovascular disorders in older adults. All chapters have been thoroughly updated by recognized experts to incorporate the most recent knowledge in the field. To the extent possible, clinical recommendations are "evidence based," but it is also acknowledged that existing data are often very limited or nonexistent in the very elderly (persons 85 years of age or older), and especially in older adults with multiple coexisting conditions and/or frailty. Thus, careful consideration of each patient's unique clinical and psychosocial circumstances, medical and nonmedical needs, and personal preferences is required in designing an individualized care plan. Indeed, it is perhaps in the compassionate management of these challenging patients where the "art of medicine" most clearly flourishes.

This edition appears 5 years after the fourth edition, which was released in 2008. During the intervening period, an extensive body of new research relevant to the diagnosis and treatment of cardiovascular disorders in older adults has been published. It is noteworthy that the number of articles posted on Medline at the intersection of "cardiovascular disease" and "age greater than 65 years" increased from 1391 for the three-year period 1997–1999, to 2630 in the interval 2003–2005, and to 3668 from 2009 to 2011—a 2.6-fold increase in the number of citations over a 15-year period. In further recognition of the growing importance of the elderly population in cardiovascular medicine, an increasing number of clinical trials focusing on older adults have been undertaken, practice guidelines are increasingly providing explicit commentary on the diagnosis and management of older adults, and both the American College of Cardiology and the American Heart Association

---

[1]U.S. Census Bureau. Projections of the population by selected age groups and sex for the United States: 2015–2060. Available at: http://www.census.gov/population/projections/data/national/2012.html (accessed December 19, 2012).

have established sections focusing on issues relevant to older adults with cardiovascular disease.

With the fifth edition of this work, the editors have chosen to rename the volume *Tresch & Aronow's Cardiovascular Disease in the Elderly* in honor of the late Donald D. Tresch and the book's senior editor Wilbert S. Aronow, whose vision, pioneering work, and numerous contributions have played a fundamental role in the emergence of geriatric cardiology as a discrete discipline. The total number of chapters has been reduced by one, as one chapter from the fourth edition has been omitted, two chapters have been combined into a single chapter, and one new chapter, "Pericardial Disease in the Elderly," has been added.

We would like to thank all of the contributors for their outstanding work. We also wish to express our gratitude to Claire Bonnett and Emily Pither at CRC Press for their dedication and support in bringing this fifth edition to fruition. Finally, we want to thank you, the reader, for your commitment to providing the best possible care for your older patients with cardiovascular disease. We hope you will find this volume to be a valuable resource as you strive to help your older patients enjoy both longer and fuller lives. We welcome any comments you may have.

Wilbert S. Aronow, MD, FACC, FAHA
Jerome L. Fleg, MD, FACC, FAHA
Michael W. Rich, MD, FACC, AGSF

1

Age-associated changes in the cardiovascular system

Jerome L. Fleg

SUMMARY

Multiple cardiovascular changes occur with advancing age, even in apparently healthy adults. Thickening and stiffening of the large arteries cause systolic blood pressure to rise with age while diastolic blood pressure generally declines after the sixth decade. Modest concentric wall thickening occurs in the left ventricle due to cellular hypertrophy, but cavity size does not change. Whereas left ventricular systolic function is preserved across the age span, early diastolic filling rate declines 30–50% between the third and ninth decades. However, an age-associated increase in late diastolic filling preserves end-diastolic volume. Aerobic exercise capacity declines approximately 10% per decade in cross-sectional studies; in longitudinal studies, this decline is accelerated in the elderly. Reductions in peak heart rate and peripheral oxygen utilization but not stroke volume mediate the age-associated decline in aerobic capacity. Deficits in both cardiac β-adrenergic receptor density and in the efficiency of postsynaptic β-adrenergic signaling contribute significantly to the reduced cardiovascular performance during exercise in older adults. Conduction disorders, including sinus node and atrioventricular dysfunction and bundle branch blocks, and both supraventricular and ventricular arrhythmias become more common with age. The prognostic significance of any arrhythmia or conduction disturbance depends primarily on the presence and severity of associated heart disease. Although many of these cardiovascular aging changes are considered "normative," they lower the threshold for development of cardiovascular disease.

INTRODUCTION

As longevity increases throughout the world, disorders and diseases associated with aging assume increasing importance. In the USA, approximately 13% of the population is 65 years and older; this proportion is expected to reach nearly 20% by the year 2030, comprising over 70 million people (1). Furthermore, the fastest-growing age group, comprising those aged 85 years or older, has quadrupled since 1960 and will reach 19.5 million by 2030 (Fig. 1.1). Because both the prevalence and incidence of cardiovascular (CV) disease increase dramatically with age, this "graying" of the population has created a huge number of elderly patients requiring treatment. It must be emphasized, however, that aging per se is not necessarily accompanied by CV disease. This chapter will set the stage for those that follow by delineating the changes in the CV system, which occur during the aging process in the absence of detectible CV disease. This is a challenging task, given the many factors that blur their separation. Nevertheless, it is important to define normal CV structure and

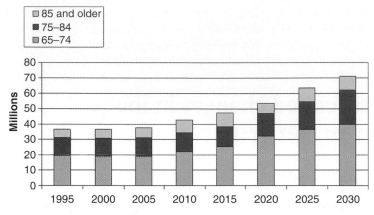
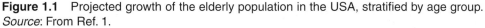

Figure 1.1   Projected growth of the elderly population in the USA, stratified by age group. *Source*: From Ref. 1.

function in older adults to facilitate the accurate diagnosis of CV disease in this rapidly growing age group.

A further goal of this chapter will be to demonstrate how aging changes in the CV system may themselves predispose to the development of CV disease. The enhanced CV risk associated with age indicates important interactions between mechanisms that underlie aging and those that underlie diseases. The nature of these interactions is complex and involves not only mechanisms of aging but also multiple defined and undefined (e.g., genetic) risk factors. Yet quantitative information on age-associated alterations in CV structure and function is essential to define and target the specific characteristics of CV aging, which render it such a major risk factor. Such information is also required to differentiate between the limitations of an elderly person that relate to disease and those that are within expected normal limits.

METHODOLOGICAL ISSUES

Numerous methodological issues must be addressed in attempting to define "normal" aging. Because the population sample from which norms are derived will strongly influence the results obtained, it should be representative of the general population. For example, neither a seniors running club nor nursing home residents would yield an appropriate estimate of maximal exercise capacity that could be applied to the majority of elders. Additionally, the degree of screening used to define a normal population can profoundly influence the results. In clinically healthy older adults, a resting electrocardiogram (ECG), echocardiogram, or exercise perfusion imaging study will often identify silent CV disease, especially coronary artery disease (CAD). If several such screening tests are used, only a small proportion of the older population may qualify as normal, limiting the applicability of findings to the majority of elderly individuals. Furthermore, the inclusion limits chosen for body fatness, blood pressure, smoking status, and other constitutional or lifestyle variables will significantly influence the normal values for measuring CV variables. For example, if a systolic pressure of ≥140 mmHg is considered hypertension, and if hypertension is considered a disease, then individuals with a systolic pressure between 140 and 160 mmHg, who a decade ago were thought to be normotensive, are now identified as having CV disease. Numerous studies have shown that individuals who manifest even modest elevations in systolic and pulse pressures are more likely to develop clinical disease or die from it.

Additional methodological factors can affect the definitions of normal aging. Cross-sectional studies, which study individuals across a wide age range at one time point, may underestimate the magnitude of age-associated changes because, in such studies, older normal persons represent "survival of the fittest." True age-induced changes are better estimated by longitudinal studies, in which given individuals are examined serially over time. A reality of aging research, however, is that most data are derived from cross-sectional studies because they are easier to perform. Even longitudinal studies have their limitations—changes in methodology or measurement drift over time and development of disease in previously healthy persons. Finally, secular trends such as the downward drift in serum cholesterol or increasing obesity of Americans can alter age-related longitudinal changes.

In this chapter, emphasis will be given to data obtained from community dwelling persons screened for the absence of clinical, and in some cases subclinical, CV disease and major systemic disorders. A sizable portion of the data presented derives from studies over the past three decades in community-based volunteers from the Baltimore Longitudinal Study of Aging (BLSA).

UNSUCCESSFUL VASCULAR AGING AS THE "RISKY" COMPONENT OF AGING
Intimal Medial Thickening

Aging changes in the arterial tree of individuals who are considered healthy may have relevance to the exponential age-associated increase in CV disease. Cross-sectional studies in humans have found that wall thickening and dilatation are prominent structural changes that occur within large elastic arteries during aging (2). Postmortem studies indicate that aortic wall thickening with aging consists mainly of intimal thickening, even in populations with a low incidence of atherosclerosis (3). Noninvasive measurements made within the context of several epidemiological studies indicate that the carotid wall intimal medial (IM) thickness increases nearly threefold between 20 and 90 years of age, which is also the case in BLSA individuals rigorously screened to exclude carotid or coronary arterial disease (Fig. 1.2A).

Some investigators believe that the age-associated increase in IM thickness in humans represents an early stage of atherosclerosis (4). Indeed, excessive IM thickening at a given age predicts silent CAD (4). Since silent CAD often progresses to clinical CAD, it is not surprising that increased IM thickness (a vascular endpoint) predicts future clinical CV disease. A plethora of other epidemiological studies of individuals not initially screened to exclude the presence of occult CV disease have indicated that increased IM thickness is an independent predictor of future CV events. Note in Fig. 1.2B that the degree of risk varies with the degree of vascular thickening and that the risk gradation among quintiles of IM thickening is nonlinear, with the greatest risk occurring in the upper quintile (5). Thus, those older persons in the upper quintile of IM thickness may be considered to have aged "unsuccessfully" or to have "subclinical" vascular disease. The potency of IM thickness as a risk factor in older individuals equals or exceeds that of most other, more "traditional," risk factors.

Age-dependent IM thickening has been noted in the absence of atherosclerosis, both in laboratory animals and in humans (3). Thus, the "subclinical disease" of excessive IM thickening is not necessarily "early" atherosclerosis. Rather, "subclinical disease" is strongly correlated with arterial aging. Interpreted in this way, the increase in IM thickness with aging is analogous to the intimal hyperplasia that develops in aortocoronary saphenous vein grafts, which is independent of atherosclerosis, but predisposes for its later development (6). Age-associated endothelial dysfunction, arterial stiffening, and arterial pulse pressure widening can also be interpreted in the same way. Combinations of these processes occurring to varying degrees determine the overall vascular aging profile of a given individual (i.e., the degree of "unsuccessful" vascular aging).

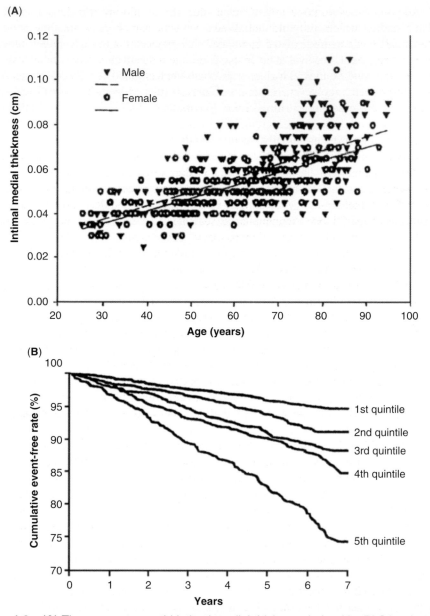

Figure 1.2 (**A**) The common carotid intimal-medial thickness in healthy BLSA volunteers as a function of age. (**B**) Common carotid intimal-medial thickness predicts future cardiovascular events in the Cardiovascular Health Study. *Abbreviation*: BLSA, Baltimore Longitudinal Study of Aging. *Source*: (**A**) from Ref. 4 and (**B**) from Ref. 5.

It is currently believed that additional risk factors (e.g., hypertension, smoking, dyslipidemia, diabetes, diet, or as-yet-unidentified genetic factors) are required to interact with vascular aging (as described above) to activate a preexisting atherosclerotic plaque. According to this view, atherosclerosis that increases with aging is not a specific disease, but an interaction between atherosclerotic plaque and intrinsic features related to vascular aging modulated by atherosclerotic risk factors. Evidence in support of this view comes from studies in which an atherogenic diet caused markedly more severe atherosclerotic lesions in older versus younger rabbits and on human primates despite similar elevations of serum lipids (7,8). Hence, it is possible that atherosclerosis occurring at younger ages may be attributable not only to exaggerated traditional CV risk factors but also to accelerated aging of the vascular wall. Of course, the traditional risk factors may themselves accelerate aging of the vascular wall. Studies in various populations with clinically defined vascular disease have demonstrated that pharmacological and lifestyle (diet, physical activity) interventions can retard the progression of IM thickening (9–14).

Endothelial Dysfunction

The endothelial monolayer that lines the luminal surface of the vascular tree plays a pivotal role in regulating multiple arterial properties, including vessel tone, permeability, response to inflammation, and angiogenesis. Several of these functions undergo important age-associated alterations. Endothelium-derived mediators such as nitric oxide (NO) and endothelin-1 are determinants of arterial tone and compliance, suggesting that endothelial cells may modulate arterial stiffness. Brachial arterial flow-mediated dilation, mediated in large part by NO, declines with age in both sexes, even in the absence of other CV risk factors (15). A decline of ~75% in this flow-mediated vasodilation occurs in men between the ages of 40 and 70 years. This decline begins approximately a decade later in women, perhaps because of the protective effect of estrogen, but is nearly 2.5 times as steep compared with men (15). The impairment of endothelial-mediated vasodilatation with aging in humans can be partially reversed by L-arginine administration, suggesting that NO production becomes reduced with aging (16). Plasma levels of asymmetric dimethyl arginine, which reduces NO synthase (NOS) activity, also increase with age in humans (16). Age-associated changes in endothelial cell integrity, shape, and surface characteristics affect the cell's physical and chemical barrier, increasing endothelial permeability, leading to aberrant macromolecular transport (17). In contrast to endothelium-mediated vasodilation, the vasodilator response to sublingual nitroglycerin is unrelated to age (15).

Several CV risk factors and disorders are associated with endothelial dysfunction, including hypertension, hypercholesterolemia, insulin resistance, cigarette smoking, CAD, and heart failure. Furthermore, impaired endothelial vasoreactivity, in both the coronary and peripheral arterial beds, is an independent predictor of future CV events (18,19). Hypertensive individuals exhibit endothelial dysfunction (20,21), and the mechanisms underlying their endothelial dysfunction are similar to those that occur with normotensive aging, albeit they appear at an earlier age (21). The normotensive offspring of hypertensives also exhibits endothelial dysfunction (22), suggesting that endothelial dysfunction may precede the development of clinical hypertension. Age-associated endothelial dysfunction, arterial stiffening, and IM thickening are risk factors for arterial diseases, even after accounting for other risk factors, such as arterial pressure, plasma lipids, smoking, etc. The interaction between arterial wall stiffening and CV diseases may set in motion a vicious cycle. In this cycle, alterations in the mechanical properties of the vessel wall contribute to endothelial cell dysfunction and, ultimately, to arterial stiffening.

Arterial Stiffness and Compliance

The increase in arterial wall thickening and reduction in endothelial function with advancing age are accompanied by an increase in arterial stiffening and a reduction in compliance. Age-associated structural changes in the arterial media that increase vascular stiffness include increased collagen content, covalent cross-linking of the collagen, reduced elastin content, elastin fracture, and calcification (23,24). In addition, there is a substantial increase in angiotensin II levels and augmented angiotensin II signaling in aged arterial walls, which may play a pivotal role in arterial aging, given the potent pressor and mitogenic effects of angiotensin II. Strictly speaking, stiffness and its inverse, distensibility, depend on intrinsic structural properties of the blood vessel wall that relate pressure change with a corresponding change in volume.

Pulse Wave Velocity

Each systolic contraction of the ventricle generates a pressure wave that propagates centrifugally down the arterial tree, slightly preceding the luminal flow wave generated during systole. The propagation velocity of this wave is proportional to the stiffness of the arterial wall. The velocity of the pulse wave in vivo is determined not only by the intrinsic stress/strain relationship (stiffness) of the vascular wall but also by the smooth muscle tone, which is reflected by the mean arterial pressure.

Noninvasive measures of the velocity of this pulse wave allow for large-scale epidemiological studies to examine its determinants and prognostic importance. In both rigorously screened normal subjects (25) and populations with varying prevalence of CV disease (26,27), a significant age-associated increase in pulse wave velocity (PWV) has been observed in men and women (Fig. 1.3A). In contrast to central arteries, the stiffness of muscular arteries does not increase with advancing age (28). Thus, the manifestations of arterial aging may vary among the different vascular beds, reflecting differences in the structural compositions of the arteries and, possibly, differences in the age-associated signaling cascades that modulate the arterial properties, or differences in the response to these signals across the arterial tree.

Increased PWV has traditionally been linked to structural alterations in the vascular media, such as those observed with aging. Prominent age-associated increases in PWV have been demonstrated in populations with little or no atherosclerosis, again indicating that these vascular parameters are not necessarily indicative of atherosclerosis (29). However, the data emerging from epidemiological studies indicate that increased large vessel stiffening also occurs in the context of atherosclerosis (30,31), metabolic syndrome (32), and diabetes (33,34). The link may be that stiffness is governed not only by the structural changes within the matrix, as noted above, but also by endothelial regulation of vascular smooth muscle tone and other aspects of vascular wall structure/function. Thus, there is evidence of a vicious cycle: altered mechanical properties of the vessel wall facilitate the development of atherosclerosis, which in turn increases arterial stiffness via endothelial cell dysfunction and other mechanisms.

Reflected Pulse Waves

In addition to the forward pulse wave, each cardiac cycle generates a reflected wave, originating at areas of arterial impedance mismatch, which travels back up the arterial tree toward the central aorta, altering the arterial pressure waveform. This reflected wave can be noninvasively assessed from recordings of the carotid (25) or radial (35) arterial pulse waveforms by arterial applanation tonometry and high-fidelity micromanometer probes. Dividing the late systolic augmentation of the arterial pulse wave by the distance from the peak to the trough of the arterial waveform (corresponding to the pulse pressure) yields the augmentation index (24). The augmentation index, like the PWV, increases with age (Fig. 1.3B) (24,25).

The velocity of the reflected flow wave is proportional to the stiffness of the arterial wall. Thus, in young individuals whose vascular wall is compliant, the reflected wave does not reach the large elastic arteries until diastole. With advancing age and increasing arterial stiffening, the velocity of the reflected wave increases, and the wave reaches the central circulation earlier in the cardiac cycle, during the systolic phase. The pressure pulse augmentation provided by the early return of the reflected wave is an added load against which the aged ventricle must contract. Furthermore, the diastolic augmentation seen in

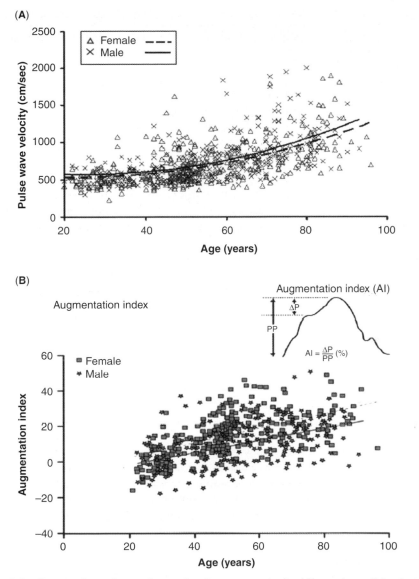

Figure 1.3 Scatterplots of aortofemoral pulse wave velocity (**A**), and carotid artery augmentation index (**B**) as a function of age in healthy non-endurance trained BLSA volunteers. A similar age-associated increase in both measures of arterial stiffness was seen in men and women. *Abbreviation*: BLSA, Baltimore Longitudinal Study of Aging. *Source*: Adapted from Ref. 25.

compliant vessels, caused by the late return of the reflected waves, is lost in the elderly, decreasing diastolic blood pressure; this decrease in diastolic pressure has the potential to reduce coronary blood flow because most coronary flow occurs during diastole.

Multiple studies (27,36–43) indicate that increased vascular stiffness, over and above blood pressure, is an independent predictor of hypertension, atherosclerosis, CV events, and mortality. Kaess et al. (38) and others have demonstrated that increased vascular stiffness precedes the development of hypertension. Thus, while a "secondary" increase in large artery stiffness is attributable to an increase in mean arterial pressure that occurs in

Table 1.1   Relationship of Cardiovascular Human Aging in Health to Cardiovascular Disease

Age-Associated Changes	Plausible Mechanisms	Possible Relation to Human Disease
Cardiovascular structural remodeling		
⇑ Vascular intimal thickness	⇑ Migration of and ⇑ matrix production by VSMC	Early stages of atherosclerosis
	Possible derivation of intimal cells from other sources	
⇑ Vascular stiffness	Elastin fragmentation ⇑ Elastase activity	Systolic hypertension
	⇑ Collagen production by VSMC and ⇑ cross-linking of collagen	Stroke
	Altered growth factor regulation/ tissue repair mechanisms	Atherosclerosis
⇑ LV wall thickness	⇑ LV myocyte size	Retarded early diastolic cardiac filling
	⇓ Myocyte number (necrotic and apoptotic death)	⇑ Cardiac filling pressure
	Altered growth factor regulation Focal collagen deposition	Lower threshold for dyspnea
⇑ Left atrial size	⇑ Left atrial pressure/volume	⇑ Prevalence of lone atrial fibrillation
Cardiovascular functional changes		
Altered regulation of vascular tone	⇓ NO production/effects	Vascular stiffening; hypertension
	⇓ β-AR responses	
⇓ Cardiovascular reserve	⇑ Vascular load	Lower threshold for, and increased severity of, heart failure
	⇓ Intrinsic myocardial Contractility	
	⇓ β-Adrenergic modulation of heart rate, myocardial contractility, and vascular tone	
Reduced physical activity	Learned lifestyle	Exaggerated age Ds in some aspects of cardiovascular structure and function; negative impact on atherosclerotic vascular disease, hypertension, and heart failure

Abbreviations: VSMC, vascular smooth muscle cell; LV, left ventricular; NO, nitric oxide; β-AR, β-adrenergic receptor.

hypertension, evidence now exists that a "primary" increase in large artery stiffness that accompanies aging gives rise to an elevation of arterial pressure. Normotensive individuals who fall within the upper quartile for measures of arterial stiffness are more likely to subsequently develop hypertension. Observations such as these reinforce the concept that hypertension, at least in part, is a disease of the arterial wall. The mechanisms of age-associated changes in vascular structure and function and the putative relationship of these changes to development of CV disease are depicted in Table 1.1.

Systolic, Diastolic, and Pulse Pressure
Arterial pressure is determined by the interplay of peripheral vascular resistance and arterial stiffness; the former raises both systolic and diastolic pressure to a similar degree,

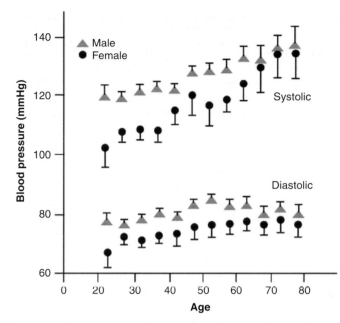

Figure 1.4 Change in blood pressure with age in healthy men (triangles) and women (circles) from the Baltimore Longitudinal Study of Aging. *Source*: From Ref. 44.

whereas the latter raises systolic but lowers diastolic pressure. A rise in average systolic blood pressure across adult age has been well documented (Fig. 1.4) (43,44). In contrast, average diastolic pressure was found to rise until about 50 years of age, level off from age 50 to 60, and decline thereafter (43,44). Thus, pulse pressure (systolic minus diastolic), a useful hemodynamic indicator of conduit artery vascular stiffness, increases with age. These age-dependent changes in systolic, diastolic, and pulse pressures are consistent with the notion that in younger people blood pressure is determined largely by peripheral vascular resistance, whereas in older individuals it is determined to a greater extent by central conduit vessel stiffness.

Because of the decline in diastolic pressure in older men and women in whom systolic pressure is increased, isolated systolic hypertension emerges as the most common form of hypertension in individuals over the age of 50 years (43). Isolated systolic hypertension, even when mild in severity, is associated with an appreciable increase in CV disease risk (45,46). On the basis of long-term follow-up of middle-aged and older subjects, however, Framingham researchers have found pulse pressure to be a better predictor of coronary disease risk than systolic or diastolic blood pressures (47). A subsequent Framingham investigation found that pulse pressure was especially informative of coronary risk in older subjects (48) because of the "J"- or "U"-shaped association between diastolic pressure and coronary risk. Thus, consideration of the systolic and diastolic pressures jointly, as reflected in pulse pressure, is preferable to consideration of either value alone.

INTERVENTIONS TO RETARD OR PREVENT ACCELERATED ARTERIAL AGING
Although the deleterious effects of aging on arterial structure and function may appear inevitable from the discussion above, it is noteworthy that the age increases in systolic and pulse pressures are markedly blunted in hunter-gatherer and forager-farmer societies

(49). Furthermore, increasing evidence is accruing that lifestyle modifications, including aerobic exercise, and dietary modifications, including reduction in sodium intake, caloric restriction, or weight loss, can prevent or retard the progression of IM thickening (50,51) or arterial stiffening (52,53) and improve endothelial function (54–57). Perhaps, the most promising of these modifications is caloric restriction, which may prolong maximal lifespan in laboratory animals when begun in youth or middle age. Limited studies in individuals have demonstrated decreases in CV risk factors and inflammatory markers with caloric restriction (51,58). In one study, 25 individuals aged 53 ± 12 years who had practiced voluntary caloric restriction of ~30% for an average of 6.5 years showed markedly lower blood pressure and inflammatory markers compared with controls matched for age and gender (58). In addition, the calorie restricted group demonstrated higher transmitral early diastolic flow measures, similar to those of younger adults (58). Whether such beneficial effects can be derived by initiating caloric restriction at older ages remains unknown.

Pharmacological interventions can also favorably modulate the elements of arterial aging. In animal models, chronic angiotensin-converting enzyme inhibition or angiotensin receptor blockade, begun at an early age, markedly delays the progression of age-associated arterial remodeling, for example, the IM thickening and rupture of internal elastic lamina (59,60), attenuates mitochondrial dysfunction, reduces reactive oxygen species, enhances NO bioavailability, reduces fibrosis, retards vascular and cardiac aging, and prolongs life (61–67). It is thus far unproven if such treatment can prevent or retard unsuccessful aging of the vasculature in animals or humans of younger to middle age who exhibit excessive subclinical evidence of accelerated arterial aging. Studies have shown that breaking nonenzymatic collagen cross-links with a novel thiazolium agent reduces arterial stiffness, both in nonhuman primates (68) and in humans (69).

CARDIAC STRUCTURE AND RESTING FUNCTION

Before the advent of echocardiography, autopsy was essentially the only method for obtaining reliable measurements of cardiac structure in normal persons. Such studies were obviously flawed by their inherent selection bias. A large autopsy series by Linsbach et al. (70) in 7112 patients demonstrated an increase in cardiac mass of 1–1.5 g/yr between the ages of 30 and 90 years. Because the study included individuals with CV disease, the age-associated increase in heart weight may derive, at least in part, from the development of cardiac pathology. An autopsy study of 765 normal hearts from persons 20 to 99 years old who were free from both hypertension and CAD showed that heart weight indexed to body surface area was not age related in men but increased with age in women, primarily between the fourth and seventh decades (71). In autopsies of hospitalized patients without evidence of CV disease, Olivetti et al. (72) observed an age-associated reduction of left ventricular (LV) mass mediated by a decrease in estimated myocyte number, although myocyte enlargement occurred with age. These investigators subsequently found a higher prevalence of apoptotic myocytes in older male than in female hearts, which paralleled a decline of LV mass with age in men but not in women (73).

The widespread application of echocardiography starting in the 1970s finally allowed accurate noninvasive assessment of age changes in cardiac structure and function. In healthy normotensive BLSA men, Gerstenblith et al. (74) observed a 25% increase in echocardiographic LV posterior wall thickness between the third and eighth decades, a finding replicated by others (75,76). Because LV diastolic cavity size was not significantly age related in the BLSA (64), calculated LV mass also increased substantially with age. Thus, an apparent discrepancy existed between the unchanged or decreased LV mass with age seen at autopsy and the increase in LV wall thickness and calculated LV mass observed by echocardiography. A study in BLSA volunteers using cardiac magnetic resonance imaging (MRI) to estimate LV mass helped to resolve these divergent findings (77). Unlike standard echocardiography, which provides one- and two-dimensional measurements, MRI assesses LV size in three dimensions. In 136 men and 200 women without CV disease, MRI-derived LV wall thickness increased with age (Fig. 1.6, upper panels), and short-axis diastolic dimension was not age related, similar to earlier echocardiographic findings. In contrast, LV length declined with age in both sexes (i.e., the LV became more spherical) (77). Thus, MRI-derived LV mass was unrelated to age in women and demonstrated an age-associated decline in men (because of their lesser age-related increase in wall thickness), similar to autopsy findings (73). Three-dimensional echocardiography has confirmed this preservation of LV mass across age in women and a reduction of LV mass in older men (78). In 5004 healthy volunteers from the CARDIA study, cardiac MRI revealed age-related declines in both LV diastolic and systolic volumes and increase in the LV mass/volume ratio in both sexes (79). With advancing age, therefore, the normal LV becomes thicker and more spherical.

Although the mechanisms for the age-associated remodeling of the LV and increase in myocyte size are not clear, they may be adaptive responses to the arterial changes that accompany aging. Putative stimuli for cardiac cell enlargement with age are an increase in vascular load due to arterial stiffening and a stretching of cells due to dropout of neighboring apoptotic myocytes (80,81). Phenotypically, the age-associated increase in LV thickness resembles the LV hypertrophy (LVH) that develops from hypertension. This finding, coupled with the increase in systolic blood pressure that occurs over time even in healthy individuals, has led to consideration of aging as a muted form of hypertension. In older rodent hearts, which demonstrate a similar increase in LV mass and myocyte size as observed in humans, a stretching of cardiac myocytes and fibroblasts releases growth factors such as angiotension II, a known stimulus for apoptosis. As a result, the heart becomes stiffer, that is, less compliant, with age. In addition, enhanced secretion of atrial natriuretic (82) and opioid (83) peptides is observed.

Echocardiographic aortic root diameter dilates modestly with age, approximating 6% in BLSA men between the fourth and eighth decades (74). Similarly, the aortic knob diameter increased from 3.4 to 3.8 cm on serial chest X rays over 17 years (84). In addition, the aortic arch lengthens with age due to arch widening (85). Both greater aortic diameter and arch length were independently associated with higher aortic arch PWV and LV mass. Such aortic root dilation and lengthening provide an additional stimulus for LVH because the larger volume of blood in the proximal aorta represents a greater inertial load that must be overcome before LV ejection can begin.

Echocardiographic LV shortening fraction (74) and radionuclide LV ejection fraction (86,87), the two most common measures of global LV systolic performance, are unaffected by age at rest in healthy normotensive persons. Because LV stroke volume (SV) is the difference of LV end-diastolic volume (EDV) and end-systolic volume (ESV), the supine resting LV stroke volume is also unrelated to age (87). Prolonged contractile activation of the thickened LV wall (88) maintains a normal ejection time in the presence of the late systolic augmentation of aortic impedance, preserving systolic cardiac pump function at rest. However, a "downside" of prolonged contractile activation is that at the time of the mitral valve opening, myocardial relaxation is less complete in older than in younger individuals, contributing to a reduced early LV filling rate.

In contrast to the preservation of resting LV systolic performance across the adult age span, LV diastolic performance is profoundly altered by aging. Reduced mitral valve E–F closure slope on M-mode echocardiography first documented these age changes in diastolic performance (74,75). Pulsed Doppler (89) and radionuclide (90) techniques

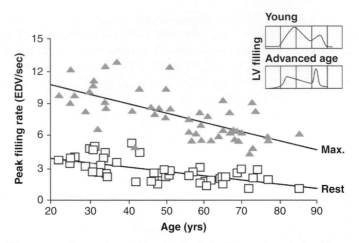

Figure 1.5 Changes with age in peak early diastolic filling rates derived from radionuclide ventriculography at rest and during maximal upright cycle ergometry. The inset shows the transmitral flow velocity profile derived from Doppler echocardiography in a young and older adult. Note the shift from a dominant early (E) filling wave in the young to a dominant late (A) filling wave in the elderly. *Source*: Adapted from Ref. 90.

confirmed that the transmitral early diastolic peak-filling rate declined by ~50% between the ages of 20 and 80 years (Fig. 1.5). Conversely, peak A-wave velocity, which represents late LV filling facilitated by atrial contraction, increases with age. This greater atrial contribution to LV filling is accomplished via a modest age-associated increase in left atrial size demonstrable on echocardiography. Tissue Doppler and color M-mode techniques, both less influenced by preload and afterload than pulsed Doppler, have confirmed the age-associated reduction in early diastolic filling rate and increased late filling (91). Because the resting LV EDV is preserved across adult age in BLSA volunteers, the augmented atrial contribution to LV filling in older adults can be considered a successful adaptation to the reduced early diastolic filling rate in the thicker, and presumably stiffer, senescent LV. Thus, the relative importance of early and late diastolic LV filling is reversed with advanced age.

Impairment of early LV filling with age may derive in part from reduced LV diastolic compliance due to the increase in LV wall thickness with age. An age-associated reduction in ventricular compliance has been shown in animals. Studies in man have confirmed an age-associated reduction in LV compliance, which was minimally changed in older adults after a full year of endurance training (92). In both intact animal hearts and isolated cardiac muscle, studies have demonstrated prolonged isovolumic relaxation and increased myocardial diastolic stiffness. The slower isovolumic relaxation observed in cardiac muscle from older animals (93) may be secondary to diminished rate of Ca^{2+} accumulation by the sarcoplasmic reticulum (94). A conceptual framework for the cardiac adaptations to age-associated arterial stiffening is shown in Figure 1.6.

Whereas the diminished early diastolic filling rate with age may not compromise resting EDV or stroke volume, an underlying reduction of LV compliance might cause a greater rise in LV diastolic pressure in older persons, especially during stress-induced tachycardia, thus causing a lower threshold for dyspnea than in the young. It might also be anticipated that the loss of atrial contribution to LV filling that occurs during atrial fibrillation would elicit a greater deterioration of diastolic performance in older than in younger individuals. Indeed, it is attractive to speculate that the frequent occurrence of heart failure

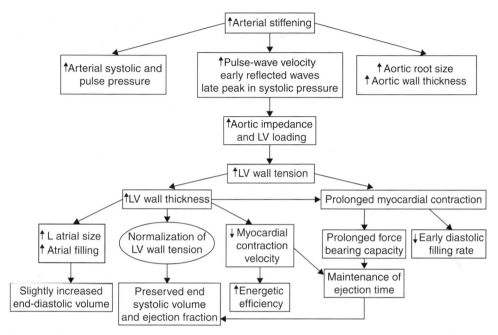

Figure 1.6   Conceptual framework for the cardiovascular adaptations to arterial stiffening that occur with aging. *Abbreviation*: LV, left ventricular.

in the elderly despite preserved LV systolic function derives, at least in part, from the age-associated impairment of early diastolic filling (Table 1.1).

Given the considerable difficulty in imaging the right ventricle by echocardiography, information regarding aging changes in right ventricular (RV) structure and function has been very limited. However, cardiac MRI can provide such information. In 4204 MESA participants aged 45–84 years who were free of clinical CV disease, cardiac MRI showed declines in both RV mass and volumes but a modest increase in RV ejection fraction with age (95). RVEDV, mass and ejection fraction were positively related to systolic blood pressure and inversely related to diastolic blood pressure. The pulmonary arteries also appear to undergo age-associated remodeling, resulting in increased pulmonary artery (PA) stiffness and PA systolic pressure. In 1413 Olmsted County, Minnesota, residents ≥45 years old, PA systolic pressure estimated by Doppler echocardiography increased modestly from 26 ± 4 mmHg in persons 45–54 years old to 30 ± 6 mmHg in those 72–96 years old. Higher PA systolic pressure was an independent mortality predictor [hazard ratio (HR) 1.46 per 10 mmHg] (96). Healthy subjects have shown an exaggerated rise in PA systolic and mean pressures with age during cycle ergometry (97).

CV Physical Findings in Older Adults
Several age-associated alterations in CV structure and function may manifest themselves during the CV examination. Because of the stiffening of the large arteries, systolic blood pressure is often elevated with a normal or low diastolic blood pressure. Therefore, the carotid artery upstroke is usually brisk in the elderly and may mask significant aortic valve stenosis. The apical cardiac impulse may be difficult to palpate secondary to senile emphysema and chest wall deformities. Respiratory splitting of the second heart sound is audible in only ~30–40% of individuals older than 60 years, presumably because of reduced compliance of the pulmonary vasculature. In contrast, an S4 gallop is commonly heard in older but not younger persons because of the age-associated increase in late diastolic filling

mediated by vigorous atrial contraction into a thicker-walled, less compliant LV. A soft basal ejection murmur occurs in 30–60% of the elderly. This murmur is thought to arise from a dilated, tortuous aorta or from sclerosis of the aortic valve.

CV RESPONSE TO STRESS

In clinical medicine, the CV response of older adults to stress (e.g., to increases in arterial pressure, to postural maneuvers, or to physical exercise) is of considerable interest. First, physicians are often called upon to provide advice and information concerning the CV potential of the elderly (e.g., the effect or importance of conditioning status on the maintenance of function). Second, the CV response to stress is important in assessing the ability of older individuals to respond to disease states. Third, the CV response to stress has considerable value in the diagnosis and management of patients with CV disease. Despite the high prevalence of CV disease among older Americans, it is important to understand the exercise capabilities of CV disease-free elders. Exercise testing is a diagnostic tool that is frequently utilized to detect and quantify the severity of CV disease. The value of such diagnostic tests and the validity of their interpretation clearly depend on precise information regarding the normal limits of such stress testing procedures relative to age.

Orthostatic Stress

Perturbations from the supine, basal state activate CV reflex mechanisms and mediate the utilization of CV reserve function. The result of these reflex mechanisms is enhanced blood flow to, and preservation of arterial pressure within, selected body organs. In response to a change from supine to upright posture, an increase in systemic vascular resistance maintains the mean arterial pressure. A change in blood flow from the heart depends on the product of changes in heart rate and LVSV, the latter being determined by the changes in EDV and end-systolic volume index (ESVI). Changes in EDV are determined, in part, by changes in venous return, which depends on the ability of the blood to flow through the vascular system, and to changes in ESV.

In healthy, community-dwelling elders, arterial pressure changes little with the assumption of upright posture, and postural hypotension or acute orthostatic intolerance (i.e., dizziness or fainting when assuming an upright from a supine position or during a passive tilt) is uncommon. Orthostatic hypotension (OH), defined by a decline of systolic blood pressure by ≥20 mmHg or diastolic blood pressure by ≥10 mmHg, occurred in 16% of volunteers aged 65 years and older from the Cardiovascular Health Study (CHS) (98) and in 7% of men aged 71–93 years from the Honolulu Heart Program (99); in both of these older cohorts, the prevalence of OH increased with age. In the former study, OH was associated with higher supine blood pressure, greater LV wall thickness, and smaller LV cavity size (100). In the latter study, OH was an independent predictor for mortality (relative risk [RR] = 1.64), and there was a linear relationship between the magnitude of orthostatic decline in systolic blood pressure and 4-year mortality rate (99). In contrast to healthy, community-dwelling older volunteers, OH and orthostatic intolerance are common in debilitated institutionalized elders with chronic illnesses. Within such populations, the likelihood for OH is increased among individuals who exhibit very low LV filling rates and small EDV and SV in the supine position (101). In such individuals, however, the effects of advanced age cannot be dissociated from those of profound deconditioning and multiple diseases and medications.

With advancing age, the acute heart rate increase to orthostatic stress decreases in magnitude and takes longer to achieve. The baroreceptor sensitivity (i.e., the slope of the relationship of the change in heart rate versus the change in arterial pressure) is negatively correlated with age and resting arterial pressure (102). The low-pressure baroreceptor, or cardiopulmonary reflex, also decreases with age in normotensives, but not in hypertensives.

Despite the lesser heart rate increase during orthostatic stress in older than in younger BLSA volunteers, the SVI reduction tends to be less in the older group; thus, the postural change in cardiac output does not vary significantly with age, because a lesser reduction in SV balances the lesser increase in heart rate in older individuals (103). Similarly, studies have found cardiac output to be reduced with age in the supine position because of a reduced SV in older versus younger men; this age effect was abolished in the sitting position because of lesser reduction in SV in the older men on sitting. Responses to gradual tilt or to graded lower body negative pressure in older individuals are similar to responses to change in body position: SV and cardiac output decrease less in older adults, offsetting their blunted heart rate increase (104). A lesser reduction in SV in older versus younger individuals following a postural stress implies either a smaller reduction in EDV or a greater reduction in ESV in older individuals. Reduced venous compliance in older versus younger individuals is a potential mechanism for a lesser peripheral fluid shift during orthostatic maneuvers, and could preserve cardiac filling volume and maintain SV in the upright position in healthy elderly individuals (105). A reduction in the venodilatory response to β-adrenergic stimulation with preservation of the α-adrenergic vasoconstrictor response may contribute to a reduced venous compliance with aging.

Pressor Stress

Acute increases in blood pressure represent another common CV stress. Sustained, isometric handgrip increases both arterial pressure and heart rate. The response varies in magnitude in proportion to the relative level and duration of effort. After sustained submaximal or maximal handgrip, heart rate was observed to increase more in younger than in older healthy individuals, whereas blood pressure increased more in older persons (106,107). In BLSA volunteers, 3 minutes of submaximal sustained handgrip elicited mild increases in echocardiographic LV diastolic and systolic dimensions and atrial filling fraction; these increases correlated positively with age (107). Thus, pressor stress accentuated the age-associated dependence on late diastolic filling.

Application of a pressor stress has also been used to assess the intrinsic myocardial reserve capacity. In healthy BLSA individuals, a 30 mmHg increase in systolic blood pressure induced by phenylephrine infusion in the presence of β-adrenergic blockade induced significant echocardiographic LV dilatation at end diastole in healthy older (60–68 years), but not in younger (18–34 years), men: the cardiac dilatation occurred in older men despite a smaller reduction in heart rate (108), analogous to the handgrip response. Thus, an apparent age-associated decrease in intrinsic myocardial contractile reserve occurs in response to an acute increase in afterload; the senescent heart dilates to preserve SV via the Frank–Starling mechanism.

Aerobic Exercise Capacity and Aging

The ability to perform oxygen-utilizing (i.e., aerobic) activities is a fundamental requirement of independent living and is probably the best-studied CV stressor. The accepted standard for aerobic fitness is maximum oxygen consumption rate (VO_2max), the product of cardiac output (the central component) and arteriovenous oxygen difference (the peripheral component). In healthy adults, VO_2max is up to 15 times greater than VO_2 at rest. This is accomplished by a four- to fivefold increase in cardiac output and up to a threefold widening of the arteriovenous oxygen difference; the latter is due to both a dramatic increase in the relative proportion of cardiac output delivered to working muscles and an increased oxygen extraction by these muscles. Because the total body VO_2max is strongly influenced by muscle mass, VO_2max is typically compared across individuals by normalizing for body weight.

Numerous studies have documented that treadmill VO_2max, adjusted for body weight, declines with age. In cross-sectional studies, the decline typically approximates 50% across the adult age span (109,110). However, the extent of the VO_2max decline with aging varies among studies, depending on age ranges, differences in body weight and composition, and differences in habitual physical activity among the individuals studied. Longitudinal studies generally report a more pronounced age-associated decline in VO_2max than do cross-sectional studies. In BLSA volunteers rigorously prescreened to exclude CV or lung disease, VO_2max declines by ~50% between the third and ninth decades by cross-sectional analysis (Fig. 1.7) (109,110).

Cross-sectional studies, such as those in Figure 1.7, are usually interpreted to indicate that VO_2max declines linearly with age. A more detailed analysis in this same population, however, demonstrated that the longitudinal decline in aerobic capacity is not constant across adulthood as assumed by cross-sectional studies, but accelerates markedly with successive age decades, especially in men, regardless of physical activity levels

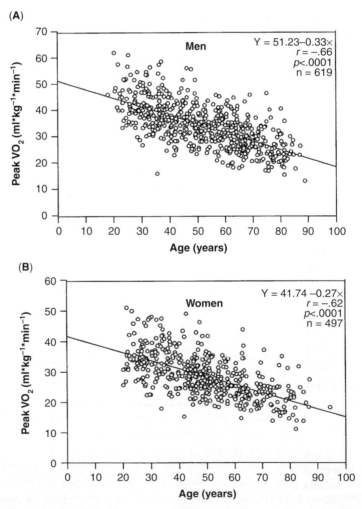

Figure 1.7   Cross-sectional declines in peak VO_2 per kg body weight in healthy BLSA men and women. *Abbreviation*: BLSA, Baltimore Longitudinal Study of Aging. *Source*: From Ref. 110.

(Fig. 1.8) (111). When the components of VO_2max were examined, the longitudinal decline in oxygen pulse (VO_2 per heart beat) mirrored that of VO_2max, whereas maximal heart rate decreased only 4–6% per decade regardless of starting age (Fig. 1.8). Although age-associated loss of muscle mass and increase in body fat also contribute to the reduction in VO_2max with aging, the pattern of accelerated VO_2max decline with age persists even after normalizing it for fat-free mass rather than body weight (111). Despite the similar rates of decline in VO_2max with age regardless of physical activity level, it should be emphasized that at any age the more active quartiles maintain a higher VO_2 max than their sedentary peers.

The accelerated decline of aerobic capacity has important implications regarding functional independence and quality of life. One should bear in mind that the data in healthy BLSA volunteers represent a "best-case scenario." The superimposition of CV or

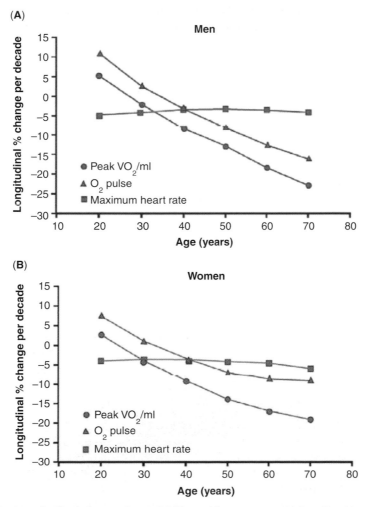

Figure 1.8 Longitudinal change in peak VO_2 and its components (maximal heart rate and O_2 pulse) in healthy BLSA volunteers. In both sexes, the decline in maximal heart rate is only ~5% per decade and is relatively constant across age. However, the decline in O_2 pulse, encompassing both stroke volume and peripheral oxygen delivery and utilization, declines more rapidly in older adults, paralleling the decline in peak VO_2. *Abbreviation*: BLSA, Baltimore Longitudinal Study of Aging. *Source*: Adapted from Ref. 111.

pulmonary disease as well as the deconditioning commonly seen in the elderly because of their sedentary lifestyle accentuate this decline in VO$_2$max. Because activities of daily living typically require a fixed aerobic expenditure, they require a significantly larger percent of VO$_2$max in an older than a younger person. Once the energy required of an activity approaches or exceeds the aerobic capacity of an elderly individual, the individual will likely be unable to perform it. Thus, it is not surprising that a low aerobic capacity comprises one of the five components of the "frailty phenotype" (112).

Another potential contributor to exercise intolerance with aging is a greater metabolic debt incurred during exercise that persists during recovery. For several minutes after a bout of aerobic exercise, the body continues to consume oxygen at a higher rate than at rest. This "oxygen debt" incurred during recovery can comprise 14–20% of the total aerobic expenditure. In one study, the VO$_2$ consumed by healthy older persons during recovery from exercise exceeded that in the young by more than 30% (113). Although the precise causes of this greater VO$_2$ use during recovery in the elderly is unclear, increased circulating catecholamine levels (114) and a higher core temperature that occur during exercise and early recovery in deconditioned older adults (115) may be contributory.

Because of the difficulty in imaging the heart during treadmill exercise, cycle ergometry has been used to dissect the relative contributions of cardiac factors in the age-associated decline in aerobic capacity (Table 1.2). During upright cycle ergometry, the peak VO$_2$ of healthy BLSA participants averages about 80% of that during treadmill exercise, regardless of age. The primary factor limiting the duration and intensity of cycle exercise is usually leg fatigue. Peak cycle work rate and VO$_2$ decline by ~50% between ages 20 and 90 years in healthy, nonathletic BLSA men and women, attributable to declines of ~30% in cardiac output and 20% in arteriovenous oxygen difference (Table 1.2) (116).

The age-associated decrease in cardiac index at maximal effort during upright cycle exercise (Fig. 1.9F) is due entirely to a reduction in heart rate (Fig. 1.9E), as the LVSVI does not decline with age in either gender (Fig. 1.9D) (114). However, the manner in which SVI is achieved during maximal exercise varies dramatically with aging. Although older

Table 1.2 Changes in Maximal Aerobic Capacity and Its Determinants Between Ages 20 and 80 Years in Healthy Volunteers

Oxygen consumption	⇓ (50%)
(A-V)O$_2$ difference	⇓ (20%)
Cardiac output	⇓ (30%)
Heart rate	⇓ (25%)
Stroke volume	no Δ
Preload	
EDV	⇑ (30%)
Afterload	⇑
Vascular (SVR)	⇑ (30%)
Cardiac (ESV)	⇑ (275%)
Cardiac (EDV)	⇑ (30%)
Contractility	⇓ (60%)
Ejection fraction	⇓ (15%)
Plasma catecholamines	⇑
Cardiac and vascular	⇓
Responses to β-adrenergic stimulation	

Abbreviations: AV, arteriovenous; EDV, end-diastolic volume; ESV, end-systolic volume; SVR, systemic vascular resistance.

individuals have a blunted capacity to reduce ESVI (Fig. 1.9B) and to increase ejection fraction (Fig. 1.9C), this deficit is offset by a larger end-diastolic volume index (EDVI) (Fig. 1.9A) (117). Thus, a "stiff heart" that prohibits sufficient filling between beats during exercise does not characterize aging in healthy individuals. The larger EDVI in healthy older versus younger individuals during vigorous aerobic exercise is due in part to a longer diastolic interval (i.e., slower heart rate) and to a greater amount of blood remaining in the heart at end systole (Fig. 1.9B) (117).

Given the accelerated decline in VO$_2$max with age, an important question is whether aerobic training of sedentary older adults can improve their CV reserve capacity. It has been amply documented that physical conditioning of older persons can substantially increase

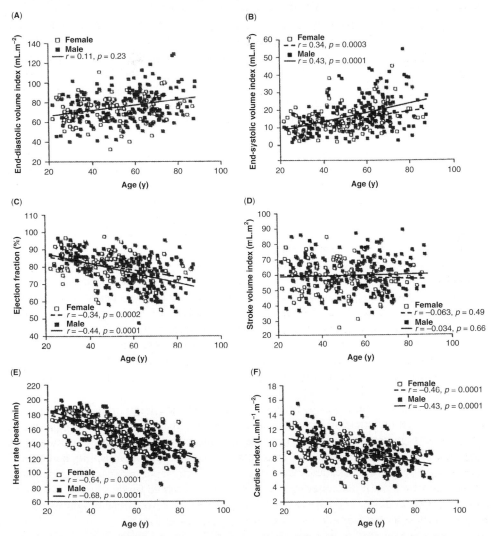

Figure 1.9 Scatter plots of left ventricular volumes (**A, B**), ejection fraction (**C**), stroke volume (**D**), heart rate (**E**), and cardiac index (**F**) during maximal graded upright cycle exercise in healthy BLSA volunteers, carefully screened to exclude silent coronary artery disease. Note the similar age changes in men and women and the increasing heterogeneity with age in the end-systolic volume index, ejection fraction, and heart rate. *Abbreviation*: BLSA, Baltimore Longitudinal Study of Aging. *Source*: Adapted from Ref. 117.

their maximum aerobic work capacity. In a meta-analysis of 41 trials in 2102 individuals aged 60 and older, aerobic training elicited a 16.3% mean increase in VO_2max (118). The extent to which this conditioning effect results from enhanced central cardiac performance versus augmented peripheral mechanisms, including changes in skeletal muscle mass, varies with the characteristics of the population studied, the type and degree of conditioning achieved, gender, body position during study, and likely genetic factors.

A longitudinal study of older men during upright cycle ergometry indicates that aerobic training enhances VO_2max in part by increases in the maximum cardiac output due to augmented maximum SV and in part by increasing the arteriovenous oxygen difference (119). The augmentation of maximum SV is due primarily to an augmented reduction of LVESV and, thus, a concomitant increase in LV ejection fraction; however, conditioning status had minimal effect on LVEDV during exercise in older adults. This contrasts with the effect of physical conditioning in younger persons, which substantially increases EDV and SV on the basis of the Frank–Starling mechanism, as well as via an enhanced LV ejection fraction. In contrast to the improved LV ejection post-training, the maximal heart rate of older (as well as younger) persons does not vary with conditioning status. Thus, physical conditioning of older persons does not appear to offset the age-associated deficiency in sympathetic modulation. Rather, increased LV ejection from aerobic training in this age group appears to derive from the reduction in vascular afterload, as reflected in a reduced PWV (120) and carotid augmentation index, with possible contribution from augmented maximum intrinsic myocardial contractility. Furthermore, aerobic training in sedentary older adults reduced their oxygen debt immediately post-exercise by nearly 30%, translating into an 18% increase in exercise efficiency; in contrast, efficiency did not change in younger persons after training (113).

MECHANISMS OF IMPAIRED LV EJECTION DURING MAXIMAL AEROBIC EXERCISE IN HEALTHY OLDER ADULTS

The ejection fraction at maximal exercise and its increase from rest are sometimes used clinically as a diagnostic tool to detect and quantify the severity of cardiac disease, particularly CAD. Exercise ejection fraction is thus of considerable clinical interest. The impaired ability of healthy older men and women to reduce LVESV during vigorous exercise accounts for their smaller increase in ejection fraction from rest and their lower maximal value compared to younger individuals (Fig. 1.9C) (117). A blunted LV ejection fraction response during exercise is even more prominent in older individuals with exercise-induced silent myocardial ischemia than in those without evident ischemia, due to a more pronounced inability to reduce ESVI (121).

The underlying mechanisms for the age-associated reduction in maximum ejection fraction are multifactorial and include (*i*) a reduction in intrinsic myocardial contractility, (*ii*) an increase in vascular afterload, (*iii*) arterial-ventricular load mismatching, and (*iv*) a diminished effectiveness of the autonomic modulation of both LV contractility and arterial afterload. Although these age-associated changes in CV reserve per se are insufficient to produce clinical heart failure, they appear to lower the threshold for developing symptoms and signs of heart failure and adversely influence its clinical severity and prognosis for any level of disease burden (Table 1.1).

Myocardial Contractility

How aging affects factors that regulate intrinsic myocardial contractility in humans is incompletely understood because the effectiveness of intrinsic myocardial contractility in the intact circulation is difficult to separate from loading and autonomic modulatory influences on contractility. Given that the heart rate per se is a determinant of the myocardial contractile state, a deficit in maximal intrinsic contractility of older persons might be expected on the basis of their reduced maximum heart rate. Supporting evidence for reduced LV contractility with aging during stress comes from a study in which the LV of older but not younger healthy BLSA men dilated at end diastole in response to a given increase in afterload during β-adrenergic blockade (108).

Myocardial systolic stiffness or elastance, one index of LV contractile performance, is best approximated by the slope of the end-systolic pressure (ESP) on ESV coordinates measured across a range of EDVs at rest; this slope cannot be accessed during exercise. A single point depicting ESP/ESV as a contractility index at each overall CV level of performance presents an age-associated pattern of myocardial contractile reserve that is nearly identical to the age-associated change in the pattern of ejection fraction in Figure 1.9C (117).

LV Afterload

Cardiac afterload has two components: one generated by the heart itself and the other by the vasculature. The cardiac component of afterload during exercise can be expected to increase slightly with age because the heart size increases in older persons throughout the cardiac cycle during exercise (117). The vascular load on the heart has four components: conduit artery compliance characteristics, reflected pulse waves, resistance, and inertance. Inertance is determined by the mass of blood in the large arteries that requires acceleration prior to LV ejection. As the central arterial diastolic diameter increases with aging (26,74), the inertance component of afterload likely increases. Thus, each of the pulsatile components of vascular load, measured at rest, increases with age.

Augmented LV afterload in older versus younger persons during exercise likely plays a major role in the failure of the acute LVESV reserve with advancing age. However, the extent to which the age-associated increases in afterload at rest becomes more pronounced during exercise is not known with certainty. Whereas the exaggerated cardiac dilation from the resting level that occurs during vigorous exercise in healthy older individuals suggests an exercise-induced increase in cardiac afterload, it has not been possible to noninvasively assess PWV, augmentation index, aortic diameter, or impedance during exercise. Although some indices of afterload, such as arterial pressure and systemic vascular resistance, have been determined during exercise, their levels are confounded by the decrease in maximum exercise capacity that occurs with age.

Arterial/Ventricular Load Matching

Optimal ejection of blood from the heart occurs when ventricular and vascular loads are matched. The precise cardiac and vascular load matching that is characteristic of younger persons is thought to be preserved at older ages, at least at rest, because the increased vascular stiffness in older persons at rest is matched by increased resting ventricular stiffness (122).

For the ejection fraction to increase during exercise, the LV end-systolic elastance (ELV), i.e., the ESP/ESV ratio, must increase to a greater extent than the effective vascular elastance (EA), i.e., ESP/stroke volume. With increasing age, however, ELV fails to increase in proportion to the increase in EA; hence, the EA/ELV during exercise in older persons decreases to a lesser extent than it does in younger persons (123). This altered arterial/ventricular load matching in older versus younger persons during exercise is a mechanism for the deficit in the acute LV ejection fraction reserve that typically accompanies advancing age. Thus, the LV ejection fraction, often considered a measure of LV pump function, is determined by both cardiac and vascular properties, each of which changes with age.

Acute pharmacological reduction in both cardiac and vascular components of LV afterload by sodium nitroprusside infusions in older, healthy BLSA volunteers augments

LV ejection fraction in these subjects at rest and throughout upright cycle exercise (124). Because of concomitant reductions in preload and afterload during sodium nitroprusside infusion, the LV of older persons delivers the same stroke volume and cardiac output as prior to infusion while working at a smaller size. In another study, acute infusion of the calcium channel blocker verapamil, which reduced exercise afterload but not preload, improved LV ejection and oxygen utilization during submaximal exercise in healthy older volunteers (122).

Sympathetic Modulation

During acute exercise and other stresses, sympathetic modulation of the CV system increases heart rate, augments myocardial contractility and relaxation, reduces LV afterload, and redistributes blood to working muscles and skin to dissipate heat. All of the factors that have been identified to play a role in the deficient CV regulation with aging—that is, heart rate, afterload (both cardiac and vascular), myocardial contractility, and redistribution of blood flow—exhibit a deficient sympathetic modulatory component.

Sympathetic Neurotransmitters

Apparent deficits in sympathetic modulation of cardiac and arterial functions with aging occur in the presence of elevated neurotransmitter levels. Plasma levels of norepinephrine and epinephrine, during any perturbation from the supine basal state, increase to a greater extent in older than in younger healthy humans (83,114). This increase appears to be a compensatory response to the reduced cardiac β-receptor density with advancing age (125). The age-associated increase in plasma levels of norepinephrine results from an increased cardiac spillover into the circulation and, to a lesser extent, to reduced plasma clearance. Deficient norepinephrine reuptake at nerve endings has been suggested as the primary mechanism for increased spillover. During prolonged submaximal exercise, however, diminished neurotransmitter reuptake might also be associated with reduced release and spillover in older adults (126), contributing to the age-associated deficit in cardioacceleration and LV systolic performance seen during such an exercise (127).

Deficits in Cardiac β-Adrenergic Receptor Signaling

The age-associated increase in neurotransmitter spillover into the circulation during acute stress implies a greater heart and vascular receptor occupancy by these substances. Experimental data indicate that this condition leads to desensitization of the postsynaptic signaling components of sympathetic modulation. The deficits in β-adrenergic signaling with aging are attributable in part to reduction in β-receptor numbers, deficient G-protein coupling of receptors to adenyl cyclase and, possibly, to age-associated reductions in the amount or activation of adenyl cyclase, leading to a relative reduction in the ability to augment cellular cyclic adenosine monophosphate (cAMP) in response to β-receptor stimulation in the older heart.

Numerous studies support the concept that the efficiency of postsynaptic β-adrenergic signaling declines with aging (125). One line of evidence derives from the observation that acute β-AR blockade changes the exercise hemodynamic profile of younger persons to resemble that of older ones. Thus, the reduction in heart rate during exhaustive aerobic exercise in the presence of acute β-adrenergic blockade is greater in younger than in older subjects, and significant β-adrenergic blockade–induced LV dilatation occurs only in the younger group (128). In addition, the age-associated deficits in early LV diastolic filling rate, both at rest and during exercise, are abolished by acute β-adrenergic blockade (89). However, acute β-adrenergic blockade causes SVI to increase to a greater extent in younger than in older individuals, due in part to the greater increase in LV filling time in the young, caused by greater reduction in their maximal heart rate (128).

When perspectives from intact humans to subcellular biochemistry in animal models are integrated, a diminished responsiveness to β-adrenergic modulation is among the most consistently observed CV changes that occur with advancing age. Age-associated alterations in CV function that exceed the identified limits for healthy elderly individuals most likely represent interactions of aging per se with severe physical deconditioning and/or CV disease, both of which are highly prevalent among older adults.

RELEVANT AGING CHANGES IN OTHER ORGAN SYSTEMS

Because of the close relationships between the CV system and other organs, it is important to recognize some of the more salient non-CV changes that occur with age. In the lungs, loss of elastic recoil causes reduced emptying and thus reduced vital capacity and minute ventilation during vigorous exercise. Plasma and total blood volumes decline moderately with age. Age-related loss of skeletal muscle mass, termed sarcopenia, is paralleled by reduced muscle strength, a major cause of disability and reduced quality of life in the elderly. A similar loss of bone occurs with age and is exacerbated by estrogen deficiency in postmenopausal women, leading to a marked increase in fracture risk. Additionally, age-associated nephrosclerosis results in loss of renal parenchyma and reductions in renal plasma flow, creatinine clearance, plasma rennin activity, and plasma aldosterone. These renal changes decrease the elimination of renally excreted drugs, attenuate responses to sodium restriction and volume expansion, and increase the risk for hyperkalemia. Although creatinine clearance typically declines by ~50% between the third and ninth decades, serum creatinine changes minimally because of the parallel loss of muscle mass.

ELECTROCARDIOGRAPHY AND ARRHYTHMIAS
Conduction System

The cardiac conduction system undergoes multiple changes with age that affect its electrical properties and, when exaggerated, cause clinical disease. A generalized increase in elastic and collagenous tissue commonly occurs. Fat accumulates around the sinoatrial node, sometimes creating partial or complete separation of the node from the atrial tissue. In extreme cases, this may contribute to the development of sick sinus syndrome. A pronounced decline in the number of pacemaker cells generally occurs after age 60; by age 75, less than 10% of the number seen in young adults remain. A variable degree of calcification of the left side of the cardiac skeleton, which includes the aortic and mitral annuli, the central fibrous body, and the summit of the interventricular system, is observed. Because of their proximity to these structures, the atrioventricular (AV) node, AV bifurcation, and proximal left and right bundle branches may be damaged or destroyed by this process, resulting in AV or intraventricular block.

ELECTROCARDIOGRAPHY

Alterations in cardiac anatomy and electrophysiology with age often manifest themselves on the ECG. Because the resting EGG remains the most widely used cardiac diagnostic test, a review of these aging changes is relevant to distinguish them from those imposed by disease.

Sinus Node Function

Whereas supine resting heart rate is unrelated to age in most studies (Fig. 1.10, upper panel), the phasic variation in R–R interval known as respiratory sinus arrhythmia declines with age (129,130). Similarly, a reduced prevalence of sinus bradycardia on resting ECG is evident by the fourth decade (126). Because both sinus arrhythmia and sinus bradycardia are indices of cardiac parasympathetic activity, the age-associated reduction in parasympathetic

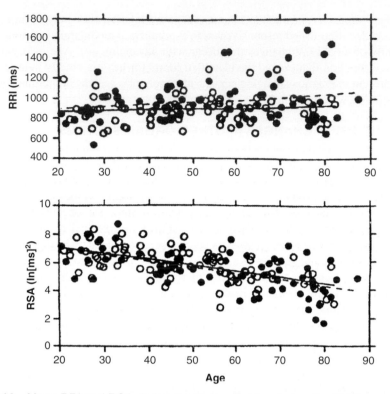

Figure 1.10 Mean RRI and RSA during 3 minutes of sitting in healthy BLSA men (closed circles and dashed line) and women (open circles and solid line). Whereas RRI (top) was unrelated to age in either sex, RSA (bottom) declined similarly with age in women ($r = 0.61$; $p < .001$) and men ($r = 0.59$; $p < .001$). *Abbreviations*: BLSA, Baltimore Longitudinal Study of Aging; RRI, RR interval; RSA, respiratory sinus arrhythmia. *Source*: From Ref. 132.

function (130) may mediate both findings. Spectral analysis of heart rate variability has confirmed an age-related reduction of high frequency (0.15–0.45 Hz) oscillations indicative of vagal efferent activity (Fig. 1.10, lower panel) (131,132). Although physical conditioning status influences autonomic tone, a cross-sectional study in BLSA volunteers demonstrated that the deconditioning that usually accompanies the aging process plays only a minor role in the age-associated blunting of these high-frequency oscillations (132). Patients with organic heart disease demonstrate a reduced respiratory sinus arrhythmia compared to age-matched normal individuals. A blunting of high-frequency oscillations in apparently healthy older volunteers is predictive of future coronary events (133) and total mortality (134). Time domain indices of heart rate variability also decline substantially with age; the pattern of decline varies with the specific time domain measure (135). Younger men generally display higher time domain indices than younger women, but this gender difference narrows or disappears at older ages. In a Swiss population of healthy persons aged 50 years and older, CV risk factors, such as hypertension, smoking, non-high-density lipoprotein cholesterol, and C-reactive protein, were each associated with reduced heart rate variability during 24-hour ECG recordings (136).

On the resting ECG, sinus bradycardia below 50 bpm was found in 4.1% of 1172 healthy, non-endurance-trained, unmedicated participants aged 40 years and older from the BLSA; the prevalence was similar in men (3.9%) and women (4.5%) (137). Individuals with unexplained sinus bradycardia (mean age 58 years) had a significantly greater prevalence of associated conduction system abnormalities than nonbradycardic age- and sex-matched controls, but there was no difference in the incidence of future coronary events [angina pectoris, myocardial infarction (MI), or cardiac death] over a 5.4-year mean follow-up period (137). Sinus bradycardia due to sick sinus syndrome is seen almost exclusively in the elderly and probably derives in part from the marked decline in the number of pacemaker cells in the sinoatrial node. In the absence of organic heart disease, such bradycardia is not associated with increased cardiac mortality (137,138).

P Waves

Paralleling the echocardiographic increase in left atrial size, the prevalence of left atrial abnormality, defined by a negative P terminal force in lead V_1 of at least 0.04 mm/s, increases with age. Among 588 institutionalized elderly, such a P terminal force was only 32% sensitive, although 94% specific, for echocardiographic left atrial enlargement (139). A small increment in P-wave duration of about 8 ms from the third to seventh decades has been observed (140), presumably secondary to the modest increase in left atrial size. There does not appear to be any increase in ECG evidence of right atrial enlargement with age when individuals with significant chronic obstructive lung disease are excluded.

P–R Interval

With advancing age, the P–R interval undergoes a modest but significant prolongation (141–143). In a database of 46,129 persons with very low probability of CV disease, mean P–R interval increased from 148 to 166 ms in women and from 153 to 182 ms in men between the third and ninth decades (141). An increase in P–R interval from 159 to 175 ms in men and from 156 to 165 ms in women occurred between the ages of 30 and 72 years in BLSA volunteers (142). By high resolution signal-averaged surface ECGs, the prolongation of AV conduction was localized proximal to the His bundle deflection, but within the P–R segment, presumably reflecting delay within the AV junction. In seven older men with first-degree AV block, there was a similarly located but more pronounced AV junctional delay (142). Using the conventional upper limit of 0.20 seconds, the prevalence of first-degree AV block in healthy older men is usually 3–4%, a prevalence several-fold greater than in young men (143). To reflect the age-associated slowing of AV conduction, a value of 0.22 seconds has been proposed for the upper limit of normal P–R interval in persons over 50 years of age (143). Although earlier studies found no correlation between first-degree AV block and cardiac disease (144) or mortality (145), 20-year follow-up of Framingham volunteers showed increased risks of atrial fibrillation, pacemaker implantation, and all-cause mortality associated with PR prolongation, even within the normal range (146).

QRS Complex

Although the QRS duration shows no significant age relationship, the QRS axis shifts progressively leftward with age. In the database of 46,129 normals, there was a shift in the mean QRS axis from 56 degrees to 8 degrees between the third and ninth decades, with no gender difference (141). The corresponding lower normal limits shifted from –30 to –60 degrees. Thus, the prevalence of left-axis deviation of less than –30 degrees increases dramatically with age, reaching 20% by the tenth decade (147). This leftward QRS axis shift may be largely due to the age-related increase in LV wall thickness (74,75). Longitudinal studies have failed to demonstrate any increase in cardiac morbidity or mortality associated with this isolated ECG finding (148,149). In patients with known organic heart disease, however, left or right bundle branch block (BBB) portends a worse CV prognosis if left-axis deviation is present (150).

Cross-sectional (151) and longitudinal (152) studies have demonstrated a decrease in R- and S-wave amplitudes with advancing age, evident by the fourth decade. At first glance, this decrease in QRS amplitude seems paradoxical, given the age-related increase in LV thickness. However, the surface ECG is influenced by extracardiac as well as cardiac factors. By increasing the distance between the heart and the chest wall, senile kyphosis and pulmonary hyperinflation in older individuals may contribute to a decrease of QRS voltage.

Despite the age-related decline in mean QRS amplitude, the prevalence of electrocardiographic LVH increases with age (153), probably secondary primarily to the high prevalence of hypertension, CAD, and degenerative aortic valvular disease in the elderly. Echocardiographic studies have demonstrated that the standard ECG is quite insensitive, although very specific, for anatomical LVH in older populations (154). In the Framingham study (153,154) and other older cohorts (155), ECG evidence of LVH was strongly related to the presence of hypertension and was a potent independent risk factor for future CV morbidity and mortality. Thus, the presence of ECG criteria for LVH in an older individual should normally trigger further diagnostic assessment, particularly echocardiography.

Left and right BBBs both increase in prevalence with age (156–158); nevertheless, these conduction defects should not be attributed to aging per se. In older populations, left BBB occurs only about half as often as right BBB. In contrast to its right-sided counterpart, left BBB is uncommon in the absence of CV disease (155). The prognosis of left BBB therefore reflects that of the underlying heart disease. Whereas left BBB portended a more ominous prognosis than right BBB in Framingham men, the two conduction defects had similar prognostic significance in women (156,157). Among 310 predominantly middle-aged individuals with BBB and no apparent heart disease, both left BBB and right BBB increased in prevalence with age, but neither was associated with increased total mortality over a 9.5-year mean follow-up (159). A nonspecific intraventricular conduction defect exceeding 120 ms occurred in only 1.9% of Framingham participants aged 70 years and older and, like left BBB, was strongly associated with clinical heart disease (160).

Complete right BBB was observed in 39 of 1142 men (3.4%) in the BLSA (161). Among the 24 individuals (mean age 64 years) without evidence of heart disease and for whom follow-up information was available, the incidence of angina, nonfatal MI, heart failure, advanced heart block, or cardiac death did not differ from those in age-matched controls over a mean observation period of 8.4 years. At long-term follow-up, maximal exercise capacity and maximal heart rate were similar to those of controls, although a higher prevalence of left-axis deviation was found in the group with right BBB (46% vs. 15%, respectively) (161). These findings suggest that right BBB in the absence of clinical heart disease is not rare in older men and reflects a primary abnormality of the cardiac conduction system.

Q waves in two or more contiguous ECG leads are generally considered evidence of prior MI. In older, as in younger, populations, such Q waves are usually associated with clinical heart disease and increased cardiac mortality. Indeed, pathological Q waves may serve as the initial clue to the presence of CAD. Prior studies have shown that 25–30% or more of acute infarctions are clinically silent (162–164). The incidence of such "silent" infarctions increases strikingly with age. Aronow et al. (160) reported that 68% of infarctions were silent in a geriatric chronic care facility. Despite the absence of symptoms, these silent MIs portend a long-term risk of mortality similar to their symptomatic counterparts.

Among the elderly, Q waves commonly occur in the absence of CAD. A QS complex in leads 3 and a VF may occasionally result from marked left-axis deviation. A pattern of poor R-wave progression in leads V_1 to V_3 is a normal age trend, because of the decrease in the initial 20 ms anterior QRS vector with age (143). Such a pattern may also result from obesity, chronic obstructive lung disease, and LVH, all of which are common in older populations.

Repolarization

Abnormalities involving the ST segment and T wave probably constitute the most prevalent age-associated findings on the ECG. In a study of 671 persons aged 70 years and older, nonspecific ST–T changes were the most common ECG abnormalities, occurring in 16% of individuals (158). In this sample and others, repolarization abnormalities were generally associated with clinical heart disease. Such an association may stem in part from the frequent use of digitalis and various antiarrhythmic drugs by elderly cardiac patients. Much of the reported increased risk attached to these nonspecific repolarization changes is undoubtedly due to the underlying heart disease that necessitated use of these cardiac medications. Even among clinically healthy older persons, however, minor ST-segment sagging or straightening is relatively common, although of questionable prognostic significance.

A decrease in the T-wave amplitude with age begins by the fourth decade (143,151). The spatial T-wave vector shifts leftward with age in concert with the leftward shift in ORS axis. Obesity magnifies these changes in the T waves, especially in men (143). The isolated presence of flattened T waves, particularly in lead a VL, does not portend increased CV risk, at least in middle-aged adults (165). In contrast, definite T-wave inversion usually occurs in patients with organic heart disease and is associated with increased mortality.

In the huge database of Mason et al. (141), the mean heart rate-corrected Q–T interval increased from 409 to 418 ms in women and from 391 to 407 ms in men between the third and the sixth decades. The prognostic significance of prolonged Q–T interval in apparently healthy older adults is controversial. Although no association between QTc prolongation and either sudden cardiac death or total mortality was found in the Framingham study (166), positive associations were reported in the CHS (167) and the Zutphen (168) and Rotterdam (169) studies. In the latter study, a QTc >456 ms in men and >470 ms in women was associated with a 2.5-fold increased risk of sudden death after adjustment for multiple CV risk factors (170). This risk was increased eightfold in persons younger than the mean age of 68 years, but only twofold in older individuals. Increased Q–T-interval dispersion, defined as the difference between the maximum and minimum QTc among the ECG leads, was also associated with a doubled risk of sudden death in this cohort (171). Table 1.3 summarizes those changes in resting ECG measurements thought to be secondary to normative aging.

Table 1.3 Normal Age-Associated Changes in Resting ECG Measurements

Measurement	Change with Age	Effect on Mortality
R–R interval	No change	
P-wave duration	Minor increase	None
P–R interval	Increase	None
QRS duration	No change	
QRS axis	Leftward shift	None
QRS voltage	Decrease	None
Q–T interval	Minor increase	Probable increase
T-wave voltage	Decrease	None

ARRHYTHMIAS

An increase in the prevalence and complexity of both supraventricular and ventricular arrhythmias, whether detected by resting ECG, ambulatory monitoring, or exercise testing, is a hallmark of normal human aging.

Atrial Arrhythmias

Isolated premature atrial ectopic beats (AEB) appear on the resting ECG in 5–10% of individuals older than 60 years and are not generally associated with heart disease. Isolated AEB were detected in 6% of healthy BLSA volunteers older than 60 years at rest, in 39% during exercise testing, and in 88% during ambulatory 24-hour monitoring (172). Such isolated AEB on ambulatory monitoring, even if frequent, were not predictive of increased cardiac risk in this sample over a 10-year mean follow-up period (173). Among 1372 predominantly healthy persons ≥65 years old in the CHS, isolated AEB were found in 97% and were frequent in 18% of women and 28% of men (Table 1.4) (174).

Atrial Fibrillation

Atrial fibrillation (AF) is found in approximately 3–4% of subjects over age 60 years (Table 1.4), a rate 10-fold higher than the general adult population (174,175); the prevalence in octogenarians approaches 10% (176). Chronic AF is most commonly due to CAD and hypertensive heart disease, mitral valvular disorders, thyrotoxicosis, and sick sinus syndrome. The association between hyperthyroidism and AF is observed almost exclusively in the elderly (177); this arrhythmia may be the sole clinical manifestation of so-called apathetic hyperthyroidism in geriatric patients. In the Framingham population, AF without identifiable cause, so-called lone AF, represented 17% of men and 6% of women with AF, with mean ages of 70.6 and 68.1 years, respectively (178). Individuals with lone AF suffered over four times as many strokes as those in sinus rhythm during long-term follow-up, although their rates of coronary events or congestive heart failure were not increased (178). Atrial flutter is a rare arrhythmia in any age group and is usually associated with organic heart disease.

Several age-associated physiological changes contribute to the high prevalence of AF among the elderly. As noted above, left atrial size increases modestly with age, providing an augmented late diastolic filling rate that appears to compensate for the age-related reduction in early filling. Among adults aged ≥65 years, in Olmsted County, Minnesota, who

Table 1.4   Arrhythmias on 24-Hour ECG in 1372 Ambulatory Persons ≥65 Years Old

Arrhythmia	Women (%)	Men (%)	Gender Difference[a]
Supraventricular			
Any	97	97	No
≥15 in any hr	18	28	Yes
PSVT (≥3 complexes)	50	48	No
Atrial fibrillation or flutter[b]	3	3	No
Ventricular			
Any	76	89	Yes
≥15 in any hr	14	25	Yes
VT (≥3 complexes)	4	13	Yes
VT (>5 complexes)	0.3	0.2	No

[a]Defined by $p < .05$.
[b]Sustained or intermittent.
Abbreviations: PSVT, paroxysmal supraventricular tachycardia; VT, ventricular tachycardia.
Source: Adapted from Ref. 170.

underwent clinically indicated echocardiography, both a larger left atrial volume and impaired early diastolic LV function were independent predictors of nonvalvular AF (179). In addition, both left and right atrial wavefront propagation velocities show strong inverse correlations with age, increasing the likelihood for intra-atrial reentry to occur in older individuals (180).

Paroxysmal AF also increases strikingly with age. Among CHS participants in sinus rhythm, short runs of AF were seen in ~3% of individuals during 24-hour ambulatory ECG monitoring (Table 1.4) (174). In a series of persons with paroxysmal AF, the number and duration of abnormal atrial electrograms recorded during sinus rhythm increased with age (181). The incidence of postoperative AF, a major cause of morbity and increased hospital costs, also rises steeply with age. Among 527 patients undergoing major elective thoracic surgery, age was the strongest predictor of postoperative AF; odds of this arrhythmia were increased 2.5-fold in persons ≥70 years old versus those <60 years (182). A study of 205 patients undergoing elective cardiac surgery demonstrated additive effects of age and left atrial volume on the seven-day incidence of postoperative AF (Fig. 1.11) (183).

Paroxysmal Supraventricular Tachycardia

Short bursts of paroxysmal supraventricular tachycardia (PSVT) on a resting ECG are found in 1–2% of normal individuals older than 65 years. Twenty-four-hour ambulatory monitoring studies have demonstrated short runs of PSVT (usually 3–5 beats) in 13–50% of clinically healthy older persons (Table 1.4) (172,174). Although the presence of nonsustained PSVT on ambulatory monitoring did not predict an increase in risk of future coronary events in BLSA participants, 2 of 13 individuals with PSVT later developed de novo AF, compared with only 1 of the 85 without PSVT (173). Exercise-induced PSVT has been observed in 3.5% of over 3000 maximal treadmill tests on apparently healthy BLSA volunteers (184). The arrhythmia increased sharply with age, from 0% in the twenties to approximately 10% in the eighties (Fig. 1.12A); similar to PSVT on ambulatory ECG, the vast majority of these episodes were asymptomatic three- to five-beat salvos. Coronary risk factors and ECG or thallium scintigraphic evidence of ischemia occurred with similar prevalence in the 85 volunteers with exercise-induced PSVT as in age- and sex-matched controls. Of importance, the group with PSVT experienced no increase in subsequent coronary events over a 5.5-year mean follow-up period. However, 10% of the individuals with PSVT later developed a spontaneous atrial tachyarrhythmia compared with only 2% of the control group, analogous to the results of the 24-hour ambulatory ECG (184).

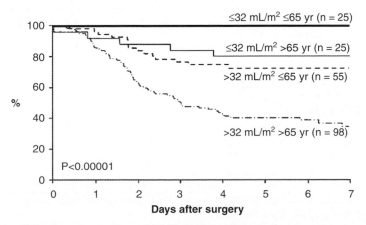

Figure 1.11 Risk of postoperative atrial fibrillation after cardiac surgery as a function of age and left atrial volume in 205 patients. *Source*: From Ref. 183.

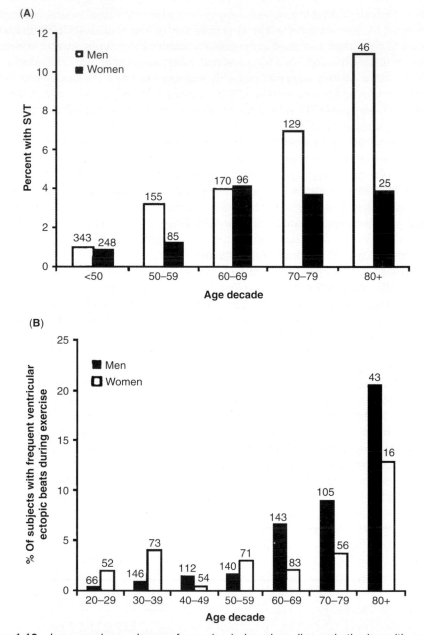

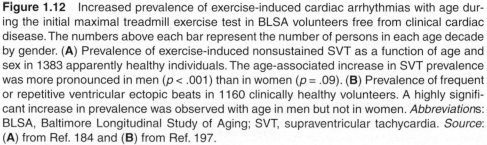

Figure 1.12   Increased prevalence of exercise-induced cardiac arrhythmias with age during the initial maximal treadmill exercise test in BLSA volunteers free from clinical cardiac disease. The numbers above each bar represent the number of persons in each age decade by gender. (**A**) Prevalence of exercise-induced nonsustained SVT as a function of age and sex in 1383 apparently healthy individuals. The age-associated increase in SVT prevalence was more pronounced in men ($p < .001$) than in women ($p = .09$). (**B**) Prevalence of frequent or repetitive ventricular ectopic beats in 1160 clinically healthy volunteers. A highly significant increase in prevalence was observed with age in men but not in women. *Abbreviations*: BLSA, Baltimore Longitudinal Study of Aging; SVT, supraventricular tachycardia. *Source*: (**A**) from Ref. 184 and (**B**) from Ref. 197.

Ventricular Arrhythmias

Both in unselected populations and in those clinically free of heart disease, an exponential increase in the prevalence of ventricular ectopic beats (VEB) occurs with advancing age. Pooled data from nearly 2500 ECGs from hospitalized patients older than 70 years revealed VEB in 8% (185). Among apparently healthy BLSA volunteers with a normal ST-segment response to treadmill exercise, isolated VEB occurred at rest in 8.6% of men over age 60 years compared with only 0.5% in those 20–40 years old (186). Of note, the prevalence of resting VEB was not age related in women.

The prognostic significance of VEB detected on the resting ECG in the general elderly population is controversial. Significant increases in cardiac mortality among persons with VEB were observed in studies from Busselton (187) and Manitoba (188), with risk ratios of 3.3 and 2.4, respectively, compared with arrhythmia-free cohorts. The Framingham community, however, demonstrated no increase in the age-adjusted risk ratio for cardiac events (189). Data from the Multiple Risk Factor Intervention Trial suggest that the prognostic significance of resting VEB may vary according to age; asymptomatic white men under 50 years with frequent or complex VEB on a 2-minute resting rhythm strip suffered a 14-fold relative risk of sudden cardiac death, while in older men the risk was not significantly increased (190).

Twenty-four-hour ambulatory ECG recordings have demonstrated the presence of VEB in 69–96% of asymptomatic elderly (173,174,191,192). Not only the prevalence but also the density and complexity of VEB increase with age. In the CHS, VEB were found in 82% of 1372 subjects aged 65 years and older, including 7% with 3- to 5-beat runs of nonsustained ventricular tachycardia (VT). The prevalence of all VEB forms was higher in men than in women (Table 1.4) (174). Among 50 individuals older than 80 years without clinical heart disease, VEB were observed in 96%, including multifocal VEB in 18%, couplets in 8%, and nonsustained VT in 2% (191). In 106 predominantly healthy patients aged 75 years and above, Camm et al. detected VEB in 69% (192); VEB were multiform in 22% and paired in 4% and occurred in short runs in 4%. Among 98 carefully screened asymptomatic BLSA participants older than 60 years, 35% had multiform VEB, 11% VEB couplets, and 4% short runs of VT on 24-hour monitoring (172). The prevalence of simple and complex VEB in all of these studies is much higher than in series of healthy younger volunteers.

The prognostic importance of VEB detected on ambulatory monitoring, like those found on the resting ECG, is unclear. Over a 10-year mean follow-up period, 14 of the 98 older, carefully screened BLSA participants who underwent ambulatory ECG developed coronary events (173). The prevalence and complexity of VEB were virtually identical in the group that experienced an event and the group that did not. However, horizontal or slowly upsloping ST-segment depression on the ambulatory ECG predicted an increased risk of such events (173). In the series of Camm et al. (192), 92% of the five-year survivors who were initially free of VEB remained without VEB on the five-year follow-up recording. In contrast to the BLSA results, an almost doubled crude mortality was found among individuals with ≥10 VEB/hr versus those with fewer VEB. It should be noted that 83% of the Camm et al. volunteers were taking medications, including several patients with known heart disease. In a cohort of 456 Swedish men aged 68 years, frequent or complex VEB on 24-hour ECG were found in 35% of those without clinical CHD and predicted increased risk of MI and CHD mortality over a 10.3-year mean follow-up (193).

Exercise testing elicits a striking increase in the prevalence and complexity of VEB with advancing age similar to that seen on the ambulatory ECG (Fig. 1.12 B). In apparently healthy BLSA volunteers, isolated VEB during or after maximal treadmill exercise increased in prevalence from 11% to 57% between the third and ninth decades (186). Although LV mass index and peak exercise systolic blood pressure were higher in subjects who developed exercise-induced VEB than in those who did not, by multivariate analysis only older age independently predicted the appearance of VEB (194). Asymptomatic exercise-induced runs of VT, all ≤6 beats in duration, were found in 4% of apparently healthy BLSA individuals aged 65 and older, a rate 25 times that of younger persons (195). Over a mean follow-up of about 2 years, however, none of these older volunteers with nonsustained VT during exercise testing developed angina, MI, syncope, or cardiac death. Extended follow-up of 81 such individuals for a mean of 12.4 years detected no adverse effect of nonsustained exercise-induced VT on mortality (196).

In a BLSA analysis of 1160 clinically healthy individuals who underwent an average of 2.4 maximal treadmill exercise tests per individual, 80 developed frequent VEB (≥10% of beats in any minute) or nonsustained VT on one or more tests (197). These 80 individuals were older than those free of such arrhythmias (64 vs. 50 years). Of note, the striking age-associated increase in occurrence of these complex exercise-induced VEB was observed only in men (Fig. 1.12B). The prevalence of coronary risk factors and exercise-induced ischemia by ECG and thallium scanning as well as the incidence of cardiac events (angina pectoris, nonfatal infarction, cardiac syncope, or cardiac death) were nearly identical in cases and controls matched for age and sex over a mean follow-up of 5.6 years without antiarrhythmic drug therapy (197). In contrast, over a 23-year follow-up of 6101 French men aged 42–53 years and initially free of clinical CV disease, frequent VEB during exercise predicted a 2.5-fold increased risk of CV death, independent of standard coronary risk factors (198). Thus, the available data available in older adults without apparent heart disease support a marked age-related increase in the prevalence and complexity of exercise-related VEB, at least in men; however, the prognosis conferred by frequent or repetitive VEB induced by exercise in such individuals is unclear.

A factor of major importance in determining the prognostic significance of VEB in the elderly is the milieu in which they occur. For example, among 467 patients aged 62–101 years in a long-term care facility, complex VEB occurred during 24-hour ambulatory monitoring in 21% (199). In the subset without clinical heart disease, future coronary events developed in an identical 4% of those individuals with or without complex VEB; among patients with CAD, however, such events developed in 46% with complex VEB but only 23% of patients without them. A similar doubling of risk was seen in patients with hypertension, valvular disease, or cardiomyopathy who demonstrated complex VEB. Table 1.5 summarizes the effect of age on the prevalence of various cardiac arrhythmias and their relationship to mortality in apparently healthy older adults (200).

In summary, aging is associated with multiple ECG changes in persons without evidence of CV disease. Such changes include a blunted respiratory sinus arrhythmia, a mild P–R interval prolongation, a leftward shift of the QRS axis, and increased prevalence, density, and complexity of ectopic beats, both atrial and ventricular. Although these

Table 1.5 Relationship of Arrhythmias to Age and Mortality

Arrhythmia	**Effect of Age on Prevalence**	**Effect on Mortality**[a]
Supraventricular ectopic beats	Increased	None
Paroxysmal supraventricular tachycardia	Increased	Probably none
Atrial fibrillation (chronic)	Increased	Increased
Ventricular ectopic beats	Increased	Probably none
Ventricular tachycardia (short runs)	Increased	Probably none

[a]In healthy elderly.

findings generally do not affect prognosis in clinically healthy older adults, other findings that become more prevalent with age, such as increased QRS voltage, Q waves, Q–T interval prolongation, and ST–T-wave abnormalities, are generally associated with increased CV risk. Abnormalities such as left BBB or AF are strongly predictive of future cardiac morbidity and mortality among older adults, even if asymptomatic. A guiding principle for the practitioner is that the prognosis associated with a given ECG abnormality in the elderly is more strongly related to the presence and severity of underlying CV disease than to the ECG finding itself.

The views expressed in this chapter are those of the author and do not necessarily represent those of the National Institutes of Health or the Department of Health and Human Services.

REFERENCES

1. United States Bureau of the Census. www.census.gov/population/www/estimates/popest.html.
2. Lakatta EG. Cardiovascular regulatory mechanisms in advanced age. Physiol Rev 1993; 73: 13.
3. Virmani R, Avolio AP, Mergner WJ, et al. Effect of aging on aortic morphology in populations with high and low prevalence of hypertension and atherosclerosis. Comparison between occidental and Chinese communities. Am J Pathol 1991; 139: 1119 29.
4. Nagai Y, Metter EJ, Earley CJ, et al. Increased carotid artery intimal-medial thickness in asymptomatic older subjects with exercise-induced myocardial ischemia. Circulation 1998; 98: 1504–9.
5. O'Leary DH, Polak JF, Kronmal RA, et al. Cardiovascular Health Study Collaborative Research Group. Carotid artery intima and media thickness as a risk factor for myocardial infarction and stroke in older adults. N Engl J Med 1999; 340: 14–22.
6. Stary HC, Blankenhorn DH, Bleakley CA, et al. A definition of the intima of human arteries and its atherosclerosis-prone regions: a report from the committee on vascular lesions of the council on arteriosclerosis, American heart association. Circulation 1992; 85: 391–405.
7. Spagnoli LG, Orlandi A, Mauriello A, et al. Aging and atherosclerosis in the rabbit. Distribution, prevalence, and morphology of atherosclerotic lesions. Atherosclerosis 1991; 89: 11–24.
8. Clarkson TB. Nonhuman primate models of atherosclerosis. Lab Animal Sci 1998; 48: 569–72.
9. Hodis HN, Mack WJ, LaBree L, et al. Reduction in carotid arterial wall thickness using lovastatin and dietary therapy. A randomized, controlled clinical trial. Ann Intern Med 1996; 124: 548–56.
10. Heblad B, Wikstrand J, Janzon L, et al. Low-dose metoprolol CR/XL and fluvastatin slow progression of carotid intima-media thickness. Main results from the b-blocker cholesterol lowering asymptomatic plaque study (BCAPS). Circulation 2001; 103: 1721–6.
11. Furberg CD, Adams HP, Applegate WB, et al. Asymptomatic Carotid Artery Progression Study (ACAPS) Research Group. Effect of lovastatin on early carotid atherosclerosis and cardiovascular events. Circulation 1994; 90: 1679–87.
12. Lonn EM, Yusuf S, Dzavik V, et al. Effects of ramipril and vitamin E on atherosclerosis. The study to evaluate carotid ultrasound changes in patients treated with ramipril and vitamin E (SECURE). For the SECURE investigators. Circulation 2001; 103: 919–25.
13. deGroot E, Jukema JW, van Swijndregt ADM, et al. B-mode ultrasound assessment of pravastatin treatment effect on carotid and femoral artery walls and its correlations with coronary arteriographic findings: a report of the regression growth evaluation statin study (REGRESS). J Am Coll Cardiol 1998; 31: 1561–7.
14. Salonen R, Nyyssönen K, Porkkala E, et al. Kuopio atherosclerosis prevention study (KAPS). A population-based primary preventive trial of the effect of LDL lowering on atherosclerosis progression in carotid and femoral arteries. Circulation 1995; 92: 1758–64.
15. Celermajer DS, Sorensen KE, Spiegelhalter DJ, et al. Aging is associated with endothelial dysfunction in healthy men years before the age-related decline in women. J Am Coll Cardiol 1994; 24: 471–6.
16. Bode-Boger SM, Muke J, Surdacki A, et al. Oral L-arginine improves endothelial function in healthy individuals older than 70 years. Vasc Med 2003; 8: 77–81.
17. Wang M, Khazan B, Lakatta EG. Central arterial aging and angiotensin II signaling. Curr Hypertens Rev 2010; 6: 266–81.
18. Halcox JP, Schenke WH, Zalos G, et al. Prognostic value of coronary vascular endothelial function. Circulation 2002; 106: 653–8.
19. Chan SY, Mancimi GBJ, Kuramoto L, et al. The prognostic importance of endothelial dysfunction and carotid atheroma burden in patients with coronary artery disease. J Am Coll Cardiol 2003; 42: 1037–43.

20. Panza JA, Casino PR, Kilcoyne CM, et al. Role of endothelium-derived nitric oxide in the abnormal endothelium-dependent vascular relaxation of patients with essential hypertension. Circulation 1993; 87: 1468–74.
21. Taddei S, Virdis A, Mattei P, et al. Hypertension causes premature aging of endothelial function in humans. Hypertension 1997; 29: 736–43.
22. Taddei S, Virdis A, Mattei P, et al. Defective L-arginine-nitric oxide pathway in offspring of essential hypertensive patients. Circulation 1996; 94: 1298–303.
23. Lakatta EG, Levy D. Arterial and cardiac aging: major shareholders in cardiovascular disease enterprises. Part I: aging arteries a "set up" for vascular disease. Circulation 2003; 107: 139–46.
24. Lakatta EG. Arterial and cardiac aging: major shareholders in cardiovascular disease enterprises. Part III: cellular and molecular clues to heart and arterial aging. Circulation 2003; 107: 49–497.
25. Vaitkcvicius PV, Fleg JL, Engel JH, et al. Effects of age and aerobic capacity on arterial stiffness in healthy adults. Circulation 1993; 88: 1456–62.
26. Kelly R, Hayward C, Avolio A, et al. Noninvasive determination of age-related changes in the human arterial pulse. Circulation 1989; 80: 1652–9.
27. Willum-Hansen T, Staessen JA, Torp-Pedersen C, et al. Prognostic value of aortic pulse wave velocity as index of arterial stiffness in the general population. Circulation 2006; 113: 664–70.
28. Yin FCP. The aging vasculature and its effect on the heart. In: Weisdfeldt ML, ed. The Aging Heart. New York: Raven Press, 1980: 137–214.
29. Avolio AP, Fa-Quan D, Wei-Qiang L, et al. Effects of aging on arterial distensibility in populations with high and low prevalence of hypertension: comparison between urban and rural communities. Circulation 1985; 71: 201–10.
30. Van Popele NM, Grobbee DE, Bots ML, et al. Association between arterial stiffness and atherosclerosis: the Rotterdam study. Stroke 2001; 32: 454–60.
31. Graner M, Varpula M, Kahri J, et al. Association of carotid intima-media thickness with angiographic severity and extent of coronary artery disease. Am J Cardiol 2006; 97: 624–9.
32. Scuteri A, Najjar SS, Muller DC, et al. Metabolic syndrome amplifies the age-associated increases in vascular thickness and stiffness. J Am Coll Cardiol 2004; 43: 1388–95.
33. Salomaa V, Riley W, Kark JD, et al. Non-insulin-dependent diabetes and fasting glucose and insulin concentrations are associated with arterial stiffness indexes. The ARIC Study. Atherosclerosis Risk in Communities Study. Circulation 1995; 91: 1432–43.
34. Schofield I, Malik R, Izzard A, et al. Vascular structural and functional changes in type 2 diabetes mellitus: evidence for the roles of abnormal myogenic responsiveness and dyslipidemia. Circulation 2002; 106: 3037–43.
35. Chen CH, Nevo E, Fetics B, et al. Estimation of central aortic pressure waveform by mathematical transformation of radial tonometry pressure. Validation of generalized transfer function. Circulation 1997; 95: 1827–36.
36. Blacher J, Asmar R, Djane S, et al. Aortic pulse wave velocity as a marker of cardiovascular risk in hypertensive patients. Hypertension 1999; 33: 1111–17.
37. Boutouyrie P, Tropeano AL, Asmar R, et al. Aortic stiffness as an independent predictor of primary coronary events in hypertensive patients: a longitudinal study. Hypertension 2002; 39: 10–15.
38. Kaess BM, Rong J, Larson MG, et al. Aortic stiffness, blood pressure progression, and incident hypertension. JAMA 2012; 308: 875–81.
39. Asmar R, Rudnichi A, Blacher J, et al. Pulse pressure and aortic pulse wave are markers of ardiovascular risk in hypertensive populations. Am J Hypertens 2001; 14: 1–97.
40. Blacher J, Pannier B, Guerin AP, et al. Carotid arterial stiffness as a predictor of cardiovascular and all-cause mortality in end-stage renal disease. Hypertension 1998; 32: 570–4.
41. van Popele NM, Grobbee DE, Bots ML, et al. Association between arterial stiffness and atherosclerosis: the Rotterdam Study. Stroke 2001; 32: 454–60.
42. Sutton-Tyrrell K, Najjar SS, Boudreau RM, et al. Health ABC Study. Elevated aortic pulse wave velocity, a marker of arterial stiffness, predicts cardiovascular events in well-functioning older adults. Circulation 2005; 111: 3384–90.
43. Franklin SS, Gustin IVW, Wong ND, et al. Hemodynamic patterns of age-related changes in blood pressure. The Framingham Heart Study. Circulation 1997; 96: 308–15.
44. Pearson JD, Morrell CH, Brant LJ, et al. Age-associated changes in blood pressure in a longitudinal study of healthy men and women. J Gerontol 1997; 52: M177–83.
45. Sagie A, Larson MG, Levy D. The natural history of borderline isolated systolic hypertension. N Engl J Med 1993; 329: 1912–17.
46. O'Donnell CJ, Ridker PM, Glynn RJ, et al. Hypertension and borderline isolated systolic hypertension increase risks of cardiovascular disease and mortality in male physicians. Circulation 1997; 95: 1132–7.

47. Franklin SS, Khan SA, Wong ND, et al. Is pulse pressure useful in predicting risk for coronary heart disease? The Framingham Heart Study. Circulation 1999; 100: 354–60.

48. Franklin SS, Larson MG, Khan SA, et al. Does the relation of blood pressure to coronary heart disease risk change with aging? The Framingham Heart Study. Circulation 2001; 103: 1245–9.

49. Gurven M, Blackwell AD, Rodriguez SJ, Kaplan H. Does blood pressure inevitably rise with age? Longitudinal evidence among forager-horticulturalists. Hypertension 2012; 60: 25–33.

50. Wildman RP, Schott LL, Brockwell S, et al. A dietary and exercise intervention slows menopause-associated progression of subclinical atherosclerosis as measured by intima-media thickness of the carotid arteries. J Am Coll Cardiol 2004; 44: 579–85.

51. Fontana L, Meyer TE, Klein S, et al. Long-term calorie restriction is highly effective in reducing the risk for atherosclerosis in humans. Proc Natl Acad Sci USA 2004; 101: 6659–63.

52. Tanaka H, Safar ME. Influence of lifestyle modification on arterial stiffness and wave reflections. Am J Hypertens 2005; 18: 137–44.

53. Avolio AP, Clyde KM, Beard TC, et al. Improved arterial distensibility in normotensive subjects on a low salt diet. Arteriosclerosis 1986; 6: 166–9.

54. Hambrecht R, Wolf A, Gielen S, et al. Effect of exercise on coronary endothelial function in patients with coronary artery disease. N Engl J Med 2000; 342: 454–60.

55. Hamdy O, Ledbury S, Mullooly C, et al. Lifestyle modification improves endothelial function in obese subjects with the insulin resistance syndrome. Diabetes Care 2003; 26: 2119–25.

56. Raitakari M, Ilvonen T, Ahotupa M, et al. Weight reduction with very-low-caloric diet and endothelial function in overweight adults: role of plasma glucose. Arterioscler Thromb Vasc Biol 2004; 24: 124–8.

57. Rywik TM, Blackman R, Yataco AR, et al. Enhanced endothelial vasoreactivity in endurance trained older men. J Appl Physiol 1999; 87: 2136–42.

58. Meyer Te, Kovacs SJ, Ehsani AA, et al. Long-term caloric restriction ameliorates the decline in diastolic function in humans. J Am Coll Cardiol 2006; 47: 398–402.

59. Huang W, Alhenc Gelas F, Osborne-Pellegrin MJ. Protection of the arterial internal elastic lamina by inhibition of the renin–angiotensin system in the rat. Circ Res 1998; 82: 879–90.

60. Michel JB, Heudes D, Michel O, et al. Effect of chronic ANG I-converting enzyme inhibition on aging processes. II. Large arteries. Am J Physiol 1994; 267: R124–35.

61. Levy BI, Michel JB, Salzmann JL, et al. Remodeling of heart and arteries by chronic converting enzyme inhibition in spontaneously hypertensive rats. Am J Hypertens 1991; 4: 240S–5S.

62. Gonzalez Bosc LV, Kurnjek ML, Muller A, et al. Effect of chronic angiotensin II inhibition on the nitric oxide synthase in the normal rat during aging. J Hypertens 2001; 19: 1403–9.

63. Moon SK, Thompson LJ, Madamanchi N, et al. Aging, oxidative responses, and proliferative capacity in cultured mouse aortic smooth muscle cells. Am J Physiol Heart Circ Physiol 2001; 280: H2779–88.

64. de Cavanagh EM, Fraga CG, Ferder L, et al. Enalapril and captopril enhance antioxidant defenses in mouse tissues. Am J Physiol 1997; 272: R514–18.

65. Inserra F, Romano L, Ercole L, et al. Cardiovascular changes by long-term inhibition of the renin-angiotensin system in aging. Hypertension 1995; 25: 437–42.

66. Ferder L, Romano LA, Ercole L, et al. Biomolecular changes in the aging myocardium: the effect of enalapril. Am J Hypertens 1998; 11: 1297–304.

67. Ferder LF, Inserra F, Basso N. Advances in our understanding of aging: role of the renin-angiotensin system. Curr Opin Pharmacol 2002; 2: 189–94.

68. Vaitkevicius PV, Lane M, Spurgeon H, et al. A cross-link breaker has sustained effects on arterial and ventricular properties in older rhesus monkeys. Proc Natl Acad Sci USA 2001; 98: 1171–5.

69. Kass DA, Shapiro EP, Kawaguchi M, et al. Improved arterial compliance by a novel advanced glycation end-product crosslink breaker. Circulation 2004; 104: 1464–70.

70. Linzbach AJ, Kuamoa-Boateng E. Die alternsveranderungen des menschlichen herzen. 1. Das herzgewicht im alter. Klin Wochenschr 1973; 51: 156–63.

71. Kitzman DW, Scholz DG, Hagen PT, et al. Age-related changes in normal human hearts during the first ten decades. Part 2 (Maturity). A quantitative anatomic study of 765 specimens from subjects 20 to 99 years old. Mayo Clin Proc 1988; 63: 137–46.

72. Olivetti G, Melissari M, Capasso JM, et al. Cardiomyopathy of the aging human heart: myocyte loss and reactive cellular hypertrophy. Circ Res 1991; 68: 1560–8.

73. Olivetti G, Giordano G, Corradi D, et al. Gender differences and aging: effects in the human heart. J Am Coll Cardiol 1995; 26: 1068–79.

74. Gerstenblith G, Frederiksen J, Yin FCP, et al. Ecliocardio-graphic assessment of a normal adult aging population. Circulation 1977; 56: 273–8.

75. Gardin JM, Henry WL, Savage DD, et al. Ecocardiographic measurements in normal subjects: evaluation of an adult population without clinically apparent heart disease. J Clin Ultrasound 1979; 7: 439–47.

76. Grandi AM, Venco A, Barzizza F, et al. Influence of age and sex on left ventricular anatomy and function in normals. Cardiology 1992; 81: 8–13.

77. Hees PS, Fleg JL, Lakatta EG, et al. Left ventricular remodeling with age in normal men versus women: novel insights using three-dimensional magnetic resonance imaging. Am J Cardiol 2002; 90: 1231–6.

78. Khouri MG, Maurer MS, Rumberger LE, et al. Assessment of age-related changes in LV structure and function by freehand three-dimensional echocardiography. Am J Geriatr Cardiol 2005; 14: 118–25.

79. Cheng S, Fernandes VRS, Bluemke DA, et al. Age-related left ventricular remodeling and associated risk for cardiovascular outcomes. The Multi-Ethnic Study of Atherosclerosis. Circ Cardiovasc Imaging 2009; 2: 191–8.

80. Anversa P, Palackal T, Sonnenblick EH, et al. Myocyte cell loss and myocyte cellular hyperplasia in the hypertrophied aging rat heart. Circ Res 1990; 67: 871–85.

81. Cheng W, Li B, Kastura J, et al. Stretch-induced programmed myocyte cell death. J Clin Invest 1995; 96: 2247–59.

82. Esler MD, Turner AG, Kaye DM, et al. Aging effects on human sympathetic neuronal function. Am J Physiol 1995; 268: R278–85.

83. Lakatta EG. Deficient neuroendocrine regulation of the cardiovascular system with advancing age in healthy humans. Circulation 1993; 87: 631–6.

84. Ensor RE, Fleg JL, Kim YC, et al. Longitudinal chest x-ray changes in normal men. J Gerontol 1983; 38: 307–14.

85. Redheuil A, Yu W-C, Mousseaux E, et al. Age-related changes in aortic arch geometry. J Am Coll Cardiol 2011; 58: 1262–70.

86. Port S, Cobb FR, Coleman RE, et al. Effect of age on the response of the left ventricular ejection fraction to exercise. N Engl J Med 1980; 303: 1133 7.

87. Rodeheffer RJ, Gerstenblith G, Becker LC, et al. Exercise cardiac output is maintained with advancing age in healthy human subjects. Circulation 1984; 69: 203–13.

88. Lakatta EG, Gerstenblith G, Angell CS, et al. Prolonged contraction duration in aged myocardium. J Clin Invest 1975; 55: 61–8.

89. Miyatake K, Okamoto J, Kimoshita N, et al. Augmentation of atrial contribution left ventricular flow with aging as assessed by intracardiac Doppler flowmetry. Am J Cardiol 1984; 53: 587 9.

90. Schulman SP, Lakatta EG, Fleg JL, et al. Age-related decline in left ventricular filling at rest and exercise. Am J Physiol 1992; 263: H1932–8.

91. Hees PS, Fleg JL, Dong S-J, et al. MRI and echocardiographic assessment of the diastolic dysfunction of normal aging: altered LV pressure decline or load? Am J Physiol Heart Circ Physiol 2004; 286: H782–8.

92. Fujimoto N, Prasad A, Hastings JL, et al. Cardiovascular effects of one year of progressive and vigorous exercise training in previously sedentary individuals older than 65 years of age. Circulation 2010; 122: 1797–805.

93. Wei JY, Spurgeon HA, Lakatta EG. Excitation-contradiction in rat myocardium: alterations with adult aging. Am J Physiol 1984; 246: H784–91.

94. Froehlich JP, Lakatta EG, Beard E, et al. Studies of sarcoplasmic reticulum function and contraction duration in young and aged rat myocardium. J Mol Cell Cardiol 1978; 10: 427–38.

95. Chahal H, Johnson C, Tandri H, et al. Relation of cardiovascular risk factors to right ventricular structure and function as determined by magnetic resonance imaging (results from the multi-ethnic study of atherosclerosis). Am J Cardiol 2010; 106: 110–16.

96. Lam CSP, Borlaug BA, Kane GC, et al. Age-associated increases in pulmonary arery systolic pressure in the general population. Circulation 2009; 119: 2663–70.

97. Kovacs G, Berghold A, Scheidl S, Olschewski H. Pulmonary artery pressure during rest and exercise in healthy subjects: a systematic review. Eur Respir J 2009; 34: 888–94.

98. Rutan GH, Hermanson B, Bild DE, et al. Orthostatic hypotension in older adults: the Cardiovascular Health Study. Hypertension 1992; 19: 508–19.

99. Masaki KH, Schatz IJ, Burchfiel CM, et al. Orthostatic hypotension predicts mortality in elderly men. The Honolulu Heart Program. Circulation 1998; 98: 2290–5.

100. Gottdiener JS, Yanez D, Rautaharju P, et al. Orthostatic hypotension in the elderly: contributions of impaired LV filling and altered sympathovagal balance. Am J Geriatr Cardiol 2000; 9: 273–80.

101. Lipsitz LA, Jonsson PV, Marks BL, et al. Reduced supine cardiac volumes and diastolic filling rates in elderly patients with chronic medical conditions: implications for postural blood pressure homeostasis. J Am Geriatr Soc 1990; 38: 103–7.

102. Gribben B, Pickering T, Sleight P, et al. Effect of age and high blood pressure on baroreflex sensitivity in man. Circ Res 1971; 29: 424.

103. Rodeheffer RJ, Gerstenblith G, Beard E, et al. Postural changes in cardiac volumes in men in relation to adult age. Exp Gerontol 1986; 21: 367–78.

104. Ebert TJ, Hughes CV, Tristani FE, et al. Effect of age and coronary heart disease on the circulatory response to graded lower body negative pressure. Cardiovasc Res 1982; 16: 663–9.

105. Olsen H, Lanne T. Reduced venous compliance in lower limbs of aging humans and its importance for capacitance function. Am J Physiol 1998; 275: H878–86.

106. Petrofsky JS, Burse RL, Lind AR. Comparison of physiologic responses of men and women to isometric exercise. J Appl Physiol 1975; 38: 863–8.

107. Swinne CJ, Shapiro EP, Lima SD, et al. Age-associated changes in cardiac performance during isometric exercise in normal subjects. Am J Cardiol 1992; 69: 823–6.

108. Yin FC, Raizes GS, Guarnieri T, et al. Age-associated decreases in ventricular response to hemodynamic stress during β-adrenergic blockade. Br Heart J 1978; 40: 1349–55.

109. Fleg JL, Lakatta EG. Role of muscle loss in the age-associated reduction in VO$_2$max. J Appl Physiol 1988; 65: 1147–51.

110. Talbot LA, Metter EJ, Fleg JL. Leisure-time physical activities and their relationship to cardiorespiratory fitness in healthy men and women 18–95 years old. Med Sci Sports Exerc 2000; 32: 417–25.

111. Fleg JL, Morrell CH, Bos AG, et al. Accelerated longitudinal decline of aerobic capacity in healthy older adults. Circulation 2005; 112: 674–82.

112. Fried LP, Taugen CM, Walston J, et al. CHS Collaborative Research Group. Frailty in older adults: evidence for a phenotype. J Gerontol 2001; 56A: M158–66.

113. Woo JS, Derleth C, Stratton JR, et al. The influence of age, gender, and training on exercise efficiency. J Am Coll Cardiol 2006; 47: 1049–57.

114. Fleg JL, Tzankoff SP, Lakatta EG. Age-related augmentation of plasma catecholamines during dynamic exercise in healthy males. J Appl Physiol 1985; 59: 1033–9.

115. Kenney WL. Thermoregulation at rest and during exercise in healthy older adults. Exerc Sport Sci Rev 1997; 25: 41–76.

116. Fleg JL, O'Connor FC, Becker LC, et al. Cardiac versus peripheral contributions to the age-associated decline in aerobic capacity. J Am Coll Cardiol 1997; 29: 269. (abstr).

117. Fleg JL, O'Connor FC, Gerstenblith G, et al. Impact of age on the cardiovascular response to dynamic upright exercise in healthy men and women. J Appl Physiol 1995; 78: 890–900.

118. Huang G, Gibson CA, Tran ZV, et al. Controlled endurance exercise traing and VO$_2$max changes in older adults: a meta-analysis. Prev Cardiol 2005; 8: 217–25.

119. Schulman SP, Fleg JL, Goldberg AP, et al. Continuum of cardiovascular performance across a broad range of fitness levels in healthy older men. Circulation 1996; 94: 359–67.

120. Tanaka H, DeSouza CA, Seals DR. Absence of age-related increase in central arterial stiffness in physically active women. Arterioscler Thromb Vasc Biol 1998; 18: 127–32.

121. Fleg JL, Schulman SP, Gerstenblith G, et al. Additive effects of age and silent myocardial ischemia on the left ventricular response to upright cycle exercise. J Appl Physiol 1993; 75: 499–504.

122. Chen C-H, Nakayama M, Talbot M, et al. Verapamil acutely reduces ventricular-vascular stiffening and improves aerobic exercise performance in elderly individuals. J Am Coll Cardiol 1999; 33: 1602–9.

123. Najjar SS, Schulman SP, Gerstenblith G, et al. Age and gender affect ventricular-vascular coupling during aerobic exercise. J Am Coll Cardiol 2004; 44: 611–17.

124. Nussbacher A, Gerstenblith G, O'Connor F, et al. Hemodynamic effects of unloading the old heart. Am J Physiol 1999; 277: H1863–71.

125. White M, Roden R, Minobe W, et al. Age-related changes in beta-adrenergic neuroeffector systems in the human heart. Circulation 1994; 90: 1225–38.

126. Seals DR, Dempsey JA. Aging, exercise and cardiopulmonary function. In: Lamb DR, Gisolfi CV, Nadel E, eds. Perspectives in Exercise Science and Sports Medicine. vol 8 Carmel: Cooper Publishing Group, 1995: 237–304.

127. Correia LCL, Lakatta EG, O'Connor FC, et al. Attenuated cardiovascular reserve during prolonged submaximal exercise in healthy older subjects. J Am Coll Cardiol 2002; 40: 1290–7.

128. Fleg JL, Schulman S, O'Connor F, et al. Effects of acute β-adrenergic receptor blockade on age-associated changes in cardiovascular performance during dynamic exercise. Circulation 1994; 90: 2333–41.

129. Hiss RG, Lamb LE. Electrocardiographic findings in 122,043 individuals. Circulation 1962; 25: 947–61.

130. Pfeifer MA, Weinberg CR, Cook D, et al. Differential changes of autonomous nervous system function with age in men. Am J Med 1983; 75: 249–58.

131. Schwartz J, Gibb WJ, Tran T. Aging effects on heart rate variation. J Gerontol 1991; 46: M99–M106.

132. Byrne EA, Fleg JL, Vaitkevicius PV, et al. Role of aerobic capacity and body mass index in the age-associated decline in heart rate variability. J Appl Physiol 1996; 81: 743–50.

133. Dekker JM, Crow RS, Folsom AA, et al. Low heart rate variability in a 2-minute rhythm strip predicts risk of coronary heart disease and mortality from several causes. The ARIC Study. Circulation 2000; 102: 1239–44.

134. Tsuji H, Vendetti FJ, Manders ES, et al. Reduced heart rate variability and mortality in an elderly cohort: the Framingham Heart Study. Circulation 1994; 90: 878–83.

135. Umetani K, Singer DH, McCraty R, et al. Twenty-four hour time domain heart rate variability and heart rate: relations to age and gender over nine decades. J Am Coll Cardiol 1998; 31: 593–601.

136. Felber-Dietrich D, Schindler C, Schwartz J, et al. Heart rate variability in an ageing population and its association with lifestyle and cardiovascular risk factors, results of the SAPALDI Study. Europace 2006; 8: 521–9.

137. Tresch DD, Fleg JL. Unexplained sinus bradycardia: clinical significance and long-term prognosis in apparently healthy persons older than 40 years. Am J Cardiol 1986; 58: 1009–13.

138. Gann D, Tolentine A, Samet P. Electrophysiologic evaluation of elderly patients with sinus bradycardia. Ann Intern Med 1979; 90: 24–9.

139. Aronow WS, Schwartz KS, Koenigsberg M. Prevalence of enlarged left atrial dimension by echocardiography and its correlation with atrial fibrillation and an abnormal P terminal force in lead VI of the electrocardiogram in 588 elderly persons. Am J Cardiol 1987; 59: 1003–4.

140. Pipberger HV, Goldman MJ, Littmann D, et al. Correlations of the orthogonal electrocardiogram and vectorcardiogram with constitutional variables in 518 normal men. Circulation 1967; 35: 536–51.

141. Mason JW, Ramseth DJ, Chanter DO, et al. Electrocardiographic reference ranges derived from 79,743 ambulatory subjects. J Electrocardiol 2007; 40: 228–34.

142. Fleg JL, Das DN, Wright J, et al. Age-associated changes in the components of atrioventricular conduction in apparently healthy volunteers. J Gerontol 1990; 45: M95–M100.

143. Simonson E. The effect of age on the electrocardiogram. Am J Cardiol 1972; 29: 64–73.

144. Rodstein M, Brown M, Wolloch L. First-degree atrioventricular heart block in the aged. Geriatrics 1968; 23: 159.

145. Mymin D, Mathewson FA, Tate RB, et al. The natural history of primary first-degree atrioventricular heart block. N Engl J Med 1986; 315: 1183–7.

146. Cheng S, Keyes MJ, Larson MG, et al. Long-term outcomes in individuals with prolonged PR interval or first-degree atriventricular block. JAMA 2009; 301: 2571–7.

147. Golden GS, Golden LH. The "nona" electrocardiogram: findings in 100 patients of the 90 age group. J Am Geriatr Soc 1974; 22: 329–31.

148. Ostrander LD. Left axis deviation: prevalence, associated conditions and prognosis. An epidemiologic study. Ann Intern Med 1971; 75: 23–8.

149. Yano K, Peskoe SM, Rhoads GG, et al. Left axis deviation and left anterior hemiblock among 8,000 Japanese and American men. Am J Cardiol 1975; 35: 809–15.

150. Pryor R, Blount SG. Clinical significance of true left-axis deviation. Am Heart J 1966; 72: 391–413.

151. Hiss RG, Lamb LE, Allen MF. Electrocardiographic findings in 67,375 asymptomatic subjects. 10. Normal values. Am J Cardiol 1960; 6: 200–31.

152. Harlan WR Jr, Graybiel A, Mitchell RE, et al. Serial electrocardiograms: their reliability and prognostic validity during a 24-yr period. J Chronic Dis 1967; 20: 853–67.

153. Kannel WB, Gordon T, Offutt D. Left ventricular hypertrophy by electrocardiogram: prevalence, incidence and mortality in the Framingham Study. Ann Intern Med 1969; 71: 89–105.

154. Levy D, Garrison RJ, Savage DD, et al. Left ventricular mass and incidence of coronary heart disease in an elderly cohort. The Framingham Heart Study. Ann Intern Med 1989; 110: 101–7.

155. Sunderstrom J, Lind L, Arnlov J. Echocardiographic and electrocardiographic diagnoses of left ventricular hypertrophy predict mortality independently of each other in a population of elderly men. Circulation 2001; 103: 2346–51.

156. Schneider JF, Thomas HE Jr, Kreger BE, et al. Newly acquired right bundle branch block: the Framingham Study. Ann Intern Med 1980; 92: 37–14.

157. Schneider JF, Thomas HE Jr, Kreger BE, et al. Newly acquired left bundle branch block: the Framingham Study. Ann Intern Med 1979; 90: 303–10.

158. Mihalick MU, Fisch C. Electrocardiographic findings in the aged. Am Heart J 1974; 87: 117–28.

159. Fahy GJ, Pinski SL, Miller DP, et al. Natural history of isolated bundle branch block. Am J Cardiol 1996; 77: 1185–90.
160. Kreger BE, Anderson KM, Kannel WB. Prevalence of intraventricular block in the general population: the Framingham Study. Am Heart J 1989; 117: 903–10.
161. Fleg JL, Das DN, Lakatta EG. Right bundle block: long-term prognosis in apparently healthy men. J Am Coll Cardiol 1983; 1: 887–92.
162. Kannel WB, Abbott RD. Incidence and prognosis of unrecognized myocardial infarction. An update on the Framingham Study. N Engl J Med 1984; 311: 1144–7.
163. Yano K, MacLean CJ. The incidence and prognosis of unrecognized myocardial infarction in the Honolulu Hawaii Heart Program. Arch Intern Med 1989; 149: 1528–32.
164. Aronow WS, Starling L, Etienne F, et al. Unrecognized Q-wave myocardial infarction in patients older than 64 years in a long-term healthcare facility. Am J Cardiol 1985; 56: 483.
165. Higgins IT, Kannel WB, Dawber TR. The electrocardiogram in epidemiological studies. reproducibility, validity and international comparison. Br J Prev Soc Med 1965; 19: 53–68.
166. Goldberg RJ, Bengston J, Chen ZY, et al. Duration of the QT interval and total and cardiovascular mortality in healthy persons (the Framingham Heart Study experience). Am J Cardiol 1991; 67: 55–8.
167. Robbins J, Nelson JC, Rautaharju PM, et al. The association between the length of the QT interval and mortality in the Cardiovascular Health Study. Am J Med 2003; 115: 689–94.
168. Dekker JM, Schouten EG, Klootwijk P, et al. Association between QT interval and coronary heart disease in middle-aged and elderly men. The Zutphen Study. Circulation 1994; 90: 779 85.
169. de Bruyne MC, Hoes AW, Kors JK, et al. Prolonged QT interval predicts cardiac and all-cause mortality in the elderly. The Rotterdam Study. Eur Heart J 1999; 20: 278–84.
170. Strauss SM, Kors JA, DeBruin ML, et al. Prolonged QTc interval and risk of sudden cardiac death in a population of older adults. J Am Coll Cardiol 2006; 47: 362–7.
171. de Bruyne MC, Hoes AW, Kors JA, et al. QTc dispersion predicts cardiac mortality in the elderly: the Rotterdam Study. Circulation 1998; 97: 467–72.
172. Fleg JL, Kennedy HL. Cardiac arrhythmias in a healthy elderly population: detection by 24-hour ambulatory electrocardiography. Chest 1982; 81: 302–7.
173. Fleg JL, Kennedy HL. Long-term prognostic significance of ambulatory electrocardiographic findings in apparently healthy subjects 60 years of age. Am J Cardiol 1992; 70: 748–51.
174. Manolio TA, Furberg CD, Rautaharju PM, et al. Cardiac arrhythmias on 24-hour ambulatory electrocardiography in older women and men: the Cardiovascular Health Study. J Am Coll Cardiol 1994; 23: 916–25.
175. Kannel WB, Abbott RD, Savage DD, et al. Epidemiologic features of chronic atrial fibrillation. N Engl J Med 1982; 306: 1018–22.
176. Wolf PA, Benjamin EJ, Belanger AJ. Secular trends in the prevalence of atrial fibrillation: the Framingham Study. Am Heart J 1996; 131: 790–5.
177. Staffurth JS, Gibberd MC, Fui SN. Arterial embolism in thyrotoxicosis with atrial fibrillation. Br Med J 1977; 2: 688–90.
178. Brand FN, Abbott RD, Kannel WB, et al. Characteristics and prognosis of lone atrial fibrillation. 30-Year follow-up in the Framingham Study. JAMA 1985; 254: 3449–53.
179. Tsang TSM, Gersh BJ, Appleton CP, et al. Left ventricular diastolic dysfunction as a predictor of the first diagnosed nonvalvular atrial fibrillation in 840 elderly men and women. J Am Coll Cardiol 2002; 40: 1636–44.
180. Kojodjojo P, Kanagaratnam P, Markides V, et al. Age-related changes in human left and right atrial conduction. J Cardiovasc Electrophysiol 2006; 17: 120–7.
181. Centurion OA, Isomoto S, Shimizu A, et al. The effects of aging on atrial endocardial electrograms in patients with paroxysmal atrial fibrillation. Clin Cardiol 2003; 26: 435–8.
182. Amar D, Zhang H, Leung DH, et al. Older age is the strongest predictor of postoperative atrial fibrillation. Anethesiology 2002; 96: 352–6.
183. Osranek M, Fatema K, Qaddoura F, et al. Left atrial volume predicts the risk of atrial fibrillation after cardiac surgery. J Am Coll Cardiol 2006; 48: 779–86.
184. Maurer MS, Shefrin EA, Fleg JL. Prevalence and prognostic significance of exercise-induced supraventricular tachycardia in apparently healthy volunteers. Am J Cardiol 1995; 75: 788–92.
185. Fisch C. Electrocardiogram in the aged. An independent marker of heart disease? Am J Med 1981; 70: 4–6.
186. Fleg JL. Epidemiology of ventricular arrhythmias in the elderly. In: Paciaroni E, ed. Proceedings of the 13th National Congress of Cardiology (Aging and Cardiac Arrhythmias) I.N.R.C.A. Ancona: Istituto a Carattere Scientifico, 1991; 26–30.

187. Cullen KJ, Stenhouse NS, Wearne KL, et al. Electrocardiograms and thirteen year cardiovascular mortality in Busselton Study. Br Heart J 1982; 47: 209–12.
188. Rabkin SW, Mathewson FAL, Tate RB. Relationship of ventricular ectopy in men without apparent heart disease to occurrence of ischemic heart disease and sudden death. Am Heart J 1981; 101: 135–42.
189. Kannel WB, Doyle JT, McNamara PM, et al. Precursors of sudden death: factors related to the incidence of sudden death. Circulation 1975; 57: 606–13.
190. Abdalla ISH, Prineas RJ, Neaton JD, et al. Relations between ventricular premature complexes and sudden cardiac death in apparently healthy men. Am J Cardiol 1987; 60: 1036–42.
191. Kantelip JP, Sage E, Duchene-Marullaz P. Findings on ambulatory electrocardiologic monitoring in subjects older than 80 years. Am J Cardiol 1986; 57: 398–401.
192. Martin A, Benbow LJ, Butrous GS, et al. Five-year follow-up of 106 elderly subjects by means of long-term ambulatory cardiac monitoring. Eur Heart J 1984; 5: 592–6.
193. Hedblad B, Janzon L, Johansson BW, et al. Survival and incidence of myocardial infarction in men with ambulatory ECG-detected frequent and complex ventricular arrhythmias. Eur Heart J 1997; 18: 1787–95.
194. Mayuga R, Arrington CT, O'Connor FC, et al. Why do exercise-induced ventricular arrhythmias increase with age? Role of M-mode echocardiographic aging changes. J Gerontol Med Sci 1996; 51A: M23–8.
195. Fleg JL, Lakatta EG. Prevalence and prognosis of exercise-induced nonsustained ventricular tachycardia in apparently healthy volunteers. Am J Cardiol 1984; 54: 762–4.
196. Marine JE, Shetty V, Chow GV, et al. Prognostic significance of exercise-induced nonsustained ventricular tachycardia in asymptomatic volunteers. J Am Coll Cardiol 2013, in press.
197. Busby MJ, Shefrin EA, Fleg JL. Prevalence and long-term prognostic significance of exercise-induced frequent or repetitive ventricular ectopic beats in apparently healthy volunteers. J Am Coll Cardiol 1989; 14: 1659–65.
198. Jouven X, Zureik M, Desnos M, et al. Long-term outcome in asymptomatic men with exercise-induced premature ventricular depolarizations. N Engl J Med 2000; 343: 826–33.
199. Aronow WS, Epstein S, Koenigsberg M, et al. Usefulness of echocardiographic abnormal left ventricular ejection fraction, paroxysmal ventricular tachycardia, and complex ventricular arrhythmias in predicting new coronary events in patients over 62 years of age. Am J Cardiol 1988; 61: 1349–51.
200. Fleg JL. Arrhythmias and conduction disorders. In: Beers MH, Berkow R, eds. The Merck Manual of Geriatrics, 3rd edn. Whitehouse Station, NJ: Merck Research Laboratories, 2000: 885–900.

2
Morphologic features and pathology of the elderly heart

Atsuko Seki, Gregory A. Fishbein, and Michael C. Fishbein

SUMMARY

As we age, many structural changes occur in the cardiovascular system that affect function and are associated with increased morbidity and mortality. Individual myocytes may undergo hypertrophy or atrophy, depending on associated conditions and the functional status of the aged individual. Major arteries become "stiffer" in the elderly, especially if other conditions common in the elderly, such as hypertension or diabetes, are present. Age is a strong risk factor for coronary atherosclerosis in both men and women, however, the burden of atherosclerosis plateaus in 60–70 year olds, but does not progress much in individuals in their 80s or 90s. Hypertension, a prevalent disorder in adulthood, results in concentric hypertrophy that increases the risk of congestive heart failure and clinically significant arrhythmias. Valvular heart disease may affect the young and old, but certain valvular diseases typically affect the elderly. Calcific aortic stenosis (AS), when severe, requires intervention by surgery or percutaneous valve replacement. Mitral valve prolapse (MVP) with myxomatous degeneration of leaflets—once thought to be a disease of young to middle age women—is probably the most common valvular cause of mitral regurgitation (MR) in the elderly. Mitral annular calcification (MAC) is also associated with aging. MAC may cause mild mitral regurgitation, and less often, mitral stenosis (MS) or atrioventricular (AV) block if the calcification encroaches on the conduction system. Age is a risk factor for infective endocarditis (IE), especially since the elderly often have pre-existing valve disease, artificial heart valves, pacemaker leads, or other intracardiac devices.

Cardiomyopathies represent another group of disorders that affect the young and the elderly. Hypertrophic cardiomyopathy (HCM)—usually inherited and a cause of sudden death in the young—may also first become manifest later in life. Indeed, in one study, one-fourth of patients with documented HCM were over 75 years old. The pathology, including asymmetric hypertrophy, myocyte disarray, and myocardial fibrosis is similar in all age groups, but subaortic obstruction is more common in older individuals with HCM. Other primary cardiomyopathies that affect the elderly include dilated cardiomyopathy (DCM) and Tako-Tsubo (stress) cardiomyopathy. One form of secondary cardiomyopathy is very prevalent in the elderly and is referred to as "senile" amyloidosis. The pathologic finding in systemic senile amyloidosis (SSA), Congo red positive birefringent interstitial material, is similar to that of other forms, but systemic senile amyloid is composed of wild type transthyretin. Since plasma cell dyscrasias often affect elderly individuals, the finding of immunoglobulin related amyloid in the heart is not unusual.

Conduction problems that often affect the elderly are associated with fibrosis at various levels of the conduction system, including the sinoatrial (SA) node, AV node, His bundle, and bundle branches. In elderly patients with atrial fibrillation (AF), the most common clinically significant arrhythmia, the atria are usually dilated and have microscopic fibrosis. The elderly may also suffer a variety of pericardial diseases that may cause tamponade or constriction, as in younger age groups.

In summary, the elderly are prone to a wide variety of cardiac disorders. It is incumbent upon those treating the elderly to be aware of the differences in pathologic processes affecting older individuals.

INTRODUCTION

Cardiovascular diseases are the leading cause of death in industrialized nations, with atherosclerotic vascular disease being the leading killer due to sudden cardiac death and/or myocardial infarction (MI). As we age, however, there are numerous other functional and structural changes that may occur in the cardiovascular system contributing to increasing morbidity and mortality. While many of these changes have been considered "degenerative", as knowledge increases it is becoming more clear that most of these processes are "regulated" and do not occur simply due to wear and tear. In this chapter, we will review the major structural abnormalities that affect the aging heart.

NONSPECIFIC CHANGES OF AGING

Some aging changes in the heart may occur in the absence of specific heart diseases. With aging there is a decrease in the functional reserve of the heart. In addition, there are major age-related cardiovascular changes, such as coronary atherosclerosis, left ventricular hypertrophy (LVH), and atrial dilatation with resulting functional changes such as heart failure and atrial fibrillation (AF) (1,2). The number of myocytes of both ventricles decreases gradually in men and is associated with hypertrophy of the remaining myocytes; notably, no similar findings occur in women (3). Loss of telomeric DNA is rather significant in the senescent heart, and apoptosis affects the aging heart (1,4). Deletions of mitochondrial DNA in human myocardial tissue have a close relationship with aging, but these DNA changes do not correlate with cardiovascular disease or heart weight (5). The so-called "aging process" of the heart is still not well-defined.

Despite the studies cited above, many consider the heart to be quite exceptional in that heart weight has been reported to be almost constant through adult life (6), while most organ weights, such as liver, kidneys and spleen, decrease significantly with advancing age. Mean heart weight has been reported to be comparable in young, middle, and older adults (7). Among individuals with no apparent cardiovascular disease, some studies indicate that total heart weight, including non-myocardial components such as pericardium, coronary arteries, and valves, does not change significantly with aging (8). However, atrophy of the heart and hypertrophy of the heart do occur in the elderly. Indeed, in one study ventricular myocardial weight gradually decreased in men, but remained constant in women with advanced age (3). There are also conflicting reports of dimensional changes with aging in the heart. Certainly, numerous conditions that may or may not be associated with aging affect cardiac dimensions.

There are definite functional and dimensional changes that occur in the cardiovascular system with aging. Left ventricular diastolic dysfunction increases after the age of 20 years. In contrast, left ventricular systolic function is preserved (2). Atrial systolic pressure increases with aging (2,4). The "normal" elderly heart, that is, the heart without any significant cardiovascular diseases, has relatively smaller ventricular cavities, and larger

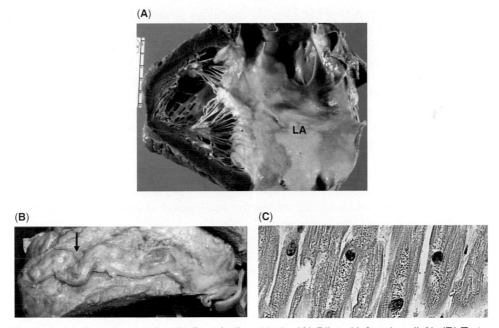

Figure 2.1 Common cardiac findings in the elderly: (**A**) Dilated left atrium (LA); (**B**) Tortuous coronary artery (arrow), and (**C**) Increased lipofuscin pigment (brown granules, H&E stain, ×400).

atria than the younger adult heart (Fig. 2.1A) (2,8–10). The valve rings dilate, the valve leaflets thicken (8), and the diameter of the aortic root increases with aging (8,9). The coronary arteries become more tortuous (Fig. 2.1B).

The prevalence of patent foramen ovale (PFO) decreases linearly with increasing age, from 34% during the first three decades to 20% during the ninth decade (11). Despite decreased prevalence with aging, PFO is independently associated with cryptogenic stroke in all age groups (11).

Undernutrition is often seen in the very elderly (6). Malnutrition is associated with a small brown heart, described as "brown atrophy". Grossly, the pericardium overlying the heart with brown atrophy has decreased adipose tissue, gelatinous degeneration of adipose tissue ("serous atrophy of fat"), and tortuous coronary arteries. As its name suggests, the myocardium in brown atrophy is brown because of increased concentration of lipofuscin pigment. Microscopically, myocytes show atrophy and increased lipofuscin granules (Fig. 2.1C). Lipofuscin is a perinuclear collection of yellowish-brown pigments (7,12). The myocardium in children under 10 years of age lacks lipofuscin (12). Lipofuscin accumulates linearly with age in man and other mammalian species. Lipofuscin also increases with hypertrophy of the myocardium (12).

VASCULAR AGING
Aged vessels "stiffen" through numerous processes occurring even in the absence of concomitant cardiovascular disease. Vascular remodeling, including intimal hyperplasia and medial hypertrophy, increases the thickness of vessel walls over time, reducing compliance. Furthermore, elastic laminae become fragmented and arterial elasticity decreases. This age-related loss of elasticity has been shown to be the result of age-associated increases in glycosylated proteins, matrix metalloproteinase activity, and trophic stimuli (13). These

processes are accelerated by other common conditions of the elderly, such as diabetes mellitus and hypertension.

Thickening of the tunica intima is seen in practically all arteries of the human body and has been described in association with aging (Fig. 2.2A). At young age, the intima consists of only a thin layer of endothelial cells, with minimal subendothelial connective tissue, lining the vascular lumen. With aging, smooth muscle cells migrate from the tunica media and accumulate in the intima. The cells undergo a switch from a differentiated contractile to a synthetic phenotype (14). Cytoskeletal markers are reduced and cell morphology becomes more rounded in shape, owing to an increase in rough endoplasmic reticulum and other cytoplasmic organelles. Proliferative behavior in response to growth factors increases. Slowly over time, this proliferation results in intimal thickening. Larger arteries, such as the aorta, are the most affected. Both peripherally and in the coronary vasculature, this phenomenon plays a significant role in the development of cardiovascular diseases such as hypertension and atherosclerosis.

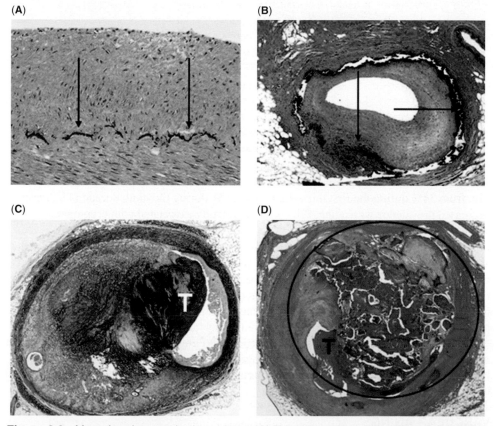

Figure 2.2 Vascular changes in the elderly: (**A**) Temporal artery with intimal hyperplasia (IH) and calcification of the internal elastic lamina (arrows) (H&E stain ×100); (**B**) Möncke-berg's sclerosis with calcification involving the internal elastic lamina and media of an artery (arrows) (H&E stain ×20); (**C**) Coronary artery with plaque rupture and luminal thrombosis (T) (trichrome/elastic stain, ×12.5), and (**D**) Coronary artery with heavily calcified athero-sclerotic plaque (calcification in circle, H&E stain ×12.5). There is an occlusive luminal thrombus (T) as well.

Like the tunica intima, the tunica media also thickens with time. However, the process is not characteristically proliferative, but rather accompanies a decrease in smooth muscle cellularity (15). Collagen accumulates, space between lamellar units increases, and elastin content decreases. Elastic laminae become encrusted in calcium. Medial smooth muscle cells increase in size (hypertrophy), but no increase in numbers (hyperplasia) is appreciable.

In addition to the age-associated alterations in wall composition described above, architectural changes are also observed in the elderly, such as vessel dilatation and tortuosity. Angiographic investigation of the relationship between coronary artery morphology, heart size, and age demonstrate that age is the best predictor of coronary artery tortuosity (16). Various studies into the relationship between age and coronary arterial lumen size have produced mixed results (8,17–19).

MEDIAL CALCIFIC SCLEROSIS (MÖNCKEBERG'S SCLEROSIS)

Medial calcific sclerosis—first described in 1903 by J.G. Mönckeberg—is a well-recognized age-related phenomenon, rarely occurring in individuals younger than 50 years. Medial calcific sclerosis is a common incidental finding in temporal arteries, arteries of the extremities, and arteries of the breast; occasionally coronary arteries are involved (20). The prevalence is notably increased in patients with other age-associated conditions, such as diabetes mellitus and osteoporosis. According to Mönckeberg, the sclerosis occur due to a calcification process limited to the tunica media of large and medium-sized arteries and does not result in luminal compromise (21). While the strict definition of Mönckeberg's sclerosis states that the process does not affect the internal elastic lamina, calcification of the internal elastic lamina is nearly always present (Fig. 2.2B) (20,22). Medial calcific sclerosis is largely considered a benign condition, usually noted as an incidental radiographic finding. However, these calcifications in arteries are a potential source of false-positive mammograms and falsely elevated electron-beam computed tomography (EBCT) calcium scores.

ATHEROSCLEROSIS

Atherosclerosis is largely considered as a disease of aging. Atherosclerosis is a process that begins in adolescence, but is not typically responsible for life-threatening disease until the fifth or sixth decade of life. Indeed, there is a close association between aging and the clinical manifestations of atherosclerotic disease (23). This association can partially be explained by associated age-related illnesses, such as hypertension, hypercholesterolemia, and diabetes. Over time these atherogenic risk factors intensify. In addition, there is evidence that components of vascular aging, particularly intimal thickening, are themselves atherogenic (14). While the burden of atherosclerosis progresses linearly during adulthood, this trend does not appear to continue in the very old. An autopsy study of 100 men between the ages of 30–89 years showed increasing atherosclerosis from ages 30 to 59 (24). However, there was no relationship between age and atherosclerotic burden in individuals age 60 and above. There is evidence that the composition of atherosclerotic plaques changes with advanced age. van Oostrom et al. (25) demonstrated more "atheromatous" plaques in subjects between the ages of 73–89 years. The lipid content of atherosclerosis increased with age. Conversely, the smooth muscle content decreased with age. This is an important finding, as the body of evidence suggests that plaques with increased lipid content and decreased smooth muscle are more vulnerable to plaque rupture and thrombosis (Fig. 2.2C) (26).

The presence of calcification in coronary arteries is used as a marker of atherosclerotic disease burden. Using EBCT, coronary artery calcium scores are calculated and used clinically for risk stratification and to guide management (27). An EBCT study of 675 men and 190 women demonstrated that the presence of calcium deposits was nearly a universal finding in elderly individuals (Fig. 2.2D) (28). After the age of 60, roughly four out of five men had detectable coronary artery calcium. The prevalence of coronary artery calcium in women was low until the age of 60, after which the prevalence approached that of men. Furthermore, the degree of calcium detected increased with age, being highest in individuals aged 70 years or older. EBCT data from patients ≥90 years are limited, but one autopsy study of such patients showed that coronary calcific deposits were grossly present in 95% of individuals (29).

The distribution of atherosclerotic disease is a relevant topic of investigation. There are numerous studies relating clinical outcomes to the location of atherosclerotic disease. Clinically, the distribution of disease may determine a patient's candidacy for percutaneous intervention after MI. The evidence suggests that coronary artery bypass graft surgery may be superior in patients with multivessel disease or left main coronary artery disease (30,31). In an autopsy study of American octogenarians, 66% had greater than 75% atherosclerotic narrowing of at least one epicardial coronary artery (32). Three or four vessel coronary artery disease was present in 24%. Left main coronary artery disease was seen in 8%. Multivessel and left main coronary artery involvement was increased in individuals who died of cardiac causes. There was no statistically significant difference in atherosclerosis distribution between both men and women. Autopsy studies of patients aged ≥90 years showed similar trends in atherosclerosis distribution (29).

Pulmonary arterial atherosclerosis may be seen in individuals of advanced age (33). This is likely due to the atherogenic properties of vascular aging (e.g., intimal thickening). Severe atherosclerosis of pulmonary arteries, however, is not typically encountered in the absence of pulmonary hypertension. Marked pulmonary artery atherosclerosis in conjunction with right ventricular hypertrophy is considered a reliable indicator of increased pulmonary artery pressure. Studies of pulmonary hemodynamics in the general population have demonstrated an age-associated increase in pulmonary arterial pressure and pulmonary vascular resistance (34). Nevertheless, even in nonagenarians, the age-associated increase in arterial pressure and vascular resistance is modest and does not qualify as pulmonary hypertension. In concordance, some autopsy studies have demonstrated no increase in right ventricular hypertrophy associated with age (8).

MYOCARDIAL INFARCTION

MI is a common manifestation of ischemic heart disease, the leading cause of death in high- and middle-income countries. The vast majority of MIs are the consequence of atherosclerotic cardiovascular disease. The morphologic appearance of MI is dependent on the acuity of the event (Fig. 2.3A). Myocardial necrosis is clearly evident grossly within two days of infarction (35). Histologically, findings are apparent within a few hours of coronary occlusion. Wavy fibers indicative of ischemic injury appear first. Then, necrotic fibers show increased eosinophilia, loss of cross-striation, loss of cytoplasmic granularity, and nuclear pyknosis or karyolysis (Fig. 2.3B). Within hours, neutrophils "marginate" in capillaries throughout the necrotic zone. Wavy fibers may be seen in infarcts only 1-hour-old. By one week, fibroblastic proliferation and collagen deposition are evident, although it is not until the third week that proliferation of connective tissue is the dominant feature. The fibrotic (or healed) MI looks the same, whether it is months or years old. If reperfusion occurs related to thrombolytic therapy or angioplasty, infarcts may become hemorrhagic (Fig. 2.3C).

In autopsy studies by Roberts et al., morphologic evidence of MI was found in half of octogenarians and 38% of individuals ≥90-years-old (29,32). In these studies, roughly half of individuals had hypertension, while approximately 60% had significant coronary

(A)

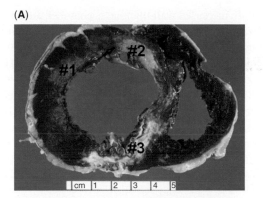

(B)   (C)

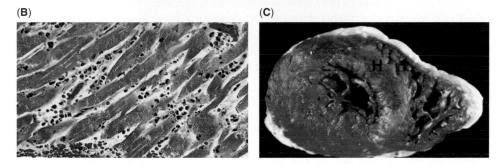

Figure 2.3 Myocardial infarction: (**A**) Tranverse slice of heart stained with triphenyltratrazolium chloride to demonstrate myocardial infarction. There are 3 infarcts of different ages #1 is about 24 hours old, #2 is days old, and #3 is months to years old; (**B**) Histologic findings in infarct that is about 24 hrs old showing hypereosinophilia and loss of nuclei in myocytes with an infiltrate of acute inflammatory cells (H&E stain, ×200), and (**C**) Myocardial infarction after reperfusion showing hemorrhage (H) in the necrotic tissue.

artery atherosclerosis (>75% stenosis) in at least one major coronary artery. Acute MI was present in 15% of those aged 90 or older. Healed MI was more prevalent, present in 27% of the ≥90 group. Similarly, Roberts's study of octogenarians showed acute MI in 24% of cases—29% of women and 19% of men. Healed MI was present in 36% of individuals—45% of men and 27% of women.

Other manifestations of MI were also noted in a subset of individuals. In octogenarians, the frequency of cardiac rupture was approximately four times greater in women than men. When cardiac rupture was found, 83% of cases involved the left ventricular free wall. The septum was involved in 29% of cases, while only 4% had rupture of a papillary muscle.

HYPERTENSION

Hypertension is a leading cause of cardiovascular disease, affecting more than one quarter of the world's population (36). More than half of the individuals with hypertension are over the age of 65 (37). As a result of age-related neurohumoral and vascular changes, systolic blood pressure (SBP) increases with advancing age. In the USA, diastolic blood pressure (DBP) peaks and plateaus in late middle age, after which it declines modestly in both men and women. As a result of the increase in SBP and decrease in DBP, pulse pressure increases with age and is a clinical marker for vascular stiffness. The morphologic changes seen in the hypertensive heart are increased wall thickness, chamber dilatation, and a combination of the two (Fig. 2.4A). Microscopically, there is evidence of myocyte hypertrophy and interstitial fibrosis (Fig. 2.4B & C).

The principle finding associated with hypertension is LVH. The classic paradigm of hypertensive heart disease teaches us that the left ventricular wall thickens in response to increased pressure (38). Through a variety of mechanisms, both mechanical and neurohumoral, cardiac myocytes increase in size resulting in an increase in left ventricular mass and wall thickness. The result is concentric LVH. However, concentric hypertrophy is not the only morphologic phenotype of hypertensive heart disease. In fact, studies of hypertensive individuals show eccentric hypertrophy is at least as common as concentric hypertrophy (39,40). Frequently, the hypertensive heart exhibits variable degrees of both concentric and eccentric LVH.

The natural history of the hypertensive patient is variable. However, it is well established that hypertensive people who develop concentric hypertrophy may subsequently develop eccentric hypertrophy through a series of events often referred to as the "transition to failure" (41). Not surprisingly, as hypertension is a significant risk factor for other cardiovascular diseases, including coronary artery disease, the progression from concentric hypertrophy to eccentric hypertrophy often involves interval MI (39,42). Particularly in the elderly, interval MI may go unrecognized. Data from a large study investigating age and MI susceptibility used cardiac magnetic resonance imaging (MRI) to demonstrate that the prevalence of unrecognized MI in individuals aged 67–93 is greater than previously

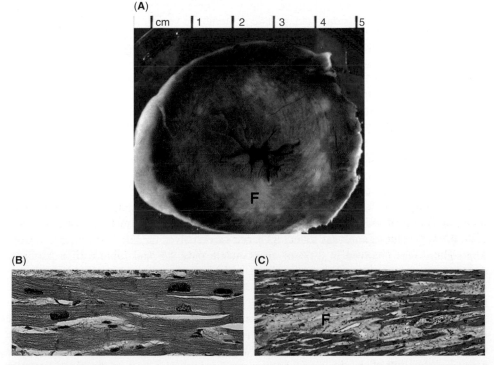

Figure 2.4 Findings in hypertrophied hypertensive hearts: (**A**) Transverse section of left ventricle showing marked concentric hypertrophy with myocardial fibrosis (white regions—F); (**B**) hypertrophic myocytes with enlarged "boxcar" nuclei (H&E stain, ×400), and (**C**) interstitial fibrosis (F) (H&E stain ×200).

estimated (43). In fact, the prevalence of unrecognized MI in that age group exceeds that of clinically recognized MI.

In an autopsy series of 490 patients 80–103 years of age, nearly half of the subjects had a clinical diagnosis of systemic hypertension (44). Increased heart weight, defined in this series as >400 g in men and >350 g in women, was found in 64% and 74% of men and women, respectively. Chamber dilatation, on the other hand, was present in only 33% of individuals. Both heart weight and chamber size tended to decrease with age.

VALVULAR HEART DISEASE

Clinically significant valvular heart disease is an increasingly common medical problem, affecting nearly 100,000 people in the USA annually (45). As one ages, the mean thickness of valve leaflets increases; of note, the thickness of valve leaflets is not significantly correlated with height, weight, heart weight, or body surface area (46).

AGING CHANGE OF VALVES

Age-related changes are seen in all of the cardiac valves, though the degree of change differs. Almost all adult aortic valves (AVs) have nodular thickenings at the centers of the free edges of the cusps—the so-called nodule of Arantii or nodule of Morgagni (47). Lambl's excrescences, hair-like projections from the nodules, are often seen in older patients (47). Fenestration of the cusps and firm ridge-like thickening at the bases of the cusps are also found in elderly AVs (47). None of these changes are functionally significant.

The mitral valve (MV) apparatus consists of the atrial wall, MV annulus, leaflets, chordae tendineae, papillary muscles, and underlying left ventricular wall. The leaflets may display thickening with degeneration of collagen fibers, lipid accumulation, and focal calcification (46). Nodular thickening of the free edge of the anterior leaflet, referred by some as "atheromatosis", is seen in all adults. Severity of the lipid deposition on the leaflet also correlates with age, but there are no gender differences (47). In addition, mitral annular calcification (MAC), small scars, diffuse opacity, or hooding of leaflets (myxomatous degeneration) are often seen in the elderly (46). MAC may be associated with mild, usually insignificant, mitral insufficiency.

Age-related changes in the pulmonary valve and tricuspid valve are minor. Nodules of Aranti and fenestrations of the cusps are sometimes present in the pulmonary valve (47).

AORTIC VALVE DISEASE

Degenerative/calcific aortic stenosis (AS) is the most common type of valvular heart disease requiring valve surgery in industrialized countries, and it is associated with significant morbidity and mortality (Fig. 2.5A) (48–51). Calcification of the AV is seen in more than one-fourth of individuals over 65 years and more than half of those over 85 years (50). AS is present in 2.4–8.1% of octogenarians (51,52).

The AV is chronically exposed to complex shear forces. Calcification primarily occurs on the aortic side of the cusps, along the line of coaptation (48). Valvular endothelium is thought to play a role in the process of calcification (48). Calcification involves the collagenous portion of the leaflets, but can erode through the endothelial surface and even embolize to other organs (53). The presence of calcification in the AV is associated with calcification at other sites, including the carotid arteries, coronary arteries, thoracic aorta, abdominal aorta, and iliac arteries (53).

Calcification of the AV and AS are associated with aging, hypertension, diabetes, elevated plasma levels of low-density lipoprotein (LDL), and smoking (48,50,51,53). AS may in part be the result of atherosclerosis—inflammation and lipid deposition on the AV (48). However, there is a discrepancy in the prevalence of coexisting calcific AS and

(A)   (B)

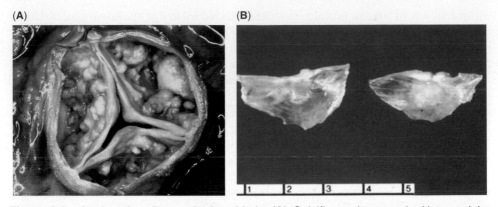

Figure 2.5   Aortic valve disease in the elderly: (**A**) Calcific aortic stenosis. Note nodular calcifications, and (**B**) Myxoid degeneration. Note thin translucent leaflets from a hypertensive elderly patient.

coronary artery disease (48,51,54). Although half of the patients with severe AS have severe coronary disease, most patients with coronary artery disease do not have AS (48,51). Therefore, the pathogenesis of AS is now recognized as a unique process (51). Indeed, calcification—once thought to be a nonspecific degenerative process—is now recognized as a highly regulated phenomenon. There are no specific or effective disease-modifying medical therapies (51). Recently, transcutaneous AV implants (TAVI) have been evaluated as a less invasive treatment for high-risk patients with AS who cannot undergo surgery (51,55–58). In such cases, TAVI has been associated with reduced mortality and hospitalizations, as well as improved symptoms but the incidence of major strokes and other vascular events appears to be higher with TAVI than with conventional surgical valve replacement (57,59,60).

Aortic regurgitation (AR) requiring surgery is less common in older adults, and usually results from infective endocarditis (IE), rheumatic fever, aortic-root dilatation or dissection, or myxoid degeneration (Fig. 2.5B) (61,62). Myxoid degeneration of the AV is seen in 36% of cases with pure AR and there is a male predominance. Long-standing hypertension is thought to be an important underlying factor (62). In contrast to myxoid degeneration of the MV, myxoid degeneration of the AV is very uncommon (62).

MITRAL VALVE DISEASE
Clinically significant MV disease affects 1–2% of the adult population, resulting in nearly 3,000 deaths in the USA each year (45). MR, mitral stenosis (MS), MAC, and mitral valve prolapse (MVP) are seen in the elderly (Fig. 2.6A). Classical MS, which primarily affects females, is usually post-inflammatory; most cases are due to rheumatic disease (45,61). In elderly patients, especially women, severe MAC with encroachment into the orifice is an uncommon cause of functional MS.

MR may be caused by myxomatous degeneration, IE, collagen vascular disease, or spontaneous rupture of the chordae tendineae (61). MVP is the most common structural valvular cause of MR in older patients (45,63). Although estimates vary, MVP has been reported in as many as 6–17% of otherwise healthy adults (45,64). Currently, the consensus of opinion is more in the range of 3–5%. Most patients with MVP are over 50 years old (64). MVP is more common in women, but clinically significant MR and chordal rupture due to MVP are more common in men. Grossly, myxomatous MVs are characterized by

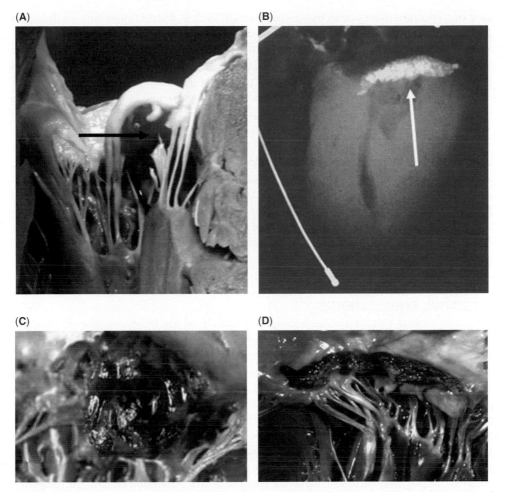

Figure 2.6 Mitral valve disease in the elderly: (**A**) Mitral valve prolapse with ruptured chordea tendinea (arrow); (**B**) Postmortem radiograph showing mitral annular calcification (arrow); (**C**) Fungal endocarditis with large vegetation on mitral valve, and (**D**) nonbacterial thrombotic endocarditis with non-destructive vegetations on valve leaflet.

floppy leaflets with elongated or ruptured chordae tendineae (Fig. 2.6A) (45,63,64). Also, the valves show an increase in leaflet thickness (65). The MV consists of a fibrosa, spongiosa, and atrialis layer. Histologically, the valve with prolapse shows collagen degeneration and disorganization, elastic fiber fragmentation, and increased thickness of the spongiosa layer (45,63). In MVP, the leaflets contain more abundant proteoglycans, biglycan, and verisican (63). Ruptured mitral chordae tendineae are seen not only in myxomatous degeneration of the MV, but also in chronic rheumatic valvulitis or endocarditis. Myxomatous degeneration mainly causes posterior chordae tendineae rupture, while anterior chordae tendineae rupture is more common in chronic rheumatic valvulitis (66). The cause and progression of myxomatous degeneration remains unclear; surgical repair is the treatment of choice in patients with severe MR (63).

The incidence and prevalence of MAC, or mitral ring calcification, show a striking increase with age. MAC is rarely found in those under the age of 40 years, except in the case of a concommitant connective tissue disorder, such as Marfan syndrome, or disorders of calcium metabolism, for example, secondary hyperparathyroidism due to severe chronic kidney disease (CKD) (53). Risk factors include advanced age, CKD, and increased mitral stress, as occurs in hypertension, AS, or MVP (47,54,67,68). The overall prevalence in individuals over 50 years is 8.5% (67). MAC is initially more common in men, but after the age of 65 the prevalence is considerably higher in women. Heavy calcification is also seen more frequently in women (Fig. 2.6B) (47,67,68). The configuration of the calcified annulus may be "J," "C," "U," or "O"-shaped (54). MAC is usually located entirely in or below the annulus of the posterior mitral leaflet (54). Although the anterior leaflet has no true annulus, there can be anterior submitral calcification, seen much less frequently than in association with the posterior leaflet (69). Ulceration and extrusion of calcium through the cusp, extensive central caseation, or endocarditis of the MV are sometimes associated with MAC (67). Microscopically, MAC shows no evidence of previous endocarditis. Nonspecific chronic inflammatory changes are seen adjacent to calcium deposition (67). Rarely MAC extends into the His bundle of the conduction system, causing atrioventricular (AV) block (68). In one autopsy study, MAC was the cause of complete AV block in 19.4% of elderly patients (70).

INFECTIVE ENDOCARDITIS

IE is a microbial infection of an endocardial surface of the heart (see also chapter 17) (71,72). The prevalence of IE ranges from 5.0 to 7.0 per 100,000 and has not changed significantly over time (73). The clinical diagnosis of IE is based on culture of organisms from the blood and visualization of cardiac vegetations (Fig. 2.6C) (74). Despite current sophisticated imaging methods, IE is frequently not diagnosed until autopsy (74). Risk factors in addition to older age include pre-existing valvular disease, artificial heart valves, intracardiac devices, and intravenous drug use (71,75). The prevalence of IE at autopsy has been reported to be 1.3% (74), and the mean age of patients is increasing (74,75). Moreover, the incidence of IE is rising steadily, commensurate with the increase in size of the elderly population (74,76). In-hospital, mortality is high—up to 20% (72). Although the most common organisms were *Streptococcus* species in the pre-antibiotic era, currently the predominant pathogen is *Staphylococcus aureus* (72–77). Endocarditis caused by *S. aureus* is associated with a poor prognosis (78). The etiologic organisms are not different between younger adults and older people (75). Fungal endocarditis is not common, but results in larger vegetations and greater destruction of tissue (75).

Left-sided endocarditis is more common, but endocarditis involving right-sided structures or both right- and left-sided valves is not rare (74,75). Right-sided endocarditis is often associated with intravenous drug use or pulmonary artery catheterization (74,75,77). Prosthetic valve endocarditis is a serious complication of valve surgery that often requires removal of the affected valve. Pathologically, bacterial colonies or fungal hyphae are demonstrated in untreated endocarditis. Gram stain for bacteria and Gomori's methenamine silver (GMS) stain for fungi are recommended (75). Infection from a native or artificial valve may spread to adjacent structures and myocardium (74). The finding of heart block indicates spread of the infection into the cardiac conduction system, and the finding of pericarditis indicates spread through the infected valve annulus—both are ominous complications. The spleen, kidneys, brain, and mesentery are common sites of embolization of infected vegetations in cases of left-sided endocarditis; lung abscesses are more common site in cases of right-sided endocarditis (74). At autopsy, gross infarction may be seen in as many as 63% of cases, the majority of which are asymptomatic (74).

Up to one third of patients with IE have cardiac disorders that are clinically silent, such as bicuspid AV or MVP (73,75). Bicuspid AV is the most common congenital cardiac abnormality (79). Patients with endocarditis and bicuspid AV are younger, have a higher frequency of aortic perivascular abscess, and usually require early surgery (79). Cardiac device-associated IE (e.g., pacemakers or ICDs) has been seen more frequently in recent years due to increased utilization of these technologies, especially in older adults (80). In one study of such patients, co-existing valve involvement was seen in 37.3%, and the most commonly infected valve was the tricuspid valve (80).

NON-BACTERIAL THROMBOTIC ENDOCARDITIS
Non-bacterial thrombotic endocarditis (NBTE) is a sterile, thrombotic vegetation of the heart valves. NBTE is found in 0.3–9.3% of autopsy patients (81,82). Thromboembolism may be the first manifestation; however, NBTE is usually asymptomatic, or at least not recognized clinically, in part because the patient has very severe underlying disease such as shock or metastatic malignancy. Accordingly, NBTE is usually first diagnosed at autopsy (82). Patients with NBTE are usually older, but NBTE is also observed in children and young adults (81). There is no gender predilection (81). NBTE is most commonly found in patients with adenocarcinomas, and it is also seen in patients with antiphospholipid syndrome (APS) or other autoimmune disorder characterized by hypercoagulability (81–83). NBTE may be seen in patients with disseminated intravascular coagulation (DIC) of any cause. NBTE occurs on the atrial surfaces of the mitral and tricuspid valves and the ventricular surfaces of the aortic and pulmonic valves (81). The mitral and AVs are most commonly involved (81). Histologically, NBTE shows agglutinated deposits of fibrin and platelets with no inflammatory reaction and no destruction of underlying valve tissue (81,83). NBTE is superficial and attached to the endocardial surface along the lines of closure of the affected valves (Fig. 2.6D) (81,83).

CARDIOMYOPATHY
According to the 2006 AHA classification scheme, cardiomyopathy is defined as a heterogenous group of diseases of the myocardium associated with mechanical and/or electrical dysfunction (84). Cardiomyopathies are divided into two major groups, primary and secondary (84). Primary cardiomyopathies are solely or predominantly confined to heart muscle, and classified as genetic, acquired, and mixed (genetic and non-genetic etiologies) (84).

HYPERTROPHIC CARDIOMYOPATHY
Hypertrophic cardiomyopathy (HCM) is a clinically heterogeneous but relatively common autosomal dominant genetic heart disease (1 in 500 individuals) characterized by unexplained hypertrophy of the left ventricle (84,85). Other causes of ventricular hypertrophy, such as hypertension or AS, must be excluded (86,87). HCM is the most common cause of sudden death in young individuals, including trained athletes (84,87,88), but HCM has been observed during all phases of life, from infancy to the advanced age (87). Males and females are equally affected (88).

HCM is not rare in the elderly. One study showed approximately one quarter of HCM patients were older than 75 years (87). However, there are substantial differences in clinical manifestations across age groups. Only a minority of aged HCM patients have severe heart failure (87). In one study, two-thirds of patients older than 75 years experienced few or no symptoms, and about 60% of those survived to age 80–96 years (89).

The clinical diagnosis of HCM is usually established by echocardiography. Although pathological findings are specific, endomyocardial biopsy is not recommended as a diagnostic tool (90). Endomyocardial biopsy is useful to exclude infiltrative or storage diseases (90). Grossly, LVH is characteristically asymmetric, with the anterior, basal interventricular septum showing the greatest wall thickness (Fig. 2.7A) (84,87,90). Subaortic obstruction is significantly more common in older HCM patients (89). Characteristic histologic features are myocyte hypertrophy, myocyte disarray, and fibrosis (Fig. 2.7B) (86,87,91). There is also wall thickening and luminal narrowing of intramyocardial arteries. In elderly patients, these morphologic features are relatively mild compared to younger patients who have died from HCM (87,89).

(A)

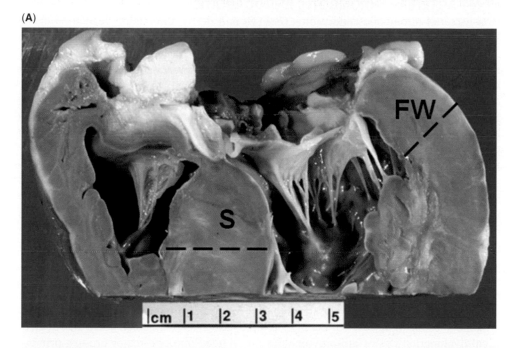

(B)   (C)

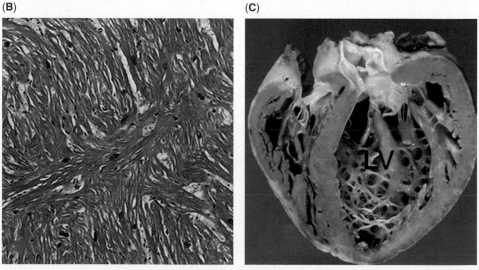

Figure 2.7 Primary cardiomyopathies: (**A**) Base of heart from a patient transplanted for hypertrophic cardiomyopathy. Note that the septum (S) is thicker than the left ventricular free wall (FW); (**B**) Characteristic myocyte disarray seen in hypertrophic cardiomyopathy, and (**C**) Heart from a patient transplanted for dilated cardiomyopathy. Note dilation of left ventricle (LV).

DILATED CARDIOMYOPATHY

Dilated cardiomyopathy (DCM) is characterized by ventricular chamber enlargement of the left or both ventricles, and systolic dysfunction in the absence of other identifiable causes of global systolic impairment (Fig. 2.7C) (84,90,92,93). DCM is the most common cardiomyopathy (92), and it is categorized as a mixed (genetic and nongenetic) cardiomyopathy in the AHA classification (84).

DCM leads to progressive biventricular heart failure, ventricular and supraventricular arrhythmias, thromboembolism due to cardiac mural thrombi, and sudden cardiac death (84,90,92,93). The 5-year survival after diagnosis is 50% (92). About 20–50% of DCM cases have been reported to be familial (84,91–93). Myocarditis is responsible for some cases of DCM, therefore viral serology and culture may be useful at the time of diagnosis (92). The cardiomyopathy may become clinically manifest long after the acute viral illness. Common organisms are parvovirus B19, coxsackie virus B3, and adenovirus (92). DCM may occur at any age, but there are onset peaks during childhood and mid-adulthood (90–92). Macroscopically, the heart often weighs two to three times normal; some hearts exceed 1000 g (92). The characteristic shape of the heart is globoid and somewhat spherical with rounding of the apex due to biventricular hypertrophy and marked dilation (92). Mural thrombi may be seen in all cardiac chambers (90,92). Histological findings are nonspecific, including interstitial fibrosis, replacement fibrosis, irregular and hyperchromatic nuclei of myocytes, and sarcoplasmic degenerative changes (90,92). Endomyocardial biopsies may be useful in order to rule out specific diseases showing similar clinical presentation, such as sarcoidosis or hemochromatosis (90,92).

TAKO-TSUBO (STRESS) CARDIOMYOPATHY

Tako-Tsubo cardiomyopathy is a relatively new form of acquired cardiomyopathy in the AHA classification (84). Tako-Tsubo cardiomyopathy refers to the shape of the heart resembling the appearance of a Japanese octopus fishing pot called a Tako (octopus)-Tsubo (pot). Synonyms include stress cardiomyopathy, transient left ventricular apical ballooning syndrome, broken-heart syndrome, and ampulla-shaped cardiomyopathy (84,93–95). Tako-Tsubo cardiomyopathy is characterized by transient regional systolic dysfunction involving the left ventricular apex and/or mid-ventricle that typically recovers within a few weeks (84,93,96,97). Diagnostic criteria include (*i*) transient left ventricular systolic dysfunction, (*ii*) the absence of obstructive coronary disease, (*iii*) new ECG abnormalities (ST-segment elevation or depression, T wave inversion, and/or Q-wave formation) or mild cardiac enzyme elevation (troponin-I, creatine kinase), and (*iv*) the absence of pheochromocytoma or myocarditis (93,94,97,98). Plasma catecholamine levels are more elevated in patients with Tako-Tsubo cardiomyopathy than in those with acute MI (93,95,98).

Gender and age discrepancies are striking. Females comprise 90–95% of reported cases. Most patients are elderly and post-menopausal (84,94,95,98). Common symptoms include abrupt onset of angina-like chest pain and dyspnea resembling an acute coronary syndrome (93–95,97). Symptoms are usually preceded by emotional or physical stress, for example, family death, abuse, a harsh argument, exhausting work, or earthquake (93,94,97). Endomyocardial biopsies obtained during the acute phase of patients with Tako-Tsubo cardiomyopathy showed contraction bands, interstitial infiltrates consisting primarily of mononuclear lymphocytes, leukocytes and macrophages, and myocardial fibrosis, but no coagulation myocardial necrosis (94,97,98). Interestingly, the pathological findings in Tako-Tsubo cardiomyopathy are similar to those seen in patients with ischemic electrocardiographic changes after an acute intracranial injury (95).

AMYLOIDOSIS

Amyloidosis may be categorized as a secondary form of cardiomyopathy, as many forms of amyloid disease are systemic. Cardiac amyloidosis is characterized by infiltration of the myocardium by one of several amyloid proteins. There are five main types of amyloidosis: primary/AL amyloidosis (amyloid light chain), familial/hereditary amyloidosis, senile systemic amyloidosis, isolated atrial amyloidosis (IAA), and secondary/AA amyloidosis (amyloid A protein) (Table 2.1) (99). Each type has different clinicopathological features including treatment and prognosis (99,100). Therefore, the identification of the specific amyloidogenic protein is essential. Cardiac involvement is primarily encountered in primary/AL amyloidosis and senile systemic amyloidosis (101). Deposition of amyloid in the heart results in a thickened heart wall with a firm and rubbery consistency (85,99). Brown "waxy" deposits may be seen in the endocardium of the atria or heart valves (Fig. 2.8A). The stiff heart worsens cardiac relaxation and compliance; therefore, cardiac manifestations of amyloidosis are dominated by diastolic heart failure resulting from restrictive cardiomyopathy (85). Right heart failure, conduction disturbances, and arrhythmias are common (85,99). When suspected clinically, the diagnosis of amyloidosis may be confirmed by biopsy. Histologically, amyloid displays an amorphous eosinophilic appearance by hematoxylin–eosin staining, and shows characteristic apple-green and yellow birefringence with polarized light following Congo Red staining (Figs. 2.8B–D) (99,101–103). After the confirmation of amyloidosis, amyloid typing may be attempted by immunohistochemistry, with antisera to amyloid A, kappa and lambda light chains, and transthyretin (Figs. 2.8E & F) (99,101,104,105). Mass spectrometry may be a more reliable but less readily available method to classify amyloid proteins (101,105). If transthyretin amyloid is detected, DNA mutational analysis may be performed to distinguish senile systemic amyloidosis from hereditary amyloidosis (101).

Primary/AL amyloidosis is the most frequent amyloid disorder in the Western world (105). Clonal plasma cells secrete monoclonal immunoglobulin light chains (99,105,106). Monoclonal plasma cell dysplasia, multiple myeloma, or lymphoproliferative disorders (e.g., Waldenstrom's macroglobulinemia) underlie most cases of AL amyloid. The kidney and heart are the major organs commonly involved by AL amyloid. Monoclonal plasma cell dysplasias are more frequent in the elderly. Cardiac involvement portends a poor prognosis (99,101,106). Right-heart failure caused by restrictive cardiomyopathy, arrhythmia, and pericardial effusion are common cardiac manifestations (85,99,102,106). Heart failure contributes to about 40–75% of deaths; however, 25% of deaths are sudden (99,101,106). Typical macroscopic findings are increased heart weight, diffuse, waxy, stiffening of tissues, and gross appearance mimicking HCM (99,102,103,107). Histologically, amyloid deposition is predominantly seen in interstitial tissue and vascular walls (108).

Other age-related amyloidoses include systemic senile amyloidosis (SSA) and IAA. Both are senescence-related and the prevalence increases with aging (101). The amyloid protein of SSA is composed of wild type transthyretin, and that of IAA is atrial natriuretic peptide (ANP) (99,101,109).

SSA is the most common form of systemic amyloidosis (99,110). SSA occurs in 11.5–25% of people over the age of 80 years (99,100,110). Wild-type transthyretin forms amyloid deposits in various organs (103), although the heart is most commonly affected (99,104,111). Both the atria and ventricles are involved (99,104,111). The extent of SSA is similar to that found in primary/AL amyloidosis; however SSA is less commonly associated with cardiomegaly, heart failure or arrhythmia than primary/AL amyloidosis (99,104,108,110). Histologically, large, diffuse or multifocal, predominantly nodular amyloid deposits are present between muscle bundles—these are nonvascular. Usually the conduction system is not affected (99,100,108).

Table 2.1 Amyloidoses Affecting the Heart (90,104,106,108,109,111,113–115)

	Age	Cardiac Manifestation	Amyloid Composition	Cause	Diagnostic Testing	Immunostains	Extra Cardiac Sites
Primary (AL) amyloidosis	Median age: 55–60 yr	CHF, arrhythmia	Monoclonal immunoglobulin light chain	Multiple myeloma, lymphoplasmacytic lymphoma	Serum/urine protein electrophoresis	κ, λ light chains	Kidney, nerve, GI tract, liver
Secondary (AA) amyloidosis		Rare	Serum AA, β2 microglobulin	Chronic inflammatory conditions, malignancy	Target organ biopsy, synovial and bone biopsy (dialysis-related), AA antiserum staining	AA protein	Kidney
Hereditary amyloidosis		Cardiomyopathy	Mutant TTR and apolipoprotein	Mutation of TTR gene	TTR antiserum staining, genetic testing	TTR	Nervous system
Senile amyloidosis	11.5–25% of people over 80-yr-old	AF, conduction abnormality, CHF	Wild type TTR	Aging	TTR antiserum staining	TTR	Aorta, pulmonary arteries, and pulmonary alveolar septa
Isolated atrial amyloidosis	80–90% of people over 90-yr-old	AF	ANP	Aging	ANP antiserum staining		None

Abbreviations: AA, amyloid A; AL, amyloid light chain; CHF, congestive heart failure; AF, atrial fibrillation; GI, gastrointestinal; TTR, transthyretin; ANP, atrial natriuretic peptide.

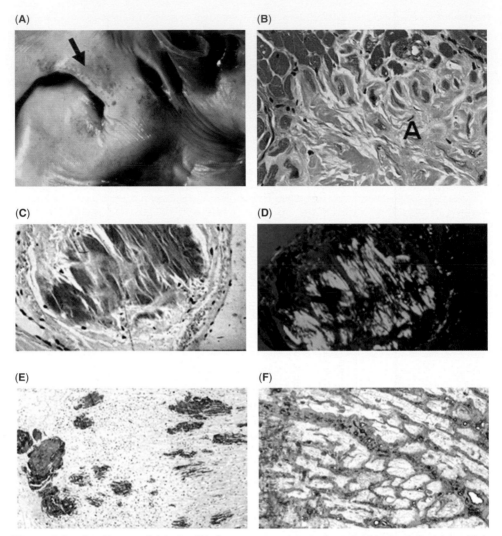

Figure 2.8 Cardiac amyloidosis: **(A)** Gross appearance of amyloid in the left atrium. Note brown "waxy" appearance (arrow); **(B)** H&E stain of amyloid (A) in the myocardium; **(C)** Congo red stain of amyloid; **(D)** Congo red stain under polarized light showing characteristic green birefringence; **(E)** Immunohistochemical staining for transthyretin from a patient with "senile" cardiac amyloidosis, ×100, and F) Immunohistochemical stain for transthyretin from a case of "senile" amyloidosis (×100), and **(F)** Immunohistochemical stain for lambda light chains from a case of immunoglobulin-related amyloidosis from a patient with multiple myeloma. Positive immunostaining is brown (×200).

IAA is a common postmortem finding in the elderly. IAA occurs in as many as 80–90% of individuals older than 90 years (99,110). IAA is associated with heart failure, AF, and conditions associated with increased plasma concentration of ANP (99,110). Grossly, deposits of amyloid are only found in the atria, predominantly in the appendages, and beneath the endocardium (99). Histologically, ANP-positive amyloid deposits surround cardiac myocytes (99,100,109,110).

Localized valvular amyloid is also predominantly found in the elderly. This amyloid deposition is associated with AV sclerosis and, less commonly, with MV dysfunction (regurgitation and stenosis) (99,112). Amyloid deposition in the valve seems to be associated with athero-inflammatory risk factors such as high shear-stress hemodynamics (112).

AGING CHANGES IN THE CONDUCTION SYSTEM AND ARRHYTHMIAS

The prevalence rates of both conduction disturbances and arrhythmias increase with age (70). The major components of the conduction system of the heart consist of the sinoatrial (SA) node, AV node, His bundle, and bundle branches. Dysfunction of the SA node progressively increases with age regardless of gender (113). Even in the healthy elderly, there is an intrinsic decline in endogenous pacemaker function (113).

In the adult SA node, the percentage of fibrosis, collagen fibers, reticular fibers, and elastic fibers increases significantly with age (10,70,114,115). Mature adipose tissue also increases with age in the conduction system (114–119). The number of SA nodal cells declines with aging (70,116,120). Nodal cells occupy 20–30% of the area of the SA node in adults 30–39 years old, but this declines to less than 10% among those older than 100 years (70). The AV node in the elderly also shows replacement by adipose tissue and an increase in elastic fibers (70,116). However, these changes are usually not extensive enough to lead to clinical problems (116). The His bundle and bundle branches also have more fibrous tissue in the aged (70).

SICK SINUS SYNDROME

Patients with sick sinus syndrome (SSS) show sinus arrest, SA exit block, or persistent sinus bradycardia. The majority of patients ultimately require a permanent pacemaker. Symptomatic SSS is mostly seen in elderly people and is the leading cause of pacemaker implantation. Reduction in the number of conduction cells, increased fibrosis, and infiltration of adipose tissue may contribute to SSS (70,116,119). In older SSS patients, there is a loss of SA node cells, resulting in decreased cellularity in the region of the SA node (70). Marked fibrosis of the SA node is found in elderly patients requiring permanent pacemakers for SSS (116). In cases without marked fibrosis, severe fatty infiltration is seen (116). Excessive fatty infiltration in the atrionodal transitional area leads to reduced atrionodal conduction with atrophy of the AV node (116). Fibrosis of right atrial muscle may also be present (70).

ATRIAL FIBRILLATION

AF is the most common clinically significant cardiac arrhythmia, and the prevalence of AF increasing markedly with increasing age. Patients with AF have higher mortality. AF in the elderly is often multifactorial or idiopathic; that is, not associated with any specific cause (118).

Macroscopically, atrial cavity dilation is seen in hearts with AF (10,70,118). Microscopic findings include SA muscle cell loss or fibrosis, disruption of the internodal atrial musculature by fibrosis and/or adipose tissue, or vascular occlusion of the SA nodal artery (70,118).

ATRIOVENTRICULAR BLOCK

AV block is defined as a delay or interruption in the transmission of an impulse from the atria to the ventricles through the conduction system. AV block can be caused by anatomical abnormalities, functional disorders, drugs, or electrolyte disturbances (121,122). Morphological changes are seen in the AV junctional area, bifurcating His bundle, or right or left bundle (121). (Fig. 2.9 A & B) In the elderly, acute and old MI, calcific valvular disease, endocarditis, myocarditis, amyloidosis, and metastatic or primary tumors may be associated with AV block (70,121,122).

(A)   (B)

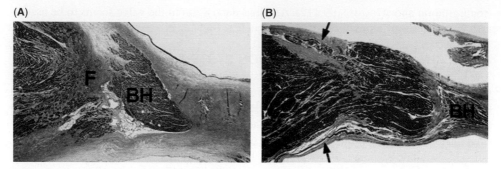

Figure 2.9 Conduction system disease in the elderly: (**A**) Section showing the bundle of His (BH) with fibrosis (F) at the base of the interventricular septum, and (**B**) Section showing bundle branches (arrows) with surrounding fibrosis (trichrome stains with which fibrous tissue stains blue and muscle red, A and B ×40).

Lev's disease and Lenègre's disease are common causes of AV block in the elderly. These disorders are characterized by idiopathic progressive cardiac conduction system disease without other evidence of organic heart disease (123). According to Lev, the heart begins to show fibrosis, hyalinization, and calcification with aging in various regions, including the conduction system (124). These age-related degenerative changes lead to interruption of the conduction fibers and AV block (123,124).

Lev reported that sclero-fibrotic changes involving the central fibrous body caused chronic AV block (124). Fibrosis and sclero-calcification is characteristically found in the bundle of His or the proximal bundle branches (124,125). In contrast, diffuse fibrotic degeneration of the conduction system is mainly seen in the distal parts of the bundle branches in the disease credited to Lenègre. A splicing mutation was found in Lenègre's disease, and the disease is now thought to be hereditary. Lenègre's disease appears to be due to a loss-of-function mutation in the gene coding the main cardiac Na channel, SCN5A (123). Whether Lev's and Lenègre's disease are the same or different entities is debatable (123–125). However, a combination of the SCN5A mutation and additional degenerative age-related changes may explain the progressive alteration of conduction velocity in both disorders (123).

In one autopsy study of elderly patients with complete AV block without any identifiable cause, the most common site of complete AV block with narrow QRS and prolonged AH interval (i.e., block proximal to the His bundle deflection) was at the branching of the His bundle (126). Complete AV block with wide QRS and prolonged HV interval (block distal to the His bundle deflection) was caused by lesions in both bundle branches (126). As the main penetrating bundle of His is located near the non-coronary cusp of the AV and near the base of the anterior leaflet of the MV, calcific deposits in either the aortic or MV may cause AV block (122).

BUNDLE-BRANCH BLOCK
Right bundle branch block (RBBB) and left bundle branch block (LBBB) occur at various levels of the branches of the His-Purkinje system. The prevalence of both RBBB and LBBB increases with age. RBBB and LBBB are associated with a wide range of diseases (122).

VENTRICULAR ARRHYTHMIAS
Ventricular arrhythmias run the gamut from asymptomatic premature ventricular complexes (PVCs) to ventricular fibrillation (VF) resulting in sudden death. Ventricular arrhythmias are particularly common in patients with acute or chronic myocardial ischemia (118).

The mechanism of ventricular tachycardia (VT) in most cases is reentry. Macro-reentry circuits result from healed myocardial infarcts and ventricular aneurysms caused by transmural MI (118). Histopathologic correlates for reentry are regions of anisotropy with mixtures of normal, ischemic, and/or fibrotic myocardium (118).

PERICARDIAL DISEASE

The human heart is surrounded by pericardial tissue. The pericardium provides structural support and reduces friction (127). There is a potential cavity between the visceral and parietal pericardium, usually containing 15–50 ml of serous fluid (127,128). In contrast to most other cardiac disorders, older adults do not seem particularly prone to pericardial disease.

Pericardial diseases include acute and recurrent pericarditis, pericardial effusion, cardiac tamponade, pericardial constriction, and pericardial tumors. Primary malignant pericardial tumors are rare, with mesothelioma being the most common type (128). In contrast, the pericardium is a common site of metastasis, especially from lung or breast primaries (128).

Acute pericarditis is caused by a wide range of disorders (127,128). The acute inflammatory response in pericarditis produces serous or purulent pericardial effusions or dense fibrinous exudate (129). Viral infection tends to cause serious, low volume pericardial effusions (129). Neoplasms and tuberculosis pericarditis cause exudative, hemorrhagic effusions (129). Bacterial infections cause purulent pericarditis (Fig. 2.10). The cause of acute pericarditis is unclear in most patients, but often presumed to be viral (127).

Pericardial constriction (less properly referred to as constrictive pericarditis) differs in developed countries and developing countries (127,130). Pericardial constriction is thought to be the result of chronic pericardial inflammation caused by any pericardial

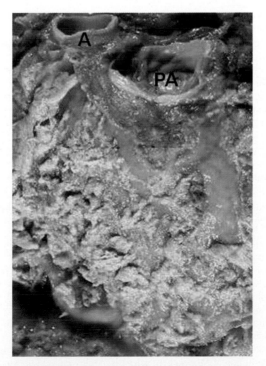

Figure 2.10   Pericarditis: fibrinopurulent pericardial exudate from a patient with bacterial pericarditis. *Abbreviations*: PA, pulmonary artery; A, aorta.

disease (127,128). However, when the pericardial tissue is examined, little if any inflammation is present. In developed countries, most cases are idiopathic (often thought to be viral), or related to previous cardiac surgery or irradiation (127). Grossly, pericardial constriction is associated with thickened pericardium, fibrosis and calcification, and adhesion to the adjacent myocardium (127,128).

In contrast, in developing countries approximately 70% of large pericardial effusions and most cases of pericardial constriction are caused by tuberculosis. Mortality of tuberculous pericarditis is high, and reported to be 17–40% (130). Tuberculous pericarditis develops by retrograde lymphatic spread; that is, neither contiguous spread from adjacent organs nor hematogenous spread (130). The early stage is characterized by fibrous exudate with high protein content. Granulomatous caseation is seen in the mid-to-late stages (130). HIV-associated tuberculous pericarditis is often associated with myopericarditis (130).

REFERENCES

1. Anversa P, Rota M, Urbanek K, et al. Myocardial aging–a stem cell problem. Basic Res Cardiol 2005; 100: 482–93.
2. Lakatta EG. Arterial and cardiac aging: major shareholders in cardiovascular disease enterprises: part II: the aging heart in health: links to heart disease. Circulation 2003; 107: 346–54.
3. Olivetti G, Giordano G, Corradi D, et al. Gender differences and aging: effects on the human heart. J Am Coll Cardiol 1995; 26: 1068–79.
4. Juhaszova M, Rabuel C, Zorov DB, et al. Protection in the aged heart: preventing the heart-break of old age? Cardiovasc Res 2005; 66: 233–44.
5. Arai T, Nakahara K. Age-related mitochondrial DNA deletion in human heart: its relationship with cardiovascular diseases. Aging Clin Exp Res 2003; 15: 1–5.
6. Sawabe M, Saito M, Naka M, et al. Standard organ weights among elderly Japanese who died in hospital, including 50 centenarians. Pathol Int 2006; 56: 315–23.
7. Okada R. Histopathological study on the effects of aging in myocardium of hypertrophied hearts. Jpn Circ J 1986; 50: 1018–22.
8. Chida K, Ohkawa S-I, Watanabe C, et al. A morphological study of the normally aging heart. Cardiovasc Pathol 1994; 3: 1–7.
9. Waller BF, Roberts WC. Cardiovascular disease in the very elderly. Analysis of 40 necropsy patients aged 90 years or over. Am J Cardiol 1983; 51: 403–21.
10. Davies MJ, Pomerance A. Quantitative study of ageing changes in the human sinoatrial node and internodal tracts. Br Heart J 1972; 34: 150–2.
11. Handke M, Harloff A, Olschewski M, et al. Patent foramen ovale and cryptogenic stroke in older patients. N Engl J Med 2007; 357: 2262–8.
12. Parson SJ, Russell SD, Bennett MK, et al. Increased lipofuscin on endomyocardial biopsy predicts greater cardiac improvement in adolescents and young adults. Cardiovasc Pathol 2012; 21: 317–23.
13. Wang JC, Bennett M. Aging and atherosclerosis: mechanisms, functional consequences, and potential therapeutics for cellular senescence. Circ Res 2012; 111: 245–59.
14. Orlandi A, Bochaton-Piallat ML, Gabbiani G, Spagnoli LG. Aging, smooth muscle cells and vascular pathobiology: implications for atherosclerosis. Atherosclerosis 2006; 188: 221–30.
15. Virmani R, Avolio AP, Mergner WJ, et al. Effect of aging on aortic morphology in populations with high and low prevalence of hypertension and atherosclerosis communities. Am J Pathol 1991; 139: 1119–29.
16. Hutchins GM, Bulkley BH, Miner MM, Boitnott JK. Correlation of age and heart weight with tortuosity and caliber of normal human coronary arteries. Am Heart J 1977; 94: 196–202.
17. Johnson MR. A normal coronary artery: what size is it? Circulation 1992; 86: 331–3.
18. Hort W, Lichti H, Kalbfleisch H, et al. The size of human coronary arteries depending on the physiological and pathological growth of the heart the age, the size of the supplying areas and the degree of coronary sclerosis. Virchows Archiv A 1982; 397: 37–59.
19. Restrepo C, Eggen DA, Guzmán MA, Tejada C. Postmortem dimensions of the coronary arteries in different geographic locations. Lab Invest 1973; 28: 244–51.
20. Micheletti RG, Fishbein GA, Currier JS, Fishbein MC. Mönckeberg sclerosis revisited: a clarification of the histologic definition of Mönckeberg sclerosis. Archiv Pathol Lab Med 2008; 132: 43–7.
21. Mönckeberg J. Über die reine Mediaverkalkung der Extremitätenarterien und ihr Verhalten zur Arteriosklerose. Virchows Arch 1903; 171: 141–67.

22. Micheletti RG, Fishbein GA, Currier JS, et al. Calcification of the internal elastic lamina of coronary arteries. Mod Pathol 2008; 21: 1019–28.
23. Bierman E. Atherosclerosis and aging. Fed Proc 1978; 37: 2832–6.
24. White NK, Edwards JE, Dry TJ. The relationship of the degree of coronary atherosclerosis with age, in men. Circulation 1950; 1: 645–54.
25. van Oostrom O, Velema E, Schoneveld AH, et al. Age-related changes in plaque composition: a study in patients suffering from carotid artery stenosis. Cardiovasc Pathol 2005; 14: 126–34.
26. Virmani R, Burke AP, Farb A, Kolodgie FD. Pathology of the vulnerable plaque. J Am Coll Cardiol 2006; 47: C13–18.
27. Raggi P, Callister TQ, Cooil B, et al. Identification of patients at increased risk of first unheralded acute myocardial infarction by electron-beam computed tomography. Circulation 2000; 101: 850–5.
28. Wong ND, Kouwabunpat D, Vo AN, et al. Coronary calcium and atherosclerosis by ultrafast computed tomography in asymptomatic men and women: relation to age and risk factors. Am Heart J 1994; 127: 422–30.
29. Roberts WC. Ninety-three hearts > or = 90 years of age. Am J Cardiol 1993; 71: 599–602.
30. Serruys P, Unger F, Sousa J, et al. Comparison of coronary-artery bypass surgery and stenting for the treatment of multivessel disease. N Engl J Med 2001; 344: 1117–24.
31. Park S, Kim Y, Park D, et al. Randomized trial of stents versus bypass surgery for left main coronary artery disease. N Engl J Med 2011; 364: 1718–27.
32. Shirani J, Yousefi J, Roberts W. Major cardiac findings at necropsy in 366 American octogenarians. Am J Cardiol 1995; 75: 151–6.
33. Wagenvoort C, Heath D, Edwards J. The Pathology of the Pulmonary Vasculature, 1st edn. Springfield, Illinois, USA: Thomas Books, 1964.
34. Lam CSP, Borlaug BA, Kane GC, et al. Age-associated increases in pulmonary artery systolic pressure in the general population. Circulation 2009; 119: 2663–70.
35. Fishbein M, Maclean D, Maroko P. The histopathologic evolution of myocardial infarction. Chest 1978; 73: 843–9.
36. Kearney PM, Whelton M, Reynolds K, et al. Global burden of hypertension: analysis of worldwide data. Lancet 2005; 365: 217–23.
37. Pestana M. Hypertension in the elderly. Int Urol Nephrol 2001; 33: 563–9.
38. Frohlich ED, Apstein C, Chobanian AV, Devereux RB. The heart in hypertension. N Engl J Med 1992; 327: 998–1008.
39. Drazner MH, Rame JE, Marino EK, et al. Increased left ventricular mass is a risk factor for the development of a depressed left ventricular ejection fraction within five years: the Cardiovascular Health Study. J Am Coll Cardiol 2004; 43: 2207–15.
40. Sehgal S, Drazner MH. Left ventricular geometry: does shape matter? Am Heart J 2007; 153: 153–5.
41. Drazner MH. The progression of hypertensive heart disease. Circulation 2011; 123: 327–34.
42. Rame JE, Ramilo M, Spencer N, et al. Development of a depressed left ventricular ejection fraction in patients with left ventricular hypertrophy and a normal ejection fraction. Am J Cardiol 2004; 93: 234–7.
43. Schelbert EB, Cao JJ, Sigurdsson S, et al. Prevalence and prognosis of unrecognized myocardial infarction determined by cardiac magnetic resonance in older adults. JAMA 2012; 308: 890–6.
44. Roberts WC. Morphological features of the elderly heart. In: Cardiovascular Disease in the Elderly. New York: Informa Healthcare, 2008: 75–98.
45. Leong SW, Soor GS, Butany J, et al. Morphological findings in 192 surgically excised native mitral valves. Can J Cardiol 2006; 22: 1055–61.
46. Sahasakul Y, Edwards WD, Naessens JM, Tajik AJ. Age-related changes in aortic and mitral valve thickness: implications for two-dimensional echocardiography based on an autopsy study of 200 normal human hearts. Am J Cardiol 1988; 62: 424–30.
47. Pomerance A. Ageing changes in human heart valves. Br Heart J 1967; 29: 222–31.
48. Goldbarg SH, Elmariah S, Miller MA, Fuster V. Insights into degenerative aortic valve disease. J Am Coll Cardiol 2007; 50: 1205–13.
49. Iung B, Cachier A, Baron G, et al. Decision-making in elderly patients with severe aortic stenosis: why are so many denied surgery? Eur Heart J 2005; 26: 2714–20.
50. O'Brien KD. Epidemiology and genetics of calcific aortic valve disease. J Investig Med 2007; 55: 284–91.
51. Shah PK. Should severe aortic stenosis be operated on before symptom onset? Severe aortic stenosis should not be operated on before symptom onset. Circulation 2012; 126: 118–25.
52. Likosky DS, Sorensen MJ, Dacey LJ, et al. Long-term survival of the very elderly undergoing aortic valve surgery. Circulation 2009; 120: S127–33.

53. Allison MA, Cheung P, Criqui MH, et al. Mitral and aortic annular calcification are highly associated with systemic calcified atherosclerosis. Circulation 2006; 113: 861–6.
54. Roberts C, Waller BF, Bethesda MD. Mitral valve "anular" calcium forming a complete circle or "O" configuration: clinical and necropsy observations. Am Heart J 1981; 101: 619–21.
55. Leon M, Smith C, Mack M. Transcatheter aortic-valve implantation for aortic stenosis in patients who cannot undergo surgery. N Engl J Med 2010; 363: 1597–607.
56. Rosengart TK, Feldman T, Borger MA, et al. Percutaneous and minimally invasive valve procedures: a scientific statement from the American Heart Association Council on Cardiovascular Surgery and Anesthesia, Council on Clinical Cardiology, Functional Genomics and Translational Biology Interdisciplin. Circulation 2008; 117: 1750–67.
57. Unbehaun A, Pasic M, Dreysse S, et al. Transapical aortic valve implantation: incidence and predictors of paravalvular leakage and transvalvular regurgitation in a series of 358 patients. J Am Coll Cardiol 2012; 59: 211–21.
58. Pasic M, Unbehaun A, Dreysse S, et al. Transapical aortic valve implantation in 175 consecutive patients: excellent outcome in very high-risk patients. J Am Coll Cardiol 2010; 56: 813–20.
59. Kalavrouziotis D, Rodés-Cabau J, Bagur R, et al. Transcatheter aortic valve implantation in patients with severe aortic stenosis and small aortic annulus. J Am Coll Cardiol 2011; 58: 1016–24.
60. Smith C, Leon M, Mack M. Transcatheter versus surgical aortic-valve replacement in high-risk patients. N Engl J Med 2011; 364: 2187–98.
61. Bekeredjian R, Grayburn P. Valvular heart disease. N Engl J Med 1997; 337: 32–41.
62. Allen WM, Matloff JM, Fishbein MC. Myxoid degeneration of the aortic valve and isolated severe aortic regurgitation. Am J Cardiol 1985; 55: 439–44.
63. Gupta V, Barzilla J, Mendez J. Abundance and location of proteoglycans and hyaluronan within normal and myxomatous mitral valves. Cardiovasc Pathol 2009; 18: 191–7.
64. Tresch DD, Doyle TP, Boncheck LI, et al. Mitral valve prolapse requiring surgery. clinical and pathologic study. Am J Med 1985; 78: 245–50.
65. Freed LA, Benjamin EJ, Levy D, et al. Mitral valve prolapse in the general population: the benign nature of echocardiographic features in the Framingham Heart Study. J Am Coll Cardiol 2002; 40: 1298–304.
66. Wu W, Luo X, Wang L, et al. The accuracy of echocardiography versus surgical and pathological classification of patients with ruptured mitral chordae tendineae: a large study in a Chinese cardiovascular center. J Cardiothorac Surg 2011; 6: 94.
67. Pomerance A. Pathological and clinical study of calcification of the mitral valve ring. J Clin Pathol 1970; 23: 354–61.
68. Fulkerson PK, Beaver BM, Auseon JC, Graber HL. Calcification of the mitral annulus: etiology, clinical associations, complications and therapy. Am J Med 1979; 66: 967–77.
69. D'Cruz I, Panetta F, Cohen H, Glick G. Submitral calcification or sclerosis in elderly patients: M mode and two dimensional echocardiography in "mitral anulus calcification". Am J Cardiol 1979; 44: 31–8.
70. Ohkawa S-I. Histopathology of the conduction system (Japanese). J Arrhythmia 2000; 16: 312–29.
71. Horstkotte D, Follath F, Gutschik E, et al. Guidelines on prevention, diagnosis and treatment of infective endocarditis executive summary; the task force on infective endocarditis of the European society of cardiology. Eur Heart J 2004; 25: 267–76.
72. Wang A. The changing epidemiology of infective endocarditis: the paradox of prophylaxis in the current and future eras. J Am Coll Cardiol 2012; 59: 1977–8.
73. Rahimtoola SH. The year in valvular heart disease. J Am Coll Cardiol 2007; 49: 361–74.
74. Fernández Guerrero ML, Álvarez B, Manzarbeitia F, Renedo G. Infective endocarditis at autopsy: a review of pathologic manifestations and clinical correlates. Medicine 2012; 91: 152–64.
75. Atkinson JB, Virmani R. Infective endocarditis: changing trends and general approach for examination. Hum Pathol 1987; 18: 603–8.
76. Watkin R, Sandoe J. British Society of Antimicrobial Chemotherapy (BSAC) guidelines for the diagnosis and treatment of endocarditis: what the cardiologist needs to know. Heart 2012; 98: 757–9.
77. Hecht SR, Berger M. Right-sided endocarditis in intravenous drug users. Prognostic features in 102 episodes. Ann Intern Med 1992; 117: 560–6.
78. Duval X, Delahaye F, Alla F, et al. Temporal trends in infective endocarditis in the context of prophylaxis guideline modifications: three successive population-based surveys. J Am Coll Cardiol 2012; 59: 1968–76.
79. Tribouilloy C, Rusinaru D, Sorel C, et al. Clinical characteristics and outcome of infective endocarditis in adults with bicuspid aortic valves: a multicentre observational study. Heart 2010; 96: 1723–9.

80. Athan E, Chu VH, Tattevin P, et al. Clinical characteristics and outcome of infective endocarditis involving implantable cardiac devices. JAMA 2012; 307: 1727–35.
81. Lopez JA, Ross RS, Fishbein MC, Siegel RJ. Nonbacterial thrombotic endocarditis: a review. Am Heart J 1987; 113: 773–84.
82. Rogers LR, Cho ES, Kempin S, Posner JB. Cerebral infarction from non-bacterial thrombotic endocarditis. Clinical and pathological study including the effects of anticoagulation. Am J Med 1987; 83: 746–56.
83. Silbiger JJ. The valvulopathy of non-bacterial thrombotic endocarditis. J Heart Valve Dis 2009; 18: 159–66.
84. Maron BJ, Towbin JA, Thiene G, et al. Contemporary definitions and classification of the cardiomyopathies: an American Heart Association Scientific Statement from the Council on Clinical Cardiology, Heart Failure and Transplantation Committee; Quality of Care and Outcomes Research and Functional Genomics and Translational Biology Interdisciplinary Working Groups; and Council on Epidemiology and Prevention. Circulation 2006; 113: 1807–16.
85. Shah KB, Inoue Y, Mehra M. Amyloidosis and the heart. Arch Intern Med 2006; 166: 1805–13.
86. Ho CY. Hypertrophic cardiomyopathy. Circulation 2012; 125: 1432–8.
87. Maron B. Hypertrophic cardiomyopathy. JAMA 2002; 287: 1308–20.
88. Semsarian C. Guidelines for the diagnosis and management of hypertrophic cardiomyopathy. Heart Lung Circ 2011; 20: 688–90.
89. Maron BJ, Casey SA, Hauser RG, Aeppli DM. Clinical course of hypertrophic cardiomyopathy with survival to advanced age. J Am Coll Cardiol 2003; 42: 882–8.
90. Leone O, Veinot JP, Angelini A, et al. 2011 consensus statement on endomyocardial biopsy from the association for european cardiovascular pathology and the society for cardiovascular pathology. Cardiovasc Pathol 2012; 21: 245–74.
91. Watkins H, Ashrafian HRC. Inherited cardiomyopathies. N Engl J Med 2011; 364: 1643–56.
92. Luk A, Ahn E, Soor GS, Butany J. Dilated cardiomyopathy: a review. J Clin Pathol 2009; 62: 219–25.
93. Elliott P, Andersson B, Arbustini E, et al. Classification of the cardiomyopathies: a position statement from the European society of cardiology working group on myocardial and pericardial diseases. Eur Heart J 2008; 29: 270–6.
94. Sinning C, Keller T, Abegunewardene N, et al. Tako-Tsubo syndrome: dying of a broken heart? Clin Res Cardiol 2010; 99: 771–80.
95. Lyon AR, Rees PSC, Prasad S, et al. Stress (Takotsubo) cardiomyopathy–a novel pathophysiological hypothesis to explain catecholamine-induced acute myocardial stunning. Nat Clin Pract Cardiovasc Med 2008; 5: 22–9.
96. Kumar S, Kaushik S, Nautiyal A, et al. Cardiac rupture in takotsubo cardiomyopathy: a systematic review. Clin Cardiol 2011; 34: 672–6.
97. Akashi YJ, Goldstein DS, Barbaro G, Ueyama T. Takotsubo cardiomyopathy: a new form of acute, reversible heart failure. Circulation 2008; 118: 2754–62.
98. Wittstein I, Thiemann D. Neurohumoral features of myocardial stunning due to sudden emotional stress. N Engl J Med 2005; 352: 539–48.
99. Kholová I, Niessen HWM. Amyloid in the cardiovascular system: a review. J Clin Pathol 2005; 58: 125–33.
100. Sawabe M, Hamamatsu A, Ito T, et al. Early pathogenesis of cardiac amyloid deposition in senile systemic amyloidosis: close relationship between amyloid deposits and the basement membranes of myocardial cells. Virchows Arch 2003; 442: 252–7.
101. Kapoor P, Thenappan T, Singh E, et al. Cardiac amyloidosis: a practical approach to diagnosis and management. Am J Med 2011; 124: 1006–15.
102. Hackel J. Clinical pathologic correlations amyloid disease of the heart. Clin Cardiol 1994; 622: 619–22.
103. Walley VM, Kisilevsky R, Young ID. Amyloid and the cardiovascular system: a review of pathogenesis and pathology with clinical correlations. Cardiovasc Pathol 1995; 4: 79–102.
104. Ueda M, Horibata Y, Shono M, et al. Clinicopathological features of senile systemic amyloidosis: an ante- and post-mortem study. Mod Pathol 2011; 24: 1533–44.
105. Schönland SO, Hegenbart U, Bochtler T, et al. Immunohistochemistry in the classification of systemic forms of amyloidosis: a systematic investigation of 117 patients. Blood 2012; 119: 488–93.
106. Falk RH. Cardiac amyloidosis: a treatable disease, often overlooked. Circulation 2011; 124: 1079–85.
107. Philippakis AA, Falk RH. Cardiac amyloidosis mimicking hypertrophic cardiomyopathy with obstruction: treatment with disopyramide. Circulation 2012; 125: 1821–4.

108. Crotty TB, Li CY, Edwards WD, Suman VJ. Amyloidosis and endomyocardial biopsy: correlation of extent and pattern of deposition with amyloid immunophenotype in 100 cases. Cardiovasc Pathol 1995; 4: 39–42.
109. Looi LM. Isolated atrial amyloidosis: a clinicopathologic study indicating increased prevalence in chronic heart disease. Hum Pathol 1993; 24: 602–7.
110. Cornwell GG, Johnson KH, Westermark P. The age related amyloids: a growing family of unique biochemical substances. J Clin Pathol 1995; 48: 984–9.
111. Rapezzi C, Merlini G, Quarta CC, et al. Systemic cardiac amyloidoses: disease profiles and clinical courses of the 3 main types. Circulation 2009; 120: 1203–12.
112. Kristen AV, Schnabel PA, Winter B, et al. High prevalence of amyloid in 150 surgically removed heart valves–a comparison of histological and clinical data reveals a correlation to atheroinflammatory conditions. Cardiovasc Pathol 2010; 19: 228–35.
113. Jones SA, Boyett MR, Lancaster MK. Declining into failure: the age-dependent loss of the L-type calcium channel within the sinoatrial node. Circulation 2007; 115: 1183–90.
114. Lev M. Aging changes in the human sinoatrial node. J Gerontol 1954; 9: 1–9.
115. Waller B, Gering L, Branyas N, Slack J. Anatomy, histology, and pathology of the cardiac conduction system: part I. Clin Cardiol 1993; 16: 249–52.
116. Chida K, Imai T, Taniguchi T. Implications of marked fatty infiltration around and in the atrophic atrioventricular node in elderly patients with permanent pacemaker implantation for symptomatic sick. Jpn Circ J 1999; 63: 343–9.
117. Shiraishi I, Takamatsu T, Minamikawa T, et al. Quantitative histological analysis of the human sino-atrial node during growth and aging. Circulation 1992; 85: 2176–84.
118. Waller B, Gering L. Anatomy, histology, and pathology of the cardiac conduction system—part III. Clin Cardiol 1993; 16: 436–42.
119. Bharati S, Lev M. The pathologic changes in the conduction system beyond the age of ninety. Am Heart J 1992; 124: 486–96.
120. Okada R. Pathological substrates of arrhythmias (Japanese). Sogo-rinsyo 1996; 45: 433–41.
121. Waller B, Gering L. Anatomy, histology, and pathology of the cardiac conduction system—Part V. Clin Cardiol 1993; 16: 565–9.
122. Waller B, Gering L. Anatomy, histology, and pathology of the cardiac conduction system—Part VI. Clin Cardiol 1993; 16: 623–8.
123. Royer A, van Veen T a B, Le Bouter S, et al. Mouse model of SCN5A-linked hereditary Lenègre's disease: age-related conduction slowing and myocardial fibrosis. Circulation 2005; 111: 1738–46.
124. Lev M. The normal anatomy of the conduction system in man and its pathology in atrioventricular block. Ann New York Acad Sci 1964; 111: 817–29.
125. Stéphan E, Aftimos G, Allam C. Familial fascicular block: histologic features of Lev's disease. Am Heart J 1985; 109: 1399–401.
126. Ohkawa S, Sugiura M, Itoh Y, et al. Electrophysiologic and histologic correlations in chronic complete atrioventricular block. Circulation 1981; 64: 215–31.
127. Khandaker MH, Espinosa RE, Nishimura RA, et al. Pericardial disease: diagnosis and management. Mayo Clinic Proc 2010; 85: 572–93.
128. Peebles CR, Shambrook JS, Harden SP. Pericardial disease–anatomy and function. Br J Radiol 2011; 84: S324–37.
129. Tingle LE, Molina D, Calvert CW. Acute pericarditis. Am Fam Physician 2007; 76: 1509–14.
130. Syed FF, Mayosi BM. A modern approach to tuberculous pericarditis. Prog Cardiovasc Dis 2007; 50: 218–36.

3

Cardiovascular drug therapy in the elderly

William H. Frishman, Wilbert S. Aronow, and Angela Cheng-Lai

SUMMARY

Cardiovascular disease is the greatest cause of morbidity and mortality in the elderly, and cardiovascular drugs are the most widely prescribed drugs in this population. Since many cardiovascular drugs have narrow therapeutic windows in the elderly, the incidence of adverse effects from using these drugs is also highest in the elderly. The appropriate use of cardiovascular drugs in the elderly requires knowledge of age-related physiologic changes, the effects of concomitant diseases that alter the pharmacokinetic and pharmacodynamic effects of cardiovascular drugs, and drug interactions.

PHARMACOKINETIC CONSIDERATIONS IN THE ELDERLY
Absorption
Age-related physiologic changes that may affect absorption include reduced gastric secretion of acid, decreased gastric emptying rate, reduced splanchnic blood flow, and decreased mucosal absorptive surface area (Table 3.1). Despite these physiologic changes, the oral absorption of cardiovascular drugs is not significantly affected by aging, probably because most drugs are absorbed passively (1).

Bioavailability
There are almost no data available for age-related changes in drug bioavailability for routes of administration other than the oral route (2). The bioavailability of cardiovascular drugs depends on the extent of drug absorption and on first-pass metabolism by the liver and/or the wall of the gastrointestinal (GI) tract. In the elderly, the absolute bioavailability of drugs such as propranolol, verapamil, and labetalol is increased because of reduced first-pass hepatic extraction (3). However, the absolute bioavailability of prazosin in the elderly is reduced (4).

Drug Distribution
With aging there is a reduction in lean body mass (5) and in total body water (6), causing a decrease in volume of distribution (V_d) of hydrophilic drugs. This leads to higher plasma concentrations of hydrophilic drugs such as digoxin and angiotensin-converting enzyme (ACE) inhibitors with the first dose in the elderly (7). The increased proportion of body fat that occurs with aging also causes an increased V_d for lipophilic drugs. This leads to lower initial plasma concentrations for lipophilic drugs such as most β-blockers, antihypertensive drugs, and central α-agonists.

Table 3.1   Physiologic Changes with Aging Potentially Affecting Cardiovascular Drug

Process	Physiologic Change	Result	Drugs Affected
Absorption	Reduced gastric acid production	Reduced tablet dissolution and decreased solubility of basic drugs	
	Reduced gastric emptying rate	Decreased absorption for acidic drugs	
	Reduced GI mobility, GI blood flow, absorptive surface	Less opportunity for drug absorption	
Distribution	Decreased total body mass, Increased proportion of body fat	Increased V_d of highly lipid-soluble drugs	↓ β blockers, central α agonists
	Decreased proportion of body water	Decreased V_d of hydrophilic drugs	↑ digoxin & ACE inhibitors
	Decreased plasma albumin, disease-related increased α_1-acid glycoprotein, altered relative tissue perfusion	Changed % of free drug, V_d, and measured levels of bound drugs	↑ disopyramide and warfarin, lidocaine, propranolol
Metabolism	Reduced liver mass, liver blood flow, and hepatic metabolic capacity	Accumulation of metabolized drugs	↑ propranolol, nitrates, lidocaine, diltiazem, warfarin, labetalol, verapamil, mexiletine
Excretion	Reduced glomerular filtration, renal tubular function, and renal blood flow	Accumulation of renally cleared drugs	Digoxin, ACE inhibitors, antiarrhythmic drugs, atenolol, sotalol, nadolol

Abbreviations: ACE, angiotensin converting enzyme; GI, gastrointestinal; V_d, volume of distribution.
Source: Adapted from Ref. 188.

The level of α-1-acid glycoprotein increases in the elderly (8). Weak bases such as disopyramide, lidocaine, and propranolol bind to α-1-acid glycoprotein. This may cause a reduction in the free fraction of these drugs in the circulation, a decreased V_d, and a higher initial plasma concentration (9). In the elderly, there is also a tendency for plasma albumin concentration to be reduced (10). Weak acids, such as salicylates and warfarin, bind extensively to albumin. Decreased binding of drugs such as warfarin to plasma albumin may result in increased free-drug concentrations, resulting in more intense drug effects (11).

Half-Life
The half-life of a drug (or of its major metabolite) is the length of time in hours that it takes for the serum concentration of that drug to decrease to half of its peak level. This can be described by the kinetic equation: $t_{1/2} = 0.693\, V_d/\mathrm{Cl}$, where $t_{1/2}$ is directly related to drug distribution and inversely to clearance. Therefore, changes in V_d and/or Cl due to aging, as previously mentioned, can affect the half-life of a drug. In elderly patients, an increased half-life of a drug means a longer time until steady-state conditions are achieved. With a prolonged half-life of a drug, there may be an initial delay in maximum effects of the drug and prolonged adverse effects. Table 3.2 lists the pharmacokinetic changes, routes of elimination, and dosage adjustment for common cardiovascular drugs used in the elderly.

Table 3.2 Pharmacokinetic Changes, Route of Elimination, and Dosage Adjustment of Selected Cardiovascular Drugs in the Elderly

Drug	$t_{1/2}$	V_d	Cl	Primary Route(s) of Elimination	Dosage Adjustment
α-adrenergic agonists centrally acting					
Clonidine	–	–	–	Hepatic/renal	Initiate at lowest dose; titrate to response
Guanabenz	–	–	–	Hepatic	Initiate at lowest dose; titrate to response
Guanfacine	↑	–	↓	Hepatic/renal	Initiate at lowest dose; titrate to response
Methyldopa	–	–	–	Hepatic	Initiate at lowest dose; titrate to response
α-1 Selective adrenergic antagonists peripherally acting					
Doxazosin	↑	↑	↑[a]	Hepatic	Initiate at lowest dose; titrate to response
Prazosin	↑	–	–	Hepatic	Initiate at lowest dose; titrate to response
Terazosin	–	–	–	Hepatic	Initiate at lowest dose; titrate to response
Angiotensin-Converting enzyme inhibitors					
Benazepril	↑	–	↓	Renal	No adjustment needed
Captopril	NS	–	↓	Renal	Initiate at lowest dose; titrate to response
Enalapril	–	–	–	Renal	Initiate at lowest dose; titrate to response
Fosinopril	–	–	–	Hepatic/renal	No adjustment needed
Lisinopril	↑	NS	↓	Renal	Initiate at lowest dose; titrate to response
Moexipril	–	–	–	Hepatic/renal	Initiate at lowest dose; titrate to response
Perindopril	–	–	↓	Renal	Initiate at lowest dose; titrate to response
Quinapril	–	–	–	Renal	Initiate at lowest dose; titrate to response
Ramipril	–	–	–	Renal	Initiate at lowest dose; titrate to response
Trandolapril	–	–	–	Hepatic/renal	Initiate at lowest dose; titrate to response
Angiotensin-II receptor–blockers					
Azilsartan	–	–	–	Hepatic/renal	No adjustment needed
Candesartan	–	–	–	Hepatic/renal	No adjustment needed
Eprosartan	–	–	↓	Hepatic/biliary/renal	No adjustment needed
Irbesartan	NS	–	–	Hepatic	No adjustment needed
Losartan	–	–	–	Hepatic	No adjustment needed
Olmesartan	–	–	–	Renal/biliary	No adjustment needed
Telmisartan	–	–	–	Hepatic/biliary	No adjustment needed
Valsartan	↑	–	–	Hepatic	No adjustment needed
Antianginal agent					
Ranolazine	NS	NS	NS	Hepatic	Initiate at lowest dose; titrate to response

(Continued)

Table 3.2 Pharmacokinetic Changes, Route of Elimination, and Dosage Adjustment of Selected Cardiovascular Drugs in the Elderly (*Continued*)

Drug	$t_{1/2}$	V_d	Cl	Primary Route(s) of Elimination	Dosage Adjustment
Antiarrhythmic agents					
Class I					
Disopyramide	↑	–	↓	Renal	Initiate at lowest dose; titrate to response
Flecainide	↑	↑	↓	Hepatic/renal	Initiate at lowest dose; titrate to response
Lidocaine	↑	↑	NS	Hepatic	Initiate at lowest dose; titrate to response
Mexilitine	–	–	–	Hepatic	No adjustment needed
Moricizine	–	–	–	Hepatic	No adjustment needed
Procainamide	–	–	↓	Renal	Initiate at lowest dose; titrate to response
Propafenone	–	–	–	Hepatic	No adjustment needed
Quinidine	↑	NS	↓	Hepatic	Initiate at lowest dose; titrate to response
Tocainide	↑	-	↓	Hepatic/renal	No adjustment needed
Class II (see β-Blockers)					
Class III					
Amiodarone	–	–	–	Hepatic/biliary	No adjustment needed
Bretylium	–	–	–	Renal	Initiate at lowest dose; titrate to response
Dofetilide	–	–	–	Renal	Adjust dose based on renal function
Dronedarone	–	–	–	Hepatic	No adjustment needed
Ibutilide	–	–	–	Hepatic	No adjustment needed
Sotalol	–	–	–	Renal	Adjust dose based on renal function
Class IV (see calcium channel blockers)					
Other antiarrhythmics					
Adenosine	–	–	–	Erythrocytes/vascular endothelial cells	No adjustment needed
Atropine	–	–	–	Hepatic/renal	Use usual dose with caution
Antithrombotics					
Anticoagulants					
Apixaban	–	–	–	Hepatic/renal	Use usual dose with caution
Argatroban	–	–	–	Hepatic/biliary	Use usual dose with caution
Bivalirudin	–	–	–	Renal/proteo-lytic cleavage	Adjust dose based on renal function
Dabigatran	–	–	–	Renal	No adjustment needed unless renal impairment
Dalteparin	–	–	–	Renal	Use usual dose with caution
Desirudin	–	–	–	Renal	Adjust dose based on renal function
Enoxaparin	–	–	–	Renal	Adjust dose based on renal function
Fondaparinux	↑	-	↓	Renal	Use usual dose with caution
Heparin	–	–	–	Hepatic/ reticuloendothelial system	Use usual dose with caution

Table 3.2 Pharmacokinetic Changes, Route of Elimination, and Dosage Adjustment of Selected Cardiovascular Drugs in the Elderly (*Continued*)

Drug	$t_{1/2}$	V_d	Cl	Primary Route(s) of Elimination	Dosage Adjustment
Lepirudin	↑	–	↓	Renal	Adjust dose based on renal function
Rivaroxaban	–	–	–	Renal/hepatic	No adjustment needed unless renal impairment
Tinzaparin	–		–	Renal	Use usual dose with caution
Warfarin	NS	NS	NS	Hepatic	Initiate at lowest dose; titrate to response
Antiplatelets					
Abciximab	–	–	–	Unknown	Use usual dose with Caution
Aspirin	–	–	↓	Hepatic/renal	Use usual dose with Caution
Clopidogrel	NS	–	–	Hepatic	Use usual dose with Caution
Dipyridamole	–	–	–	Hepatic/biliary	Use usual dose with caution
Eptifibatide	–	–	–	Renal/plasma	Use usual dose with caution
Prasugrel	–	–	–	Hepatic	Use usual dose with caution
Ticagrelor	–	–	–	Hepatic	Use usual dose with caution
Ticlopidine	–	–	↓	Hepatic	Use usual dose with caution
Tirofiban	↑	–	↓	Renal	Use usual dose with caution
Thrombolytics					
Alteplase	–	–	–	Hepatic	Use usual dose with caution
Anistreplase	–	–	–	Unknown	Use usual dose with caution
Reteplase	–	–	–	Hepatic	Use usual dose with caution
Streptokinase	–	–	–	Circulating antibodies/ reticuloen-dothelial system	Use usual dose with caution
Tenecteplase	–	–	–	Hepatic	Use usual dose with caution
Urokinase	–	–	–	Hepatic	Use usual dose with caution
β-adrenergic blockers					
Nonselective without ISA					
Nadolol	NS	–	–	Renal	Initiate at lowest dose; titrate to response
Propranolol	↑	NS	↓	Hepatic	Initiate at lowest dose; titrate to response
Timolol	–	–	–	Hepatic	Initiate at lowest dose; titrate to response
β1 selective without ISA					
Atenolol	↑	NS	↓	Renal	Initiate at lowest dose; titrate to response
Betaxolol	–	–	–	Hepatic	Initiate at lowest dose; titrate to response
Bisoprolol	–	–	–	Hepatic/renal	Initiate at lowest dose; titrate to response
Esmolol	–	–	–	Erythrocytes	Use usual dose with caution
Metoprolol	NS	NS	NS	Hepatic	Initiate at lowest dose; titrate to response
Nebivolol	–	–	–	Hepatic/renal	No adjustment necessary

(Continued)

Table 3.2 Pharmacokinetic Changes, Route of Elimination, and Dosage Adjustment of Selected Cardiovascular Drugs in the Elderly (*Continued*)

Drug	$t_{1/2}$	V_d	Cl	Primary Route(s) of Elimination	Dosage Adjustment
β1 selective with ISA					
Acebutolol	↑	↓	–	Hepatic/Biliary	Initiate at lowest dose; titrate to response
Nonselective with ISA					
Carteolol	–	–	–	Renal	Initiate at lowest dose; titrate to response
Penbutolol	–	–	–	Hepatic	Initiate at lowest dose; titrate to response
Pindolol	–	–	–	Hepatic/renal	Initiate at lowest dose; titrate to response
Dual acting					
Carvedilol	–	–	–	Hepatic/biliary	Initiate at lowest dose; titrate to response
Labetalol	–	–	NS	Hepatic	Initiate at lowest dose; titrate to response
Calcium channel blockers					
Amlodipine	↑	–	↓	Hepatic	Initiate at lowest dose; titrate to response
Clevidipine	–	–	–	Blood/extravascular tissue	Use usual dose with caution
Diltiazem	↑	NS	↓	Hepatic	Initiate at lowest dose; titrate to response
Felodipine	–	NS	↓	Hepatic	Initiate at lowest dose; titrate to response
Isradipine	–	–	–	Hepatic	Initiate at lowest dose; titrate to response
Nicardipine	NS	–	–	Hepatic	No initial adjustment needed
Nifedipine	↑	NS	↓	Hepatic	Initiate at lowest dose; titrate to response
Nimodipine	–	–	–	Hepatic	Use usual dose with caution
Nisoldipine	–	–	–	Hepatic	Initiate at lowest dose; titrate to response
Verapamil	↑	NS	↓	Hepatic	Initiate at lowest dose; titrate to response
Direct renin inhibitor					
Aliskiren	–	–	–	Renal/biliary	No initial dosage adjustment is needed
Diuretics					
Loop					
Bumetanide	–	NS	–	Renal/hepatic	No initial adjustment needed
Ethacrynic Acid	–	–	–	Hepatic	No initial adjustment needed
Furosemide	↑	NS	↓	Renal	No initial adjustment needed
Torsemide	–	–	–	Hepatic	No initial adjustment needed
Thiazides					
Bendroflumethiazide	–	–	–	Renal	No initial adjustment needed
Benzthiazide	–	–	–	Unknown	No initial adjustment needed
Chlorothiazide	–	–	–	Renal	No initial adjustment needed
Chlorthalidone	–	–	–	Renal	No initial adjustment needed
Hydrochlorothiazide	–	–	↓	Renal	No initial adjustment needed

Table 3.2 Pharmacokinetic Changes, Route of Elimination, and Dosage Adjustment of Selected Cardiovascular Drugs in the Elderly (*Continued*)

Drug	$t_{1/2}$	V_d	Cl	Primary Route(s) of Elimination	Dosage Adjustment
Hydroflumethiazide	–	–	–	Unknown	No initial adjustment needed
Indapamide	–	–	–	Hepatic	No initial adjustment needed
Methyclothiazide	–	–	–	Renal	No initial adjustment needed
Metolazone	–	–	–	Renal	No initial adjustment needed
Polythiazide	–	–	–	Unknown	No initial adjustment needed
Quinethazone	–	–	–	Unknown	No initial adjustment needed
Trichlormethiazide	–	–	–	Unknown	No initial adjustment needed
Potassium-sparing					
Amiloride	–	–	↓	Renal	No initial adjustment needed
Spironolactone	–	–	–	Hepatic/biliary/renal	No initial adjustment needed
Triamterene	↑	–	–	Hepatic/renal	Initiate at lowest dose; titrate to response
Aldosterone receptor antagonist					
Eplerenone	–	–	–	Hepatic	No initial adjustment needed
Endothelin receptor antagonist					
Ambrisentan	–	–	–	Hepatic/biliary	Use usual dose with caution
Bosentan	–	–	–	Hepatic/biliary	Use usual dose with caution
Human B-type natriuretic peptide					
Nesiritide	–	–	–	Cellular internalization and lysosomal proteoly-sis/ proteolytic cleavage/ renal filtration	Use usual dose with caution
Inotropic and vasopressor agents					
Inamrinone	–	–	–	Hepatic/renal	Initiate at lowest dose; titrate to response
Digoxin	↑	↓	↓	Renal	Initiate at lowest dose; titrate to response
Dobutamine	–	–	–	Hepatic/tissue	Initiate at lowest dose; titrate to response
Dopamine	–	–	–	Renal/hepatic/ plasma	Initiate at lowest dose; titrate to response
Epinephrine	–	–	–	Sympathetic nerve endings/plasma	Initiate at lowest dose; titrate to response
Isoproterenol	–	–	–	Renal	Initiate at lowest dose; titrate to response
Metaraminol	–	–	–	Hepatic/biliary/renal	Initiate at lowest dose; titrate to response
Methoxamine	–	–	–	Unknown	Initiate at lowest dose; titrate to response
Midodrine	–	–	–	Tissue/hepatic/renal	No initial adjustment needed
Milrinone	–	–	–	Renal	Adjust based on renal function
Norepinephrine	–	–	–	Sympathetic nerve endings/hepatic	Initiate at lowest dose; titrate to response
Phenylephrine	–	–	–	Hepatic/intestinal	Initiate at lowest dose; titrate to response
Vasopressin	–	–	–	Hepatic/renal	Use usual dose with caution

(*Continued*)

Table 3.2 Pharmacokinetic Changes, Route of Elimination, and Dosage Adjustment of Selected Cardiovascular Drugs in the Elderly (*Continued*)

Drug	$t_{1/2}$	V_d	Cl	Primary Route(s) of Elimination	Dosage Adjustment
Lipid-lowering agents					
BAS					
Cholestyramine	–	–	–	Not absorbed in GI tract	No adjustment needed
Colestipol	–	–	–	Not absorbed in GI tract	No adjustment needed
Colesevelam	–	–	–	Not absorbed in GI tract	No adjustment needed
Cholesterol absorption inhibitor					
Ezetimibe	–	–	–	Small intestine/ hepatic/biliary	No adjustment needed
FADS					
Bezafibrate	–	–	↓	Renal	Avoid use in patients <70 years due to declining renal function
Fenofibrate	–	–	–	Renal	Initiate at lowest dose; titrate to response
Gemfibrozil	–	–	–	Hepatic/renal	No adjustment necessary
Nicotinic Acid	–	–	–	Hepatic/renal	No initial adjustment needed
HMG CoA reductase inhibitors					
Atorvastatin	–	–	–	Hepatic/biliary	No initial adjustment needed
Fluvastatin	–	–	–	Hepatic	No initial adjustment needed
Lovastatin	–	–	–	Hepatic/fecal	No initial adjustment needed
Pitavastatin	–	–	–	Hepatic/fecal/renal	No initial adjustment needed
Pravastatin	–	–	–	Hepatic	No initial adjustment needed
Rosuvastatin	–	–	–	Hepatic/fecal	No initial adjustment needed
Simvastatin	–	–	–	Hepatic/fecal	Initiate at lowest dose; titrate to response
Omega 3 fatty acids					
Omega 3 acid ethyl esters	–	–	–	–	No adjustment needed
Neuronal and ganglionic blockers					
Guanadrel	–	–	–	Hepatic/renal	Initiate at lowest dose; titrate to response
Guanethidine	–	–	–	Hepatic/renal	Initiate at lowest dose; titrate to response
Mecamylamine	–		–	Renal	Initiate at lowest dose; titrate to response
Reserpine	–	–	–	Hepatic/fecal	Initiate at lowest dose; titrate to response
PDE5 enzyme inhibitors					
Sildenafil	–	–	↓	Hepatic/fecal	Use usual dose with caution
Tadalafil	–	–	↓	Hepatic/fecal/renal	No adjustment needed
Vasodilators					
Alprostadil	–	–	–	Pulmonary/renal	Initiate at lowest dose; titrate to response
Cilostazol	–	–	–	Hepatic/renal	No adjustment necessary
Diazoxide	–	–	–	Hepatic/renal	Initiate at lowest dose; titrate to response

Table 3.2 Pharmacokinetic Changes, Route of Elimination, and Dosage Adjustment of Selected Cardiovascular Drugs in the Elderly (*Continued*)

Drug	$t_{1/2}$	V_d	Cl	Primary Route(s) of Elimination	Dosage Adjustment
Epoprostenol	–	–	–	Hepatic/renal	Initiate at usual dose with caution
Fenoldopam	–	–	–	Hepatic	No adjustment necessary
Hydralazine	–	–	–	Hepatic	Initiate at lowest dose; titrate to response
ISDN	–	–	–	Hepatic	Initiate at lowest dose; titrate to response
ISMN	NS	–	NS	Hepatic	No adjustment necessary
Isoxsuprine	–	–	–	Renal	Initiate at lowest dose; titrate to response
Minoxidil	–	–	–	Hepatic	Initiate at lowest dose; titrate to response
Nitroglycerin	–	–	–	Hepatic	Initiate at lowest dose; titrate to response
Nitroprusside	–	–	–	Hepatic/renal/ erythrocytes	Use usual dose with caution
Papaverine	–	–	–	Hepatic	Initiate at lowest dose; titrate to response
Pentoxifylline	–	–	↓	Hepatic/renal	Use usual dose with caution; dose reduction may be needed
Vasopressin antagonists					
Conivaptan	–	–	–	Hepatic	No adjustment needed
Tolvaptan	–	–	–	Hepatic	No adjustment needed

[a]Increase in Cl is small compared to increase in V_d. *Abbreviations*: $t_{1/2}$, half-life; V_d, volume of distribution; Cl, clearance; ↑, increase; ↓, decrease; –, no information or not relevant; NS, no significant change; LMWH, low molecular weight heparin; ISA, intrinsic sympathomimetic activity; GI, gastrointestinal; BAS, bile acid sequestrants; FADS, fibric acid derivatives; HMG CoA, hydroxymethylglutaryl coenzyme A; PDE5 – phosphodiesterase 5; ISDN, isosorbide dinitrate; ISMN, isosorbide mononitrate.
Source: From Ref. 189.

Drug Metabolism

Decreased hepatic blood flow, liver mass, liver volume, and hepatic metabolic capacity occur in the elderly (12). There is a reduction in the rate of many drug oxidation reactions (phase 1) and little change in drug conjugation reactions (phase 2). These changes in the elderly may result in higher serum concentrations of cardiovascular drugs that are metabolized in the liver, including propranolol, lidocaine, labetalol, verapamil, diltiazem, nitrates, warfarin, and mexiletine.

Drug Excretion

With aging, there is a reduction in the total numbers of functioning nephrons and thereby a parallel decline in both glomerular filtration rate and renal plasma flow (13,14). The age-related decline in renal function is likely the single most important physiologic change causing pharmacokinetic alterations in the elderly. The change in renal function with aging is insidious and poorly characterized by serum creatinine determinations, although serum creatinine measurements remain one of the most widely used tests for gauging renal function. To estimate renal function from a serum creatinine value requires its being indexed for muscle mass, which is difficult in even the most skilled hands. Creatinine is a byproduct of creatine metabolism in muscle and its daily production correlates closely with muscle mass. Thus, the greater the muscle mass, the higher the "normal serum creatinine." For example, in a heavily muscled male, a serum creatinine value of 1.4 mg/dL might be considered normal, though such a value may be considered grossly abnormal in an individual with less muscle, such as an aged individual. A safer way to estimate renal function in the elderly is by use of a urine-free formula such as the Cockcroft–Gault formula (15):

$$\text{Creatinine clearance (mL/min)} = (140 - \text{age}) \times \text{body weight (kg)}/72 \times S_{creat} \text{ (mg/dL)}$$

For females, the results of this equation can be multiplied by 0.85 to account for the small muscle mass in most females. It should be appreciated that creatinine clearance is reciprocally related to serum creatinine concentrations, such that a doubling of serum creatinine represents an approximate halving of renal function. The axiom that glomerular filtration rate is reciprocally related to serum creatinine is most important with the first doubling of serum creatinine. For example, a serum creatinine value of 0.6 mg/dl in an elderly subject doubles to 1.2 mg/dl and with this doubling creatinine clearance falls from 80 to about 40 cc/min.

The National Kidney Foundation guidelines use the Modification of Diet in Renal Disease (MDRD) study equation to estimate glomerular filtration rate (16). The MDRD equation is as follows:

$$\text{Glomerular filtration rate (mL/min/1.73 m}^2)$$
$$= 186 \times S_{creat}^{-1.154} \times \text{age}^{-0.203} \times 0.742 \text{ if female} \times 1.210 \text{ if black}$$

The reduced clearance of many drugs primarily excreted by the kidneys causes their half-life to be increased in the elderly. Cardiovascular drugs known to be excreted by the kidney, via various degrees of filtration and tubular secretion, include digoxin, diuretics, ACE inhibitors, antiarrhythmic medications (bretylium, disopyramide, flecainide, procainamide, and tocainide), and the β-blockers (atenolol, bisoprolol, carteolol, nadolol, and sotalol). Typically, a renally cleared compound begins to accumulate when creatinine clearance values drop below 60 cc/min. An example of this phenomenon can be seen with ACE inhibitors (17), wherein accumulation begins early in the course of renal functional decline. Moreover, ACE inhibitor accumulation in the elderly is poorly studied in the case of many of the ACE inhibitors particularly as related to the "true level of renal function" when an otherwise healthy elderly subject undergoes formal pharmacokinetic testing. Thus, it has not been uncommon for elderly subjects with serum creatinine values as high as 2.0 mg/dl to be allowed entry into a study whose primary purpose is to determine the difference in drug handling of a renally cleared compound in young versus elderly subjects.

PHARMACODYNAMICS

There are numerous physiologic changes with aging which affect pharmacodynamics with alterations in end-organ responsiveness (Table 3.3). Increased peripheral vascular resistance is the cause of systolic and diastolic hypertension in the elderly (18). Inappropriate sodium intake and retention may contribute to increased arteriolar resistance and/or plasma volume. Cardiac output, heart rate, renal blood flow, glomerular filtration rate, and renin levels decline with aging. Increased arterial stiffness, resulting from changes in the arterial media and an increase in arterial tonus and arterial impedance, increases systolic blood pressure and contributes to a widened pulse pressure. Maintenance of α-adrenergic vasoconstriction with impaired β-adrenergic-mediated vasodilation may be an additional contributory factor to increased peripheral vascular resistance. The cardiovascular response to catecholamines as well as carotid arterial baroreflex sensitivity are both decreased in the

Table 3.3 Characteristics of the Elderly Relative to Drug Response

Physiologic Changes	Changes in Response
Decreased cardiac reserve	Potential for heart failure
Decreased LV compliance due to thickened ventricular wall, increased blood viscosity, decreased aortic compliance, increased total and peripheral resistance	Decrease of cardiac output
Decreased baroreceptor sensitivity	Tendency to orthostatic hypotension
Diminished cardiac and vascular responsiveness to β-agonists and antagonists	Decreased sensitivity to β-agonists and antagonists
Suppressed rennin–angiotensin–aldosterone system	Theoretically decreased response to ACE inhibitors, but not observed
Increased sensitivity to anticoagulant agents	Increased effects of warfarin
Concurrent illnesses	Increased drug–disease interactions
Multiple drugs	Increased drug–drug interactions
Sinus and AV node dysfunction	Potential for heart block

Abbreviations: ACE, angiotensin-converting enzyme; AV, atrioventricular; LV, left ventricular.
Source: Adapted from Ref. 188.

elderly. Left ventricular (LV) mass and left atrial dimension are increased, and there is a reduction in both the LV early diastolic filling rate and volume (18).

The pharmacodynamic, chronotropic, and inotropic effects of β-agonists and β-blockers on β-1 adrenergic receptors are diminished in the elderly (19–21). The density of β-receptors in the heart is unchanged in the elderly, but there is a decrease in the ability of β-receptor agonists to stimulate cyclic adenosine monophosphate production (22). There are also age-related changes in the cardiac conduction system, as well as an increase in arrhythmias in the elderly. In the Framingham study, the prevalence of atrial fibrillation was 1.8% in persons 60–69 years old, 4.8% in those 70–79 years old, and 8.8% in those 80–89 years old (23). In a study of 3624 elderly patients (mean age 81 years), the prevalence of atrial fibrillation was 16% (1160) in elderly men and 13% (2464) in elderly women (24).

In elderly patients with unexplained syncope, a 24-hour ambulatory electrocardiogram (ECG) should be obtained to rule out the presence of second-degree or third-degree atrioventricular (AV) block or sinus node dysfunction with pauses >3 seconds not seen on the resting ECG. These phenomena were observed in 21 of 148 patients (14%) with unexplained syncope (25). These 21 patients included 8 with sinus arrest, 7 with advanced second-degree AV block, and 6 with atrial fibrillation with a slow ventricular rate not drug induced. Unrecognized sinus node or AV node dysfunction may become evident in elderly persons after drugs such as amiodarone, β-blockers, digoxin, diltiazem, procainamide, quinidine, or verapamil are administered. Clinical use of these drugs in the elderly, therefore, must be carefully monitored.

USE OF CARDIOVASCULAR DRUGS IN THE ELDERLY
Digoxin
Digoxin has a narrow toxic-therapeutic ratio, especially in the elderly (26). Decreased renal function and lean body mass may increase serum digoxin levels in this population. Serum creatinine may be normal in elderly persons despite a marked reduction in creatinine clearance, thereby decreasing digoxin clearance and increasing serum digoxin levels. Older persons are also more likely to take drugs which interact with digoxin by interfering with bioavailability and/or elimination. Quinidine, cyclosporin, itraconazole, calcium preparations, verapamil, amiodarone, diltiazem, triamterene, spironolactone, tetracycline,

erythromycin, propafenone, and propantheline can increase serum digoxin levels. Hypokalemia, hypomagnesemia, hypercalcemia, hypoxia, acidosis, acute and chronic lung disease, hypothyroidism, and myocardial ischemia may also cause digitalis toxicity despite normal serum digoxin levels. Digoxin may also cause visual disturbances (27), depression, and confusional states in older persons, even with therapeutic blood levels.

Indications for using digoxin are slowing a rapid ventricular rate in patients with supraventricular tachyarrhythmias such as atrial fibrillation, and treating patients with congestive heart failure (CHF) in sinus rhythm associated with abnormal LV ejection fraction (LVEF) that does not respond to diuretics, ACE inhibitors, and β-blockers with a class IIa indication (28). Digoxin should not be used to treat patients with CHF in sinus rhythm associated with normal LVEF. By increasing contractility through increasing intracellular calcium ion concentration, digoxin may increase LV stiffness and increase LV filling pressures, adversely affecting LV diastolic dysfunction. Since almost half the elderly patients with CHF have normal LVEFs (29,30), LVEF should be measured in all older patients with CHF so that appropriate therapy may be given (31). Many older patients with compensated CHF who are in sinus rhythm and are on digoxin may have digoxin withdrawn without decompensation in cardiac function (32,33).

A post hoc subgroup analysis of data from women with an LVEF <45% in the Digitalis Investigation Group (DIG) study showed by multivariate analysis that digoxin significantly increased the risk of death among women by 23% (absolute increase of 4.2%) (34). A post hoc subgroup analysis of data from men with an LVEF <45% in the DIG study showed that digoxin significantly reduced mortality by 6% if the serum digoxin level was 0.5–0.8 ng/mL, insignificantly increased mortality by 3% if the serum digoxin level was 0.8–1.1 ng/mL, and significantly increased mortality by 12% if the serum digoxin level was ≥1.2 ng/mL (35).

Another post hoc subgroup analysis of data from all 1926 women with systolic or diastolic HF in the DIG study showed that digoxin significantly increased mortality by 20% in women (36). However, digoxin did not increase mortality in women with an LVEF <35% and a serum digoxin level of 0.5–1.1 ng/mL (37). In women with an LVEF <35% and a serum digoxin level ≥1.2 ng/mL, digoxin significantly increased mortality 1.83 times (37).

Therapeutic levels of digoxin do not reduce the frequency or duration of episodes of paroxysmal atrial fibrillation detected by 24-hour ambulatory ECGs (38). In addition, therapeutic concentrations of digoxin do not prevent the occurrence of a rapid ventricular rate in patients with paroxysmal atrial fibrillation (38,39). Many elderly patients are able to tolerate atrial fibrillation without the need for digoxin therapy because the ventricular rate is slow as a result of concomitant AV nodal disease.

Some studies have suggested that digoxin may decrease survival after acute myocardial infarction (MI) in patients with LV dysfunction (40,41). Leor et al. (42) showed that digoxin may exert a dose-dependent deleterious effect on survival in patients after acute MI, although other studies have not confirmed this finding (43,44). Eberhardt et al. (45) demonstrated in the Bronx Longitudinal Aging Study that digoxin use in the elderly without evidence of CHF was an independent predictor of mortality. The results of the DIG study trial demonstrated that digoxin could be used in older subjects with CHF, but in lower doses than that previously employed in clinical practice (46).

Diuretics

The Joint National Committee on Detection, Evaluation and Treatment of High Blood Pressure recommended as initial drug treatment of hypertension thiazide-like diuretics or β-blockers because these drugs had been demonstrated to reduce cardiovascular morbidity and mortality in controlled clinical trials (47). Moreover, the results of the Systolic

Hypertension in the Elderly (SHEP) trial specifically show the safety and efficacy of a diuretic and β-blocker in the treatment of isolated systolic hypertension in the elderly (48). In the elderly, a blanket recommendation for the starting medication in the treatment of hypertension is ill-advised, in part, because of the presence of comorbid conditions. For example, in older elderly hypertensive patients with CHF and a reduced LVEF (49–53) or in those elderly patients with CHF with a normal LVEF (53–55), therapy should include a diuretic, an ACE inhibitor, and a β-blocker.

Loop diuretics remain first-line drug therapy in the treatment of patients with decompensated CHF. Diuretics are multi-faceted in their effect in CHF. First, they effect a reduction in plasma volume by triggering a time-dependent natriuretic response. This drop in plasma volume reduces venous return and thereby decreases ventricular filling pressures. These volume changes facilitate relief of congestive symptomatology, such as peripheral and/or pulmonary edema. Intravenous loop-diuretic therapy has also been shown to increase central venous capacitance, which may further contribute to improvement in congestive symptomatology. Both loop and thiazide-like diuretics undergo a mixed pattern of renal/hepatic elimination with the component of renal clearance being responsible for diuresis (56). Age-related decreases in renal function may reduce the efficacy of conventional doses of diuretics in elderly patients. This "renal function-related resistance" can be easily overcome, if recognized, by careful upward titration of the diuretic dose. Resistance to diuretic effect in CHF may also derive from a pattern of variable and unpredictable absorption, particularly with the loop diuretic furosemide. This issue is resolvable with the use of a predictably absorbed loop diuretic, such as torsemide (57).

A thiazide-like diuretic, such as hydrochlorothiazide, may be used in the occasional older patient with mild CHF. However, thiazide-like diuretics have diminished effectiveness at conventional doses when the glomerular filtration rate falls below 30 mL/min; accordingly, older patients with moderate-to-severe CHF should be treated with a loop diuretic, such as furosemide. Older patients with severe CHF or concomitant significant renal insufficiency may need combination diuretic therapy employing a loop diuretic together with the thiazide-like diuretic metolazone (56). The slowly and erratically absorbed form of metolazone (Zaroxylyn®) is the preferred form when combination therapy is being considered. Non-steroidal antiinflammatory drugs (NSAIDs) may decrease both the antihypertensive and natriuretic effect of loop diuretics (56). This is a particular problem when loop diuretics are being employed to manage CHF-related congestive symptomatology (58). A final consideration is the sometimes insidious manner by which NSAIDs can interact with diuretics in that several commonly used NSAIDs are now available over-the-counter.

Serum electrolytes need to be closely monitored in older patients treated with diuretics. Hypokalemia and/or hypomagnesemia, both of which may precipitate ventricular arrhythmias and/or digitalis toxicity, can occur with diuretic therapy (59). Hyponatremia is not uncommon in the elderly treated with diuretics, particularly when thiazide-like diuretics are being employed (60). Older patients with CHF are especially sensitive to volume depletion with dehydration, hypotension, and prerenal azotemia occurring in the face of excessive diuretic effect. Older patients with CHF and normal LVEF should receive diuretics more cautiously.

β-Adrenergic Blockers

β-blockers are used in various cardiovascular disorders, with resultant beneficial and adverse effects (61). β-blockers are very effective antianginal agents in older, as well as younger, patients. Combined therapy with β-blockers and nitrates may be more beneficial in the treatment of angina pectoris than either drug alone (61).

Diuretics or β-blockers have been recommended as initial drug therapy for hypertension in older persons because these drugs have been shown to decrease cardiovascular morbidity and mortality in controlled clinical trials (47,62). β-blockers are especially useful in the treatment of hypertension in older patients who have had a prior MI, angina pectoris, silent myocardial ischemia, complex ventricular arrhythmias, supra-ventricular tachyarrhythmias, or hypertrophic cardiomyopathy.

Teo et al. (63) analyzed 55 randomized controlled trials that investigated the use of β-blockers in patients after MI. Mortality was significantly decreased (19%) in patients receiving β-blockers, compared with control patients. In the β-Blocker Heart Attack Trial (BHAT), propranolol significantly decreased total mortality by 34% in patients aged 60–69 years, and insignificantly reduced total mortality by 19% in patients aged 30–59 years (64). In the Norwegian Timolol Study, timolol significantly decreased total mortality by 43% in postinfarction patients aged 65–75 years, and significantly reduced total mortality by 34% in postinfarction patients <65 years of age (65). Despite the utility of β-blockers in post-MI patients, they are still being underutilized in older patients (66–68).

β-blockers decrease complex ventricular arrhythmias including ventricular tachycardia (69–72). β-blockers also increase the ventricular fibrillation threshold in animal models, and have been shown to reduce the incidence of ventricular fibrillation in patients with acute MI (73). A randomized, double-blind, placebo-controlled study of propranolol in high-risk survivors of acute MI at 12 Norwegian hospitals demonstrated that patients treated with propranolol for 1 year had a statistically significant 52% decrease in sudden cardiac death (70).

In addition, β-blockers decrease myocardial ischemia (71,72,74), which may reduce the likelihood of ventricular fibrillation. Stone et al. (74) demonstrated by 48-hour ambulatory ECGs in 50 patients with stable angina pectoris that propranolol, not diltiazem or nifedipine, caused a significant decrease in the mean number of episodes of myocardial ischemia and in the mean duration of myocardial ischemia compared with placebo. Furthermore, β-blockers reduce sympathetic tone.

Studies have demonstrated that β-blockers reduce mortality in older and younger patients with complex ventricular arrhythmias and heart disease (Table 3.4) (64,71,72,75–77). In the BHAT of 3290 patients comparing propranolol with placebo, propranolol reduced sudden cardiac death by 28% in patients with complex ventricular arrhythmias and by 16% in patients without ventricular arrhythmias (64).

Hallstrom et al. (75) did a retrospective analysis of the effect of antiarrhythmic drug use in 941 patients resuscitated from prehospital cardiac arrest due to ventricular fibrillation between the years 1970 and 1985. β-blockers were administered to 28% of the patients, and no antiarrhythmic drug to 39%. There was a reduced incidence of death or recurrent cardiac arrest in patients treated with β-blockers versus no antiarrhythmic drug (relative risk 0.47; adjusted relative risk 0.62).

Aronow et al. (71) performed a prospective study in 245 elderly patients (mean age 81 years) with heart disease (64% with prior MI and 36% with hypertensive heart disease), complex ventricular arrhythmias diagnosed by 24-hour ambulatory ECGs, and LVEF >40%. Nonsustained ventricular tachycardia occurred in 32% of patients. Myocardial ischemia occurred in 33% of patients. Mean follow-up was 30 months in patients randomized to propranolol and 28 months in patients randomized to no antiarrhythmic drug. Propranolol was discontinued because of adverse effects in 11% of patients. Follow-up 24-hour ambulatory ECGs showed that propranolol was significantly more effective than no antiarrhythmic drug in reducing ventricular tachycardia (>90%), in decreasing the average number of ventricular premature complexes per hour (>70%), and in abolishing silent ischemia.

Table 3.4 Effect of β-Blockers on Mortality in Elderly Patients with Complex Ventricular Arrhythmias and Heart Disease

Study	Age (yrs)	Mean Follow-Up (mos)	Results
BHAT (64)	60–69(33%)	25	Compared with placebo, propranolol reduced sudden cardiac death by 28% in patients with complex VA and 16% in patients without VA.
Hallstrom (75)	62 (mean)	108	Reduced incidence of death or recurrent cardiac arrest in patients treated with β-blockers vs. no antiarrhythmic drug (adjusted relative risk 0.62).
Aronow, et al. (71)	62–96 (mean 81)	29	Compared with no antiarrhythmic drug, propranolol caused a 47% significant decrease in sudden cardiac death, a 37% significant reduction in total cardiac death, and a 20% insignificant decrease in total death.
Aronow, et al. (72)	62–96 (mean 81)	29	Among patients taking propranolol, suppression of complex VA caused a 33% reduction in sudden cardiac death, a 27% decrease in total cardiac death, and a 30% reduction in total death; abolition of silent ischemia caused a 70% decrease in sudden cardiac death, a 72% reduction in total cardiac death, and a 69% decrease in total death.
Aronow, et al. (76)	62–96 (mean 81)	29	Incidence of sudden cardiac death or fatal myocardial infarction was significantly increased between 6 am and 12 am, with peak hour at 8 a.m. and secondary peak at 7 p.m. in patients with no antiarrhythmic drug; propranolol abolished the circadian distribution of sudden cardiac death or fatal myocardial infarction.
CAST (77)	66–79 (40%)	12	Patients on β-blockers (30% of study group) had a significant reduction in all-cause mortality of 43% at 30 days, 46% at 1 year, and 33% at 2 years: in patients on β-blockers, arrhythmic death or cardiac arrest was significantly reduced by 66% at 30 days, 53% at 1 year, and 36% at 2 years; multivariate analysis showed β-blockers to be an independent factor for reduced arrhythmic death or cardiac arrest by 40% and for all-cause mortality by 33%.

Abbreviations: BHAT, β-blocker heart attack trial; VA, ventricular arrhythmias; CAST, cardiac arrhythmia suppression trial.
Source: From Ref. 190.

Multivariate Cox regression analysis showed that propranolol caused a significant 47% decrease in sudden cardiac death, a significant 37% reduction in total cardiac death, and an insignificant 20% decrease in total death (71). Univariate Cox regression analysis showed that the reduction in mortality and complex ventricular arrhythmias in elderly patients with heart disease taking propranolol was due more to an anti-ischemic effect than to an antiarrhythmic effect (72). Table 3.4 also shows that there was a circadian distribution of sudden cardiac death or fatal MI, with the peak incidence occurring from 6 a.m. to 12 a.m. (peak hour 8 a.m. and secondary peak around 7 p.m.) in patients treated with no antiarrhythmic drug (76). Propranolol abolished this circadian distribution of sudden cardiac death or fatal MI (76).

In a retrospective analysis of data from the Cardiac Arrhythmia Suppression Trial (CAST), Kennedy et al. (77) found that 30% of patients with an LVEF <40% were receiving β-blockers. Forty percent of these 1735 patients were between 66 and 79 years of age. Patients on β-blockers had a significant reduction in all-cause mortality of 43% within 30 days, 46% at 1 year, and 33% at 2 years. Patients receiving β-blockers also had a significant decrease in arrhythmic death or cardiac arrest of 66% at 30 days, 53% at 1 year, and 36% at 2 years. Multivariate analysis showed that β-blockers were an independent factor for reducing arrhythmic death or cardiac arrest by 40%, for decreasing all-cause mortality by 33%, and for reducing the occurrence of new or worsening CHF by 32%. On the basis of these data (64,71,72,75–77), β-blockers can be utilized in the treatment of older and younger patients with ventricular tachycardia or complex ventricular arrhythmias associated with ischemic or nonischemic heart disease, and with normal or abnormal LVEF, if there are no absolute contraindications to the drugs.

β-blockers are also useful in the treatment of supraventricular tachyarrhythmias in older and younger patients (78,79). If a rapid ventricular rate associated with atrial fibrillation persists at rest or during exercise despite digoxin therapy, then verapamil (80), diltiazem (81), or a β-blocker (82) should be added to the therapeutic regimen. These drugs act synergistically with digoxin to depress conduction through the AV junction. The initial oral dose of propranolol is 10 mg q6h, which can be increased to a maximum of 80 mg q6h if necessary.

β-blockers have been demonstrated to reduce mortality in older persons with New York Heart Association (NYHA) Class II–IV CHF and abnormal LVEF treated with diuretics and ACE inhibitors with or without digoxin (52,53,83–87). β-blockers have also been shown to reduce mortality in older persons with NYHA Class II–III CHF and normal LVEF treated with diuretics plus ACE inhibitors (53,55,86,87).

Numerous drug interactions have been reported with β-blockers in the elderly (61). Quinidine, a known inhibitor of CYP2D6, was shown to decrease the hepatic metabolism of topically applied ophthalmic timolol, with resultant exaggeration of the β-blocking effect of timolol (88).

ACE Inhibitors

ACE inhibitors are effective antihypertensive agents. A meta-analysis of 109 treatment studies showed that ACE inhibitors are more effective than other antihypertensive drugs in decreasing LV mass (89). Older hypertensive patients with CHF associated with abnormal (49–51) or normal (54) LVEF, LV hypertrophy, or diabetes mellitus should initially be treated with an ACE inhibitor. ACE inhibitors reduce mortality in patients with CHF associated with abnormal LVEF (49–51). The Survival and Ventricular Enlargement (SAVE) trial (90) and the combined Studies of Left Ventricular Dysfunction (SOLVD) treatment and prevention trials (91) also demonstrated that ACE inhibitors such as captopril or enalapril should be standard therapy for most patients with significant LV systolic dysfunction with or without CHF. In addition, ACE inhibitor therapy has been shown to be beneficial in the treatment of elderly patients (mean age 80 years) with CHF caused by prior MI associated with normal LVEF (54). High-dose ACE inhibitor therapy remains the standard of care in the management of CHF. Low-dose ACE inhibitor therapy has been studied in CHF, but with less favorable results. For example, a trial compared low (2.5–5.0 mg/day) with high-dose lisinopril (32.5–35.0 mg/day), with the latter being associated with a more significant reduction in mortality and all-cause hospitalization rate (92).

An observational prospective study was performed in 477 patients, mean age 79 years, with prior MI and an asymptomatic LVEF <40% (mean LVEF 31%) (93). At 34-month follow-up, patients treated with ACE inhibitors without β-blockers had a 17% significant reduction in new coronary events and a 32% significant reduction in CHF. At 34-month follow-up, patients treated with β-blockers without ACE inhibitors had a 25% significant reduction in new coronary events and a 41% significant reduction in CHF. At 41-month follow-up, patients treated with both β-blockers and ACE inhibitors had a significant 37% reduction in new coronary events and a significant 60% reduction in CHF.

Treatment with ACE inhibitors should be initiated in elderly patients in low doses after correction of hyponatremia or volume depletion. It is important to avoid overdiuresis before beginning therapy with ACE inhibitors since volume depletion may cause hypotension or renal insufficiency when ACE inhibitors are begun or when the dose of these drugs is increased to full therapeutic levels. After the maintenance dose of ACE inhibitor is reached, it may be necessary to increase the dose of diuretics. The initial dose of enalapril is 2.5 mg daily and of captopril is 6.25 mg TID. The maintenance doses are 5–20 mg daily and 25–50 mg TID, and the maximum doses are 20 mg BID and 150 mg TID, respectively.

Older patients at risk for excessive hypotension should have their blood pressure monitored closely for the first 2 weeks of ACE inhibitor or angiotensin-II receptor-blocking therapy, and thereafter whenever the dose of ACE inhibitor or diuretic is increased. Renal function should be monitored in patients on ACE inhibitors to detect increases in blood urea nitrogen and serum creatinine, especially in older patients with renal artery stenosis. A rise in serum creatinine in an ACE inhibitor treated CHF patient is not uncommonly the result of ACE inhibitor-induced alterations in renal hemodynamics. There is no specific rise in serum creatinine where corrective actions need be taken though logic would suggest the greater the increment in serum creatinine the more important the intervention. Typically, reducing or temporarily discontinuing diuretics and/or liberalizing sodium intake are sufficient measures to return renal function to baseline. Not uncommonly though, the administered ACE inhibitor is either stopped or the dose reduced. In most instances, ACE inhibitor therapy can be safely resumed as long as careful attention is paid to patient volume status (94). Potassium-sparing diuretics or potassium supplements should be carefully administered to patients receiving ACE inhibitor therapy because of the attendant risk of hyperkalemia. In this regard, the Randomized Aldactone Evaluation Study (RALES) showed in persons with severe CHF treated with diuretics, ACE inhibitors, and digoxin that compared with placebo, spironolactone 25 mg/day did not carry an excessive risk of hyperkalemia while resulting in a significant reduction in mortality and hospitalization for CHF (95).

Angiotensin-II Receptor Blockers

Angiotensin-II receptor blockers (ARBs) have been studied fairly extensively in hypertension (96–99), diabetic nephropathy (100), and CHF (101), with results comparable to those seen when these disease states are treated with ACE inhibitors. Although the published experience with these drugs in the elderly is limited, the drugs appear to be safe if used with similar precautions as those recommended for ACE inhibitors, as described above (96,98). These drugs are noteworthy in that they have a more favorable side-effect profile and, in particular, are not associated with cough, a fairly common side effect with ACE inhibitor therapy (97). Likewise, in the Losartan Heart Failure Survival Study (ELITE II), losartan was associated with fewer adverse effects than was captopril (102). Outcomes studies are supportive of ARBs, such as losartan and irbesartan, being superior to conventional non-ACE-inhibitor-based therapy in decreasing end-stage renal failure event rates in patients with Type II diabetic nephropathy (103,104). In CHF, the hope that ARBs are more effective therapy than ACE inhibitors has not been realized, as of yet, though additional studies are underway to establish the positioning of ARB in current HF regimens.

Direct Renin Inhibitors

Aliskiren is a nonpeptide direct renin inhibitor, and is the first drug of this class to be approved for clinical use in systemic hypertension (see chap. 4) (105). The drug is approved for once daily use as a monotherapy and for combination use with other antihypertensive drugs.

There is no dose adjustment necessary in elderly patients or in patients with hepatic or renal insufficiency (106). The most common side effects of aliskiren are a lower incidence of headache, nasopharyngitis, dizziness, and diarrhea. The drug is not associated with an increased incidence of cough (107). Angioedema is a rare complication of therapy, and appears to occur at a lower frequency than with ACE inhibitors (107).

Pharmacokinetic studies with aliskiren have shown no relevant drug–drug interactions with warfarin, digoxin, amlodipine, valsartan, and ramipril (108,109). With the combination of aliskiren and furosemide, there are decreased levels of the diuretic (106).

Nitrates

Nitrates are effective therapies for older individuals; however, caution should always be used because of the associated dangers of orthostatic hypotension, syncope, and falls, especially if the treatment is combined with diuretics and other vasodilators. It was shown that nitrate headaches are less frequent in older patients and in individuals with renal dysfunction (110). It has also been shown that the use of the thiazolidinedione rosiglitazone may increase the risk of myocardial ischemia in patients taking concomitant nitrate therapy.

Calcium Channel Blockers

Calcium channel blockers are effective antihypertensive and antianginal drugs in older patients. Verapamil (80) and diltiazem (81) are especially valuable in treating hypertensive patients who also have supraventricular tachyarrhythmias. However, later reports have suggested an increased mortality risk with calcium channel blockers, especially with the use of short-acting dihydropyridines in older subjects (111–113). With the use of longer-acting calcium blockers, such as the dihydropyridine nitrendipine, a strong mortality benefit was seen in patients with isolated systolic hypertension (114), although many were receiving concurrent β-blocker therapy. In contrast, nisoldipine was shown to be less effective in protecting against cardiovascular mortality in diabetic patients with hypertension when compared to an enalapril-treated group (115).

Verapamil improved exercise capacity, peak LV filling rate, and a clinicoradiographic HF score in patients with CHF, normal LVEF, and impaired LV diastolic filling (116). However, calcium channel blockers such as verapamil, diltiazem, and nifedipine may exacerbate CHF in patients with associated abnormal LVEF (117). In addition, some calcium channel blockers have been shown to increase mortality in patients with CHF and abnormal LVEF after MI (118). Therefore, calcium channel blockers such as verapamil, diltiazem, and nifedipine may be used to treat older patients with CHF associated with normal LVEF, but are contraindicated in treating older patients with CHF associated with abnormal LVEF.

Amlodipine and felodipine are two vasculospecific dihydropyridine agents that appear to be safer in patients having CHF, although neither of these drugs should be used to treat CHF (28).

The age-associated decrease in hepatic blood flow and hepatic metabolic capacity may result in higher serum concentrations of verapamil, diltiazem, and nifedipine (119). Therefore, these drugs should be given to older persons in lower starting doses and titrated carefully.

α-Adrenergic Blockers

α-adrenergic blockers are effective treatments for patients with hypertension and have become first-line treatments for males with symptomatic prostatism. Caution should be exercised when using these agents because of a significant incidence of postural hypotension, especially in patients receiving diuretics or other vasodilator drugs (78,120). A more selective α-1 blocker, tamsulosin, has become available, which improves prostatism symptoms without having vasodilator effects (121). However, the National Heart, Lung and Blood Institute withdrew doxazosin from the Antihypertensive and Lipid-Lowering Treatment to Prevent Heart Attack Trial (ALLHAT) after an interim analysis showed a 25% greater rate of a secondary endpoint, combined cardiovascular disease, in patients on doxazosin than in those on chlorthalidone, largely driven by the increased risk of CHF (122). These findings have cast a shroud over the use of doxazosin in the elderly particularly if it is being contemplated as monotherapy in a hypertensive elderly patient.

Lidocaine

IV lidocaine may be used to treat complex ventricular arrhythmias during acute MI (78). Lidocaine toxicity is more common in the elderly and older patients should be monitored for dose-related confusion, tinnitus, paresthesias, slurred speech, tremors, seizures, delirium, respiratory depression, and hypotension. Older patients with CHF or impaired liver function are at increased risk for developing central nervous system adverse effects from lidocaine (123). In these patients, the loading dose should be decreased by 25–50%, and any maintenance infusion should be initiated at a rate of 0.5–2.5 mg/min, with the patient monitored closely for adverse effects. The dose of lidocaine should also be reduced if the patient is receiving β-blockers (124) or cimetidine, since these drugs reduce the metabolism of lidocaine.

Other Antiarrhythmic Drugs

The use of antiarrhythmic drugs in the elderly is extensively discussed elsewhere (79,125). In the CAST I trial, encainide and flecainide significantly increased mortality in survivors of MI with asymptomatic or mildly symptomatic ventricular arrhythmias, when compared to placebo (126). In the CAST II, moricizine insignificantly increased mortality when compared to placebo (127). Akiyama et al. (128) found that older age increased the likelihood of adverse events, including death, in patients treated with encainide, flecainide, or moricizine in these two studies.

In a retrospective analysis of the effect of empirical antiarrhythmic treatment in 209 cardiac arrest patients who were resuscitated out of hospital, Moosvi et al. (129) found that the 2-year mortality was significantly lower for patients treated with no antiarrhythmic drug than for patients treated with quinidine or procainamide. Hallstrom et al. (75) showed an increased incidence of death or recurrent cardiac arrest in patients treated with quinidine or procainamide versus no antiarrhythmic drug.

In a prospective study of 406 elderly subjects (mean age 82 years) with heart disease (58% with prior MI) and asymptomatic complex ventricular arrhythmias, the incidence of sudden cardiac death, total cardiac death, and total mortality were not significantly different in patients treated with quinidine or procainamide or with no antiarrhythmic drug (130). In this study, quinidine or procainamide did not reduce mortality in comparison with no antiarrhythmic drug in elderly patients with presence versus absence of ventricular tachycardia, ischemic or nonischemic heart disease, and abnormal or normal LVEF. The incidence of adverse events causing drug cessation in elderly patients in this study was 48% for quinidine and 55% for procainamide.

A meta-analysis of 6 double-blind studies of 808 patients with chronic atrial fibrillation who underwent direct current cardioversion to sinus rhythm demonstrated that the 1-year mortality was significantly higher in patients treated with quinidine than in patients treated with no antiarrhythmic drug (131). In the Stroke Prevention in Atrial Fibrillation Study, arrhythmic death and cardiac mortality were also significantly increased in patients receiving antiarrhythmic drugs compared with patients not receiving antiarrhythmic drugs, especially in patients with a history of CHF (132).

Teo et al. (63) analyzed 59 randomized controlled trials comprising 23,229 patients which investigated the use of class I antiarrhythmic drugs after MI. Patients receiving class I antiarrhythmic drugs had a significantly higher mortality than patients receiving no antiarrhythmic drugs. None of the 59 trials demonstrated that a class I antiarrhythmic drug decreased mortality in postinfarction patients. Therefore, it is not recommended that class I antiarrhythmic drugs be used for the treatment of ventricular tachycardia or complex ventricular arrhythmias associated with heart disease.

Amiodarone is very effective in suppressing ventricular tachycardia and complex ventricular arrhythmias. However, there are conflicting data about the effect of amiodarone on mortality (133–140). The Veterans Administration Cooperative Study comparing amiodarone versus placebo in HF patients with malignant ventricular arrhythmias showed that amiodarone was very effective in decreasing ventricular tachycardia and complex ventricular arrhythmias, but it did not affect mortality (139).

In the Sudden Cardiac Death in Heart Failure Trial (SCD-HEFT), 2521 patients, mean age 60 years, with NYHA class II or III HF, an LVEF of 35% or less, and a mean QRS duration on the resting ECG of 120 ms, were randomized to placebo, amiodarone or an ICD (140). At 46-month median follow-up, compared with placebo, amiodarone insignificantly increased mortality by 6%, but ICD therapy significantly reduced all-cause mortality by 23% (140).

The incidence of adverse effects from amiodarone has been reported to approach 90% after 5 years of treatment (141). In the Cardiac Arrest in Seattle: Conventional Versus Amiodarone Drug Evaluation Study, the incidence of pulmonary toxicity was 10% at 2 years in patients receiving an amiodarone dose of 158 mg daily (142). On the basis of these data, one should reserve the use of amiodarone for the treatment of life-threatening ventricular tachyarrhythmias or in patients who cannot tolerate or who do not respond to β-blocker therapy.

Amiodarone is also the most effective drug for treating refractory atrial fibrillation in terms of converting atrial fibrillation to sinus rhythm and slowing a rapid ventricular rate. However, because of the high incidence of adverse effects caused by amiodarone, amiodarone should be used in low doses in patients with atrial fibrillation when life-threatening atrial fibrillation is refractory to other therapy (143).

Dronedarone was introduced to provide the same antiarrhythmic efficacy of amiodarone with less toxicity. However, there is an increased mortality rate when the drug is used in patients with HF (144).

Lipid-Lowering Drugs

The safety of lipid-lowering drugs, specifically 3-hydroxy-3-methylglutaryl-coenzyme A (HMG CoA) reductase inhibitors (statins), was demonstrated in the Cholesterol Reduction in Seniors Program (CRISP) (145). Furthermore, a meta-analysis of 14 randomized trials of statins from 90,056 participants confirmed the safety and efficacy of statins (146).

In the Scandinavian Simvastatin Survival Study (147), 1,464,444 men and women with coronary artery disease were treated with double-blind simvastatin or placebo. At 5.4 years follow up, patients treated with simvastatin had a 35% decrease in serum low-density lipoprotein (LDL)-cholesterol, a 25% reduction in serum total cholesterol, an 8% increase in serum high-density lipoprotein (HDL) cholesterol, a 34% decrease in major coronary events, a 42% reduction in coronary deaths, and a 30% decrease in total mortality. In patients aged 65–70 years, simvastatin reduced all-cause mortality 35%, coronary artery disease mortality 43%, major coronary events 34%, nonfatal MI 33%, any atherosclerosis-related endpoint 34% and coronary revascularization 41% (148). The absolute risk reduction for both all-cause mortality and coronary artery disease mortality was approximately twice as great in persons aged 65–70 years compared to persons younger than 65 years.

In the cholesterol and recurrent events trial (149), 4159 men and women aged 21–75 years (1283 aged 65–75 years) with MI, serum total cholesterol levels <250 mg/dL, and serum LDL-cholesterol levels ≥115 mg/dL were treated with double-blind pravastatin and placebo. At 5 year follow-up, patients treated with pravastatin had a 32% reduction in serum LDL-cholesterol, a 20% decrease in serum total cholesterol and a 5% increase in serum HDL-cholesterol. Pravastatin reduced coronary artery disease death or nonfatal MI significantly by 39% in persons aged 65–75 years, and insignificantly by 13% in persons younger than 65 years (149). Pravastatin decreased major coronary events significantly by 32% in persons aged 65–75 years, and significantly by 19% in persons younger than 65 years. It also reduced stroke significantly by 40% in persons aged 65–75 years, and insignificantly by 20% in persons younger than 65 years. Pravastatin decreased coronary revascularization significantly by 32% in persons aged 65–75 years, and significantly by 25% in persons younger than 65 years. For every 1000 persons treated with pravastatin for 5 years, 225 cardiovascular events would be prevented in persons aged 65–75 years and 121 cardiovascular events would be prevented in persons younger than 65 years (149).

In the Prospective Study of Pravastatin in the Elderly at Risk (PROSPER) trial, a randomized, placebo-controlled study of 5804 men and 3000 women, pravastatin 40 mg/day was shown to lower LDL concentrations by 34% in subjects 70–82 years of age (150). In this study, drug treatment reduced coronary heart disease death and nonfatal MI. No benefit on stroke prevention was seen, and there were more cancer diagnoses with pravastatin. However, incorporation of this latter finding in a meta-analysis showed no overall increase in cancer risk.

The Long-Term Intervention with Pravastatin in Ischaemic Disease study randomized 9014 persons with a history of MI or unstable angina who had initial serum total cholesterol levels of 155–271 mg/dL to pravastatin 40 mg daily or placebo (151). At 8-year follow-up of 3514 persons aged 65–75 years at study entry, compared with placebo, pravastatin significantly reduced all-cause mortality by 21%, death from CHD by 24%, fatal and nonfatal MI by 26%, death from cardiovascular disease by 26%, need for coronary artery bypass graft surgery by 26%, and need for coronary angioplasty by 34% (151).

The Heart Protection Study randomized 20,536 men and women (5806 of whom were aged 70–80 years) with prior MI (8510 persons), other CHD (4876 persons), and no

CHD (7150 persons) and a serum total cholesterol level of 135 mg/dL or higher to simvastatin 40 mg daily or to placebo (152). Of the 7150 persons without CHD, 25% had cerebrovascular disease, 38% had PAD, 56% had diabetes mellitus, and 3% had only treated hypertension without atherosclerotic vascular disease or diabetes mellitus. At 5-year follow-up, compared to placebo, simvastatin significantly reduced all-cause mortality by 13%, any cardiovascular death by 17%, major coronary events by 27%, any stroke by 25%, coronary or noncoronary revascularization by 24%, and any major cardiovascular event by 24% (152). These significant reductions in mortality and in cardiovascular events occurred regardless of initial levels of serum lipids, age, or gender. First major cardiovascular event was significantly reduced by simvastatin by 24% in persons younger than 65 years, by 23% in persons aged 65–69 years, and by 18% in persons aged 70–80 years at study entry. Five years of simvastatin treatment prevented MI, stroke, and revascularization in 70–100 persons per 1000 treated persons (152).

Sixty-nine elderly patients, mean age 75 years, with intermittent claudication due to peripheral arterial disease (PAD) were randomized to simvastatin 40 mg daily or placebo (153). Compared with placebo, simvastatin significantly increased treadmill exercise time until the onset of intermittent claudication by 24% at 6 months after treatment and by 42% at 1 year after treatment.

Observational data have also demonstrated in 1410 men and women, mean age 81 years, with CHD and hypercholesterolemia that at 3-year follow-up, use of statins significantly reduced CHD death or nonfatal MI by 50% (154), stroke by 60% (155), and CHF by 48% (156). The lower the reduction in serum LDL cholesterol, the greater the reduction in coronary events (154) and in stroke (155). Statins also significantly reduced new coronary events by 37% and new stroke by 47% in 529 men and women, mean age 79 years, with diabetes mellitus, prior MI, and hypercholes-terolemia at 29-month follow-up (157). In addition, statins significantly reduced in 660 men and women with PAD and hypercholesterolemia at 39-month follow-up new coronary events by 52% in persons with prior MI and by 59% in persons with no prior MI (158).

On the basis of the available data showing increased risk of cardiovascular disease from abnormal lipoprotein patterns (159), dietary therapy for older patients with dyslipidemia, regardless of age, in the absence of other serious life-limiting illnesses such as cancer, dementia or malnutrition, is recommended (160). If hyperlipidemia persists after 3 months of dietary therapy, hypolipidemic drugs should be considered, depending on serum lipid levels, presence or absence of coronary artery disease, presence or absence of other coronary risk factors, and the patient's overall clinical status. This approach is consistent with the National Cholesterol Education Program (NCEP) Expert Panel on Detection, Evaluation, and Treatment of High Blood Cholesterol in Adults recommendations in males ≥65 years and females ≥75 years (161). In older men and women, the HMG-CoA reductase inhibitors would be the drugs of choice for treating a high serum LDL-cholesterol level (162).

Previous data have demonstrated that the serum LDL cholesterol should be reduced to <70 mg/dl in high-risk persons regardless of age or gender (163–165). The updated NCEP III guidelines state that in very high-risk patients, a serum LDL cholesterol level of less than 70 mg/dl is a reasonable clinical strategy (166). When a high-risk person has hypertriglyceridemia or low serum HDL cholesterol, consideration can be given to combining a fibrate or nicotinic acid with an LDL cholesterol-lowering drug (166). For moderately high-risk persons (2 or more risk factors and a 10-year risk for CHD of 10–20%), the serum LDL cholesterol should be reduced to less than 100 mg/dl. When LDL cholesterol-lowering drug therapy is used to treat high-risk persons or moderately high-risk persons, the serum LDL cholesterol should be reduced at least 30–40%.

Anticoagulants

Anticoagulant therapy in the elderly is discussed extensively elsewhere (79,167). Antico-agulants are effective in the prevention and treatment of many thromboembolic disorders, including venous thromboembolism and pulmonary embolism, acute MI, and embolism associated with prosthetic heart valves or atrial fibrillation. These conditions, necessitating the use of anticoagulants, are more common in elderly than in younger patients. In the report from the Sixty Plus Reinfarction Group who evaluated the effects of oral anticoagu-lant therapy on total mortality after MI in patients older than 60 years, it was shown that active therapy lowered both mortality and reinfarction compared with placebo (168). However, the treatment group also had more major bleeding complications.

The anticoagulant response to warfarin is increased with age (169). Chronic diseases that increase the risk for bleeding during anticoagulant therapy are also more common in elderly patients than in younger patients. In addition, elderly patients are at higher risk for bleeding during anticoagulant therapy because of increased vascular or endothelial fragil-ity (170). Furthermore, older patients may be at increased risk for bleeding due to antico-agulant therapy because they may be taking other drugs which potentiate the anticoagulant effect. Drugs such as aspirin, cephalosporins and penicillins increase the risk of bleeding in patients treated with heparin. Drugs such as allopurinol, amiodarone, aspirin, cimetidine, ciprofloxacin, clofibrate, cotrimoxazole, dextropropoxyphene, disulfiram, erythromycin, fluconazole, isoniazid, ketoconazole, meclofenamic acid, metronidazole, miconazole, nor-floxacin, phenylbutazone, phenytoin, quinidine, sulfinpyrazone, sulindac, thyroxine and trimethoprim-sulfamethoxazole potentiate the effect of warfarin, causing an increased prothrombin time and risk of bleeding.

In past few years, two new antiplatelet drugs, prasugrel and ticagrelor, were approved for clinical use by the FDA (171). Prasugrel is relatively contraindicated in elderly patients (172).

Two new anticoagulants, dabigatran and rivaroxaban, were approved for clinical use in patients at risk for thromboembolic complications from atrial fibrillation (173,174). Apixaban, a factor Xa inhibitor, is about to be approved by the FDA (175). Since there are no anticoagulation tests available with these drugs to monitor their efficacy, they should be used with caution in the elderly.

Herbal Remedies

The use of herbal substances for various cardiovascular indications has increased in the elderly patient (176). The issue with these herbal remedies is not their efficacy, but the herbal–drug interaction that can occur (Table 3.5). It is important that clinicians ask about herbal medication use in their history taking.

Table 3.5 Potential and Documented Interactions of Herbs with Warfarin

Potential increase in risk of bleeding	
Chamomile	Gingko
Feverfew	Horse chestnut
Garlic	Licorice root
Ginger	
Documented reports of possible decrease in warfarin's effects	
Ginseng	
Green tea	

Source: From Ref. 176.

ADVERSE EFFECTS OF DRUGS IN THE ELDERLY

Cardiovascular drugs are often associated with adverse effects which simulate common disorders of the elderly (Table 3.6). In addition, there are important drug–disease interactions (Table 3.7), drug–drug interactions (Table 3.8), drug–alcohol interactions (Table 3.9), and drug–herbal interactions (Table 3.5), which occur in older patients.

Table 3.6 Cardiovascular Drugs Regularly Detected as the Culprit in Some Common Disorders of the Elderly

Disorder	Drugs
Confusion states	β-blockers, digoxin, methyldopa and related drugs, quinidine
Tinnitus, vertigo	Aspirin, furosemide, ethacrynic acid
Depression	β-blockers, methyldopa, reserpine
Falls	All drugs liable to produce postural hypotension, glycerol trinitrates
Postural hypotension	All antihypertensives, antianginal drugs, β-blockers, diuretics
Constipation	Anticholinergics, clonidine, diltiazem, diuretics, verapamil
Urinary retention	Disopyramide, midodrine
Urinary incontinence	β-blockers, diuretics, labetalol, prazosin

Source: Adapted from Ref. 188.

Table 3.7 Important Drug–Disease Interactions in Geriatric Patients

Underlying Disease	Drugs	Adverse Effect
Congestive heart failure	β-blockers, verapamil	Acute cardiac decompensation
Cardiac conduction disorders	Tricyclic antidepressants	Heart block
Hypertension	NSAIDs	Increased blood pressure
Peripheral vascular disease	β-blockers	Intermittent claudication
Chronic obstructive pulmonary disease	β-blockers	Bronchoconstriction
Chronic renal impairment	NSAIDs, contrast agents, aminoglycosides, ACE inhibitors	Acute renal failure
Diabetes mellitus	Diuretics	Hyperglycemia
Prostatic hypertrophy	Drugs with antimuscarinic side effects	Urinary retention
Depression	β-blockers, centrally acting antihypertensives	Precipitation or exacerbation of depression
Hypokalemia	Digoxin	Cardiac arrhythmias
Peptic ulcer disease	Anticoagulants, salicylates	GI hemorrhage

Abbreviations: GI, gastrointestinal; NSAIDs, nonsteroidal anti-inflammatory drugs.
Source: Adapted from Ref. 191.

Table 3.8 Selected Clinically Significant Drug–Drug Interactions in Geriatric Patients

Primary Drugs	Interacting Drugs	Mechanism of Interaction	Possible Effects
Augmented Drug Effects			
Antidiabetic sulfonylureas	Chloramphenicol, warfarin	IM	Hypoglycemia
(tolbutamide,	Phenylbutazone	IM, DP, IE	
chlorpropamide)	Quinidine	OM	
Azathioprine	Allopurinol	IM	Bone marrow suppression
Carbamazepine	Diltiazem, verapamil	IM	Increase serum carbamazepine concentration and risk of toxicity (e.g., nausea, ataxia, nystagmus)
Cyclosporine	Diltiazem, verapamil	IM	Increase serum cyclosporine concentration and risk of toxicity (e.g., hepato- and nephrotoxicity)
Digoxin	Amiodarone, diuretics, Quinidine, verapamil	OM	Increase serum digoxin concentration and risk of toxicity (e.g., nausea, confusion, cardiotoxicity)
Disopyramide	Diltiazem, verapamil	OM	Bradycardia
Lidocaine	β-blockers, cimetidine	HBF	Increase serum lidocaine concentration and risk of toxicity (e.g. sedation, seizures, cardiotoxicity)
Methotrexate	Aspirin, indomethacin, phenylbutazone	DP, IE	Bone marrow suppression
	Probenecid	IE	
	Sulfisoxazole	DP	
Procainamide	Diltiazem, verapamil	OM	Bradycardia
Propranolol	Cimetidine	HBF	Bradycardia
	Diltiazem, verapamil	OM	Bradycardia, hypotension
Phenytoin	Amiodarone, chloram-phenicol, cimetidine, fluconazole, isoniazid,	IM	Increase serum phenytoin concentration and risk of toxicity (e.g., nystagmus, sedation)
	Phenylbutazone valproic acid, warfarin	DP, IM	
Quinidine	Diltiazem, verapamil	IM	Increase serum quinidine concentration and risk of toxicity (e.g., nausea, cinchonism, arrhythmias)
Warfarin	Aspirin, Indomethacin	DP	Hemorrhage
	Amiodarone, cimetidine, metronidazole	IM	
	phenylbutazone, sulfonamides	DP, IM	
Decreased drug effects			
All medications	Cholestyramine	IA	Delay or reduce absorption of other drugs. Administer other drugs 1–2 hr before or 4–6 hr after cholestyramine

(Continued)

Table 3.8 Selected Clinically Significant Drug–Drug Interactions in Geriatric Patients (*Continued*)

Primary Drugs	Interacting Drugs	Mechanism of Interaction	Possible Effects
Antidiabetic sulfonylureas (tolbutamide, chlorpropamide)	β-blockers (nonselective)	IIS, MCM, IIR	Decrease hypoglycemic effects
	Corticosteroids, thiazide diuretics	OM	
Digoxin	Sucralfate	IA	Reduce absorption of digoxin. Administer sucralfate at least 2 hr apart from digoxin.
Lincomycin	Kaolin-pectin	IA	Decrease drug bioavailability
Phenytoin	Calcium, sucralfate	IA	Decrease serum phenytoin
	Rifampin	SM	concentration and anticonvulsant effect
Prednisone	Barbiturates	SM	Decreased steroid effects
Quinidine	Barbiturates, rifampin	SM	Decrease antiarrhythmic effect
Tetracycline	Antacids–iron	IA	Decrease drug bioavailability
Warfarin	Barbiturates, carbamazepine, glutethimide, rifampin	SM	Loss of anticoagulant control
	Vitamin K	SP	
Other drug effects			
ACE inhibitors	Potassium-sparing diuretics, potassium-containing medications	RAP	Hyperkalemia
HMG-CoA reductase inhibitors	Cyclosporine, gemfibrozil, and niacin	Unknown	Rhabdomyolysis, acute renal failure
	Erythromycin	IM	

Abbreviations: DP, displacement of protein binding; HBF, decreased hepatic blood flow; HMG-CoA, 3-hydroxy-3-methylglutaryl-coenzyme A; IA, inhibition of drug absorption; IE, inhibition of renal excretion; IM, inhibition of drug metabolism; IIR, increased peripheral insulin resistance; IIS, inhibition of insulin; MCM, modification of carbohydrate metabolism; OM, other mechanisms (pharmacodynamic effects of drugs on tissue responses); RAP, reduction of aldosterone production; SM, stimulation of drug metabolism; SP, increased hepatic synthesis of procoagulant factors.
Source: Adapted from Ref. 192.

Table 3.9 Selected Clinically Significant Drug–Alcohol Interactions in Geriatric Patients

Primary Drugs	Interacting Drug	Possible Effects
Antidiabetic sulfonylureas	Alcohol	Disulfiram-like reactions (especially with chlorpropamide)
ACE inhibitors	Alcohol	Hypotension
Isoniazid	Alcohol	Decreased therapeutic effect of isoniazid, increased risk of hepatic toxicity
Nitrates	Alcohol	Hypotension
Phenytoin	Alcohol	Decreased serum phenytoin concentration and effectiveness (chronic use of alcohol); increased serum phenytoin concentration and risk of toxicity (acute intake of alcohol)

(*Continued*)

Table 3.9 Selected Clinically Significant Drug–Alcohol Interactions in Geriatric Patients (*Continued*)

Primary Drugs	Interacting Drug	Possible Effects
Rifampin	Alcohol	Decreased therapeutic effect of rifampin, increased risk of hepatic toxicity
Sedatives–hypnotics	Alcohol	Excessive sedation
Vitamins	Alcohol	Decreased absorption and storage of folic acid and thiamine
Warfarin	Alcohol	Increased anticoagulant activity (acute intoxication); decreased anticoagulant activity (chronic abuse)

Abbreviation: ACE, angiotensin-converting enzyme.
Source: From Ref. 193,194.

MEDICATIONS BEST TO AVOID IN THE ELDERLY

Careful selection of drugs and dosages of drugs in the elderly can minimize adverse outcomes while maximizing clinical improvement. In their first attempt to identify medications and doses of medication which may be best to avoid in the elderly, Beers and colleagues developed a set of explicit criteria after an extensive review of the literature and assistance from 13 well-recognized experts in geriatric medicine and pharmacology (177). These criteria included 30 statements which described medications that should generally be avoided in nursing home residents as well as statements which described doses, frequencies, and duration of medications that should generally not be exceeded. Since the publication of the explicit criteria, several research studies have utilized these criteria to evaluate the appropriateness of medication prescribing in the elderly (178–181). The most striking study of this type was performed by Willcox and colleagues (181) who reported a potentially inappropriate medication prescription in 23.5% of elderly in the community. Willcox and colleagues were criticized, however, for applying criteria that were designed for frail elderly patients in nursing homes to healthier elderly residents in the community, along with criteria that need to be updated (182).

Acknowledging the limitation of this first set of criteria, Beers updated and expanded it to encompass elderly patients who are in the ambulatory setting, as well as medications that should be avoided in elderly known to have certain conditions (183). With the assistance of six nationally recognized experts in geriatric medicine and pharmacology, a set of 63 criteria was developed using the first set of criteria plus a more recent literature review. Out of the 63 criteria, 28 criteria described medications or categories of medication that were considered to be potentially inappropriate when used by all older patients, 35 criteria described medications or categories of medications that were considered to be potentially inappropriate when used by elderly patients with any of 15 known medical conditions such as HF, diabetes, hypertension, asthma, and arrhythmias. These criteria were further rated by the six panelists regarding their importance. The panelists considered a criterion to be severe when an adverse outcome was both likely to occur and, if it did occur, would likely lead to a clinically significant event (182). Table 3.10 lists some cardiac medications that were recognized by the expert panel as having the highest severity of potential problems occurring from their use and the reasons for their avoidance. Table 3.11 lists medications that were identified by the expert panel as having the highest severity of potential problems and the reasons for their avoidance in the elderly when certain cardiac-related conditions exist.

Table 3.10　Some Medications to Avoid in Older Patients

Medications	Prescribing Concerns
Disopyramide	Of all antiarrhythmics, disopyramide is the most potent negative inotrope, and therefore may induce heart failure in the elderly. It is also strongly anticholinergic. When appropriate, other antiarrhythmic drugs should be used.
Digoxin[a]	Because of decreased renal clearance of digoxin, doses in the elderly should rarely exceed 0.125 mg daily, except when treating atrial arrhythmias.
Methyldopa[a] & methyldopa/ HCTZ[a]	Methyldopa may cause bradycardia and exacerbate depression in the elderly. Alternate treatments for hypertension are generally preferred.
Ticlopidine	Ticlopidine has been shown to be no better than aspirin in preventing clotting and is considerably more toxic. Avoid in the elderly.
Verapamil and diltiazem	May cause sinus bradycardia and/or heart block in the elderly, especially when used with β-blockers.

[a]Panelists believed that the severity of adverse reaction would be substantially greater when these drugs were recently started. In general, the greatest risk would be within about a 1-month period.
Abbreviation: HCTZ, hydrochlorothiazide.
Source: Adapted from Ref. 195.

Table 3.11　Medications to Avoid in Older Patients with Specific Diseases and Conditions

Diseases/Conditions	Medications	Prescribing Concerns
Heart Failure	Disopyramide, NSAIDs	Negative inotrope; may worsen heart failure
Hypertension	Diet pills; NSAIDs amphetamines	May elevate blood pressure
Blood-clotting disorders, limited to those receiving anticoagulant	Aspirin, NSAIDS, dipyridamole, prasugrel and ticlopidine	May cause bleeding in those using anticoagulant therapy
Syncope or falls	Long-acting benzodiazepine drugs	May contribute to falls
Arrhythmias	Tricyclic antidepressant drugs[a]	May induce arrhythmias

[a]Panelists believed that the severity of adverse reaction would be substantially greater when these drugs were recently started. In general, the greatest risk would be within about a 1-month period.
Abbreviation: NSAIDS, nonsteroidal antiinflammatory drugs.
Source: Adapted from Ref. 195.

Although these criteria serve as useful tools for assessing the quality of prescribing to the elderly, they do not identify all cases of potentially inappropriate prescribing. In fact, these criteria may identify appropriate prescribing as inappropriate at times. The latter case may particularly be likely when physicians and pharmacists carefully adjust medication regimens for specific needs of individual patients (183).

PRUDENT USE OF MEDICATION IN THE ELDERLY

Although the elderly make up only 14% of our population, they receive more than 30% of all prescribed medication (184). The increased exposure of medications in the elderly may lead to higher incidence of adverse drug reactions and drug–drug interactions in this population (185).

Physiologic changes with aging may also alter the elimination of drugs, which can contribute to adverse outcomes with medication usage. With these concerns in mind, several authors have suggested some steps, which clinicians may employ to ensure safe prescribing (184,186,187). These suggestions include the following:

- Acquire a full history of the patient's habits and medication use.
- Evaluate the need for drug therapy. Consider alternative nondrug approaches when appropriate.
- Know the pharmacology of the drugs prescribed.
- Start with low dose of medication and titrate up slowly.
- Titrate medication dosage according to the patient's response.
- Minimize the number of medications used.
- Educate patients regarding proper usage of medications.
- Be aware of medication cost, which may have an impact on compliance.
- Provide patient with a portable prescription record.
- Review the treatment plan regularly and discontinue medications no longer needed.

With proper monitoring and adequate understanding of the effects of medications in the elderly, the use of medication can be a positive experience for both the elderly patient and the clinician.

REFERENCES

1. Fleg JL, Aronow WS, Frishman WF. Cardiovascular drug therapy in the elderly: benefits and challenges. Nat Rev Cardiol 2011; 8: 13–28.
2. Frishman WH. Basic principles of clinical pharmacology relevant to cardiology. In: Frishman WH, Sonnenblick EH, Sica D, eds. Cardiovascular Pharmacotherapeutics, 3rd edn. Minneapolis: Cardiotext, 2011: 3–15.
3. Castleden CM, George CF. The effect of aging on the hepatic clearance of propranolol. Br J Clin Pharmacol 1979; 7: 49–54.
4. Rubin PC, Scott PJW, Reid JL. Prazosin disposition in young and elderly subjects. Br J Clin Pharmacol 1981; 12: 401–4.
5. Novak LP. Aging, total body potassium, fat-free mass and cell mass in males and females between the ages of 18 and 85 years. J Gerontol 1972; 27: 438–43.
6. Vestal RE, Norris AH, Tobin JD, et al. Antipyrine metabolism in man: influence of age, alcohol, caffeine and smoking. Clin Pharmacol Ther 1975; 18: 425–32.
7. Cusack B, Kelly J, O'Malley K, et al. Digoxin in the elderly: pharmacokinetic consequences of old age. Clin Pharmacol 1979; 2: 722–6.
8. Abernethy DR, Kerzner L. Age effects on alpha-1 acid glycoprotein concentration and imipramine plasma protein binding. J Am Geriatr Soc 1984; 32: 705–8.
9. Holt DW, Hayler AM, Healey GF. Effect of age and plasma concentrations of albumin and alpha-1 acid glycoprotein on protein binding of disopyramide. Br J Clin Pharmacol 1983; 16: 344–5.
10. Schmucker DL. Aging and drug disposition: an update. Pharmacol Rev 1985; 37: 133–48.
11. Hayes MJ, Langman MJS, Short AH. Changes in drug metabolism with increasing age. II. Phenytoin clearance and protein binding. Br J Clin Pharmacol 1975; 2: 73–9.
12. Wynne HA, Cope LH, Mutch E, et al. The effect of age upon liver volume and apparent liver blood flow in healthy man. Hepatology 1989; 9: 297–301.
13. Rowe JW, Andres R, Tobin JD, et al. The effect of age on creatinine clearance in man: a cross-sectional and longitudinal study. J Gerontol 1976; 31: 155–63.
14. Bender AD. The effect of increasing age on the distribution of peripheral blood flow in man. J Am Geriatr Soc 1965; 13: 192–8.
15. Cockcroft DW, Gault MH. Prediction of creatinine clearance from serum creatinine. Nephron 1976; 16: 31–41.
16. Levey AS, Coresh J, Balk E, et al. National Kidney Foundation practice guidelines for chronic kidney disease: evaluation, classification, and stratification. Ann Intern Med 2003; 139: 137–47.
17. Sica DA. Kinetics of angiotensin converting enzyme inhibitors in renal failure. J Cardiovasc Pharmacol 1992; 20: S13–20.
18. Aronow WS, Fleg JL, Pepine CJ, et al. ACCF/AHA 2011 Expert consensus document on hypertension in the elderly. A report of the American college of cardiology foundation task force on clinical expert consensus documents. J Am Coll Cardiol 2011; 57: 2037–114.

19. Abernethy DR, Schwartz JB, Plachetka JR, et al. Comparison of young and elderly patients of phar-macodynamics and disposition of labetalol in systemic hypertension. Am J Cardiol 1987; 60: 697–702.
20. Dillon N, Chung S, Kelly J, O'Malley K. Age and beta-adrenoceptor mediated function. Clin Pharmacol Ther 1980; 27: 769–72.
21. Vestal RE, Wood AJJ, Shand DG. Reduced beta-adrenoceptor sensitivity in the elderly. Clin Pharmacol Ther 1979; 26: 181–6.
22. Scarpace PJ, Armbrecht HJ. Adenylate cyclase in senescence: catecholamine and parathyroid hormone pathways. Rev Clin Basic Pharmacol 1987; 6: 105–18.
23. Wolf PA, Abbott RD, Kannel WB. Atrial fibrillation as an independent risk factor for stroke: the Framingham Study. Stroke 1991; 22: 983–8.
24. Aronow WS, Ahn C, Gutstein H. Prevalence and incidence of cardiovascular disease in 1160 older men and 2464 women in a long-term health care facility. J Gerontol Med Sci 2002; 57A: M45–6.
25. Aronow WS, Mercando AD, Epstein S. Prevalence of arrhythmias detected by 24 hour ambulatory electrocardiography and value of antiarrhythmic therapy in elderly patients with unexplained syn-cope. Am J Cardiol 1992; 70: 408–10.
26. Aronow WS. Digoxin or angiotensin converting enzyme inhibitors for congestive heart failure in geriatric patients: which is the preferred treatment? Drugs Aging 1991; 1: 98–103.
27. Butler VP Jr, Odel JG, Rath E, et al. Digitalis-induced visual disturbances with therapeutic serum digitalis concentrations. Ann Intern Med 1995; 123: 676–80.
28. Hunt SA, Abraham WT, Feldman AM, et al. ACC/AHA 2005 guideline update for the diagnosis and management of chronic heart failure in the adult. A report of the American College of Cardiology/American Heart Association Task Force on Practice Guidelines (Writing Committee to Update the 2001 Guidelines for the Evaluation and Management of Heart Failure). Developed in collaboration with the American College of Chest Physicians and the International Society for Heart and Lung Transplantation. Endorsed by the Heart Rhythm Society. Circulation 2005; 112: 1825–52.
29. Aronow WS, Ahn C, Kronzon I. Comparison of incidences of congestive heart failure in older African-Americans, Hispanics, and whites. Am J Cardiol 1999; 84: 611–12.
30. Gottdiener JS, McClelland RL, Marshall R, et al. Outcome of congestive heart failure in elderly persons: influence of left ventricular systolic function. The Cardiovascular Health Study. Ann Intern Med 2002; 137: 631–9.
31. Aronow WS. Echocardiography should be performed in all elderly patients with congestive heart failure. J Am Geriatr Soc 1994; 42: 1300–2.
32. Fleg JL, Gottlieb SH, Lakatta EG. Is digoxin really important in treatment of compensated heart failure? A placebo-controlled crossover study in patients with sinus rhythm. Am J Med 1982; 73: 244–50.
33. Aronow WS, Starling L, Etienne F. Lack of efficacy of digoxin in treatment of compensated congestive heart failure with third heart sound and sinus rhythm in elderly patients receiving diuretic therapy. Am J Cardiol 1986; 58: 168–9.
34. Rathore SS, Wang Y, Krumholz HM. Sex-based differences in the effect of digoxin for the treatment of heart failure. N Engl J Med 2002; 347: 1403–11.
35. Rathore SS, Curtis JP, Wang Y, et al. Association of serum digoxin concentration and outcomes in patients with heart failure. JAMA 2003; 289: 871–8.
36. Ahmed A, Aronow WS, Fleg JL. Predictors of mortality and hospitalization in women with heart failure in the Digitalis Investigation Group trial. Am J Ther 2006; 13: 325–31.
37. Ahmed A, Aban IB, Weaver MT, et al. Serum digoxin concentration and outcomes in women with heart failure: a bi-directional effect and a possible effect modification by ejection fraction. Eur J Heart Failure 2006; 8: 409–19.
38. LeJemtel TH, Klapholz M, Frishman WH. Inotropic agents. In: Frishman WH, Sica DA, eds. Cardiovascular Pharmacotherapeutics, 3rd edn. Minneapolis: Cardiotext, 2011: 189–203.
39. Galun E, Flugelman MY, Glickson M, Eliakim M. Failure of long-term digitalization to prevent rapid ventricular response in patients with paroxysmal atrial fibrillation. Chest 1991; 99: 1038–40.
40. Moss AJ, Davis HT, Conard DL, et al. Digitalis-associated cardiac mortality after myocardial infarc-tion. Circulation 1981; 64: 1150–6.
41. Bigger JT Jr, Fleiss JL, Rolnitzky LM, et al. Effect of digitalis treatment on survival after acute myocardial infarction. Am J Cardiol 1985; 55: 623–30.
42. Leor J, Goldbourt U, Rabinowitz B, et al. Does digoxin exert adverse effects on survivors of myocardial infarction? The importance of digoxin dose (abst). J Am Coll Cardiol 1994; 23: 113A.
43. Byington R, Goldstein S; BHAT Research Group. Association of digitalis therapy with mortality in survivors of acute myocardial infarction: observation of the Beta Blocker Heart Attack Trial. J Am Coll Cardiol 1985; 6: 976–82.

44. Muller JE, Turi ZG, Stone PH, et al. Digoxin therapy and mortality after myocardial infarction: experience in the MILIS study. N Engl J Med 1986; 314: 265–71.

45. Eberhardt RT, Frishman WH, Landau A, et al. Increased mortality incidence in elderly individuals receiving digoxin therapy: results from the Bronx Longitudinal Aging Study. Cardiol Elderly 1995; 3: 177–82.

46. Digitalis Investigation Group. The effect of digoxin on mortality and morbidity in patients with heart failure. N Engl J Med 1997; 336: 525–33.

47. Chobanian AV, Bakris GL, Black HR, et al. The seventh report of the joint national committee on prevention, detection, evaluation, and treatment of high blood pressure. The JNC 7 report. JAMA 2003; 289: 2560–72.

48. SHEP Cooperative Research Study Group. Prevention of stroke by antihypertensive drug treatment in older persons with isolated systolic hypertension: final results of the systolic hypertension in the elderly program (SHEP). J Am Med Assoc 1991; 265: 3255–64.

49. The CONSENSUS Study Group. Effect of enalapril on mortality in severe congestive heart failure: results of the cooperative north scandinavian enalapril survival study (CONSENSUS). N Engl J Med 1987; 316: 1429–35.

50. Sica DA, Gehr TWB, Frishman WH. Diuretic therapy in cardiovascular disease. In: Frishman WH, Sica DA, eds. Cardiovascular Pharmacotherapeutics, 3rd edn. Minneapolis: Cardiotext, 2011: 157–75.

51. The SOLVD Investigators. Effect of enalapril on survival in patients with reduced left ventricular ejection fractions and congestive heart failure. N Engl J Med 1991; 325: 293–302.

52. MERIT-HF Study Group. Effect of metoprolol CR/XL in chronic heart failure: metoprolol CR/XL randomised intervention trial in congestive heart failure (MERIT-HF). Lancet 1999; 353: 2001–7.

53. Flather MD, Shibata MC, Coats AJS, et al. Randomized trial to determine the effect of nevibilol on mortality and cardiovascular hospital admission in elderly patients with heart failure (SENIORS). Eur Heart J 2005; 26: 215–25.

54. Aronow WS, Kronzon I. Effect of enalapril on congestive heart failure treated with diuretics in elderly patients with prior myocardial infarction and normal left ventricular ejection fraction. Am J Cardiol 1993; 71: 602–4.

55. Aronow WS, Ahn C, Kronzon I. Effect of propranolol versus no propranolol on total mortality plus nonfatal myocardial infarction in older patients with prior myocardial infarction, congestive heart failure, and left ventricular ejection fraction ≥40% treated with diuretics plus angiotensin-converting-enzyme inhibitors. Am J Cardiol 1997; 80: 207–9.

56. Sica DA, Gehr TW. Diuretic combinations in refractory edema states: pharmacokinetic-pharmacodynamic relationships. Clin Pharmacokinet 1996; 30: 229–49.

57. Sica DA, Gehr TWB. Drug absorption in congestive heart failure: loop diuretics. Congestive Heart Failure 1998; 5: 37–43.

58. Page J, Henry D. Consumption of NSAIDs and the development of congestive heart failure in elderly patients: an underrecognized public health problem. Arch Intern Med 2000; 160: 777–84.

59. Franse LV, Pahor M, Di Bari M, et al. Hypokalemia associated with diuretic use and cardiovascular events in the Systolic Hypertension in the Elderly Program. Hypertension 2000; 35: 1025–30.

60. Baglin A, Boulard JC, Hanslik T, Prinseau J. Metabolic adverse reactions to diuretics. Clinical relevance to elderly patients. Drug Safety 1995; 12: 161–7.

61. Frishman WH, Sonnenblick EH. Beta-adrenergic blocking drugs and calcium channel blockers. In: Alexander RW, Schlant RC, Fuster V, eds. The Heart, 9th edn. New York: McGraw Hill, 1998: 1583–618.

62. Sica DA. Old antihypertensive agents – diuretics and β-blockers – do we know how and in whom they lower blood pressure. Curr Hypertens Rep 1999; 1: 296–304.

63. Teo KK, Yusuf S, Furberg CD. Effects of prophylactic antiarrhythmic drug therapy in acute myocardial infarction: an overview of results from randomized controlled trials. J Am Med Assoc 1993; 270: 1589–95.

64. Hawkins CM, Richardson DW, Vokonas PS; BHAT Research Group. Effect of propranolol in reducing mortality in older myocardial infarction patients: the Beta Blocker Heart Attack Trial experience. Circulation 1983; 67: I-94–I97.

65. Gundersen T, Abrahamsen AM, Kjekshus J, et al. Timolol-related reduction in mortality and reinfarction in patients aged 65–75 years surviving acute myocardial infarction. Circulation 1982; 66: 1179–84.

66. Park KC, Forman DE, Wei JY. Utility of β blocker treatment for older post-infarction patients. J Am Geriatr Soc 1995; 43: 751–5.

67. Gurwitz JH, Goldberg RJ, Chen Z, et al. Beta blocker therapy in acute myocardial infarction: evidence for underutilization in the elderly. Am J Med 1992; 93: 605–10.

68. Mendelson G, Aronow WS. Underutilization of beta blockers in older patients with prior myocardial infarction or coronary artery disease in an academic hospital-based geriatrics practice. J Am Geriatr Soc 1997; 45: 1360–1.

69. Frishman WH. β-Adrenergic blockers: a 50 year historical perspective. Am J Ther 2008; 15: 565–76.

70. Hansteen V. Beta blockade after myocardial infarction: the norwegian propranolol study in high-risk patients. Circulation 1983; 67: I-57–60.

71. Aronow WS, Ahn C, Mercando AD, et al. Effect of propranolol versus no antiarrhythmic drug on sudden cardiac death, total cardiac death, and total death in patients >62 years of age with heart disease, complex ventricular arrhythmias, and left ventricular ejection fraction >40%. Am J Cardiol 1994; 74: 267–70.

72. Aronow WS, Ahn C, Mercando AD, et al. Decrease of mortality by propranolol in patients with heart disease and complex ventricular arrhythmias is more an anti-ischemic than an antiarrhythmic effect. Am J Cardiol 1994; 74: 613–15.

73. Norris RM, Barnaby PF, Brown MA, et al. Prevention of ventricular fibrillation during acute myocardial infarction by intravenous propranolol. Lancet 1984; 2: 883–6.

74. Stone PH, Gibson RS, Glasser SP, et al. Comparison of propranolol, diltiazem and nifedipine in the treatment of ambulatory ischemia in patients with stable angina: differential effects on ambulatory ischemia, exercise performance, and anginal symptoms. Circulation 1990; 82: 1962–72.

75. Hallstrom AP, Cobb LA, Yu BH, et al. An antiarrhythmic drug experience in 941 patients resuscitated from an initial cardiac arrest between 1970 and 1985. Am J Cardiol 1991; 68: 1025–31.

76. Aronow WS, Ahn C, Mercando AD, Epstein S. Circadian variation of sudden cardiac death or fatal myocardial infarction is abolished by propranolol in patients with heart disease and complex ventricular arrhythmias. Am J Cardiol 1994; 74: 819–21.

77. Kennedy HL, Brooks MM, Barker AH, et al. Beta blocker therapy in the Cardiac Arrhythmia Suppression Trial. Am J Cardiol 1994; 74: 674–80.

78. Frishman WH. Alpha- and beta-adrenergic blocking drugs. In: Frishman WH, Sica DA, eds. Cardiovascular Pharmacotherapeutics, 3rd edn. Minneapolis: Cardiotext, 2011: 57–85.

79. Aronow WS. Management of the older person with atrial fibrillation. J Gerontol Med Sci 2002; 57A: M352–63.

80. Lang R, Klein HO, Weiss E, et al. Superiority of oral verapamil therapy to digoxin in treatment of chronic atrial fibrillation. Chest 1983; 83: 491–9.

81. Roth A, Harrison E, Mitani G, et al. Efficacy and safety of medium and high-dose diltiazem alone and in combination with digoxin for control of heart rate at rest and during exercise in patients with chronic atrial fibrillation. Circulation 1986; 73: 316–24.

82. David D, DiSegni E, Klein HO, Kaplinsky E. Inefficacy of digitalis in the control of heart rate in patients with chronic atrial fibrillation: beneficial effect of an added beta-adrenergic blocking agent. Am J Cardiol 1979; 44: 1378–82.

83. Packer M, Bristow MR, Cohn JN, et al. The effect of carvedilol on morbidity and mortality in patients with chronic heart failure. N Engl J Med 1996; 334: 1349–55.

84. CIBIS-II Investigators and Committees. The Cardiac Insufficiency Bisoprolol Study II (CIBIS-II): a randomised trial. Lancet 1999; 353: 9–13.

85. Packer M, Coats AJS, Fowler MB, et al. Effect of carvedilol on survival in chronic heart failure. N Engl J Med 2001; 344: 651–8.

86. Frishman WH. Carvedilol: a new alpha- and beta-adrenoceptor blocker for the treatment of congestive heart failure. N Engl J Med 1998; 339: 1759–65.

87. Aronow WS. Effect of beta blockers on mortality and morbidity in persons treated for congestive heart failure. J Am Geriatr Soc 2001; 49: 331–3.

88. Edeki TI, He H, Wood AJJ. Pharmacogenetic explanation for excessive β blockade following timolol eye drops: potential for oral-ophthalmic drug interaction. JAMA 1995; 274: 1611–13.

89. Dahlof B, Pennert K, Hansson L. Reversal of left ventricular hypertrophy in hypertensive patients: a meta-analysis of 109 treatment studies. Am J Hypertens 1992; 5: 95–110.

90. Pfeffer MA, Braunwald E, Moye LA, et al. On Behalf of the SAVE Investigators. Effect of captopril on mortality and morbidity of patients with left ventricular dysfunction after myocardial infarction: results of the survival and ventricular enlargement trial. N Engl J Med 1992; 327: 669–77.

91. Yusuf S, Pepine CJ, Garces C, et al. Effect of enalapril on myocardial infarction and unstable angina in patients with low ejection fractions. Lancet 1992; 340: 1173–8.

92. Packer M, Poole-Wilson PA, Armstrong PW, et al. Comparative effects of low and high doses of the angiotensin-converting enzyme inhibitor, lisinopril, on morbidity and mortality in chronic heart failure. Circulation 1999; 100: 2312–18.

93. Aronow WS, Ahn C, Kronzon I. Effect of beta blockers alone, of angiotensin-converting enzyme inhibitors alone, and of beta blockers plus angiotensin-converting enzyme inhibitors on new coronary events and on congestive heart failure in older persons with healed myocardial infarcts and asymptomatic left ventricular systolic dysfunction. Am J Cardiol 2001; 88: 1298–300.

94. Schoolwerth A, Sica DA, Ballermann BJ, Wilcox CS. Renal considerations in angiotensin converting enzyme inhibitor therapy. Circulation 2001; 104: 1985–91.

95. Pitt B, Zannad F, Remme WJ, et al. The effect of spironolactone on morbidity and mortality in patients with severe heart failure. N Engl J Med 1999; 341: 709–17.

96. Okereke CE, Messerli FH. Efficacy and safety of angiotensin II receptor blockers in elderly patients with mild to moderate hypertension. Am J Geriatr Cardiol 2001; 10: 424–9.

97. Elliott WJ. Therapeutic trials comparing angiotensin converting enzyme inhibitors and angiotensin II receptor blockers. Curr Hypertens Rep 2000; 2: 402–11.

98. Grossman E, Messerli FH, Neutel JM. Angiotensin II receptor blockers: equal or preferred substitutes for ACE inhibitors? Arch Intern Med 2000; 160: 1905–11.

99. Lam S. Azilsartan: a newly approved angiotensin II receptor blocker. Cardiol Rev 2011; 19: 300–4.

100. Toto R. Angiotensin II subtype 1-receptor blockers and renal function. Arch Intern Med 2001; 161: 1492–9.

101. Jamali AH, Tang WH, Khot UN, Fowler MB. The role of angiotensin receptor blockers in the management of chronic heart failure. Arch Intern Med 2001; 161: 667–72.

102. Pitt B, Poole-Wilson PA, Segal R, et al. Effect of losartan compared with captopril on mortality in patients with symptomatic heart failure: randomised trial—the Losartan Heart Failure Survival Study ELITE II. Lancet 2000; 355: 1582–7.

103. Brenner BM, Cooper ME, de Zeeuw D, et al. Effects of losartan on renal and cardiovascular outcomes in patients with type 2 diabetes and nephropathy. N Engl J Med 2001; 345: 861–9.

104. Lewis EJ, Hunsicker LG, Clarke WR, et al. Renoprotective effect of the angiotensin-receptor antagonist irbesartan in patients with nephropathy due to type 2 diabetes. N Engl J Med 2001; 345: 851–60.

105. Sepehrdad R, Stier CT Jr, Frishman WH, Sica DA. Specific inhibition of renin as a cardiovascular pharmacotherapy: focus on Aliskiren. Cardiol Rev 2007; 15: 242–56.

106. Aliskiren (Tekturna) for hypertension. Med Lett Drugs Ther 2007; 49: 29–31.

107. Frampton JE, Curran MP. Aliskiren: a review of its use in the management of hypertension. Drugs 2007; 67: 1767–92.

108. Dieterich H, Kemp C, Vaidyanathan S, Yeh C. Aliskiren, the first in a new class of orally effective renin inhibitors, has no clinically significant drug interactions with digoxin in healthy volunteers. Clin Pharmacol Ther 2006; 79: 64(PIII-24).

109. Dieterle W, Corynen S, Mann J. Effect of the oral renin inhibitor aliskiren on the pharmacokinetics and pharmacodynamics of a single dose of warfarin in healthy subjects. Br J Clin Pharmacol 2004; 58: 433–6.

110. Pahor M, Cecchi E, Fumagalli S, et al. Association of serum creatinine and age with headache caused by nitrates. Gruppo Italiano di Farmacovigilanza nell' Anziano. Clin Pharmacol Ther 1995; 59: 470–81.

111. Furberg CD, Psaty BM. Should dihydropyridines be used as first-line drugs in the treatment of hypertension? Arch Intern Med 1995; 155: 2157–61.

112. Pahor M, Guralnik JM, Corti MC, et al. Long-term survival and use of antihypertensive medications in older persons. J Am Geriatr Soc 1995; 43: 1191–7.

113. Furberg CD, Psaty BM. Calcium antagonists: antagonists or protagonists of mortality in elderly hypertensives? J Am Geriatr Soc 1995; 43: 1309–10.

114. Staessen JA, Fagard R, Thijs L, et al. Randomized double-blind comparison of placebo vs active treatment for older patients with isolated systolic hypertension: the Systolic Hypertension in Europe (SYST-EUR) Trial Investigators. Lancet 1997; 350: 757–64.

115. Estacio RO, Jeffers BW, Hiatt WR, et al. The effect of nisoldipine as compared with enalapril on cardiovascular outcomes in patients with non-insulin-dependent diabetes and hypertension. N Engl J Med 1998; 338: 645–52.

116. Setaro JF, Zaret BL, Schulman DS, et al. Usefulness of verapamil for congestive heart failure associated with abnormal left ventricular diastolic filling and normal left ventricular systolic performance. Am J Cardiol 1990; 66: 981–6.

117. Elkayam U, Amin J, Mehra A, et al. A prospective, randomized, double-blind, crossover study to compare the efficacy and safety of chronic nifedipine therapy with that of isosorbide dinitrate and their combination in the treatment of chronic congestive heart failure. Circulation 1990; 82: 1954–61.

118. The Multicenter Diltiazem Post Infarction Trial Research Group. Effect of diltiazem on mortality and reinfarction after myocardial infarction. N Engl J Med 1988; 319: 385–92.

119. Kelly JG, O'Malley K. Clinical pharmacokinetics of calcium antagonists. Clin Pharmacokinet 1992; 22: 416–33.

120. Frishman WH. Alpha- and beta adrenergic blocking drugs. In: Frishman WH, Sonnenblick EH. Cardiovascular Pharmacotherapeutics, Companion Handbook. New York: McGraw Hill, 1998: 23–64.

121. Frishman WH, Kotob F. Alpha-adrenergic blocking drugs in clinical practice. J Clin Pharmacol 1999; 39: 7–16.

122. The ALLHAT Officers and Coordinators for the ALLHAT Collaborative Research Group. Major cardiovascular events in hypertensive patients randomized to doxazosin vs chlorthalidone: the Anti-hypertensive and Lipid-Lowering Treatment to Prevent Heart Attack Trial (ALLHAT). JAMA 2000; 283: 1967–75.

123. Zimethaum P, Kowey PR, Michelson EL. Antiarrhythmic drugs. In: Frishman WH, Sica DA, eds. Cardiovascular Pharmacotherapeutics, 3rd edn. Minneapolis: Cardiotext, 2011: 227–56.

124. Ochs HR, Carstens G, Greenblatt DJ. Reduction of lidocaine clearance during continuous infusion and by coadministration of propranolol. N Engl J Med 1980; 303: 373–7.

125. Aronow WS. Management of the person with ventricular arrhythmias. J Am Geriatr Soc 1999; 47: 886–95.

126. The Cardiac Arrhythmia Suppression Trial (CAST) Investigators. Preliminary report: effect of encainide and flecainide on mortality in a randomized trial of arrhythmia suppression after myocardial infarction. N Engl J Med 1989; 321: 406–12.

127. The Cardiac Arrhythmia Suppression Trial II Investigators. Effect of the antiarrhythmic agent moricizine on survival after myocardial infarction. N Engl J Med 1992; 327: 227–33.

128. Akiyama T, Pawitan Y, Campbell WB, et al. Effects of advancing age on the efficacy and side effects of antiarrhythmic drugs in post-myocardial infarction patients with ventricular arrhythmias. J Am Geriatr Soc 1992; 40: 666–72.

129. Moosvi AR, Goldstein S, Vanderbrug Mcdendorp S, et al. Effect of empiric antiarrhythmic therapy in resuscitated out-of-hospital cardiac arrest victims with coronary artery disease. Am J Cardiol 1990; 65: 1192–7.

130. Aronow WS, Mercando AD, Epstein S, Kronzon I. Effect of quinidine and procainamide versus no antiarrhythmic drug on sudden cardiac death, total cardiac death, and total death in elderly patients with heart disease and complex ventricular arrhythmias. Am J Cardiol 1990; 66: 423–8.

131. Coplen SE, Antman EM, Berlin JA, et al. Efficacy and safety of quinidine therapy for maintenance of sinus rhythm after cardioversion: a meta-analysis of randomized control trials. Circulation 1990; 82: 1106–16.

132. Flaker GC, Blackshear JL, McBride R, et al. Antiarrhythmic drug therapy and cardiac mortality in atrial fibrillation. J Am Coll Cardiol 1992; 20: 527–32.

133. Nicklas JM, McKenna WJ, Stewart RA, et al. Prospective, double-blind, placebo-controlled trial of low dose amiodarone in patients with severe heart failure and asymptomatic frequent ventricular ectopy. Am Heart J 1991; 122: 1016–21.

134. Hockings B, George T, Mahrous F, et al. Effectiveness of amiodarone on ventricular arrhythmias during and after acute myocardial infarction. Am J Cardiol 1987; 60: 967–70.

135. Pfisterer M, Kiowski W, Burckhardt D, et al. Beneficial effect of amiodarone on cardiac mortality in patients with asymptomatic complex ventricular arrhythmias after acute myocardial infarction and preserved but not impaired left ventricular function. Am J Cardiol 1992; 69: 1399–402.

136. Julian DG, Camm AJ, Frangin G, et al. Randomised trial of effect of amiodarone on mortality in patients with left-ventricular dysfunction after recent myocardial infarction: EMIAT. Lancet 1997; 349: 667–74.

137. Cairns JA, Connolly SJ, Roberts R, et al. Randomised trial of outcome after myocardial infarction in patients with frequent or repetitive ventricular premature depolarisations: CAMIAT. Lancet 1997; 349: 675–82.

138. Doval HC, Nul DR, Grancelli HO, et al. Randomised trial of low dose amiodarone in severe congestive heart failure. Lancet 1994; 344: 493–8.

139. Singh SN, Fletcher RD, Fisher SG, et al. Amiodarone in patients with congestive heart failure and asymptomatic ventricular arrhythmias. N Engl J Med 1995; 333: 77–82.

140. Bardy GH, Lee KL, Mark DB, et al. Amiodarone or an implantable cardioverter-defibrillator for congestive heart failure. N Engl J Med 2005; 352: 225–37.

141. Herre J, Sauve M, Malone P, et al. Long-term results of amiodarone therapy in patients with recurrent sustained ventricular tachycardia or ventricular fibrillation. J Am Coll Cardiol 1989; 13: 442–9.

142. Greene HL for the CASCADE Investigators. The CASCADE study: randomized anti-arrhythmic drug therapy in survivors of cardiac arrest in Seattle. Am J Cardiol 1993; 72: 70F–4F.

143. Gold RL, Haffajee CI, Charos G, et al. Amiodarone for refractory atrial fibrillation. Am J Cardiol 1986; 57: 124–7.

144. Chatterjee S, Ghosh J, Lichstein E, et al. Meta-analysis of cardiovascular outcomes with dronedarone in patients with atrial fibrillation or heart failure. Am J Cardiol 2012; 110: 607–13.

145. LaRosa JC, Applegate W, Crouse JR III, et al. Cholesterol lowering in the elderly: results of the Cholesterol Reduction in Seniors Program (CRISP) pilot study. Arch Intern Med 1994; 154: 529–39.

146. Cholesterol Treatment Trialists' Collaborators. Efficacy and safety of cholesterol-lowering treatment: prospective meta-analysis of data from 90 056 participantys in 14 randomised trials of statins. Lancet 2005; 366: 1267–78.

147. Scandinavian Simvastatin Survival Study Group. Randomised trial of cholesterol lowering in 4444 patients with coronary heart disease: The Scandinavian Simvastatin Survival Study (4S). Lancet 1994; 344: 1383–9.

148. Miettinen TA, Pyorala K, Olsson AG, et al. Cholesterol-lowering therapy in women and elderly patients with myocardial infarction or angina pectoris. Findings from the Scandinavian Simvastatin Survival Study (4S). Circulation 1997; 96: 4211–18.

149. Lewis SJ, Moye LA, Sacks FM, et al. Effect of pravastatin on cardiovascular events in older patients with myocardial infarction and cholesterol levels in the average range. Results of the Cholesterol and Recurrent Events (CARE) trial. Ann Intern Med 1998; 129: 681–9.

150. Shepherd J, Blauw GJ, Murphy MB, et al. Pravastatin in elderly individuals at risk of vascular disease (PROSPER): a randomised controlled trial. Lancet 2002; 360: 1623–30.

151. The LIPID Study Group. Long-term effectiveness and safety of pravastatin in 9014 patients with coronary heart disease and average cholesterol concentrations: the LIPID trial follow-up. Lancet 2002; 359: 1379–87.

152. Heart Protection Study Collaborative Group. MRC/BHF Heart Protection Study of cholesterol lowering with simvastatin in 20,536 high-risk individuals: a randomised placebo-controlled trial. Lancet 2002; 360: 7–22.

153. Aronow WS, Nayak D, Woodworth S, Ahn C. Effect of simvastatin versus placebo on treadmill exercise time until the onset of intermittent claudication in older patients with peripheral arterial disease at six months and at one year after treatment. Am J Cardiol 2003; 92: 711–12.

154. Aronow WS, Ahn C. Incidence of new coronary events in older persons with prior myocardial infarction and serum low-density lipoprotein cholesterol ≥125 mg/dL treated with statins versus no lipid-lowering drug. Am J Cardiol 2002; 89: 67–9.

155. Aronow WS, Ahn C, Gutstein H. Incidence of new atherothrombotic brain infarction in older persons with prior myocardial infarction and serum low-density lipoprotein cholesterol ≥125 mg/dL treated with statins versus no lipid-lowering drug. J Gerontol Med Sci 2002; 57A: M333–5.

156. Aronow WS, Ahn C. Frequency of congestive heart failure in older persons with prior myocardial infarction and serum low-density lipoprotein cholesterol ≥125 mg/dl treated with statins versus no lipid-lowering drug. Am J Cardiol 2002; 90: 147–9.

157. Aronow WS, Ahn C, Gutstein H. Reduction of new coronary events and of new atherothrombotic brain infarction in older persons with diabetes mellitus, prior myocardial infarction, and serum low-density lipoprotein cholesterol ≥125 mg/dL treated with statins. J Gerontol Med Sci 2002; 57A: M747–50.

158. Aronow WS, Ahn C. Frequency of new coronary events in older persons with peripheral arterial disease and serum low-density lipoprotein cholesterol ≥125 mg/dl treated with statins versus no lipid-lowering drug. Am J Cardiol 2002; 90: 789–91.

159. Zimetbaum P, Frishman WH, Ooi WL, et al. Plasma lipids and lipoproteins and the incidence of cardiovascular disease in the old old: Bronx Longitudinal Aging Study. Arterio Thrombo 1992; 12: 416–23.

160. Collins R, Armitage J. High-risk elderly patients PROSPER from cholesterol-lowering therapy (commentary). Lancet 2002; 360: 1618–19.

161. Executive Summary of The Third Report of The National Cholesterol Education Program (NCEP). Expert panel on detection, evaluation, and treatment of high blood cholesterol in adults (adult treatment panel III). JAMA 2001; 285: 2486–97.

162. Frishman WH, Aronow WS. Lipid-lowering drugs. In: Frishman WH, Sica DA, eds. Cardiovascular Pharmacotherapeutics, 3rd edn. Minneapolis: Cardiotext, 2011: 323–75.

163. Nissen SE, Tuzcu EM, Schoenhagen P, et al. Effect of intensive compared with moderate lipid-lowering therapy on progression of coronary atherosclerosis. A randomized controlled trial. JAMA 2004; 291: 1071–80.

164. Cannon CP, Braunwald E, McCabe CH, et al. Comparison of intensive and moderate lipid lowering with statins after acute coronary syndromes. N Engl J Med 2004; 350: 1495–504.

165. LaRosa JC, Grundy SM, Waters DD, et al. Intensive lipid lowering with atorvastatin in patients with stable coronary disease. N Engl J Med 2005; 352: 1425–35.

166. Grundy SM, Cleeman JI, Merz CNB, et al. Implications of recent clinical trials for the National Cholesterol Education Program Adult Treatment Panel III guidelines. Circulation 2004; 110: 227–39.

167. Sebastian JL, Tresch D. Anticoagulation therapy in the elderly. In: Fresch DD, Aronow WS, eds. Cardiovascular Disease in the Elderly Patient. New York: Marcel Dekker Inc, 1994: 213–61.

168. The Sixty Plus Reinfarction Study Research Group. A double-blind trial to assess long-term anticoagulation therapy in elderly patients after myocardial infarction: report of the sixty plus reinfarction study research group. Lancet 1980; 2: 989–94.

169. Shepherd AMM, Hewick DS, Moreland TA, Stevenson TH. Age as a determinant of sensitivity to warfarin. Br J Clin Pharmacol 1977; 4: 315–20.

170. Hylek EM, Singer DE. Risk factors for intracranial hemorrhage in outpatients taking warfarin. Ann Intern Med 1994; 120: 897–902.

171. Frishman WH, Lerner RG, Desai H. Antiplatelet and other antithrombotic drugs. In: Frishman WH, Sica DA, eds. Cardiovascular Pharmacotherapeutics, 3rd edn. Minneapolis: Cardiotext, 2011: 257–304.

172. Bhatt DL. Prasugrel in clinical practice (perspective). N Engl J Med 2009; 361: 940–2.

173. Connolly SJ, Ezekowitz MD, Yusuf S, et al. RE-LY Steering committee and investigators. Dabigatran versus warfarin in patients with atrial fibrillation. N Engl J Med 2009; 361: 1139–51.

174. Patel MR, Mahaffey KW, Garg J, et al. ROCKET AF Investigators. Rivaroxaban versus warfarin in nonvalvular atrial fibrillation. N Engl J Med 2011; 365: 883–91.

175. Connolly SJ, Eikelboom J, Joyner C, et al. AVERROES Steering Committee and Investigators. Apixaban in patients with atrial fibrillation. N Engl J Med 2011; 364: 806–17.

176. Frishman WH, Sinatra ST, Moizuddin M. Herbal approach to cardiac disease. In: Frishman WH, Weintraub MI, Micozzi MS, eds. Complementary and Integrative Therapies for Cardiovascular Disease. St. Louis: Elsevier/Mosby, 2005: 86–106.

177. Beers MH, Ouslander JG, Rollingher I, et al. Explicit criteria for determining inappropriate medication use in nursing home residents. Arch Intern Med 1991; 151: 1825–32.

178. Beers MH, Ouslander JG, Fingold SF, et al. Inappropriate medication prescribing in skilled-nursing facilities. Ann Intern Med 1992; 117: 684–9.

179. Beers MH, Fingold SF, Ouslander JG, et al. Characteristics and quality of prescribing by doctors practicing in nursing homes. J Am Geriatr Soc 1993; 41: 802–7.

180. Stuck AE, Beers MH, Steiner A, et al. Inappropriate medication use in community-residing older persons. Arch Intern Med 1994; 154: 2195–200.

181. Willcox SM, Himmelstein DU, Woolhandler S. Inappropriate drug prescribing for the community-dwelling elderly. JAMA 1994; 272: 292–6.

182. Gurwitz JH. Suboptimal medication use in the elderly: the tip of the iceberg. JAMA 1994; 272: 316–17.

183. Beers MH. Explicit criteria for determining potentially inappropriate medication use by the elderly: an update. Arch Intern Med 1997; 157: 1531–6.

184. Johnson JF. Considerations in Prescribing for the Older Patient. Arizona: PCS Health Systems, Inc, 1998; 1/98.

185. Abrams WB. Cardiovascular drugs in the elderly. Chest 1990; 98: 9809–86.

186. Stein BE. Avoiding drug reactions: seven steps to writing safe prescriptions. Geriatrics 1994; 49: 28–36.

187. Nagle BA, Erwin WG. Geriatrics. In: DiPiro JT, Talbert RL, Yee GC, et al. eds. Pharmacotherapy. A Patho-physiologic Approach, 3rd edn. Stamford: Appleton and Lange, 1997: 87–100.

188. Hui KK. Gerontologic considerations in cardiovascular pharmacology and therapeutics. In: Singh BN, Dzau VJ, Vanhoutte PM, et al. eds. Cardiovascular Pharmacology and Therapeutics. New York: Churchill-Livingstone, 1994: 1130.

189. Cheng-Lai A, Frishman WH. Appendices. Cardiovascular Pharmacotherapeutics, 3rd edn. Minneapolis: Cardiotext, 2011: 745–9.

190. Aronow WS. Cardiovascular drug therapy in the elderly. In: Frishman WH, Sonnenblick EH, eds. Cardiovascular Pharmacotherapeutics. New York: McGraw-Hill, 1997: 1273.

191. Parker BM, Cusack BJ. Pharmacology and appropriate prescribing. In: Reuben DB, Yoshikawa TT, Besdine RW, eds. Geriatric Review Syllabus: A Core Curriculum in Geriatric Medicine, 3rd edn. Iowa: Kendall/Hunt Publishers, Am Geriatric Soc, 1996: 33.

192. Bressler R. Adverse drug reactions. In: Bressler R, Katz MD, eds. Geriatric Pharmacology. New York: McGraw-Hill, 1993: 54.

193. Fraser AG. Pharmacokinetic interactions between alcohol and other drugs. Clin Pharmacokinet 1997; 33: 79–90.

194. Frishman WH, Aronow WS, Cheng-Lai A. Cardiovascular drug therapy in the elderly. In: Aronow WS, Fleg JL, Rich MW. Cardiovascular Disease in the Elderly, 4th edn. New York: Informa, 2008: 99–135.

195. Beers MH. Explicit criteria for determining potentially inappropriate medication use by the elderly: an update. Arch Intern Med 1997; 157: 1531–6.

4

Systemic hypertension in the elderly

William H. Frishman and Wilbert S. Aronow

SUMMARY

Hypertension is a major risk factor for cardiovascular disease and is present in 69% of patients with a first myocardial infarction (MI), in 77% of patients with a first stroke, in 74% of patients with chronic heart failure, and in 60% of patients with peripheral arterial disease. Double-blind, randomized, placebo-controlled trials have demonstrated that antihypertensive drug therapy reduces cardiovascular events in patients aged between 65 and 79 years and also in patients aged 80 years and older. Although the optimal blood pressure (BP) treatment goal in the elderly has not been determined, existing epidemiologic and clinical trial data suggest that a reasonable therapeutic BP goal should be <140/90 mm Hg in persons aged 65–79 years and a systolic BP of 140–145 mm Hg if tolerated in persons aged 80 years and older. Non-pharmacologic lifestyle measures should be encouraged both to prevent the development of hypertension and as adjunctive therapy in persons with hypertension. Diuretics, angiotensin-converting enzyme (ACE) inhibitors, angiotensin receptor blockers (ARBs), β blockers, and calcium channel blockers have all shown benefit in reducing cardiovascular events in randomized trials. The choice of specific drugs depends mainly on efficacy, tolerability, presence of specific comorbidities, and cost.

INTRODUCTION

Hypertension in older persons is a systolic blood pressure (BP) ≥140 mm Hg or a diastolic BP ≥90 mm Hg based on the mean of two or more properly measured seated BP readings on each of two or more office visits (1,2). Isolated systolic hypertension (ISH) is a systolic BP ≥140 mm Hg with a diastolic BP <90 mm Hg (1,2). Stage 1 hypertension is a systolic BP of 140–159 mm Hg or a diastolic BP of 90–99 mm Hg. Stage 2 hypertension is a systolic BP ≥160 mm Hg or a diastolic BP ≥100 mm Hg. Prehypertension is a systolic BP of 120–139 mm Hg or a diastolic BP of 80–89 mm Hg (1).

Pseudohypertension in the elderly is a falsely increased systolic BP resulting from markedly sclerotic arteries that do not collapse during inflation of the BP cuff (1,2). Suspect pseudohypertension is seen in elderly patients with refractory hypertension, no target organ damage, and/or symptoms of overmedication, and the diagnosis is confirmed by measuring intra-arterial pressure (2). White coat hypertension is diagnosed when the physician's office BP measurement is persistently high but daytime ambulatory BP readings are normal (1,2). Ambulatory BP monitoring should be performed to confirm white coat hypertension in persons with office hypertension with no target organ damage (1–3).

Ambulatory BP monitoring in the elderly is also indicated when the response to therapy is unclear from office visits, when syncope or hypotensive disorders are suspected, and for evaluation of vertigo and dizziness (2). Home recordings of BP should also be obtained to ensure adequate control of BP in the elderly, to avoid excessive BP reduction in the elderly, and for better prognostic accuracy versus office BP (2).

A physical exam and complete history should be performed in patients with hypertension, to know: What is the duration and severity of hypertension? What are the causes or exacerbations of hypertension? What are the current and previous treatments of hypertension? What are the adverse effects from antihypertensive drugs taken? (2)

Patients with hypertension should be evaluated for other cardiovascular risk factors including smoking, dyslipidemia, diabetes mellitus (DM), age >55 years for men and 65 years for women, body mass index ≥ 30 kg/m^2, physical inactivity, microalbuminuria, an estimated glomerular filtration rate <60 ml/min/1.73 m^2, and for a family history of premature cardiovascular disease (<55 years in fathers or brothers and <65 years in mothers or sisters) (2). Patients with hypertension should also be evaluated for target organ damage and clinical cardiovascular disease, including left ventricular hypertrophy (LVH), prior myocardial infarction (MI), angina pectoris, prior coronary revascularization, congestive heart failure (CHF), stroke or transient ischemic attack, peripheral arterial disease (PAD), nephropathy, and retinopathy (2).

Routine laboratory tests that should be obtained in older patients with hypertension include a urinalysis to look for renal damage, especially albuminuria/microalbuminuria, serum electrolytes, especially serum potassium, serum creatinine, and estimated glomerular filtration rate, fasting serum total cholesterol, low-density lipoprotein cholesterol, high-density lipoprotein cholesterol, and triglycerides, fasting blood sugar, a hemoglobin A$_{1c}$ in diabetics, and a 12-lead electrocardiogram (2). In selected elderly patients with hypertension, a 2-dimensional echocardiogram should be obtained to look for LVH and for an abnormal LV ejection fraction.

Interarm differences of ≥ 10 mm Hg in systolic BP were present in 14% of 528 older adults (4), and appear to be an independent risk factor for cardiovascular disease (5,6). Interarm differences of ≥ 10 mm Hg in diastolic BP were present in 5% of 528 older adults (4). The BP should be measured in both arms in the sitting position with the arm with the highest BP used for future measurements (2). The BP must also be measured with the patient standing for 1–3 minutes to evaluate for postural hypotension or hypertension (2).

Orthostatic hypotension is defined as a decrease in systolic BP of ≥ 20 mm Hg or in diastolic BP of ≥ 10 mm Hg within 3 minutes of standing and can result from blunting the carotid baroflex due to increased stiffness of the carotid arteries (7). Orthostatic hypotension may result in falls and syncope (2,7).

PATHOPHYSIOLOGY

An increase in systolic BP in elderly persons is related to an age-associated increase in arterial stiffness due to structural changes within the arterial media (a change in the amount or nature of collagen, interstitial fibrosis, and calcification, and degradation of elastin fibers) (Fig. 4.1) (8). The increased wall stiffness and tortuosity of the aorta and large arteries with aging is often reflected by an increased systolic BP and widened pulse pressure. Older persons with hypertension are more likely to have increased LV mass, increased peripheral resistance, reduced baroreceptor sensitivity, increased characteristic aortic impedance at rest, decreased LV early diastolic filling rate, decreased LV early diastolic filling volume, increased left atrial dimension, and decreased cardiovascular response to catecholamines (8).

Flow-mediated arterial dilation, primarily mediated by endothelium-derived nitric oxide, decreases markedly with aging (2). The neurohormonal profile of older adults is characterized by increased plasma norepinephrine, low renin, and low aldosterone levels (2).

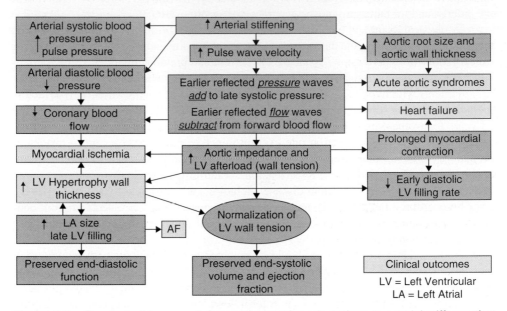

Figure 4.1   Conceptual framework for cardiovascular adaptations to arterial stiffness that occur with aging. *Abbreviations*: CBF, coronary blood flow; DBP, diastolic blood pressure; EF, ejection fraction; LA, left atrial; LV, left ventricular; SBP, systolic blood pressure; ↓ = decrease; ↑ = increased. *Source*: Adapted from Ref. 133.

Many so-called normal aging changes in arterial structure and function are blunted or absent in populations not chronically exposed to high sodium/calorie diets, low physical activity levels, and high rates of obesity (2).

The decrease in baroreflex sensitivity with age and with hypertension leads to impaired baroreflex-mediated increase in total systemic vascular resistance and to an inability to increase heart rate in response to decreased BP (9). Therefore, older persons with hypertension have a greater impairment in baroreflex sensitivity and are more likely to develop orthostatic and postprandial hypotension on antihypertensive drug therapy (10).

Hypertension in the elderly also increases the age-dependent decline in renal function. Of 143 older persons, mean age 73 years, with hypertension in an academic nursing home, 60 (42%) had moderate (33%) or severe (9%) renal insufficiency with an estimated glomerular filtration rate <60 ml/min/1.73 m² (11). Renal artery stenosis is also an important cause of secondary hypertension in the elderly (12).

PREVALENCE

Hypertension occurs in more than two-thirds of persons >65 years (13). Hypertension was present in 57% of 1160 older men, mean age 80 years, and in 60% of 2464 older women, mean age 81 years, with two-thirds of these older persons having ISH (14). Of 1819 older persons, mean age 80 years, living in the community and seen in an academic geriatrics practice, 58% had hypertension (37% with ISH) (15). In this study, hypertension was present in 52% of older whites, 71% of older blacks, 61% of older Hispanics, and 64% of older Asians (15). Target organ damage, clinical cardiovascular disease, or DM was present in 70% of these older persons with hypertension (15). The prevalence of hypertension in older persons in an academic nursing home was 71% (16). The prevalence of hypertension in older persons with DM in an academic nursing home was 76% (17). The age-adjusted prevalence of hypertension in the USA is 64% of elderly men and 78% of elderly women according to the American Heart Association (AHA) Statistics Committee and Stroke Statistics Committee (18).

HYPERTENSION AND RISK OF CARDIOVASCULAR DISEASE

The higher the systolic or diastolic BP in older persons, the higher the risk of cardiovascular morbidity and mortality (19). Increased systolic BP and pulse pressure are stronger risk factors for cardiovascular morbidity and mortality in older persons than is increased diastolic BP (20–22). An increased pulse pressure found in older persons with ISH indicates decreased vascular compliance in the large arteries and is even a better marker of risk than is systolic or diastolic BP (20–22). The Cardiovascular Health Study found that in 5202 older men and women that a brachial systolic BP >169 mm Hg increased the mortality rate 2.4 times (23).

Hypertension in older persons is a major risk factor for coronary events (1,2,24–28), for stroke (1,2,24,28–31), for CHF (1,2,23,32,33), and for PAD (2,34–38). Hypertension is present in approximately 69% of patients with a first MI (18), in approximately 77% of patients with a first stroke (18), in approximately 74% of patients with CHF (18), and in 60% of patients with PAD (38). Hypertension is also a major risk factor for a dissecting aortic aneurysm, sudden cardiac death, angina pectoris, atrial fibrillation, DM, the metabolic syndrome, chronic kidney disease, thoracic and abdominal aortic aneurysms, LV hypertrophy, vascular dementia, Alzheimer's disease, and ophthalmologic disorders (2).

At 40-month follow-up of 664 men, mean age 80 years, and at 48-month follow-up of 1488 women, mean age 82 years, hypertension increased the incidence of new coronary events in men (relative risk = 2.0, $p = 0.0001$) and in women (relative risk = 1.6, $p = 0.0001$) (25). At 42-month follow-up of 664 men, mean age 80 years, and at 48-month follow-up of 1488 women, mean age 82 years, hypertension increased the incidence of new stroke in men (relative risk = 2.2, $p = 0.0001$) and in women (relative risk = 2.4, $p = 0.0001$) (29). Hypertension was an independent risk factor for PAD in 467 men, mean age 80 years, with an odds ratio of 2.2 ($p = 0.023$) and in 1444 women, mean age 81 years, with an odds ratio of 2.8 ($p = 0.001$) (36). Hypertension was an independent risk factor for CHF in 2902 patients (926 men and 1976 women), mean age 81 years, with a risk ratio of 2.5 ($p = 0.0001$) (32). In 61 prospective studies of 1 million adults, coronary heart disease mortality increased with each decade from ages 40–49 to 80–89 and with each increase in systolic BP from 120–140 to 160–180 mm Hg (39). Of interest is the observation that an increased heart rate remains a long-term predictor of cardiovascular events, even in those patients with good BP control on medication (40).

Older persons are more likely to have hypertension and ISH, to have target organ damage and clinical cardiovascular disease, and to develop new cardiovascular events. Older persons also have the lowest rates of BP control (1,2,41,42). BP is adequately controlled in 36% of men and 28% of women aged 60–79 years and in 38% of men and 23% of women aged 80 years and older (42).

Barriers to treatment of hypertension include physicians not understanding that frail elderly persons should be treated according to recommended guidelines to decrease cardiovascular morbidity and mortality. Prevalent comorbidities, polypharmacy, an asymptomatic state, side effects from medications, and high cost of medications contribute to lower BP control rates in older persons (2,43). A BP <140/90 mm Hg was achieved in 70% of 492 Medicaid or private insurance patients versus 38% of 122 patients who had to pay for their antihypertensive medications ($p < 0.001$) (43). This problem needs to be addressed if we are to reduce the great amount of cardiovascular events and mortality caused by inadequate treatment of hypertension.

EFFECT OF ANTIHYPERTENSIVE THERAPY IN LOWERING CARDIOVASCULAR EVENTS

Numerous prospective, double-blind, randomized, placebo-controlled studies have shown that antihypertensive drug therapy reduces the development of new coronary events, stroke, and CHF in older persons (1,2,44–55). Older persons with hypertension, if treated appropriately, will have a greater absolute reduction in cardiovascular events such as major coronary events, stroke, CHF, and renal insufficiency, and a greater reduction in dementia (56) than in younger persons.

Therapy with antihypertensive drugs reduces the incidence of all strokes: 38% in women, 34% in men, 36% in older persons, and 34% in persons >80 years (30). The overall data suggest that the decrease of stroke in older persons with hypertension is related more to a reduction in BP than to the type of antihypertensive drugs used (30).

In the Perindopril Protection Against Recurrent Stroke Study (57), perindopril plus indapamide reduced stroke-related dementia by 34% and cognitive decline by 45%. In the Systolic Hypertension in Europe trial (58), nitrendipine reduced dementia by 55% at 3.9-year follow-up. In 1900 older African-Americans, antihypertensive drug treatment reduced cognitive impairment by 38% (59). In the Rotterdam Study (60), antihypertensive drugs decreased vascular dementia by 70%.

On the basis of data available at the time, Aronow (61) proposed in an editorial that unless the Hypertension in the Very Elderly Trial (HYVET) (55) found that antihypertensive drug therapy was not beneficial in patients aged 80 years and older, this group should receive antihypertensive drug treatment. Goodwin (62) disagreed with this approach, and his response to Aronow's editorial was accompanied by eight commentaries, some of which supported the treatment of very older hypertensive patients and some of which did not.

In HYVET, 3845 persons aged 80 years and older (mean age 83.6 years) with a sustained systolic BP ≥160 mm Hg were randomized to indapmide (sustained release 1.5 mg) or matching placebo (55). Perindopril 2 or 4 mg, or matching placebo, was added if needed to achieve the target BP of 150/80 mm Hg. Median follow-up was 1.8 years. Antihypertensive drug treatment reduced the incidence of the primary end point (fatal or nonfatal stroke) by 30% ($p = 0.06$). Antihypertensive drug treatment reduced fatal stroke by 39% ($p = 0.05$), all-cause mortality by 21% ($p = 0.02$), death from cardiovascular causes by 23% ($p = 0.06$), and heart failure by 64% ($p < 0.001$). The significant 21% reduction in all-cause mortality by antihypertensive drug treatment was unexpected. The benefits of antihypertensive drug treatment began to be apparent during the first year of follow-up.

The prevalence of baseline cardiovascular disease was only 12% in the patients in HYVET. In a cohort of patients, mean age 80 years, with hypertension seen in a university geriatrics practice, 70% had baseline cardiovascular disease, target organ damage, or DM (15). An older population such as this one with a high prevalence of cardiovascular disease would be expected to have a greater absolute reduction in cardiovascular events resulting from antihypertensive drug therapy.

Although the results of HYVET clearly indicate that hypertensive patients aged ≥80 years should be treated with antihypertensive drug therapy, the study does not give us data on target BP (63). Further research is needed to answer this question (2).

Although the optimal BP treatment goal has not been determined, a therapeutic target of <140/90 mm Hg in persons <80 years and a systolic BP of 140–145 mm Hg if tolerated in persons aged ≥80 years is reasonable (2). We should also be careful to avoid intensive lowering of the BP, especially in older persons with DM and coronary artery disease, as this might be poorly tolerated and might increase cardiovascular events (the J-curve phenomenon) (2,64–69). However, until additional data from randomized controlled trials (including the Systolic BP INtervention Trial—SPRINT) comparing various BP targets in the elderly and younger become available, existing epidemiologic and clinical trial data suggest a diagnostic and therapeutic threshold for hypertension of 140/90 mm Hg remains reasonable in adults 65–79 years of age and younger and of 150 mm Hg of systolic BP in adults >80 years of age (2).

LIFESTYLE MEASURES

Lifestyle modification should be used in older persons to prevent mild hypertension and to decrease the dose levels of drugs needed to control hypertension. Weight reduction, consuming a diet rich in fruits, vegetables, and low-fat dairy products with a reduced amount of saturated fat and total fat, sodium reduction to not exceed 1.5 grams daily, smoking cessation, regular aerobic physical activity, avoidance of excessive alcohol intake, avoidance of excessive caffeine, and avoidance of drugs which can increase BP, including nonsteroidal anti-inflammatory drugs, glucocorticoids, and sympathomimetics, are recommended (1,2). Implementing a national salt reduction program is likely a simple and cost effective way of improving public health (70,71).

Long-term observational follow-up was performed in 744 persons in the trial of hypertension prevention (TOHP) I (10 years after its end) and in 2382 persons in TOHP II (5 years after its end), in which persons with prehypertension were randomized to sodium reduction or usual diet (25–35% greater sodium intake) (72). In these studies, sodium reduction decreased cardiovascular events by 25% ($p = 0.04$). At 31-month follow-up of 1981 Taiwanese veterans, mean age 75 years, living in a retirement home, those randomized to a potassium enriched diet with 50% less sodium had a 41% reduction in cardiovascular mortality (95% CI, 0.37, 0.95) compared with those randomized to a regular salt diet (73).

At 14.8-year follow-up of 12,267 adults in the Third National Health and Nutrition Examination Survey, a higher sodium intake was associated with a 20% increase in all-cause mortality per 1000 mg of sodium intake per day ($p = 0.02$), whereas a higher potassium intake was associated with a 20% reduction in mortality per 1000 mg of potassium intake per day ($p = 0.01$) (74). For the sodium–potassium ratio, compared with the lowest quartile, the highest quartile increased all-cause mortality 46% ($p < 0.001$), cardiovascular mortality 46% ($p < 0.001$), and ischemic heart disease mortality 215% ($p < 0.001$) (74). Current guidelines suggest no more than 2300 mg of sodium daily in the general population and no more than 1500 mg of sodium daily in the elderly, in blacks, and in persons with hypertension, DM, chronic kidney disease, or CHF (75,76).

USE OF ANTIHYPERTENSIVE DRUG THERAPY IN OLDER PERSONS

A meta-analysis of 147 randomized trials including 464,000 persons with hypertension showed that except for the extra protective effect of β blockers given after MI and a minor additional effect of calcium channel blockers in preventing stroke, the use of β blockers, angiotensin-converting enzyme (ACE) inhibitors, angiotensin receptor blockers (ARBs), diuretics, and calcium channel blockers cause a similar reduction in coronary events and stroke for a given decrease in BP (77,78). The proportionate decrease in cardiovascular events was the same or similar regardless of pretreatment BP and the presence or absence of cardiovascular events (77,78). Diuretics, ACE inhibitors, ARBs, calcium channel blockers, or β blockers may be used as initial therapy in the treatment of primary hypertension in older and in younger persons. Atenolol should not be used (79–81). β Blockers such as carvedilol, nebivolol, and bisoprolol are preferred (81).

Table 4.1 Rationale for Combination Drug
Therapy for Hypertension

Increased antihypertensive efficacy
   Additive effects
   Synergistic effects
Reduced adverse events
   Low-dose strategy
   Drugs with offsetting actions
Enhanced convenience and compliance
Prolonged duration of action
Potential for additive target organ protection

Source: From Ref. 134.

Centrally acting agents, such as clonidine, reserpine, and guanethidine, should not be used as monotherapy in older persons because they have been associated with a high incidence of significant side effects, including sedation, depression, and constipation

Mostly older persons with hypertension will need two or more antihypertensive drugs to control their BP (1,2). If the BP is >20/10 mm Hg above the goal BP, drug therapy should be initiated with two antihypertensive drugs (Table 4.1) (1,2). The initial antihypertensive drug should be given at the lowest dose and gradually increased to the maximum dose. If the antihypertensive response to the initial drug is inadequate after reaching the full dose, a second drug from another class should be given if the person is tolerating the initial drug. If there is no therapeutic response or if there are significant adverse effects, a drug from another class should be substituted. If the antihypertensive response is inadequate after reaching the full dose of two classes of drugs, a third drug from another class should be added.

Before adding new antihypertensive drugs, the physician should consider possible reasons for inadequate response to antihypertensive drug therapy, including nonadherence to therapy, volume overload, drug interactions (use of nonsteroidal anti-inflammatory drugs, caffeine, antidepressants, nasal decongestants, sympathomimetics, etc.), and associated conditions such as increasing obesity, smoking, excessive ethanol intake, and insulin resistance (1,2). Causes of secondary hypertension should be identified and treated in accordance with current guidelines (1,2,12).

Elderly persons with hypertension have a very high prevalence of associated medical conditions (1,2). The selection of antihypertensive drug therapy in these persons depends on their associated medical conditions (1,2).

Falls or syncope in elderly persons may be due to orthostatic or postprandial hypotension (10). Management of orthostatic and postprandial hypotension in elderly persons is discussed in detail elsewhere (10). The dose of antihypertensive drug may need to be decreased or another antihypertensive drug given. Elderly frail persons are most susceptible to orthostatic and postprandial hypotension (10). Measurements of BP in the upright position, especially after eating, are indicated in these persons.

ADVERSE EFFECTS OF ANTIHYPERTENSIVE DRUG THERAPY

All antihypertensive drugs may predispose older persons to develop symptomatic orthostatic hypotension and postprandial hypotension, and syncope or falls (10). Diuretics may cause volume depletion. Vasodilators such as ACE inhibitors, ARBs, calcium channel blockers, hydralazine, nitrates, and prazosin may cause a reduction in systemic vascular resistance and venodilation (Table 4.2).

Table 4.2 Adverse Effects of Antihypertensive Therapy in the Elderly

Drug Class	Adverse Effect
Thiazide and loop diuretics	Hypokalemia, hyponatremia, hypomagnesemia, volume depletion hypotension, renal impairment, hyperuricemia, gout, hyperglycemia
Potassium-sparing diuretics	Hyperkalemia, hypotension
β-adrenergic blockers	Sinus bradycardia, fatigue, AV nodal heart block, bronchospasm, intermittent claudication, confusion, aggravation of acute heart failure, hyperglycemia
α–β adrenergic blockers (vasodilator-β-adrenergic blockers)	Hypotension, heart block, sinus bradycardia, bronchospasm
α 1-adrenergic antagonists	Orthostatic hypotension
ACE inhibitors	Cough, hyperkalemia (only with eGFR <50 ml/min), angioneurotic edema, rash, altered taste sensation, renal impairment
ARBs	Hyperkalemia, renal impairment
Central-acting drugs	Sedation, constipation, dry mouth
Calcium antagonists	
Non-dihydropyridines	Rash, exacerbation of GERD symptoms, sinus bradycardia, heart block, heart failure, constipation (verapamil), gingival hyperplasia
Dihydropyridines	Peripheral edema, heart failure, tachycardia, aggravation of angina pectoris (short-acting agents)
Direct vasodilators	Tachycardia, fluid retention, angina pectoris

Abbreviations: ACE, angiotension converting enzyme; ARBs, angiotensin receptor blockers; AV, atrioventricular; eGFR, estimated glomerular filtration rate; GERD, gastrocsophageal reflux disease.
Source: From Ref. 2.

Compared with amlodipine, ramipril significantly reduced progression of renal disease in 1094 African-Americans with hypertensive nephrosclerosis (82). If the older person cannot tolerate an ACE inhibitor because of cough, angioneurotic edema, rash, or altered taste sensation, an ARB should be administered (83). In the Ongoing Telmisartan Alone and in Combination With Ramipril Global Endpoint Trial (ONTARGET) (84), when compared to ramipril alone, the addition of telmisartan to ramipril in patients, mean age 67 years, with vascular disease or high-risk DM, did not decrease cardiovascular events but increased hypotensive symptoms (4.8% vs. 1.7%,) syncope (0.3% vs. 0.2%), and renal dysfunction (1.1% vs. 0.7%) (85).

Potassium-sparing diuretics should not be given to elderly persons taking ACE inhibitors or ARBs to avoid hyperkalemia. Risk factors for renal insufficiency in older persons receiving ACE inhibitors or ARBs include renal artery stenosis (usually bilateral), polycystic renal disease, reduced absolute or effective arterial blood volume, use of nonsteroidal anti-inflammatory drugs, cyclosporine or tacrolimus, and sepsis (86,87). However, reversible renal failure may occur in older persons treated with ACE inhibitors or ARBs who are dehydrated or salt depleted. ACE inhibitors or ARBs can cause an azotemic response when there is an absolute decrease in intravascular volume due to aggressive diuresis, poor oral intake, or gastroenteritis or an effective reduction in intravascular volume in patients with severe CHF (87).

β Blockers depress the sinus node and the atrioventricular node and are contraindicated in patients with severe sinus bradycardia, sinoatrial disease, and marked first-degree, second-degree, and third-degree atrioventricular block (88). β Blockers should also not be given to patients with bronchial asthma or to patients with lung disease with severe bronchospasm (88). β Blockers may also cause depression or confusion in eldelry persons.

Short-acting dihydropyridine calcium channel blockers have the potential to increase cardiovascular events and should be avoided (89). Verapamil and diltiazem depress the sinus node and the atrioventricular node and are contraindicated in patients with severe sinus bradycardia, sinoatrial disease, and marked first-degree, second-degree, and third-degree atrioventricular block (89,90).

Diltiazem and verapamil are contraindicated in treating postinfarction patients with an abnormal LV ejection fraction because they will increase coronary events and mortality as well as CHF (91–93). Calcium channel blockers such as nifedipine, diltiazem, and verapamil exacerbate CHF in patients with CHF and abnormal LV ejection fraction (94).

In the Antihypertensive and Lipid-Lowering Treatment to Prevent Heart Attack Trial (ALLHAT), the doxazosin arm involving 9067 patients was prematurely stopped at a median of 3.3 years (95). Compared with the diuretic chlorthalidone, the α blocker doxazosin significantly increased CHF 204%, stroke 19%, and combined cardiovascular disease (coronary heart disease death, nonfatal MI, stroke, angina pectoris, coronary revascularization, CHF, or PAD) 25%, angina pectoris 16%, and coronary revascularization 15%.

In an observational study of older persons, mean age 80 years, with prior MI and hypertension, those treated with α blockers had a significant increase in new coronary events at 40-month mean follow-up, of 1.69 times compared with β blockers, of 1.50 times compared with ACE inhibitors, and of 1.35 times compared with diuretics (93). α blockers cause a high incidence of orthostatic hypotension, especially in patients receiving diuretics or other vasodilator drugs (96).

Centrally acting drugs should not be used as monotherapy in older persons because they cause a high incidence of sedation, precipitate or exacerbate depression, and cause constipation (96). Direct vasodilators may cause headache, fluid retention, tachycardia, and aggravate angina pectoris. Hydralazine caused a lupus-like syndrome in 6.7% of 281 patients treated with hydralazine for 3 years (97). Minoxidil may cause hirsutism and a pericardial effusion (98).

USE OF ANTIHYPERTENSIVE DRUGS IN PERSONS WITH ASSOCIATED MEDICAL CONDITIONS

Older persons with prior MI should be treated with β blockers and ACE inhibitors (1,2,93,99–103). In an observational prospective study of 1212 older men and women with prior MI and hypertension treated with β blockers, ACE inhibitors, diuretics, calcium channel blockers, or α blockers, at 40-month follow-up, the incidence of new coronary events in older persons treated with one antihypertensive drug was lowest in those treated with β blockers or ACE inhibitors (93). In older persons treated with two antihypertensive drugs, the incidence of new coronary events was lowest in those treated with β blockers plus ACE inhibitors.

β Blockers should be used to treat older patients with complex ventricular arrhythmias with abnormal (104) or normal (105) LV ejection fraction and with CHF with abnormal (106,107) or normal (107,108) LV ejection fraction. β Blockers should also be used to treat elderly patients with hypertension who have angina pectoris (109), myocardial ischemia (110), supraventricular tachyarrhythmias such as atrial fibrillation with a rapid ventricular rate (111,112), hyperthyroidism (113), preoperative hypertension (1), migraine (1), or essential tremor (1).

In addition to β blockers, older persons with CHF should be treated with diuretics and ACE inhibitors and with aldosterone antagonists if needed (114). ACE inhibitors or ARBs should be administered to older persons with DM, chronic renal disease, or proteinuria (1,2,82,83,100). Diuretics and ACE inhibitors are recommended by JNC 7 to prevent recurrent stroke in older persons with hypertension (1,57). Thiazide diuretics should be used to treat elderly persons with osteoporosis (1).

It is also very important to treat other cardiovascular risk factors in older persons with hypertension to reduce cardiovascular events and mortality (2). Smoking must be stopped (115). Dyslipidemia must be treated (64,115,116). DM must be controlled (17,117–120).

The more aggressive control of BP among persons at high risk for coronary artery disease, such as those with DM, chronic kidney disease, coronary artery disease or coronary artery risk equivalent, or a 10-year Framingham risk score $\geq 10\%$ with maintenance of the BP $<130/80$ mm Hg and $<120/80$ mm Hg in patients with LV dysfunction recommended by the AHA Task Force scientific statement in 2007 (88), was based upon expert medical opinion at that time, not on prospective, randomized, adequately controlled trial data (65).

The Pravastatin or Atorvastatin Evaluation and Infection Therapy-Thrombolysis in Myocardial Infarction (PROVE IT-TIMI) 22 trial (121) enrolled 4162 patients with an acute coronary syndrome (acute MI with or without ST-segment elevation or high-risk unstable angina pectoris). The lowest cardiovascular event rates occurred with a systolic BP between 130 and 140 mm Hg and a diastolic BP between 80 and 90 mm Hg with a nadir of 136/85 mm.

An observational subgroup analysis was performed in 6400 of the 22,576 persons enrolled in the International Verapamil SR-Trandolapril Study (INVEST) (122). The study participants had DM and coronary artery disease. Persons were categorized as having tight control of their BP if they could maintain their systolic BP below 130 mm Hg and their diastolic BP below 85 mm Hg, usual control if they could maintain their systolic BP between 130 and 139 mm Hg, and uncontrolled if their systolic BP was ≥ 140 mm Hg. Using 16,893 patient years of follow-up, a cardiovascular event rate of 12.6% occurred in patients with usual control of BP versus 19.8% in patients with uncontrolled hypertension, $p < 0.001$ (122). The incidence of cardiovascular events was 12.6% in patients with usual control of BP versus 12.7% in patients with tight control of BP (p not significant). The all-cause mortality rate was 11.0% with tight control of BP versus 10.2% with usual control of BP ($p = 0.06$). When extended follow-up was included, the all-cause mortality rate was 22.8% with tight control of BP versus 21.8% with usual control of BP, $p = 0.04$.

The Action to Control Cardiovascular Risk in Diabetes (ACCORD) BP trial (123) randomized 4733 persons with type 2 DM to intensive BP control with a target systolic BP of <120 mm Hg or to standard BP control with a target systolic BP <140 mm Hg. The primary composite outcome was nonfatal MI, nonfatal stroke, or death from cardiovascular causes. The mean follow-up was 4.7 years. After 1 year, the mean systolic BP was 119.3 mm Hg in the intensive BP control group versus 133.5 mm Hg in the standard BP control group. The annual rate of the primary outcome was 1.87% in the intensive BP control group versus 2.09% in the standard BP control group (p not significant). The annual rate of death from any cause was 1.28% in the intensive BP control group versus 1.19% in the standard BP control group (p not significant). The annual rate of stroke, a prespecified secondary outcome, was 0.32% in the intensive BP control group versus 0.53% in the standard BP control group, $p = 0.01$. Serious adverse events attributed to antihypertensive treatment occurred in 3.3% of the intensive BP control group versus 1.3% of the standard BP control group ($p < 0.001$) (123).

We studied the impact of baseline systolic BP on outcomes in 7785 persons with mild to moderate chronic CHF in the Digitalis Investigation Group trial (124). A baseline systolic BP ≤ 120 mm Hg was associated during 5 years of follow-up with a 15% increase in cardiovascular mortality ($p = 0.032$), with a 30% increase in heart failure mortality

($p = 0.006$), with a 13% increase in cardiovascular hospitalization ($p = 0.008$), with a 10% increase in all-cause hospitalization ($p = 0.017$), and with a 21% increase in heart failure hospitalization ($p = 0.002$).

In ONTARGET, a progressive increase in the proportion of visits in which the BP was decreased to <140/90 mm Hg or to <130/80 mm Hg was associated with a progressive decrease in stroke, new onset of microalbuminuria or macroalbuminuria, and a return to normo-albuminuria in persons with albuminuria (125). However, the adjusted risk of cardiovascular events was reduced by increasing the frequency of BP control to <140/90 mm Hg but not to <130/80 mm Hg.

In ONTARGET, 9603 of 25,584 patients had DM (126). DM increased the primary outcome of cardiovascular death, nonfatal MI or stroke, or hospitalization for CHF by 48% (95% CI, 1.38–1.57). In both diabetics and non-diabetics, antihypertensive treatment reduced the primary outcome if baseline systolic BP levels ranged from 143 to 155 mm Hg. Except for stroke, there was no benefit in fatal or nonfatal outcomes by lowering systolic BP below 130 mm Hg.

During >12 years of median follow-up in the Cardiovascular Health Study, we found that isolated diastolic hypotension (a diastolic BP <60 mm Hg with a systolic BP ≥100 mm Hg) was associated with a 29% significant independent increase in incident CHF ($p = 0.003$) (127). Therefore, ISH and isolated diastolic hypotension are significant risk factors for CHF in community-dwelling older persons.

Three trials including 2272 patients with chronic kidney disease and proteinuria without DM showed that a BP target of <130/80 mm Hg did not improve clinical outcomes more than a BP target of <140/90 mm Hg (128).

At 2.5-year follow-up of 20,330 patients with a noncardioembolic stroke (129), compared with a systolic BP of 130–139 mm Hg, the incidence of the primary outcome of cardiovascular death, MI, or stroke was increased 29% (95% CI, 1.07–1.56) by a systolic BP <120 mm Hg, 23% (95% CI, 1.07–1.41) by a systolic BP of 140–149 mm Hg, and 208% (95% CI by a systolic BP of ≥150 mm Hg.

Finally, although the optimal BP treatment goal in the elderly has not been determined, a therapeutic target of <140/90 mm Hg in persons aged 65–79 years and a systolic BP of 140–145 mm Hg if tolerated in persons aged 80 years and older is reasonable (2,64–69). We should also be careful to avoid intensive lowering of the BP in elderly persons, especially those with diabetes and coronary artery disease, as this might be poorly tolerated and might increase cardiovascular events (the J-curve phenomenon).

TREATMENT OF DRUG REFRACTORY HYPERTENSION

Despite the availability of numerous effective pharmacologic agents for hypertensive patients, control of BP in the elderly is achieved in <50% of patients (1,2,41,42) Alternative approaches to achieving additional BP control that are under investigation in drug refractory patients include the use of implantable carotid stimulation devices (130), devices to control the respiratory rate that can indirectly reduce BP (131), and the use of catheter-based renal sympathetic denervation (132). As of now, there are limited data available with these approaches in the elderly regarding both efficacy and safety.

REFERENCES

1. Chobanian AV, Bakris GL, Black HR, et al. The seventh report of the joint national committee on prevention, detection, evaluation, and treatment of high BP. The JNC 7 Report. JAMA 2003; 289: 2560–72.
2. Aronow WS, Fleg JL, Pepine CJ, et al. ACCF/AHA 2011 expert consensus document on hypertension in the elderly: a report of the American College of Cardiology Foundation Task Force on Clinical Expert Consensus Documents. J Am Coll Cardiol 2011; 57: 2037–114.

3. Waeber B, Banegas JR, Mancia G, Ruilope LM. BP control based on office and ambulatory BP monitoring: the European experience in hypertensive patients treated in clinical practice. Arch Med Sci 2009; 5: 351–8.

4. Mendelson G, Nassimiha D, Aronow WS. Simultaneous measurements of BPs in right and left brachial arteries. Cardiol Rev 2004; 12: 276–8.

5. Clark CE, Taylor RS, Shore AC, et al. Association of a difference in systolic blood pressure between arms with vascular disease and mortality: a systematic review and meta-analysis. Lancet 2012; 379: 905–14.

6. McManus RJ, Mant J. Do differences in blood pressure between arms matter? Lancet 2012; 379: 872–3.

7. Aronow WS, Lee NH, Sales FF, Etienne F. Prevalence of postural hypotension in elderly patients in a long-term health care facility. Am J Cardiol 1988; 62: 336.

8. Lakatta EG. Mechanisms of hypertension in the elderly. J Am Geriatr Soc 1989; 37: 780–90.

9. Gribbin B, Pickering GT, Sleight P, Peto R. Effect of age and high BP on baroreflex sensitivity in man. Circ Res 1971; 29: 424–31.

10. Aronow WS. Dizziness and syncope. In: Hazzard WR, Blass JP, Ettinger WH Jr, Halter JB, Ouslander JG, eds. Principles of Geriatric Medicine and Gerontology, 4th edn. New York: McGraw-Hill, Inc, 1998: 1519–34.

11. Joseph J, Koka M, Aronow WS. Prevalence of moderate and severe renal insufficiency in older persons with hypertension, DM, coronary artery disease, PAD, ischemic stroke, or congestive heart failure in an academic nursing home. J Am Med Dir Assoc 2008; 9: 257–9.

12. Chiong JR, Aronow WS, Khan IA, et al. Secondary hypertension: current diagnosis and treatment. Int J Cardiol 2008; 124: 6–21.

13. Joint National Committee on Prevention, Detection, Evaluation, and Treatment of High BP. The sixth report of the Joint National committee on prevention, detection, evaluation, and treatment of high BP. Arch Intern Med 1997; 157: 2413–46.

14. Aronow WS, Ahn C, Gutstein H. Prevalence and incidence of cardiovascular disease in 1160 older men and 2464 older women in a long-term health care facility. J Gerontol Med Sci 2002; 57A: M45–6.

15. Mendelson G, Ness J, Aronow WS. Drug treatment of hypertension in older persons in an academic hospital-based geriatrics practice. J Am Geriatr Soc 1999; 47: 597–9.

16. Koka M, Joseph J, Aronow WS. Adequacy of control of hypertension in an academic nursing home. J Am Med Dir Assoc 2007; 8: 538–40.

17. Joseph J, Koka M, Aronow WS. Prevalence of a hemoglobin A_{1c} <7.0%, of a BP <130/80 mm Hg, and of a serum low-density lipoprotein cholesterol <100 mg/dl in older patients with DM in an academic nursing home. J Am Med Dir Assoc 2008; 9: 51–4.

18. Lloyd-Jones D, Adams R, Carnethon M, et al. Heart disease and stroke statistics-2009 update: a report from the American Heart Association Statistics Committee and Stroke Statistics Subcommittee. Circulation 2009; 119: e21–181.

19. National High BP Education Program Working Group. National high BP education program working group report on hypertension in the elderly. Hypertension 1994; 23: 275–85.

20. Madhavan S, Ooi WL, Cohen H, Alderman MH. Relation of pulse pressure and BP reduction to the incidence of myocardial infarction. Hypertension 1994; 23: 395–401.

21. Rigaud AS, Forette B. Hypertension in older adults. J Gerontol Med Sci 2001; 56A: M217–25.

22. Franklin SS, Khan SA, Wong ND, et al. Is pulse pressure useful in predicting risk for coronary heart disease? The framingham heart study. Circulation 1999; 100: 354–60.

23. Fried LP, Kronmal RA, Newman AB, et al. Risk factors for 5-year mortality in older adults. The Cardiovascular Health Study. JAMA 1998; 279: 585–92.

24. Aronow WS, Ahn C, Kronzon I, Koenigsberg M. Congestive heart failure, coronary events and atherothrombotic brain infarction in elderly blacks and whites with systemic hypertension and with and without echocardiographic and electrocardiographic evidence of left ventricular hypertrophy. Am J Cardiol 1991; 67: 295–9.

25. Aronow WS, Ahn C. Risk factors for new coronary events in a large cohort of very elderly patients with and without coronary artery disease. Am J Cardiol 1996; 77: 864–6.

26. Vokonas PS, Kannel WB. Epidemiology of coronary heart disease in the elderly. In: Aronow WS, Fleg JL, Rich MW, eds. Cardiovascular Disease in the Elderly, 4th edn. New York: Informa Healthcare, 2008: 15–241.

27. Franklin SS, Larson MG, Khan SA, et al. Does the relation of BP to coronary heart disease risk change with aging? The Framingham Heart Study. Circulation 2001; 103: 1245–9.

28. Psaty BM, Furberg CD, Kuller LH, et al. Association between BP level and the risk of myocardial infarction, stroke, and total mortality: the cardiovascular health study. Arch Intern Med 2001; 161: 1183–92.

29. Aronow WS, Ahn C, Gutstein H. Risk factors for new atherothrombotic brain infarction in 664 older men and 1,488 older women. Am J Cardiol 1996; 77: 1381–3.

30. Aronow WS, Frishman WH. Treatment of hypertension and prevention of ischemic stroke. Curr Cardiol Rep 2004; 6: 124–9.

31. Wolf PA. Cerebrovascular disease in the elderly. In: Tresch DD, Aronow WS, eds. Cardiovascular Disease in the Elderly Patient. New York: Marcel Dekker, Inc, 1994: 125–47.

32. Aronow WS, Ahn C, Kronzon I. Comparison of incidences of congestive heart failure in older African-Americans, Hispanics, and whites. Am J Cardiol 1999; 84: 611–12.

33. Levy D, Larson MG, Vasan RS, Kannel WB, Ho KKL. The progression from hypertension to congestive heart failure. JAMA 1996; 275: 1557–62.

34. Stokes J III, Kannel WB, Wolf PA, et al. The relative importance of selected risk factors for various manifestations of cardiovascular disease among men and women from 35 to 64 years old: 30 years of follow-up in the Framingham Study. Circulation 1987; 75: V-65–73.

35. Aronow WS, Sales FF, Etienne F, Lee NH. Prevalence of PAD and its correlation with risk factors for PAD in elderly patients in a long-term health care facility. Am J Cardiol 1988; 62: 644–6.

36. Ness J, Aronow WS, Ahn C. Risk factors for PAD in an academic hospital-based geriatrics practice. J Am Geriatr Soc 2000; 48: 312–14.

37. Ness J, Aronow WS, Newkirk E, McDanel D. Prevalence of symptomatic PAD, modifiable risk factors, and appropriate use of drugs in the treatment of PAD in older persons seen in a university general medicine clinic. J Gerontol Med Sci 2005; 60A: M255–7.

38. Aronow WS, Ahmed MI, Ekundayo OJ, et al. A propensity-matched study of the association of PAD with cardiovascular outcomes in community-dwelling older adults. Am J Cardiol 2009; 103: 130–5.

39. Lewington S, Clarke R, Qizilbash N, et al. Age-specific relevance of usual BP to vascular mortality: a meta-analysis of individual data for one million adults in 6 prospective studies. Lancet 2002; 360: 1903–13.

40. Julius S, Palatini P, Kjeldsen SE, et al. Usefulness of heart rate to predict cardiac events in treated patients with high-risk systemic hypertension. Am J Cardiol 2012; 109: 685–92.

41. Hyman DJ, Pavlik VN. Characteristics of patients with uncontrolled hypertension in the United States. N Engl J Med 2001; 345: 479–86.

42. Lloyd-Jones DM, Evans JC, Levy D. Hypertension in adults across the age spectrum: current outcomes and control in the community. JAMA 2005; 294: 466–72.

43. Gandelman G, Aronow WS, Varma R. Prevalence of adequate BP control in self-pay or Medicare patients versus Medicaid or private insurance patients with systemic hypertension followed in a university cardiology or general medicine clinic. Am J Cardiol 2004; 94: 815–16.

44. Report by the Management Committee. The Australian therapeutic trial in mild hypertension. Lancet 1980; 1: 1261–7.

45. Medical Research Council Working Party. MRC trial of mild hypertension: principal results. Br Med J 1985; 291: 97–104.

46. MRC Working Party. Medical research council trial of treatment of hypertension in older adults: Principal results. Br Med J 1992; 304: 405–12.

47. Amery A, Birkenhager W, Brixko P, et al. Morbidity and mortality results from the European working party on high BP in the elderly trial. Lancet 1985; 1: 1349–54.

48. Coope J, Warrender TS. Randomised trial of the treatment of hypertension in elderly patients in primary care. Br Med J 1986; 293: 1145–51.

49. Dahlof B, Lindholm LH, Hansson L, et al. Morbidity and mortality in the Swedish Trial in Old Patients With Hypertension (STOP Hypertension). Lancet 1991; 338: 1281–5.

50. SHEP Cooperative Research Group. Prevention of stroke by antihypertensive drug treatment in older persons with ISH. Final results of the Systolic Hypertension in the Elderly Program (SHEP). JAMA 1991; 265: 3255–64.

51. Kostis JB, Davis BR, Cutler J, et al. Prevention of heart failure by antihypertensive drug treatment in older persons with ISH. JAMA 1997; 278: 212–16.

52. Perry HM Jr, Davis BR, Price TR, et al. Effect of treating ISH on the risk of developing various types and subtypes of stroke. The Systolic Hypertension in the Elderly Program (SHEP). JAMA 2000; 284: 465–71.

53. Staessen JA, Fagard R, Thijs L, et al. Randomised double-blind comparison of placebo and active treatment for older patients with ISH. Lancet 1997; 350: 757–64.

54. Wang JG, Staessen JA, Gong L, Liu L. Chinese trial on ISH in the elderly. Arch Intern Med 2000; 160: 211–20.
55. Beckett NS, Peters R, Fletcher AE, et al. Treatment of hypertension in patients 80 years of age or older. N Engl J Med 2008; 358: 1887–98.
56. Aronow WS, Frishman WH. Effect of antihypertensive drug treatment on cognitive function. Clin Geriatr 2006; 14: 25–8.
57. Progress Collaborative Group. Randomised trial of a perindopril-based blood-pressure-lowering regimen among 6105 individuals with previous stroke or transient ischaemic attack. Lancet 2001; 358: 1033–41.
58. Forette F, Seux ML, Staessen JA, et al. The prevention of dementia with antihypertensive treatment. New evidence from the Systolic Hypertension in Europe (Syst-Eur) study. Arch Intern Med 2002; 162: 2046–52.
59. Murray MD, Lane KA, Gao S, et al. Preservation of cognitive function with antihypertensive medications. A longitudinal analysis of a community-based sample of African Americans. Arch Intern Med 2002; 162: 2090–6.
60. Veld BA, Ruitenberg A, Hofman A, Stricker BH, Breteler MM. Antihypertensive drugs and incidence of dementia: the Rotterdam Study. Neurobiol Aging 2001; 22: 407–12.
61. Aronow WS. What is the appropriate treatment of hypertension in elders? J Gerontol A Biol Sci Med Sci 2002; 57: M483–6.
62. Goodwin JS. Embracing complexity: a consideration of hypertension in the very old. J Gerontol Med Sci 2003; 58A: M653–8.
63. Aronow WS. Older age should not be a barrier to the treatment of hypertension. Nat Clin Pract Cardiovasc Med 2008; 5: 514–15.
64. Fleg JL, Aronow WS, Frishman WH. Cardiovascular drug therapy in the elderly. Nat Rev Cardiol 2011; 8: 13–28.
65. Aronow WS. Hypertension guidelines. Hypertension 2011; 58: 347–8.
66. Banach M, Michalska M, Kjeldsen SE, et al. What should be the optimal levels of BP: does the J-curve phenomenon really exist? Expert Opin Pharmacother 2011; 12: 1835–44.
67. Banach M, Aronow WS. Should we have any doubts about hypertension therapy in elderly patients. ACCF/AHA 2011 expert consensus document on hypertension in the elderly. Pol Arch Med Wewn 2011; 121: 253–8.
68. Aronow WS, Banach M. Ten most important things to learn from the ACCF/AHA 2011 expert consensus document on hypertension in the elderly. Blood Press 2012; 21: 3–5.
69. Banach M, Aronow WS. Hypertension therapy in the elderly-do we know the answers to all the questions? The status after publication of the ACCF/AHA 2011 expert consensus document on hypertension in the elderly. J Hum Hypertens 2012; 26: 641–3.
70. Webster JL, Dunford EK, Hawkes C, Neal BC. Salt reduction initiatives around the world. J Hypertens 2011; 29: 1043–50.
71. Frohlich ED, Susic D. Sodium and its multiorgan targets. Circulation 2011; 124: 1882–5.
72. Cook NR, Cutler JA, Obarzanek E, et al. Long term effects of dietary sodium reduction on cardiovascular disease outcomes: observational follow-up of the trials of hypertension prevention (TOHP). BMJ 2007; 334: 885–8.
73. Chang HY, Hu YVV, Yue CS, et al. Effect of potassium-enriched salt on cardiovascular mortality and medical expenses of elderly men. Am J Clin Nutr 2006; 83: 1289–96.
74. Yang Q, Liu T, Kuklina EV, et al. Sodium and potassium intake and mortality among US adults: prospective data from the Third National Health and Nutrition Examination Survey. Arch Intern Med 2011; 171: 1183–91.
75. US Department of Health and Human Services and US Department of Agriculture. Dietary Guidelines for Americans, 2010, 7th edn. Washington, DC: US Government Printing Office, 2011.
76. Whelton PK. Urinary sodium and cardiovascular disease risk. Informing guidelines for sodium consumption. JAMA 2011; 306: 2262–4.
77. Mancia G, Laurent S, Agabiti-Rosei E, et al. Reappraisal of European guidelines on hypertension management: a European society of hypertension task force document. Blood Press 2009; 18: 308–47.
78. Law MR, Morris JK, Wald NJ. Use of BP lowering drugs in the prevention of cardiovascular disease: meta-analysis of 147 randomised trials in the context of expectations from prospective epidemiological studies. BMJ 2009; 338: b1665. doi.10.1136/bmj.b1665.
79. Aronow WS. Might losartan reduce sudden cardiac death in diabetic patients with hypertension? Lancet 2003; 362: 591–2.

80. Carlberg B, Samuelson O, Lindholm LH. Atenolol in hypertension: is it a wise choice? Lancet 2004; 364: 1684–9.
81. Aronow WS. Current role of beta blockers in the treatment of hypertension. Exp Opin Pharmacother 2010; 11: 2599–607.
82. Agodoa LY, Appel L, Bakris GL, et al. Effect of ramipril versus amlodipine on renal outcomes in hypertensive nephrosclerosis. A randomized controlled trial. JAMA 2001; 285: 2719–28.
83. Brenner BM, Cooper ME, de Zeeuw D, et al. Effects of losartan on renal and cardiovascular outcomes in patients with type 2 diabetes and nephropathy. N Engl J Med 2001; 345: 861–9.
84. The ONTARGET Investigators. Telmisartan, ramipril, or both in patients at high risk for vascular events. N Engl J Med 2008; 358: 1547–59.
85. Palmer BF. Renal dysfunction complicating the treatment of hypertension. N Engl J Med 2002; 347: 1256–61.
86. Hricick DE, Browning PJ, Kopelman R, et al. Captopril-induced functional renal insufficiency in patients with bilateral renal artery stenosis or renal artery stenosis in a solitary kidney. N Engl J Med 1983; 308: 373–6.
87. Toto RD, Mitchell HC, Lee HC, Milam C, Pettinger WA. Reversible renal insufficiency due to angiotensin-converting enzyme inhibitorsin hypertensive nephrosclerosis. Ann Intern Med 1991; 115: 513–19.
88. Rosendorff C, Black HR, Cannon CP, et al. Treatment of hypertension in the prevention and management of ischemic heart disease. A scientific statement from the American heart association council for high BP research and the councils on clinical cardiology and epidemiology and prevention. Circulation 2007; 115: 2761–88.
89. Pahor M, Guralnik JM, Corti C, et al. Long-term survival and use of antihypertensive medications in older persons. J Am Geriatr Soc 1995; 43: 1191–7.
90. Aronow WS. Verapamil as an antiarrhythmic agent. In: Gould LA, ed. Drug Treatment of Cardiac Arrhythmias. Mount Kisco, New York: Futura Publishing Company, Inc, 1983: 325–41.
91. The Multicenter Diltiazem Postinfarction Trial Research Group. The effect of diltiazem on mortality and reinfarction after myocardial infarction. N Engl J Med 1988; 319: 385–92.
92. Goldstein RE, Boccuzzi SJ, Cruess D, Nattel S. Diltiazem increases late-onset congestive heart failure in postinfarction patients with early reduction in ejection fraction. Circulation 1991; 83: 52–60.
93. Aronow WS, Ahn C. Incidence of new coronary events in older persons with prior myocardial infarction and systemic hypertension treated with beta blockers, angiotensin-converting enzyme inhibitors, diuretics, calcium antagonists, and alpha blockers. Am J Cardiol 2002; 89: 1207–9.
94. Elkayam U, Amin J, Mehra A, et al. A prospective, randomized, double-blind, crossover study to compare the efficacy and safety of chronic nifedipine therapy with that of isosorbide dinitrate and their combination in the treatment of chronic congestive heart failure. Circulation 1990; 82: 1954–61.
95. ALLHAT Officers and Coordinators for the ALLHAT Collaborative Research Group. Major cardiovascular events in hypertensive patients randomized to doxazosin vs chlorthalidone. The Antihypertensive and Lipid-Lowering Treatment to Prevent Heart Attack Trial (ALLHAT). JAMA 2000; 283: 1967–75.
96. Frishman WH, Aronow WS, Cheng-Lai A. Cardiovascular drug therapy in the elderly. In: Aronow WS, Fleg JL, Rich MW, eds. Cardiovascular Disease in the Elderly, 4th edn. New York: Informa Healthcare, 2008: 99–135.
97. Cameron HA, Ramsay LE. The lupus syndrome induced by hydralazine: a common complication with low dose treatment. Br Med J (Clin Res Ed) 1984; 289: 410–12.
98. Krehlik JM, Hindson DA, Crowley JJ Jr, Knight LL. Minoxidil-associated pericarditis and fatal cardiac tamponade. West J Med 1986; 143: 527–9.
99. Ryan TJ, Antman EM, Brooks NH, et al. 1999 update: ACC/AHA guidelines for the management of patients with acute myocardial infarction: executive summary and recommendations. A report of the American college of cardiology/American heart association task force on practice guidelines (committee on management of acute myocardial infarction). Circulation 1999; 100: 1016–30.
100. The Heart Outcomes Prevention Evaluation Study Investigators. Effects of an angiotensin-converting-enzyme inhibitor, ramipril on cardiovascular events in high-risk patients. N Engl J Med 2000; 342: 145–53.
101. Aronow WS, Ahn C, Kronzon I. Effect of beta blockers alone, of angiotensin-converting enzyme inhibitors alone, and of beta blockers plus angiotensin-converting enzyme inhibitors on new coronary events and on congestive heart failure in older persons with healed myocardial infarcts and asymptomatic left ventricular systolic dysfunction. Am J Cardiol 2001; 88: 1298–300.

102. Aronow WS, Ahn C. Effect of beta blockers on incidence of new coronary events in older persons with prior myocardial infarction and DM. Am J Cardiol 2001; 87: 780–1.

103. Aronow WS, Ahn C. Effect of beta blockers on incidence of new coronary events in older persons with prior myocardial infarction and symptomatic PAD. Am J Cardiol 2001; 87: 1284–6.

104. Kennedy HL, Brooks MM, Barker AH, et al. Beta-blocker therapy in the Cardiac Arrhythmia Suppression Trial. Am J Cardiol 1994; 74: 674–80.

105. Aronow WS, Ahn C, Mercando AD, Epstein S, Kronzon I. Effect of propranolol versus no antiar-rhythmic drug on sudden cardiac death, total cardiac death, and total death in patients ≥62 years of age with heart disease, complex ventricular arrhythmias, and left ventricular ejection fraction ≥40%. Am J Cardiol 1994; 74: 267–70.

106. MERIT-HF Study Group. Effect of metoprolol CR/XL in chronic heart failure: Metoprolol CR/XL Randomised Intervention Trial in Congestive Heart Failure (MERIT-HF). Lancet 1999; 353: 2001–7.

107. Flather MD, Shibata MC, Coats AJS, et al. Randomized trial to determine the effect of nebivolol on mortality and cardiovascular hospital admission in elderly patients with heart failure (SENIORS). Eur Heart J 2005; 26: 215–25.

108. Aronow WS, Ahn C, Kronzon I. Effect of propranolol versus no propranolol on total mortality plus nonfatal myocardial infarction in older patients with prior myocardial infarction, congestive heart failure, and left ventricular ejection fraction ≥40% treated with diuretics plus angiotensin-converting-enzyme inhibitors. Am J Cardiol 1997; 80: 207–9.

109. Aronow WS, Frishman WH. Angina in the elderly. In: Aronow WS, Fleg JL, Rich MW, eds. Cardio-vascular Disease in the Elderly, 4th edn. New York: Informa Healthcare, 2008: 269–92.

110. Aronow WS, Ahn C, Mercando AD, Epstein S, Kronzon I. Decrease of mortality by propranolol in patients with heart disease and complex ventricular arrhythmias is more an anti-ischemic than an antiarrhythmic effect. Am J Cardiol 1994; 74: 613–15.

111. Aronow WS. Treatment of atrial fibrillation. Part 1. Cardiol Rev 2008; 16: 181–8.

112. Aronow WS. Treatment of atrial fibrillation and atrial flutter Part 2. Cardiol Rev 2008; 16: 230–9.

113. Aronow WS. The heart and thyroid disease. In: Gambert SR, ed. Clinics in Geriatric Medicine. Thyroid Disease. Philadelphia: W. B. Saunders Co, 1995: 219–29.

114. Hunt SA, Baker DW, Chin MH, et al. ACC/AHA guidelines for the evaluation and management of chronic heart failure in the adult: executive summary. A report of the American college of cardiology/ American heart association task force on practice guidelines (committee to revise the 1995 guidelines for the evaluation and management of heart failure). Developed in collaboration with the international society for heart and lung transplantation. Endorsed by the heart failure society of America. J Am Coll Cardiol 2001; 38: 2101–13.

115. Smith SC Jr, Benjamin EJ, Bonow RO, et al. AHA/ACCF secondary prevention and risk reduction therapy for patients with coronary and other atherosclerotic vascular disease: 2011 update. A guideline from the American Heart Association and American College of Cardiology Foundation. J Am Coll Cardiol 2011; 58: 2432–46.

116. Grundy SM, Cleeman JI, Merz CNB, et al. Implications of recent clinical trials for the National Cholesterol Education Program Adult Treatment Panel III guidelines. Circulation 2004; 110: 227–39.

117. American Diabetes Association. Standards of medical care for patients with DM. Diabetes Care 2003; 26: 533–50.

118. Stratton IM, Adler AI, Neil HA, et al. Association of glycaemia with macrovascular and microvascular complications of type 2 diabetes (UKPDS 35): prospective observational study. Br Med J 2000; 321: 405–12.

119. Ravipati G, Aronow WS, Ahn C, et al. Association of hemoglobin A_{1c} level with the severity of coronary artery disease in patients with DM. Am J Cardiol 2006; 97: 968–9.

120. Aronow WS, Ahn C, Weiss MB, Babu S. Relation of hemoglobin A_{1c} levels to severity of PAD in patients with DM. Am J Cardiol 2007; 99: 1468–9.

121. Bangalore S, Qin J, Sloan S, Murphy SA, Cannon CP; PROVE-IT -TIMI 22 Trial Investigators. What is the optimal BP in patients after acute coronary syndromes? Relationship of BP and cardiovascular events in the Pravastatin or Atorvastatin Evaluation and Infection Therapy-Thrombolysis in Myocar-dial Infarction (PROVE IT-TIMI) 22 trial. Circulation 2010; 122: 2142–51.

122. Cooper-DeHoff RM, Gong Y, Handberg EM, et al. Tight BP control and cardiovascular outcomes among hypertensive patients with diabetes and coronary artery disease. JAMA 2010; 304: 61–8.

123. The ACCORD Study Group. Effects of intensive blood-pressure control in type 2 DM. N Engl J Med 2010; 362: 1575–85.

124. Banach M, Bhatia V, Feller MA, et al. Relation of baseline systolic BP and long-term outcomes in ambulatory patients with chronic mild to moderate heart failure. Am J Cardiol 2011; 107: 1208–14.

125. Mancia G, Schumacher H, Redon J, et al. BP targets recommended by guidelines and incidence of cardiovascular and renal events in the Ongoing Telmisartan Alone and in Combination With Ramipril Global Endpoint Trial (ONTARGET). Circulation 2011; 124: 1727–36.
126. Redon J, Mancia G, Sleight P, et al. Safety and efficacy of low BPs among patients with diabetes. Subgroup analyses from the ONTARGET (ONgoing Telmisartan and in combination with Ramipril Endpoint trial). J Am Coll Cardiol 2012; 59: 74–83.
127. Guichard JL, Desai RV, Ahmed MI, et al. Isolated diastolic hypotension and incident heart failure in older adults. Hypertension 2011; 58: 895–901.
128. Upadhyay A, Earley A, Haynes SM, Uhlig K. Systematic review: BP target in chronic kidney disease and proteinuria as an effect modifier. Ann intern Med 2011; 154: 541–8.
129. Ovbiagele B, Diener HC, Yusuf S, et al. Level of systolic BP within the normal range and risk of recurrent stroke. JAMA 2011; 306: 2137–44.
130. Ng MM, Sica DA, Frishman WH. Rheos: an implantable carotid sinus stimulation device for the nonpharmacologic treatment of resistant hypertension. Cardiol Rev 2011; 19: 52–7.
131. Sharma M, Frishman WH, Gandhi K. Resperate: nonpharmacological treatment of hypertension. Cardiol Rev 2011; 19: 47–51.
132. Burke GM, Sica DA, Frishman WH. Renal sympathetic denervation for the treatment of systemic hypertension. Cardiol Rev 2012; 20: 274–8.
133. Fleg JL. Effects of aging on the cardiovascular system. In: Lewis RP, ed. Adult Clinical Cardiology Self-Assessment Program (ACCSAP 6). Bethesda, Md: American College of Cardiology Foundation, 2005: 6–20.
134. Weber MA, Neutel JM, Frishman WH. Combination drug therapy. In: Frishman WH, Sonnenblick EH, Sica DA, eds. Cardiovascular Pharmacotherapeutics, 2nd edn. New York: McGraw Hill, 2003: 355–68.

5
Disorders of lipid metabolism

Seth S. Martin and Roger S. Blumenthal

SUMMARY

With increases in life expectancy and growth of the elderly population, including the very old, the topic of dyslipidemia in the elderly is becoming increasingly important. Although the relative risk associated with dyslipidemia may decrease with age, because the absolute risk increases, the risk of cardiovascular events attributable to elevated cholesterol is higher. A large pool of data has proven that statin treatment reduces atherogenic lipid levels and the risk of atherosclerotic cardiovascular disease as effectively in older high-risk individuals as in younger individuals. Indeed, clinical guideline statements support treatment of high risk elderly patients with statins. Yet, despite these benefits, many high risk older individuals are not receiving statins and other evidence-based therapies. Physicians must engage patients in discussions about the benefits and risks of therapy. Physicians must use the evidence-base, their knowledge of the patient, experience and clinical judgment in deciding who to offer statins or other lipid-lowering treatments. Of course the decision will also need to incorporate patient preferences for another medication and overall healthcare goals, competing risks and life expectancy, and possible side effects and quality of life. Put simply, patients should not be denied statin therapy and other dyslipidemia interventions solely on the basis of age, but therapy should reflect a careful risk/benefit analysis.

INTRODUCTION

Elderly persons are a rapidly growing segment of the population, and most heart attacks and strokes occur among them (1). The most likely reason for death in an elderly person is cardiovascular disease (CVD) (1). In the pathophysiology of the atherosclerotic process underlying these clinical outcomes, disorders of lipid metabolism play a central role. Atherosclerosis is a systemic disease that accumulates over a lifetime and, therefore, addressing disorders of lipid metabolism in the elderly is an important endeavor. Prevention remains paramount, especially given the elderly may be prone to suffering disability following a cardiovascular event. Lack of independence with activities following a stroke or heart failure following a myocardial infarction are particularly devastating outcomes in the elderly.

An increase in age strongly increases both the global risk of CVD and absolute benefit from risk reduction therapies. Paradoxically the elderly are less likely to receive aggressive primary and secondary prevention therapies (2–4). Whether or not an elderly person has established CVD, many will be at high risk over the next decade, and many will likely benefit from statins and other cardiovascular risk reduction therapies. Nevertheless, the increased risks of side effects, and competing risks from other comorbidities, can decrease

Table 5.1   Risk Factors for Myopathy

Medication Factors	Clinical Factors
Lipophilic statin	Elderly
Fibrate	Small body frame, low body mass, frailty
Nicotinic acid (rarely)	Liver, renal, or multisystem disease
Cyclosporin	Hypothyroidism
Macrolides (erythromycin, clarithromycin)	Surgery or trauma
Antifungal azole	Rheumatologic disease
HIV antiviral (protease inhibitor)	Severe illness
Amiodarone	Excessive intake of alcohol or grapefruit juice
Verapamil and diltiazem	Heavy exercise
Proton pump inhibitors	Stress or sleep deprivation

the net benefits of intervention. In this regard, treatment decision making in the elderly is different than in younger patients (Table 5.1). A balanced, personalized treatment approach for each elderly individual is indicated.

More informed treatment of dyslipidemia in the elderly could help promote more successful aging in this population. The purpose of this chapter is to discuss the topic of disorders of lipid metabolism in the elderly, with a look at risk attributable to dyslipidemia, an emphasis on the preventive treatments, and special considerations for dyslipidemia management in the elderly.

DYSLIPIDEMIA AND CARDIOVASCULAR RISK IN THE ELDERLY

There is no question that dyslipidemia confers higher risk for CVD over the lifetime of an individual. However, there is some degree of disagreement among various studies in the literature about whether lipid-related measures retain their expected epidemiologic associations with CVD risk in elderly individuals. In the general population, cholesterol levels are tightly linked to coronary heart disease (CHD). Cholesterol levels are also associated with stroke; however, the relationship is less robust than with CHD (5) as some strokes are embolic and, therefore, may not be primarily driven by atherosclerosis.

A number of studies have demonstrated the expected graded, positive relationship of atherogenic cholesterol levels with CVD in the elderly. In the Kaiser Permanente Coronary Heart Disease in the Elderly Study, 2746 white men aged 60–79 years and free of CHD at enrollment were followed for an average of 10 years (6). CHD risk was higher in those with higher cholesterol concentrations. Moreover, the excess mortality attributable to elevated total cholesterol levels increased with age, from 2.2 deaths per 1000 person-years in those 60–64 years of age to 11.3 deaths per 1000 person-years in men aged 75–79 years.

In an elderly sample of men and women with a mean age of 72 years from the Systolic Hypertension in the Elderly Program (SHEP), baseline total cholesterol, non-high-density lipoprotein cholesterol (HDL-C), and low-density lipoprotein cholesterol (LDL-C) levels and the ratios of total cholesterol, non-HDL-C, and LDL-C to HDL-C were significantly related to CHD incidence over approximately 4 years of follow-up (7). Furthermore, a National Heart Lung and Blood Institute review found that total cholesterol and LDL-C levels were significantly correlated with fatal CHD in both men and women across a broad range of age groups including patients older than 65 years (8), at least up to 75 years of age. Even into the ninth decade of life, a cohort of both men and women with a mean age of 82 years living in a long-term health-care facility still demonstrated an association of total cholesterol levels (over 200 mg/dL in men and over 250 mg/dL in women) with an increase in coronary events (9).

Of course, in elderly patients, competing risks from other diseases, such as cancer, are more important, and can confound the association of lipids with clinical outcomes in observational studies (10). In this context, an analysis from the Established Populations for the Epidemiologic Studies of the Elderly failed to detect an association of total cholesterol, HDL-C, or the total to HDL cholesterol ratio with cardiovascular outcomes and mortality in the elderly in 997 patients (11). Men aged 65–74 years in the Honolulu Heart Program also did not show a relationship between lipid levels and mortality (12). In the Framingham Heart Study, age-specific analyses suggested that as age increased, the relative risk for CHD mortality associated with a high total cholesterol level decreased (13). The relationship with CHD mortality was significantly positive at ages 40, 50, and 60 years but was attenuated with age until the relationship was positive but not significant at age 70 years, and negative but not significant at age 80 years. Other studies have shown a differential effect in men versus women. For example, in the Bronx Aging Study, lower HDL-C levels were linked to CHD in elderly men, whereas higher LDL-C levels were linked to myocardial infarction in elderly women (14).

Perhaps differences in the populations studied, lipid-related measures examined, length of follow-up, or clinical endpoints evaluated explain part of the disagreement in the observational studies. Nevertheless, it is a key point that although the relative risk associated with dyslipidemia may decrease with age, because the absolute risk increases, the risk of cardiovascular events attributable to elevated cholesterol is higher. In this sense, dyslipidemia is more, not less, important to CVD risk in the elderly. Moreover, beyond epidemiologic associations, the more directly relevant clinical question is whether dyslipidemia interventions are efficacious in reducing CVD risk in the elderly, which is the topic of the next section of this chapter.

EFFICACY OF DYSLIPIDEMIA INTERVENTIONS IN THE ELDERLY
Lifestyle Interventions

As in the young, a heart healthy diet is a central component of a comprehensive approach to dyslipidemia and risk reduction therapy. An evidence-based diet is the Dietary Approaches to Stop Hypertension (DASH) diet, which is a Mediterranean-style diet that is low in salt (<2 grams of salt/day), low in saturated and trans fat, high in fiber, and high in fruits and vegetables. When alcohol is part of one's diet, the amount of consumption should be limited to moderate (≤2 servings a day for men, ≤1 serving a day for women; 1 serving = 12 oz of beer, 5 oz of wine, 1.5 oz liquor).

There is not a strong evidence base to support any recommendations for dietary supplements, such as omega-3 fatty acid supplements, vitamin A, B, C, E, antioxidants, folic acid, flax seed, garlic, magnesium, saw palmetto, zinc, coenzyme Q10, or ginko biloba. When discussing dietary approaches with an elderly person, recommendations will certainly need to be individualized to the patient. Some elderly patients will be prone to malnutrition, and in this setting, a more liberalized diet is warranted.

Regular exercise is also important for the maintenance of cardiovascular health in the elderly. Moderate intensity exercise is recommended for a minimum of 30 minutes 5 times per week or more. Muscle-strengthening exercises are recommended 2 days a week or more. Elderly patients may find it beneficial to wear a pedometer to monitor their walking. Exercise interventions improve functional capacity, raise HDL-C, and lower triglyceride levels, thereby favorably altering the cardiovascular risk profile. Moreover, cardiac rehabilitation reduces the risk of recurrent CVD events including death, following acute myocardial infarction or coronary bypass surgery, and should be recommended to such patients, as well as those with heart failure.

Overall, making changes toward a heart healthy lifestyle changes are the first line of treatment for dyslipidemia and CVD risk in any patient, including the elderly. Nevertheless, in many patients, an improvement in lifestyle alone will not be an adequate intervention.

Statins

Statins (3-hydroxy-3-methylglutaryl coenzyme A reductase inhibitors) are the most robustly studied class of medications for the reduction of atherogenic lipoprotein cholesterol and CVD prevention. Guidelines from the American Heart Association/American College of Cardiology and other societies recommend statins as first-line therapy for the management of dyslipidemia in elderly patients meeting the risk threshold for therapy. The data in support of these recommendations include multiple prospective observational studies and randomized clinical trials, which in total, have collected data on large numbers of older persons at high risk for CVD events, including coronary, cerebrovascular, and peripheral vascular events. Nevertheless, evidence at the extreme of old age is limited by relatively lower numbers of patients studied.

Prospective Studies of Statin Therapy

In a prospective study of 1410 long-term health-care facility residents aged 60–100 years (mean age 81 years) with LDL-C ≥125 mg/dL and a history of a myocardial infarction, statin therapy was associated with a 36% reduction in the incidence of new coronary events, with consistent benefits observed across all age ranges (15). Another prospective observational study of statin therapy in the elderly, the Cardiovascular Health Study, recorded relative risk reductions for all-cause mortality on the order of 40–50% in patients aged 65 years and older without any history of CVD (16). Results were consistent in participants who were 74 years of age or older at baseline.

In a secondary prevention setting, a similar relationship between statin therapy and morality was observed in the Intermountain Heart Collaborative Study (17). In this study, mortality was lower among statin recipients in all age groups, including those 80 years or above, in which the mortality rate was 29.5% among patients not taking a statin versus 8.5% of those taking a statin (adjusted hazard ratio [HR] 0.50, $p = 0.04$). Registries of patients hospitalized for myocardial infarction have shown a similar association with mortality. In an analysis of more than 40,000 Medicare beneficiaries (18) and a registry of 14,907 patients in Sweden (19), statins were associated with a mortality benefit and the benefits of statin therapy appeared to outweigh potential toxicities.

Clinical Trials of Statin Therapy

Statin therapy provided a benefit to the elderly subgroup in multiple primary prevention trials. The Anglo-Scandinavian Cardiac Outcomes Trial Lipid Lowering Arm (ASCOT-LLA) of 10,305 patients aged 40–79 years with nonfasting total cholesterol concentrations of 6.5 mmol/L or less, hypertension, and other cardiovascular risk factors, randomly assigned patients to atorvastatin 10 mg or placebo. Atorvastatin reduced the risk of nonfatal myocardial infraction or fatal CHD by 36%, and benefit was similar in patients older than 60 years (HR estimate 0.64; $p = 0.003$) and those 60 years and younger (0.66; $p = 0.09$) (20).

The Justification for the Use of statins in Prevention: An Intervention Trial Evaluating Rosuvastatin (JUPITER) was an even larger primary prevention trial that randomly assigned 17,802 apparently healthy men and women with LDL-C levels <130 mg/dL and high-sensitivity C-reactive protein levels of ≥2.0 mg/l to rosuvastatin 20 mg daily or placebo (21). After a median follow-up of 1.9 years (maximum, 5.0), the rates of the primary composite point (myocardial infarction, stroke, arterial revascularization, hospitalization for unstable angina, or death from cardiovascular causes) were 0.77 and 1.36 per 100 person-years of follow-up in the rosuvastatin and placebo groups, respectively (hazard ratio for rosuvastatin, 0.56; 95% confidence interval [CI], 0.46–0.69; $p < 0.00001$).

There was a significant reduction in all components of the primary composite endpoint. There was also a reduction in death from any cause (HR, 0.80; 95% CI, 0.67–0.97; $p = 0.02$). Among JUPITER participants, there were 5695 subjects who were 70 years or older at enrollment. This group accrued 49% of confirmed primary end point events in the trial, and rates of the primary end point in this age group were 1.22 and 1.99 per 100 person-years of follow-up in the rosuvastatin and placebo groups, respectively (hazard ratio, 0.61 [95% CI, 0.46–0.82]; $p < 0.001$) (22).

Multiple clinical trials have demonstrated improved outcomes of lipid-lowering therapy in elderly patients with established CHD. The Scandinavian Simvastatin Survival Study (4S) enrolled 4444 men and women who had CHD and an age up to 70 years. In 4S, simvastatin decreased total mortality by 35% and coronary mortality by 42% in participants aged ≥60 years over 5 years (23). Additionally, coronary procedures and cerebrovascular events were reduced in patients receiving simvastatin. Similar proportional reductions in these cardiovascular endpoints were seen in the elderly 4S participants and younger participants (24). The absolute risk reduction for all-cause mortality and CHD mortality for statin allocated patients was about twice as great in the elderly versus younger patients due to higher overall mortality rates in the elderly group.

Similarly, a consistent effect across age strata was shown in the Cholesterol and Recurrent Events (CARE) study (25). CARE enrolled 4129 patients up to the age of 75 years with average cholesterol levels and a history of a prior myocardial infarction. CARE found that elderly patients benefitted from a 32% reduction in major coronary events, 45% reduction in coronary death, and 40% reduction in stroke with pravastatin. Elderly patients with established CVD are at particularly high risk for future events, and therefore even the short-term number needed to treat to prevent an event can be quite low. In CARE, the number needed to treat for 5 years to prevent a major coronary event was 11. Large randomized trials of more intensive statin therapy with atorvastatin 80 mg per day, namely Pravastatin or Atorvastatin Evaluation and Infection Therapy–Thrombolysis in Myocardial Infarction 22 (PROVE-IT) (26) and Treating to New Targets (TNT) (27), showed a benefit of the more aggressive lipid-lowering irrespective of age.

In addition to subgroup analyses from broader clinical trial populations, randomized clinical trials have specifically investigated the benefits of statin treatment in the elderly. The Prospective Study of Pravastatin in the Elderly at Risk (PROSPER) enrolled 5804 elderly patients aged 70–82 years with established CVD or high risk for CVD (28). After 3.2 years of follow-up, pravastatin 40 mg per day reduced LDL-C levels by 34% and triglycerides by 13%. Pravastatin treatment reduced the incidence of the composite primary endpoint of coronary death, nonfatal myocardial infarction, and fatal or nonfatal stroke by 15% and reduced CHD mortality by 24% (Fig. 5.1). While an increased incidence of cancer was noted in PROSPER, this has not been confirmed in numerous other trials, and when the PROSPER investigators pooled their data with other trials in a meta-analysis, there was no risk of cancer (Fig. 5.2).

The question of whether more intensive statin therapy is beneficial in the elderly was addressed in the Study Assessing Goals in the Elderly (SAGE) (29). In SAGE, 893 patients aged 65–85 years (mean 73 years) with CHD were randomized to atorvastatin 80 mg or pravastatin 40 mg per day and followed for 12 months. More intensive therapy with atorvastatin produced a nonsignificant 29% reduction in major cardiovascular events ($p = 0.11$) and 67% reduction in all-cause mortality ($p = 0.01$).

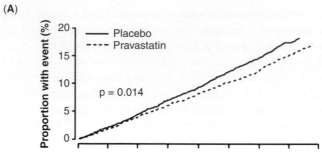

Number at risk

| Placebo | 2913 | 2832 | 2748 | 2651 | 2560 | 2458 | 2128 | 730 | 44 |
| Pravastatin | 2891 | 2812 | 2738 | 2655 | 2562 | 2483 | 2167 | 770 | 40 |

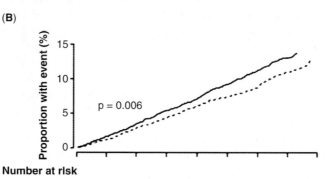

Number at risk

| Placebo | 2913 | 2847 | 2775 | 2692 | 2614 | 2535 | 2208 | 766 | 46 |
| Pravastatin | 2891 | 2827 | 2768 | 2696 | 2608 | 2544 | 2237 | 797 | 40 |

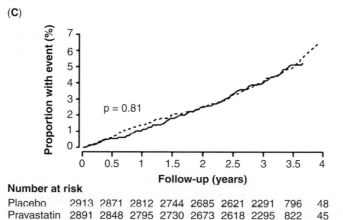

Number at risk

| Placebo | 2913 | 2871 | 2812 | 2744 | 2685 | 2621 | 2291 | 796 | 48 |
| Pravastatin | 2891 | 2848 | 2795 | 2730 | 2673 | 2618 | 2295 | 822 | 45 |

Figure 5.1 Kaplan–Meier analysis of time to primary and secondary endpoints in the PROSPER randomized clinical trial of statin therapy in the elderly. (**A**) coronary heart disease death, nonfatal myocardial infarction, or fatal or nonfatal stroke. (**B**) coronary heart disease death or nonfatal myocardial infarction. (**C**) fatal or nonfatal stroke. *Source*: From Ref. 28.

The totality of evidence from randomized clinical statin trials of primary and secondary prevention was recently summarized in the Cholesterol Treatment Trialists' prospective meta-analysis of data from 170,000 participants treated over an average of 5 years in 26 randomized clinical trials (30). In this analysis, the proportional benefit of therapy, or relative risk reduction, was relatively constant across a wide array of patient

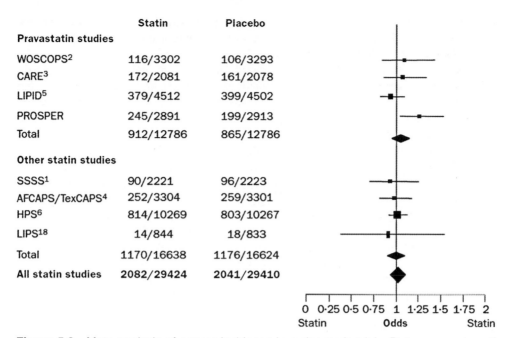

	Statin	Placebo
Pravastatin studies		
WOSCOPS[2]	116/3302	106/3293
CARE[3]	172/2081	161/2078
LIPID[5]	379/4512	399/4502
PROSPER	245/2891	199/2913
Total	912/12786	865/12786
Other statin studies		
SSSS[1]	90/2221	96/2223
AFCAPS/TexCAPS[4]	252/3304	259/3301
HPS[6]	814/10269	803/10267
LIPS[18]	14/844	18/833
Total	1170/16638	1176/16624
All statin studies	2082/29424	2041/29410

Figure 5.2 Meta-analysis of cancer incidence in major statin trials. Data are number of individuals with cancer/number of individuals in treatment group for each treatment group with odds ratio (95% CI) for risk of cancer in statin treated group relative to placebo. *Source*: From Ref. 28.

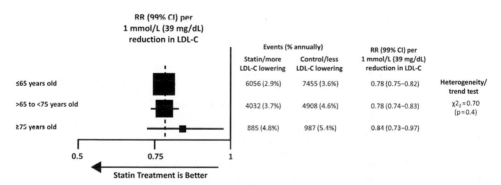

Figure 5.3 CTT meta-analysis showing similar relative risk reduction for major vascular events with statin therapy in the elderly compared with younger patients. Rate ratios (RRs) are plotted for each comparison of first event rates between treatment groups, and are weighted per 1.0 mmol/L (39 mg/dL) LDL cholesterol (LDL-C) difference at 1 year. Missing data are not plotted. RRs are shown with horizontal lines denoting 99% CIs or with open diamonds showing 95% CIs. *Source*: Adapted from Ref. 30.

subgroups, including the elderly (Fig. 5.3). Of 24,323 cardiovascular events in this meta-analysis, 8940 of them occurred in individuals aged 65–75 years, while 1872 of them occurred in those over the age of 75 years. Overall, lipid lowering with statin therapy produced proportional reductions in major cardiovascular events per each 1.0 mmol/L (39 mg/dL) LDL-C reduction of 13% reduction in coronary death or nonfatal myocardial infarction (95% CI 7–19; $p < 0.0001$), 19% reduction in coronary revascularization (95% CI 15–24; $p < 0.0001$), and 16% reduction in ischemic stroke (95% CI 5–26; $p = 0.005$).

All-cause mortality was reduced by 10% per 1.0 mmol/L LDL-C reduction (relative risk [RR] 0.90, 95% CI 0.87–0.93; $p < 0.0001$) primarily due to protection from cardiovascular death (RR 0.80, 99% CI 0.74–0.87; $p < 0.0001$).

Another meta-analysis specifically focused on secondary prevention in the elderly (31). The investigators included 9 trials ≥6 months of follow-up with 19,569 patients ranging in age from 65 to 82 years. All-cause mortality occurred in 15.6% of elderly patients treated with statins and 18.7% given placebo. There was a 22% relative risk reduction in all-cause mortality over 5 years (relative risk [RR] 0.78; 95% CI 0.65–0.89) (Fig. 5.4). Statins also reduced CHD mortality by 30% (RR 0.70; 95% CI 0.53–0.83), nonfatal myocardial infarction by 26% (RR 0.74; 95% CI 0.60–0.89), need for revascularization by 30% (RR 0.70; 95% CI 0.53–0.83), and stroke by 25% (RR 0.75; 95% CI 0.56–0.94). The estimated number needed to treat to save 1 life was 28 (95% CI 15–56).

Like any drug, statins have side effects. Nevertheless, statins have an excellent overall safety profile and side effects that are rarely irreversible. Very low levels of LDL-C by modern standards are generally within the evolutionarily normal range and safe. A systematic overview of risks associated with statin therapy from 35 randomized clinical trials including 74,102 participants with a mean follow-up of 17 months (range 1.5–64.8 months) found no significant increase in the risk of myalgias, creatine kinase elevations, rhabdomyolysis or discontinuation of statin therapy due to any adverse event (32). In JUPITER, those participants attaining LDL-C levels <50 mg/dL experienced a reduction in CVD events and all-cause mortality without a systematic increase in reported adverse events (33).

While randomized controlled trials utilize run-in phases to select out patients who are prone to early adverse effects from statin therapy, a relatively small proportion of patients were generally excluded for side effects, and the above data indicate that statin therapy is extremely safe in those who initially tolerate therapy. What follows here is an extended general discussion of statin safety, however, the chance of side effects may

	No. Events/ Total No. of Patients		Posterior Median Relative Risk	Favors Statin	Favors Placebo
Study	Statin	Placebo	(95% Credible Interval)		
4S	67 / 518	96 / 503	0.75 (0.59 , 0.89)		
CARE	77 / 640	108 / 643	0.76 (0.61 , 0.90)		
FLARE	2 / 179	6 / 187	0.74 (0.47 , 0.97)		
HPS	963 / 5366	1089 / 5331	0.87 (0.80 , 0.93)		
LIPID	287 / 1741	365 / 1773	0.80 (0.71 , 0.90)		
LIPS	23 / 324	32 / 299	0.75 (0.55 , 0.94)		
PLAC I	1 / 42	2 / 52	0.76 (0.51 , 1.00)		
PROSPER	110 / 934	128 / 899	0.82 (0.69 , 0.98)		
REGRESS	1 / 75	1 / 63	0.75 (0.49 , 0.99)		
Pooled (5 year)	1531 / 9819	1827 / 9750	0.78 (0.65 , 0.89)		

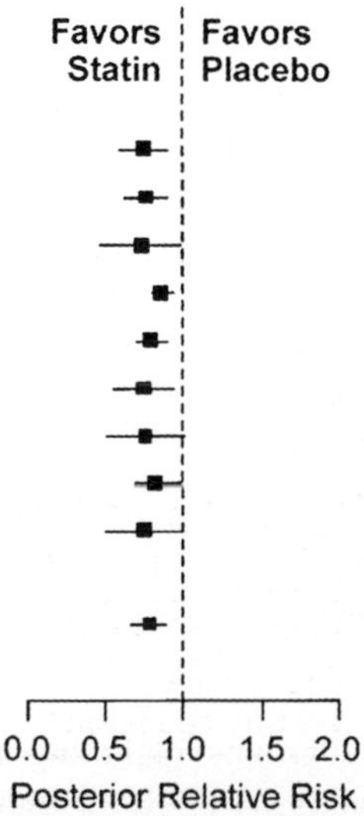

0.0   0.5   1.0   1.5   2.0
Posterior Relative Risk

Figure 5.4 Bayesian forest plot for all-cause mortality with statin treatment in the elderly. Statin therapy reduced the incidence of all-cause mortality by 22% over 5 years as compared to placebo. The posterior median estimate of the number need to treat was 28. *Source*: Adapted from Ref. 31.

increase in certain elderly patients with comorbidities (see section "Special Considerations for Dyslipidemia Management in the Elderly").

Myopathy is the most common concern with statins. In daily clinical practice, 8–9% of statin treated versus 4–6% of untreated patients develop myopathy, of which 95% are myalgias or mild myositis (34). Rhabdomyolysis is a rare, severe form of myopathy, with systemic myoglobin release and risk of renal failure, occurring in fewer than 1 in 10,000 patients on statin therapy (35). Risk factors for myopathy and rhabdomyolysis on statin therapy include being elderly, as well as interacting medications and other clinical factors (Table 5.2; also see section "Special Considerations for Dyslipidemia Management in the Elderly"). Statin risk may be increased with concomitant use of P450 inhibitors, including macrolides (erythromycin, clarithromycin), antiviral drugs (protease inhibitors), systemic antifungals (itraconazole and ketoconazole), verapamil (for simvastatin), diltiazem (for lovastatin, atorvastatin), amiodarone (for simvastatin), and grapefruit juice consumption exceeding 1 quart per day can also significantly inhibit P450. The risk of myopathy may also be increased for statin use in the setting of chronic immunosuppressive therapy

Table 5.2 Major Safety and Efficacy Outcomes Across Strata of Achieved LDL Cholesterol (Percent of Subjects)

Safety Measure	Achieved LDL Cholesterol (mg/dL)				
	>80–100 $n = 256$	>60–80 $n = 576$	>40–60 $n = 631$	<40 $n = 193$	p Trend
Muscle side effects[a]					
Myalgia	6.4	4.3	6.2	5.7	0.75
Myositis	0.4	0.6	0.6	0	0.64
CK >3 × ULN	2.3	0.7	1.9	1.0	0.18
CK >10 × ULN	0	0	0.3	0	0.45
Rh abdomyolvsis	0	0	0	0	1.0
Liver side effects					
ALT >3 × ULN	3.2	3.0	3.2	2.6	0.98
Study drug discontinued because of LIT	2.0	2.6	2.4	1.6	0.83
Other					
Hemorrhagic stroke	0.4	0.2	0	0	0.12
Retinal AE	0.4	0.9	1.0	0	0.48
Suicide/trauma death	0	0	0	0	1.0
Study drug discontinued because of any AE	10.2	9.4	9.7	9.8	0.99
Major efficacy measures					
Death	1.1	1.4	1.3	0.5	0.59
CHD death	0.5	0.5	0.6	0.0	0.06
Myocardial infarction	1.0	0.7	0.5	9.6	0.009
Any stroke	0.8	0.9	0.6	1.6	0.32
Primary composite[a]	26.1	22.2	20.4	20.4	0.10

[a]Primary composite = percent of subjects with any of the following: death, myocardial infarction, stroke, unstable angina requiring rehospitalization, and revascularization. Myalgia = muscle symptoms without CK elevation; myositis = muscle symptoms with CK elevation; rhabdomyolysis = muscle symptoms with CK >10 × ULN and evidence of renal dysfunction.

Abbreviations: AE, adverse event; ALT, alanine aminotransferase; CHD, coronary heart disease; CK, creatine kinase; LFT, liver function test; LDL, low-density lipoprotein; ULN, upper limit of normal. *Source*: From Ref. 94.

Table 5.3   Statin Therapy in the Elderly Versus Younger Patients

Relative risk reduction	Similar
Absolute risk reduction	Higher
Number needed to treat	Lower
Competing risks	Higher
Chance of adverse effects	Higher

(Cyclosporine), fibrates (Gemfibrozil), niacin, or alcohol intake exceeding 2 drinks per day. Adverse reactions to statin treatment, including muscle toxicity, are not significantly associated with on-treatment LDL-C (Table 5.3) (36). Reassuringly, if myopathy occurs, statin discontinuation generally leads to full recovery.

Asymptomatic transaminitis occurs with statins, but statins are not strongly tied to an increased risk of liver disease (35). Alanine transaminase elevations exceeding three times the upper limit of normal have occurred in 0.11–3.3% of patients on statin therapy (35). Other systematic reviews have not found an increased risk of transaminase elevations with statin therapy (32). In patients with mild-to-moderately elevated baseline liver tests, statins are safe and can actually lead to improvement in liver tests of many patients, perhaps explained by nonalcoholic fatty liver disease (37).

Statins are associated with a modest increase in the incidence of diabetes mellitus. There was a 9% increase (odds ratio [OD] 1.09; 95% CI 1.02–1.17) in the incidence of diabetes in a meta-analysis of 13 trials including 91,140 participants (38). Approximately 1 new case of diabetes occurred per 1000 person-years of treatment; thus, the risk of diabetes mellitus is low in absolute terms and relative to the reduction in CVD events. Moreover, it is not known to what degree statin-related hyperglycemia actually confers risk in the future. Indeed, in the trials in which diabetes occurred, there was a net cardiovascular benefit with statin therapy.

Overall, the potential harms of treating with a statin are usually outweighed by their benefits in the vast majority of statin treated patients (for circumstances where this may not be the case, see section "Special Considerations for Dyslipidemia Management in the Elderly"). Framing the well-established benefits of LDL-C lowering with statin therapy against their risks, the National Lipid Association Statin Safety Task Force stated, "For every 1 million high risk persons treated with a statin over 100,000 heart attacks, strokes or other major adverse cardiac event will be prevented for every 1 serious side effect. Therefore, the person should fear the heart attack not the statin" (39).

Nonstatin Drugs

In combination with statin therapy, or as monotherapy in patients who are not candidates for statins, additional lipid lowering agents are available including, bile acid sequestrants, fibrates, niacin, and ezetimibe. Each has a unique mechanism of action and side effect profile in elderly persons. Favorable outcomes data for nonstatin lipid lowering agents generally preceded the statin era with more recent studies focused on surrogate endpoints, and thus their efficacy as add-on therapy compared with maximal statin therapy alone has not been firmly established in large randomized clinical outcomes trials.

Bile acid sequestrants favorably redirect enterohepatic exchange of bile acids, increasing hepatic LDL-C receptor expression and clearance of circulating LDL-C, leading to a 5–30% dose-dependent reduction in LDL-C levels. The Lipid Research Clinics Coronary Primary Prevention Trial (LRC-CPPT) showed significant reductions in myocardial infarction and cardiovascular death with bile acid sequestrant monotherapy (40,41). Bile acid sequestrants remain in the gut without systemic absorption and therefore side effects are limited to gastrointestinal disturbances or impaired absorption of other drugs. Recent advances in bile acid sequestrant therapy include the introduction of a once daily cole-sevelam suspension, which may promote the ease of patient adherence to therapy.

Fibric acid derivatives (fibrates) activate lipoprotein lipase, promote hepatic bile secretion and reduce hepatic triglyceride production. The Helsinki Heart Study investigated gemfibrozil dosed at 600 mg twice daily in the primary prevention of heart disease in men (42). In subjects with the best adherence to treatment, gemfibrozil reduced, on average, triglycerides by 45%, total cholesterol by14%, and LDL-C by 15% while raising HDL-C by 14%. The lipid changes seen in the gemfibrozil group were associated with a significantly lower risk of coronary events.

In the secondary prevention arena, gemfibrozil was studied in men with low levels of HDL-C in the Veterans Affairs High-Density Lipoprotein Cholesterol Intervention Trial (43). The study included 2531 male participants who were randomized to gemfibrozil 1200 mg per day versus placebo and followed for a median of 5.1 years. Gemfibrozil therapy significantly reduced the risk of major cardiovascular events. A clinical benefit of fibrates was also seen in the Bezafibrate Infarction Prevention trial in patients with CHD (44).

Fibrates are generally well tolerated. However, they have important interactions with other drugs that are of particular relevance in the elderly. Due to increased risk of myopathy in combination with statins, fibrates should be used in this setting with only the utmost caution, and probably avoided in those with risk factors for myopathy. An interaction of warfarin with fibrates leads to an increase in warfarin levels and the international normalized ratio. Thus, warfarin is typically dosed at one-third its standard dose when administered with fenofibrate and careful follow-up of the international normalized ratio is needed. Given fibric acid derivatives are excreted primarily through the kidney, if they are used in the setting of chronic kidney disease, then dose adjustment is necessary. Gastrointestinal side effects are common in patients taking fibrate therapy, including mild nausea during the first week of therapy. To reduce this potential side effect, it can be useful to start treatment with one-half the normal dose for several days before increasing to a full dose.

Nicotinic acid (niacin) is a B vitamin that inhibits adenylate cyclase (45), and in daily doses of 1500–3000 mg, increases HDL-C levels by 15–30%, reduces total cholesterol and LDL-C levels by about 10–25%, and reduces triglyceride levels by up to 50%. In the Coronary Drug Project, niacin monotherapy provided protection from myocardial infarction and reduced long-term mortality by 11% at 15 years (46). A series of Arterial Biology for the Investigation of the Treatment Effects of Reducing Cholesterol (ARBITER) studies have examined the effects of adding niacin on top of background statin therapy (47,48). In these studies, niacin has led to slowing and even regression of atherosclerosis, as measured by carotid intima-media thickness (47,48). Nevertheless, the absolute impact on carotid intima-media thickness was modest on average, and the clinical significance of these changes is uncertain.

From a clinical outcomes standpoint, the results for niacin as an add-on therapy to statins were disappointing from the Atherothrombosis Intervention in Metabolic Syndrome with Low HDL/High Triglycerides: Impact on Global Health Outcomes (AIM-HIGH) trial. In a secondary prevention setting, with statin and ezetimibe titrated to LDL-C levels of less than 70 mg per deciliter, there was no incremental clinical benefit from the addition of niacin during a 36-month follow-up period in AIM-HIGH (49). While the study did not meet its primary endpoint for efficacy, the trial was stopped early and there were a number of issues with the trial (e.g., change in end-point during trial; low-dose niacin use in control group). In the larger Heart Protection Study 2-Treatment of HDL to Reduce the Incidence of Vascular

Events (HPS2-THRIVE), in 25,673 patients with well-controlled LDL-C levels, the investigators have announced that the combination of niacin and laropiprant did not reduce a composite CVD endpoint. HPS2-THRIVE recorded a significantly increased risk of adverse events with niacin/laropiprant, with approximately 30 adverse events per 1000 treated.

Laropiprant was used in HPS2-THRIVE to inhibit the most common side effect of niacin: prostaglandin-mediated flushing. The extent of off-target effects of laropiprant is uncertain. Flushing may also be prevented or minimized by aspirin, avoidance of alcohol, monosodium glutamate, hot beverages, and spicy foods. Other side effects from high-dose niacin include a small increase in the serum glucose, a moderate increase in the serum uric acid level, and a small reduction in the serum phosphorus level.

Ezetimibe reduces LDL-C 15–20% primarily by selectively inhibiting cholesterol absorption at the intestinal brush border. This is mechanistically attractive in combination with a statin, and safe and efficacious in the reduction of atherogenic cholesterol levels (50,51). However, limited data are available on the use of ezetimibe in the elderly, either as a single agent or in combination with a statin. Surrogate endpoint trials, limited by the lack of a reliable correlation with clinical outcomes, have introduced doubt surrounding ezetimibe's clinical efficacy.

In the Ezetimibe and Simvastatin in Hypercholesterolemia Enhances Atherosclerosis Regression (ENHANCE) trial, involving 720 patients with heterozygous familial hypercholesterolemia, adding ezetimibe to maximal simvstatin therapy yielded greater LDL-C reduction (56% vs. 39%), but there was no difference in carotid intima-media thickness at 2 years (52). Surprisingly, the Arterial Biology for the Investigation of the Treatment Effects of Reducing Cholesterol 6–HDL and LDL Treatment Strategies (ARBITER 6–HALTS) study observed a paradoxical increase in carotid intima-media thickness with LDL-C lowering by ezetimibe (53). Such findings may be related to off-target effects of ezetimibe, or more likely, limitations of carotid intima-media thickness as a surrogate endpoint or chance findings.

Indeed, the Study of Heart and Renal Protection (SHARP) trial provided the first look at an ezetimibe trial powered for clinical outcomes and found that the drug added to simvastatin reduced CVD events though the comparator group was allocated placebo, not statin monotherapy (54). A large ongoing secondary prevention trial, Improved Reduction of Outcomes: Vytorin Efficacy International Trial (IMPROVE-IT), will address the question of benefit from adding ezetimibe to simvastatin monotherapy, anticipating completion in 2013 or 2014.

Ezetimibe is generally well tolerated. When coadministered with a statin, elevations in serum transaminases may occur slightly more frequently than with a statin alone. Rhabdomyolysis has been reported very rarely with ezetimibe monotherapy or when ezetimibe has been added to a statin.

DYSLIPIDEMIA INTERVENTION AS ONE COMPONENT OF A GLOBAL ABC APPROACH

Ultimately, dyslipidemia interventions are one component of a multifactorial, or global, approach to CVD prevention. The important lifestyle changes that help to lower cholesterol also tend to produce benefits for other components of the cardiovascular risk profile, including body mass index and blood pressure. Regarding pharmacotherapy for risk reduction, even if optimal lipid lowering is achieved in high risk patients, the overall prognosis will remain suboptimal if other risk factors are not simultaneously addressed. In this respect, anytime dyslipidemia interventions are employed, it is imperative for providers to consider the other components of the global approach to risk reduction. An "ABC" or "ABCDE" approach can be practically applied in clinic, and includes (A) Anti platelet and anti thrombotic agents; (B) Blood pressure control; (C) Cigarettes smoking and cholesterol; (D) Diet and diabetes control; (E) Exercise.

The benefits associated with achieving optimal global risk factor control in the primary prevention of CVD in elderly men was demonstrated in the Physicians' Health Study (55). There were 4182 male physicians ≥65 years of age (mean age was 73 years) who enrolled in 1997. The physicians were free of CVD and diabetes at enrollment and followed for an average of 9 years. Adjusting for competing causes of mortality, a multifactorial prevention strategy was associated with considerable cardiovascular protection. Compared with control of 4 of 4 risk factors (smoking avoidance, control of non-HDL-C and blood pressure, and aspirin use) were controlled (only 6.0% of participants), control of 0 of 4 risk factors almost quadrupled the risk of CVD (0.4% of participants; event rate 41.2%; HR 3.83, 95% CI 1.72–8.55). Control of 1 of 4 risk factors more than doubled the risk (14.2% of participants; HR 2.53, 95% CI 1.80–3.57). Most patients had partial risk factor control; with control of 2 of 4 risk factors, risk was nearly doubled (43.8% of participants; HR 1.94, 95% CI 1.41–2.69), and those with control of 3 of 4 risk factors also were at increased risk (35.6% of participants; HR 1.80, 95% CI 1.30–2.50). Depending on the number of risk factors controlled, the number-needed to control to prevent one CVD event ranged from 5 to 22.

SPECIAL CONSIDERATIONS FOR DYSLIPIDEMIA MANAGEMENT IN THE ELDERLY
Increased Near-Term Efficacy with Increased Age
Age is a dominant factor in risk prediction models used in dyslipidemia guidelines and therefore a key determinant of whether a patient qualifies for treatment. Moreover, given higher absolute risk with age, even small relative risk reductions can translate into large absolute benefits in the elderly (24). Although relative risk reductions were similar in patients ≥65 years compared with those <65 years treated with pravastatin, absolute risk reductions were 1.5–2 times greater in the elderly patients (56). The short-term benefit of statins is greatest in populations with the greatest cardiovascular risk, and even in the setting of high risk primary prevention, the totality of evidence supports the use of statin therapy (57). We have not yet identified an age above which, or atherogenic cholesterol level below which, patients no longer benefit from statin therapy.

Noncoronary Outcomes
Multiple noncoronary outcomes are of particular interest in the elderly. As noted in this chapter, noncoronary CVD is also linked to dyslipidemia and responsive to interventions including statin therapy. Some of the nuances of these noncoronary outcomes warrant additional discussion.

First, while many strokes are attributable to atherosclerotic vascular disease, a considerable portion is also thromboembolic, such as those related to atrial fibrillation, a disease concentrated in the elderly. There is some suggestion in the literature that statin therapy is associated with protection against atrial fibrillation in patients with coronary artery disease (58) as well as prevention of recurrence of atrial fibrillation in patients with lone atrial fibrillation after successful cardioversion (59). In major trials of statin therapy of patients both with and without known CHD, statin therapy has reduced the future incidence of stroke, which typically has been captured as a secondary outcome or component of the primary outcome.

In PROSPER, there was a trend toward reduction in transient ischemic attacks by 25% ($p = 0.05$). The Stroke Prevention by Aggressive Reduction in Cholesterol Levels (SPARCL) trial examined intensive statin therapy for protection from recurrent stroke in

Study	No. Events/ Total No. of Patients		Posterior Median Relative Risk	Favors Statin	Favors Placebo
	Statin	Placebo	(95% Credible Interval)		
CARE	29 / 640	47 / 643	0.72 (0.51 , 0.92)		
HPS	280 / 5366	390 / 5331	0.73 (0.64 , 0.84)		
LIPID	104 / 1741	119 / 1773	0.80 (0.66 , 1.01)		
PLAC I	0 / 42	2 / 52	0.72 (0.35 , 1.04)		
PROSPER	45 / 934	53 / 899	0.77 (0.60 , 1.02)		
Pooled (5 year)	**458 / 8723**	**611 / 8698**	**0.75 (0.56 , 0.94)**		

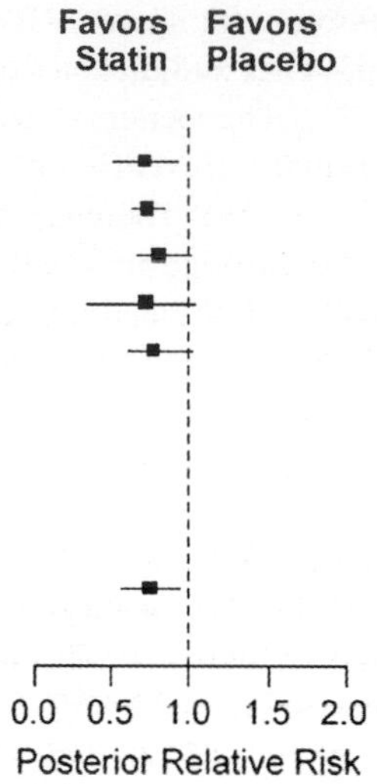

```
          0.0  0.5  1.0  1.5  2.0
          Posterior Relative Risk
```

Figure 5.5   Bayesian forest plot for stroke with statin treatment in the elderly. Statin therapy reduced the incidence of stroke by 25% over 5 years as compared to placebo. The posterior median estimate of the number need to treat was 58. *Source*: From Ref. 31.

stroke survivors without CHD (60). In SPARCL, statin intervention led to a 16% reduction in the risk of fatal or nonfatal stroke [HR 0.84 (0.71–0.99), $p = 0.03$]. When recurrent strokes did occur, they were generally less severe in patients who were allocated statin therapy. When the data were viewed collectively, meta-analyses have found a beneficial effect of statin therapy on stroke prevention (61,62), including in the elderly (Fig. 5.5) (31).

Atherosclerosis affects many arterial regions throughout the body, and, therefore, beyond coronary and cerebrovascular disease, dyslipidemia may play a role in abdominal aortic aneurysm (AAA), renal artery stenosis, and peripheral arterial disease of the extremities. Accumulating evidence supports statin treatment in these settings as well. For example, in the Heart Protection Study of simvastatin, patients with peripheral arterial disease benefitted from a 19% reduction in the rate of new vascular events (63).

Moreover, a frequent end-stage disease process for many patients with atherosclerosis is heart failure. Observational studies suggest a potential value of statins in patients who have heart failure with reduced systolic function (64–66). In a small single center study, statin therapy was associated with lower mortality in patients with heart failure with preserved ejection fraction after accounting for baseline differences in hypertension, diabetes, coronary artery disease, and creatinine (67). Mechanisms beyond effects on atherosclerosis may explain how statin therapy could produce beneficial effects in heart failure patients. For example, statin therapy has been shown to reduce myocardial necrosis and preserve myocardial viability (68).

Nevertheless, randomized trials of initiating statin therapy in more advanced heart failure have been negative. In the Controlled Rosuvastatin Multinational Trial in Heart Failure (CORONA), 5011 older patients (≥60 years of age; mean age 73 years) with New York Heart Association class II–IV ischemic, systolic heart failure [mean left ventricular ejection fraction (LVEF) 31%] were randomly assigned to receive 10 mg of rosuvastatin or placebo per day (69). At baseline, the mean LDL-C was 137 mg/dL and an entry requirement was that the investigator thought that the patient did not need a cholesterol lowering drug. After a median follow-up of 33 months, rosuvastatin reduced LDL-C to 76 mg/dL in the intervention group versus 138 mg/dL in the control group; however, there was not a significant reduction in the primary composite outcome of death from cardiovascular causes, nonfatal myocardial infarction, or nonfatal stroke (11.4 vs. 12.3% with placebo, HR 0.92, 95% CI 0.83–1.02), or secondary outcomes such as cardiovascular mortality (9.3 vs. 9.6%, HR 0.97), or coronary events (9.3 vs. 10.0 percent, HR 0.92).

Similarly, the Gruppo Italiano per lo Studio della Sopravvivenza nell'Insuffi cienza cardiac (GISSI-HF trial) (70) did not show a benefit of rosuvastatin 10 mg per day in 4574 patients (mean age 68 years) with ischemic or nonischemic New York Heart Association class II–IV heart failure (mean LVEF 33%). While LDL-C was reduced from 122 to 89 mg/dL, after a median follow-up of 47 months, there was no significant difference in deaths from any cause or in the combined end point of death or admission to the hospital for cardiovascular causes in both ischemic and nonischemic cardiomyopathy. Thus, together the CORONA and GISSI-HF trials suggest that initiating statin therapy is not generally useful in patients with more advanced systolic heart failure who would not have otherwise met criteria for initiation of statin therapy for the purpose of primary or secondary prevention. Nevertheless, there may be more to the story—a retrospective hypothesis-generating analysis of CORONA found an interaction between high-sensitivity C-reactive protein levels and the effect of rosuvastatin on outcomes such that rosuvastatin treatment was associated with better outcomes in patients with high-sensitivity C-reactive protein levels > or = 2.0 mg/L (71).

Also, of particular consideration in the elderly is calcific aortic stenosis, a disease that is associated with older age and dyslipidemia. While observational studies have suggested that statin therapy can slow the progression of aortic stenosis as measured by aortic valve area (72) or accumulation of aortic calcium (73), randomized trials have not confirmed this effect (74,75). The prospective Simvastatin and Ezetimibe in Aortic Stenosis (SEAS) trial enrolled 1873 adults (mean age 68) with mild to moderate aortic stenosis (mean aortic jet velocity 3.1 m/s) and randomly assigned them to treatment with simvastatin plus ezetimibe or placebo (75).

After an average follow-up of 52 months, there was no difference between groups in the primary composite endpoint of cardiovascular death, aortic valve replacement, nonfatal myocardial infarction, hospitalized unstable angina pectoris, heart failure as a result of progression of AS, coronary artery bypass grafting, percutaneous coronary interventions, and nonhemorrhagic stroke. There was also no difference in the rate of aortic valve replacement (28% vs. 30%) or in the rate of hemodynamic progression of aortic stenosis.

A Note on the Term Elderly in the Context of Dyslipidemia and CVD Risk

The medical literature often defines an elderly person as someone who is 65 years of age or older. This is a convenient cut-point to stratify populations of individuals and helps to assess for differences by age at the population scale. However, of course it is an artificial cut-point when applied to an individual patient. A patient who is 64 years, 11 months, and 30 days old, becomes "elderly" on his or her 65th birthday, but this binary distinction suggests much more of a change than has occurred.

In addition, patients age differently. For clinical purposes, it is potentially useful to consider physiologic age, in addition to chronologic age. From a cardiovascular standpoint, the concept of "physiologic age" or "heart age" may be useful in understanding the absolute cardiovascular risk of a patient, and therefore the patient's potential to benefit from statins and other risk reduction therapies. A patient who is 65 years old with cardiac risk factors may have a heart age in the 80s, and therefore, can be considered more elderly from a risk standpoint, with a larger potential role for risk reducing therapies including statins. If the patient does not have many noncardiovascular comorbidities, the patient may be younger from the standpoint of potential statin side effects and competing risks. If so, intervention seems like a more attractive option and in understanding that the patient's heart age is older than the chronologic age, the patient may buy in more to intervention.

Conversely, a patient who is also 65 years of age with multiple noncardiovascular comorbidities, such as HIV on a protease inhibitor, alcohol abuse, and atrial fibrillation on amiodarone, is at increased risk for statin side effects, perhaps on the order of a much older, frail individual, and the attractiveness of intervention is less. Therefore, one nuance in the clinical management of dyslipidemia in the elderly is that the concept of elderly is probably best viewed more broadly than simply as chronological age.

Increased Adverse Effects with Increased Age

Common adverse events for statins and other lipid lowering drugs were discussed above. It is important to consider that elderly patients are at higher risk for adverse drug effects because of the more frequent use of multiple concomitant medications, presence of multi-morbidity, and impaired ability to metabolize and excrete compounds as a result of declining renal and hepatic function with age. Consequently, the safety of lipid-lowering agents, including potential drug–drug interactions, requires increased attention in this population. Indeed, aging related changes in muscle mass, total body water and fat, first-pass metabolism, and cytochrome P450 functioning, can change the bioavailability of statins and other lipid lowering drugs, altering the risk of toxicity.

Given the chance of adverse statin effects is related to the particular statin and dose, physicians may be able to reduce the likelihood of adverse drug effects in their choice of statin and dosing. The Food and Drug Administration has issued a warning on simvastatin at a dose of 80 mg per day due to greater incidence of myopathy and serious cases of rhabdomyolysis. Therefore, this statin regimen should be avoided, especially in elderly patients. It has been suggested that the lipophilicity of statins may determine entry into muscle tissue. Hydrophilic statins, such as rosuvastatin, pravastatin, and lovastatin may penetrate muscle tissue less than lipophilic statins, such as atorvastatin, fluvastatin, and simvastatin, and may therefore be less frequently implicated in myopathic events (76).

In elderly patients at increased risk for myopathy and other adverse drug effects, including women with low body weight, or those with hepatic or renal dysfunction, providers might consider choosing hydrophilic statins and consider initiating therapy at a lower dose than they choose in younger, healthier patients. If the statin is well tolerated, the option for gradual titration remains. The highest dose of statins should be used with caution in the elderly. If severe illness, major surgery, or major trauma occur, then it is prudent discontinue statin use in an elderly patient until the patient has recovered.

Despite these potential issues, statin therapy is generally well tolerated in the elderly. For example, the Cholesterol Reduction in Seniors Program (CRISP) pilot study showed that lovastatin doses at 20–40 mg daily was associated with preserved health-related quality of life relative to placebo in a cohort of older adults with a mean age of 71 years (77). A recent post hoc analysis from the TNT study assessed more potent treatment with atorvastatin 80 mg daily and in patients 65 years of age or older with stable CHD. High-dose atorvastatin was well-tolerated and produced a 2.3% absolute reduction in major cardiovascular events and a 19% relative risk reduction compared with low-dose atorvastatin (78).

Preservation of cognitive function is a topic of particular relevance to the elderly who are at elevated risk for dementia and there has been interest in whether statins or cholesterol lowering can impact cognitive function. Cholesterol may contribute to the pathogenesis of dementia including both of the most common forms, Alzheimer's disease and vascular dementia. Increased mid-life circulating cholesterol levels are linked with subsequent development of Alzheimer's disease (79,80). In addition, increased non-HDL-C and decreased HDL-C are associated with an increased prevalence of vascular dementia (81).

Although cholesterol does not freely circulate between the systemic circulation and brain, patients with both Alzheimer's disease and coronary artery disease have increased cortical cholesterol levels (82). Moreover, atherosclerosis may play a mechanistic role in the development of cognitive impairment in some patients and cholesterol may also facilitate deposition of amyloid plaques (83). Indeed, observational studies have found an association of statin therapy with a lower rate of dementia (84–86) and higher modified Mini-Mental State Examination (MMSE) scores (87).

Cancer is another topic of special importance in the elderly. With rising statin use in the 1990s, the concern arose that statin therapy could cause cancer. The Cholesterol Treatment Trialists' set out to study this issue prospectively and the latest meta-analysis of data from clinical trials of statin therapy did not show any significant association of statin therapy with cancer. In fact, the risk estimate was exactly 1.00, indicating no effect.

In agreement, in a meta-analysis of 26 randomized controlled trials including 86,936 participants with 6662 incident cancer cases and 2407 cancer deaths, there was no association of statin therapy with the diagnosis of cancer or cancer death (88). When the data were stratified according to cancer type, statin brand, dose, or pharmacologic characteristics, the results were consistent. These results, along with longer term safety established in multiple clinical trials beyond 10 years, should reassure clinicians.

COMPETING RISKS

Even if statins do not contribute to cancer, this does not mean that cancer, and other comorbidities that are more common in the elderly, do not impact treatment decisions. While evaluating cardiovascular risk and estimating the potential benefits of cardiovascular risk reduction therapies, providers must consider the effect of competing risks and discuss the global prognosis with patients. Of course, prognosis depends not only upon a new diagnosis of dyslipidemia and/or CVD but also on risks from other causes.

Investigators have used the declining exponential approximation for life expectancy (DEALE) to provide a framework to help clinicians gauge the effect of competing risks as a function of age (10). In such modeling, the absolute effect of a new diagnosis on life expectancy is often relatively small, and therefore, the potential gain even from optimal therapy may also be small, at least for the endpoint of mortality. This point, combined with the added risks of therapy in old age reduces the net benefit of intervention in the elderly, and is a reason to exercise greater caution in initiating therapy or lower tolerance for side effects in elderly patients with such comorbidities.

UNDERTREATMENT IN THE ELDERLY

Despite the clear benefits of lipid lowering on cardiovascular outcomes in the elderly, undertreatment is especially prevalent in this patient population, even in those in the younger range of the elderly group. In a study published in 2006, examining male patients aged 60–75 years with acute myocardial infarction, only 29% of patients were on a lipid lowering drug and only 12% achieved cholesterol levels recommended by the NCEP guidelines (18). The situation has been characterized as a treatment-risk paradox (2) in which treatment is prescribed preferentially to individuals under the age of 65 years, and use is more restricted in the elderly group with higher short-term cardiovascular risk.

Recently, low use of statins was documented in elderly persons living in the United Kingdom (89). Medical records were reviewed in 41,250 patients aged ≥40 years who were seen at general medical practices. In those without known CVD, use of statins and antihypertensives were assessed across age categories. Whereas antihypertensive use increased with age, as expected, statin use peaked in the 70–74 age group and then declined. Compared to a reference group aged 40–44 years, the odds ratio for taking a statin was 10.9 in the

65–69-year-old group, and similar at 10.1 for antihypertensive use. The odds ratios in the 70–74-year-old group increased to 13.6 for statins and 16.2 for antihypertensives. However, thereafter use for statins dropped off, with an odds ratio down to 10.3 in the group aged over 80–84 years, whereas the odds ratio for antihypertensive use continued to increase up to 25.8.

Several factors might explain lower statin prescription rates in the elderly. First, the higher potential for adverse effects likely translates into a higher threshold for initiating therapy as physicians weigh the potential benefits and risks. Second, physicians may be less inclined to prescribe additional drugs to an elderly patient due the potential for lower adherence to therapy in the setting of polypharmacy, medication costs, and cognitive decline. Third, physicians may be swayed by the potential for lower net benefits of intervention due to competing risk from multiple other comorbidities. Fourth, statins may be avoided due to shifting clinical priorities and patient preference. Fifth, clinicians may hesitate to prescribe statin therapy in very old patients (i.e., >75) for primary prevention because of the perception of too little clinical trial evidence (90) in this population and lack of clear benefit for functional status (91,92). Ultimately, it is difficult to know for certain what portion of lack of treatment of dyslipidemia in the elderly is due to undertreatment and what portion is due to reasonable withholding of therapy.

GUIDELINE RECOMMENDATIONS

Clinical guideline statements support treatment of high risk elderly patients with statins. Recently, the European guidelines state (93), as a class IB recommendation, "Treatment with statins is recommended for elderly patients with established CVD in the same way as for younger patients." Consistent with the evidence above, they also indicate that statin therapy for primary prevention can be appropriate in the elderly. The European guidelines state, as a Class IIb recommendation, "Statin therapy may be considered in elderly subjects free of CVD, particularly in the presence of at least one other CV risk factors besides age." Though based on expert opinion only (level of evidence C), the European guidelines do recommend greater caution in treating the elderly, stating, "Since elderly people often have comorbidities and have altered pharmacokinetics, it is recommended to start lipid-lowering medication at a low dose and then titrate with caution to achieve target lipid levels which are the same as in the younger subjects."

CONCLUSION

With increases in life expectancy and growth of the elderly population, including the very old, the topic of dyslipidemia in the elderly is becoming increasingly important. The growth of this population also gives the opportunity for further research to incorporate these patients in even greater numbers. Ensuring informed clinicians and patients, and appropriate use of risk reduction therapies for dyslipidemia in the elderly is vital to maintaining quality of life and avoiding preventable morbidity. A large pool of data has proven that statin treatment reduces atherogenic lipid levels and the risk of CVD as effectively in older high-risk individuals as in younger individuals. Yet, despite these benefits, many high risk older individuals are not receiving statins and other evidence-based therapies.

Physicians must engage patients in discussions about the benefits and risks of therapy. Physicians must use the evidence-base, their knowledge of the patient, experience and clinical judgment in deciding who to offer statins or other lipid-lowering treatments. Of course the decision will also need to incorporate patient preferences for another medication and overall healthcare goals, competing risks and life expectancy, and possible side effects and quality of life. Put simply, patients should not be denied statin therapy and other dyslipidemia interventions solely on the basis of age, but therapy should reflect a careful risk/benefit analysis.

REFERENCES

1. Rosamond W, Flegal K, Friday G, et al. Heart disease and stroke statistics-2007 update: a report from the American Heart Association Statistics Committee and Stroke Statistics Subcommittee. Circulation 2007; 115: e69–171.
2. Ko DT, Mamdani M, Alter DA. Lipid-lowering therapy with statins in high-risk elderly patients: the treatment-risk paradox. JAMA 2004; 291: 1864–70.
3. Alexander KP, Roe MT, Chen AY, et al. Evolution in cardiovascular care for elderly patients with non-ST-segment elevation acute coronary syndromes: results from the CRUSADE National Quality Improvement Initiative. J Am Coll Cardiol 2005; 46: 1479–87.
4. Grundy SM, Cleeman JI, Rifkind BM, Kuller LH. Cholesterol lowering in the elderly population. Coordinating Committee of the National Cholesterol Education Program. Arch Intern Med 1999; 159: 1670–8.
5. Blood pressure, cholesterol, and stroke in eastern Asia. Eastern Stroke and Coronary Heart Disease Collaborative Research Group. Lancet 1998; 352: 1801–7.
6. Rubin SM, Sidney S, Black DM, et al. High blood cholesterol in elderly men and the excess risk for coronary heart disease. Ann Intern Med 1990; 113: 916–20.
7. Frost PH, Davis BR, Burlando AJ, et al. Serum lipids and incidence of coronary heart disease. Findings from the Systolic Hypertension in the Elderly Program (SHEP). Circulation 1996; 94: 2381–8.
8. Manolio TA, Pearson TA, Wenger NK, et al. Cholesterol and heart disease in older persons and women. Review of an NHLBI workshop. Ann Epidemiol 1992; 2: 161–76.
9. Aronow WS, Starling L, Etienne F, et al. Risk factors for coronary artery disease in persons older than 62 years in a long-term health care facility. Am J Cardiol 1986; 57: 518–20.
10. Welch HG, Albertsen PC, Nease RF, Bubolz TA, Wasson JH. Estimating treatment benefits for the elderly: the effect of competing risks. Ann Intern Med 1996; 124: 577–84.
11. Krumholz HM, Seeman TE, Merrill SS, et al. Lack of association between cholesterol and coronary heart disease mortality and morbidity and all-cause mortality in persons older than 70 years. JAMA 1994; 272: 1335–40.
12. Schatz IJ, Masaki K, Yano K, et al. Cholesterol and all-cause mortality in elderly people from the Honolulu Heart Program: a cohort study. Lancet 2001; 358: 351–5.
13. Kronmal RA, Cain KC, Ye Z, Omenn GS. Total serum cholesterol levels and mortality risk as a function of age. A report based on the Framingham data. Arch Intern Med 1993; 153: 1065–73.
14. Zimetbaum P, Frishman WH, Ooi WL, et al. Plasma lipids and lipoproteins and the incidence of cardiovascular disease in the very elderly. The Bronx Aging Study. Arterioscler Thromb 1992; 12: 416–23.
15. Aronow WS, Ahn C. Incidence of new coronary events in older persons with prior myocardial infarction and serum low-density lipoprotein cholesterol > or = 125 mg/dl treated with statins versus no lipid-lowering drug. Am J Cardiol 2002; 89: 67–9.
16. Lemaitre RN, Psaty BM, Heckbert SR, et al. Therapy with hydroxymethylglutaryl coenzyme a reductase inhibitors (statins) and associated risk of incident cardiovascular events in older adults: evidence from the Cardiovascular Health Study. Arch Intern Med 2002; 162: 1395–400.
17. Allen Maycock CA, Muhlestein JB, Horne BD, et al. Statin therapy is associated with reduced mortality across all age groups of individuals with significant coronary disease, including very elderly patients. J Am Coll Cardiol 2002; 40: 1777–85.
18. Foody JM, Rathore SS, Galusha D, et al. Hydroxymethylglutaryl-CoA reductase inhibitors in older persons with acute myocardial infarction: evidence for an age-statin interaction. J Am Geriatr Soc 2006; 54: 421–30.
19. Gransbo K, Melander O, Wallentin L, et al. Cardiovascular and cancer mortality in very elderly post-myocardial infarction patients receiving statin treatment. J Am Coll Cardiol 2010; 55: 1362–9.
20. Sever PS, Dahlof B, Poulter NR, et al. Prevention of coronary and stroke events with atorvastatin in hypertensive patients who have average or lower-than-average cholesterol concentrations, in the Anglo-Scandinavian Cardiac Outcomes Trial–Lipid Lowering Arm (ASCOT-LLA): a multicentre randomised controlled trial. Lancet 2003; 361: 1149–58.
21. Ridker PM, Danielson E, Fonseca FA, et al. Rosuvastatin to prevent vascular events in men and women with elevated C-reactive protein. N Engl J Med 2008; 359: 2195–207.
22. Glynn RJ, Koenig W, Nordestgaard BG, Shepherd J, Ridker PM. Rosuvastatin for primary prevention in older persons with elevated C-reactive protein and low to average low-density lipoprotein cholesterol levels: exploratory analysis of a randomized trial. Ann Intern Med 2010; 152: 488–96, W174.
23. Randomised trial of cholesterol lowering in 4444 patients with coronary heart disease: the Scandinavian Simvastatin Survival Study (4S). Lancet 1994; 344: 1383–9.

24. Miettinen TA, Pyorala K, Olsson AG, et al. Cholesterol-lowering therapy in women and elderly patients with myocardial infarction or angina pectoris: findings from the Scandinavian Simvastatin Survival Study (4S). Circulation 1997; 96: 4211–18.

25. Sacks FM, Pfeffer MA, Moye LA, et al. The effect of pravastatin on coronary events after myocardial infarction in patients with average cholesterol levels. Cholesterol and Recurrent Events Trial investigators. N Engl J Med 1996; 335: 1001–9.

26. Cannon CP, Braunwald E, McCabe CH, et al. Intensive versus moderate lipid lowering with statins after acute coronary syndromes. N Engl J Med 2004; 350: 1495–504.

27. LaRosa JC, Grundy SM, Waters DD, et al. Intensive lipid lowering with atorvastatin in patients with stable coronary disease. N Engl J Med 2005; 352: 1425–35.

28. Shepherd J, Blauw GJ, Murphy MB, et al. Pravastatin in elderly individuals at risk of vascular disease (PROSPER): a randomised controlled trial. Lancet 2002; 360: 1623–30.

29. Deedwania P, Stone PH, Bairey Merz CN, et al. Effects of intensive versus moderate lipid-lowering therapy on myocardial ischemia in older patients with coronary heart disease: results of the Study Assessing Goals in the Elderly (SAGE). Circulation 2007; 115: 700–7.

30. Baigent C, Blackwell L, Emberson J, et al. Efficacy and safety of more intensive lowering of LDL cholesterol: a meta-analysis of data from 170,000 participants in 26 randomised trials. Lancet 2010; 376: 1670 81.

31. Afilalo J, Duque G, Steele R, et al. Statins for secondary prevention in elderly patients: a hierarchical bayesian meta-analysis. J Am Coll Cardiol 2008; 51: 37–45.

32. Kashani A, Phillips CO, Foody JM, et al. Risks associated with statin therapy: a systematic overview of randomized clinical trials. Circulation 2006; 114: 2788–97.

33. Hsia J, MacFadyen JG, Monyak J, Ridker PM. Cardiovascular event reduction and adverse events among subjects attaining low-density lipoprotein cholesterol <50 mg/dl with rosuvastatin. The JUPITER trial (Justification for the Use of Statins in Prevention: an Intervention Trial Evaluating Rosuvastatin). J Am Coll Cardiol 2011; 57: 1666–75.

34. Nichols GA, Koro CE. Does statin therapy initiation increase the risk for myopathy? An observational study of 32,225 diabetic and nondiabetic patients. Clin Ther 2007; 29: 1761–70.

35. Armitage J. The safety of statins in clinical practice. Lancet 2007; 370: 1781–90.

36. O'Keefe JH Jr, Cordain L, Harris WH, Moe RM, Vogel R. Optimal low-density lipoprotein is 50–70 mg/dl: lower is better and physiologically normal. J Am Coll Cardiol 2004; 43: 2142–6.

37. Athyros VG, Tziomalos K, Gossios TD, et al. Safety and efficacy of long-term statin treatment for cardiovascular events in patients with coronary heart disease and abnormal liver tests in the Greek Atorvastatin and Coronary Heart Disease Evaluation (GREACE) Study: a post-hoc analysis. Lancet 2010; 376: 1916–22.

38. Sattar N, Preiss D, Murray HM, et al. Statins and risk of incident diabetes: a collaborative meta-analysis of randomised statin trials. Lancet 2010; 375: 735–42.

39. McKenney JM, Davidson MH, Jacobson TA, Guyton JR. Final conclusions and recommendations of the National Lipid Association Statin Safety Assessment Task Force. Am J Cardiol 2006; 97: 89C–94C.

40. The Lipid Research Clinics Coronary Primary Prevention Trial results. I. Reduction in incidence of coronary heart disease. JAMA 1984; 251: 351 64.

41. The Lipid Research Clinics Coronary Primary Prevention Trial results. II. The relationship of reduction in incidence of coronary heart disease to cholesterol lowering. JAMA 1984; 251: 365–74.

42. Manttari M, Huttunen JK, Koskinen P, et al. Lipoproteins and coronary heart disease in the helsinki heart study. Eur Heart J 1990; 11: 26–31.

43. Rubins HB, Robins SJ, Collins D, et al. Gemfibrozil for the secondary prevention of coronary heart disease in men with low levels of high-density lipoprotein cholesterol. Veterans Affairs High-Density Lipoprotein Cholesterol Intervention Trial Study Group. N Engl J Med 1999; 341: 410–18.

44. Goldenberg I, Goldbourt U, Boyko V, Behar S, Reicher-Reiss H. Relation between on-treatment increments in serum high-density lipoprotein cholesterol levels and cardiac mortality in patients with coronary heart disease (from the Bezafibrate Infarction Prevention trial). Am J Cardiol 2006; 97: 466–71.

45. Guyton JR. Niacin in cardiovascular prevention: mechanisms, efficacy, and safety. Curr Opin Lipidol 2007; 18: 415–20.

46. Canner PL, Berge KG, Wenger NK, et al. Fifteen year mortality in Coronary Drug Project patients: long-term benefit with niacin. J Am Coll Cardiol 1986; 8: 1245–55.

47. Taylor AJ, Sullenberger LE, Lee HJ, Lee JK, Grace KA. Arterial biology for the investigation of the treatment effects of reducing cholesterol (ARBITER) 2: a double-blind, placebo-controlled study of extended-release niacin on atherosclerosis progression in secondary prevention patients treated with statins. Circulation 2004; 110: 3512–17.

48. Taylor AJ, Villines TC, Stanek EJ, et al. Extended-release niacin or ezetimibe and carotid intima-media thickness. N Engl J Med 2009; 361: 2113–22.
49. Boden WE, Probstfield JL, Anderson T, et al. Niacin in patients with low HDL cholesterol levels receiving intensive statin therapy. N Engl J Med 2011; 365: 2255–67.
50. Goldberg AC, Sapre A, Liu J, Capece R, Mitchel YB. Efficacy and safety of ezetimibe coadministered with simvastatin in patients with primary hypercholesterolemia: a randomized, double-blind, placebo-controlled trial. Mayo Clin Proc 2004; 79: 620–9.
51. Feldman T, Koren M, Insull W Jr, et al. Treatment of high-risk patients with ezetimibe plus simvastatin co-administration versus simvastatin alone to attain National Cholesterol Education Program Adult Treatment Panel III low-density lipoprotein cholesterol goals. Am J Cardiol 2004; 93: 1481–6.
52. Kastelein JJ, Akdim F, Stroes ES, et al. Simvastatin with or without ezetimibe in familial hypercholesterolemia. N Engl J Med 2008; 358: 1431–43.
53. Taylor AJ, Villines TC, Stanek EJ. Paradoxical progression of atherosclerosis related to low-density lipoprotein reduction and exposure to ezetimibe. Eur Heart J 2012.
54. Baigent C, Landray MJ, Reith C, et al. The effects of lowering LDL cholesterol with simvastatin plus ezetimibe in patients with chronic kidney disease (Study of Heart and Renal Protection): a randomised placebo-controlled trial. Lancet 2011; 377: 2181–92.
55. Robinson JG, Rahilly-Tierney C, Lawler E, Gaziano JM. Benefits associated with achieving optimal risk factor levels for the primary prevention of cardiovascular disease in older men. J Clin Lipidol 2012; 6: 58–65.
56. Hunt D, Young P, Simes J, et al. Benefits of pravastatin on cardiovascular events and mortality in older patients with coronary heart disease are equal to or exceed those seen in younger patients: results from the LIPID trial. Ann Intern Med 2001; 134: 931–40.
57. Ali R, Alexander KP. Statins for the primary prevention of cardiovascular events in older adults: a review of the evidence. Am J Geriatr Pharmacother 2007; 5: 52–63.
58. Young-Xu Y, Jabbour S, Goldberg R, et al. Usefulness of statin drugs in protecting against atrial fibrillation in patients with coronary artery disease. Am J Cardiol 2003; 92: 1379–83.
59. Siu CW, Lau CP, Tse HF. Prevention of atrial fibrillation recurrence by statin therapy in patients with lone atrial fibrillation after successful cardioversion. Am J Cardiol 2003; 92: 1343–5.
60. Amarenco P, Bogousslavsky J, Callahan A III, et al. High-dose atorvastatin after stroke or transient ischemic attack. N Engl J Med 2006; 355: 549–59.
61. Briel M, Studer M, Glass TR, Bucher HC. Effects of statins on stroke prevention in patients with and without coronary heart disease: a meta-analysis of randomized controlled trials. Am J Med 2004; 117: 596–606.
62. Anand SS. Quantifying effect of statins on low density lipoprotein cholesterol, ischaemic heart disease, and stroke: systematic review and meta-analysis. Law MR, Wald NJ, Rudnicka AR. BMJ 2003; 326: 1407–408. Vasc Med 2003; 8: 289–90.
63. MRC/BHF Heart Protection Study of cholesterol lowering with simvastatin in 20,536 high-risk individuals: a randomised placebo-controlled trial. Lancet 2002; 360: 7–22.
64. Go AS, Lee WY, Yang J, Lo JC, Gurwitz JH. Statin therapy and risks for death and hospitalization in chronic heart failure. JAMA 2006; 296: 2105–11.
65. Ray JG, Gong Y, Sykora K, Tu JV. Statin use and survival outcomes in elderly patients with heart failure. Arch Intern Med 2005; 165: 62–7.
66. Horwich TB, MacLellan WR, Fonarow GC. Statin therapy is associated with improved survival in ischemic and non-ischemic heart failure. J Am Coll Cardiol 2004; 43: 642–8.
67. Fukuta H, Sane DC, Brucks S, Little WC. Statin therapy may be associated with lower mortality in patients with diastolic heart failure: a preliminary report. Circulation 2005; 112: 357–63.
68. Bauersachs J, Galuppo P, Fraccarollo D, Christ M, Ertl G. Improvement of left ventricular remodeling and function by hydroxymethylglutaryl coenzyme a reductase inhibition with cerivastatin in rats with heart failure after myocardial infarction. Circulation 2001; 104: 982–5.
69. Kjekshus J, Apetrei E, Barrios V, et al. Rosuvastatin in older patients with systolic heart failure. N Engl J Med 2007; 357: 2248–61.
70. Tavazzi L, Maggioni AP, Marchioli R, et al. Effect of rosuvastatin in patients with chronic heart failure (the GISSI-HF trial): a randomised, double-blind, placebo-controlled trial. Lancet 2008; 372: 1231–9.
71. McMurray JJ, Kjekshus J, Gullestad L, et al. Effects of statin therapy according to plasma high-sensitivity C-reactive protein concentration in the Controlled Rosuvastatin Multinational Trial in Heart Failure (CORONA): a retrospective analysis. Circulation 2009; 120: 2188–96.
72. Novaro GM, Tiong IY, Pearce GL, et al. Effect of hydroxymethylglutaryl coenzyme a reductase inhibitors on the progression of calcific aortic stenosis. Circulation 2001; 104: 2205–9.

73. Shavelle DM, Takasu J, Budoff MJ, et al. HMG CoA reductase inhibitor (statin) and aortic valve calcium. Lancet 2002; 359: 1125–6.
74. Cowell SJ, Newby DE, Prescott RJ, et al. A randomized trial of intensive lipid-lowering therapy in calcific aortic stenosis. N Engl J Med 2005; 352: 389–97.
75. Rossebo AB, Pedersen TR, Boman K, et al. Intensive lipid lowering with simvastatin and ezetimibe in aortic stenosis. N Engl J Med 2008; 359: 1343–56.
76. Sica DA, Gehr TW. Rhabdomyolysis and statin therapy: relevance to the elderly. Am J Geriatr Cardiol 2002; 11: 48–55.
77. Santanello NC, Barber BL, Applegate WB, et al. Effect of pharmacologic lipid lowering on health-related quality of life in older persons: results from the Cholesterol Reduction in Seniors Program (CRISP) Pilot Study. J Am Geriatr Soc 1997; 45: 8–14.
78. Wenger NK, Lewis SJ, Herrington DM, Bittner V, Welty FK. Outcomes of using high- or low dose atorvastatin in patients 65 years of age or older with stable coronary heart disease. Ann Intern Med 2007; 147: 1–9.
79. Notkola IL, Sulkava R, Pekkanen J, et al. Serum total cholesterol, apolipoprotein E epsilon 4 allele, and Alzheimer's disease. Neuroepidemiology 1998; 17: 14–20.
80. Kivipelto M, Helkala EL, Hanninen T, et al. Midlife vascular risk factors and late-life mild cognitive impairment: a population-based study. Neurology 2001; 56: 1683–9.
81. Reitz C, Tang MX, Luchsinger J, Mayeux R. Relation of plasma lipids to Alzheimer disease and vascular dementia. Arch Neurol 2004; 61: 705–14.
82. Sparks DL. Coronary artery disease, hypertension, ApoE, and cholesterol: a link to Alzheimer's disease? Ann N Y Acad Sci 1997; 826: 128–46.
83. Hofman A, Ott A, Breteler MM, et al. Atherosclerosis, apolipoprotein E, and prevalence of dementia and Alzheimer's disease in the Rotterdam Study. Lancet 1997; 349: 151–4.
84. Wolozin B, Kellman W, Ruosseau P, Celesia GG, Siegel G. Decreased prevalence of Alzheimer disease associated with 3-hydroxy-3-methyglutaryl coenzyme A reductase inhibitors. Arch Neurol 2000; 57: 1439–43.
85. Hajjar I, Schumpert J, Hirth V, Wieland D, Eleazer GP. The impact of the use of statins on the prevalence of dementia and the progression of cognitive impairment. J Gerontol A Biol Sci Med Sci 2002; 57: M414–18.
86. Rockwood K, Kirkland S, Hogan DB, et al. Use of lipid-lowering agents, indication bias, and the risk of dementia in community-dwelling elderly people. Arch Neurol 2002; 59: 223–7.
87. Yaffe K, Barrett-Connor E, Lin F, Grady D. Serum lipoprotein levels, statin use, and cognitive function in older women. Arch Neurol 2002; 59: 378–84.
88. Dale KM, Coleman CI, Henyan NN, Kluger J, White CM. Statins and cancer risk: a meta-analysis. JAMA 2006; 295: 74–80.
89. Sheppard JP, Singh S, Fletcher K, McManus RJ, Mant J. Impact of age and sex on primary preventive treatment for cardiovascular disease in the West Midlands, UK: cross sectional study. BMJ 2012; 345: e4535.
90. Forman DE, Rich MW, Alexander KP, et al. Cardiac care for older adults. Time for a new paradigm. J Am Coll Cardiol 2011; 57: 1801–10.
91. LaCroix AZ, Gray SL, Aragaki A, et al. Statin use and incident frailty in women aged 65 years or older: prospective findings from the Women's Health Initiative Observational Study. J Gerontol A Biol Sci Med Sci 2008; 63: 369–75.
92. Gray SL, Boudreau RM, Newman AB, et al. Angiotensin-converting enzyme inhibitor and statin use and incident mobility limitation in community-dwelling older adults: the Health, Aging and Body Composition study. J Am Geriatr Soc 2011; 59: 2226–32.
93. Reiner Z, Catapano AL, De Backer G, et al. ESC/EAS Guidelines for the management of dyslipidae-mias: the Task Force for the management of dyslipidaemias of the European Society of Cardiology (ESC) and the European Atherosclerosis Society (EAS). Eur Heart J 2011; 32: 1769–818.
94. Wiviott SD, Cannon CP, Morrow DA, et al. PROVE IT-TIMI 22 Investigators. Can low-density lipoprotein be too low? The safety and efficacy of achieving very low low-density lipoprotein with intensive statin therapy: a PROVE IT-TIMI 22 substudy. J Am Coll Cardiol 2005; 46: 1414.

6
Diabetes mellitus and cardiovascular disease in the elderly

Mark D. Corriere, Rita Rastogi Kalyani, and Samuel C. Durso

SUMMARY

Type 2 diabetes is increasing worldwide and is frequent among older patients. Special care and consideration should be given when caring for older patients with diabetes. Comorbid illness, functional status, and shortened life expectancy are additional considerations that may significantly affect the benefits of diabetes treatments in this population. Poorly controlled diabetes leads to microvascular and macrovascular complications which can both result in significant morbidity and mortality. Evidence shows that tight glycemic control lowers the risk of microvascular complications. Similar findings have not been as definitively shown with macrovascular outcomes. Trials investigating macrovascular outcomes in older patients treated with more aggressive glycemic goals have not shown clear benefit and suggested potential harm. Multiple options exist for the treatment of hyperglycemia in type 2 diabetes. These include oral agents, non-insulin injectables, and insulin therapy. In addition to controlling hyperglycemia, these agents may have positive, negative or neutral cardiovascular-related effects. With an aging population, diabetes among older adults will continue to represent a growing problem. Individualized goals of care for glycemia are often appropriate in this population. It is also important to address cardiovascular risk factor reduction (including anti-platelet therapy, lipid-lowering, and blood pressure control) when managing diabetes in the older patient.

INTRODUCTION

Diabetes mellitus is a growing worldwide concern. In the USA, studies suggest that 12.9% of people aged 20 years and older have diabetes. More concerning is that nearly 40% of these people are unaware of their diagnosis (1). Prevalence is particularly high in older patients. Diabetes prevalence is 30% in people aged 60–74 years and 29.1% in people aged 75 years and older (2). These numbers will continue to grow worldwide. In 2000, it was estimated that the worldwide prevalence of diabetes for all age groups was 2.8%. This number is expected to rise to 4.4% by 2030. Worldwide, 366 million people could be affected at that time with the largest demographic change being the increase in proportion of people >65 years of age with diabetes (3).

In parallel to the rising prevalence of diabetes, the cost of caring for patients with diabetes is also rising. Estimates from 2010 put the average annual cost per case of undiagnosed diabetes at nearly $3000 and of diagnosed diabetes at nearly $10,000 (2). Overall cost estimates for annual diabetes related spending in the USA in 2009 was $113 billion.

Annual spending is expected to nearly triple to an estimation of $336 billion (US) by 2034 (4). A large portion of this spending goes toward treating diabetes related complications, of which cardiovascular complications are a major component. Diabetes confers a nearly twofold excess risk for a wide range of macrovascular diseases. This includes risk of coronary artery disease, ischemic stroke, hemorrhagic stroke, and peripheral vascular disease (5).Cardiovascular complications are associated with both increased morbidity and mortality. This is especially true for older patients who account for more than 70% of diabetes associated deaths (6). With the rising prevalence of diabetes mellitus in older adults, optimally preventing and treating cardiovascular complications in this patient population becomes even more critical.

CLINICAL GUIDELINES FOR MANAGEMENT OF DIABETES IN OLDER ADULTS

Special care and consideration needs to be taken when applying clinical guidelines for diabetes to older patients. The American Geriatrics Society (AGS) guidelines (7) seek to recognize that elderly patients have marked functional and medical heterogeneity that can alter their potential treatment benefits.

The use of a patient-centered care plan for older adults with diabetes has been proposed to address some of the special conditions that make this population unique (8). An initial step includes considering a patient's life expectancy in the presence or absence of unusually good or poor health and function, which may help the clinician and patient assess the likely benefits and risks of different therapeutic choices over time. A second step includes establishing the patient's preferences and goals of care. Many older patients may prefer to maintain independence and perform activities of daily living. This may affect their view of intensive insulin therapy. Multiple injections and self glucose monitoring are required to achieve tight glycemic control, which may be perceived as a threat to the patient's independence and also may not be feasible. Discussions regarding the goals of care early in the course of treatment can help to avoid treatment failures.

Evaluating and managing comorbid geriatric syndromes are important. The AGS guidelines recommend that elderly patients with diabetes be screened for depression within 3 months of diagnosis and again if there is an unexplained decline in clinical status. This recognizes the increased prevalence of depression in older patients and its potential negative effect on diabetes care. Similarly, screening for cognitive impairment is recommended soon after the diagnosis of diabetes and again if a decline in health status occurs. Polypharmacy is a frequent problem for older patients with multiple medical problems and drug–drug interactions frequently need to be considered. Diabetes is associated with a higher prevalence of other common geriatric syndromes such as incontinence, falls, and persistent pain that may affect treatment outcomes (7). Diabetes and insulin resistance are also associated with frailty, a geriatric syndrome of physiological vulnerability to stressors associated with adverse outcomes such as disability, hospitalization, and death (9–14). Evidence suggests that older individuals with severe hyperglycemia and/or insulin resistance are more likely to develop frailty up to a decade later (10,15).

Older patients with diabetes are a unique population for whom an individualized approach to management may be most appropriate. Most clinical guidelines in diabetes are based on studies that have not included older adults. Patient preference, comorbid illness, and functional status should all be taken into account when choosing therapy for the older patient with diabetes. These important factors can help guide intensity of therapy for glycemic control, blood pressure, lipid status, and modification of other cardiovascular risk factors. In older patients, an individualized approach to setting glycemic goals is important. For active, highly functioning older patients with few comorbidities and a life expectancy of greater than 10 years, motivation to achieve a hemoglobin A1C of 7% may be appropriate. However, for older patients with multiple comorbidities, limited functional capacity, and/ or barriers to self management, higher hemoglobin A1C goals may be sufficient to prevent symptoms of hyperglycemia while avoiding the adverse consequences of hypoglycemia. An evolving area of research is exploring the association of hyperglycemia with the development of geriatric syndromes such as frailty, but more studies are needed.

PATHOPHYSIOLOGY OF DIABETES MELLITUS AND INSULIN RESISTANCE

Diabetes mellitus is classified as type 1 (formerly called juvenile onset or insulin dependent diabetes mellitus) and type 2 (formerly called adult onset or noninsulin dependent diabetes mellitus).

Type 1 Diabetes Mellitus

Type 1 diabetes accounts for 5–10% of all patients with diabetes. It results from a cellular mediated autoimmune destruction of the β cells of the pancreas. The disease has a strong HLA association with linkage to the DQA and DQB genes. The immune mediated process generally occurs in childhood and adolescence but can occur as late as the eighth decade of life. Patients with type 1 diabetes are at risk for other autoimmune diseases such as Addison's disease, Graves' disease, Hashimoto's thyroiditis, celiac sprue, vitiligo, and pernicious anemia (16). The importance of genetics in the development of type 1 diabetes is supported by the observation that the incidence is increased in relatives of patients with type 1 diabetes. For children of patients with type 1 diabetes, the lifetime risk for type 1 diabetes is 6%. In families with no history of type 1 diabetes, the risk is only 0.4%. An identical twin has a 30% lifetime risk of developing diabetes, while a sibling or fraternal twin has a 5% risk (17).

Type 2 Diabetes Mellitus

Type 2 diabetes accounts for 90–95% of all patients with diabetes. The pathogenesis of type 2 diabetes is multifactorial. Environmental factors such as diet, obesity, visceral fat, and sedentary lifestyle play a key role in type 2 diabetes. There is also a strong genetic predisposition with first-degree family members (children, siblings) having up to a six times increased risk for developing type 2 diabetes compared to those with a negative family history (18). However, the genetic factors are complex and not clearly defined. Type 2 diabetes results from a combination of insulin resistance (exacerbated by obesity and sedentary lifestyle) and relative insulin deficiency. Unlike type 1 diabetes, there is no pancreatic β cell destruction and patients with type 2 diabetes do not require insulin therapy to survive (at least not initially). Over time, and with increasing insulin resistance, β cell function worsens and can no longer compensate in the majority of patients. This leads to relative insulin deficiency and ultimately requires exogenous insulin therapy. Ketoacidosis rarely occurs in this type of diabetes. This form of diabetes may go undiagnosed for many years because the hyperglycemia develops gradually (16).

COMPLICATIONS OF DIABETES MELLITUS
Pathophysiologic Changes

The complications of diabetes mellitus have been traditionally divided into two major categories: (*i*) microvascular complications including retinopathy, neuropathy, and nephropathy and (*ii*) macrovascular complications including coronary artery disease, cerebrovascular disease, and peripheral vascular disease.

Microvascular Complications

Diabetic microvascular complications lead to significant morbidity and cost. Diabetes mellitus is the leading cause of chronic kidney disease and can lead to the need for dialysis. Diabetic retinopathy is a leading cause of potentially reversible blindness. Further, diabetic neuropathy can lead to chronic pain, infections, and limb loss or even amputations in severe cases. However, microvascular complications are avoidable with optimal diabetic care.

The Diabetes Control and Complications Trial (DCCT) (19) demonstrated a delay in the onset and progression of diabetic neuropathy, retinopathy, and nephropathy by up to 70% with intensive treatment of type 1 diabetes. The United Kingdom Prospective Diabetes Study (UKPDS) evaluated intensive blood glucose control in patients with new onset of type 2 diabetes (20). The intensive blood glucose control group in UKPDS achieved a mean glycosylated hemoglobin of 7%, compared to the standard therapy group value of 7.9%, and showed a reduction in the risk of microvascular complications, principally through a reduction in incident photocoagulation of retinopathy and in reduction of progression to albuminuria (21,22). An important limitation of both the DCCT and UKPDS studies is that older persons with diabetes were excluded, which some authors argue may affect generalizability of these findings to the elderly population (23).

Macrovascular Complications

Diabetes mellitus is associated with atherosclerosis which is likely related to the presence of chronic hyperglycemia, insulin resistance, and dyslipidemia. Both hyperglycemia and insulin resistance impair endothelium-dependent vasodilation by decreasing nitric oxide formation (24). Increased levels of endothelin-1 in patients with diabetes stimulate vasoconstriction, induce vascular smooth muscle hypertrophy, and activate the renin–angiotensin system (25). Diabetes promotes the accumulation of foam cells in the subendothelial space by increasing the production of leukocyte adhesion molecules and proinflammatory mediators (26). Plaque instability and rupture is increased in diabetes as a result of decreased synthesis and increased breakdown of the collagen that plays a critical role in reinforcing the fibrous cap of vulnerable plaques (27,28).

In addition to the atherosclerotic effects of diabetes upon the arterial wall, the hematologic system is adversely affected. Diabetes promotes platelet activation by increasing platelet-surface expression of glycoprotein Ib that mediates binding to the glycoprotein IIb/IIIa (GPIIb/IIIa) receptor and to the von Willebrand factor (29). Inhibitors of platelet activity, including platelet-derived nitric oxide and endothelial prostacyclin, are decreased in diabetes. Diabetes also increases coagulation activity by stimulating production of procoagulants such as tissue factor and by reducing levels of anticoagulants such as protein C and antithrombin III (30,31). Furthermore, decreased levels of plasminogen activator type 1 in diabetes result in impaired fibrinolysis (32).

The clinical consequences of these blood vessel changes are an increase in the incidence of atherosclerotic disease in the form of coronary artery disease, stroke, and peripheral vascular disease. Despite the risk associated with hyperglycemia, the relationship of intensive glucose control to reduction of macrovascular events has not been established. Both the DCCT and UKPDS did not demonstrate a significant reduction in macrovascular events at the time of their initial reports. However, long-term follow up of these cohorts has provided data on macrovascular outcomes. The DCCT/Epidemiology of Diabetes Interventions and Complications Study (EDICS) was an observational study that followed participants from the initial DCCT (33). After a mean of 6.5 years of intensive versus standard glucose control during the DCCT, the standard glucose control group participants were offered intensive treatment and all participants returned to their own health care providers. The difference in hemoglobin A1C dissipated in the 11 years of follow up to 8% in the previous intensively treated group and 8.2% in the previous standard treatment group. During follow up, there was a significant 42% relative risk reduction of any cardiovascular disease event in the intensively treated group. The mean age of participants at follow-up was 45 years.

Similar findings with regard to cardiovascular complications were seen in the 10-year follow-up of the UKPDS (34). One year after the original UKPDS was completed, the hemoglobin A1C differences between the intensively treated and conventional therapy groups had dissipated. At 10-year follow-up, the intensively treated insulin/sulfonylurea arm had a significant 15% relative risk reduction for myocardial infarction compared to the conventional treatment group. A significant 33% relative risk reduction of myocardial infarction was found in the intensively treated metformin arm compared to the conventional treatment group. Of note, the mean ages of participants in the UKPDS follow-up study was 63 years.

GLYCEMIC CONTROL FOR MACROVASCULAR AND MICROVASCULAR RISK REDUCTION

Long-term data from the DCCT and UKPDS suggest that intensive glycemic control, for at least a period of time, may lower the risk of diabetic related cardiovascular disease events. Additionally, epidemiologic and meta-analyses showed a direct relationship between hemoglobin A1C and cardiovascular disease (35,36). Three clinical trials (ACCORD, ADVANCE, and VADT) were undertaken in an attempt to demonstrate prospectively that intensive glycemic control in type 2 diabetes decreases cardiovascular events (Table 6.1). In contrast to the older studies, these newer trials did not exclude older persons with diabetes.

The Action to Control Cardiovascular Risk in Diabetes (ACCORD) study investigated 10,252 older patients with type 2 diabetes (mean age 62 years) (37). These patients

Table 6.1 Findings from Clinical Trials Investigating the Benefits of Intensive Glycemic Control in Older Adults

	ACCORD	ADVANCE	VADT
Mean age (yr)	62	66	60
Duration of diabetes (yr)	10	8	11.5
History of CV disease	35%	32%	40%
Median baseline A1C	8.1%	7.2%	9.4%
Median duration of follow up (yr)	3.5 (terminated early)	5	5.6
Achieved median A1C intensive versus standard	6.4% vs. 7.5%	6.3% vs. 7.0%	6.9% vs. 8.5%
Definition of primary outcome	Nonfatal MI, nonfatal stroke, CVD death	Microvascular plus macrovascular (nonfatal MI, nonfatal stroke, CVD death) outcomes	Nonfatal MI, nonfatal stroke, CVD death, hospitalization for heart failure, revascularization
HR for primary outcome (95% CI)	0.90 (0.78–1.04)	0.9 (0.82–0.98); macrovascular 0.94 (0.84–1.06)	0.88 (0.74–1.05)
HR for mortality findings (95% CI)	1.22 (1.01–1.46)	0.93 (0.83–1.06)	1.07 (0.81–1.42)

Abbreviations: CVD, cardiovascular disease; A1C, hemoglobin A1C; MI, myocardial infarction; HR, hazard ratio; CI, confidence interval.
Source: Adapted from Ref. 41.

were at high risk for cardiovascular disease with 35% having a history of previous cardio-vascular event and the remaining patients having at least two cardiovascular risk factors. Study participants had a history of type 2 diabetes for a mean of 10 years and a mean base-line hemoglobin A1C of 8.2%. They were randomized to an intensive glycemic control group targeting an A1C of <6% or standard glycemic control group targeting an A1C of 7–7.9%. At 1 year, the intensive glycemic control group had achieved a hemoglobin A1C of 6.4% compared to 7.5% in the standard glycemic control group. The study was halted at a mean of 3.5-years follow-up due to the finding of overall increased mortality in the inten-sively treated group. At the time the study was stopped, the primary composite outcome (nonfatal myocardial infarction, nonfatal stroke, or death from cardiovascular cause) occurred in similar numbers in both groups. However, the overall number of deaths was significantly higher in the intensively treated group compared to the standard glycemic control group (257 deaths intensive group vs. 203 deaths standard care group, hazard ratio, 1.22; 95% CI, 1.01–1.46; $p = 0.04$). As expected, episodes of hypoglycemia were more common in the intensively treated group. Unrecognized and untreated hypoglycemia and its sequalae have been proposed as a potential mechanism to explain the excess mortality. A follow up to the ACCORD study reported findings of 5 years from randomization (38). After the study was halted, the intensive and standard glycemic control groups reached similar hemoglobin A1C values and had similar frequencies of hypoglycemia. However, the finding of increased overall mortality in the intensive glycemic control group persisted through this follow-up period.

Similarly, the Veterans Affairs Diabetes Trial (VADT) was designed to evaluate intensive versus standard glycemic control on cardiovascular events in type 2 diabetes (39). The study population was 1791 predominantly older men (mean age 60.4 years) with sig-nificant cardiovascular risk (40% already had a cardiovascular event). The intensive glyce-mic control group achieved a hemoglobin A1C of 6.9% compared to 8.4% in the standard glycemic control group. After a mean of 5.6 years of follow up, no difference between the groups was seen regarding cardiovascular events. Unlike the ACCORD study, no differ-ence in overall mortality was seen between the two groups. There were 95 deaths in the standard glycemic control group compared to 102 in the intensive therapy group (hazard ratio, 1.07; 95% CI, 0.81–1.42; $p = 0.62$).

The Action in Diabetes and Vascular Disease (ADVANCE) study looked at a similar population of 11,140 patients with type 2 diabetes (40). Study participants were older (mean age 66 years) with a mean baseline hemoglobin A1C of 7.2%. One-third of the population had a history of vascular disease at baseline with the remaining two thirds having multiple risk factors. Patients were randomized to intensive glycemic control or standard glycemic control. The groups achieved mean hemoglobin A1Cs of 6.5% and 7.3% respectively. After a mean follow-up of 5 years, there was no difference between the two groups in the rate of macrovascular events or death from cardiovascular causes. Similar to the VADT, there was no difference in overall mortality between the intensive and standard glycemic control groups. A total of 1031 deaths occurred, including 8.9% in the intensive control group and 9.6% in the standard control group (hazard ratio, 0.93; 95% CI, 0.83–1.06; $p = 0.28$).

Given the findings of the ACCORD, VADT, and ADVANCE studies, the clinical prac-tice of intensive glycemic control for the prevention of cardiovascular disease in type 2 dia-betes has been debated. The American Diabetes Association (ADA), American College of Cardiologists, and American Heart Association published a joint statement on this topic (41). Subset analyses of ACCORD, VADT, and ADVANCE suggest that patients with a shorter duration of type 2 diabetes and without history of cardiovascular disease might gain greatest benefit in macrovascular disease risk reduction from intensive control. Alternatively, the risks of intensive glycemic control (hypoglycemia in particular) may outweigh benefits in patients with a long standing history of diabetes, frequent hypoglycemia, advanced cardiovascular disease, or older age. Recent recommendations from the ADA recognize the decision to achieve intensive control is not always clear (42). The guidelines recommend achieving a hemoglobin A1C <7% in adults to reduce microvascular complications and particularly in patients recently diagnosed due to association with long-term reduction in macrovascular disease. A less stringent hemoglobin A1C goal of <8% may be appropriate for patients with a history of severe hypoglycemia, advanced microvascular or macrovascular complications, or with limited life expectancy. Findings from trials suggest that too aggressive glucose control (i.e., <6%) may not be beneficial and, in fact, may be harmful.

VASCULAR CONSEQUENCES OF DIABETES MELLITUS
Coronary Artery Disease
The Framingham Study demonstrated that diabetes is a powerful predictor of Coronary Artery Disease (CAD) (43). The older patient with diabetes is at particularly high risk for CAD; in one study 44% of octogenarians with diabetes were found to have CAD (44).

Many patients with diabetes have CAD that is clinically unapparent. This was demonstrated in a population based autopsy series that characterized coronary atherosclerosis in 293 persons with diabetes (mean age of 73 years), without clinically known CAD. Nearly 75% had high grade coronary atherosclerosis and more than half had multivessel disease (45). In addition to clinically undiagnosed CAD, there is an increased prevalence of silent ischemia and unrecognized MI with diabetes. In a French study, the prevalence of silent ischemia was found to be approximately 30% in men with type 2 diabetes and established CAD, while the prevalence in patients without diabetes was 1–4% (46). Specifically looking at older patients, the Framingham epidemiological study reports an increased incidence of asymptomatic MI in this population (47). A study by Aronow and Epstein demonstrated silent ischemia through Holter monitoring in about one-third of older patients (48). Given the high prevalence of silent ischemia in the elderly and in diabetes, older patients with diabetes present a particularly high-risk population for silent ischemia.

However, at this time, the ADA recommends against routine screening for CAD in asymptomatic patients. Screening has not been shown to improve outcomes in patients who are already being treated with optimized cardiovascular risk factor modifications (42).

Acute Coronary Syndromes
MI rates are increased among people with diabetes of all ages (49). For example, in a population based study the 7-year incidence of first MI was 20% for type 2 diabetes but only 3.5% for people without diabetes (50). Short- and long-term outcomes following MI are worsened in patients with diabetes (51). The Framingham Study determined that the overall risk of cardiac mortality, particularly post-MI, was two to three times higher in people with diabetes compared to those without diabetes.

The explanation for the worse prognosis among people with diabetes is not entirely clear. Diabetes is associated with complicated metabolic changes and alterations in coagulation parameters that may predispose to worse outcomes (52). People with diabetes tend to have fewer collateral vessels compared to those without diabetes and may have more diffuse coronary disease (53).

Stroke
The Framingham Study and others have demonstrated that the risk of stroke is increased 1.5–4 times for patients with diabetes (54). Hypertension, a frequent comorbidity with diabetes, additionally increases the risk for stroke. A Finnish study prospectively followed nearly 50,000 patients without a history of stroke or CAD for incident stroke over a mean

follow-up of 19 years (55). The hazard ratio for stroke was 1.98 for patients with stage II hypertension, 2.54 for patients with diabetes, and 4.50 for patients with both stage II hypertension and diabetes. Similar to post-MI prognosis, diabetes is also associated with a worse prognosis after stroke. In the same Finnish study, the hazard ratio for stroke mortality was 3.06 for patients with diabetes. This hazard ratio climbed to 9.27 in patients with both diabetes and stage II hypertension.

HEART FAILURE AND LEFT VENTRICULAR DYSFUNCTION

The importance of diabetes as a risk factor for heart failure (HF) was first established in the Framingham Heart Study. Among participants between the ages of 45 and 75 years, the frequency of HF was increased in both men and women with diabetes (56). Approximately 15–25% of HF patients in large clinical trials and up to 30% of hospitalized HF patients have diabetes as a comorbid condition (57,58). Traditional risk factors for HF (hypertension and coronary artery disease) have a high prevalence among patients with diabetes. However, even people with diabetes who lack these other traditional risk factors have a higher incidence of HF.

The term "diabetic cardiomyopathy" is defined as ventricular dysfunction occurring independently of a recognized cause such as coronary artery disease or hypertension (59). The Strong Heart Study demonstrated some of the structural changes that patients with diabetes experience. Patients with diabetes had higher left ventricular mass, wall thickness, and arterial stiffness compared to patients without diabetes. These findings were independent of body mass index or blood pressure (60). Additionally, a large epidemiologic study involving over 800,000 patients showed diabetes to be independently associated with the occurrence of HF after adjusting for left ventricular hypertrophy, hypertension, coronary artery disease, and atrial fibrillation (61).

Traditional therapies for HF used in patients without diabetes are appropriate for patients with diabetes. This includes use of angiotensin-converting enzyme (ACE) inhibitors, β-blockers, and statins (59). Additionally, glycemic control is a potential therapeutic avenue to prevent and treat HF. For each 1% elevation in hemoglobin A1C, the risk of developing HF increases by 8% (62). Early in the course of cardiomyopathy, good glycemic control can improve diastolic function and myocardial perfusion (63).

PERIPHERAL ARTERY DISEASE

Peripheral artery disease (PAD) is common among patients with diabetes. The Hoorn Study found the prevalence of ankle brachial index <0.9 in patients with normal glucose tolerance to be 7% compared to 20.9% in patients with diabetes (64). PAD presents at an earlier age and progresses more rapidly in patients with diabetes compared to patients without diabetes. Patients with diabetes may not be offered revascularization procedures as readily as those without diabetes and when they do undergo procedures, they tend to have a poorer prognosis and a higher risk of undergoing amputation (65). PAD may also go largely undiagnosed and untreated in diabetes until the late stages. This is due to a potential lack of claudication symptoms which can be masked by diabetic neuropathy. One of the most important risk factors for PAD in patients with diabetes is increasing age. This has been correlated with PAD in both type 1 and type 2 diabetes (66).

Treatment and management of PAD in diabetes is largely similar to treatment in the non-diabetes population. Hallmarks of therapy should include lifestyle and risk factor modification. Smoking cessation, blood pressure control, and treatment of dyslipidemia have all been shown to be effective therapies. Tight glycemic control has been investigated as a potential therapeutic method but has not been conclusively shown to lower the risk of PAD (34). Antiplatelet therapy with aspirin or clopidogrel is usually indicated. Regular walking to the point of calf discomfort is the primary treatment for symptomatic claudication. Cilostazol is also effective in reducing symptoms, either alone or in combination with walking. Finally, revascularization such as stenting or bypass grafting should be considered for disabling claudication or critical limb ischemia (66).

MANAGEMENT OF ACUTE CORONARY SYNDROMES IN PATIENTS WITH DIABETES MELLITUS

Few studies have addressed specifically the impact of modern medical therapies for acute coronary syndromes (ACS) in patients with diabetes. Subgroup analyses, however, of several clinical trials suggest a generally consistent beneficial effect of modern therapies in this population. The management of ACS is similar for older patients with and without diabetes with a few considerations, as noted below. Three major issues will be considered here: (*i*) optimal reperfusion therapy for ST-elevation MI (STEMI), (*ii*) early invasive versus early conservative management of unstable angina and non-ST-elevation MI (UA/NSTEMI), and (*iii*) adjunctive antiplatelet pharmacotherapy and its applicability to older patients with diabetes and ACS.

REPERFUSION THERAPY FOR STEMI
Thrombolytic Therapy

Thrombolytic therapy (TT) for STEMI has been shown to be equally or more beneficial in patients with diabetes compared to those without diabetes. The Fibrinolytic Therapy Trialists (FTT) overview found a statistically greater mortality benefit in the diabetes group: 37 lives saved per 1000 treated patients with diabetes compared with 15 lives saved per 1000 treated patients without diabetes (67). Concerns about possible TT related increased ocular hemorrhagic complications because of underlying diabetic retinopathy have not been substantiated (68). The beneficial effects of TT in the elderly (>75 years of age) are uncertain with conflicting results showing potential benefit and harm in this population (67,69–71). The use of this form of reperfusion therapy in elderly patients with and without diabetes remains controversial.

Primary Percutaneous Coronary Intervention

Acute success rates with primary percutaneous coronary intervention (PCI) are comparable in the presence or absence of diabetes, although the restenosis and long-term mortality rates may be higher in patients with diabetes (72,73). An observational study comparing early and late outcomes of PCI and TT of patients with diabetes and STEMI concluded that PCI was associated with reduced early and late adverse outcomes relative to TT (74). However, mortality was similar in both groups. In this study, over one-third of the patients were 65 years or older.

Management of UA/NSTEMI

Beginning with the Thrombolysis in MI (TIMI) III study of early invasive versus early conservative management of UA, subgroup analyses of several randomized controlled trials have demonstrated a consistent, modest benefit of early invasive therapy in older patients (aged >65 years) and patients with diabetes. In the Fast Revascularization During Instability in Coronary Artery Disease (FRISC) II trial (75), reduction in the composite endpoint of death and nonfatal MI among those assigned to the early invasive group resulted entirely from the benefit realized by the subgroup over age 65. The TIMI 18 study compared outcomes of ACS patients treated with an early invasive strategy or a more conservative strategy of catheterization only if the patient demonstrated ischemia. Although no clear survival benefit was demonstrated, subgroup analysis showed that both patients over age 65 and patients with diabetes assigned to the early invasive strategy realized significant risk reductions in endpoints (76).

Adjunctive Antiplatelet Therapies in ACS

The beneficial effects of aspirin in ACS have been conclusively demonstrated in many studies. Several studies have shown that patients with either type 1 or type 2 diabetes mellitus have a prothrombotic state including enhanced platelet aggregation in response to various stimuli (77,78), and that agents that inhibit platelet aggregation in vivo consistently reduce the incidence of thrombotic events.

Platelet aggregation is enhanced in patients with diabetes and GPIIb/IIIa inhibitors given in addition to aspirin have been shown to improve outcomes in UA/NSTEMI. These agents have been shown to be particularly effective in patients with diabetes, likely owing to the enhanced platelet aggregation of this population. Clopidogrel was shown in the Clopidogrel in Unstable Angina to Prevent Recurrent Ischemic Events (CURE) trial to improve long-term outcomes when administered for 3–9 months to patients with UA/NSTEMI who did not undergo PCI (79). Improved outcomes were demonstrated in patients over the age of 65 years and in patients with diabetes.

The use of triple antiplatelet therapy (aspirin–clopidogrel–GPIIb/IIIa inhibitors) in older diabetes patients with ACS has raised concerns because of the increased risk of bleeding. Despite these concerns, results obtained in patients with diabetes undergoing PCI and receiving triple antiplatelet therapy in clinical trials suggest that such therapy is probably warranted in older patients with diabetes and ACS unless major contraindications exist (80).

MANAGEMENT OF CHRONIC ISCHEMIC HEART DISEASE
Medical Therapy Vs. Revascularization

All patients with diabetes and chronic ischemia are recommended to receive maximal medical therapy. However, controversy exists regarding if and when revascularization should be performed in these patients. Considering high-risk patients with severe angina, early revascularization has been shown to be beneficial (81). Appropriate management of patients with less severe disease is not as clear. The Clinical Outcomes Utilizing Revascularization and Aggressive Drug Evaluation (COURAGE) trial showed that in patients with stable coronary artery disease, initial management by PCI did not improve outcomes when added to optimal medical therapy (82). These results were similar in prespecified subgroups of patients with and without diabetes. The Bypass Angioplasty Revascularization Investigation 2 Diabetes Study (BARI-2D) study was designed in part to help answer the question if and when to revascularize, specifically in patients with diabetes. BARI 2D enrolled patients with type 2 diabetes who had documented coronary ischemia and at least one significant angiographic stenosis (83). Participants were evaluated prior to randomization by a local cardiologist to determine if they could be managed by initial medical therapy alone or by revascularization plus medical therapy. This led to the exclusion of patients with severe unstable angina or left main disease with left ventricular dysfunction that required immediate revascularization and for whom medical therapy alone was not an option. Once enrolled in the study and randomized, cardiologists selected the most appropriate revascularization method [PCI or coronary artery bypass grafting (CABG)] based on clinical and angiographic features for the group randomized to medical therapy plus revascularization. Comparing the medical therapy and medical therapy/revascularization groups, 5 year mortality (12% vs. 12%, $p = 0.97$) and cardiovascular event rates (23% vs. 24%, $p = 0.70$) were similar. The findings in type 2 diabetes patients were similar to the overall results from the COURAGE trial where early revascularization was not better than intensive medical management.

Revascularization: CABG Vs. PCI

Revascularization for the management of patients with diabetes and high-risk coronary anatomy or severe angina may be necessary. Debate exists over which type of revascularization, CABG versus PCI, should be utilized in treating these patients.

The original BARI study provided guidance to this important clinical question. The study randomly assigned 1829 patients (most with unstable angina and multivessel disease) to CABG or PCI. In 1996, this trial reported no overall difference in the rates of death and MI when comparing the two treatment arms (84). However, in the diabetes subgroup analysis, there was a better 5.4 year survival with CABG versus PCI (76% vs. 56%; $p = 0.0011$). This was due to reduced cardiac mortality with CABG versus PCI (5.8% vs. 20.6%, $p = 0.0003$). The beneficial findings from CABG were largely confined to patients who received at least one internal mammary artery graft (85). The improved survival among patients with diabetes treated with CABG persisted at 10-year follow-up (CABG 57.8% vs. PCI 45.5%, $p = 0.025$) (86).

Two studies have reported initial 1 year outcome data comparing CABG versus PCI in diabetes. The Coronary Artery Revascularization in Diabetes (CARDia) study randomized 510 patients with diabetes and multivessel or complex single vessel CAD to CABG or PCI (87). At 1 year, the composite rates for death, stroke, or MI were similar in the CABG versus PCI groups (10.5% vs. 13%, $p = 0.39$). However, the PCI group experienced a higher rate of late MI (1.2% CABG vs. 5.5% PCI, $p = 0.016$) and a higher rate of revascularization at 1 year (2% CABG vs. 11.8% PCI, $p \leq 0.001$). The Synergy between Percutaneous Coronary Intervention with Taxus and Cardiac Surgery (SYNTAX) study compared 1 year outcomes among CABG and PCI (with paclitaxel stents) in 1800 patients (88). These patients had complex left main or three vessel disease. There was a mix of patients with and without diabetes. In subgroup analysis of the 452 patients with diabetes, the composite end point of death, stroke, and MI at 1 year was comparable between the CABG and PCI treated groups. Even though the groups were similar for the composite endpoint, the PCI group had a higher 1 year major adverse cardiac and cerebrovascular event rate (26% PCI vs. 14% CABG, $p = 0.003$). This was driven by an increased rate of repeat revascularization with PCI compared to CABG (20.3% PCI vs. 6.4% CABG, $p < 0.001$).

Taken together, these studies suggest that CABG may have some advantages over PCI in patients with diabetes. Longer term follow up from studies such as CARDia and SYNTAX will likely help further delineate advantages and disadvantages of both types of revascularization in patients with diabetes

MEDICAL THERAPY FOR CARDIOVASCULAR DISEASE
Aspirin for Primary Prevention
Aspirin has been shown to have beneficial effects for primary prevention of cardiovascular disease among the general population. The Antithrombotic Trialist's (ATT) Collaboration meta-analysis (89), which included over 95,000 patients, demonstrated a 12% reduction in risk of vascular events (Relative Risk 0.88, 95% CI 0.82–0.94). The ATT meta-analysis included only a modest number of patients with diabetes (~4000), but risk reduction was similar for both diabetic and non-diabetic patients. Conversely, two randomized placebo-controlled trials examined the role of aspirin for primary prevention of cardiovascular disease in patients with diabetes (90,91), but neither trial demonstrated an overall benefit for preventing CAD or stroke.

Aspirin is also a drug that has the potential to cause harm. In patients with and without diabetes, low dose aspirin (75–162 mg/daily) is associated with an absolute risk of hemorrhagic stroke of ~1 in 10,000 people annually (92). Additional risk for gastrointestinal bleeding exists with the use of aspirin.

Given the potential risks of aspirin and negative findings in primary prevention studies in patients with diabetes, caution should be exercised when deciding which patients with diabetes should be treated with aspirin for primary prevention. The American Diabetes Association, American Heart Association, and American College of Cardiology

Foundation addressed this question with a consensus position statement (93). As an initial step, assessment of the 10-year risk of developing cardiovascular disease is recommended prior to deciding whether to prescribe aspirin for primary prevention. Risk assessment can be performed using Framingham risk calculators or other risk calculators (i.e., UKPDS Risk Engine: http://www.dtu.ox.ac.uk/riskengine/index.php or the Atherosclerosis Risk in Communities CAD Risk Calculator: http://www.aricnews.net/riskcalc/html/RC1.html).

Patients with a 10-year risk of cardiovascular disease >10% and no increased risk of bleeding (no previous gastrointestinal bleed, peptic ulcer disease, or concurrent use of high-risk medicines such as NSAIDs or warfarin) should be treated with low dose aspirin (75–162 mg/daily). This encompasses most men over age 50 and women over age 60 with one additional major risk factor such as smoking, hypertension, hyperlipidemia, albuminuria, or family history of premature cardiovascular disease.

In considering the older patient with diabetes, caution should be exercised prior to the initiation of aspirin. A thorough history should be taken to assess the risk for gastrointestinal bleeding. The prevalence of atrial fibrillation rises with age, and concurrent use of warfarin and aspirin places these patients at increased risk for bleeding. Older patients may also be prone to falls and dual therapy anticoagulation such as aspirin and warfarin could have adverse effects in an older patient after a fall. These factors should be considered prior to initiation of aspirin in the elderly patient with diabetes.

Hypertension and Diabetes Mellitus

Patients with diabetes have an increased prevalence of hypertension and, conversely, hypertensive patients have an increased incidence of impaired glucose tolerance and demonstrate increased insulin release following an oral glucose load (42,94). More than seven million people in the USA have both hypertension and diabetes, and the association between these risk factors and cardiovascular disease becomes stronger with advancing age. Epidemiological studies have demonstrated that hypertension increases the risk of atherosclerotic vascular disease in patients with diabetes more than in patients without diabetics. The Systolic Hypertension in the Elderly Program (SHEP) found almost twofold increases in the 5-year rates of major cardiovascular events, coronary events, and strokes among patients with versus without diabetes in the placebo group (95). Randomized controlled trials have shown benefit with reduction in cardiovascular events, stroke, and nephropathy with treatment of hypertension in both patients with and without diabetes (96,97).

Because of the high prevalence, increased morbidity, and apparent benefits of treatment, patients with diabetes should be aggressively screened and treated for hypertension. The ADA recommends that blood pressure be measured at every clinic visit with a goal blood pressure of <130/80 (42). Lifestyle modifications such as exercise and the Dietary Approach to Stop Hypertension (DASH) diet may be effective for patients in the pre-hypertensive range (120–139/80–89). Generally, patients with blood pressures >140/90 require drug therapy and the majority of patients require multidrug therapy to achieve adequate control.

Drug therapy regimens often include ACE inhibitors or angiotensin II receptor blockers (ARB). The Heart Outcomes Prevention Evaluation (HOPE) trial investigated the effect of ramipril versus placebo in 9297 high-risk patients of 55 years or older with evidence of vascular disease or diabetes plus one other cardiovascular risk factor (98). Patients with diabetes made up 38% and 39% of the treatment and placebo groups, respectively. Ramipril was found to significantly reduce the rate of MI, stroke, or death from cardiovascular causes compared to placebo. The beneficial effects of treatment with ramipril were consistently observed in patient both with and without diabetes. In patients unable to tolerate ACE inhibitors due to cough, ARBs are an appropriate substitute. Similar to ACE inhibitors, ARBs provide protection from diabetic nephropathy. The Ongoing Telmisartan Alone and in Combination with Ramipril Trial

(ONTARGET) evaluated a high risk patient population with underlying vascular disease or diabetes with end organ damage that was similar to the HOPE trial population (99). The effects of telmisartan versus ramipril versus combination telmisartan/ramipril were compared. The impact of therapy on patients with diabetes was not a primary outcome in ONTARGET but of the 25,620 individuals enrolled in the study, 38% ($n = 9612$) had diabetes. In the overall population, the primary end point of CV death, MI, stroke, or hospitalization for HF was reached by 1412 patients in the ramipril group (16.5%), compared with 1423 patients in the telmisartan group (16.7%; risk ratio: 1.01; 95% CI: 0.94–1.09). Combination therapy of ramipril and telmisartan increased the rate of the primary end points. These data suggest that ARBs are a viable alternative to ACE inhibitors for providing cardiovascular protection to patients with diabetes.

Other agents are also useful for treatment of hypertension in diabetes. The Antihypertensive and Lipid Lowering Treatment to Prevent Heart Attack (ALLHAT) trial included over 33,000 patients among whom over 35% had type 2 diabetes (100). This large trial compared a thiazide diuretic (chlorthalidone), calcium channel blocker (amlodipine), and ACE inhibitor (lisinopril). Because chlorthalidone was at least as effective as the other agents in preventing cardiovascular events and is less costly, ALLHAT supports the use of this agent as first line therapy for hypertension. In general, the drugs commonly used to treat hypertension (β-blockers, calcium channel blockers, ACE inhibitors, and diuretics) are effective in patients with diabetes (101).

Although treating hypertension in patients with diabetes is beneficial, the degree to which blood pressure should be lowered is not clear. The ADA guidelines recommend a blood pressure goal of <130/80. To explore whether more intensive blood pressure control is associated with proportionally greater cardiovascular benefits, the ACCORD Study group followed 4733 patients with type 2 diabetes at high risk for cardiovascular disease (102). Participants were randomized to intensive blood pressure control (target systolic <120 mm Hg) or standard blood pressure control (target systolic <140 mm Hg). By 1 year the intensive therapy group had achieved a systolic pressure of 119.3 mm Hg compared to 133.5 mm Hg in the standard therapy arm. Over a mean follow-up of 4.7 years, no difference was seen between the two groups in the rate of fatal and nonfatal cardiovascular events. However, the intensive therapy group experienced significantly more adverse events (hypotension, hyperkalemia, and bradycardia) compared to the standard therapy group.

When treating hypertension in older patients with diabetes, consideration should be given to their increased risk of falls and potential adverse reactions to antihypertensive medications. Autonomic dysfunction is a common complication of diabetes. Cardiovascular autonomic dysfunction may be present in up to one-third of patients with type 2 diabetes (103). This can manifest clinically as abnormal heart rate fluctuations with variations in peripheral vascular tone, ultimately contributing to orthostatic hypotension. As a result, antihypertensive therapy should be titrated gradually to minimize complications (7). Screening for falls and orthostasis is important before and during antihypertensive treatment. Given the lack of additional benefit seen in the ACCORD Study to intensive blood pressure control, a target of <140/80 seem appropriate for most older patients. The American College of Cardiology Foundation and American Heart Association published consensus guidelines for hypertension in the elderly (104). Their recommendations included less stringent goals (BP < 145/90) in patients >80 years of age recognizing a potential harm with more aggressive treatment.

Lipid Disorders and Diabetes Mellitus

Patients with diabetes commonly have two lipid disorders that must be considered. The first is an elevated low-density lipoprotein (LDL) cholesterol level. This leads to atherogenesis and contributes to plaque rupture and acute coronary events. The second is atherogenic dyslipidemia, which is characterized by increased triglyceride levels, depressed high-density lipoprotein (HDL) levels, and normal to mildly increased LDL levels but increased levels of small dense (easily oxidizable) LDL particles. Both these disorders are associated with progressive atherosclerosis and increased incidence of cardiovascular events (105,106).

Multiple clinical trials have demonstrated the beneficial effects of statin therapy on CV outcomes in patients with diabetes and history of CAD and have suggested potential benefits in primary prevention for CV disease (107). The Collaborative Atorvastatin Diabetes Study evaluated the use of atorvastatin for primary prevention of CV disease in patients with type 2 diabetes. The trial was stopped 2 years early when a prespecified early stopping rule for efficacy was met. The atorvastatin treated patients demonstrated a 37% relative risk reduction in major cardiovascular events compared to placebo. This trial and others support the use of statin therapy in patients with diabetes to lower their LDL. The use of HDL raising therapies (specifically niacin) is less promising. A systematic review in 2007 evaluated 31 trials looking at therapies to raise HDL and found only modest evidence to support aggressively raising HDL beyond what can be achieved with lifestyle modifications alone (108). Fibrates have also been evaluated as potential therapeutic agents to treat dyslipidemia in patients with diabetes. The Fenofibrate Intervention and Event Lowering in Diabetes (FIELD) study examined the long-term use of fenofibrate in patients with type 2 diabetes. Use of fenofibrate in this population with diabetes and no statin use at entry was not associated with a reduction in overall cardiovascular outcomes (109).

Because of the high prevalence of dyslipidemia and the proven benefits of statin therapy, the ADA recommends measuring a fasting lipid profile at least annually in patients with diabetes (42). Lifestyle modifications that include nutritional changes (i.e., reducing saturated fats, trans fats, and cholesterol intake) and increases in physical activity should be initial therapy for all patients with diabetes and dyslipidemia. Pharmacotherapy is warranted in specific populations. Patients with known CAD should receive statin therapy if no contraindications exist. In addition, patients with diabetes, age >40 years, and one other CV risk factor should also be considered for treatment. Goals of therapy for those without known CAD include a target LDL <100 mg/dL. More aggressive therapeutic goals (LDL <70 mg/dL) may be indicated in patients with ACS or known CAD (110,111). In addition to the LDL cholesterol goals, patients with diabetes have goals to target triglycerides <150 mg/dL and HDL >40 mg/dL in men and >50 mg/dL in women.

Combination statin and other lipid-lowering therapy has not necessarily been shown to be more efficacious than statin monotherapy. The ACCORD study group investigated the effect of combination statin and fenofibrate therapy in patients with type 2 diabetes (112). All patients were treated with simvastatin and then were randomized to additional placebo or fenofibrate. Combination therapy with statin and fenofibrate did not reduce the rate of fatal CV events, nonfatal MI, or nonfatal stroke when compared to the statin and placebo group. Combination statin and extended release niacin therapy was studied in the Atherthrombosis Intervention in Metabolic Syndrome with Low HDL/High Triglycerides (AIM-HIGH) study (113). A total of 3414 patients (1158 with diabetes) who had established cardiovascular disease were treated with statins for a goal LDL <70 mg/dL. Patients were then randomized to the addition of placebo or extended release niacin. The study was halted early when no between-group difference was seen in the primary outcome of CV events.

Other studies have suggested that statins, particularly at higher doses, can lead to elevations in blood glucose; however, the potential cardiovascular benefits seem to outweigh these minor risks (114,115). Although niacin has been shown, in short-term trials, to exacerbate insulin resistance, the glycemic response in patients with and without diabetes is usually mild. Niacin can be used safely in patients with diabetes (116). Combination therapy of statins and fibrates can also increase the risk for adverse reactions such as transaminitis, myositis, and rhabdomyolysis (116). The risk of rhabdomyolysis is higher in patients with chronic kidney disease. Given the age related reduction in glomerular filtration rate, special consideration should be given when using combination therapy in older patients.

LIFESTYLE MODIFICATIONS

The importance of lifestyle modifications in the management of diabetes as a way to improve glycemic control and modify cardiovascular risk factors cannot be overstated. The Diabetes Prevention Program demonstrated that in patients with prediabetes, intensive lifestyle modification with diet, exercise, and weight loss was more effective than standard care or metformin at reducing the incidence of type 2 diabetes (117). Among patients already diagnosed with type 2 diabetes, the Look Action for Health in Diabetes (AHEAD) trial provided insight into the benefits of intensive lifestyle modification. This study included 5145 patients aged 45–74 years with type 2 diabetes who were also overweight. Participants were randomized to an Intense Lifestyle Intervention (ILI) group or Diabetes Support and Education (DSE) group. The ILI group participated in group and individual meetings to achieve and maintain weight loss through decreased caloric intake and increased physical activity. At 1 year, the ILI group had lost an average of 8.6% of their initial weight versus 0.7% in the DSE group ($p < 0.001$). The mean A1C in the ILI group also dropped from 7.4% to 6.6% compared to the change in the DSE group of 7.3% to 7.2% ($p < 0.001$). Accompanying these improvements in weight and glycemic control, patients in the ILI group experienced reductions in blood pressure, dyslipidemia (i.e., increased HDL and decreased triglyceride levels), and microalbuminuria (118) that persisted after 4 years of follow up (119).

The ADA recommends that all individuals with diabetes receive individualized nutritional therapy (120). Ideally this is done by a registered dietician familiar with diabetes nutritional therapy. Weight loss is recommended for all overweight or obese individuals with type 2 diabetes. Saturated fats should be limited to <7% of total calories and trans fat intake should be minimized to help with LDL and HDL control. In type 2 diabetes, moderate weight loss (5% of body weight) has been associated with decreased insulin resistance, improved glycemic and lipid control, and reduced blood pressure (121).

It is recommended that patients with diabetes should perform at least 150 minutes per week of moderate intensity aerobic exercise. This should be supplemented by resistance exercises at least two to three times per week, as resistance training has been shown to exert favorable effects on insulin resistance (42). Prior to starting an exercise regimen, clinicians should assess patients with multiple cardiovascular risk factors, but the role of stress testing and other imaging modalities (e.g., coronary artery calcium scans) to screen asymptomatic patients with diabetes for CAD remains unclear (122).

Treatment of Diabetes Mellitus

The current approach to the treatment of type 2 diabetes mellitus focuses heavily on the combination of lifestyle modifications and metformin as initial therapy (123). All patients are encouraged to modify lifestyle with dietary changes, weight loss, and exercise. Metformin therapy is often initiated and titrated at the time of diagnosis. If the goal hemoglobin A1C is not achieved after 3 months of therapy, well validated therapies include the addition of basal insulin or sulfonylurea to continued metformin use and lifestyle changes. Other options that are less well validated include the addition of thiazolidinediones, Dipeptidyl peptidase IV (DPP-IV) inhibitors, or glucagon like peptide-1 (GLP-1) agonists (124). If the goal hemoglobin A1C still has not been met after an additional 3 months, therapy can be escalated. If basal insulin has not been tried, it can be added. Other options include the use of an additional oral agent, although this option is less preferred due to concerns about polypharmacy. If the patient does not achieve the goal hemoglobin A1C with oral agents and basal insulin, the use of a more complex/intensive multi-shot insulin regimen is usually considered. The therapies used in the management of type 2 diabetes are described below and additional cardiovascular considerations are noted (Table 6.2).

Metformin

Metformin is a biguanide that remains the most widely used first line drug for type 2 diabetes. The mechanism of action is suppression of hepatic gluconeogenesis through reduction in hepatic insulin resistance, leading primarily to reduction of fasting blood glucose. Metformin can lower hemoglobin A1C by ~1.5% when used as monotherapy or in combination (125). It does not cause weight gain and may actually help promote mild weight loss. Hypoglycemia is not a known side effect.

Aside from improved glycemic control, metformin has been shown to improve some cardiovascular risk factors. Metformin has a positive effect on arterial vasculature through lowering inflammatory markers and improving platelet, endothelial, and hemostatic functions. These effects are independent of the glycemic effects of metformin (126). Further supporting the use of metformin as first line therapy in type 2 diabetes is the UKPDS study (127). This study enrolled at 753 overweight patients with newly diagnosed type 2 diabetes. Patients were randomized to intensive therapy (with metformin) versus conventional therapy (with diet). The metformin treated group achieved a median hemoglobin A1C of 7.4% compared to 8.0% in the control group. Comparing the two groups, metformin-treated patients had a 42% risk reduction for diabetes related death (95% CI 9–63%, $p = 0.017$) and a 36% risk reduction for all cause mortality (95% CI 9–55%, $p = 0.011$). Comparing the intensively treated metformin group to intensive glycemic control using other agents (chlorpropamide, glibenclamide, or insulin), metformin showed a greater effect for all cause mortality ($p = 0.021$) and stroke ($p = 0.032$).

Potential drawbacks from the use of metformin include adverse gastrointestinal effects such as diarrhea, nausea, and abdominal cramping. These adverse reactions can largely be mitigated using a slow titration process that begins with 500–1000 mg daily followed by gradual increases to a target dose of 2000 mg daily (123). Other clinical considerations include the rare risk of lactic acidosis in patients with renal dysfunction (128). Current US prescribing guidelines warn against the use of metformin with a serum creatinine ≥1.5 mg/dl in men and ≥1.4 mg/dl in women. However, alternative recommendations have suggested glomerular filtration rate based dosing criteria that allows for a dose reduction with frequent monitoring when the GFR is <45 ml/min/1.73 m^2. Metformin is contraindicated if the GFR is <30 ml/min/1.73 m^2 (129).

Sulfonylureas

The sulfonylureas have been used for management of diabetes longer than any other oral hypoglycemic agents. The drug class has wide variability from early developed ("first generation") drugs like chlorpropamide to the most recent ("third generation") agents like glimepiride. Newer third generation drugs are associated with less fasting insulin secretory stimulation and hypoglycemia compared to first generation sulfonylureas (130). The drugs bind to receptors on the ATP dependent potassium channel on β cells leading to an influx of calcium which stimulates insulin secretion (131). Reductions in hemoglobin A1C of 1–2% can be seen when using sulfonylureas as monotherapy.

The overall effect of sulfonylureas on cardiovascular risk appears to be neutral. Available data suggest no significant effects on blood pressure, lipid profiles, or coagulant factors. Concern for potential adverse cardiovascular outcomes from sulfonylureas dates back to the University Group Diabetes Program in the 1970s (132). This trial was halted early when participants treated with the first generation sulfonylurea tolbutamide were

Table 6.2 Brief Summary of Cardiovascular Risks and Benefits of Noninsulin Pharmacologic Therapies for Diabetes

Class	Example	Mode of Action	CV Risk/Benefit	Special Consideration for Elderly Patients
Biguanides	Metformin	Suppression of hepatic gluconeogenesis	Improves arterial vasculature, platelet function, and inflammatory markers (126). Improved CV outcomes in UKPDS (127).	Renal insufficiency limits use due to risk of lactic acidosis. Careful attention to declining GFR as patient's age.
Sulfonylureas	Glipizide, Glimepiride, Glyburide	β Cell Secretagogue	Adverse outcomes in University Group Diabetes Program (132) but not replicated in other studies. ADOPT (133) demonstrates potential benefit.	Risk for hypoglycemia. Use with caution in patients with renal or hepatic impairment, especially glyburide.
Meglitinides	Repaglinide, Nateglinide	Sulfonylurea-Like β Cell Secretagogue	No data to suggest CV benefits beyond improvements in surrogate markers (135).	Risk for hypoglycemia. Use with caution in patients with renal or hepatic impairment. Potential dosing convenience to match to meals and limit hypoglycemia in patients with erratic dietary intake.
Thiazolinediones	Pioglitazone Rosiglitazone	Peripheral insulin sensitizers working via P-PAR gamma receptors	Rosiglitazone not routinely available in U.S. due to reports of increased risk for MI. Pioglitazone has not been found to raise risk of MI (144) and may have potential benefits, (i.e., PROactive) and studies are ongoing Both drugs increase risk of HF.	Caution in patients with a history of HF, fluid retention, hepatic or renal impairment. May also be associated with bone fractures.

(Continued)

Table 6.2 Brief Summary of Cardiovascular Risks and Benefits of Noninsulin Pharmacologic Therapies for Diabetes (*Continued*)

Class	Example	Mode of Action	CV Risk/Benefit	Special Consideration for Elderly Patients
GLP-1 analogs	Exenatide Liraglutide	Slow gastric emptying, decrease hepatic gluconeogenesis, and improve glucose dependent β cell insulin release	Associated weight loss may improve CV risk factor of obesity. Long-term CV outcome studies are needed and studies are ongoing	Injectable medications that require patient dexterity or assistance to deliver.
DPP-IV inhibitors	Sitagliptin Saxagliptin Linagliptin	Inhibit endogenous DPP-IV from enzymatic breakdown of GLP-1 extending time course of glucose lowering effects of GLP-1	Long-term CV outcome studies are needed and studies are ongoing	Can be used in patients with renal impairment but dosing reductions may be required.
α glucosidase inhibitors	Acarbose Miglitol	Inhibit α glucosidase enzymatic breakdown of carbohydrates in gut leading to malabsorption of carbohydrates	Encouraging findings reported in STOP-NIDDM (137) trial but conflicting data in meta analyses (138,139).	Adverse gastrointestinal side effects.

Abbreviations: CV, cardiovascular; UKPDS, United Kingdom Prospective Diabetes Study; GFR, Glomerular Filtration Rate; P-PAR, peroxisome proliferator activated receptor; PROactive, Prospective Pioglitazone Clinical Trial in Macrovascular Events; HF, heart failure; GLP-1, glucagon like peptide 1; DPP-IV, dipeptidyl peptidase IV; STOP NIDDM, Study to Prevent Non Insulin Dependent Diabetes Mellitus.
Source: Modified from Ref. 130.

found to have excess cardiovascular mortality compared to diet alone. This finding resulted in a black box warning for sulfonylureas noting an increased risk of cardiovascular events. Subsequent trials have not shown similar results. Notably, the UKPDS trial was able to demonstrate a reduction in all endpoints in the intensive treatment groups (sulfonylureas or insulin) compared to conventional therapy groups. Within the intensively treated group (sulfonylureas vs. insulin) there was no difference in any of the end points (20).

In 2006, A Diabetes Outcome Progression Trial (ADOPT) studied 4360 patients previously untreated with oral agents. Participants were randomized to glyburide, metformin, or rosiglitazone. The study was designed to evaluate a primary outcome of time to monotherapy failure. However, there were fewer serious cardiovascular events in the glyburide group compared to the rosiglitazone group (1.8% vs. 3.4%, $p < 0.05$). There was no difference in cardiovascular events comparing glyburide and metformin treated patients (133).

In older patients, renal and hepatic impairment can affect clearance of sulfonylureas and lead to hypoglycemia. Poor nutritional status, anorexia, or concurrent illnesses limiting nutritional intake can commonly occur in older patients with comorbidities making them more vulnerable to adverse side effects. Nonetheless, sulfonylureas can be useful agents in selected patients, and newer generation sulfonylureas may be preferable in older patients who may be susceptible to hypoglycemia. However, there is conflicting evidence regarding the effects of sulfonylureas on cardiovascular outcomes.

Meglitinides

Meglitinides produce an insulin secretory effect through action on the β cell sulfonylurea receptor at a unique site from sulfonylureas. The different activation of this ATP dependent potassium channel causes a more rapid onset of action and shorter half life allowing these drugs to be taken before meals to control postprandial hyperglycemia. This may be particularly helpful as postprandial hyperglycemia has been suggested as an independent risk factor for cardiovascular disease (134). In general, this class of medicines modestly lowers hemoglobin A1C levels 0.5–1.0%.

Using surrogate markers, meglitinides have shown promise as a class of agents that may have beneficial effects on cardiovascular risk factors. A study comparing the effects of repaglinide (a meglitnide) versus glimepiride on cardiovascular risk factors after a test meal showed repaglinide to be more efficient than the sulfonylurea in lowering plasma free fatty acids, fibrinogen, thrombin–antithrombin complex, and plasminogen activator 1 levels (135). However, when studied in a large cardiovascular outcomes trial, meglitinides did not show benefit in an at risk population with impaired glucose tolerance. The Nateglinide and Valsartan in Impaired Glucose Tolerance Outcomes Research (NAVIGATOR) trial included 9306 patients with impaired glucose tolerance and cardiovascular disease or risk factors. Participants received nateglinide versus placebo and valsartan versus placebo in a 2 × 2 factorial design. They were followed for a median of 5 years with primary endpoints of incident diabetes, core cardiovascular outcome (death from cardiovascular cause, nonfatal MI, nonfatal stroke, or hospitalization for HF) and an extended cardiovascular outcome (composite of core outcome components plus hospitalization for unstable angina or arterial revascularization). Nateglinide compared to placebo did not reduce the incidence of diabetes or the composite cardiovascular outcomes (136).

For older patients with type 2 diabetes, the meglitinides may be useful agents for glycemic control. They are helpful in reducing postprandial hyperglycemia. They also offer flexibility in dosing to match a patient's dietary intake and reduce the risk of hypoglycemia that can occur with longer acting sulfonylureas. To date, they have not been shown to reduce cardiovascular events.

α Glucosidase Inhibitors

α glucosidase inhibitors competitively block the action of α glucosidase in the gut. This enzyme is important for the enzymatic breakdown of carbohydrates. This class of agents interferes with carbohydrate digestion and absorption resulting in a blunting of postprandial glucose levels. The glucose lowering effect of α glucosidase inhibitors is mild with hemoglobin A1C reductions of ~0.5%. Common side effects include gastrointestinal bloating, diarrhea, and flatulence.

The cardiovascular effects of α glucosidase inhibitors were evaluated in the Study to Prevent-Noninsulin-Dependent Diabetes Mellitus (STOP-NIDDM) trial. This study randomized 1429 patients with impaired glucose tolerance to placebo or acarbose 100 mg thrice daily for prevention of type 2 diabetes. A substudy assessed the development of major cardiovascular events and hypertension. Acarbose was associated with a 49% relative risk reduction (hazard ratio 0.51; 95% CI; 0.28–0.95; $p = 0.03$) and 2.5% absolute risk reduction of incident cardiovascular events (137).

Other studies have shown inconsistent findings with regard to cardiovascular effects of α glucosidase inhibitors. A meta-analysis of seven studies with a minimum treatment time of 1 year included over 2000 patients with type 2 diabetes randomized to acarbose or placebo. This meta-analysis showed a reduced risk of myocardial infarction (HR 0.36, 95% CI, 0.16–0.8, $p = 0.012$) and cardiovascular events (HR 0.65, 95% CI, 0.48–0.88, $p = 0.006$) (138). Conversely, a Cochrane review and meta-analysis evaluated 42 studies. Although α glucosidase inhibitors decreased BMI by 0.17 kg/m^2 (95% CI 0.08–0.26), there was no effect on plasma lipids and no evidence of improvement in morbidity or mortality (139).

Thiazolinediones

Thiazolinediones (TZDs) are peripheral insulin sensitizers that work through the peroxisome proliferator-activated receptors (PPARs) to improve peripheral insulin sensitivity in skeletal muscle. The two available drugs in this class are rosiglitazone and pioglitazone which have divergent cardiovascular effects. TZDs reduce hemoglobin A1C by ~1 to 1.5%.

This drug class does not usually cause hypoglycemia. Major adverse effects include fluid retention, weight gain, HF, and bone fractures. More recent data suggest an association of pioglitazone with bladder cancer but this has not been definitely demonstrated (140).

Pioglitazone's cardiovascular disease effects were highlighted in the PROspective pioglitAzone Clinical Trial In macroVascular Events (PROactive study), (141) in which 5238 patients with type 2 diabetes were prospectively followed after receiving pioglitazone or placebo in addition to their regular glucose lowering drugs. The primary endpoint was the composite of all cause mortality, nonfatal MI, stroke, ACS, endovascular, or surgical intervention in the coronary or leg arteries, and amputation above the ankles. The primary endpoint occurred in 19.7% of the pioglitazone group and 21.7% of the placebo group ($p = 0.095$). There was a significant reduction in the secondary composite outcome of all cause mortality, nonfatal MI, and stroke, which occurred less frequently in the pioglitazone group than in the placebo group (HR 0.84, 95% CI 0.72–0.98, $p = 0.027$). However, there were significantly more HF events and HF admissions in the pioglitazone group, although there was no difference between groups in HF mortality.

In 2011, the FDA restricted the use of rosiglitazone due to reports of an increased risk for myocardial infarction, and the drug is now only available in the USA through a special access program. A meta-analysis of 35,531 patients, including 19,509 who received rosiglitazone and 16,022 who received control therapy (142), found that rosiglitazone significantly increased the risk for MI (OR, 1.28, 95% CI 1.02–1.63, $p = 0.04$). However, there was no difference between rosiglitazone and control for all cause or cardiovascular mortality.

In summary, rosiglitazone is associated with an increased risk for MI and has been restricted by the FDA, but pioglitazone does not seem to carry the same adverse ischemic cardiovascular risks. Both drugs are associated with an increased risk of HF.

INCRETIN BASED THERAPY: DPP-IV INHIBITORS AND GLP-1 ANALOGS

Incretins are gut hormones that are released in response to oral but not intravenous glucose loads. Two known human incretins are GLP-1 and gastric inhibitory peptide (GIP). They have glucose dependent action allowing their release to be augmented in the prandial period when glucose levels are rising. GLP-1 stimulates pancreatic β cell release, inhibits hepatic gluconeogenesis, and slows gastric emptying. This combination of actions works to lower glucose levels. Because the incretins are stimulated in response to a glucose load, they are not associated with hypoglycemia.

DPP-IV is an endogenous enzyme that degrades GLP-1 and limits the time course of glucose lowering actions of GLP-1. Inhibitors of DPP-IV have been developed. These are orally available agents that block the action of DPP-IV and allow endogenous GLP-1 to have a prolonged course of action. These agents modestly lower hemoglobin A1C levels 0.5–1%. Analogs of GLP-1 are also available. Exanatide and liraglutide are GLP-1 analogs given as subcutaneous injections. They can be used in combination with other oral agents and typically lower hemoglobin A1C levels by ~1%.

The slowed gastric emptying effect of GLP-1 analogs is thought to be responsible for the common side effects of gastrointestinal symptoms such as nausea, vomiting, and diarrhea. GLP-1 analogs also frequently lead to early satiety and, as a consequence, weight loss is frequently seen. A meta-analysis evaluated the weight loss effects in patients receiving GLP-1 analogs compared to a control population treated with placebo, oral glycemic drugs, or insulin (143). The analysis included 6411 participants and demonstrated a weighted mean weight loss difference of −2.9 kg favoring GLP-1 analogs over controls (95% CI −3.6 to −2.2). Other cardiovascular risk factor benefits from GLP-1 analogs included decreased systolic blood pressure of 3.6 mm Hg (95% CI 1.7–5.5 mm Hg), decreased diastolic blood pressure of 1.4 mm Hg (95% CI 0.7–2.0 mm Hg), and a decrease in total cholesterol of 0.1 mmol/L (95% CI 0.04–0.16 mmol/L). In contrast to the GLP-1 analogs, the DPP-IV inhibitors are weight neutral and have not been shown to reduce cardiovascular risk factors. Data from ongoing trials are needed to determine if GLP-1 analogs or DPP-IV inhibitors improve cardiovascular outcomes.

For older patients with diabetes, the GLP-1 analogs and DPP-IV inhibitors offer favorable profiles. These drug classes do not predispose patients to hypoglycemia, and DPP-IV inhibitors can be renally dosed for use in patients with chronic kidney disease.

Insulin

The natural history of type 2 diabetes leads to progressive β-cell dysfunction in the setting of insulin resistance. Insulin replacement therapy often becomes necessary to achieve appropriate glycemic control that cannot be garnered with oral agents alone. Additionally, comorbidities such as liver or renal dysfunction can sometimes limit the use of oral agents necessitating the use of insulin therapy for type 2 diabetes.

Initial management with insulin typically involves a basal, long acting insulin to provide steady levels of insulin during the day and night. This can be achieved with intermediate acting insulins such as neutral protamine Hagedorn (NPH) or long acting insulin analogs (glargine or detemir). These insulins are usually dosed at night and titrated to achieve a target morning glucose level. Oral agents such as metformin, sulfonylureas, pioglitazone, or DPP-IV inhibitors can be continued while basal insulin therapy is used but dose reductions of oral agents may be necessary. β-cell dysfunction may become so severe that basal insulin alone is not sufficient to achieve desired glycemic control. Short acting insulins given at meal times to assist with prandial rises in glucose may be necessary. This can be achieved with rapid acting insulin analogs such as lispro, aspart, or glulisine (123,124).

The advantages of insulin use include established efficacy and the ability to titrate the dosage to achieve desired glycemic control. Inherent disadvantages include weight gain and a high risk of hypoglycemia. The risk of hypoglycemia can be substantial in vulnerable older patients. Additionally, multiple daily injections of insulin require frequent self-monitoring of glucose levels for safe use. Patients must also have adequate hand–eye coordination to appropriately dose and inject insulin. This can be a potential problem in some older patients with common comorbidities, such as visual impairment or tremor.

CONCLUSION

The burden of diabetes mellitus continues to grow. In addition, as our population ages, older adults with type 2 diabetes mellitus will remain the fastest growing subgroup. Diabetes mellitus increases the risk of cardiovascular disease, which in turn is associated with significant morbidity and mortality. Therefore, management of older adults with diabetes mellitus should focus on cardiovascular risk reduction through control of hypertension, lipid management, antiplatelet therapy, and lifestyle modifications to include smoking cessation, weight reduction, and exercise. While tight glycemic control in non-elderly adults with type 1 and type 2 diabetes mellitus has been shown to reduce microvascular complications, a comparable benefit has not been demonstrated in elderly patients and there is significant potential for harm associated with hypoglycemia. Similarly, tight glycemic control has not been shown to reduce macrovascular complications for elderly patients with type 1 or type 2 diabetes mellitus. Comorbidities, functional status, and life expectancy should be taken into account when setting glycemic goals for older patients, and therapy should be individualized to account for patient preferences and health status. For most elderly patients with diabetes mellitus, a hemoglobin A1C target <8% is usually sufficient to control symptomatic hyperglycemia while avoiding hypoglycemia. For older adults with multimorbidity or limited life expectancy, an even less stringent A1C target may be appropriate. Ongoing studies are investigating the effects of newer hypoglycemic agents on cardiovascular outcomes and the role of hyperglycemia in the development of geriatric syndromes. Additional research is needed to develop more effective strategies for the prevention and management of diabetes mellitus in older adults.

REFERENCES

1. American Diabetes Association. Diagnosis and classification of diabetes mellitus. Diabetes Care 2010; 33: S62–9.
2. Cowie CC, Rust KF, Ford ES, et al. Full accounting of diabetes and pre-diabetes in the U.S. population in 1988–1994 and 2005–2006. Diabetes Care 2009; 32: 287–94.
3. American Diabetes Association. Economic costs of diabetes in the U.S. In 2007. Diabetes Care 2008; 31: 596–615.
4. Dall TM, Zhang Y, Chen YJ, et al. The economic burden of diabetes. Health Aff (Millwood) 2010; 29: 297–303.
5. Sarwar N, Gao P, Seshasai SR, et al. Emerging Risk Factors Collaboration. Diabetes mellitus, fasting blood glucose concentration, and risk of vascular disease: a collaborative meta-analysis of 102 prospective studies. Lancet 2010; 375: 2215–22.
6. Huang ES, Basu A, O'Grady M, Capretta JC. Projecting the future diabetes population size and related costs for the U.S. Diabetes Care 2009; 32: 2225–9.
7. Brown AF, Mangione CM, Saliba D, Sarkisian CA; California Healthcare Foundation/American Geriatrics Society Panel on Improving Care for Elders with Diabetes. Guidelines for improving the care of the older person with diabetes mellitus. J Am Geriatr Soc 2003; 51: S265–80.

8. Durso SC. Using clinical guidelines designed for older adults with diabetes mellitus and complex health status. JAMA 2006; 295: 1935–40.

9. Bandeen-Roche K, Xue QL, Ferrucci L, et al. Phenotype of frailty: characterization in the women's health and aging studies. J Gerontol A Biol Sci Med Sci 2006; 61: 262–6.

10. Barzilay JI, Blaum C, Moore T, et al. Insulin resistance and inflammation as precursors of frailty: the Cardiovascular Health Study. Arch Intern Med 2007; 167: 635–41.

11. Blaum CS, Xue QL, Tian J, et al. Is hyperglycemia associated with frailty status in older women? J Am Geriatr Soc 2009; 57: 840–7.

12. Fried LP, Tangen CM, Walston J, et al. Frailty in older adults: evidence for a phenotype. J Gerontol A Biol Sci Med Sci 2001; 56: M146–56.

13. Kalyani RR, Varadhan R, Weiss CO, Fried LP, Cappola AR. Frailty status and altered glucose-insulin dynamics. J Gerontol A Biol Sci Med Sci 2011.

14. Walston J, McBurnie MA, Newman A, et al. Frailty and activation of the inflammation and coagulation systems with and without clinical comorbidities: results from the Cardiovascular Health Study. Arch Intern Med 2002; 162: 2333–41.

15. Kalyani RR, Tian J, Xue QL, et al. Hyperglycemia and incidence of frailty and lower extremity mobility limitations in older women. J Am Geriatr Soc 2012.

16. Kaprio J, Tuomilehto J, Koskenvuo M, et al. Concordance for type 1 (insulin-dependent) and type 2 (non-insulin-dependent) diabetes mellitus in a population-based cohort of twins in Finland. Diabetologia 1992; 35: 1060–7.

17. Wild S, Roglic G, Green A, Sicree R, King H. Global prevalence of diabetes: estimates for the year 2000 and projections for 2030. Diabetes Care 2004; 27: 1047–53.

18. Harrison TA, Hindorff LA, Kim H, et al. Family history of diabetes as a potential public health tool. Am J Prev Med 2003; 24: 152–9.

19. The Diabetes Control and Complications Trial Research Group. The effect of intensive treatment of diabetes on the development and progression of long-term complications in insulin-dependent diabetes mellitus. N Engl J Med 1993; 329: 977–86.

20. UK Prospective Diabetes Study (UKPDS) Group. Intensive blood-glucose control with sulphonylureas or insulin compared with conventional treatment and risk of complications in patients with type 2 diabetes (UKPDS 33). Lancet 1998; 352: 837–53.

21. Bilous R. Microvascular disease: what does the UKPDS tell us about diabetic nephropathy? Diabet Med 2008; 25: 25–9.

22. Kohner EM. Microvascular disease: what does the UKPDS tell us about diabetic retinopathy? Diabet Med 2008; 25: 20–4.

23. Finucane TE. Tight control in geriatrics: the emperor wears a thong. J Am Geriatr Soc 2012; 60: 1571–5.

24. De Vriese AS, Verbeuren TJ, Van de Voorde J, Lameire NH, Vanhoutte PM. Endothelial dysfunction in diabetes. Br J Pharmacol 2000; 130: 963–74.

25. Hopfner RL, Gopalakrishnan V. Endothelin: emerging role in diabetic vascular complications. Diabetologia 1999; 42: 1383–94.

26. Beckman JA, Creager MA, Libby P. Diabetes and atherosclerosis: epidemiology, pathophysiology, and management. JAMA 2002; 287: 2570–81.

27. Hussain MJ, Peakman M, Gallati H, et al. Elevated serum levels of macrophage-derived cytokines precede and accompany the onset of IDDM. Diabetologia 1996; 39: 60–9.

28. Uemura S, Matsushita H, Li W, et al. Diabetes mellitus enhances vascular matrix metalloproteinase activity: role of oxidative stress. Circ Res 2001; 88: 1291–8.

29. Vinik AI, Erbas T, Park TS, Nolan R, Pittenger GL. Platelet dysfunction in type 2 diabetes. Diabetes Care 2001; 24: 1476–85.

30. Ceriello A, Giacomello R, Stel G, et al. Hyperglycemia-induced thrombin formation in diabetes. The possible role of oxidative stress. Diabetes 1995; 44: 924–8.

31. Ceriello A, Giugliano D, Quatraro A, et al. Evidence for a hyperglycaemia-dependent decrease of antithrombin III-thrombin complex formation in humans. Diabetologia 1990; 33: 163–7.

32. Carr ME. Diabetes mellitus: a hypercoagulable state. J Diabetes Complications 2001; 15: 44–54.

33. Nathan DM, Cleary PA, Backlund JY, et al. Intensive diabetes treatment and cardiovascular disease in patients with type 1 diabetes. N Engl J Med 2005; 353: 2643–53.

34. Holman RR, Paul SK, Bethel MA, Matthews DR, Neil HA. 10-year follow-up of intensive glucose control in type 2 diabetes. N Engl J Med 2008; 359: 1577–89.

35. Selvin E, Marinopoulos S, Berkenblit G, et al. Meta-analysis: glycosylated hemoglobin and cardiovascular disease in diabetes mellitus. Ann Intern Med 2004; 141: 421–31.

36. Stettler C, Allemann S, Juni P, et al. Glycemic control and macrovascular disease in types 1 and 2 diabetes mellitus: meta-analysis of randomized trials. Am Heart J 2006; 152: 27–38.

37. Gerstein HC, Miller ME, Byington RP, Goff DC Jr, Bigger JT, et al. Action to Control Cardiovascular Risk in Diabetes Study Group. Effects of intensive glucose lowering in type 2 diabetes. N Engl J Med 2008; 358: 2545–59.

38. Gerstein HC, Miller ME, Genuth S, Ismail-Beigi F, Buse JB, et al. ACCORD Study Group. Long-term effects of intensive glucose lowering on cardiovascular outcomes. N Engl J Med 2011; 364: 818–28.

39. Duckworth W, Abraira C, Moritz T, et al. Glucose control and vascular complications in veterans with type 2 diabetes. N Engl J Med 2009; 360: 129–39.

40. Patel A, MacMahon S, Chalmers J, Neal B, Billot L, et al. ADVANCE Collaborative Group. Intensive blood glucose control and vascular outcomes in patients with type 2 diabetes. N Engl J Med 2008; 358: 2560–72.

41. Skyler JS, Bergenstal R, Bonow RO, et al. Intensive glycemic control and the prevention of cardiovascular events: implications of the ACCORD, ADVANCE, and VA Diabetes Trials: a position statement of the American Diabetes Association and a Scientific Statement of the American College of Cardiology Foundation and the American Heart Association. J Am Coll Cardiol 2009; 53: 298–304.

42. Introduction: the American Diabetes Association's (ADA) evidence-based practice guidelines, standards, and related recommendations and documents for diabetes care. Diabetes Care 2012; 35: S1–2.

43. Kannel WB, McGee DL. Diabetes and cardiovascular risk factors: the Framingham study. Circulation 1979; 59: 8–13.

44. Ness J, Nassimiha D, Feria MI, Aronow WS. Diabetes mellitus in older African-Americans, Hispanics, and whites in an academic hospital-based geriatrics practice. Coron Artery Dis 1999; 10: 343–6.

45. Goraya TY, Leibson CL, Palumbo PJ, et al. Coronary atherosclerosis in diabetes mellitus: a population-based autopsy study. J Am Coll Cardiol 2002; 40: 946–53.

46. Janand-Delenne B, Savin B, Habib G, et al. Silent myocardial ischemia in patients with diabetes: who to screen. Diabetes Care 1999; 1396–400.

47. Kannel WB, Abbott RD. Incidence and prognosis of unrecognized myocardial infarction. An update on the Framingham study. N Engl J Med 1984; 311: 1144–7.

48. Aronow WS, Epstein S. Usefulness of silent myocardial ischemia detected by ambulatory electrocardiographic monitoring in predicting new coronary events in elderly patients. Am J Cardiol 1988; 62: 1295–6.

49. Weitzman S, Wagner GS, Heiss G, Haney TL, Slome C. Myocardial infarction site and mortality in diabetes. Diabetes Care 1982; 5: 31–5.

50. Haffner SM, Lehto S, Ronnemaa T, Pyorala K, Laakso M. Mortality from coronary heart disease in subjects with type 2 diabetes and in nondiabetic subjects with and without prior myocardial infarction. N Engl J Med 1998; 339: 229–34.

51. Miettinen H, Lehto S, Salomaa V, et al. The FINMONICA Myocardial Infarction Register Study Group. Impact of diabetes on mortality after the first myocardial infarction. Diabetes Care 1998; 21: 69–75.

52. Jacoby RM, Nesto RW. Acute myocardial infarction in the diabetic patient: pathophysiology, clinical course and prognosis. J Am Coll Cardiol 1992; 20: 736–44.

53. Abaci A, Oguzhan A, Kahraman S, et al. Effect of diabetes mellitus on formation of coronary collateral vessels. Circulation 1999; 99: 2239–42.

54. Currie CJ, Morgan CL, Gill L, Stott NC, Peters JR. Epidemiology and costs of acute hospital care for cerebrovascular disease in diabetic and nondiabetic populations. Stroke 1997; 28: 1142–6.

55. Hu G, Sarti C, Jousilahti P, et al. The impact of history of hypertension and type 2 diabetes at baseline on the incidence of stroke and stroke mortality. Stroke 2005; 36: 2538–43.

56. Kannel WB, Hjortland M, Castelli WP. Role of diabetes in congestive heart failure: the Framingham study. Am J Cardiol 1974; 34: 29–34.

57. Croft JB, Giles WH, Pollard RA, et al. National trends in the initial hospitalization for heart failure. J Am Geriatr Soc 1997; 45: 270–5.

58. Polanczyk CA, Rohde LE, Dec GW, DiSalvo T. Ten-year trends in hospital care for congestive heart failure: improved outcomes and increased use of resources. Arch Intern Med 2000; 160: 325–32.

59. Murarka S, Movahed MR. Diabetic cardiomyopathy. J Card Fail 2010; 16: 971–9.

60. Devereux RB, Roman MJ, Paranicas M, et al. Impact of diabetes on cardiac structure and function: the strong heart study. Circulation 2000; 101: 2271–6.

61. Movahed MR, Hashemzadeh M, Jamal MM. Diabetes mellitus is a strong, independent risk for atrial fibrillation and flutter in addition to other cardiovascular disease. Int J Cardiol 2005; 105: 315–18.

62. Iribarren C, Karter AJ, Go AS, et al. Glycemic control and heart failure among adult patients with diabetes. Circulation 2001; 103: 2668–73.

63. von Bibra H, Hansen A, Dounis V, et al. Augmented metabolic control improves myocardial diastolic function and perfusion in patients with non-insulin dependent diabetes. Heart 2004; 90: 1483–4.

64. Beks PJ, Mackaay AJ, de Neeling JN, et al. Peripheral arterial disease in relation to glycaemic level in an elderly Caucasian population: the Hoorn study. Diabetologia 1995; 38: 86–96.

65. Jude EB, Oyibo SO, Chalmers N, Boulton AJ. Peripheral arterial disease in diabetic and nondiabetic patients: a comparison of severity and outcome. Diabetes Care 2001; 24: 1433–7.

66. Jude EB, Eleftheriadou I, Tentolouris N. Peripheral arterial disease in diabetes–a review. Diabet Med 2010; 27: 4–14.

67. Fibrinolytic Therapy Trialists' (FTT) Collaborative Group. Indications for fibrinolytic therapy in suspected acute myocardial infarction: collaborative overview of early mortality and major morbidity results from all randomised trials of more than 1000 patients. Lancet 1994; 343: 311–22.

68. Mahaffey KW, Granger CB, Toth CA, et al. Diabetic retinopathy should not be a contraindication to thrombolytic therapy for acute myocardial infarction: review of ocular hemorrhage incidence and location in the GUSTO-I trial. Global Utilization of Streptokinase and t-PA for Occluded Coronary Arteries. J Am Coll Cardiol 1997; 30: 1606–10.

69. Berger AK, Radford MJ, Wang Y, Krumholz HM. Thrombolytic therapy in older patients. J Am Coll Cardiol 2000; 36: 366–74.

70. Thiemann DR, Coresh J, Schulman SP, et al. Lack of benefit for intravenous thrombolysis in patients with myocardial infarction who are older than 75 years. Circulation 2000; 101: 2239–46.

71. White HD. Thrombolytic therapy in the elderly. Lancet 2000; 356: 2028–30.

72. Elezi S, Kastrati A, Pache J, et al. Diabetes mellitus and the clinical and angiographic outcome after coronary stent placement. J Am Coll Cardiol 1998; 32: 1866–73.

73. Abizaid A, Kornowski R, Mintz GS, et al. The influence of diabetes mellitus on acute and late clinical outcomes following coronary stent implantation. J Am Coll Cardiol 1998; 32: 584–9.

74. Hsu LF, Mak KH, Lau KW, et al. Clinical outcomes of patients with diabetes mellitus and acute myocardial infarction treated with primary angioplasty or fibrinolysis. Heart 2002; 88: 260–5.

75. FRagmin and Fast Revascularisation during InStability in Coronary artery disease Investigators. Invasive compared with non-invasive treatment in unstable coronary-artery disease: FRISC II prospective randomised multicentre study. Lancet 1999; 354: 708–15.

76. Cannon CP, Weintraub WS, Demopoulos LA, et al. Comparison of early invasive and conservative strategies in patients with unstable coronary syndromes treated with the glycoprotein IIb/IIIa inhibitor tirofiban. N Engl J Med 2001; 344: 1879–87.

77. Colwell JA, Nesto RW. The platelet in diabetes: focus on prevention of ischemic events. Diabetes Care 2003; 26: 2181–8.

78. Colwell JA. Antiplatelet agents for the prevention of cardiovascular disease in diabetes mellitus. Am J Cardiovasc Drugs 2004; 4: 87–106.

79. Yusuf S, Zhao F, Mehta SR, et al. Effects of clopidogrel in addition to aspirin in patients with acute coronary syndromes without ST-segment elevation. N Engl J Med 2001; 345: 494–502.

80. Roffi M, Moliterno DJ, Meier B, et al. Impact of different platelet glycoprotein IIb/IIIa receptor inhibitors among diabetic patients undergoing percutaneous coronary intervention: do Tirofiban and ReoPro Give Similar Efficacy Outcomes Trial (TARGET) 1-year follow-up. Circulation 2002; 105: 2730–6.

81. RITA-2 trial participants. Coronary angioplasty versus medical therapy for angina: the second Randomised Intervention Treatment of Angina (RITA-2) trial. Lancet 1997; 350: 461–8.

82. Boden WE, O'Rourke RA, Teo KK, et al. Optimal medical therapy with or without PCI for stable coronary disease. N Engl J Med 2007; 356: 1503–16.

83. Frye RL, August P, Brooks MM, Hardison RM, Kelsey SF, et al. BARI 2D Study Group. A randomized trial of therapies for type 2 diabetes and coronary artery disease. N Engl J Med 2009; 360: 2503–15.

84. The Bypass Angioplasty Revascularization Investigation (BARI) Investigators. Comparison of coronary bypass surgery with angioplasty in patients with multivessel disease. N Engl J Med 1996; 335: 217–25.

85. BARI Investigators. Influence of diabetes on 5-year mortality and morbidity in a randomized trial comparing CABG and PTCA in patients with multivessel disease: the Bypass Angioplasty Revascularization Investigation (BARI). Circulation 1997; 96: 1761–9.

86. BARI Investigators. The final 10-year follow-up results from the BARI randomized trial. J Am Coll Cardiol 2007; 49: 1600–6.

87. Kapur A, Hall RJ, Malik IS, et al. Randomized comparison of percutaneous coronary intervention with coronary artery bypass grafting in diabetic patients. 1-year results of the CARDia (Coronary Artery Revascularization in Diabetes) trial. J Am Coll Cardiol 2010; 55: 432–40.

88. Banning AP, Westaby S, Morice MC, et al. Diabetic and nondiabetic patients with left main and/or 3-vessel coronary artery disease: comparison of outcomes with cardiac surgery and paclitaxel-eluting stents. J Am Coll Cardiol 2010; 55: 1067–75.

89. Baigent C, Blackwell L, Collins R, et al. Antithrombotic Trialists' (ATT) Collaboration, Aspirin in the primary and secondary prevention of vascular disease: collaborative meta-analysis of individual participant data from randomised trials. Lancet 2009; 373: 1849–60.

90. Ogawa H, Nakayama M, Morimoto T, et al. Low-dose aspirin for primary prevention of atherosclerotic events in patients with type 2 diabetes: a randomized controlled trial. JAMA 2008; 300: 2134–41.

91. Belch J, MacCuish A, Campbell I, et al. The prevention of progression of arterial disease and diabetes (POPADAD) trial: factorial randomised placebo controlled trial of aspirin and antioxidants in patients with diabetes and asymptomatic peripheral arterial disease. BMJ 2008; 337: a1840.

92. He J, Whelton PK, Vu B, Klag MJ. Aspirin and risk of hemorrhagic stroke: a meta-analysis of randomized controlled trials. JAMA 1998; 280: 1930–5.

93. Pignone M, Alberts MJ, Colwell JA, et al. Aspirin for primary prevention of cardiovascular events in people with diabetes: a position statement of the American Diabetes Association, a scientific statement of the American Heart Association, and an expert consensus document of the American College of Cardiology Foundation. Diabetes Care 2010; 33: 1395–402.

94. Oldridge NB, Stump TE, Nothwehr FK, Clark DO. Prevalence and outcomes of comorbid metabolic and cardiovascular conditions in middle- and older-age adults. J Clin Epidemiol 2001; 54: 928–34.

95. Curb JD, Pressel SL, Cutler JA, et al. Systolic Hypertension in the Elderly Program Cooperative Research Group. Effect of diuretic-based antihypertensive treatment on cardiovascular disease risk in older diabetic patients with isolated systolic hypertension. JAMA 1996; 276: 1886–92.

96. Lewington S, Clarke R, Qizilbash N, Peto R, Collins R; Prospective Studies Collaboration. Age-specific relevance of usual blood pressure to vascular mortality: a meta-analysis of individual data for one million adults in 61 prospective studies. Lancet 2002; 360: 1903–13.

97. UK Prospective Diabetes Study Group. Tight blood pressure control and risk of macrovascular and microvascular complications in type 2 diabetes: UKPDS 38. BMJ 1998; 317: 703–13.

98. Yusuf S, Sleight P, Pogue J, et al. The Heart Outcomes Prevention Evaluation Study Investigators. Effects of an angiotensin-converting-enzyme inhibitor, ramipril, on cardiovascular events in high-risk patients. N Engl J Med 2000; 342: 145–53.

99. Yusuf S, Teo KK, Pogue J, Dyal L, Copland I, et al. ONTARGET Investigators. Telmisartan, ramipril, or both in patients at high risk for vascular events. N Engl J Med 2008; 358: 1547–59.

100. ALLHAT Officers and Coordinators for the ALLHAT Collaborative Research Group. The Antihypertensive and Lipid-Lowering Treatment to Prevent Heart Attack Trial. Major outcomes in high-risk hypertensive patients randomized to angiotensin-converting enzyme inhibitor or calcium channel blocker vs diuretic: The Antihypertensive and Lipid-Lowering Treatment to Prevent Heart Attack Trial (ALLHAT). JAMA 2002; 288: 2981–97.

101. Chobanian AV, Bakris GL, Black HR, et al. Seventh report of the joint National committee on prevention, detection, evaluation, and treatment of high blood pressure. Hypertension 2003; 42: 1206–52.

102. Cushman WC, Evans GW, Byington RP, Goff DC Jr, Grimm RH Jr, et al. ACCORD Study Group. Effects of intensive blood-pressure control in type 2 diabetes mellitus. N Engl J Med 2010; 362: 1575–85.

103. Ziegler D, Gries FA, Spuler M, Lessmann F. Diabetic Cardiovascular Autonomic Neuropathy Multicenter Study Group. The epidemiology of diabetic neuropathy. J Diabetes Complications 1992; 6: 49–57.

104. Aronow WS, Fleg JL, Pepine CJ, et al. ACCF/AHA 2011 expert consensus document on hypertension in the elderly: a report of the American College of Cardiology Foundation Task Force on Clinical Expert Consensus Documents. Circulation 2011; 123: 2434–506.

105. Laakso M. Insulin resistance and coronary heart disease. Curr Opin Lipidol 1996; 7: 217–26.

106. Grundy SM. Small LDL, atherogenic dyslipidemia, and the metabolic syndrome. Circulation 1997; 95: 1–4.

107. Baigent C, Keech A, Kearney PM, et al. Efficacy and safety of cholesterol-lowering treatment: prospective meta-analysis of data from 90,056 participants in 14 randomised trials of statins. Lancet 2005; 366: 1267–78.

108. Singh IM, Shishehbor MH, Ansell BJ. High-density lipoprotein as a therapeutic target: a systematic review. JAMA 2007; 298: 786–98.

109. Keech A, Simes RJ, Barter P, et al. Effects of long-term fenofibrate therapy on cardiovascular events in 9795 people with type 2 diabetes mellitus (the FIELD study): randomised controlled trial. Lancet 2005; 366: 1849–61.

110. Cannon CP, Braunwald E, McCabe CH, et al. Intensive versus moderate lipid lowering with statins after acute coronary syndromes. N Engl J Med 2004; 350: 1495–504.

111. Nissen SE, Tuzcu EM, Schoenhagen P, et al. Effect of intensive compared with moderate lipid-lowering therapy on progression of coronary atherosclerosis: a randomized controlled trial. JAMA 2004; 291: 1071–80.

112. Ginsberg HN, Elam MB, Lovato LC, Crouse JR III, Leiter LA, et al. ACCORD Study Group. Effects of combination lipid therapy in type 2 diabetes mellitus. N Engl J Med 2010; 362: 1563–74.

113. Boden WE, Probstfield JL, Anderson T, Chaitman BR, Desvignes-Nickens P, et al. AIM-HIGH Investigators. Niacin in patients with low HDL cholesterol levels receiving intensive statin therapy. N Engl J Med 2011; 365: 2255–67.

114. Preiss D, Seshasai SR, Welsh P, et al. Risk of incident diabetes with intensive-dose compared with moderate-dose statin therapy: a meta-analysis. JAMA 2011; 305: 2556–64.

115. Sattar N, Preiss D, Murray HM, et al. Statins and risk of incident diabetes: a collaborative meta-analysis of randomised statin trials. Lancet 2010; 375: 735–42.

116. Guyton JR, Bays HE. Safety considerations with niacin therapy. Am J Cardiol 2007; 99: 22C–31C.

117. Knowler WC, Barrett-Connor E, Fowler SE, et al. Reduction in the incidence of type 2 diabetes with lifestyle intervention or metformin. N Engl J Med 2002; 346: 393–403.

118. Pi-Sunyer X, Blackburn G, Brancati FL, Bray GA, Bright R, et al. Look AHEAD Research Group. Reduction in weight and cardiovascular disease risk factors in individuals with type 2 diabetes: one-year results of the look AHEAD trial. Diabetes Care 2007; 30: 1374–83.

119. Wing RR. Look AHEAD Research Group. Long-term effects of a lifestyle intervention on weight and cardiovascular risk factors in individuals with type 2 diabetes mellitus: four-year results of the Look AHEAD trial. Arch Intern Med 2010; 170: 1566–75.

120. Bantle JP, Wylie-Rosett J, Albright AL, Apovian CM, Clark NG, et al. American Diabetes Association. Nutrition recommendations and interventions for diabetes: a position statement of the American Diabetes Association. Diabetes Care 2008; 31: S61–78.

121. Klein S, Sheard NF, Pi-Sunyer X, et al. Weight management through lifestyle modification for the prevention and management of type 2 diabetes: rationale and strategies: a statement of the American Diabetes Association, the North American Association for the Study of Obesity, and the American Society for Clinical Nutrition. Diabetes Care 2004; 27: 2067–73.

122. Colberg SR, Sigal RJ, Fernhall B, et al. Exercise and type 2 diabetes: the American College of Sports Medicine and the American Diabetes Association: joint position statement executive summary. Diabetes Care 2010; 33: 2692–6.

123. Nathan DM, Buse JB, Davidson MB, et al. Medical management of hyperglycemia in type 2 diabetes: a consensus algorithm for the initiation and adjustment of therapy: a consensus statement of the American Diabetes Association and the European Association for the Study of Diabetes. Diabetes Care 2009; 32: 193–203.

124. Inzucchi SE, Bergenstal RM, Buse JB, et al. Management of hyperglycemia in type 2 diabetes: a patient-centered approach: position statement of the American Diabetes Association (ADA) and the European Association for the Study of Diabetes (EASD). Diabetes Care 2012; 35: 1364–79.

125. DeFronzo RA, Goodman AM. The Multicenter Metformin Study Group. Efficacy of metformin in patients with non-insulin-dependent diabetes mellitus. N Engl J Med 1995; 333: 541–9.

126. Anfossi G, Russo I, Bonomo K, Trovati M. The cardiovascular effects of metformin: further reasons to consider an old drug as a cornerstone in the therapy of type 2 diabetes mellitus. Curr Vasc Pharmacol 2010; 8: 327–37.

127. UK Prospective Diabetes Study (UKPDS) Group. Effect of intensive blood-glucose control with metformin on complications in overweight patients with type 2 diabetes (UKPDS 34). Lancet 1998; 352: 854–65.

128. Salpeter S, Greyber E, Pasternak G, Salpeter E. Risk of fatal and nonfatal lactic acidosis with metformin use in type 2 diabetes mellitus. Cochrane Database Syst Rev 2006: CD002967.

129. Lipska KJ, Bailey CJ, Inzucchi SE. Use of metformin in the setting of mild-to-moderate renal insufficiency. Diabetes Care 2011; 34: 1431–7.

130. Uwaifo GI, Ratner RE. Differential effects of oral hypoglycemic agents on glucose control and cardiovascular risk. Am J Cardiol 2007; 99: 51B–67B.

131. Bryan J, Crane A, Vila-Carriles WH, Babenko AP, Aguilar-Bryan L. Insulin secretagogues, sulfonylurea receptors and K(ATP) channels. Curr Pharm Des 2005; 11: 2699–716.

132. The University Group Diabetes Program. A study of the effects of hypoglycemic agents on vascular complications in patients with adult-onset diabetes. V. Evaluation of pheniformin therapy. Diabetes 1975; 24: 65–184.

133. Kahn SE, Haffner SM, Heise MA, et al. Glycemic durability of rosiglitazone, metformin, or gly-buride monotherapy. N Engl J Med 2006; 355: 2427–43.

134. Haffner SJ, Cassells H. Hyperglycemia as a cardiovascular risk factor. Am J Med 2003; 115: 6S–11S.

135. Rizzo MR, Barbieri M, Grella R, Passariello N, Paolisso G. Repaglinide has more beneficial effect on cardiovascular risk factors than glimepiride: data from meal-test study. Diabetes Metab 2005; 31: 255–60.

136. Holman RR, Haffner SM, McMurray JJ, Bethel MA, Holzhauer B, et al. NAVIGATOR Study Group. Effect of nateglinide on the incidence of diabetes and cardiovascular events. N Engl J Med 2010; 362: 1463–76.

137. Chiasson JL, Josse RG, Gomis R, et al. Acarbose treatment and the risk of cardiovascular disease and hypertension in patients with impaired glucose tolerance: The STOP-NIDDM trial. JAMA 2003; 290: 486–94.

138. Hanefeld M, Cagatay M, Petrowitsch T, et al. Acarbose reduces the risk for myocardial infarction in type 2 diabetic patients: meta-analysis of seven long-term studies. Eur Heart J 2004; 25: 10–16.

139. van de Laar FA, Lucassen PL, Akkermans RP, et al. Alpha-glucosidase inhibitors for patients with type 2 diabetes: results from a Cochrane systematic review and meta-analysis. Diabetes Care 2005; 28: 154–63.

140. Colmers IN, Bowker SL, Majumdar SR, Johnson JA. Use of thiazolidinediones and the risk of blad-der cancer among people with type 2 diabetes: a meta-analysis. CMAJ 2012.

141. Dormandy JA, Charbonnel B, Eckland DJ, et al. Secondary prevention of macrovascular events in patients with type 2 diabetes in the PROactive Study (PROspective pioglitAzone Clinical Trial In macroVascular Events): a randomised controlled trial. Lancet 2005; 366: 1279–89.

142. Nissen SE, Wolski K. Rosiglitazone revisited: an updated meta-analysis of risk for myocardial infarc-tion and cardiovascular mortality. Arch Intern Med 2010; 170: 1191–201.

143. Vilsboll T, Christensen M, Junker AE, Knop FK, Gluud LL. Effects of glucagon-like peptide-1 receptor agonists on weight loss: systematic review and meta-analyses of randomised controlled trials. BMJ 2012; 344: d7771.

144. Nagajothi N, Adigopula S, Balamuthusamy S, et al. Pioglitazone and the risk of myocardial infarction and other major adverse cardiac events: a meta-analysis of randomized, controlled trials. Am J Ther 2008; 15: 506–11.

7
Epidemiology of coronary heart disease in the elderly

Nathan D. Wong, David M. Tehrani, and Stanley S. Franklin

SUMMARY

The majority of the burden of coronary heart disease occurs in persons aged 60 and over. While certain risk factors such as systolic blood pressure and blood glucose remain strongly predictive in older persons, other risk factors such as cholesterol and cigarette smoking have less consistent relationships in older persons. The efficacy of key risk factor interventions, in particular hypertension control and lipid management remain crucial for the prevention of cardiac events in older persons especially because the absolute risk in such persons is substantial. Continued efforts to address the myriad of coronary risk factors common in older persons are crucial to reduce their burden of coronary heart disease.

INTRODUCTION

With more than 70% of cardiovascular diseases (CVD) occurring among developing countries (1), where people are living to an older age due to reduced communicable diseases and improved health care, the burden of CVD, including coronary heart disease (CHD) affecting mainly those aged 65 years and over is rapidly becoming a global problem. There are more than 35 million persons aged 65 years and over in the USA, and this is expected to double by the year 2030, hence the need to better address primary and secondary prevention in this age group is critical (2,3). With approximately 83 million American adults with CVD, approximately 40 million are aged 60 years or greater (4). Twenty-three percent of men and 14% of women aged 60–79 years have CHD and among those 80 years and over, 36% of men and 21% of women in the USA have CHD (Fig. 7.1).

While atherosclerosis begins at an early age, its prevalence is nearly universal by the age of 65 both in men and women (5). With age being the most important risk factor for CVD, the clinical and economic implications of the demographic shift in age distribution not only in the USA, but throughout the developing world are dramatic. The estimated economic costs of CHD are currently over $400 billion annually, and expected to rise to more than $1 trillion by the year 2030 and nearly half of these costs are in those aged 65 years and over (4).

This chapter on the epidemiology of CHD in the elderly will focus on the disease burden and its manifestations, including the extent of subclinical atherosclerosis, as well as the key risk factors for CHD in the elderly and the evidence for managing these risk factors both in primary and in secondary prevention.

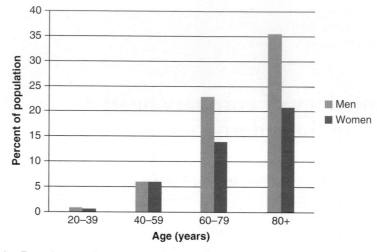

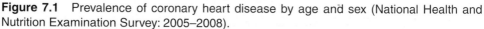

Figure 7.1 Prevalence of coronary heart disease by age and sex (National Health and Nutrition Examination Survey: 2005–2008).

PRESENTATION OF CORONARY HEART DISEASE

The lifetime risk of CHD is substantial; even at age 70, the lifetime risk of a first CHD event is 34.9% in men and 24.2% in women (6). While the average age of a heart attack is 64.5 years in men, it is 70.3 years in women; however, early prognosis is worse for men in part because they have heart attacks at an older age. Eighty-one percent of people overall who die of CHD are aged 65 years and over (4). There is also variation within older individuals. In the Cardiovascular Health Study (CHS), the prevalence of any CHD ranged from 28.4% in men aged 65–74 years to 35.2% in those aged 75–84 years, but in women ranged from 19.2% in those aged 65.74 years to 36.7% in those aged 85 years and over; the large proportion of CHD was due to angina, followed by myocardial infarction (MI), treatment by bypass, and angioplasty (7). The prognosis associated with MI in the elderly is also worse than for younger persons, with recurrent MI being 1.5–3-fold greater in those aged 70 years and over compared to those aged 40–69; death within one year is also 2- to 3-fold higher (8). One-year death rates from MI are 27% in white men, 32% in white women, 26% in black men, and 28% in black women aged 70 years and greater (3). The Atherosclerosis Risk in Communities Study has demonstrated rates of MI to increase approximately 10-fold between the ages of 35–44 and 65–74 years (Fig. 7.2). Annually in the USA, 275,000 adults aged 65–74 years and more than a half million aged 75 years and over suffer an MI or fatal CHD (Fig. 7.3).

The Framingham Heart Study has previously demonstrated that among persons aged 65 years and over experiencing CHD, among men the most common presentation is MI (55%) followed by angina pectoris (30%), and sudden death (15%); however, in women, angina pectoris is most common (45%) followed by MI (40%) and sudden death (12%). Of particular note is the fact that with increasing age, there is a greater proportion of MIs that are clinically unrecognized, being as high as 42% in men aged 75–84 years and 46% among women aged 85 years and over (9).

SUBCLINICAL DISEASE

While many older persons live with no apparent evidence of clinical CVD, evidence of subclinical CVD is common. In the CHS of adults aged 65 years and over without known CVD, carotid artery stenosis >50% was shown to be present in 4.3% of men aged 65–74 years increasing to 10.9% by age 85 years and over, and in women ranged from 3.4% to 11.8%,

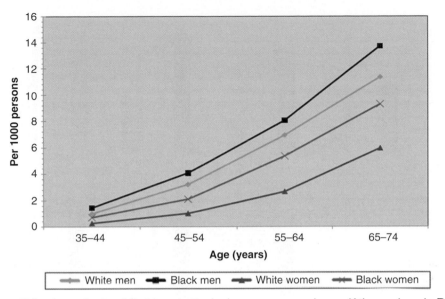

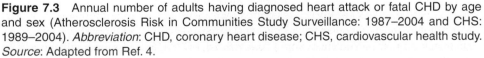

Figure 7.2 Annual rate of first heart attacks by age, sex, and race (Atherosclerosis Risk in Communities Study Surveillance, 1987–2004). *Source*: National Heart Lung and Blood Institute. Adapted from Ref. 4.

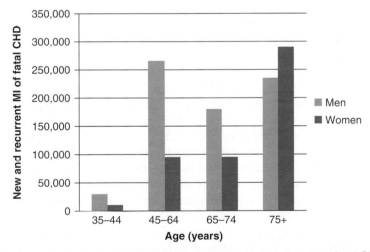

Figure 7.3 Annual number of adults having diagnosed heart attack or fatal CHD by age and sex (Atherosclerosis Risk in Communities Study Surveillance: 1987–2004 and CHS: 1989–2004). *Abbreviation*: CHD, coronary heart disease; CHS, cardiovascular health study. *Source*: Adapted from Ref. 4.

respectively. Moreover, the prevalence of electrocardiographic left ventricular hypertrophy ranged from 2.1% to 6.3% in men and 1.9% to 5.2% in women within these age groups (7). Kuller et al. showed the prevalence of subclinical CVD measured by several characteristics (composite of electrocardiographic abnormalities, ABI<0.9, increased carotid intimal-media thickness (CIMT), echocardiographic abnormalities, angina or claudication) to be 61% with such persons at increased risk of future CVD events (8). Additionally, Wong et al. (5), have shown in the Multiethnic Study of Atherosclerosis the prevalence

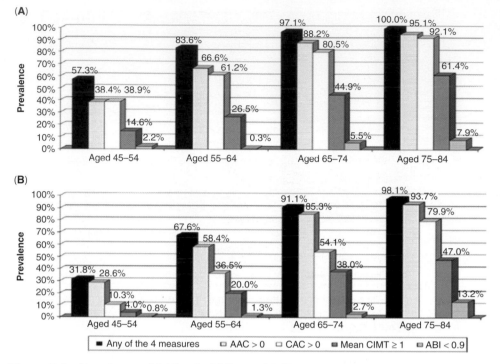

Figure 7.4   Prevalence of AAC > 0, CAC > 0, CIMT ≥ 1 mm, ABI < 0.9, or any of the four measures: Multiethnic Study of Atherosclerosis. *p* < 0.001 across age categories for men and women for each of the measures. *Source*: Adapted from Ref. 5.

of subclinical atherosclerosis measured by either increased CIMT, low ankle-brachial index, or the presence of coronary or abdominal aortic calcification to range from 55% in men aged 45–54 years to 100% among those aged 75–84 years (and 32% to 98% in women, respectively) with abdominal aortic calcification the most common subclinical disease measure, which in fact, unlike coronary calcification, occurs with nearly as high a prevalence in women as in men at most age groups (Fig. 7.4). The presence and extent of abdominal aortic calcification was in particular a strong predictor of the presence of other subclinical measures of atherosclerosis (increased CIMT, low ABI, or coronary artery calcium).

RISK FACTORS

The distribution of risk for CVD rises dramatically with age with more than half of men and nearly one-third of women by the age of 70 being at ≥10% 10-year CVD risk (Fig. 7.5). Data from the Framingham Heart Study show the risk of CHD increases more than five-fold according to the number of risk factors present (Fig. 7.6). In general, as shown by the Framingham Heart Study, most risk factors for younger persons also hold for those in older age groups, but not consistently in both genders. While systolic blood pressure (SBP) is strongly associated with CHD both in younger and older persons in both genders, diastolic blood pressure (DBP) appears to be weaker in older women and while total cholesterol is strongly associated with CHD in younger men and women, it loses its importance in older men. Blood glucose is a power predictor both in older and younger women, and older men, but not younger men. In addition, cigarette smoking appears to be less important of a predictor in older persons of both genders than in younger persons (9).

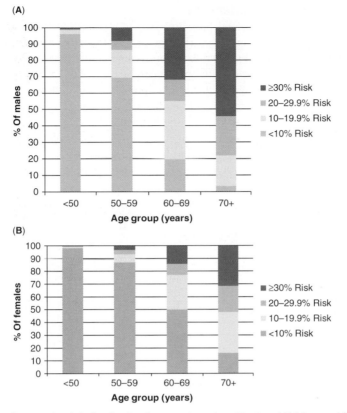

Figure 7.5 Cardiovascular risk distribution by age, Americas Region: (**A**) Men and (**B**) Women. *Source*: From Ref. 1.

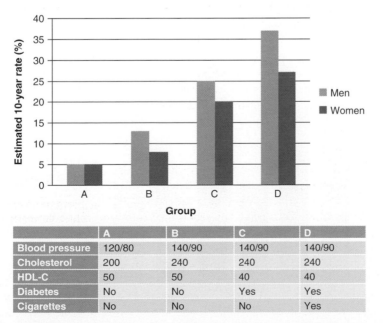

Figure 7.6 Estimated 10-year coronary heart disease risk in adults 55 years of age according to levels of various risk factors (Framingham Heart Study). *Source*: Adapted from Ref. 4.

Blood Pressure and Hypertension

On a global basis, elevated blood pressure (BP) is responsible for more than 7 million deaths annually, more than any other risk factor (1). Hypertension among US adults is more prevalent than any other CVD risk factor in older adults, present on two-third of men aged 65 years and over, and nearly 80% of women by the age of 75 (Fig. 7.7). Among those with hypertension, we have shown that while under the age of 40 years isolated diastolic hypertension (systolic <140 mg/dL while diastolic ≥90 mmHg) is the most common subtype, by the fifth decade of life systolic hypertension (isolated systolic and systolic diastolic combined) becomes predominant, and by the sixth decade of life, isolated systolic hypertension (ISH) becomes the most predominant subtype (10). By ages 60–69, more than 80% are of the ISH (Fig. 7.8), due to large artery stiffness increasing with advancing

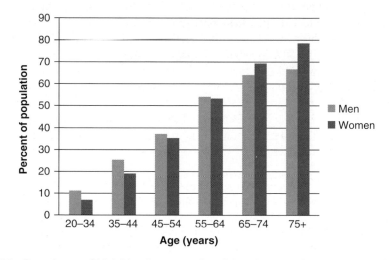

Figure 7.7   Prevalence of high blood pressure in adults ≥20 years by age and sex (NHANES: 2005–2008). *Source*: Adapted from Ref. 4.

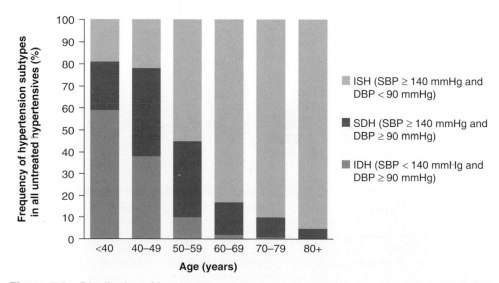

Figure 7.8   Distribution of hypertension subtype in the untreated hypertensive population in NHANES III by age. *Source*: Adapted from Ref. 10.

age. Moreover, in the presence of diseases that accelerate arterial stiffness, such as diabetes or chronic renal disease, ISH can develop at an earlier age (11). Furthermore, a Framingham study showed that normotensive persons reaching age 65 years had a 90% lifetime risk of developing hypertension—almost exclusively of the ISH subtype—if they lived another 20–25 years (12).

Considerable evidence, including a series of Framingham Heart studies, now favors the superiority of increased pulse pressure and decreased DBP to that of elevated SBP alone in predicting cardiovascular risk in the elderly. After age 50, SBP increases disproportionately to DBP, and after 60 years of age DBP falls, resulting in a further widening of pulse pressure (13). In the age range of 50–79 years, SBP was positively related to the incidence of CHD risk and DBP was inversely related to risk, therefore supporting pulse pressure as a stronger CHD risk factor than SBP (14). Age is an important effect-modifier in influencing BP components that predict CHD risk. Indeed, with advancing age, there is a gradual shift from DBP to SBP and eventually to pulse pressure as predictors of CHD risk (15). Additionally, it was shown that combining SBP and DBP was superior to SBP alone in predicting CVD risk (16). SBP is usually superior to DBP as a predictor of CVD risk from the age of 50 years onward; however, very high or very low DBP add to the SBP risk (16). For example, a DBP <70 mmHg can add approximately 20 mmHg of SBP risk to subjects with high-normal or stage 1 hypertension (Table 7.1). Importantly, data from the National Health and Nutrition Examination Survey (NHANES) confirmed that DBP <70 mmHg, with a prevalence of 30% among untreated persons with ISH, was associated with increased CVD risk; advanced age, female sex, and diabetes mellitus, but not treatment status, were associated with low DBP (17).

While those aged 60–69 and 70 years and over have high treatment rates for hypertension (81–65%), control rates are poor (54 and 33% among those treated), largely due to SBP being far from target. Among most persons with cardiovascular comorbidities, mean age exceeds 65 years and ISH is the most predominant subtype, with SBP averaging 20 mmHg or more away from goal (18). Analyzing treatment failures by age revealed in the

Table 7.1 Prediction of CVD events by ESH & JNC-6 Stages

JNC-6 Group	BP Limits	SBP/DBP	OR (95% CI)
Optimal	SBP < 120 DBP < 80	109/69	Ref. = 1.0
"Pre-HTN"	SBP 120–139 DBP < 70	127/65	2.0 (1.5–2.6)[a]
Stage 1 ISH	SBP 140–159 DBP 70–89	147/81	2.0 (1.6–2.5)[a]
Stage 1 ISH	SBP 140–159 DBP < 70	147/64	3.0 (2.1–4.3)[a]
Stage 2 ISH	SBP ≥ 160 DBP < 90	171/81	3.1 (2.4–4.1)[a]
Stage 2 SDH	SBP ≥ 160 DBP 90–99	172/94	2.7 (2.0–3.6)[a]
Stage 2 SDH	SBP 160–179 DBP ≥ 100	168/106	3.6 (2.5–5.1)[a]

[a]$p < 0.0001$.
Abbreviations: DBP, diastolic blood pressure; HTN, hypertension; ISH, isolated systolic hypertension; JNC-6, Sixth Joint National Committee; SBP, systolic blood pressure; SDH, systolic-diastolic hypertension; ESH, European Society of Hypertension.
Source: Adapted from Ref. 16.

NHANES III subjects an age-related discrepancy in the successful control of BP (10). Approximately 50% of younger patients who failed treatment had both SBP and DBP that were not at target goals, representing a concordant failure in this younger population (10). In contrast, older patients who failed to achieve treatment goals had discordant failure: Only 17% of patients aged 50 or over were above their DBP goal, but fully 82% were above their SBP target goal and by a significantly greater SBP margin (10).

While several aspects involving treatment approaches may explain the failure to optimally control ISH overall, including physician inertia and patient nonadherence, one must conclude that there exists a substantial number of patients with systolic hypertension that are truly resistant to currently available medications, even when used properly. That the target SBP apparently becomes more difficult to achieve with aging might be explained by the presence of advanced large artery stiffness.

Numerous antihypertensive clinical trials have also shown important reductions in CVD events in older men and women. This includes the Swedish Trial in Old Patients with Hypertension among those aged 70–84 years, demonstrating a 25% reduction in fatal MI and a 67% reduction in sudden deaths and 73% reduction in fatal stroke (19), the Medical Research Council trial among those aged 65–74 years showing a 25% reduction in stroke (20), the Systolic Hypertension in the Elderly study (21) among those aged 72 years on average showing a 27% reduction in nonfatal MIs and coronary death, 36% reduction in stroke and a 49% reduction in heart failure, and in the Systolic Hypertension in Europe study (mean age 70) (22) showing a 42% reduction in stroke, but smaller nonsignificant reductions in MI and coronary mortality. Moreover, a meta-analysis of 1670 persons aged 80 years and over with hypertension showed drug therapy to reduce stroke 34%, major CVD events 22% and heart failure 39% (23). In the largest single antihypertensive clinical trial, the Antihypertensive and Lipid-Lowering Treatment to Prevent Heart Attack Trial (ALLHAT) consisting of over 40,000 patients of mean age 67 years with hypertension showed after 5 years of follow-up that compared with chlorthalidone, amlodipine increased heart failure 38% and lisinopril combined CVD 10%, stroke 15% and heart failure 19%, despite no statistically significant difference between the drugs in the primary endpoint of fatal CHD or nonfatal MI (relative risks of 0.98–0.99) (24). Also, in the Second Australian National Blood Pressure Study, 6083 patients with mean age 72 years were randomized to hydrochlorothiazide or to the angiotensin-converting enzyme (ACE) inhibitor enalapril and after 4.1 years the latter resulted in a significant 11% reduction in all CVD or death from any cause (25).

Finally, with the lack of clinical trials done in those aged 80 years and older, the Hypertension in the Very Elderly Trial (HYVET) study randomized over 3800 persons with a SBP of 160 mmHg or higher to the diuretic indapamide (sustained release, 1.5 mg) or matching placebo for 2 years and found the active treatment was associated with a 30% reduction in the rate of fatal or nonfatal stroke ($p = 0.06$), a 39% reduction in the rate of death from stroke ($p = 0.05$), and a 21% reduction in the rate of death from any cause ($p = 0.02$), with a 64% reduction in the rate of heart failure ($p < 0.001$) (Fig. 7.9) (26). On the other hand, there are questions that remain unanswered in the HYVET study, which was stopped prematurely at 18 months. The majority of recruited subjects for HYVET were healthy and robust; would an increasing number of frail elderly give different results? Secondly, what is the optimal BP target goal for maximizing therapeutic benefit in the HYVET study?

To date, there have been no intervention trials involving the elderly that used SBP target goals of <160 mmHg. However, national and international guidelines used target goals of <140 mmHg for all ages, largely on the basis of expert opinion rather than on outcome of randomized controlled trials. There is a new US consensus statement (27) that

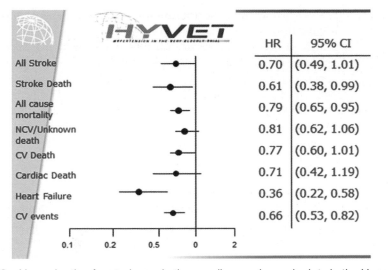

	HR	95% CI
All Stroke	0.70	(0.49, 1.01)
Stroke Death	0.61	(0.38, 0.99)
All cause mortality	0.79	(0.65, 0.95)
NCV/Unknown death	0.81	(0.62, 1.06)
CV Death	0.77	(0.60, 1.01)
Cardiac Death	0.71	(0.42, 1.19)
Heart Failure	0.36	(0.22, 0.58)
CV events	0.66	(0.53, 0.82)

Figure 7.9 Hazard ratios for stroke and other cardiovascular endpoints in the Hypertension in the Very Elderly Trial (HYVET). *Source*: Adapted from Ref. 26.

confirms antihypertensive therapy should be started in uncomplicated hypertension in persons aged 65–79 years with a SBP of ≥140 mmHg or a DBP of ≥90 mmHg with a target goal of <140/90 mmHg; however, in persons ≥80 years of age, the threshold for starting therapy and target goal was raised to a SBP of ≥150 mmHg (27). Unfortunately, there is no agreement on how to define elderly. Should it be based on chronological or physiological age? Are we dealing with vigorous or frail elderly with competing illnesses? Thus, there are no firm randomized controlled trial outcomes that provide a basis of using geriatric chronological age cut-points versus overall general health of the patient for a guide as how low to go with antihypertensive therapy. Furthermore, the Blood Pressure Treatment Trialists' Collaboration studies have not shown major significant differences between drug classes in treating the elderly on the basis of differences in major events; therefore, factors such as tolerability and cost can be used to determine choice (28).

Controversy persists regarding the presence and significance of BP "J-curves" of increased cardiovascular disease risk as they relate to older people with ISH (29). A solitary DBP J-curve, noted in the Framingham Heart Study with elevated SBP and pulse pressure, strongly suggests increased large artery stiffness (16); risk is defined by increased pulse pressure that results in decreased DBP and increased SBP. In contrast, the combination of J-curves of SBP and DBP, with normal-to-low pulse pressure and low MAP, strongly suggest reverse causality (29); risk is defined by decreased DBP and decreased SBP, rather than by increased pulse pressure. Finally, in the presence of high-grade stenosis of coronary arteries, increased risk of MI with antihypertensive therapy-induced decrease in BP may well occur (30), but is by far the least common occurrence of the J-curve phenomenon. Indeed, the risk of plaque disruption that leads to acute coronary syndromes depends more on plaque composition, plaque vulnerability (plaque type), and the degree of pulsatile stress than on the degree of coronary artery stenosis (plaque size) (31), Not surprisingly, therefore, the majority of MIs (>70%) occur from plaque rupture in coronary arteries that have <50% stenosis (31). Because of the many factors that result in J-curve risks, only a prospective trial with baseline and pre-event BP determinations can establish the presence and frequency of treatment-induced increase risk. On the other hand, the optimal therapeutic reduction in SBP and DBP in elderly subjects with ISH that maximizes benefit is a separate question from the presence of a therapeutic J-curve of increased cardiovascular risk.

In summary, there is overwhelming evidence that middle-aged and elderly persons have the highest prevalence of hypertension, predominantly of the ISH subtype, and this represents a significant burden for future CVD events. Paradoxically, ISH in the elderly remains more difficult to control than diastolic hypertension in younger adults. The therapeutic target goal in reducing SBP and DBP depends in part on competing comorbidities, disabilities, and the presence of possible orthostatic hypotension. Future randomized controlled trials based on out-of-office BP monitoring are necessary to determine how low to go for maximum benefit of antihypertensive therapy.

Dyslipidemia

While the Framingham Heart Study initially showed that serum cholesterol loses its predictive value in older men (9), other cohorts have shown it remains a risk factor for new or recurrent events in both older men and women (32–35). Aronow et al. have demonstrated among 644 elderly men and 1488 elderly women with 40–48 month follow-up a 12% increase in risk for every 10 mg/dL increment in total cholesterol (32). In a large meta-analysis among 22 US and international cohort studies, serum cholesterol appears to be a weaker predictor in both older men and women (36), although this is confounded by frailty and other comorbid conditions that when adjusted for appears to strength it as a predictor of CHD death (37).

Castelli et al. also showed an important inverse relation of low High Density Lipoprotein-Cholesterol (HDL-C) cholesterol with new coronary events (33), and Aronow et al., showed a 70% increased risk in men and 95% increased risk in women for every decrement of 10 mg/dL in HDL-C among the large elderly cohort described above (32). This study also showed hypertriglyceridemia not to be a risk factor in men and a weak risk factor for CHD events in women. While total cholesterol (whose measurement alone is obsolete) is not a consistent predictor of risk, HDL-C or use of the total cholesterol/HDL-C ratio, in particular, appears to be an important indicator of risk from several studies (38–40).

In several major clinical trials, the efficacy of lipid intervention has been shown to be similar when comparing older persons to younger persons. In the Scandanavian Simvastatin Survival Study (4S), a placebo-controlled trial among high risk persons, mostly with pre-existing CHD, the statin treated group shows a 43% reduction in CHD mortality among those aged 65 and over versus under age 65 (41). Moreover, in the Cholesterol and Recurrent Events (CARE) study, statin therapy was actually somewhat more effective for reducing major recurrent coronary events in those aged 65 years and over (32% risk reduction) compared to those under age 65 (19% risk reduction) (42). Few trials of lipid intervention have been done specifically in the elderly. In the Prosper trial (43), men and women aged 70–82 years with a history of, or risk factors for, vascular disease were randomized to pravastatin (40 mg per day; $n = 2891$) or placebo ($n = 2913$). Follow-up was 3.2 years on average with the primary endpoint a composite of coronary death, nonfatal MI, and fatal or nonfatal stroke. Pravastatin lowered LDL cholesterol concentrations by 34% and reduced the incidence of the primary endpoint (hazard ratio 0.85, 95% CI 0.74–0.97, $p = 0.014$). CHD death and nonfatal MI risk was also reduced (0.81, 0.69–0.94, $p = 0.006$). However, new cancer diagnoses were more frequent on pravastatin than on placebo (1.25, 1.04–1.51, $p = 0.020$) although incorporation of this finding in a meta-analysis of all pravastatin and statin trials showed no overall increase in risk. Importantly, the Cholesterol Treatment Trialists' collaboration (44) of over 170,000 subjects among 26 trials showed an overall benefit of lipid-lowering therapy to reduce CHD event risk by 22% with no significant differences across age groups <65 years, 65–74 years, and 75 years and over, although the benefit appeared a bit weaker (16% risk reduction) in the latter group.

Metabolic Syndrome and Diabetes

Metabolic syndrome as defined by the American Heart Association/National Heart, Lung, and Blood Institute (NHLBI) definition (45) as the presence of three or more of the following factors: (*i*) abdominal obesity defined as a waist circumference >102 cm in men or >88 cm in women, (*ii*) increased BP of ≥130 mmHg systolic or ≥85 mmHg diastolic or on therapy for BP, (*iii*) impaired fasting glucose of 100 mg/dL or higher or on hypoglycemic therapy, (*iv*) HDL-cholesterol <40 mg/dL in men or <50 mg/dL in women or on medication for low HDL-C, and/or (*v*) fasting triglycerides of 150 mg/dL or higher or on medication for triglycerides. The prevalence of metabolic syndrome in US adults increases dramatically with age, exceeding 50% by the age of 65 (46). Moreover, diabetes, defined by a fasting glucose or ≥126 mg/dL or higher or on hypoglycemic therapy, also increases in prevalence with age, approaching 20% by the age of 65 (47), with a lifetime risk of 25–45% in females and 30–55% in males that varies substantially according to ethnicity, being highest in Hispanics and lowest in non-Hispanic whites (48) (Fig. 7.10). Importantly, with the burden of CVD risk factors increasing as well with age, estimated short-term (10-year) risk of CHD or CVD increases with age, with many persons with metabolic syndrome or DM who already either have CHD or CVD or are at >20% 10-year risk of these conditions by the age of 65 (49,50). 80% or more of those with diabetes over the age of 60 are at either >20% CVD risk or have pre-existing CVD (50) (Fig. 7.11).

Diabetes is clearly a risk factor for CHD events in older men and women (32,40) and has been associated with an approximate two-fold increase in risk of new coronary events in a large study of 644 elderly men and 1488 elderly women followed for 40–48 months (32). In the Framingham Heart Study, increased blood glucose as well as composite of glucose intolerance and diabetes was a powerful risk factor for incident CHD events in 30-year follow-up (9); it is also a stronger risk factor in women, both among younger and older adults (51).

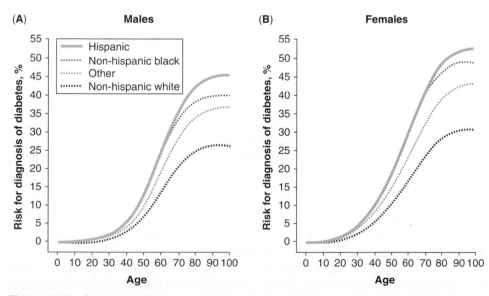

Figure 7.10 Cumulative lifetime risk of developing diabetes by age and ethnicity. *Source*: Adapted from Ref. 48.

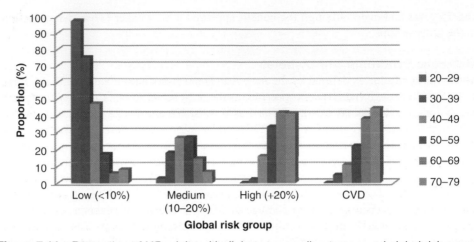

Figure 7.11   Proportion of US adults with diabetes according to age and global risk group. *Source*: Adapted from Ref. 50.

There have not been any large clinical trials examining the impact of intensive glycemic control in older persons with diabetes; however, several large trials have examined stratification of their key results according to age groups. For example, the Action in Diabetes and Vascular Disease: Preterax and Diamicron MR Controlled Evaluation (ADVANCE) Study of intensive blood glucose control and vascular outcomes in 11,140 persons with type-2 diabetes showed intensive control to an HbA1c to ≤6.5% showed a similar 30% reduction in combined major microvascular and macrovascular events in both those aged <65 and 65 and over, although the finding did not reach statistical significance in the older subgroup and overall this study did not show a risk reduction in major macrovascular events (52). The Action to Control Cardiovascular Risk in Diabetes (ACCORD) Study Group similarly showed no beneficial effect of intensive glucose control among 10,251 patients randomized to standard or intensive therapy to achieve an HbA1c <6.0% in either younger or older (age 65 years or greater) subgroups (53). Given that these trials tended to show benefit in persons with less advanced diabetes (shorter duration and without prior macrovascular disease), the benefit of intensive glycemic control in older persons is doubtful because of their high prevalence of pre-existing CVD and/or long standing type-2 diabetes in general.

Cigarette Smoking

The Framingham Heart Study initially demonstrated that cigarette smoking was not associated with incident CHD in persons aged 65 and over; however, approximate 2-fold greater risks of CHD among smokers have been observed both among men aged 65–74 years in the Honolulu Heart Study (54) as well as in 40–48 month follow-up of 644 men and 1488 women with a mean age of 80 years (32). Among secondary prevention studies, the Coronary Artery Surgery Study (CASS) showed a 1.5-fold greater risk of MI or death in those aged 65–69 years of age, which increased to 2.9-fold for those aged 70 and over among those who continued to smoke compared to quitters (55). CASS data additionally showed that the 6-year mortality rate (relative risk of 1.7) was greater among continuing smokers as compared to those who quit smoking a year prior to the study and abstained from smoking throughout the study. Importantly, there was no diminution of the beneficial effects of smoking cessation by age. This indicates that smoking cessation lessens the risk of MI and improves survival rates in both older and younger individuals.

Overweight and Obesity

It has been well established that obesity is a risk factor for second coronary events in older adults with CHD. While past prospective studies have shown that general and central adiposity are risk factors for CHD incidence in middle-aged men and women, fewer studies have focused on CHD in the elderly population. Data from the Framingham Heart Study suggest that older persons have similar risk factors for coronary artery disease as younger adults (56).While true, studies of data from both the Honolulu Heart Program and the Health Professionals Follow-Up Study (HPFS) have shown that weight gain in adults younger than 65 years of age are more strongly correlated with CHD risk than weight gain in those older than 65 years (57,58). The different correlations of weight gain to CHD in younger and older adults may be attributable to the phenomenon of gradual fat replacement of muscle in older adults. This phenomenon explains why past cohort studies in the elderly have found weak to no correlation of BMI with CHD (57,58). However, these same studies did show waist circumference and fat distribution are strong predictor of CVD and CHD events (59). Rimm et al. using HPFS data showed that among men ≥65 years of age despite a weak association between BMI and risk of CHD, waist-to-hip ratio showed a relative risk of 2.76 when comparing extreme quintiles (57). This is most likely due to increased body fat in the abdominal cavity with increased age, causing body mass index (BMI) to become a worse indicator of overall fat in older persons (60).

Villareal et al. used a randomized control trial to show that lifestyle interventions of diet induced weight loss and exercise training improved obesity related CHD risk factors in obese older adults (61). These results indicate that CHD risk factors, including waist circumference, BP, circulating inflammatory markers, oral glucose tolerance, insulin resistance, plasma glucose, triglycerides, and FFA concentrations, were reversible not only in younger obese adults but also in older obese adults.

Physical Activity

Decreased fitness and physical activity has been shown to be a predictor of mortality in older adults (62). These findings, independent of overall or abdominal adiposity, have led to recommendations for regular physical activity in older adults. Physical activity is additionally a significant predictor of CHD risk. Data from the Honolulu Heart Program show a 2.2 relative risk of developing a coronary event for those who walked less than 0.25 miles a day as compared to those who walked more than 1.5 miles a day (63). Similar results were found from the Harvard Alumni Study, in which men with a starting mean age of 66 who expended 4000 kcal/week in physical activities through recreational sports, stairs climbing, and walking found a relative risk reduction of 38% for CHD as compared to those expending less than 1000 kcal/week (64). The study found that the duration of physical activity did not have a different effect on relative risk as long as energy expended was the same. Such physical activity has proven beneficial for total cardiovascular health in the elderly. Data from 1645 men and women older than 65 years old showed that walking more than 4 hours/week was associated significantly with a reduced risk of cardiovascular disease hospitalization (relative risk of 0.69) compared to those walking less than 1 hour/ week after adjusting for baseline cardiovascular risk factors and general health (65). Of note in all these studies of older cohorts, smaller proportions of individuals were older than 80 years of age. Nonetheless, data from these studies suggest that exercise in older adults have similar magnitudes of benefits of CHD risk reduction as seen in those who are younger.

Secondary prevention through physical activity has additionally been proven effective for reduction of mortality secondary to CHD. A study of the British Regional Heart Study showed that of those patients diagnosed with CHD, lowest risk for all-cause cardiovascular mortality were seen in patients with light and moderate physical activity (relative risks of 0.42 and 0.47 respectively) as compared to those patients who were inactive or occasionally active (66). Nonsporting activities such as heavy gardening and regular walking were seen to be more beneficial than sporting activities.

Inflammatory Risk Factors

Inflammatory makers increase with age, due to declining levels of sex hormones and increases in visceral adipose tissue (67). Thus, whether these inflammatory markers can be categorized as independent risk factors for CHD has become of high interest for early screening. C-reactive protein (CRP) has been established as an acute inflammatory marker that plays a significant role in cardiovascular health. In 2002, American Heart Association and Center for Disease Control suggested that CRP may be a useful screening mechanism for 10-year risk of CHD between 10% and 20% (68). However, not based on data from elderly population, these recommendations would have applied to the vast majority of American men and women over the age of 65 who have a 10-year CHD risk of at least 10% (69). Inflammatory markers have been shown to have association with CHD risk prediction for older adults; however there added benefit over other traditional risk factors are controversial. Cesari et al. used data from patients aged 70–79 in the Health, Aging, and Body Composition Study (Health ABC) to be one of the first to predict cardiovascular events using a broad spectrum of inflammatory markers in an older population (70). This study showed that interleukin-6 (IL-6) and tumor necrosis factor-alpha (TNF-α), but not CRP were associated with CHD events. However, a subsequent analysis of the ABC study showed that only the IL-6 increased risk of incident CHD beyond traditional risk factors (71). Using IL-6 6.6% of participants could accurately reclassify those at risk for CHD incidence.

Lipoprotein-associated phospholipase A2 (Lp-PLA2), a proatherogenic inflammatory marker, has been shown to been strongly associated with risk of incident CHD in middle age populations (72,73). Data from the Rancho Bernardo Study showed that Lp-PLA2 mass has demonstrated capabilities for predicting risk of CHD independent of traditional risk factors of CHD in healthy older adults (74). Hazard ratios ranging between 1.89 and 1.75 were calculated for the highest Lp-PLA2 quartile when compared to the lowest quartile after adjusting for cumulative traditional CHD risk factors.

PREVENTIVE STRATEGIES
Primordial and Primary Prevention

Preventing CHD in the elderly involves not only primary and secondary prevention approaches but also primordial prevention approaches, that is preventing the major CHD risk factors from developing in the first place. The construct of the American Heart Association's Life's Simple Seven (75) calls for maintaining normal cholesterol, BP, glucose, body fat, being a nonsmoker, and following a heart healthy diet and getting regular physical activity. Of interest are data from the NHANES 2007–2008, which shows that older persons adhered least to meeting these important criteria for heart health; those aged 60 years and over had the lowest proportion of any age group meeting four or more criteria; barely 10% had four criteria met and less than 5% had five or six of the heart healthy criteria met (Fig. 7.12).

While the relative benefits of BP lowering and lipid intervention, in particular have been shown to be consistent across all age groups, such interventions are of particular importance in the elderly where the absolute risk for CHD events is dramatically higher than in younger persons. Thus, the absolute risk reduction resulting from risk factor interventions is dramatic and number of preventable CHD events substantial. For example,

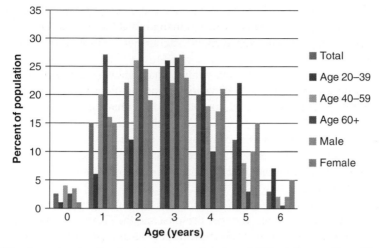

Figure 7.12 Age-standardized prevalence estimates of US adults meeting different numbers of criteria for Ideal Cardiovascular Health, overall and by age and sex subgroups, National Health and Nutrition Examination Survey (NHANES) 2007–2008. *Source*: Adapted from Ref. 4.

we have previously demonstrated among US adults with the metabolic syndrome that optimal management of dyslipidemia (LDL-C and HDL-C) and BP could potentially prevent up to 80% of CHD events, a finding that is consistent across age groups. This translates to preventing about 1.3 million CHD events in men and 530,000 CHD events in women; however, of these, approximately 600,000 of those events in men and 300,000 in women are among those aged 60 years and over (76). In the same study, optimal management of BP to <120/80 mmHg would be projected to prevent up to 29% of CHD events in older men and 48% of CHD events in older women.

Given that hypertension is the single greatest cause of mortality globally (1), its prevention and control is especially among the elderly who have the highest absolute risks due to CHD, is essential. Besides sodium restriction, achieving ideal body weight, moderation of alcohol consumption and getting regular physical activity, which each can lower SBP 5 mmHg or more, together can have a significant impact on controlling elevated BP. Achieving better adherence to these means to lower BP is crucial given that many older persons still have SBP averaging 20 mmHg or more away from goal despite being on treatment (10).

Tobacco use, high blood glucose, physical inactivity, overweight/obesity, and elevated cholesterol levels being the second through sixth top risk factors for death globally make these important targets for primary prevention of CHD in the elderly as well given their predominance in older adults. The benefits of tobacco cessation and lipid intervention are well demonstrated in the elderly and improved weight control and physical activity will have benefits also in helping to maintain healthy blood glucose levels and prevention of diabetes.

Secondary Prevention

Secondary prevention of CHD in the elderly involves intervention on many of the same risk factors although there is a lack of studies that have described these interventions in older persons (77). Smoking cessation can reduce overall mortality by 25–50% in those who have suffered a MI with much of this decline in the first year (78).

Smoking cessation rates in middle-aged and older persons range from 20% to 70% after 1 year (79); multiple component programs combine strong physician advice with behavioral counseling, nicotine replacement therapy and nurse case management for follow-up (80).

For antihypertensive therapy, meta-analyses have shown the efficacy of treatment to be particularly high in those aged 60–80 years (81) and in older persons, more strokes and heart failure are generally prevented compared to coronary events. While the general target of <140/90 mmHg holds, a lower target such as <130 in those with heart failure, renal insufficiency of diabetes is recommended (82); however, subsequent guidelines have suggest more lenient targets in less complicated patients (such as a systolic BP <150 mmHg) may be appropriate given the lack of rigorous clinical trial evidence in the elderly population (27).

For lipid-lowering therapy, given the consistency of statin therapy to impact on reducing CHD events both in older and younger persons, and the greater absolute baseline CHD risk makes appropriate achievement of lipid targets an important measure in secondary prevention. It is estimated from the CARE study where statin therapy was shown to be even a bit more effective in older patients with known CHD (32% risk reduction compared with 19% risk reduction) where total cholesterol <240 mg/dL that for every 1000 older patients treated, 225 CVD hospitalizations could be prevented compared with 121 for 1000 younger patients (83). Statin therapy in the elderly has been shown to be cost-effective, with an incremental cost per quality-adjusted life year being $18,800 which will be even lower if estimated based on the cost of now widely available generic statins (82).

The control of obesity, which is an important risk factor for secondary CHD events in older persons with CHD from the Framingham Heart Study (83) can have important benefits on several important risk factors including dyslipidemia, hypertension, and insulin resistance, which all impact on CHD risk. It is well-established that exercise training alone without a nutritional approach has only a minimal effect, thus a multidiscliplinary approach combining the two, along with other behavioral intervention as needed is critically important. There are relatively few studies specifically among the elderly in those with CHD that have documented the effects of weight loss. In one study of obese patients of mean age 60 who had CHD, a mean weight loss of 11 kg was associated with a 10% reduction in total and LDL-cholesterol, 24% reduction in triglycerides, and an 8% increase in HDL-C as a result of a hypocaloric diet (84).

While there is a lack of data on the efficacy of diabetes interventions in elderly persons with CHD, the management of diabetes, which is often accompanied by dyslipidemia and hypertension, particularly in the elderly, is crucial to preventing microvascular complications and also reduces the attributable risk of CHD events especially due to dyslipidemia and hypertension. While an official goal A1c <7% is generally recommended, especially in those with relatively uncomplicated diabetes, most older persons have had long-standing diabetes and/or macrovascular disease; such subgroups of persons had an increased risk of cardiovascular mortality in ACCORD and thus less stringent A1c goals may be appropriate in many such elderly patients.

CONCLUSIONS

Much of the burden and costs due to hospitalizations from CHD are borne by those aged 65 years and over. With key lifestyle recommendations that we know can help to prevent or reduce the development of important risk factors such as hypertension, dyslipidemia, and diabetes, as well as known pharmacologic interventions to address hypertension, dyslipidemia and other risk factors whose effects have been demonstrated to be consistent in older populations, we have a significant opportunity in this decade to keep older persons healthier and free of CHD longer; this represents the concept of healthy aging. The clear guidelines we have for secondary prevention of CHD and efficacy of risk factor interventions in this group as well can have a significant impact on reducing risk of recurrent events as well. What is now known about prevention that was not known or accepted a generation ago can help keep our current young and middle-aged adult populations healthier into their senior years, hopefully having a dramatic effect on increasing the CVD-free life expectancy.

REFERENCES

1. Mendis S, Puska P, Norvving B, eds. Global Atlas on Cardiovascular Disease Prevention and Control. Geneva: World Health Organization, 2011.
2. US Census Bureau. US Population Projects: 2010–2050. Washington, DC: US Dept of Commerce, 2008: [Available from: www.census.gov/population/www/projections/summarytables.html]
3. Najjar SS, Lakatta EG, Gerstenblith G. Cardiovascular aging: the next frontier in cardiovascular prevention. In: Blumenthal RS, Foody JM, Wong ND, eds. Preventive Cardiology: A Companion to Braunwald's Heart Disease. New York: Elsevier, 2011.
4. Roger VL, Go AS, Lloyd-Jones DM, et al. Heart disease and stroke statistics-2012 update: a report from the American Heart Association. Circulation 2012; 125: e2–e220; published online before print December 15, 2011, 10.11/CIR.0b013e31823ac046.
5. Wong ND, Lopez VA, Allison M, et al. Abdominal aortic calcium and multi-site atherosclerosis: the Multiethnic Study of Atherosclerosis. Atherosclerosis 2011; 214: 436–41.
6. Lloyd-Jones D, Larson MG, Beiser A, et al. Lifetime risk of developing coronary heart disease. Lancet 1999; 353: 89–92.
7. Bild DE, Fitzpatrick A, Fried LP, et al. Age-related trends in cardiovascular morbidity and physical functioning in the elderly: the Cardiovascular Health Study. J Am Geriatr Soc 1993; 41: 1047–56.
8. Kuller LH, Arnold AM, Psaty BM, et al. 10-year follow-up of subclinical cardiovascular disease and risk of coronary heart disease in the cardiovascular health study. Arch Intern Med 2006; 166: 71–8.
9. Cupples LA, D'Agostino RB. Section 34. Some risk factors related to the annual incidence of cardiovascular disease and death using pooled repeated biennial measurements: Framingham Heart Study, 30-year follow-up. In: Kannel WB, Wolf PA, Garrison RJ, eds. The Framingham Study: An Epidemiological Investigation of Cardiovascular Disease. Bethesda, MD: National Heart, Lung and Blood Institute, publication No. (NIH), 1987: 87–2703.
10. Franklin SS, Jacobs MJ, Wong ND, et al. Predominance of isolated systolic hypertension among middle-aged and elderly US hypertensives. Hypertension 2001; 37: 869–74.
11. Ronnback M, Fagerudd J, Forsblom C, et al. Altered age-related blood pressure pattern in type 1 diabetes. Circulation 2004; 110: 1076–108.
12. Vasan RS, Beiser A, Seshadri S, et al. Residual lifetime risk for developing hypertension in middle-aged women and women: the Framingham Heart Study. JAMA 2002; 287: 1003–10.
13. Franklin SS, Gustin W, Wong ND, et al. Hemodynamic patterns of age-related changes in blood pressure. The Framingham Heart Study. Circulation 1997; 96: 308–15.
14. Franklin SS, Khan SA, Wong ND, et al. Is pulse pressure useful in predicting risk for coronary heart disease? The Framingham Heart Study. Circulation 1999; 100: 354–60.
15. Franklin SS, Larson MG, Khan SA, et al. Does the relation of blood pressure to coronary heart disease risk change with aging? The Framingham Heart Study. Circulation 2001; 103: 1245–9.
16. Franklin SS, Lopez VA, Wong ND, et al. Single versus combined blood pressure components and risk for cardiovascular disease. The Framingham Heart Study. Circulation 2009; 119: 243–50.
17. Franklin SS, Chow VH, Mori A, et al. The significance of low DBP in US adults with isolated systolic hypertension. J Hypertens 2011; 29: 1101–8.
18. Wong ND, Lopez VA, L'Italien G, et al. Inadequate control of hypertension in U.S. adults with cardiovascular disease comorbidities in 2003–2004. Arch Intern Med 2007; 167: 2437–42.
19. Dalhof B, Lindholm LH, Hansson L, et al. Morbidity and mortality in the Swedish Trail in Old Patients with Hypetension (STOP Hypertension). Lancet 1991; 338: 1281–5.
20. MRC Working Party. Medical Research Council Trial of treatment of hypertension in older adults: principal results. BMJ 1992; 304: 405–12.
21. SHEP Cooperative Research Group. Prevention of stroke by antihypertensive drug treatment in older persons with isolated systolic hypertension: final results of the Systolic Hypertension in the Elderly Program (SHEP). JAMA 1991; 265: 3255–64.
22. Staessen JA, Fagard R, Thijs L, et al. Randomised double-blind comparison of placebo and active treatment for older patients with isolated systolic hypertension. Lancet 1997; 350: 757–64.

23. Gueyffier F, Bulpitt C, Boissel J-P, et al. Antihypertensive drugs in very old people: a subgroup meta-analysis of randomized controlled trials. Lancet 1999; 353: 793–6.
24. ALLHAT Officers and Coordinators for the ALLHAT Collaborative Research Group. Major outcomes in high-risk hypertensive patients randomized to angiotensin-converting enzyme inhibitor or calcium channel blocker vs. diuretics: the Antihypertensive and Lipid-Lowering Treatment to Prevent Heart Attack Trial (ALLHAT). JAMA 2002; 288: 2981–97.
25. Wing LMH, Reid CM, Ryan P, et al. A comparison of outcomes with angiotrension-coverting enzyme inhibitors and diuretics for hypertension in the elderly. N Engl J Med 2003; 348: 583–92.
26. Beckett NS, Peters R, Fletcher AE, et al. HYVET Study Group. Treatment of hypertension in patients 80 years of age or older. N Engl J Med 2008; 358: 1887–98.
27. Aronow WS, Fleg JL, Pepine CJ. ACCF/AHA 2011 expert consensus document on hypertension in the elderly: a report of the American College of Cardiology Foundation Task Force on Clinical Expert Consensus documents developed in collaboration with the American Academy of Neurology, American Geriatrics Society, American Society for Preventive Cardiology, American Society of Hypertension, American Society of Nephrology, Association of Black Cardiologists, and European Society of Hypertension. J Am CollCardiol 2011; 57: 2037–114.
28. Blood Pressure Lowering Treatment Trialists' Collaboration. Effects of different regimens to lower blood pressure on major cardiovascular events in older and younger adults: meta-analysis of randomized trials. BMJ 2008; 336: 1121–3.
29. Franklin SS. Isolated systolic hypertension and the J-curve of cardiovascular disease risk. Artery Res 2010; 4: 1–6.
30. Messerli FH, Mancia G, Conti CR, et al. Dogma disputed: can aggressively lowering blood pressure in hypertensive patients with coronary artery disease be dangerous? Ann Intern Med 2006; 144: 884–993.
31. Falk E, Shah PK, Fuster V. Coronary plaque disruption. Circulation 1995; 92: 657–61.
32. Aronow WS, Ahn C. Risk factors for new coronary events in a large cohort of very elderly patients with and without coronary artery disease. Am J Cardiol 1996; 77: 864–6.
33. Castelli WP, Wilson PWF, Levy D, Anderson K. Cardiovascular disease in the elderly. Am J Cardiol 1989; 63: 12H–9H.
34. Wong ND, Wilson PWF, Kannel WB. Serum cholesterol as a prognostic factor after myocardial infarction: the Framingham Study. Ann Intern Med 1991; 115: 697–3.
35. Belfante R, Reed D. Is elevated serum cholesterol level a factor for coronary heart disease in the elderly? JAMA 1990; 263: 393–6.
36. Manolio TA, Pearson TA, Wenger NK, et al. Cholesterol and heart disease in older persons and women: review of an NHLBI Workshop. Ann Epidemiol 1992; 2: 161–76.
37. Corti MC, Guralnik JM, Salive ME, et al. Clarifying the direct relation between total cholesterol levels and death from coronary heart disease in older persons. Ann Intern Med 1997; 126: 753–60.
38. Corti MC, Guralnik JM, Salive ME, et al. HDL cholesterol predicts coronary heart disease mortality in older adults. JAMA 1995; 274: 539–44.
39. Castelli WP, Anderson K, Wilson PWF, et al. Lipids and risk of coronary heart disease. The Framingham Study. Ann Epidemiol 1992; 2: 23–8.
40. Hong MK, Romm PA, Reagan K, et al. Total cholesterol/HDL ratio is the best predictor of anatomic coronary artery disease among elderly patients. J Am Coll Cardiol 1991; 17. 151A; abstract.
41. Miettinen TA, Pyorala K, Olsson AG, et al. Cholesterol-lowering therapy in women and elderly patients with myocardial infarction or angina pectoris: findings from the Scandinavian Simvastatin Survival Study (4S). Circulation 1997; 96: 4211–18.
42. Lewis SJ, Moye LA, Sacks FM, et al. Effect of pravastatin on cardiovascular events in older persons with myocardial infarction and cholesterol levels in the average age range: results from the Cholesterol and Recurrent Events (CARE) trial. Ann Intern Med 1998; 129: 681–9.
43. Cholesterol Trialists' Collaboration. Efficacy and safety of more intensive lowering of LDL cholesterol: a meta analysis of data from 170 000 participants in 26 randomised trials. Lancet 2010; 376: 1670–81.
44. Shepherd J, Blauw GJ, Murphy MB, et al. PROSPER study group. PROspective Study of Pravastatin in the Elderly at Risk. Pravastatin in elderly individuals at risk of vascular disease (PROSPER): a randomised controlled trial. Lancet 2002; 360: 1623–30.
45. Grundy SM, Cleeman JI, Daniels SR, et al. American Heart Association/ National Heart, Lung, and Blood Institute. Diagnosis and management of the metabolic syndrome: an American Heart Association/National Heart Lung and Blood Institute Scientific Statement. Circulation 2005; 112: 2735–52.
46. Ford ES, Giles WH, Mokdad AH. Increasing prevalenceof the metabolic syndrome among US adults. Diabetes Care 2004; 27: 2444.

47. Wild S, Rogic G, Green A, et al. Global prevalence of diabetes: estimates for the year 2000 and projections or 2030. Diabetes Care 2004; 27: 1047.

48. Narayan KM, Boyle JP, Thompson TJ, Sorensen SW, Williamson DF. Lifetime risk for diabetes mellitus in the United States. JAMA 2003; 290: 1884–90.

49. Hoang K, Ghandehari H, Lopez VA, Barboza MG, Wong ND. Global coronary heart disease risk assessment of individuals with the metabolic syndrome in the U.S. Diabetes Care 2008; 31: 1405–9.

50. Wong ND, Glovaci D, Wong K, et al. Global cardiovascular disease risk assessment in United States adults with diabetes. Diab Vasc Dis Res 2012; 9: 146–52.

51. Aronow WS, Ahn C. Association of diabetes mellitus using old and new diagnostic criteria with incidence of new coronary events in older men and women. Am J Cardiol 2000; 85: 104–5.

52. The ADVANCE Collaborative Group. Intensive blood glucose control and vascular outcomes in patients with type 2 diabetes. N Engl J Med 2008; 358: 2560–72.

53. The Action to Control Cardiovascular Risk in Diabetes Study Group. Effects of intensive glucose lowering in type 2 diabetes. N Engl J Med 2008; 358: 2545–59.

54. Belfante R, Reed D, Frank J. Does cigarette smoking have an independent effect on coronary heart disease incidence in the elderly? Am J Public Health 1991; 81: 897–9.

55. Hermanson B, Omenn GS, Kronmal RA, Gersh BJ. Beneficial six-year outcome of smoking cessation in older men and women with coronary artery disease: results of the CASS registry. N Engl J Med 1988; 319: 1365–9.

56. Harris T, Cook EF, Kannel WB, Goldman L. Proportional hazards analysis of risk factors for coronary heart disease in individuals aged 65 or older. The Framingham Heart Study. J Am Geriatr Soc 1988; 36: 1023–8.

57. Rimm EB, Stampfer MJ, Giovannucci E, et al. Body size and fat distribution as predictors of coronary heart disease among middle-aged and older US men. Am J Epidemiol 1995; 141: 1117–27.

58. Galanis DJ, Harris T, Sharp DS, Petrovitch H. Relative weight, weight change, and risk of coronary heart disease in the Honolulu Heart Program. Am J Epidemiol 1998; 147: 379–86.

59. Dey DK, Lissner L. Obesity in 70-year-old subjects as a risk factor for 15-year coronary heart disease incidence. Obes Res 2003; 11: 817–27.

60. Seidell JC, Visscher TL. Body weight and weight change and their health implications for the elderly. Eur J Clin Nutr 2000; 54: S33–9.

61. Villareal DT, Miller BV III, Banks M, et al. Effect of lifestyle intervention on metabolic coronary heart disease risk factors in obese older adults. Am J Clin Nutr 2006; 84: 1317–23.

62. Sui X, LaMonte MJ, Laditka JN, et al. Cardiorespiratory fitness and adiposity as mortality predictors in older adults. JAMA 2007; 298: 2507–16.

63. Hakim AA, Curb JD, Petrovitch H, et al. Effects of walking on coronary heart disease in elderly men: the Honolulu Heart Program. Circulation 1999; 100: 9–13.

64. Lee IM, Sesso HD, Paffenbarger RS Jr. Physical activity and coronary heart disease risk in men: does the duration of exercise episodes predict risk? Circulation 2000; 102: 981–6.

65. LaCroix AZ, Leveille SG, Hecht JA, Grothaus LC, Wagner EH. Does walking decrease the risk of cardiovascular disease hospitalizations and death in older adults? J Am Geriatr Soc 1996; 44: 113–20.

66. Wannamethee SG, Shaper AG, Walker M. Physical activity and mortality in older men with diagnosed coronary heart disease. Circulation 2000; 102: 1358–63.

67. Singh T, Newman AB. Inflammatory markers in population studies of aging. Ageing Res Rev 2011; 10: 319–29.

68. Pearson TA, Mensah GA, Alexander RW, et al. Markers of inflammation and cardiovascular disease: application to clinical and public health practice: a statement for healthcare professionals from the Centers for Disease Control and Prevention and the American Heart Association. Circulation 2003; 107: 499–511.

69. Kritchevsky SB, Cesari M, Pahor M. Inflammatory markers and cardiovascular health in older adults. Cardiovasc Res 2005; 66: 265–75.

70. Cesari M, Penninx BW, Newman AB, et al. Inflammatory markers and onset of cardiovascular events: results from the Health ABC study. Circulation 2003; 108: 2317–22.

71. Rodondi N, Marques-Vidal P, Butler J, et al. Markers of atherosclerosis and inflammation for prediction of coronary heart disease in older adults. Am J Epidemiol 2010; 171: 540–9.

72. Packard CJ, O'Reilly DS, Caslake MJ, et al. West of Scotland Coronary Prevention Study Group. Lipoprotein-associated phospholipase A2 as an independent predictor of coronary heart disease. N Engl J Med 2000; 343: 1148–55.

73. Koenig W, Khuseyinova N, Lowel H, Trischler G, Meisinger C. Lipoprotein-associated phospholipase A2 adds to risk prediction of incident coronary events by C-reactive protein in apparently healthy

middle-aged men from the general population: results from the 14-year follow-up of a large cohort from southern Germany. Circulation 2004; 110: 1903–8.

74. Daniels LB, Laughlin GA, Sarno MJ, et al. Lipoprotein-associated phospholipase A2 is an independent predictor of incident coronary heart disease in an apparently healthy older population: the Rancho Bernardo Study. J Am Coll Cardiol 2008; 51: 913–19.

75. American Heart Association. Life's simple seven. [Available from: http://www.mylifecheck.org/] [accessed 25 September 2012].

76. Wong ND, Pio J, Franklin SS, et al. Preventing coronary events by optimal control of blood pressure and lipids in patients with the metabolic syndrome. Am J Cardiol 2003; 91: 1421–6.

77. Williams MA, Fleg JL, Ades PA, et al. Secondary prevention of coronary heart disease in the elderly (with emphasis of patients ≥75 years of age). Circulation 2002; 105: 1735–43.

78. Sparrow D, Dawber T, Colton T. The influence of cigarette smoking on prognosis after first myocardial infarction. J Chronic Dis 1978; 31: 415–22.

79. Taylor CB, Miller NH, Killen JD, et al. Smoking cessation after myocardial infarction: effects of a nurse-managed intervention. Ann Intern Med 1990; 113: 118–23.

80. DeBusk RF, Houston Miller N, Superko HR, et al. A case management system for coronary risk factor modification after acute myocardial infarction. Ann Intern Med 1994; 120: 721–9.

81. Lewis SJ, Moye LA, Sacks FM, et al. Effect of pravastatin on cardiovascular events in older patients with myocardial infarction or angina pectoris: findings from the Scandinavian Simvastatin Survival Study (4S). Circulation 1997; 96: 4211–18.

82. Ganz DA, Kuntz KM, Jacobson GA, et al. Cost-effectiveness of 3-hydrozy-3-methylglutaryl coenzyme A reductase inhibitor therapy in older patients with myocardial infarction. Ann Intern Med 2000; 132: 780–7.

83. Vokonas PS, Kannel WB. Epidemiology of coronary heart disease in the elderly. In: Tresch DD, Aronow WS, eds. Cardiovascular Disease in the Elderly Patient. New York: Marcel Dekker, 1994: 91–123.

84. Katzel LI, Coon PJ, Dengel J, et al. Effects of an American Heart Association step I diet and weight loss on lipoprotein levels in obese men with silent myocardial ischemia and reduce HDL-C. Metabolism 1995; 44: 307–14.

8
Diagnosis of coronary heart disease in the elderly

Wilbert S. Aronow and Jerome L. Fleg

SUMMARY

This chapter discusses the diagnosis of coronary heart disease in the elderly. Diagnostic tests for diagnosing coronary heart disease in the elderly include the resting electrocardiogram, ambulatory electrocardiography, signal-averaged electrocardiography, echocardiography, exercise and pharmacological stress testing, multislice computed tomography, magnetic resonance imaging, and coronary arteriography.

INTRODUCTION

Coronary heart disease (CHD) is very common in the elderly population, with autopsy studies demonstrating a prevalence of at least 70% in persons over the age of 70 years (1,2). These autopsy findings may be coincidental, with the disease clinically silent throughout the person's life; however, only 15–30% of persons over the age of 65 years show clinical manifestations of CHD. In the National Health and Nutrition Examination Survey (NHANES) 2005–2008, the prevalence of clinical CHD rose progressively with age, reaching 35.5% in men and 20.8% in women aged 80 years and above (3). Clinical CHD was present in 502 of 1160 men (43%) of mean age 80 years, and in 1019 of 2464 women (41%), of mean age 81 years in a long-term care facility (4). The marked discrepancy between the clinical and autopsy prevalence of CHD in the elderly indicates that CHD is often silent in this age group. Studies employing exercise testing and myocardial perfusion imaging in asymptomatic volunteers have demonstrated a striking age-related increase in silent myocardial ischemia, helping to reconcile differences in CHD prevalence between clinical and autopsy studies (5).

Though CHD is widely prevalent among the elderly, the disease is often undiagnosed or misdiagnosed in this age group. Failure to correctly diagnose the disease in the elderly may be due to a difference in clinical manifestations in this age group compared with that of younger patients. Such differences may reflect a difference in the disease process between older and younger patients, or it may be related to the superimposition of normal aging changes on those of concomitant diseases that may mask the usual clinical manifestations.

Both the prevalence and extent of CHD increase with age. In the Coronary Artery Surgery Study, the prevalence of three-vessel CHD was 61% in patients aged 65 years and

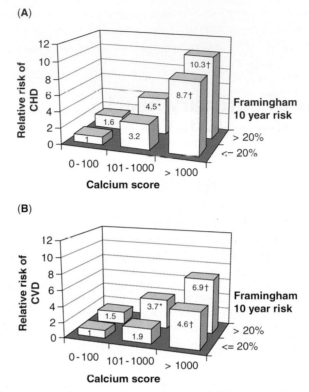

Figure 8.1   Relative risks of coronary heart disease (CHD) events (**A**) and cardiovascular (CVD) events (**B**) in older volunteers by coronary artery calcium score and Framingham risk categories. *Source*: From Ref. 8.

older versus 46% in those younger than 65 years; left main coronary artery stenosis was seen in 13% versus 9%, respectively (6). In a database of 21,573 patients undergoing cardiac catheterization between 1995 and 1998, left main coronary artery disease (CAD) increased in prevalence from 6.3% below the age of 70 years to 13.9% in those of 80 years and older (7). Multiple studies of patients undergoing percutaneous coronary interventions have also found higher prevalence of multivessel and left main disease in the elderly.

Coronary artery calcium is also more common in the elderly than in younger populations. In the community-based Rotterdam Study, 1795 volunteers (mean age 71 years) with no history of CHD underwent electron beam computed tomography to detect coronary artery calcium (8). Calcium scores greater than 100 were observed in 49% and scores greater than 400 in 25%, both markedly higher than in younger populations. In this study, scores of 401–1000 were associated with a fourfold risk of hard CHD events compared with those with scores less than or equal to 100 even after adjustment for standard CHD risk factors; scores greater than 1000 increased CHD risk more than eightfold (Fig. 8.1) (8). Thus, coronary artery calcium is highly prevalent in older volunteers free of clinical CHD and has similar adverse prognostic significance as in younger populations.

MYOCARDIAL ISCHEMIA
In young and middle-aged individuals, exertional angina pectoris caused by myocardial ischemia is commonly the first manifestation of CHD. It is usually easy to recognize because of its typical features; however, in the elderly, this may not be the case. Because of limited physical activity, many elderly persons with CHD will not experience

exertional angina pectoris. Even when angina pectoris does occur, the patient and physician may often attribute it to a cause other than CHD. For example, myocardial ischemia, appearing as shoulder or back pain, may be misdiagnosed as degenerative joint disease or, if the pain is located in the epigastric area, it may be ascribed to peptic ulcer disease. Nocturnal or postprandial epigastric discomfort is often attributed to hiatus hernia or esophageal reflux instead of CHD. Postprandial angina pectoris tends to occur among elderly and hypertensive patients with severe CHD and a markedly reduced ischemic threshold (9). Furthermore, the presence of comorbid conditions, so frequent in the elderly, adds to the confusion and may lead to misdiagnosis of the patient's symptoms, which are actually due to myocardial ischemia.

Myocardial ischemia in elderly patients is commonly manifested as dyspnea rather than chest tightness, and is referred to as an "angina equivalent". Usually the dyspnea is exertional and is thought to be related to a transient rise in left ventricular (LV) end-diastolic pressure caused by myocardial ischemia superimposed on reduced ventricular compliance. Reduction in LV compliance may reflect normal aging changes or, more likely, is caused by the presence of coexisting hypertension and LV hypertrophy, disorders commonly present in elderly patients. Not infrequently, the dyspnea will occur in combination with angina pectoris, although the angina may be mild and of little concern to the patient.

In other elderly individuals, myocardial ischemia is manifested clinically as frank heart failure, with some patients presenting with acute pulmonary edema. Chest pain may not be present, although the myocardial ischemia is severe enough to produce a combination of diastolic and systolic LV dysfunction.

Several studies have described the presentation of older patients with CHD in acute pulmonary edema caused by myocardial ischemia without infarction (10–15). Graham and Vetrovec (15) compared patients with CHD hospitalized with acute pulmonary edema with patients hospitalized with angina pectoris without heart failure. The patients with acute pulmonary edema were older and most of them had pre-existing hypertension. Three-vessel CHD was common in both groups, although angina pectoris was infrequent in patients with pulmonary edema. LV ejection fraction was more depressed in patients with pulmonary edema (42%) than in the angina pectoris group (59%). In another study, Kunis and associates (13) reported findings of a small group of elderly patients with CHD who had recurrent pulmonary edema that could not be prevented with medical therapy. Angiographic studies demonstrated three-vessel coronary disease with preserved LV systolic function. Only after undergoing coronary bypass surgery, the recurrent pulmonary edema was prevented in these very elderly patients (13).

Another subset of elderly patients with CHD who present with acute pulmonary edema will demonstrate mitral valvular regurgitation that may be secondary to papillary muscle ischemia. In a study of 40 patients with acute pulmonary edema who had CHD, Stone and associates (16) found that 67% of the patients demonstrated moderate to severe mitral regurgitation on Doppler echocardiographic examination. The mean age of the patients was 76 years. In majority of the patients (74%), a murmur of mitral regurgitation was not detected despite examination by multiple observers. The authors concluded that mitral valve regurgitation is not uncommon in elderly patients with CHD who present with acute LV failure and may contribute to the genesis of pulmonary edema.

In addition to having more severe CHD than younger patients, the elderly demonstrate greater clinical instability, CHD complications, and comorbidities. In 21,573 patients in a Canadian registry, unstable angina pectoris was the indication for arteriography in 38% of persons aged 80 years and above versus 28% in those younger than 70 years (7). A history of heart failure was present, respectively, in 31% versus 11% of patients. Furthermore, comorbidities such as cerebrovascular and peripheral vascular disease, and chronic obstructive lung disease were two to three times more common in the elderly (7). A single-center study by Tresch et al. (17) in a group of elderly patients (mean age 71 years) who underwent coronary arteriography showed similar findings. The initial manifestation in the majority of patients was unstable ischemic chest pain; 34% of the patients presented with an acute myocardial infarction. In 8% of these elderly patients, the initial manifestation was acute heart failure unassociated with an acute myocardial infarction. On cardiac catheterization, multivessel disease was common, although LV systolic function was often normal. Only 9% of the patient had an LV ejection fraction of less than 35%. In contrast, patients younger than 65 years more commonly sustained an acute myocardial infarction as the initial manifestation of CHD, were less likely to present with heart failure, and had less multivessel CHD (17).

Cardiac arrhythmias, particularly complex ventricular arrhythmias, may be a manifestation of myocardial ischemia in elderly patients with CHD. In the study of Tresch' et al. (17), 14% of elderly patients had arrhythmias as the initial manifestation of CHD. Sudden death may be the initial manifestation of CHD in older adults; in Framingham volunteers, 65–94 years old, CHD was manifest as sudden death in 15% of men and 12% of women (18).

Silent or asymptomatic myocardial ischemia is a common problem in elderly patients with CHD. In a study of 185 nursing home patients with CHD, mean age 83 years, silent myocardial ischemia (SI) was detected by 24-hour ambulatory electrocardiography (AECG) in 34% (19). SI was detected by 24-hour AECG in 51 of 117 (44%) similar patients with CHD or hypertension and an abnormal LV ejection fraction (20). In a community-based sample of men 68-years old, Hedblad et al. (21) detected SI by 24-hour AECG in 25%. The risk of subsequent myocardial infarction was 4.4-fold higher in men with SI but no clinical CHD compared to similar men without SI; those with both clinical CHD and SI experienced a 16-fold higher risk.

The reason for the frequent absence of chest pain in elderly patients with CAD is unclear. Various speculations have included (1) mental deterioration with inability to verbalize a sensation of pain, (2) better myocardial collateral circulation related to gradual progressive coronary artery narrowing, and (3) a decreased sensitivity to pain because of aging changes. Ambepitiya and associates (22) investigated the issue of age-associated changes in pain perception by comparing the time delay between the onset of 1 mm of electrocardiographic ST-segment depression and the onset of angina pectoris during exercise stress testing. The mean delay was 49 seconds in patients aged 70–82 years compared with 30 seconds in patients aged 42–59 years. The reason for this delay in perception of myocardial ischemia in the elderly is unexplained. The authors postulated that the impairment is most likely multifactorial in origin, involving peripheral mechanisms such as changes in the myocardial autonomic nerve endings with blunting of the perception of ischemic pain, as well as changes in central mechanisms. Another theory has suggested that the increase in SI and infarction in elderly patients with CHD is related to increased levels of, or receptor sensitivity to, endogenous opioids (23). This explanation does not appear likely because studies have demonstrated a similar increase in response of β-endorphin levels to exercise in both elderly and younger patients (24), and animal studies show a decrease in opioid receptor responsivity with advancing age (25).

MYOCARDIAL INFARCTION

Some older patients with acute myocardial infarction may be completely asymptomatic or the symptoms may be so vague that they are unrecognized by the patient or physician as an acute myocardial infarction. The Framingham Heart Study (26) found that in the general population, approximately 25% of myocardial infarctions diagnosed by pathological Q-waves on ECG were clinically unrecognized and, of these, 48% were truly silent. The incidence of silent infarction increased with age, with 42% of infarctions clinically silent in men aged 75–84 years. In women, the proportion of unrecognized myocardial infarctions was greater than in men, but the incidence was unaffected by increasing age. Other studies (27–34) have also reported a high prevalence of silent or unrecognized myocardial infarction in elderly patients, with rates from 21% to 68% (Table 8.1). These studies also demonstrated that the incidence of new coronary events, including recurrent myocardial infarction, ventricular fibrillation, and sudden death, in patients with unrecognized myocardial infarction is similar to (26,31–33,35) or higher (34) than in patients with recognized myocardial infarction.

In elderly patients with an acute myocardial infarction, symptoms may be extremely vague when present and, as with myocardial ischemia, the diagnosis may be easily missed. Numerous studies have demonstrated the atypical features and wide variability of symptoms in elderly patients with acute myocardial infarction (Table 8.2) (27–29,36–40). Rodstein (27) found that in 52 elderly patients with acute myocardial infarction, 31% had no symptoms, 29% had chest pain, and 38% had dyspnea, neurological symptoms, or gastrointestinal symptoms (Tables 8.1 and 8.2). Pathy (36) demonstrated in 387 elderly patients with acute myocardial infarction that 19% had chest pain, 56% had dyspnea, neurological, or gastrointestinal symptoms, 8% had sudden death, and 17% had other symptoms (Table 8.2). In 110 elderly patients with acute myocardial infarction, Aronow (29) showed

Table 8.1   Prevalance of Silent or Unrecognized Q-Wave Myocardial Infarction in Elderly Patients

		Unrecognized MI	
Study (Reference)	Age (yr)	Number	Age (%)
Rodstein (*n* = 52) (27)	61–92	16	31
Aronow et al. (*n* = 115) (28)	mean, 82	78	68
Aronow (*n* = 110) (29)	mean, 82	23	21
Kannel et al. (*n* = 199 men) (26)	65–94	66	33
Kannel et al. (*n* = 162 women) (26)	65–94	58	36
Muller et al. (*n* = 46 men) (30)	65–95	14	30
Muller et al. (*n* = 67 women) (30)	65–95	34	51
Nadelmann et al. (*n* = 115) (31)	75–85	50	43
Sigurdsson et al. (*n* = 237) (32)	58–62	83	35
Sheifer et al. (*n* = 901) (33)	mean, 72	201	22

Abbreviation: MI, myocardial infarction.

Table 8.2   Prevalence of Dyspnea, Chest Pain, Neurological Symptoms, and Gastrointestinal Symptoms Associated with Acute Myocardial Infarction in Elderly Patients

Study (Reference)	Age (yr)	Dyspnea	Chest Pain	Neurological Symptoms	GI Symptoms
Rodstein (*n* = 52) (27)	61–92	10 (19%)	15 (29%)	7 (13%)	3 (6%)
Pathy (*n* = 387) (36)	>65	77 (20%)	75 (19%)	126 (33%)	10 (3%)
Tinker (*n* = 87) (37)	mean, 74	19 (22%)	51 (59%)	14 (16%)	0 (0%)
Bayer et al. (*n* = 777) (38)	65–100	329 (42%)	515 (66%)	232 (30%)	145 (19%)
Aronow (*n* = 110) (29)	mean, 82	38 (35%)	24 (22%)	20 (18%)	5 (4%)
Wroblewski (*n* = 96) (39)	mean, 84	57 (59%)	19 (20%)	33 (34%)	24 (25%)

Abbreviation: GI, gastrointestinal.

that 21% had no symptoms, 22% had chest pain, 35% had dyspnea, 18% had neurological symptoms, and 4% had gastrointestinal symptoms (Tables 8.1 and 8.2).

Other studies have also shown a high prevalence of dyspnea and neurological symptoms in elderly patients with acute myocardial infarction (37–39). In these studies, dyspnea was present in 22% of 87 patients (37), 42% of 777 patients (38), and 57% of 96 patients (39). Neurological symptoms were present in 16% (37), 30% (38), and 34% (39) of patients, respectively. In 777 elderly patients with acute myocardial infarction, Bayer and associates (38) reported that with increasing age, the prevalence of chest pain decreased whereas the prevalence of dyspnea increased. In the Multicenter Chest Pain Study, the clinical presentation of acute myocardial infarction was compared in 1615 patients older than 65 years to 5109 younger patients (41). Because of the decreased prevalence in elderly patients of some typical features of acute myocardial infarction present in younger patients, such as pressure-like chest pain, the initial symptoms, and signs had a lower predictive value for diagnosing acute myocardial infarction in the older group (41). Thus, the clinician should maintain a high index of suspicion for acute myocardial infarction in elderly patients with acute onset of dyspnea, or unexplained neurological symptoms.

Another important age difference in myocardial infarction presentation is that elderly patients delay longer in seeking medical assistance after the onset of chest pain (42–44). In a study of out-of-hospital chest pain, Tresch et al. (42) reported that patients 80 years or older delayed more than 6.5 hours in calling paramedics, compared with a 3.9 hours delay in patients younger than 70 years. Interestingly, this prolonged delay occurred even though more than 50% of the elderly patients had a past history of either a myocardial infarction or coronary bypass surgery. Such delay may partially explain the lesser use of thrombolytic therapy or primary coronary angioplasty in elderly patients with acute myocardial infarction compared with younger patients. Among 102,339 patients older than 65 years with confirmed acute myocardial infarction in the Cooperative Cardiovascular Project, 29.4% arrived at the hospital 6 hours or later after onset of symptoms (44).

Another important age difference found in several studies (42,45,46) is the greater incidence of non-Q-wave myocardial infarctions in the elderly; In one study, 40% of elderly patients with acute myocardial infarction demonstrated non-Q-wave infarction compared with only 20% of the younger patients with infarction (42). Of 91 consecutive patients aged 70 years and older, mean age 78 years, with acute myocardial infarction, 61 (75%) had non-Q-wave myocardial infarction (46). Though non-Q-wave myocardial infarctions in younger patients are usually associated with a more benign hospital course than Q-wave myocardial infarctions, this does not pertain to elderly patients. Chung and associates (47) reported a 10% hospital mortality and 36% 1-year mortality in a group of elderly patients sustaining acute non-Q-wave myocardial infarction. In contrast, the acute hospital and 1-year mortality in younger patients was 3% and 16%, respectively. Moreover, 23% of the elderly patients with non-Q-wave myocardial infarction developed atrial fibrillation, and 53% had congestive heart failure.

Regardless of the type of myocardial infarction, elderly patients with acute myocardial infarction usually demonstrate more LV dysfunction than younger patients upon hospital admission and have a more complicated hospital course. Complications are common in elderly patients (48) including heart failure, ventricular rupture, shock, and death; and, not infrequently, the elderly patient's initial complaints will reflect these complications instead of chest pain. Fedullo and Swinburne (49) compared complications from acute myocardial infarction in 104 patients aged 70 years and older with 157 patients 70 years or younger. Mortality was 22% in the older group versus 5% in the younger group. Cardiogenic shock occurred in 7% of the older group versus 1% of the younger group. Pulmonary edema occurred in 18% of the older group versus 4% of the younger group. Heart failure occurred in 29% of the older group versus 14% of the younger group. A rhythm disturbance requiring pacemaker implantation occurred in 5% of the older group versus 2% of the younger group (49). The increased mortality and complication rates in older patients with acute myocardial infarction suggest that an aggressive diagnostic and therapeutic approach may be beneficial in these patients (48). More aggressive therapy, including use of aspirin, β-blockers, angiotensin-converting enzyme inhibitors, statins, thrombolytic therapy, and coronary revascularization by percutaneous transluminal coronary angioplasty or by coronary bypass surgery, should be considered (see chap. 11).

DIAGNOSTIC TECHNIQUES
Resting ECG

Despite the advent of sophisticated cardiac imaging techniques, the ECG remains a cornerstone for diagnosing recent or previous myocardial infarction. In addition, the resting ECG may show ischemic ST-segment depression, arrhythmias, conduction defects, and LV hypertrophy that have prognostic value for subsequent coronary events. Over an 8 year follow-up of 2192 ambulatory volunteers 70–79 years old without known CHD, major baseline ECG abnormaities (Q waves, bundle branch block, atrial fibrillation or flutter, or major ST-T wave changes) were associated with a 50% increased risk of CHD events, independent of conventional risk factors. Even minor ST-T changes were associated with a 35% increased CHD event risk (50). Elderly nursing home patients with ischemic ST-segment depression 1 mm or greater on the resting ECG were 3.1 times more likely to develop new coronary events (myocardial infarction, primary ventricular fibrillation, or sudden cardiac death) than were those with no significant ST-segment depression over 37 months of mean follow-up (51). In this population, patients with ischemic ST-segment depression 0.5–0.9 mm on the resting ECG were 1.9 times more likely to develop new coronary events during the 37-month follow-up than were those with no significant ST-segment depression (51). At 45-month mean follow-up, pacemaker rhythm, atrial fibrillation, premature ventricular complexes, left bundle branch block, intraventricular conduction defect, and type II second-degree atrioventricular (AV) block were all associated with a higher incidence of new coronary events in such elderly patients (52).

Numerous studies have documented that older adults with ECG LV hypertrophy have an increased incidence of new cardiovascular events. Men and women, 65–94 years of age, participating in the Framingham Heart Study who had ECG LV hypertrophy had an increased incidence of new coronary events, atherothrombotic brain infarction, chronic heart failure (CHF), and peripheral arterial disease compared with persons without ECG LV hypertrophy (53). Aronow et al. (54) also found that elderly patients with hypertension or CHD and ECG LV hypertrophy had an increased incidence of new coronary events, atherothrombotic brain infarction, and heart failure.

Ambulatory Electrocardiography

Multiple studies have demonstrated that complex ventricular arrhythmias in older adults without underlying cardiovascular disease are not associated with an increased incidence of new coronary events (Table 8.3) (55–61). In contrast, complex ventricular arrhythmias in elderly persons with underlying cardiovascular disease are associated with an increased incidence of new coronary events, including sudden cardiac death (Table 8.3) (57–61). The incidence of new coronary events is especially increased in elderly patients with complex ventricular arrhythmias and abnormal LV ejection fraction (58) or LV hypertrophy (59). In elderly nursing home patients with heart disease, complex ventricular arrhythmias detected by 24-hour AECG predicted a 2.5 times greater incidence of new coronary events at a 2-year follow-up in persons with normal LV ejection fraction and 7.6 times greater

Table 8.3 Association of Complex Ventricular Arrhythmias and Ventricular Tachycardia with New Coronary Events in Elderly Patients

Study (Reference)	Mean Age (yr)	Cardiac Status	Follow-up (mo)	Incidence of New Coronary Events
Fleg et al. (n = 98) (55)	69	No heart disease	120	No association
Kirkland et al. (n = 30) (56)	79	No heart disease	29	No association
Aronow et al. (n = 843) (58)	82	Heart disease	39	Increased 1.7 times by complex VA
Aronow et al. (n = 391) (59)	82	Heart disease	24	With normal LVEF, increased 2.5 times by complex VA and 3.2 times by VT; increased 7.6 times by complex VA plus abnormal LVEF and increased 6.8 times by VT plus abnormal LVEF
Martin et al. (n = 106)(57)	75–95	No heart disease	60	Total mortality increased 1.9 times by frequent VA
Aronow et al. (n = 468) (60)	82	Heart disease	27	With no LVH, SCD or VF increased 2.4 times by complex VA and 1.8 times by VT; SCD or VF increased 7.3 times by complex VA plus LVH and increased 7.1 times by VT plus LVH
Aronow et al. (n = 395 men) (61)	80	CAD	45	Increased 2.4 times by complex VA and 1.7 times by VT
Aronow et al. (n = 385 men) (61)	80	HT, VD, or CMP	45	Increased 1.9 times by complex VA and 1.9 times by VT
Aronow et al. (n = 135 men) (61)	80	No heart disease	45	No association
Aronow et al. (n = 771 women) (61)	81	CAD	47	Increased 2.5 times by complex VA and 1.7 times by VT
Aronow et al. (n = 806 women) (61)	81	HT, VD, or CMP	47	Increased 2.2 times by complex VA and 2.0 times by VT
Aronow et al. (n = 297 women) (61)	81	No heart disease	47	No association

Abbreviations: VA, ventricular arrhythmias; VT, ventricular tachycardia; LVEF, left ventricular ejection fraction; LVH, left ventricular hypertrophy; SCD, sudden coronary death; VF, primary ventricular fibrillation; CAD, coronary artery disease; HT, hypertension; VD, valvular heart disease; CMP, cardiomyopathy.

incidence in those with abnormal LV ejection fraction (Table 8.3) (60). In elderly persons with heart disease, non-sustained ventricular tachycardia detected by 24-hour AECG was associated with a 3.2 times increased incidence of new coronary events at a 2-year follow-up in persons with normal LV ejection fraction, and 6.8-fold higher incidence in those with abnormal LV ejection fraction (Table 8.3) (59). Those with heart disease, normal LV mass, and complex ventricular arrhythmias detected by 24-hour AECG experienced a 2.4-fold greater incidence of primary ventricular fibrillation or sudden cardiac death at a 27-month follow-up than those without such arrhythmias. This risk was 7.3 times higher in persons with both complex ventricular arrhythmias and echocardiographic LV hypertrophy (60).

AECG performed for 24 hour is also useful in detecting myocardial ischemia in elderly persons with suspected CHD who cannot perform treadmill or bicycle exercise stress testing because of advanced age, intermittent claudication, musculoskeletal disorders, heart failure, or pulmonary disease. Ischemic ST-segment changes demonstrated on the 24-hour AECG correlate with transient abnormalities in myocardial perfusion and LV systolic dysfunction. The changes may be associated with symptoms, or symptoms may be completely absent, which is referred to as SI. SI is predictive of future coronary events, including cardiovascular mortality in older persons with CHD (19–21,62–66) and in those with no clinical heart disease (21,55,67).

The incidence of new coronary events is especially increased in elderly individuals with SI plus complex ventricular arrhythmias (62), abnormal LV ejection fraction (20), or echocardiographic LV hypertrophy (68). In a population of institutionalized elderly with CHD or hypertension, at a 40-month follow-up, SI predicted a doubled incidence of new coronary events in persons with normal LV ejection fraction and a 3.2-fold increase in those with abnormal LV ejection fraction (Table 8.4) (20). The combination of complex ventricular arrhythmias plus SI was associated with a fourfold higher incidence of new coronary events (Table 8.4) (20); echocardiographic LV hypertrophy plus SI predicted a 3.4-fold greater incidence of new coronary events at a 31-month follow-up (68). SI was associated with approximately a doubled incidence of new coronary events over nearly 4 years of follow-up in both elderly men and women with CHD, hypertension, valvular heart disease, or cardiomyopathy. Among those without clinical heart disease, SI predicted an incidence of new coronary events 6.3-fold higher in men and 4.4-fold higher in women (Table 8.4) (67). Other studies have shown similarly increased incidence of new coronary events over long-term follow-up of elderly persons with SI on AECG but without clinical heart disease (21,55).

SI detected by 24-hour AECG identifies older individuals at higher risk of CHD events after non-cardiac surgery. Such use of 24-hour AECG may be especially beneficial in elderly persons, who are frequently at high surgical risk and may not be able to undergo preoperative exercise stress testing because of concomitant illness. No study, however, has shown SI detected by 24-hour AECG to be more accurate than pharmacological stress testing in stratifying preoperative elderly patients into high- and low-risk groups.

Among 176 older patients who underwent 24-hour AECG before peripheral vascular surgery, 18% had myocardial ischemia on their preoperative 24-hour AECG, with the ischemia silent in the majority (69). Preoperative myocardial ischemia was highly predictive of postoperative cardiac events. The sensitivity of preoperative myocardial ischemia for postoperative cardiac events in this study was 92%, the specificity 88%, the positive predictive value 38%, and the negative predictive value 99% (69). Multivariate analysis showed preoperative myocardial ischemia to be the most significant variable correlating with postoperative cardiac events. A follow-up study by these investigators determined that preoperative myocardial ischemia strongly correlated with intraoperative and postoperative ischemia, and perioperative myocardial ischemia commonly preceded clinical cardiac events (70).

Table 8.4   Association of SI with New Coronary Events in Elderly Patients

Study (Reference)	Mean Age (yr)	Cardiac Status	Follow-up (mo)	Incidence of New Coronary Events
Fleg et al. (*n* = 98) (55)	69	No heart disease	120	Increased 3.8 times by SI
Aronow et al. (*n* = 393) (20)	82	CAD or HT	40	Increased 2.0 times by SI; increased 2.4 times by SI with normal LVEF; increased 3.2 times by SI with abnormal LVEF
Aronow et al. (*n* = 404) (62)	82	CAD or HT	37	Increased 2.0 times by SI; increased 4.0 times by SI plus complex VA; increased 2.5 times by SI plus VT
Hedblad et al. (*n* = 39 men) (21)	68	CAD	43	Increased 16.0 times by SI
Hedblad et al. (*n* = 385 men) (21)	68	No CAD	43	Increased 4.4 times by SI
Aronow et al. (*n* = 395 men) (67)	80	CAD	45	Increased 2.1 times by SI
Aronow et al. (*n* = 385 men) (67)	80	HT, VD, or CMP	45	Increased 1.8 times by SI
Aronow et al. (*n* = 135 men) (67)	80	No heart disease	45	Increased 6.3 times by SI
Aronow et al. (*n* = 771 women) (67)	81	CAD	47	Increased 2.1 times by SI
Aronow et al. (*n* = 806 women) (67)	81	HT, VD, or CMP	47	Increased 1.7 times by SI
Aronow et al. (*n* = 297 women) (67)	81	No heart disease	47	Increased 4.4 times by SI

Abbreviations: SI, silent myocardial ischemia; CAD, coronary artery disease; HT, hypertension; LVEF, left ventricular ejection fraction; VA, ventricular arrhythmias; VT, ventricular tachycardia; VD, valvular heart disease; CMP, cardiomyopathy.

Signal-Averaged Electrocardiography

Signal-averaged electrocardiography (SAECG) was performed in 121 elderly postinfarction patients with asymptomatic complex ventricular arrhythmias detected by 24-hour AECG and a LV ejection fraction greater than or equal to 40% (71). At 29-month follow-up, the sensitivity, specificity, positive predictive value, and negative predictive value for predicting sudden cardiac death were 52%, 68%, 32%, and 83%, respectively, for a positive SAECG; 63%, 70%, 38%, and 87%, respectively, for non-sustained ventricular tachycardia; and 26%, 89%, 41%, and 81%, respectively, for a positive SAECG plus non-sustained ventricular tachycardia (71).

Echocardiography

Echocardiography is useful in detecting regional LV wall motion abnormalities, acute myocardial ischemia, and complications secondary to acute myocardial infarction, LV aneurysm, cardiac thrombi, left main CAD, LV hypertrophy, and associated valvular heart disease. Echocardiography is useful in evaluating LV function and cardiac chamber size in elderly persons with CHD. Echocardiographic LV ejection fraction is also important in predicting new coronary events in elderly persons with CHD (20,59,72). New coronary events developed at a 2-year follow-up in 30 of 45 elderly nursing home patients with CHD and abnormal LV ejection fraction (<50%) and in 24 of 90 such patients with CHD and normal LV ejection fraction (relative risk = 2.5) (59). In this population of older adults with CHD and heart failure, cardiovascular mortality is higher among individuals with abnormal than those with normal LV ejection fraction (72,73). Multivariate analysis showed that LV ejection fraction was the most important prognostic variable for mortality in elderly persons with CHF associated with CHD; those with abnormal LV ejection fraction had approximately twice the mortality of persons with normal LV ejection fraction (72,73).

Numerous studies have demonstrated that elderly patients with echocardiographic LV hypertrophy have an increased incidence of new cardiovascular events (53,54,60,68,74,75). At 4-year follow-up, elderly men and women in the Framingham Study with echocardiographic LV hypertrophy had a relative risk for new coronary events of 1.67 for men and of 1.60 for women per 50 g/m increase in LV mass/height (Table 8.5) (74). In these volunteers,

Table 8.5 Association of Echocardiographic LVH with New Cardiovascular Events in Elderly Persons

Population (Reference)	Mean Age (yr)	Follow-up (yr)	Incidence of New Cardiovascular Events
Framingham Study (n = 406 men) (74)	65–94	4	Coronary events increased 1.67 times per 50 g/m increase in LV mass/height
Framingham Study (n = 735 women) (74)	65–94	4	Coronary events increased 1.60 times per 50 g/m increase in LV mass/height
Cardiovascular disease (n = 557) (75)	82	2.3	LVH increased coronary events 2.7 times and ABI 3.7 times
Hypertension or CHD (n = 360) (59)	82	3.1	LVH increased coronary events 2.0 times and ABI 2.8 times
Heart disease (n = 468) (60)	82	2.3	LVH increased primary ventricular fibrillation or sudden cardiac death 3.3 times
African-Americans with hypertension (n = 84) (54)	78	3.1	LV increased coronary events 3.3 times, ABI 2.8 times, and CHF 3.7 times
Whites with hypertension (n = 326) (54)	82	3.6	LV increased coronary events 2.7 times, ABI 3.3 times, and CHF 3.5 times

Abbreviations: LVH, left ventricular hypertrophy; CHD, coronary heart disease; ABI, atherothrombotic brain infarction; CHF, chronic heart failure.

echocardiographic LV hypertrophy was 15.3 times more sensitive than ECG LV hypertrophy in predicting new coronary events in elderly men and 4.3 times more sensitive than ECG LV hypertrophy in predicting new coronary events in elderly women (74). Other studies in institutionalized elders have consistently shown echocardiographic LVH to predict increased rates of coronary events and thrombotic stroke (Table 8.5)

Exercise and Pharmacological Stress Testing

Although age per se significantly influences the cardiovascular response to aerobic exercise, treadmill, or cycle ergometer exercise testing remains a useful diagnostic and prognostic tool for evaluating older patients with suspected or documented CHD. Exercise ECG is also a useful prognostic indicator of subsequent coronary events in patients with documented CHD, with or without previous myocardial infarction. Exercise testing in elderly patients should evaluate symptoms that develop during exercise (especially angina pectoris or dyspnea, which may be an anginal equivalent), the maximal workload achieved, the heart rate and blood pressure response, the presence, magnitude, and onset time of ischemic ST-segment depression or elevation, and the presence of exercise-induced arrhythmias. These variables must be interpreted in light of normative age-associated changes including a decline of maximal aerobic capacity averaging 8–10% per decade (76,77), a reduced maximal heart rate of approximately 1 beat/min/yr, and an exaggerated rise in systolic blood pressure (78,79). Maximal LV systolic emptying is impaired in older adults, resulting in a higher end-systolic volume and lower ejection fraction compared with younger individuals (78–80); stroke volume is preserved, however, by a greater reliance on the Frank–Starling mechanism to augment LV end-diastolic volume (79,80). Both the exercise-induced supraventricular (81) and ventricular arrhythmias (82) increase exponentially with age in clinically healthy volunteers but do not increase the risk for future CHD events in such a population.

Given the cardiovascular and noncardiovascular limitations to exercise in older adults, exercise-testing protocols should employ low starting work rates and smaller work increments than in younger patients. Thus, protocols such as the Naughton or Balke, in which the speed is held constant and only the elevation is increased, are ideal for the elderly. Individuals with gait disturbances can often be tested on a cycle ergometer, although their aerobic capacity and peak heart rate are usually lower than those achieved with treadmill exercise.

Diagnostic sensitivity of the exercise ECG for CHD appears to increase with age at the expense of a modest reduction in specificity. Hlatky et al. (83) found the exercise ECG to have a sensitivity of 84% and a specificity of 70% for the diagnosis of CHD in patients 60 years or older. In contrast, sensitivity was only 56% in patients younger than 40 years, although specificity was 84%. In patients aged 65 years and older, Newman and Phillips (84) found a sensitivity of 85%, a specificity of 56%, and a positive predictive value of 86% for the exercise ECG in diagnosing CHD. The increased sensitivity and high positive predictive value of the exercise ECG with increasing age found in these two treadmill exercise studies was probably due to the increased prevalence and severity of CHD in elderly persons (85). Reduced specificity is largely explained by a higher prevalence of ST-T-wave abnormalities on the pre-exercise ECG.

Prognostic Utility of the Exercise ECG

Numerous studies in patients with known or suspected CHD have shown that the standard treadmill exercise test provides valuable prognostic information. In a sample of 2632 patients 65 years or older undergoing clinically indicated exercise testing, a lower peak treadmill workload was a strong independent predictor of cardiac death over the subsequent 2.9-year mean follow-up period (86). Of note, neither ischemic ST changes nor angina were predictive. In a similar population, however, Glover et al. demonstrated that an ischemic ST-segment response to exercise predicted an eightfold cardiovascular mortality (17% vs. 2%) over a 2-year follow-up (87). The Duke treadmill score, which incorporates exercise duration, magnitude of ischemic ST-segment depression, and presence of exercise-induced angina, has demonstrated prognostic utility in younger populations (88,89), but appears to be less useful in patients aged 75 years or older (89). A large study of male veterans reported similar prognostic utility of the exercise ECG in those aged 65 years and older compared to younger men (90). In both age groups, exercise-induced ST segment depression predicted cardiovascular death whereas peak exercise metabolic equivalents achieved best predicted all-cause mortality (90).

Exercise testing after myocardial infarction has prognostic value in older patients, as it does in younger ones. Identification of jeopardized myocardium in such post-myocardial infarction patients may be useful because recurrent infarction and sudden cardiac death are the most common causes of 1-year mortality post-hospital discharge (91). In 188 patients aged 70 years or older who underwent exercise testing a mean of 14 days' postinfarction, Ciaroni et al. (92) found that a rise in systolic blood pressure of less than 30 mmHg, a maximal cycle workrate less than 60 W, and an exercise duration less than 5 minutes predicted cardiovascular death; whereas ST-segment depression and ventricular arrhythmias predicted reinfarction and the need for coronary revascularization. Similar to the general postinfarction population, older patients excluded from exercise testing after myocardial infarction have the highest cardiovascular risk. For example, Deckers et al. (93) found a mortality of 4% for patients 65 years or older who were able to perform a cycle exercise test postinfarction versus a mortality of 37% for those excluded.

Though the diagnostic and prognostic utility of exercise testing in general population is modest, such testing may have greater value in asymptomatic older persons with multiple CHD risks factors. Older subjects embarking on a vigorous training program or those entrusted with the safety of others, such as school bus drivers, are appropriate candidates for testing.

Exercise Cardiac Imaging

Exercise stress testing incorporating thallium perfusion scintigraphy, radionuclide ventriculography, or echocardiography provides additional value in the diagnosis and prognosis of CHD compared with the exercise ECG alone. Iskandrian et al. (94) showed that exercise thallium-201 imaging can be used for risk stratification of elderly patients with CHD. The risk for cardiac death or nonfatal myocardial infarction at a 25-month follow-up in 449 patients 60 years or older was less than 1% in patients with normal images, 5% in patients with single-vessel thallium-201 abnormality, and 13% in patients with multivessel thallium-201 abnormality. In 120 patients 70 years or older with known or suspected CHD who underwent exercise thallium-201 scintigraphy, Hilton et al. (95) showed that the combination of low peak exercise capacity and any thallium-201 perfusion defect was the most powerful predictor of new cardiac events (relative risk, 5.3 at 1 year). Individuals with an ischemic ST-segment depression more than 2 mm and a thallium defect who failed to complete stage 1 of a Bruce protocol suffered a 47% event rate. Exercise single-photon emission computed tomography (SPECT) was performed in 247 elderly patients aged 75 years and older (108 women and 139 men) and classified 49% of the patients as low risk and 35% of the patients as high risk by a summed stress score (96). At 6.4-year follow-up, patients classified as low risk had an annual cardiac mortality rate of 0.8%, and those classified as high risk had an annual cardiac mortality rate of 5.8%. In this study, the Duke treadmill score was not significantly associated with cardiac death (96).

Fleg et al. (5) performed maximal treadmill exercise ECGs and thallium scintigraphy in 407 asymptomatic volunteers aged between 40 and 96 years from the Baltimore Longitudinal Study on Aging. At 4.6 years of follow-up, new cardiac events developed in 7% of patients who had negative results on both tests, 8% of patients with a single positive result, and 48% of patients with both results positive. Persons with both a positive exercise ECG and a thallium perfusion defect averaged 69 years of age and had 3.6 times the relative risk for new coronary events as those with negative results, independent of standard coronary risk factors (5).

Echocardiography during, or more commonly, immediately after treadmill or cycle exercise has also proven useful in the detection and prognostication of CHD. Overall sensitivity of exercise-induced wall motion abnormalities for CHD using this technique is 74–97% with specificity of 64–88%, similar to values of exercise thallium scintigraphy (97,98). As with other diagnostic modalities, the sensitivity of exercise echocardiography increases with the extent of CHD, which should result in a high sensitivity in the elderly. Though a lower technical success of echocardiographic imaging in older versus younger patients is probably responsible for a lesser utilization of exercise echocardiography in the elderly, advances in echocardiographic equipment have largely overcome this deficiency. In 2632 patients, aged 65 years or older, referred for clinically indicated exercise echocardiography, the exercise-induced changes in LV end-systolic volume and the exercise LV ejection fraction or wall motion score were predictors of cardiac events and cardiac death, independent of clinical status, resting echocardiography, and exercise duration (86) (Fig. 8.2).

At 2.8-year follow-up of 1268 patients of mean age 60 years, nonfatal myocardial infarction or cardiac death occurred in 1.1% patients per year with a normal stress echocardiogram and in 3.6% patients per year with a normal stress ECG ($p < 0.001$) (99). Peak wall motion score index (hazard ratio = 2.55) and LV ejection fraction (hazard ratio = 0.99) were independent and incremental prognostic markers for stress echocardiography (99). In 2159 patients aged ≥70 years with known or suspected CHD undergoing stress echocardiography, 844 patients (38.6%) developed ischemia during exercise (100). The

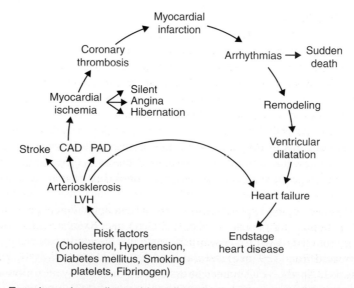

Figure 8.2   Exercise echocardiographic wall motion score as a predictor of survival free of cardiac events in 2632 patients aged 65 years or older referred for exercise testing. A higher wall motion score index (WMSI) denotes worse LV function. *Source*: From Ref. 86.

cumulative 5-year mortality was 29.3% in those with ischemia versus 16.8% in those without ischemia (100).

Older patients with diabetes mellitus (mean age 63 years) had a significantly higher prevalence of unrecognized myocardial infarction (18% of 287 patients) detected by a treadmill exercise sestamibi stress test than age-matched and gender-matched patients without diabetes mellitus (7% of 292 patients) ($p < 0.001$) (101). Patients with diabetes mellitus also had a higher prevalence of SI without a history of angina pectoris (33%) than patients without diabetes mellitus (18%) ($p < 0.001$) (101).

Pharmacological Stress Testing

The greatest advancement in stress testing over the past decade has been the widespread application of pharmacological stress testing on populations unable to perform diagnostically adequate exercise tests. The elderly are clearly the greatest beneficiaries of pharmacological stress testing because of the high prevalence of exercise-limiting conditions among them, such as obstructive lung disease, peripheral arterial insufficiency, arthritis, and neuromuscular disorders. The agents most commonly used for this purpose are the vasodilators, dipyridamole, and adenosine, and the synthetic catecholamine, dobutamine, in conjunction with either radionuclide or echocardiographic imaging.

Dipyridamole is a phosphodiesterase inhibitor that blocks degradation of adenosine, thereby increasing plasma adenosine, which is a potent arteriolar dilator. Both dipyridamole and adenosine dilate normal coronary arteries more than stenotic vessels, creating a coronary steal that causes a myocardial perfusion defect or wall motion abnormality. With either drug, serious side effects, including bronchospasm, hypotension, and arrhythmias, occur in 2–3% of patients but do not appear to be age-related (102–104). In 101 subjects older than 70 years, the sensitivity and specificity of dipyridamole thallium imaging for CHD were 86% and 75%, respectively, compared with corresponding values of 83% and 70% in younger patients (105). In 92 patients aged 65 years and older who had undergone prior coronary artery bypass grafting, the dipyridamole sestamibi stress test had a sensitivity of 95%, a specificity of 50%, a positive predictive value of 96%, and a negative predictive value of 43% for graft occlusion or 50% or more new native CAD (106); these values were similar to those in younger patients (105).

Prognostic utility of dipyridamole in combination with echocardiography was shown in 190 patients aged 65 years and above (mean, 68 + 3), evaluated at a mean of 10 days after uncomplicated myocardial infarction. Patients with a positive test experienced a threefold risk of future cardiac events and 4.4-fold risk of death compared with those with negative, i.e., normal results (106). An abnormal dipyridamole thallium scan was the best predictor of subsequent events in 348 patients aged 70 years and older with known or suspected CHD conferring a relative risk of 7.2 on multivariate analysis (107). Dipyridamole stress imaging has also been used to identify patients at high cardiovascular risk prior to vascular surgery. Hendel et al. (108) observed that a reversible thallium perfusion defect conferred a ninefold risk of perioperative myocardial infarction or cardiac death in 360 such patients whose mean age was 65 years.

Adenosine echocardiography has also demonstrated both diagnostic and prognostic utility in older patients with known or suspected CHD. In 120 such patients 70 years or older, sensitivity for CHD was 66%, specificity 90%, and diagnostic accuracy 73% (104). Sensitivity increased from 42% in patients with single-vessel CHD to 73% in those with multivessel disease. An abnormal adenosine echocardiogram predicted a threefold risk of future cardiac events, independent of clinical CHD risk factors. The only serious effect was transient AV block, which occurred in 6% of patients, but was asymptomatic and self limited in all (104). In another study, the risk of such transient AV block after adenosine infusion was 18% in patients 75 years or older versus 8% in younger patients (109). Combining adenosine infusion with symptom-limited treadmill exercise reduced the incidence of premature infusion termination from 15% to 5%.

A potential advantage of adenosine, and probably dipyridamole, stress testing over exercise is the ability to continue β-blockers without compromising on diagnostic yield. In a study of 158 consecutive patients (mean age 66 years) who had adenosine SPECT myocardial perfusion imaging, β-blocker therapy was continued through the test in 82 patients and stopped 48 hours prior to the test in 76 patients (110). β-Blocker therapy did not affect the extent, severity, and reversibility of perfusion defects on adenosine SPECT myocardial perfusion imaging. However, patients who stopped β-blockers for 48 hours had a higher incidence of angina pectoris (10%) than those who continued β-blocker therapy through the test (2%) (110).

Dobutamine is a synthetic catecholamine that is frequently used as a pharmacological stressor in older patients, in combination with echocardiography or thallium imaging. Dobutamine produces dose-related increases in heart rate and inotropy that augment coronary artery blood flow, thereby inducing ischemia by a mechanism similar to exercise in patients with CHD. Atropine is frequently combined with dobutamine to help insure an adequate chronotropic response. The classic ischemic response induced by dobutamine is characterized by improved wall motion at low doses but worsening wall motion at high doses. Dobutamine is particularly useful in older patients with obstructive lung disease, in whom both dipyridamole and adenosine are contraindicated. In 120 patients aged 70 years or older with known or suspected CHD, dobutamine echocardiography had a sensitivity of 87%, a specificity of 84%, and an accuracy of 86%, all higher than corresponding figures for adenosine in the same patients (Table 8.6) (104). Patients with a positive dobutamine stress test had a 7.3-fold risk for a future cardiac event compared with those with a normal test. Dobutamine thallium scintigraphy demonstrated sensitivity of 86% and specificity of 90% in 144 patients aged 65 ± 10 years (111), numbers very similar to the echocardiographic data with this drug. Dobutamine has also been used to predict perioperative coronary events in older patients undergoing vascular surgery (112). Though dobutamine is generally well tolerated in all age groups, higher rates of asymptomatic hypotension and both supraventricular and ventricular arrhythmias, but a lower rate of chest pain, were reported in patients older versus younger than 70 years (113,114).

Several large series have confirmed the prognostic value of dobutamine stress testing. At 6.5-year follow-up of 1434 patients older than 65 years who had dobutamine stress echocardiography, resting wall abnormalities (hazard ratio = 1.13) and inducible ischemia (hazard ratio = 2.1) were significant independent predictors of cardiac death or nonfatal myocardial infarction (115). At 2.6-year follow-up of 7333 patients, mean age 59 years,

Table 8.6   Comparison of Dobutamine and Adenosine Echocardiography in Detection of CAD in Patients Aged 70 Years or Older

	Dobutamine (%)	**Adenosine (%)**	*p* **Value**
Sensitivity			
Overall	87	66	<0.001
1-vessel CHD	74	42	NS
2-vessel CHD	88	76	NS
3-vessel CHD	91	71	0.02
Specificity	84	90	NS
Accuracy	86	73	0.01

Abbreviations: CHD, coronary heart disease; NS, not significant.
Source: Adapted from Ref. 104.

who had stress echocardiography with either dipyridamole or dobutamine, the cardiac mortality was 29% in patients with a positive test versus 8% in those with a negative test (116). Older age remained a strong independent predictor of cardiac death. Among 931 patients (mean age 61 years) with inducible myocardial ischemia during dobutamine stress echocardiography, ischemia was silent in 69% and symptomatic in 31% (117). At 5.5-year follow-up, cardiac death or nonfatal myocardial infarction occurred in 3% of patients with symptomatic myocardial ischemia and in 4.6% of patients with SI ($p < 0.01$). SI predicted a 70% higher risk of cardiac death or nonfatal myocardial infarction, perhaps because such patients were less likely to be treated with cardioprotective therapy and coronary revascularization than patients with symptomatic myocardial ischemia (117). Dobutamine stress echocardiography showed a significant prognostic value in 227 octogenarians in predicting at three-year follow-up an increase in all-cause mortality ($p = 0.002$) and in major cardiac events ($p = 0.02$) (118).

Multislice Computed Tomography and Magnetic Resonance Imaging

Over the past several years, multislice computed tomography (MSCT) and magnetic resonance imaging (MRI) have become increasingly used to detect CHD. Both techniques allow direct visualization of the coronary arteries rather than relying on their functional consequences. Since their introduction for coronary artery imaging in 2000, CT scanners have increased from 4 to 16 detectors and advanced to 64 or more detectors. Thus, new generation scanners acquire more imaging slices per rotation, allowing faster image acquisition and improved temporal and spatial resolution. As a result, these scanners require a shorter period of breath holding by the patient, allow a wider range of acceptable heart rates, and the ability to image very obese patients and those with moderate coronary artery calcium, using lower contrast volumes. All of these advances in CT imaging facilitate the imaging of older patients with suspected CHD.

A meta-analysis of 24 studies using 4, 8, and 16 slice scanners revealed a per artery sensitivity of 85% and specificity of 95% for detecting obstructive CHD (119). However, that the mean age of patients in the 24 studies included ranged from 56 to 65 years; no separate analyses were performed in the elderly. In another pooled analysis, MSCT detected occluded coronary artery bypass grafts with a sensitivity of 84% and a specificity of 95% (120). In 145 patients, mean age 67 ± 10 years, 64-slice MSCT had a 98% sensitivity, a 74% specificity, a 90% positive predictive value, and a 94% negative predictive value in diagnosing obstructive CHD (121). In 2538 patients undergoing MSCT, at 78-month follow-up, MSCT provided independent and incremental value in predicting all-cause mortality in symptomatic patients independent of age, gender, conventional risk factors, and coronary artery calcium score (122). A consecutive cohort of 24,775 patients without known CHD underwent MSCT angiography between 2005 and 2009 using scanners with 64 or more detector rows. Over a 2.3 year mean follow-up, mortality increased in proportion to the number of coronary arteries with ≥50% stenosis. When stratified by age <65 years versus ≥65 years, younger patients experienced higher relative hazards for death from 2-vessel disease (hazard ratio (HR) 4.0 vs. 2.5) and 3-vessel disease (HR 6.2 vs. 3.1). However, the adverse prognosis associated with both 2- and 3-vessel disease remained highly significant in both age groups (123). Artifacts from heavily calcified coronary arteries, more common in the elderly, and metal surgical clips remain an important limitation of MSCT; only about 80% of grafts can be evaluated. Significant drawbacks of MSCT are the contrast dye load and the radiation exposure, both similar to those from conventional invasive coronary angiography. The ability to estimate myocardial blood flow and fractional flow reserve with MSCT may allow more accurate assessment of hemodynamically significant coronary lesions without the need for invasive coronary angiography (124).

Cardiac MRI has also become an attractive method for noninvasive coronary artery imaging. This technique avoids the use of ionizing radiation and iodinated intravenous contrast material as well as the need for breath holding. Faster MRI techniques and more powerful magnets have improved the quality of coronary arterial images. A meta-analysis of 28 studies using MRI coronary angiography found a per-artery sensitivity of 72% and a specificity of 87%; 86% of the coronary arterial segments were assessable (119). However, the mean age of the patients in this analysis was 63 years, with only one very small study having a mean patient age over 65 years. As with MSCT, therefore, age-specific diagnostic accuracy is not available.

Dewey et al. performed a direct comparison of MSCT with MRI for noninvasive coronary arteriography in 129 patients (mean age, 64 years) with suspected CHD (125). Sensitivity for coronary stenoses greater than 50% of lumimal diameter was 82% for MSCT versus 54% for MRI; the respective specificities were 90% and 87%. Negative predictive value was slightly higher for CT (95% vs. 90%). In this study, 74% of patients preferred MSCT to MRI. The greater diagnostic accuracy of MSCT over MRI in this study is consistent with the meta-analytic findings noted above. Thus, MSCT currently has a higher accuracy than MRI to detect or exclude significant CHD, although data specific to the elderly are lacking. As both techniques may miss significant coronary artery stenoses, they are best used in patients with a pretest probability of CHD less than 50%. In such patients, a normal coronary arteriogram by MSCT or MRI would reduce the post-test probability of CHD to less than 10%, avoiding the need for invasive coronary arteriography (126). Both techniques are thus attractive for use in emergency room settings in determining which low-to-intermediate risk patients presenting with acute chest pain should be admitted. Cardiac MRI perfusion imaging with vasodilator stress can detect myocardial ischemia and infarction with high accuracy and provide valuable prognostic information similar to that from other pharmacological stress imaging modalities (127). The 2010 American College of Cardiology Foundation/American College of Radiology/American Heart Association/North American Society for Cardiovascular Imaging/Society for Cardiovascular Magnetic Resonance expert consensus document on MRI states that the combination of MRI stress perfusion, function, and late gadolinium enhancement may be used to (i) identify patients with ischemic heart disease with resting ECG abnormalities or an inability to exercise; (ii) define patients with large vessel CAD who are candidates for interventional procedures; and (iii) determine patients who are appropriate candidates for interventional procedures (128).

Coronary Arteriography

Despite the advances in noninvasive cardiac imaging discussed above, invasive coronary arteriography remains the accepted standard for detection and quantitation of CHD, although it may underestimate the extent of coronary atherosclerosis compared with intravascular ultrasound. Major complications of coronary arteriography include myocardial infarction, stroke, and death. In the Coronary Artery Surgery Study (CASS) registry, each of these endpoints was approximately three times as common in patients aged 65 and above than in younger individuals (6). A single center study between 1980 and 1990 in 242 patients 80–92 years old reported a mortality of 0.8% and nonfatal complication rate of 5%, compared with respective rates of 0.15% and 1.5% in patients younger than 80 years (129). Niebauer et al. reported a hospital mortality of 2.1% in 1085 octogenarians after coronary angiography (130). The increased risk in the elderly is largely explained by their generally greater severity of underlying cardiac and non-cardiac disease. Although major complication rates from cardiac catheterization and coronary arteriography continued to decline through the 1990s (131), the elderly should still be considered at higher risk, especially those aged 80 years and beyond.

REFERENCES

1. White NK, Edwards JE, Dry TJ. The relationship of the degree of coronary atherosclerosis with age. Circulation 1950; 1: 645–54.
2. Elveback L, Lie JT. Continued high prevalence of coronary artery disease at autopsy in Olmstead County, Minnesota, 1950 to 1970. Circulation 1984; 70: 345–9.
3. Center for Disease Control and Prevention/National center for Health Statistics. National Health and Nutrition Examination Survey (NHANES). 2005–2008.
4. Aronow WS, Ahn C, Gutstein H. Prevalence and incidence of cardiovascular disease in 1160 older men and 2464 older women in a long-term health care facility. J Gerontol Med Sci 2002; 57A: M45–6.
5. Fleg JL, Gerstenblith G, Zonderman AB, et al. Prevalence and prognostic significance of exercise-induced silent myocardial ischemia detected by thallium scintigraphy and electro-cardigraphy in asymptomatic volunteers. Circulation 1990; 81: 428–36.
6. Gersh BJ, Kronmal RA, Frye RL, et al. Coronary arteriography and coronary artery bypass surgery: morbidity and mortality in patients ages 65 years or older. A report from the Coronary Artery Surgery Study. Circulation 1983; 67: 483–91.
7. Graham MM, Ghali WA, Faris PD, et al. Alberta Provincial Project for Outcomes Assessment in Coronary Heart Disease Investigators. Survival after coronary revascularization in the elderly. Circulation 2002; 105: 2378–84.
8. Vliegenthart R, Oudkerk M, Hofman A, et al. Coronary calcification improves cardiovascular risk prediction in the elderly. Circulation 2005; 112: 572–7.
9. Figueras J, Domingo E. Fasting and postprandial ischemic threshold in patients with unstable angina with and without postprandial angina at rest. Am Heart J 1998; 136: 252–8.
10. Wiener RS, Moses HW, Richeson F, Gatewood RP. Hospital and long-term survival of patients with acute pulmonary edema associated with coronary artery disease. Am J Cardiol 1987; 60: 33–5.
11. Clark LT, Garfein OB, Dwyer EM. Acute pulmonary edema due to ischemic heart disease without accompanying myocardial infarction. Am J Med 1983; 75: 332–6.
12. Dodek A, Kassembaum DG, Bristow JD. Pulmonary edema in coronary artery disease without cardiomegaly: paradox of the stiff heart. N Engl J Med 1972; 286: 1347–50.
13. Kunis R, Greenberg H, Yeoh CG, et al. Coronary revascularization of recurrent pulmonary edema in elderly patients with ischemic heart disease and preserved ventricular function. N Engl J Med 1985; 313: 1207–10.
14. Setaro JF, Soufer R, Remetz MS, et al. Long-term outcome in patients with congestive heart failure and intact systolic left ventricular performance. Am J Cardiol 1992; 69: 1212–16.
15. Graham SP, Vetrovec GW. Comparison of angiographic findings and demographic variables in patients with coronary artery disease presenting with acute pulmonary edema versus those presenting with chest pain. Am J Cardiol 1991; 68: 1614–18.
16. Stone GW, Griffin B, Shah PK, et al. Prevalence of unsuspected mitral regurgitation and left ventricular diastolic dysfunction in patients with coronary artery disease and acute pulmonary edema associated with normal or depressed left ventricular systolic function. Am J Cardiol 1991; 67: 37–41.
17. Tresch DD, Saeian K, Hoffman R. Elderly patients with late onset of coronary artery disease: clinical and angiographic findings. Am J Geriatr Cardiol 1992; 1: 14–25.
18. Cupples LA, D'Agostino RB. Some risk factors related to the annual incidence of cardiovascular disease and death using pooled repeated biennial measurements: Framingham Heart Study, 30-year follow-up. In: Kannel WB, Wolf PA, Garrison RJ, eds. The Framingham Heart Study: An Epidemiological Investigation of Cardiovascular Disease. Bethesda, MD, National Heart, Lung, and Blood Institute, Publication No. (NIH): 1987: 87–2703.
19. Aronow WS, Epstein S. Usefulness of silent myocardial ischemia detected by ambulatory electrocardiographic monitoring in predicting new coronary events in elderly patients. Am J Cardiol 1988; 62: 1295–6.
20. Aronow WS, Epstein S, Koenigsberg M. Usefulness of echocardiographic left ventricular ejection fraction and silent myocardial ischemia in predicting new coronary events in elderly patients with coronary artery disease or systemic hypertension. Am J Cardiol 1990; 65: 811–12.
21. Hedblad B, Juul-Moller S, Svensson K, et al. Increased mortality in men with ST segment depression during 24 h ambulatory long-term ECG recording. Results from prospective population study 'Men born in 1914,' from Malmo, Sweden. Eur Heart J 1989; 10: 149–58.
22. Ambepitiya G, Roberts M, Ranjadayalan K, et al. Silent exertional myocardial ischemia in the elderly. A quantitative analysis of angina perceptual threshold and the influence of autonomic function. J Am Geriatr Soc 1994; 42: 732–7.
23. Ellestad MH, Kaun P. Naloxone and asymptomatic ischemia: failure to induce angina during exercise testing. Am J Cardiol 1984; 54: 982–4.

24. Hatfield BD, Goldfarb AH, Sporzo GA, et al. Serum beta-endorphin and affective response to graded exercise in young and elderly men. J Gerontol 1987; 42: 429–31.

25. Morley JE. Neuropeptides: behavior and aging. J Am Geriatr Soc 1986; 34: 52–61.

26. Kannel WB, Abbott RD. Incidence and prognosis of unrecognized myocardial infarction: an update on the Framingham Study. N Engl J Med 1984; 311: 1144–7.

27. Rodstein M. The characteristics on non-fatal myocardial infarction in the aged. Arch Intern Med 1956; 98: 84–90.

28. Aronow WS, Starling L, Etienne F, et al. Unrecognized Q-wave myocardial infarction in patients older than 64 years in a long-term health care facility. Am J Cardiol 1985; 56: 483.

29. Aronow WS. Prevalence of presenting symptoms of recognized acute myocardial infarction and of unrecognized healed myocardial infarction in elderly patients. Am J Cardiol 1987; 60: 1182.

30. Muller RT, Gould LA, Betzu R, et al. Painless myocardial infarction in the elderly. Am Heart J 1990; 119: 202–4.

31. Nadelmann J, Frishman WH, Ooi WL, et al. Prevalence, incidence, and prognosis of recognized and unrecognized myocardial infarction in persons aged 75 years or older: the Bronx aging study. Am J Cardiol 1990; 66: 533–7.

32. Sigurdsson E, Thorgeirsson G, Sigvaldason H, et al. Unrecognized myocardial infarction: epidemiology, clinical characteristics, and the prognostic role of angina pectoris: the Reykjavik study. Ann Intern Med 1995; 22: 96–102.

33. Sheifer SE, Gersh BJ, Yanez ND, et al. Prevalence, predisposing factors, and prognosis of clinically unrecognized myocardial infarction in the elderly. J Am Coll Cardiol 2000; 35: 119–26.

34. Yano K, MacLean CJ. The incidence and prognosis of unrecognized myocardial infarction in the Honolulu, Hawaii, Heart Program. Arch Intern Med 1989; 149: 1528–32.

35. Aronow WS. New coronary events at four-year follow-up in elderly patients with recognized or unrecognized myocardial infarction. Am J Cardiol 1989; 63: 621–2.

36. Pathy MS. Clinical presentation of myocardial infarction in the elderly. Br Heart J 1967; 29: 190–9.

37. Tinker GM. Clinical presentation of myocardial infarction in the elderly. Age Aging 1981; 10: 237–40.

38. Bayer AJ, Chadha JS, Farag RR, et al. Changing presentation of myocardial infarction with increasing old age. J Am Geriatr Soc 1986; 23: 263–6.

39. Wroblewski M, Mikulowski P, Steen B. Symptoms of myocardial infarction in old age: clinical case, retrospective and prospective studies. Age Aging 1986; 15: 99–104.

40. MacDonald JB. Presentation of acute myocardial infarction in the elderly: a review. Age Aging 1980; 13: 196–204.

41. Solomon CG, Lee TH, Cook EF, et al. Comparison of clinical presentation of acute myocardial infarction in patients older than 65 years of age to younger patients: the multicenter pain study experience. Am J Cardiol 1989; 63: 772–6.

42. Tresch DD, Brady WF, Aufderheide TP, et al. Comparison of elderly and younger patients with out-of-hospital chest pain. Arch Intern Med 1996; 156: 1089–93.

43. Weaver WD, Litwin PE, Martin JS, et al. Effect of age on use of thrombolytic therapy and mortality in acute myocardial infarction. J Am Coll Cardiol 1991; 18: 657–62.

44. Sheifer SE, Rathore SS, Gersh BJ, et al. Time to presentation with acute myocardial infarction in the elderly. Associations with race, sex, and socioeconomic characteristics. Circulation 2000; 102: 1651–6.

45. Nicod P, Gilpin E, Dittrich H, et al. Short- and long-term clinical outcome after Q-wave, and non-Q-wave myocardial infarction in a large patient population. Circulation 1989; 79: 528–36.

46. Woodworth S, Nayak D, Aronow WS, et al. Comparison of acute coronary syndromes in men versus women >70 years of age. Am J Cardiol 2002; 90: 1145–7.

47. Chung MK, Bosner MS, McKenzie JP, et al. Prognosis of patients ≥70 years of age with non-Q-wave acute myocardial infarction compared with younger patients with similar infarcts and with patients ≥70 years of age with Q-wave acute myocardial infarction. Am J Cardiol 1995; 75: 18–22.

48. Rich MW, Bosner MS, Chung MK, et al. Is age an independent predictor of early and late mortality in patients with acute myocardial infarction? Am J Med 1992; 92: 7–13.

49. Fedullo AJ, Swinburne AJ. Intensive care for elderly patients with myocardial infarction: age-related comparison of clinical features and outcome. J Intens Care Med 1988; 3: 265–71.

50. Auer R, Bauer DC, Marques-Vida l P, et al. Association of major and minor ECG abnormalities with coronary heart disease events. JAMA 2012; 307: 1497–505.

51. Aronow WS. Correlation of ischemic ST-segment depression on the resting electrocardiogram with new cardiac event in 1,106 patients over 62 years of age. Am J Cardiol 1989; 64: 232–3.

52. Aronow WS. Correlation of arrhythmias and conduction defects on the resting electrocardiogram with new cardiac events in 1,153 elderly patients. Am J Noninvas Cardiol 1991; 5: 88–90.

53. Kannel WB, Dannenberg AL, Levy D. Population implications of electrocardiographic left ventricular hypertrophy. Am J Cardiol 1987; 60: 851–931.

54. Aronow WS, Ahn C, Kronzon I, et al. Congestive heart failure, coronary events, and atherothrombotic brain infarction in elderly blacks and whites with systemic hypertension and with and without echocardiographic and electrocardiographic evidence of left ventricular hypertrophy. Am J Cardiol 1991; 67: 295–9.

55. Fleg JL, Kennedy HL. Long-term prognostic significance of ambulatory electrocardographic findings in apparently healthy subjects ≥60 years of age. Am J Cardiol 1992; 90: 748–51.

56. Kirkland JL, Lye M, Faragher EB, et al. A longitudinal study of the prognostic significance of ventricular ectopic beats in the elderly. Gerontology 1983; 29: 199–201.

57. Martin A, Benbow LJ, Butrous GS, et al. Five-year follow-up of 106 elderly subjects by means of long-term ambulatory cardiac monitoring. Eur Heart J 1984; 5: 592–6.

58. Aronow WS, Epstein S, Mercando AD. Usefulness of complex ventricular arrhythmias detected by 24-hour ambulatory electrocardiogram and by electrocardiograms with one-minute rhythm strips in predicting new coronary events in elderly patients with and without heart disease. J Cardiovasc Technol 1991; 10: 21–5.

59. Aronow WS, Epstein S, Koenigsberg M, et al. Usefulness of echocardiographic abnormal left ventricular ejection fraction, paroxysmal ventricular tachycardia, and complex ventricular arrhythmias in predicting new coronary events in patients over 62 years of age. Am J Cardiol 1988; 61: 1349–51.

60. Aronow WS, Epstein S, Koenigsberg M, et al. Usefulness of echocardiographic left ventricular hypertrophy, ventricular tachycardia and complex ventricular arrhythmias in predicting ventricular fibrillation or sudden cardiac death in elderly patients. Am J Cardiol 1988; 62: 1124–5.

61. Aronow WS, Ahn C, Mercando A, et al. Prevalence and association of ventricular tachycardia and complex ventricular arrhythmias with new coronary events in older men and women with and without cardiovascular disease. J Gerontol Med Sci 2002; 57A: M178–80.

62. Aronow WS, Epstein S. Usefulness of silent ischemia, ventricular tachycardia, and complex ventricular arrhythmias in predicting new coronary events in elderly patients with coronary artery disease or systemic hypertension. Am J Cardiol 1990; 65: 511–12.

63. Dicker RC, Han LF, Mancone JJ. Quality of Care Surveillance Using Administrative Data, 1996. Baltimore, MD: Health Care Financing Administration, 1998.

64. Gottlieb SO, Weisfeldt ML, Ouyang P, et al. Silent ischemia as a marker for early unfavorable outcomes in patients with unstable angina. N Engl J Med 1986; 314: 1214–19.

65. Gottlieb SO, Gottlieb SH, Achuff SC, et al. Silent ischemia on Holter monitoring predicts mortality in high-risk postinfarction patients. JAMA 1988; 259: 1030–5.

66. Gottlieb SO, Weisfeldt ML, Ouyang P, et al. Silent ischemia predicts infarction and death during 2-year follow-up on unstable angina. J Am Coll Cardiol 1987; 10: 756–60.

67. Aronow WS, Ahn C, Mercando AD, et al. Prevalence and association of silent myocardial ischemia with new coronary events in older men and women with and without cardiovascular disease. J Am Geriatr Soc 2002; 50: 1075–8.

68. Aronow WS, Epstein S, Koenigsberg M. Usefulness of echocardiographic left ventricular hypertrophy and silent ischemia in predicting new cardiac events in elderly patients with systemic hypertension or coronary artery disease. Angiology 1990; 41: 189–93.

69. Raby KE, Goldman L, Creager MA, et al. Correlation between preoperative ischemia and major cardiac events after peripheral vascular surgery. N Engl J Med 1989; 321: 1296–300.

70. Raby KE, Barry J, Creager MA, et al. Detection and significance of intraoperative and postoperative myocardial ischemia in peripheral vascular surgery. JAMA 1992; 268: 222–7.

71. Mercando AD, Aronow WS, Epstein S, et al. Signal-averaged electrocardiography and ventricular tachycardia as predictors of mortality after acute myocardial infarction in elderly patients. Am J Cardiol 1995; 76: 436–40.

72. Aronow WS, Ahn C, Kronzon I. Prognosis of congestive heart failure in elderly patients with normal versus abnormal left ventricular systolic function associated with coronary artery disease. Am J Cardiol 1990; 66: 1256–9.

73. Aronow WS, Ahn C, Kronzon I. Prognosis of congestive heart failure after prior myocardial infarction in older men and women with abnormal versus normal left ventricular ejection fraction. Am J Cardiol 2000; 85: 1382–4.

74. Levy D, Garrison RJ, Savage DD, et al. Left ventricular mass and incidence of coronary heart disease in an elderly cohort: the Framingham Heart Study. Ann Intern Med 1989; 110: 101–7.

75. Aronow WS, Koenigsberg M, Schwartz KS. Usefulness of echocardiographic left ventricular hypertrophy in predicting new coronary events and atherothrombotic brain infarction in patients over 62 years of age. Am J Cardiol 1988; 61: 1130–2.

76. Buskirk ER, Hodgson JL. Age and aerobic power. The rate of change in men and women. Fed Proc 1987; 46: 1824–9.
77. Talbot LA, Metter EJ, Fleg JL. Leisure-time physical activities and their relationship to cardiorespiratory fitness in healthy men and women 18–95 years old. Med Sci Sports Exerc 2000; 32: 417–25.
78. Stratton JR, Levy WC, Cerqueira MD, et al. Cardiovascular responses to exercise. Effects of aging and exercise training in healthy men. Circulation 1994; 89: 1648–55.
79. Fleg JL, O'Connor F, Gerstenblith G, et al. Impact of age on the cardiovascular response to dynamic upright exercise in healthy men and women. J Appl Physiol 1995; 78: 890–900.
80. Fleg JL, Schulman S, O'Connor F, et al. Effects of acute beta-adrenergic receptor blockade on age-associated changes in cardiovascular performance during dynamic exercise. Circulation 1994; 90: 2333–41.
81. Maurer MS, Shefrin EA, Fleg JL. Prevalence and prognostic significance of exercise-induced supraventricular tachycardia in apparently healthy volunteers. Am J Cardiol 1995; 75: 788–92.
82. Busby MJ, Shefrin EA, Fleg JL. Prevalence and long-term significance of exercise-induced frequent or repetitive ventricular ectopic beats in apparently healthy volunteers. J Am Coll Cardiol 1989; 14: 1659–65.
83. Hlatky MA, Pryor DB, Harrell FE, et al. Factors affecting sensitivity and specificity of exercise electrocardiography: multivariable analysis. Am J Med 1984; 77: 64–71.
84. Newman KP, Phillips JH. Gradual exercise testing for diagnosis of coronary artery disease in elderly patients. South Med J 1988; 81: 430–2.
85. Chaitman BR, Bourassa MG, Davis K, et al. Angiographic prevalence of high-risk coronary artery disease in patient subsets (CASS). Circulation 1981; 64: 360–7.
86. Arruda AM, Das MK, Roger VL, et al. prognostic value of exercise echocardiography in 2,632 patients ≥65 years of age. J Am Coll Cardiol 2001; 37: 1036–41.
87. Glover DR, Robinson CS, Murray RG. Diagnostic exercise testing in 104 patients over 65 years of age. Eur Heart J 1984; 5: 59–61.
88. Mark DB, Shaw L, Harrell FE, et al. Prognostic value of a treadmill exercise score in outpatients with suspected coronary artery disease. N Engl J Med 1991; 325: 849–53.
89. Kwok JM, Miller TD, Hodge DO, et al. Prognostic value of the Duke treadmill score in the elderly. J Am Coll Cardiol 2002; 39: 1475–81.
90. Lai S, Kayha A, Yamazaki T, et al. Treadmill scores in elderly men. J Am Coll Cardiol 2004; 43: 606–15.
91. Smith SC Jr, Gilpin E, Ahnve S, et al. Outlook after acute myocardial infarction in the very elderly compared with that in patients aged 65 to 75 years. J Am Coll Cardiol 1990; 16: 784–92.
92. Ciaroni S, Delonca J, Righetti A. Early exercise testing after acute myocardial infarction in the elderly: clinical evaluation and prognostic significance. Am Heart J 1993; 126: 304–11.
93. Deckers JW, Fioretti P, Brower RW, et al. Ineligibility for predischarge exercise testing after myocardial infarction in the elderly: implications for prognosis. Eur Heart J 1984; 5: 97–100.
94. Iskandrian AS, Heo J, Decoskey D, et al. Use of exercise, thallium-201 imaging for risk stratification of elderly patients with coronary artery disease. Am J Cardiol 1988; 61: 269–72.
95. Hilton TC, Shaw LJ, Chaitman BR, et al. Prognostic significance of exercise thallium-201 testing in patients aged ≥70 years with known or suspected coronary artery disease. Am J Cardiol 1992; 69: 45–50.
96. Valeti US, Miller TD, Hodge DO, et al. Exercise single-photon emission computed tomography provides effective risk stratification of elderly men and elderly women. Circulation 2005; 111: 1771–6.
97. Quinones MA, Verani MS, Haichin RM, et al. Exercise echocardiography versus 102 Tl single-photon emission computed tomography in evaluation of coronary artery disease. Analysis of 292 patients. Circulation 1992; 85: 1026–31.
98. Crouse LJ, Harbrecht JJ, Vacek JL, et al. Exercise echocardiography as a screening test for coronary artery disease and correlation with coronary arteriography. Am J Cardiol 1991; 67: 1213–18.
99. Mahenthiran J, Bangalore S, Yao SS, et al. Comparison of prognostic value of stress echocardiography versus stress electrocardiography in patients with suspected coronary artery disease. Am J Cardiol 2005; 96: 628–34.
100. Bouzas-Mosquera A, Peteiro J, Broullon FJ, et al. Value of exercise echocardiography for predicting mortality in elderly patients. Eur J Clin Invest 2010; 40: 1122–30.
101. DeLuca AJ, Kaplan S, Aronow WS, et al. Comparison of prevalence of unrecognized myocardial infarction and of silent myocardial ischemia detected by a treadmill exercise sestamibi stress test in patients with versus without diabetes mellitus. Am J Cardiol 2006; 98: 1045–6.
102. Ranhosky A, Kempthorne-Rawson J; Intravenous Dipyridamole Thallium-Imaging Study Group. The safety of intravenous dipyridamole thallium myocardial perfusion imaging. Circulation 1990; 81: 1205–9.

103. Lam JY, Chaitman BR, Glaenzer M, et al. Safety and diagnostic accuracy of dipyridamole- thallium imaging in the elderly. J Am Coll Cardiol 1988; 11: 585–9.
104. Anthopoulos LP, Bonou MS, Kardaras FG, et al. Stress echocardiography in elderly patients with coronary artery disease: applicability, safety and prognostic value of dobutamine and adenosine echocardiography in elderly patients. J Am Coll Cardiol 1996; 28: 52–9.
105. DeLuca AJ, Cusack E, Aronow WS, et al. Sensitivity, specificity, positive predictive value, and negative predictive value of the dipyridamole sestamibi stress test in predicting draft occlusion or ≥50% new native coronary artery disease in men versus women and in patients aged ≥65 years versus <65 years who had prior coronary artery bypass grafting. Am J Cardiol 2004; 94: 625–6.
106. Camerieri A, Picano E, Landi P, et al. Prognostic value of dipyridamole echocardiography early after myocardial infarction in elderly patients. Echo Persantine Italian Cooperative (EPIC) Study Group. J Am Coll Cardiol 1993; 22: 1809–15.
107. Shaw L, Chaitman BR, Hilton TC, et al. Prognostic value of dipyridamole thallium-201 imaging in elderly patients. J Am Coll Cardiol 1992; 19: 1390–8.
108. Hendel RC, Whitfield SS, Villegas BJ, et al. Prediction of late cardiac events by dipyridamole thallium imaging in patients undergoing elective vascular surgery. Am J Cardiol 1992; 70: 1243–9.
109. Hashimoto A, Palmer EL, Scott JA. Complications of exercise and pharmacologic stress tests: differences in younger and elderly patients. J Nucl Cardiol 1999; 6: 612–19.
110. Lakkireddy D, Aronow WS, Bateman T, et al. Does beta blocker therapy affect the diagnostic accuracy of adenosine single photon emission computed tomographic myocardial perfusion imaging? Am J Therap 2008; 15: 19–23.
111. Hays JT, Mahmarian JJ, Cochran AJ, et al. Dobutamine thallium-201 tomography for evaluating patients with suspected coronary artery disease unable to undergo exercise or vasodilator pharmacologic stress testing. J Am Coll Cardiol 1993; 21: 1583–90.
112. Eichelberger JP, Schwarz KQ, Black ER, et al. Predictive value of dobutamine echocardiography just before noncardiac vascular surgery. Am J Cardiol 1993; 72: 602–7.
113. Elhendy A, van Domburg RT, Bax JJ, et al. Safety, hemodynamic profile, and feasibility of dobutamine stress technitium myocardial perfusion single-photon emission CT imaging for evaluation of coronary artery disease in the elderly. Chest 2000; 117: 649–56.
114. Hiro J, Hiro T, Reid CL, et al. Safety and results of dobutamine stress echocardiography in women versus men and in patients older and younger than 75 years of age. Am J Cardiol 1997; 80: 1014–20.
115. Sicari R, Pasanisi E, Venneri L, et al. Stress echo results predict mortality: a large-scale multicenter prospective international study. J Am Coll Cardiol 2003; 41: 589–95.
116. Biagini E, Elhendy A, Schinkel AF, et al. Long-term prediction of mortality in elderly persons by dobutamine stress echocardiography. J Gerontol A Biol Sci Med Sci 2005; 60: 1333–8.
117. Biagini E, Schinkel AFL, Bax JJ, et al. Long-term outcome in patients with silent versus symptomatic ischaemia during dobutamine stress echocardiography. Heart 2005; 91: 737–42.
118. Innocenti F, Totti A, Baroncini C, et al. Prognostic value of dobutamine stress echocardiography in octogenarians. Int J Cardiovasc Imaging 2011; 27: 65–74.
119. Schuijf JD, Bax JJ, Shaw LJ, et al. Meta-analysis of comparative diagnostic performance of magnetic resonance imaging and multislice computed tomography for noninvasive coronary angiography. Am Heart J 2006; 151: 404–11.
120. Cademartiri F, Schuijf JD, Mollet NR, et al. Multislice CT coronary angiography: how to do it and what is the current clinical performance? Eur J Nucl Med Mol Imaging 2005; 32: 1337–47.
121. Ravipati G, Aronow WS, Lai H, et al. Comparison of sensitivity, specificity, positive predictive value, and negative predictive value of stress testing versus 64-multislice coronary computed tomography angiography in predicting obstructive coronary artery disease diagnosed by coronary angiography. Am J Cardiol 2008; 101: 774–5.
122. Ostrom MP, Gopal A, Ahmadi N, et al. Mortality incidence and the severity of coronary atherosclerosis assessed by computed tomography angiography. J Am Coll Cardiol 2008; 52: 1335–43.
123. Min JK, Dunning A, Lin FY, et al. Age-and sex-related differences in all-cause mortality risk based on coronary computed tomography angiography findings: results from the International Multicenter CONFIRM (Coronary CT Angiography Evaluation for Clinical Outcomes: an International multicenter Registry of 23,854 patients without known coronary arery disease. J Am Coll Cardiol 2011; 58: 849–60.
124. Bamberg F, Becker A, Schwarz F, et al. Detection of hemodynamically significant coronary stenosis: incremental diagnostic value of dynamic CT-based myocardial perfusion imaging. Radiology 2011; 260: 689–98.
125. Dewey M, Teige F, Schnapauff D, et al. Noninvasive detection of coronary artery stenosis with multislice computer tomography or magnetic resonance imaging. Ann Intern Med 2006; 145: 407–15.

126. Greenland P. Who is a candidate for noninvasive coronary angiography? Ann Intern Med 2006; 145: 466–7.
127. Coelho-Fihlho OR, Seabra LF, Mongeon FP, et al. Stress myocardial perfusion imaging by CR provides strong prognostic value to cardiac events regardless of patient's sex. JACC Cardiovasc Imgging 2011; 4: 850–61.
128. Hundley WG, Bluemke DA, Finn JP, et al. ACCF/ACR/NASCI/SCMR 2010 expert consensus document on cardiovascular magnetic resonance. A report of the American College of Cardiology Foundation Task Force on Expert Consensus Documents. Circulation 2010; 121: 2462–508.
129. Clark VL, Khaja F. Risk of cardiac catheterization in patients ≥80 years without previous cardiac surgery. Am J Cardiol 1994; 74: 1076–7.
130. Niebauer J, Sixt S, Zhang F, et al. Contemporary outcome of cardiac catheterization in 1085 consecutive octogenarians. Int UJ Cardiol 2004; 93: 225–30.
131. West R, Ellis G, Brooks N. Complications of diagnostic cardiac catheterisation: results from a confidential inquiry into cardiac catheter complications. Heart 2006; 92: 810–14.

9
Angina pectoris in the elderly

Wilbert S. Aronow and William H. Frishman

SUMMARY

Patients with stable angina pectoris should be treated with antianginal drug therapy and with secondary prevention therapies to reduce cardiovascular events and mortality. β-Blockers, nitrates, calcium channel blockers, and ranolazine are clinically effective antianginal drugs. Refractory angina pectoris should be treated with coronary revascularization. Patients with unstable angina pectoris should be treated according to the 2011 updated American College of Cardiology (ACC) Foundation/American Heart Association (AHA) guidelines for treating unstable angina pectoris. High-risk unstable angina patients should be treated with early coronary revascularization rather than with an early conservative strategy. Other treatments for angina pectoris, including other antianginal drugs, cell therapy, transmyocardial laser revascularization, enhanced external counterpulsation, spinal cord stimulation, and the use of a coronary sinus reducer stent, are discussed.

Coronary artery disease (CAD) is the number one cause of death in elderly patients and also the major cause of hospitalization and rehospitalizations in this age group. Clinically, CAD manifests as both acute and chronic ischemic syndromes, and it is important that the practicing physician have an understanding of the pathophysiology of these syndromes, as well as confidence in the management of these syndromes in elderly patients. This chapter will discuss the evaluation and management of elderly patients who demonstrate two of these ischemic syndromes—stable and unstable angina.

Advances in cellular and molecular biology have provided a better understanding of coronary atherosclerosis, the underlying disease process causing myocardial ischemia. Due to these advances and the development of new therapies, we are now not only able to relieve the patient's symptoms but are also able to modify the underlying pathophysiology.

Evaluation and treatment of myocardial ischemia in elderly patients pose unique challenges to the physician. Although the pathophysiology of myocardial ischemia and the treatment options are similar in elderly and younger patients, there are significant differences in presentation and response to treatment between the age groups. Elderly CAD patients with myocardial ischemia often present with "atypical" symptoms, and have more comorbid illnesses, a greater number of vessels involved, and worse left ventricular (LV) function (1–6). The pharmacokinetics of medications are altered in elderly patients, and there is often a greater sensitivity to medication and a greater potential for side effects and drug–drug interactions. Since elderly patients often present with more advanced CAD and their prognosis is often worse, there is a greater potential for gain from aggressive interventions, such as percutaneous coronary intervention (PCI) and coronary artery bypass surgery (CABG), although the risks are greater compared to younger patients. Finally, elderly patients and their families may place different values on risk, quality of life, and the importance of prognosis, all of which must be considered by the practicing physician.

EVALUATION AND MANAGEMENT

The most common symptom of myocardial ischemia in elderly patients as well as in younger patients is exertional chest pain (angina); however, in many older patients, instead of chest pain, exertional dyspnea may be the initial manifestation of ischemia. Other common symptoms experienced by elderly patients with myocardial ischemia are dizziness, mental confusion, or easy fatigability. In some elderly patients with myocardial ischemia, the presentation will be the sudden onset of heart failure ("flash" pulmonary edema) (7–9) or arrhythmias, including sudden death (10). Silent ischemia is particularly common in elderly patients with CAD, occurring in up to one-third of elderly patients, as documented by ambulatory electrocardiographic (ECG) monitoring (11,12).

The initial evaluation of the elderly patient with possible myocardial ischemia should begin with a thorough history and complete physical examination, and determination of coronary risk factors and comorbid illnesses. The assessment should determine if the patient is stable or unstable and the risk stratification of the patient. In addition to advanced age, morbidity and mortality in elderly patients with acute myocardial ischemia are directly related to LV function, the extent of CAD, and the presence of comorbidity. During the evaluation, the physician caring for elderly patients with myocardial ischemia will need to consider the effects of the disease on the whole person (including physical, psychosocial, and economic aspects) and the impact of the disease on the patient's family.

Angina pectoris is a clinical syndrome reflecting inadequate oxygen supply for myocardial metabolic demands with resultant ischemia. Depending upon the underlying pathophysiology, the patient will present with stable or unstable angina. The goals of therapy in elderly patients with angina (ischemic syndromes) are to (*i*) relieve the acute symptoms and stabilize the acute pathophysiological process; (*ii*) minimize the frequency and severity of recurrent anginal attacks; and (*iii*) prevent progression, plus cause regression of the underlying pathophysiological process. Therapeutic measures are directed at modifying the underlying pathophysiology with therapeutic agents and reducing myocardial ischemia by (*i*) reducing myocardial oxygen demand and (*ii*) increasing coronary blood flow.

The main underlying pathological process in patients with angina is coronary atherosclerosis with plaque formation and narrowing of the vessel luminal diameter, plus intermittent rupture of the atherosclerotic plaque. Because thrombus formation is an important factor in the progression of atherosclerotic lesions and in the conversion of clinical to acute events after plaque rupture, antiplatelet and anticoagulant therapy is important in the management of elderly CAD patients. In addition, stabilization and regression of the atherosclerotic lesions are possible by vigorous control of the patient's serum lipids, particularly with hydroxymethylglutaryl coenzyme A (HMG-CoA)-reductase inhibitors (statins), and treatment of other risk factors, such as systemic hypertension, smoking, and diabetes mellitus.

The main determinants of myocardial oxygen demand are heart rate, myocardial contractility, and intramyocardial tension, which is a function of systemic pressure and ventricular volume. Reduction of the myocardial oxygen demand includes correction of potentially reversible factors, such as heart failure, hyperthyroidism, valvular heart disorders (particularly aortic stenosis), obesity, emotional stress, hypertension, and arrhythmias, such as atrial fibrillation. Drug therapy to reduce myocardial oxygen demand is directed at reducing myocardial contractility, slowing heart rate, and limiting myocardial tension by reducing systemic pressure (afterload) and preload.

Coronary blood flow is dependent upon the duration of cardiac diastole, coronary arterial resistance, aortic diastolic pressure, and the availability of coronary collateral vessels. Improvement in coronary blood flow can be accomplished by those drugs that increase the duration of diastole, that decrease coronary artery resistance by vasodilatation, by reducing intramyocardial tension, and that stimulate the development of and flow through collateral vessels.

SPECIFIC DRUG THERAPIES

The principles of drug therapy for treating angina in elderly patients are the same as those for younger patients (13). The physician treating elderly patients, however, must be aware that the pharmacokinetics of drugs may be different in this age group. Gastrointestinal disorders may potentially interfere with drug absorption, although drug bioavailability is usually unaffected by the aging process (14). The decrease in lean body mass and increase in adipose tissue associated with aging affects the volume of drug distribution. Hepatic blood flow and hepatic oxidation (phase I reactions) decrease with aging, whereas hepatic conjugation is unchanged. Not only is renal dysfunction common in elderly patients, but aging is associated with a decline in glomerular filtration rate of 30% between the fifth and ninth decades in normal patients (14). The elderly often demonstrate increased sensitivity to drugs at any given dosage and may tolerate side effects less well. The presence of comorbid conditions increases the potential for adverse drug reactions. The axiom to remember when prescribing drugs in elderly patients is to start low and titrate up slowly.

Given the pharmacological considerations of drug therapy in elderly patients, the specific antianginal drugs can be very effective in controlling symptoms and modifying the underlying pathophysiological process in elderly patients with angina. The classes of drugs commonly used include (*i*) nitrates, (*ii*) β-blockers, (*iii*) calcium channel blockers, and (*iv*) antiplatelet and/or anticoagulant agents.

Nitrates

Nitrates are safe, effective, and usually the first choice for treatment of angina. Denitration of the organic nitrate with the subsequent liberation of nitric oxide (NO) is necessary for the drug to have therapeutic effects. Nitric oxide stimulates guanylyl cyclase, which leads to the conversion of guanosine triphosphate to cyclic guanosine monophosphate, which causes relaxation of vascular smooth muscle with vasodilatation (15,16). The exact mechanism by which the organic nitrates undergo denitration and thus liberate NO remains controversial (17,18).

The active metabolite, NO, is also known as the endothelium-derived relaxing factor (EDRF) (19) which, in addition to relaxing vascular smooth muscle, reduces platelet adhesion and aggregation (20). In vessels with atherosclerosis, it has been shown that the endothelium is dysfunctional with attenuation of EDRF activity (21). Such attenuation of EDRF has been found in patients with hypercholesterolemia without overt coronary atherosclerosis (22). Due to this attenuated activity of EDRF, vascular vasoconstriction is predominant in patients with CAD. Therefore, nitrates as exogenous donors of NO would appear to be the ideal drug to use in elderly patients with angina (myocardial ischemia).

The mechanisms by which nitrates relieve and prevent myocardial ischemia include both a reduction in myocardial oxygen demand and an increase in myocardial oxygen supply due to the drug's potent vasodilator properties (Table 9.1). Dilatation of capacitance veins reduces ventricular volume and preload, thus lowering myocardial oxygen requirement and improving subendocardial blood flow. Dilatation of systemic conductive arteries decreases afterload, another determinant of oxygen consumption. Nitrates dilate epicardial

Table 9.1   Cardiovascular Effects of Nitrates and Mechanisms to Relieve Angina (Ischemia)

Decreased myocardial O_2 demand
    Venodilatation $\rightarrow \downarrow$ preload $\rightarrow \downarrow$ wall tension
    Arteriolar dilatation $\rightarrow \downarrow$ afterload $\rightarrow \downarrow$ wall tension
Increase myocardial blood flow (O_2)
    Coronary dilatation $\rightarrow \uparrow$ coronary flow $\rightarrow \uparrow$ regional myocardial perfusion (subendocardial)
    Increase collateral flow $\rightarrow \uparrow$ myocardial perfusion (subendocardial)
    Decrease coronary resistance $\rightarrow \uparrow$ coronary flow

coronary arteries with an increase in coronary flow and an improvement in subendocardial perfusion. Nitrates also dilate collateral vessels, which can improve blood flow to the areas of ischemia (23). In the doses used clinically, nitrates do not affect coronary resistance vessels (24). Thus, the risk of myocardial ischemia due to coronary steal is minimal, which has been shown to occur with drugs such as dipyridamole and short-acting calcium channel blockers that cause arteriolar dilatation (25).

Nitrate Preparations

Short-Acting Nitrates. Nitroglycerin is the drug most frequently used for relief of the acute anginal attack. It is given either as a sublingual tablet or as a sublingual spray and is absorbed rapidly with hemodynamic effects occurring within 2 minutes after drug administration. The advantage of the spray is that sublingual tablets deteriorate when exposed to light and will need to be renewed every 4–6 months to ensure complete bioavailability. The other advantage of nitroglycerin spray is that it may be easier to administer in elderly patients who have difficulty with the fine motor skills necessary to administer sublingual tablets. An inhalational form of nitroglycerin has just been approved for the management of acute anginal attacks. Orally nitrates are also available to abort acute anginal attacks that are not relieved with sublingual tablets or spray, and to prevent recurrent anginal attacks. Table 9.2 lists the different nitrate preparations and dosages (26).

Long-Acting Nitrates

Nitrates have been proven not only effective in relieving acute anginal pain but also beneficial in preventing recurrent anginal attacks. Long-acting nitrates also improve exercise time until the onset of angina and reduce exercise-induced ischemic ST-segment depression (27,28). The oral preparation is usually the nitrate of choice in the prevention of angina. Standard-formulation isosorbide dinitrate is rapidly absorbed and is typically administered three times a day with a 14-hour nitrate-free interval. Sustained-release isosorbide dinitrate has a slower rate of absorption and results in a therapeutic plasma concentration for 12 hours. The usual dosage schedule is twice daily in doses of 20–80 mg.

An isosorbide mononitrate is also available for the prevention of angina. The major advantage of the mononitrate preparation is that it is completely bioavailable because it does not undergo first-pass hepatic metabolism. To avoid drug tolerance, it is recommended that the 20- to 40-mg tablets be given twice daily with 7 hours between doses. A sustained-release formulation of isosorbide mononitrate is also available that provides therapeutic plasma drug concentrations for up to 12 hours each day and low concentrations during the latter part of the 24-hour period. The drug dose range is 30–240 mg given once daily.

Transdermal nitroglycerin is a topical nitroglycerin preparation that is effective in preventing angina, and may be particularly beneficial in elderly patients who are taking numerous pills and have difficulty in remembering drug schedules. Moreover, transdermal nitrate preparations will be more effective than oral preparations in elderly patients who

Table 9.2   Different Nitrate Preparations and Dosages

Medication	Usual Dose (mg)	Onset of Action (min)	Duration of Action
Short-acting			
Sublingual nitroglycerin	0.3–0.6	2–5	10–30 min
Aerosol nitroglycerin	0.4	2–5	10–30 min
Sublingual and chewable isosorbide dinitrate	2.5–10	3–15	1–2 hr
Intravenous	5 µg/min to 30–80 µg/min	1	Sustained during infusion
Long-acting			
Oral isosorbide dinitrate	5–40	15–30	3–6 hr
Oral isosorbide dinitrate (SR)	40	30–60	6–10 hr
Oral erythrityl tetranitrate	10	30	Variable
Oral isosorbide mononitrate	5–60	30	6–8 hr
Transdermal nitroglycerin	5–15	30–60	8–14 hr

Abbreviation: SR, sustained release.
Source: Adapted from Ref. 26.

have problems with gastrointestinal malabsorption. Transdermal nitroglycerin is available as an ointment or patch preparation. Both preparations are effective, although the patch obviates some of the inherent messiness of the ointment. As with the oral preparation, a 12- to 14-hour nitrate-free interval is necessary to avoid tolerance when using nitroglycerin ointment or patches.

Adverse Effects

Elderly patients in general tolerate nitrates without significant adverse effects, although the two major side effects, hypotension and headaches, can be extremely bothersome in certain patients. Hypotension may occur within minutes after sublingual administration of a nitrate or 1–2 hours after oral ingestion and is caused by the reduction in preload and afterload caused by the vasodilator effect of the drug. Symptoms may range from light headedness to syncope and are commonly positional, precipitated by standing. The hypotension related to nitrates more commonly occurs following the initial use of the drug, when hypovolemia is present, or with concomitant vasodilator therapy use, such as calcium channel blockers or other antihypertensive drugs. The hypotension episode may also be potentiated by alcohol. The episodes can be alleviated by reduction of the dose of nitrate, by correction of hypovolemia, and by avoiding an upright position after sublingual use of the drug. In certain elderly patients, the hypotension will be associated with bradycardia, similar to a typical vasovagal reaction. The hypotension associated with nitrate use will usually be alleviated by the patients lying down; in certain patients with a severe hypotensive reaction, elevation of the legs plus administration of fluid will be necessary.

The headache associated with nitrates can be a significant problem in certain elderly patients. It may be a mild, transient frontal headache, although in other patients the headache will be diffuse and throbbing, with persistent head and neck pain associated with nausea or vomiting. Such severe headaches are more common with the use of intravenous or transdermal nitrates. Nitrates may also aggravate vascular headaches and even initiate episodes of "cluster headaches." As in the management of hypotension related to nitrates, the best approach to alleviate or prevent headaches is to use the lowest doses of nitrates possible and titrate slowly upward if necessary. The use of an analgesic such as aspirin or acetaminophen in conjunction with the nitrate administration may prevent the associated headache. Commonly, due to vascular adaptation, within 7–10 days after initiation of nitrate use, the headache will diminish and subside. However, while waiting for adaptation to occur, elderly patients will require much reassurance to continue using the drug; and in certain elderly patients, a different antianginal drug will have to be substituted for the nitrate because the patient will not be able to tolerate the recurrent headaches.

Nitrate tolerance, defined as the loss of hemodynamic and antianginal effects during sustained therapy (29), is another consideration when treating elderly CAD patients. Tolerance has been shown to occur, regardless of the nitrate preparation, if the patient is continuously exposed to nitrates throughout a 24-hour period. The clinical impact of nitrate tolerance, however, is unknown, and the mechanism of nitrate tolerance remains unclear (29,30). Various possible hypotheses include (*i*) increased intravascular blood volume; (*ii*) depletion of sulfhydryl groups, which are needed for conversion of nitrates to NO; (*iii*) activation of vasoconstriction hormones; and (*iv*) an increased free radical production by the endothelium during nitrate therapy (31–33). To prevent tolerance, it is recommended that a 12- to 14-hour nitrate-free interval be established when using long-acting nitrate preparations. During the nitrate-free interval, the use of another antianginal drug will be necessary. In elderly patients with unstable angina who are receiving continuous intravenous nitrates, tolerance is not a consideration; if tolerance develops in this setting, the dose of the nitrate should be increased.

Studies have demonstrated that abrupt withdrawal of nitrate exposure may produce nonatherosclerotic ischemic cardiac events, including myocardial infarction (MI) (34,35). Such events are presumably due to coronary artery spasm. Therefore, caution should be exercised when high-dose nitrate therapy is discontinued in elderly patients; if possible, the nitrate dose should be slowly tapered downward before discontinuation. Phosphodiesterase inhibitors, such as sildenafil, vardenafil, and tadalafil, used in the treatment of erectile dysfunction, can be safely prescribed to men with CAD, but should not be used in men receiving long-acting nitrates (36).

β-Adrenergic Blockers

β-Adrenergic blocking agents are effective in preventing angina and are considered by many authorities to be the drug of choice to prevent ischemic events. β-Blockers also improve exercise time until the onset of angina and reduce exercise-induced ischemic ST-segment depression (37). β-Blockers prevent angina mainly by causing a reduction in myocardial oxygen demand related to slowing of the heart rate, by depressing myocardial contractility, and by reducing blood pressure (Table 9.3). These effects are particularly impressive in the setting of increased emotional and physical stress, such as during exercise and high anxiety states. In addition to the reduction of myocardial oxygen demand, β-blockers will increase myocardial oxygen supply by slowing the heart rate and extending the period of diastole.

Table 9.3 Cardiovascular Effects of β-Blockers and Mechanisms to Relieve Angina (Ischemia)

Decrease myocardial O_2 demand
Decrease contractility $\rightarrow$ $\downarrow$ blood pressure and $\downarrow$ CO
Decrease heart rate $\rightarrow$ $\downarrow$ blood pressure and $\downarrow$ CO
Increase myocardial blood flow (O_2)
Decrease heart rate $\rightarrow$ $\uparrow$ diastolic perfusion time

Abbreviation: CO, cardiac output.

β-Adrenergic blocking agents can be classified according to (*i*) β-1 selectivity, (*ii*) intrinsic sympathomimetic activity; and (*iii*) lipophilic activity (Table 9.4). Consideration of these specific properties is important when using the drug in elderly CAD patients. β-1 Selectivity is determined by the extent the agent is capable of blocking β_1-receptors and not β_2-receptors (38). Certain agents, such as metoprolol and atenolol, are relatively more β-1 selective than propranolol, which makes these drugs less prone to inducing bronchospasm or peripheral arterial vasoconstriction, as compared to the nonselective agents. At higher doses, however, β-1 selective β-blockers react like nonselective agents with full potential for bronchospasm and peripheral arterial constriction.

Some β-blockers, such as pindolol and acebutolol, in addition to blocking β-adrenergic receptors, possess partial agonist properties and, therefore, are capable of producing intrinsic sympathetic stimulation (ISA) (39). The degree to which sympathomimetic activity is clinically apparent depends upon the underlying sympathetic activity of the patient receiving the drugs. β-Blockers with ISA may prevent slowing of the heart rate, depression of atrioventricular conduction, and a decrease in myocardial contractility in the setting of a low sympathetic state, such as when the patient is resting. When the sympathetic state is high, however, the effect of β-blockers with ISA is similar to that of the usual β-blockers, with a slowing of heart rate and a decrease of blood pressure and ventricular contractility. It should be emphasized that β-blockers with ISA do not prevent sudden death in post-MI patients, which has been demonstrated with the use of the usual β-blockers; therefore, these agents are not recommended in elderly patients who have had a MI (40).

The various β-blockers differ with regard to their lipophilic properties. Some β-blockers, such as propranolol and metoprolol, are highly lipophilic, which facilitates transfer of the drug across the blood–brain barrier and, therefore, the lipophilic agents are more likely to produce central nervous system side effects, including mood changes, depression, and sleeping disturbances (41). In contrast, the hydrophilic β-blockers, such as atenolol and nadolol, are less likely to produce central nervous system side effects.

In general, β-blockers are well tolerated in elderly patients, and some studies have not shown any difference in prevalence of drug side effects between older and younger patients (42). However, significant drug side effects may occur in elderly patients and may be life-threatening. Bradycardia, secondary to the drug effects upon the sinus node and atrioventricular conduction may occur, and, due to attenuation of bronchodilatation,

Table 9.4 Pharmacology of β-Blockers and Dosage

Generic Drug (Brand)	Cardioselectivity (Relative B_1-Sensitivity)	ISA	Lipophilic Properties	Usual Maintenance Dose
Propranolol (Inderal)	0	0	High	10–40 mg, q.i.d.
Propranolol LA (Inderal LA)	0	0	high	40–240 mg, q.d.
Atenolol (Tenormin)	+	0	low	25–100 mg, q.d.
Metoprolol (Lopressor)	+	0	moderate	25–100 mg, b.i.d.
Metroprolol ER (Toprol XL)	+	0	moderate	50–200 mg, q.d.
Timolol (Blocadren)	0	0	low	10–20 mg, b.i.d.
Carvedilol	0	0	low	25mg b.i.d.
Acebutolol (Sectral)	+	+	low	200–600 mg, b.i.d.
Pindolol (Visken)	0	+	moderate	5–2 mg, t.i.d.
Labetalol (Normadyne)	0	0	low	100–600 mg, b.i.d.
Nadolol (Corgard)	0	0	low	40–80 mg, q.d.
Esmolol (Brevibloc injection)	+	0	low	0.10–0.15 μg/kg/min

Abbreviations: ER, extended release; ISA, intrinsic sympathomimetic activity; LA, long-acting.

asthmatic attacks may be precipitated by the drugs. Therefore, β-blockers are contraindicated in patients with significant bradycardia, unless a pacemaker is inserted, and in persons with a history of bronchospasm. The drugs should also be avoided, or used with caution, in persons with hypotension, hypoglycemic reactions, severe peripheral vascular disease with gangrene, mental depression, and severe heart failure secondary to severe LV systolic dysfunction. The possibility of a withdrawal rebound phenomenon with activation of acute ischemic events should be considered when discontinuing β-blockers in elderly patients. Accordingly, if possible, the dose of β-blockers should slowly be tapered downward before discontinuation while another antianginal drug should be started; in addition, the patient should be advised to avoid strenuous activities during the tapering period.

β-Blockers do have effects on serum lipids, which need to be considered when managing elderly CAD patients. Some studies have shown β-blockers to increase triglycerides and to decrease HDL cholesterol, although no significant change was noted in total cholesterol or LDL cholesterol (43). Other studies have not demonstrated a significant effect of long-term propranolol use in serum lipids in elderly persons (44). Patients with angina pectoris should be treated with β-blockers (45,46).

Calcium Channel Blockers

Calcium channel blockers are usually not considered as first-line drugs in elderly patients with acute coronary artery syndromes. Unlike β-blockers, their effects are less predictable, and they have not been shown to reduce mortality, sudden death, or reinfarction in post-MI patients (47). The studies that have shown increase in morbidity and mortality with the use of these drugs in treating hypertension or CAD are also disturbing (48,49). In turn, calcium blockers have cardiovascular effects that can be beneficial in preventing and controlling angina. In general, the calcium blockers exert their effect by inhibiting influx of calcium ions through calcium channels of cardiac and vascular smooth muscle cells. Due to this inhibition of calcium influx, myocardial contractility is decreased, dilatation of the peripheral and coronary vasculature occurs, and sinus node and atrioventricular conduction function are suppressed. Therefore, myocardial oxygen demand is reduced by the decrease in preload and afterload and the decrease in myocardial contractility. Slowing of heart rate, which occurs with the use of nondihydropyridine calcium blockers, such as verapamil and diltiazem, is also effective in decreasing myocardial oxygen demand. In addition to reducing myocardial oxygen demand, calcium blockers can improve myocardial oxygen supply by relaxing the tone of coronary arteries and by promoting the development of coronary collaterals (Table 9.5). This property of relaxing coronary vasculature tone is particularly beneficial when Prinzmetal's angina (vasospasm) is present.

Calcium channel blockers are usually divided into the dihydropyridine and nondihydropyridine groups (Table 9.6). Nifedipine was the first dihydropyridine made available for the treatment of angina, but newer generations of dihydropyridine agents are now available, including nicardipine, nisoldipine, nimodipine, felodipine, amlodipine, and isradipine.

Table 9.5 Cardiovascular Effects of Calcium Blockers and Mechanisms to Relieve Angina

---

Decreased myocardial O_2 demand
    Arteriolar vasodilatation → ↓ afterload → ↓ wall tension
    Decrease contractility
    Decrease heart rate
Increase myocardial blood flow (O_2)
    Decrease heart rate → ↑diastolic perfusion time
    Coronary vasodilatation → ↑ flow

Nifedipine is a potent coronary and peripheral artery vasodilator with negative inotropic properties. Significant afterload reduction occurs due to the vasodilation. At therapeutic doses, nifedipine has only a minor effect on the sinus and atrioventricular nodes; thus due to the decrease in afterload, sympathetic reflex increases in heart rate commonly occur when the drug is administered. The increased heart rate may ameliorate the negative inotropic effect, and clinically hemodynamic indices of contractility generally are unaffected. Due to intense vasodilation of the peripheral coronary circulation, however, the possibility of a coronary steal phenomenon has to be considered when using the drug (50). Such a phenomenon is more common when using a short-acting drug preparation and in patients with severe three-vessel CAD. Therefore, a β-blocker should be added if nifedipine is used to treat elderly patients with acute ischemic syndromes. A sustained-release preparation of nifedipine is available, which results in less sympathetic activity and is considered to be a safer agent than the shorter-acting preparations. Nevertheless, the addition of a β-blocker with nifedipine, regardless of the type of preparation, is considered the best approach when managing elderly patients with acute ischemic syndromes. The second-generation dihydropyridines, such as amlodipine and felodipine, have greater vascular selectivity and less negative inotropy and have no clinical effect on the sinus or atrioventricular nodes. Therefore, coronary artery steal does not appear to be a major concern with these drugs, and the drugs can be used in elderly patients with LV systolic dysfunction.

Verapamil and diltiazem, two nondihydropyridine agents, are both potent inhibitors of sinus node activity and atrioventricular node conduction, in addition to being peripheral vasodilators (Table 9.6). Both drugs have significant negative inotropic effects. Due to these effects, the drugs are effective antianginal agents; however, caution is necessary when using the drugs in elderly patients with bradycardia and depressed LV systolic function. These drugs are contraindicated in patients with LV systolic dysfunction with or without clinical heart failure, in patients with disorders of the sinus node, and in patients with heart block. The Multicenter Diltiazem Post-Infarction study reported an increased mortality in postinfarction patients with heart failure or abnormal LV ejection fraction who were

Table 9.6 Calcium Channel Blocker Preparations and Dosage

Generic Drug (Brand)	Potential for SA Node and AV Node Depression	Potential for Depression of Myocardial Contractility	Usual Adult Oral Dosage (mg)
Nifedipine (Procardia) (Adalat)	0	0 to +	10–30, t.i.d.
Nifedipine GITS (Procardia XL)	0	0 to +	30–90, q.d.
Nicardipine (Cardene)	0	0 to +	20–30, t.i.d.
Amlodipine (Norvasc)	0	0	2.5–10, q.d.
Felodipine (Plendil)	0	0	2.5–20, q.d.
Diltiazem (Cardizem)	+ +	+	30–90, t.i.d.
Diltiazem CD (Cardizem CD)	+ +	+	120–300, q.d.
Verapamil (Isoptin) (Calan) (Verelan)	+ +	+ +	40–120, t.i.d.
Verapamil SR (Isoptin SR) (Calan SR)	+ +	+ +	120–240, q.d.

Abbreviations: CD; GITS, gastrointestinal therapeutic system; SR, sustained release.
Source: Adapted from Ref. 26.

randomized to diltiazem therapy (51). Therefore, if a calcium channel blocker is necessary to control angina in elderly postinfarction patients with depressed LV systolic function, second-generation dihydropyridines, such as amlodipine and felodipine, should be used instead of diltiazem or verapamil.

Extreme caution is required when using diltiazem or verapamil in combination with a β-blocker, particularly in elderly patients who demonstrate sinus node or atrioventricular conduction dysfunction, or in elderly patients who have depressed LV systolic function. Some authorities recommend ECG monitoring when initiating these drugs, particularly verapamil, in combination with β-blockers.

It should be emphasized that the American College of Cardiology/American Heart Association guidelines state that there are no Class I indications for using calcium channel blockers during or after MI (52). However, if angina pectoris persists despite the use of β-blockers and nitrates, long-acting calcium channel blockers such as dilatiazem or verapamil should be used as antianginal agents in elderly patients with CAD and normal LV systolic function and amlodipine or felodipine in patients with CAD and abnormal LV systolic function.

Aspirin

The knowledge of the importance of thrombus formation in acute coronary syndromes and the results of studies demonstrate a decreased incidence of MI in patients taking daily aspirin compared with patients receiving placebo (53). The updated ACC/AHA guidelines for the management of patients with stable angina pectoris (45) and the American College of Physicians (ACP) clinical practice guidelines (46) recommend treating all patients with CAD with aspirin in a dose of 75 to 325 mg daily unless there are contraindications to the use of this drug. The use of enteric low-dose aspirin may be associated with aspirin resistance (a lack of an antiplatelet effect) and a 160 mg aspirin dose may need to be prescribed.

In an observational prospective study of 1410 patients, mean age 81 years, with prior MI and hypercholesterolemia, 59% of patients were treated with aspirin (51), and at 36-month follow-up, the use of aspirin was associated with a 52% reduction in new coronary events (54).

Clopidogrel

Not all patients can tolerate aspirin, and later an aspirin-resistance phenomenon has been described in patients where there is little to no antiplatelet effect from the drug. Clopidogrel is a useful alternative to aspirin when the drug is not tolerated, although it has its own associated toxicities (55). This may, however, be dose related in most situations.

Clopidogrel in a dose of 75 mg daily is recommended in patients who cannot tolerate aspirin (45,46,53,56). Dipyridamole should not be used in patients with angina pectoris since it can cause a coronary steal syndrome and increase exercise-induced myocardial ischemia (57).

Other Adjunctive Treatments
Angiotensin-Converting-Enzyme Inhibitors and Angiotensin Receptor Blockers
Based on the results of various clinical trials, there is now strong evidence that angiotensin-converting-enzyme (ACE) inhibitors can reduce the frequency of new cardiovascular events in both normotensive and hypertensive patients with known vascular disease and in patients with diabetes mellitus. If tolerated, ACE inhibitors should be part of a medical regimen to treat chronic ischemic heart disease (58). Angiotensin I receptor blockers are now being studied in patients with known ischemic heart disease who have no history of a previous MI or LV dysfunction.

Statins

Numerous studies have demonstrated that statins reduce cardiovascular morbidity and mortality in elderly patients with CAD including those with stable angina pectoris (59–66). The low-density lipoprotein cholesterol should be reduced to less than 70 mg/dl in patients with stable angina pectoris (64,65). The updated ACC/AHA guidelines for management of patients with chronic stable angina pectoris (45) and the ACP clinical practice guidelines (46) both recommend treating patients with chronic stable angina pectoris with lipid-lowering drug therapy.

STABLE CORONARY ARTERY DISEASE

In the Clinical Outcomes Utilizing Revascularization and Aggressive druG Evaluation (COURAGE) trial, 904 of the 2085 patients with stable CAD randomized to optimal medical therapy or optimal medical therapy plus PCI were aged 65 years and older (mean age 72 years) (67). The addition of PCI to optimal medical therapy in these older patients did not improve or worsen clinical outcomes during a median follow-up of 4.6 years (67).

AN APPROACH TO MANAGEMENT: SPECIFIC PRACTICE CONSIDERATIONS
Unstable Angina

Unstable angina is a transitory syndrome that results from disruption of a coronary atherosclerotic plaque with the subsequent cascade of pathological processes, including thrombosis formation that critically decreases coronary blood flow resulting in new onset or exacerbation of angina (ischemia) (68). Transient episodes of vessel occlusion or near occlusion by thrombus at the site of plaque injury may occur and lead to angina at rest. The thrombus may be labile and result in temporary obstruction to flow. Release of vasoconstrictive substances by platelets and vasoconstriction secondary to endothelial vasodilator dysfunction can contribute to further reduction in blood flow (69), and in some patients myocardial necrosis (non-Q-wave infarction) is documented. Table 9.7 lists the various clinical presentations that are classified as unstable angina.

In contrast to elderly patients with stable angina who do not require hospitalization, elderly patients with unstable angina are usually hospitalized and, depending upon their risk stratification, may require monitoring in an intensive care unit. Severe classification schemes of risk stratification have been developed. Table 9.8 lists a classification that subdivides patients into high-, intermediate- and low-risk groups (70). As noted by this classification, clinical characteristics are readily identifiable on the initial patient evaluation that stratifies the patient into low-, intermediate-, or high-risk subgroups for hospital complications. For example, acute resting ischemic ECG abnormalities markedly worsen the prognosis. Other characteristics that identify the high-risk patient include prolonged ongoing rest pain longer than 20 minutes and signs of LV dysfunction (S_3, rales, new murmur, or mitral regurgitation). Within each subgroup of unstable angina, it is important to

Table 9.7 Unstable Angina Presentations

Rest angina within 1 wk of presentation
New-onset angina of Canadian Cardiovascular Society Classification
    (CCSC) class III or IV within 2 mo of presentation
Angina increasing in CCSC class to at least CCSC III or IV
Variant angina
Non-Q-wave myocardial infarction
Postmyocardial infarction angina (>24 hr)

Table 9.8 Risk Stratification Scheme of Unstable Angina Based on Presenting Clinical Characteristics

Risk Class[a]	Clinical Characteristics
IA	Acceleration of previous exertional angina without ECG changes
IB	Acceleration of previous exertional angina with ECG changes
II	New onset of exertional angina
III	New onset of rest angina
IV	Coronary insufficiency syndrome; protracted chest pain >20 min with persistent ECG changes

[a]IA = lowest risk for in-hospital complications; IV = highest risk for in-hospital complications.
Source: Adapted from Ref. 70.

recognize certain elderly patients who have specific characteristics that will influence therapy. Recurrent angina after percutaneous transluminal coronary angioplasty (PTCA) is a common clinical event related to partial artery restenosis and occurs in as many as 40% of patients within the first 3–6 months post-PCI, regardless of the patient's age. The prognosis is favorable, and the elderly patient can usually be stabilized medically prior to a scheduled repeat angiogram and a possible repeat PCI. Angina after intracoronary stent placement occurs less frequently than after an isolated angioplasty and is often the result of subacute closure due to thrombus formation. These patients are at higher risk for MI and are usually managed as higher risk patients (71). Patient with angina following CABG are another subgroup of elderly patients who require specific considerations. Since the risk of reoperation is higher than that of the initial surgery, surgeons are often reluctant to reoperate in elderly patients, especially on those elderly patients who have undergone internal mammary grafting. Medical therapy is usually the first approach to this subgroup of elderly patients with unstable angina. Other clinical subgroups of elderly patients with unstable angina who require special considerations are the patient with a non-Q-wave infarct, variant angina, and cocaine intoxication.

Table 9.9 lists the ACC/AHA stratification of patients with unstable angina into high-risk, intermediate-risk, and low-risk groups for short-term risk of death or nonfatal MI (72). Following risk stratification of the elderly patient with unstable angina, therapy should be initiated. The initial goals of therapy should be to alleviate symptoms by decreasing myocardial oxygen demand and increasing myocardial blood flow and to stabilize the atherosclerotic plaque. Furthermore, a plan to promote regression of the atherosclerotic lesion should be initiated during the patient's hospitalization.

Therapy, including drug therapy, should be started in the emergency department; it should not be delayed until hospital admission. Reversible factors causing angina should be identified and corrected, including anemia, which may require packed red cell transfusion. ECG monitoring is important since arrhythmias can occur and ST-T changes are a marker for an increased risk of complications. The aggressiveness of the drug dosage will depend upon the severity of symptoms and will need modification through the elderly patient's hospitalization. Oxygen should be given to patients with cyanosis, respiratory distress, heart failure, or high-risk factors. Oxygen therapy should be guided by arterial saturation; its use when the baseline saturation is more than 94% is questionable. Morphine sulfate should be administered intravenously when symptoms are not immediately relieved with nitroglycerin or when acute pulmonary congestion and/or severe agitation is present.

Aspirin should be given to all patients with unstable angina unless contraindicated and continued indefinitely. Clopidogrel should be administered to patients who are unable

Table 9.9   Risk Stratification of Patients with Unstable Angina for Short-Term Risk of Death or Nonfatal Myocardial Infarction

High Risk (at least one of the following factors)	Intermediate Risk (no high-risk feature but one of the following features)	Low Risk (no high or intermediate risk feature)
Accelerating tempo of ischemic symptoms in prior 48 hr	Prior MI or CABG; peripheral or cerebrovascular disease; prior aspirin use	—
Prolonged ongoing (>20 min) rest pain	Prolonged (>20 min) rest angina, now resolved, with moderate or high likelihood of CAD; rest angina (<20 min or relieved with rest or sublingual NTG)	New-onset CCS Class III or IV angina in past 2 wk with moderate or high likelihood of CAD
Pulmonary edema; new or worsening MR murmur; S_3 or new/worsening rales; hypotension, tachycardia, bradycardia; age >75 yr	Age >70 yr	—
Angina at rest with transient ST-segment changes >0.05 mV; bundle branch block, new or presumed new; sustained ventricular tachycardia	T-wave inversions >0.2 mV; pathological Q-waves	Normal or unchanged ECG during episode of chest discomfort
Markedly elevated troponin T or I (>0.1 ng/mL)	Slightly elevated troponin T or I (>0.01 but <0.1 ng/mL)	Normal

Abbreviations: CAD, coronary artery disease; CABG, coronary artery bypass graft surgery; CCS, Canadian Cardiovascular Society; MI, myocardial infarction; MR, mitral regurgitation; NTG, nitroglycerin.
Source: Adapted from Ref. 72.

to tolerate aspirin because of hypersensitivity or major gastrointestinal intolerance. Data from the Clopidogrel in Unstable Angina to Prevent Recurrent Events (CURE) trial favors the use of aspirin plus the use of clopidogrel for 9 months in patients with unstable angina (73). The ACC/AHA guidelines for unstable angina support the use of aspirin plus clopidogrel in high-risk and intermediate-risk patients with unstable angina, with clopidogrel withheld for 5–7 days if CABG is planned (74).

Prasugrel is a thienopyridine that requires conversion to an active metabolite before binding to the platelet P2Y12 receptor. Compared to clopidogrel, it is metabolized more efficiently, has greater bioavailability, and produces a greater antiplatelet effect. In the Trial to Assess Improvement in Therapeutic Outcomes by Optimizing Platelet Inhibition with Prasugrel–Thrombolysis in Myocardial Infarction (TRITON–TIMI) 38 (75), prasugrel significantly lowered the rates of ischemic events in the prasugrel group, with a 2.3% absolute reduction and a 24% relative reduction of MI. There was also a 52% relative reduction for stent thrombosis. These benefits were seen irrespective of the type of stent used. However, patients with a prior history of stroke or transient ischemic attack (TIA) had poor clinical outcomes with a net harm from prasugrel (hazard ratio 1.54), and there was a 32% increase in relative TIMI major hemorrhage with prasugrel. Therefore prasugrel is contraindicated in patients with history of prior stroke or TIA, while for patients weighing <60 kg and those >75 years of age, a reduced dose of the drug is suggested (75). The 2011 ACCF/AHA guidelines support the use of prasugrel or clopidogrel as an addition to aspirin in patients with acute coronary syndromes (74).

Ticagrelor is a nonthienopyridine with a plasma half-life of 12 hours. It is a reversible and direct-acting oral antagonist of the ADP receptor P2Y12. In the Study of Platelet Inhibition and Patient Outcomes (PLATO) trial (76), when compared with clopidogrel, ticagrelor significantly lowered at 1 year the rate of death from vascular causes, MI, or stroke from 11.7% to 9.8% ($p < 0.001$) in patients with acute coronary syndromes. However, the drug seemed to work better at preventing clinical events when accompanied by low-dose as opposed to high-dose aspirin based on the findings that the outcomes were superior with the new drug across the entire international trial but not in North America, where the aspirin doses were generally higher. It was approved by the US Food and Drug Administration (FDA) provided a low dose of aspirin ≤100 mg was coadministered.

Parenteral anticoagulation with intravenous unfractionated heparin or preferably with subcutaneous low-molecular-weight heparin (77–80) should be added to antiplatelet therapy in patients with high-risk or intermediate-risk unstable angina. The revised ACC/AHA guidelines for unstable angina also recommend adding a platelet glycoprotein IIb/IIIa inhibitor in addition to aspirin, clopidogrel or prasugrel, and low-molecular-weight heparin in patients with continuing ischemia or with other high-risk features, and to patients in whom PCI is planned. Eptifibatide and tirofiban are approved for this use (74). Abciximab can also be used for 12–24 hours in patients with unstable angina in whom PCI is planned within the next 24 hours (74).

As with the use of aspirin, nitrates should be instituted quickly in the emergency department. Patients whose symptoms are not fully relieved with three sublingual nitroglycerin tablets should receive continuous intravenous nitroglycerin. The initial dose is of 5–10 mg/min, and the dose should be titrated every 3–5 minutes to relieve symptoms or associated hypertension. If angina is relieved, then an oral or transdermal preparation can be started after 24 hours of intravenous therapy. β-Blockers (in addition to aspirin, heparin, and nitrates) should also be started in the emergency room unless there are contraindications. Intravenous loading (e.g., metoprolol 5 mg for 5 minutes, repeated every 15 minutes for a total of 15 mg) or propranolol followed by oral therapy is recommended. A continuous β-blocker intravenous infusion may be used (esmolol, starting maintenance dose of 0.1 g/kg/min intravenously with titration upward in increments of 0.5 g/kg/min every 10–15 minutes as tolerated by blood pressure until the desired response has been obtained, limiting symptoms develop, or a dose of 0.20 mg/min is reached). An oral ACE inhibitor and a statins drug should also be administered unless there are contraindications.

Interventional Therapy

The majority of elderly patients with stable and unstable angina can be stabilized with medical management. Patients who continue to have unstable angina 30 minutes after initiation of therapy or who have recurrent unstable angina during the hospitalization are at increased risk for MI or cardiac death. In addition, patients who demonstrate major ischemic complications, such as pulmonary edema, ventricular arrhythmias, or cardiogenic shock associated with unstable angina also have a poor prognosis. In these patients, emergency cardiac catheterization should be performed with the consideration of interventional therapy (CABG or PCI). Insertion of an intra-aortic balloon pump may be necessary in some of these elderly patients.

For the majority of elderly patients whose angina is stabilized, two alternate strategies for definitive treatment of angina need to be considered: "early invasive" and "early conservative" (81). The "early invasive strategy" approach is to perform cardiac catheterization in all patients after 48 hours of presentation unless interventional therapy is contraindicated due to extensive comorbidities. In contrast, the "early conservative" strategy is to perform cardiac catherization only in patients who have one or more of the following high-risk indicators: prior revascularization, associated congestive heart failure or depressed LV ejection fraction (<50%) by noninvasive study, malignant ventricular arrhythmia, persistent or recurrent pain/ischemia, and/or a functional study (stress test) indicating high risk. On the basis of data from the TACTICS—Thrombolysis in Myocardial Infarction 18 study, an early invasive strategy is superior to a conservative strategy in high-risk unstable angina patients (82). The revised ACC/AHA guidelines recommend an early invasive strategy for all high-risk patients with unstable angina.

A stress test can be performed 48–72 hours after the patient has stabilized. The choice of the type of stress testing (exercise, exercise with imaging, or pharmacological) will depend upon the resting ECG findings and the patient's ability to exercise.

Myocardial revascularization is indicated in patients who at catheterization are found to have significant left main CAD (≥50%) or significant (≥70%) three-vessel disease with depressed LV function (LV ejection fraction <50%); patients with two-vessel disease with proximal severe subtotal stenosis (≥95%) of the left anterior descending coronary artery and depressed LV ejection fraction; and patients with significant CAD if they fail to stabilize with medical treatment have recurrent angina/ischemia at rest or with low-level activities, and/or if ischemia is accompanied by congestive heart failure symptoms, an S3 gallop, new or worsening mitral regurgitation, or definite ECG changes (81).

The ACC/AHA guidelines recommend CABG for patients with unstable angina with significant left main CAD, three-vessel CAD, and for two-vessel CAD with significant proximal left anterior descending CAD and either abnormal LV function (ejection fraction <50%) or demonstrable ischemia on noninvasive testing (74). PCI or CABG is recommended for patients with one-vessel or two-vessel CAD without significant proximal left anterior descending CAD, but with a large area of viable myocardium and high-risk criteria on noninvasive testing. PTCA is recommended for patients with multivessel CAD with a suitable coronary anatomy with normal LV function and without diabetes mellitus (74).

For some patients without these high-risk features, revascularization may still be an option, depending on recurrent symptoms, test results, and patient preferences. The healthcare team should educate the patient and his or her family or advocate about the expected risks and benefits of revascularization and determine individual patient preferences and fears that may affect the selection of therapy. CABG with or without cardiopulmonary bypass causes a high incidence of cognitive decline (83).

Interventional therapy with PTCA, atherectomy, and/or some combination of PCI and coronary artery stenting has increased in usage in patients with CAD, diminishing the frequency of CABG. Studies comparing PCI and CABG have been performed, and generally the results of PCI and CABG are similar in reference to mortality. However, an increased incidence of recurrent angina and need for revascularization procedure occurs with PCI (84–86). On the other hand, the incidence of cognitive decline is high in older persons undergoing CABG with no difference seen when comparing the incidence of cognitive dysfunction in on-pump and off-pump bypass procedures (83).

Stable Angina

Elderly patients with stable angina who are at "low risk" (preserved LV function and no left main CAD) can be treated as effectively with medical therapy as with interventional therapy. In patients with stable angina, the atherosclerotic lesions are predominantly advanced fibrolipid plaques or fibrotic lesions (87). Usually no plaque ulceration or thrombosis is present, and the main cause of angina is the reduction of luminal diameter of the coronary vessel due to chronic atherosclerosis. Therefore, therapy is directed at decreasing myocardial oxygen demand and increasing coronary blood flow. In addition, prevention of plaque instability and initiation of therapy to cause regression of the atherosclerotic lesion are necessary.

Studies have not demonstrated any significant benefit of a specific class of antianginal drugs compared to other classes in treatment of stable angina. Therefore, the choice of a single antianginal drug will depend upon the clinical situation, contraindications, and the physician's preference. Surely a β-blocker should be the first choice in elderly patients who have a history of MI or demonstrate ECG evidence of silent infarction or silent myocardial ischemia (88).

Combination drug therapy, in which a β-blocker and a vasodilator are used, is highly advantageous in treating elderly patients with angina. Studies have shown that combination therapy with a nitrate and β-blocker decreases the number of anginal attacks and increases the duration of time of treadmill stress testing as compared to either nitrates or β-blockers alone (89). The combination of a β-blocker and a calcium channel blocker has also been shown to be more effective in reducing angina and extending exercise time than monotherapy (89). Such a combination can be very beneficial when attempting to control both hypertension and angina in elderly patients. In turn, caution is necessary when using β-blockers in combination with diltiazem or verapamil due to the potential risk of provoking serious bradycardia or precipitating heart failure. This is particularly a concern when verapamil and a β-blocker are used in combination, and when underlying sinus or atrioventricular nodal disease or LV systolic dysfunction is present. In elderly patients whose angina is refractory to double drug therapy, triple drug therapy may be necessary. Such therapy would include a β-blocker, a long-acting nitrate, and a calcium channel blocker. Such therapy may be beneficial in preventing anginal attacks. However, elderly patients taking these multiple dugs will need to be monitored closely for side effects, and the drugs should be started at low doses. Patients aged 75 years or older with angina despite standard drug therapy benefit more from coronary revascularization (90,91).

A preventive program in elderly patients with angina is mandatory, including abstinence from smoking, treatment of hypertension, use of aspirin and ACE inhibitors, an exercise program, and control of lipids and weight (92). Treatment of associated heart failure and anemia can also prevent or relieve symptoms of angina. The previous studies that have demonstrated the efficacy of statin therapy in lowering serum lipids and in preventing future coronary events in elderly patients with CAD (59–66) compel physicians to screen elderly anginal patients for elevated serum lipids and to be aggressive in their treatment of lipid abnormalities. In the Heart Protection Study, 20,536 adults up to age 80 years with CAD, other occlusive arterial disease, or diabetes mellitus were randomized to simvastatin 40 mg daily or double-blind placebo and followed for a mean of 5 years (63). All-cause mortality, coronary events, stroke, and coronary and noncoronary revascularization were significantly reduced by simvastatin, regardless of age and initial serum lipids (63).

In addition, elderly patients will require counseling in reference to lifestyle, with avoidance of activities that "trigger" ischemic attacks (93). The physician will need to be aware of the potential for the development of mental depression in elderly CAD patients. The symptoms of depression may be subtle in elderly patients and will progress unless the disease is treated. Depression has also been shown to be a risk factor for future coronary events in patients with CAD (94).

The role of exercise should be emphasized when managing elderly patients with angina. Exercise programs that progressively increase physical endurance and reduce the heart rate and cardiac work at any given level of activity lead to improvement in cardiac performance and prolong exercise time before onset of angina (95). In addition, some studies have shown stress-induced myocardial ischemia (as assessed by thallium 201 scintigraphy) to be significantly decreased after a 1-year program of supervised exercise and low cholesterol diet in patients with stable angina (96). Caution is necessary, however, when initiating an exercise program in elderly CAD patients. Elderly patients should be screened for high-risk characteristics, including results of a stress test, before starting an exercise program since exercise can provoke serious arrhythmias in high-risk patients, especially in poorly conditioned patients. Other exercise programs can be advised according to the patient's needs and preference, such as swimming or stationary cycling.

New Approaches for the Management of Angina

Over the years, the management of patients with angina has changed, and new approaches have developed. Some of these changes are due to increased knowledge of the underlying pathophysiology of myocardial ischemia with the development of new drugs. Other changes are related to the development of innovative mechanical devices and techniques that theoretically should relieve angina.

Ranolazine

Ranolazine is a piperazine derivative and a partial fatty acid oxidation inhibitor which reduced calcium overload in the ischemic myocyte by inhibition of the late sodium current (97,98). This action decreases the magnitude of ischemia-induced sodium and calcium overload, improving myocardial function as well as myocardial perfusion. Four randomized, double-blind trials have demonstrated that ranolazine reduces frequency of angina episodes and nitroglycerin consumption and improves exercise duration and time to anginal attacks without clinically significant effects on heart rate or blood pressure (99–102). Ranolazine's anti-ischemic mechanism is most likely due to an improvement in regional coronary blood flow in areas of myocardial ischemia (103).

Ranolazine was approved by the US FDA for treatment of patients with chronic stable angina pectoris in January 2006. Ranolazine was approved for use as combination therapy when angina is not adequately controlled with other antianginal drugs. The recommended dose of sustained release ranolazine is 750 mg or 1000 mg twice daily.

Other Pharmacologic Approaches

Other drugs under investigation and being considered for FDA approval include nicorandil and ivabradine. Nicorandil is a coronary vasodilator with a unique dual mechanism of action that involves a nitrate-like effect and a potassium ion channel opening action (97,104). The Impact of Nicorandil in Angina (IONA) study showed at 1.6-year follow-up in patients with stable angina pectoris that 2565 patients randomized to nicorandil 20 mg twice daily had a 17% significant reduction in CAD death, nonfatal MI, or unplanned hospital admission for cardiac chest pain compared with 2561 patients randomized to placebo (105).

Ivabradine is a heart rate lowering drug that acts specifically on the sinoatrial node (106). Ivabradine caused dose-dependent improvements in exercise tolerance and time to development of ischemia during exercise (107). In a subgroup of patients with heart rate of 70 beats per min or higher, ivabradine did not affect the primary endpoint of cardiovascular death or hospital admission for fatal and nonfatal MI (108). However, ivabradine did reduce the secondary endpoint of hospital admission for fatal and nonfatal MI by 36% ($p = 0.001$) and coronary revascularization by 30% ($p = 0.016$) (108).

Cell Therapy

Innovative approaches for the management of drug resistant angina pectoris include the use of vascular growth factors to induce myocardial angiogenesis (108,109). Granulocyte macrophage colony stimulating factor has been used to mobilize bone marrow stem cells to induce angiogenesis. In addition, stem cells are being used by direct injection to affect new vascular growth (109).

Other Mechanical Approaches

Mechanical techniques for the treatment of angina include transmyocardial laser revascularization (TMLR), enhanced external counter pulsation (EECP), and spinal cord stimulation (110). These approaches have been used in patients with severe angina who are not candidates for PTCA or CABG, usually due to diffuse CAD or extreme comorbidities. Such approaches would appear to be suitable for many elderly CAD patients who may have inoperable CAD and multiple comorbidities plus angina that is difficult to control with medical therapy.

TMLR employs a high-energy laser beam to create channels in the myocardium from the epicardial to the endocardial surface (111). The channels allow oxygenated LV blood to perfuse ischemic myocardial zones (112). The human myocardium contains an extensive network of sinusoids, and TMLR theoretically delivers oxygenated blood to these sinusoids with improved myocardial oxygen delivery to the ischemic region. Data on the efficacy of TMLR in improving anginal symptoms and exercise capacity are controversial (113–115).

EECP is a noninvasive outpatient treatment designed to increase coronary flow in the treatment of angina (116,117). This treatment involves wrapping the calves, thighs, and buttocks with pneumatic cuffs. Synchronized pulsatory pressure is applied sequentially from calves to thighs during diastole, returning arterial blood to the heart to increase diastolic pressure in the coronary vessels. Pressure is relieved during systole, reducing afterload and cardiac work, thus decreasing myocardial oxygen demand. The typical course of treatment is 35 1-hour sessions over a period of 7 weeks. EECP has been shown to improve ischemia in patients who have thallium reperfusion evidence of ischemia. In one study of patients who received EECP, 75% of subjects had resolution of ischemia, demonstrated by improved thallium scintigraphy with normal thallium stress tests, except for areas scarred by previous MIs (118). In addition, the subjects showed exercise improvement. A controlled study of 139 patients showed a reduction in anginal episodes, an increase in the time to 1-mm ischemic ST-segment depression, and a trend toward reduced nitroglycerin use in the EECP group but a similar increase in exercise duration in both groups (119). In a prospective study of 47 patients with chronic refractory angina pectoris, EECP improved anginal symptoms, dyspnea on exertion, quality of life, and 6-minute walking distance at 1 year ($p < 0.001$) (120).

Spinal cord stimulation (SCS) has been demonstrated to cause clinical improvement in patients with refractory angina pectoris in the number of anginal episodes, in nitroglycerin consumption, in maximal exercise time, in exercise time until angina, in the number of episodes of myocardial ischemia, in the duration of episodes of myocardial ischemia, and in ischemic ST-segment depression at a comparable workload (121,122). Double-blind, randomized, placebo-controlled studies have not been performed with SCS. The clinical improvement from SCS occurred despite no evidence of improvement in regional myocardial blood flow during exercise or in myocardial oxygen consumption as assessed by the heart rate times systolic pressure product at maximal exercise. The mechanisms of clinical improvement by SCS are unclear. SCS must be considered experimental at this time and is a therapeutic option for the treatment of refractory angina pectoris in patients unable to have coronary revascularization or at very high risk for coronary revascularization.

A coronary sinus reducer stent has also been found to clinically improve patients with refractory angina pectoris (123). However, randomized, placebo-controlled data are necessary to evaluate this form of therapy in treating patients with refractory angina pectoris who are not candidates for coronary revascularization.

Based on the results of these preliminary studies, these new techniques may have a role in the management of certain elderly patients with angina. Further studies are necessary, however, before these new approaches can be recommended as therapy for the management of elderly patients with severe angina refractory to conventional medical therapy.

REFERENCES

1. Toffler G, Muller FE, Stone PH; MILIS Study Group. Factors leading to shorter survival after acute myocardial infarction in patients ages 65 to 75 years compared with younger patients. Am J Cardiol 1988; 62: 860–7.
2. Tresch D, Aronow W. Clinical manifestations and diagnosis of coronary artery disease. Clin Geriatr Med 1996; 12: 89–100.
3. Wei J. Heart disease in the elderly. Cardiol Med 1984; 9: 971–82.
4. ten berg J, Bal E, Gin T, et al. Initial and long-term results of percutaneous transluminal coronary angioplasty in patients 75 years of age and older. Cathet Cardiovasc Diagn 1992; 26: 165–70.
5. Kelsey SF, Miller DP, Holubkov R, et al. Results of percutaneous transluminal coronary angioplasty in patients 65 years of age (from the 1985 to 1986 National Heart, Lung, and Blood Institute's Coronary Angioplasty Registry). Am J Cardiol 1990; 66: 1033–8.
6. Thompson RC, Holmes DR Jr, Gersh BJ, Bailey KR. Percutaneous transluminal coronary angioplasty in the elderly: early and long-term results. Circulation 1992; 88: 1579–87.
7. Siegel R, Clemens T, Wingo M, Tresch DD. Acute heart failure: another manifestation of unstable angina [abstr]. J Am Coll Cardiol 1991; 17: 149.
8. Clark LT, Garfein OB, Dwyer EM. Acute pulmonary edema due to ischemic heart disease without accompanying myocardial infarction. Am J Med 1983; 75: 332–6.
9. Kunis R, Greenberg H, Yeoh CB, et al. Coronary revascularization of recurrent pulmonary edema in elderly patients with ischemic heart disease and preserved ventricular function. N Engl J Med 1985; 313: 1207–10.
10. Tresch D, Saeian K, Hoffman R. Elderly patients with late onset of coronary artery disease: clinical and angiographic findings. Am J Geriatr Cardiol 1992; 1: 14–25.
11. Aronow WS, Epstein S. Usefulness of silent myocardial ischemia detected by ambulatory electrocardiographic monitoring in predicting new coronary events in elderly patients. Am J Cardiol 1988; 62: 1295–6.
12. Hedblad B, Juul-Moller S, Svensson K, et al. Increased mortality in men with ST segment depression during 14 h ambulatory long-term ECG recording Results from prospective population study 'Men born in 1914', from Malmo, Sweden. Eur Heart J 1989; 10: 149–58.
13. Aronow WS, Frishman WH. Angina in the elderly. In: Aronow WS, Fleg JF, Rich MW, eds. Cardiovascular Disease in the Elderly, 4th edn. New York: Informa, 2008: 269–92.
14. Everitt D, Avorn J. Drug prescribing for the elderly. Arch Intern Med 1986; 146: 2393–6.
15. Katsuki S, Murad F. Regulation of adenosine cycli 3',5'-monophosphate and guanosine cyclic 3'5'-monophosphate levels and contractility in bovine tracheal smooth muscle. Mol Pharmacol 1977; 13: 330–41.
16. Axelsson KL, Wikberg JES, Andersson RGG. Relationship between nitroglycerin, cyclic GMP and relaxation of vascular smooth muscle. Life Sci 1979; 24: 1779–86.
17. Fung HL, Chung SJ, Bauer JA, et al. Biochemical mechanism of organic nitrate action. Am J Cardiol 1992; 70: 4B–10B.
18. Abrams J, Frishman WH. The organic nitrates and nitroprusside. In: Frishman WH, Sica DA, eds. Cardiovascular Pharmacotherapeutics, 3rd edn. Minneapolis: Cardiotext, 2011: 205–15.
19. Moncada S, Higgs A. The L-arginine-nitric oxide pathway. N Engl J Med 1993; 329: 2002–12.
20. Diodati J, Cannon RO. Effect of nitroglycerin on platelet activation in patients with stable coronary disease. Circulation 1991; 84: 731.
21. Hansson GK. Immune and inflammatory mechanisms of monocyte recruitment and accumulation. Br Heart J 1993; 69: 9S–29S.
22. Flavahan NA. Atherosclerosis or lipoprotein induced endothelial dysfunction. Potential mechanism underlying reduction in EDRF/nitric oxide activity. Circulation 1985; 85: 1927–38.
23. Goldstein RE, Stinison EB, Scherer JL, et al. Intraoperative coronary collateral function in patients with coronary occlusive disease: nitroglycerin responsiveness and angiographic correlations. Circulation 1974; 49: 298–308.
24. Harrison DG, Bates JN. The nitrovasodilators: new ideas about old drugs. Circulation 1993; 87: 1461–7.
25. Nifedipine/Metoprolol Trial (HINT) Research Group. Early treatment of unstable angina in the coronary care unit: a randomized, double blind, placebo controlled comparison of recurrent ischaemia in patients treated with nifedipine or metoprolol or both: report of the Holland Interuniversity Nifedipine/Metoprolol Trial (HINT). Br Heart J 1986; 56: 400–13.
26. Olson HG, Aronow WS. Medical management of stable angina and unstable angina in the elderly with coronary artery disease. In: Aronow WS, Tresch DD, eds. Clinics in Geriatric Medicine: Coronary Artery Disease in the Elderly. Philadelphia: WB Saunders, 1996: 121–40.

27. Danahy DT, Burwell DT, Aronow WS, Prakash R. Sustained hemodynamic and antianginal effect of high-dose oral isosorbide dinitrate. Circulation 1977; 55: 381–7.
28. Danahy DT, Aronow WS. Hemodynamics and antianginal effects of high dose oral isosorbide dinitrate after chronic use. Circulation 1977; 56: 205–12.
29. Parker JD, Parker JO. Nitrate therapy for stable angina pectoris. N Engl J Med 1998; 337: 520–31.
30. Elkayam U. Tolerance to organic nitrates: evidence, mechanisms, clinical relevance and strategies for prevention. Ann Intern Med 1991; 114: 667–77.
31. Needleman P, Johnson EM. Mechanism of tolerance development of organic nitrates. J Pharmacol Exp Ther 1973; 84: 709–15.
32. Munzel T, Giaid A, Kurz S, et al. Evidence for enhanced vascular superoxide anion production in nitrate tolerance: a novel mechanism underlying tolerance and cross-tolerance. J Clin Invest 1995; 95: 187–94.
33. Munzel T, Giaid A, Kurz S, et al. Evidence for a role of endothelin 1 and protein kinase C in nitroglycerin tolerance. Proc Natl Acad Sci USA 1995; 92: 5244–8.
34. Lange RL, Reid MS, Tresch DD, et al. Nonatheromatous ischemic heart disease following withdrawal from chronic industrial nitroglycerin exposure. Circulation 1972; 466: 666–78.
35. Klock JC. Nonocclusive coronary disease after chronic exposure to nitrate. Evidence for physiologic nitrate dependence. Am Heart J 1975; 89: 510–13.
36. Ravipati G, McClung JA, Aronow WS, et al. Type 5 phosphodiesterase inhibitors and cardiovascular disease. Cardiol Rev 2007; 15: 76–86.
37. Aronow WS, Turbow M, Van Camp S, et al. The effect of timolol vs. placebo an angina pectoris. Circulation 1980; 61: 66–9.
38. Frishman WH. Alpha- and beta-adrenergic blocking drugs. In: Frishman WH, Sica DA, eds. Cardiovascular Pharmacotherapeutics, 3rd edn. Minneapolis: Cardiotext, 2011: 57–85.
39. Cocco G, Burkart F, Chu D, Follath F. Intrinsic sympathomimetic activity of beta-adreno-receptor blocking agents. Eur J Clin Pharmacol 1978; 13: 1–4.
40. Yusuf S, Peto R, Lewis J, et al. Beta blockade during and after myocardial infarction: an overview of the randomized trials. Prog Cardiovasc Dis 1985; 27: 335–71.
41. Westerlund A. Central nervous system side effects with hydrophilic and lipophilic beta blockers. Eur J Clin Pharmacol 1985; 28(Suppl): 73–6.
42. Hjalmarson A, Herlitz J, Waagstein F. Treatment of myocardial infarction with beta blockers in elderly patients. In: Lang E, Sorgel F, Blaha L, eds. Beta-Blockers in the Elderly. New York: Springer-Verlag, 1982: 47–55.
43. Lehtonen A. Effect of beta blockers on blood lipid profile. Am Heart J 1985; 109: 1192–6.
44. Aronow WS, Ahn C, Mercando AD, Epstein S. Effect of propranolol versus no antiarrhythmic drug on serum lipids in patients with heart disease and complex ventricular arrhythmias. Curr Ther Res 1994; 55: 1442–5.
45. Fraker TD Jr, Fihn SD, Gibbons RJ, et al. 2007 chronic angina focused update of the ACC/AHA 2002 guidelines for the management of patients with chronic stable angina. A report of the American College of Cardiology/American Heart Association Task Force on Practice Guidelines Writing Group to Develop the Focused Update of the 2002 Guidelines for the Management of Patients With Chronic Stable Angina. Circulation 2007; 116: 2762–72.
46. Snow V, Barry P, Fihn SD, et al. Primary care management of chronic stable angina and asymptomatic suspected or known coronary artery disease: a clinical practice guideline from the American College of Physicians. Ann Intern Med 2004; 141: 562–7.
47. Frishman WH, Sica DA. Calcium channel blockers. In: Frishman WH, Sica DA, eds. Cardiovascular Pharmacotherapeutics, 3rd edn. Minneapolis: Cardiotext, 2011: 99–120.
48. Psaty MD, Heckbert SR, Koepsell MD, et al. The risk of myocardial infarction associated with antihypertensive drug therapies. JAMA 1995; 274: 620–5.
49. Furberg CD, Psaty BM, Meyer JV. Nifedipine: dose-related increase in mortality in patients with coronary heart disease. Circulation 1995; 92: 1326–31.
50. Boden WE, Korr KS, Bough KW. Nifedipine-induced hypotension and myocardial ischemia in refractory angina pectoris. JAMA 1985; 253: 1131–5.
51. The Multicenter Diltiazem Post Infarction Trial Research Group. The effect of diltiazem on mortality and reinfarction after myocardial infarction. N Engl J Med 1988; 319: 385–92.
52. Ryan TJ, Antman EM, Brooks NH, et al. 1999 update: ACC/AHA guidelines for the management of patients with acute myocardial infarction: executive summary and recommendations, a report of the American College of Cardiology/American Heart Association Task Force on Practice Guidelines (Committee on Management of Acute Myocardial Infarction). Circulation 1999; 100: 1016–30.

53. Antithrombotic Trialists' Collaboration. Collaborative meta-analysis of randomised trials of anti-platelet therapy for prevention of death, myocardial infarction, and stroke in high risk patients. Br Med J 2002; 324: 71–86.
54. Aronow WS, Ahn C. Reduction of coronary events with aspirin in older patients with prior myocar-dial infarction treated with and without statins. Heart Dis 2002; 4: 159–61.
55. Lerner RG, Frishman WH, Mohan KT. Clopidogrel. A new antiplatelet drug. Heart Dis 2000; 2: 168–73.
56. CAPRIE Steering Committee. A randomised, blinded, trial of clopidogrel versus aspirin in patients at risk of ischaemic events (CAPRIE). Lancet 1996; 348: 1329–39.
57. Tsuya T, Okada M, Horie H, Ishikawa K. Effect of dipyridamole at the usual oral dose on exercise-induced myocardial ischemia in stabl;e angina pectoris. Am J Cardiol 1990; 66: 275–8.
58. Yusuf S, Sleight P, Pogue J, et al. The Heart Outcomes Prevention Evaluation Study Investigators: effects of an angiotensin converting enzyme inhibitor, ramipril, on cardiovascular events and stroke in high-risk patients. N Engl J Med 2000; 342: 145–53.
59. Miettinen TA, Pyorala K, Olsson AG, et al. Cholesterol-lowering therapy in women and elderly patients with myocardial infarction or angina pectoris. Findings from the Scandinavian Simvastatin Survival Study (4S). Circulation 1997; 96: 4211–18.
60. Lewis SJ, Moye LA, Sacks FM, et al. Effect of pravastatin on cardiovascular events in older patients with myocardial infarction and cholesterol levels in the average range. Results of the Cholesterol and Recurrent Events (CARE) Trial. Ann Intern Med 1998; 129: 681–9.
61. The Long-Term Intervention With Pravastatin in Ischaemic Disease (LIPID) Study Group. Prevention of cardiovascular events and death with pravastatin in patients with coronary heart disease and a broad range of initial cholesterol levels. N Engl J Med 1998; 339: 1349–57.
62. Aronow WS, Ahn C. Incidence of new coronary events in older persons with prior myocardial infarc-tion and serum low-density lipoprotein cholesterol 125 mg/dL treated with statins versus no lipid-lowering drug. Am J Cardiol 2002; 89: 67–9.
63. Heart Protection Study Collaborative Group. MRC/BHF Heart Protection Study of cholesterol lower-ing with Simvastatin in 20,536 high-risk individuals: a randomised placebo-controlled trial. Lancet 2002; 360: 7–22.
64. LaRosa JC, Grundy SM, Waters DD, et al. Intensive lipid lowering with atorvastatin in patients with stable coronary disease. N Engl J Med 2005; 352: 1425–35.
65. Grundy SM, Cleeman JI, Merz CNB, et al. Implications of recent clinical trials for the National Cholesterol Education Program Adult Treatment Panel III guidelines. Circulation 2004; 110: 227 39.
66. Deedwania P, Stone Ph, Merz CNB, et al. Effects of intensive versus moderate lipid-lowering therapy on myocardial ischemia in older patients with coronary heart disease. Results of the Study Assessing Goals in the Elderly (SAGE). Circulation 2007; 115: 700–7.
67. Teo KK, Sedlis SP, Boden WE, et al. Optimal medical therapy with or without percutaneous coronary intervention in older patients with stable coronary disease: a pre-specified subset analysis of the COURAGE (Clinical Outcomes Utilizing Revascularization and Aggressive druG Evaluation) trial. J Am Coll Cardiol 2009; 54: 1303–8.
68. Theroux P, Lidon R. Unstable angina: pathogenesis, diagnosis, and treatment. Curr Probl Cardiol 1993; 3: 162–231.
69. Chesebro JH, Fuster V. Thrombosis in unstable angina. N Engl J Med 1992; 327: 192–4.
70. Rizik D, Healy S, Margulis A, et al. A new clinical classification for hospital prognosis of unstable angina pectoris. Am J Cardiol 1995; 75: 993–7.
71. Mark K, Belli G, Ellis S, Moliterno D. Subacute stent thrombosis: evolving issues and current con-cepts. J Am Coll Cardiol 1996; 27: 494–503.
72. Braunwald E, Antman EM, Beasle JW, et al. ACC/AHA guidelines for the management of patients with unstable angina and non-ST-segment elevation myocardial infarction: executive summary and recommendations. A report of the American College of Cardiology/American Heart Association Task Force on Practice Guidelines (Committee on the Management of Patients With Unstable Angina). J Am Coll Cardiol 2000; 36: 970–1056.
73. The Clopidogrel in Unstable Angina to Prevent Recurrent Events Trial Investigators. Effects of clop-idogrel in addition to aspirin in patients with acute coronary syndromes without ST-segment eleva-tion. N Engl J Med 2001; 345: 494–502.
74. Wright RS, Anderson JL, Adams CD, et al. 2011 ACCF/AHA focused update of the guidelines for the management of patients with unstable angina/non-ST- elevation myocardial infarction (updating the 2007 guideline). A report of the American College of Cardiology Foundation/American Heart Asso-ciation Task Force on Practice Guidelines. J Am Coll Cardiol 2011; 57: 1920–59.

75. e Wiviott SD, Braunwald E, McCabe t al. Prasugrel versus clopidogrel in patients with acute coronary syndromes. N Engl J Med 2007; 357: 2001–15.

76. Wallentin L, Becker RC, Budaj A, et al. Ticagrelor versus clopidogrel in patients with acute coronary syndromes. N Engl J Med 2009; 361: 1045–57.

77. Antman EM, McCabe CH, Garfinkel EP, et al. Enoxaparin prevents death and cardiac ischemic events in unstable angina/non-Q-wave myocardial infarction. Results of the Thrombolysis in Myocardial Infarction (TIMI) 11B Trial. Circulation 1999; 100: 1593–601.

78. Antman EM, Cohen M, Radley D, et al. Assessment of the treatment effect of enoxaparin for unstable angina/non-Q-wave myocardial infarction TIMI IIB-ESSENCE meta-analysis. Circulation 1999; 100: 1602–8.

79. Goodman SG, Cohen M, Bigonzi F, et al. Randomized trial of low molecular weight heparin (enoxaparin) versus unfractionated heparin for unstable coronary artery disease. One-year results of the ESSENCE study. J Am Coll Cardiol 2000; 36: 693–8.

80. Goodman SG, Barr A, Sobtchouk A, et al. Low molecular weight heparin decreases rebound ischemia in unstable angina or non-Q-wave myocardial infarction: the Canadian ESSENCE ST Segment Monitoring Substudy. J Am Coll Cardiol 2000; 36: 1507–13.

81. Braunwald E, Jones RH, Mark DB, et al. Diagnosing and managing unstable angina. Circulation 1994; 90: 613–22.

82. Cannon CP, Weintraub WS, Demopoulo LA, et al. Comparison of early invasive and conservative strategies in patients with unstable coronary syndromes treated with the glycoprotein IIb/IIIa inhibitor tirofiban. N Engl J Med 2001; 344: 1879–87.

83. van Dijk D, Spoor M, Hijman R, et al. Cognitive and cardiac outcomes 5 years after off-pump vs on-pump coronary artery bypass graft surgery. JAMA 2007; 297: 701–8.

84. CABRI Trial Participants. First-year results of CABRI (Coronary Angioplasty versus Bypass Revascularization Investigation). Lancet 1995; 346: 1179–84.

85. King SB III, Lembo NJ, Weintraub WS, et al. A randomized trial comparing coronary angioplasty with coronary bypass surgery. N Engl J Med 1994; 331: 1044–50.

86. Hamm CW, Reimers J, Ischinger T, et al. A randomized study of coronary angioplasty compared with bypass surgery in patients with symptomatic multivessel coronary disease. N Engl J Med 1994; 331: 1037–43.

87. Gallo R, Badiman JJ, Fuster V. Pathobiology of coronary ischemic events: clinical implications. Adv Intern Med 1998; 43: 203–32.

88. Aronow WS, Ahn C, Mercando AD, et al. Decrease in mortality by propranolol in patients with heart disease and complex ventricular arrhythmias is more an anti-ischemic than an antiarrhythmic effect. Am J Cardiol 1994; 74: 613–15.

89. Aronow WS. Medical management of stable angina pectoris. Comp Ther 1987; 13: 54–60.

90. The TIME Investigators. Trial of invasive versus medical therapy in elderly patients with chronic symptomatic coronary-artery disease (TIME): a randomised trial. Lancet 2001; 358: 951–7.

91. Aronow WS. Commentary Approach to symptomatic coronary disease in the elderly: TIME to change? Lancet 2001; 358: 945–6.

92. Smith SC Jr, Benjamin EJ, Bonow RO, et al. AHA/ACCF secondary prevention and risk reduction therapy for patients with coronary and other atherosclerotic vascular disease: 2011 update. A guideline from the American Heart Association and American College of Cardiology Foundation. Endorsed by the world Heart Federation and the Preventive Cardiovascular Nurses Association. J Am Coll Cardiol 2011; 58: 2432–46.

93. Willich SN, Lewis M, Lowel H, et al. Physical exertion as a trigger of acute myocardial infarction. N Engl J Med 1993; 329: 1684–90.

94. Frasure-Smith N, Lesperance F, Talajic M. Depression. following myocardial infarction. Impact on six-month survival. J Am Med Assoc 1993; 270: 1819–25.

95. Aronow WS. Exercise therapy for older persons with cardiovascular disease. Am J Geriatr Cardiol 2001; 10: 245–52.

96. Schuler G, Schlierf G, Wirth A, et al. Low-fat diet and regular supervised physical exercise in patients with symptomatic coronary artery disease: reduction of stress-induced myocardial ischemia. Circulation 1988; 77: 172–81.

97. Frishman WH, Nawarskas JJ, Anderson JR. Ranolazine: A piperazine derivative. In: Frishman WH, Sica DA, eds. Cardiovascular Pharmacotherapeutics, 3rd edn. Minneapolis: Cardiotext, 2011: 217–22.

98. Belardinelli L, Antzelevitch C, Fraser H. Inhibition of late (sustained/persistent) sodium current: a potential drug target to reduce intracellular sodium dependent calcium overload and its detrimental effects on cardiomyocyte function. Eur Heart J 1994; 9:13–17.

99. Chaitman BR, Skettino SL, Parker JO, et al. Anti-ischemic effects and long-term survival during ranolazine monotherapy in patients with chronic severe angina. J Am Coll Cardiol 2004; 43: 1375–82.

100. Chaitman BR, Pepine CJ, Parker JO, et al. Effects of ranolazine with atenolol, amlodipine, or diltiazem on exercise tolerance and angina frequency in patients with severe chronic angina: a randomized controlled trial. JAMA 2004; 291: 309–16.

101. Rousseau MF, Pouleur H, Cocco G, Wolff AA. Comparative efficacy of ranolazine for chronic angina pectoris. Am J Cardiol 2005; 95: 311–16.

102. Stone PH, Gratsiansky NA, Blokhin A, et al. Antianginal efficacy of ranolazine when added to treatment with amlodipine: the ERICA (Efficacy of Ranolazine in Chronic Angina) trial. J Am Coll Cardiol 2006; 48: 566–75.

103. Stone PH, Chaitman BR, Stocke K, et al. The anti-ischemic mechanism of action of ranolazine in stable ischemic heart disease. J Am Coll Cardiol 2010; 56: 934–42.

104. Taira N. Nicorandil as a hybrid between nitrates and potassium channel activators. J Cardiol 1989; 63: 18J–24J.

105. The IONA Study Group. Effect of nicorandil on coronary events in patients with stable angina: the Impact of Nicorandil in Angina (IONA) randomised trial. Lancet 2002; 359: 1269–75.

106. DiFrancesco CD, Camm JA. Heart rate lowering by specific and selective I_f current inhibition with ivabradine. A new therapeutic perspective in cardiovascular disease. Drugs 2004; 64: 1757–65.

107. Borer JS, Fox K, Jaillon P, et al. Antianginal and antiischemic effects of ivabradine, an I_f inhibitor, in stable angina. A randomized, double-blind, multicentered, placebo-controlled trial. Circulation 2003; 107: 817–23.

108. Fox K, Ford I, Steg G, et al. Ivabradine for patients with stable coronary artery disease and left ventricular systolic dysfunction (BEAUTIFUL): a randomised, double-blind, placebo-controlled trial. Lancet 2008; 372: 807–16.

109. Takano H, Komuro I. Cytokines and heart remodeling. In: Leri A, Anversa P, Frishman WH, eds. Cardiovascular Regeneration and Stem Cell Therapy. Malden, Massachusetts: Blackwell Futura, 2007: 139–47.

110. Deedwania PC, Chatterjere K. Current therapeutic options and evolving therapies for chronic stable angina/chronic coronary syndrome. Johns Hopkins Adv Stud Med 2006; 6: S827–36.

111. Frazier OH, Cooley DA, Kadipasaoglu KA, et al. Myocardial revascularization with laser. Preliminary findings. Circulation 1995; 92:II-58–65.

112. Donovan CL, Landolfo KP, Lowe JE, et al. Improvement in inducible ischemia during dobutamine stress echocardiography after transmyocardial laser revascularization in patients with refractory angina pectoris. J Am Coll Cardiol 1997; 30: 607–12.

113. Lauer B, Junghans U, Stahl F, et al. Catheter-based percutaneous myocardial laser revascularization in patients with end-stage coronary artery disease. J Am Coll Cardiol 1999; 34: 1663–70.

114. Schofield PM, Sharpies LD, Caine N, et al. Transmyocardial laser revascularization in patients with refractory angina: a randomised controlled trial. Lancet 1999; 353: 519–24.

115. Oesterle SN, Sanborn TA, Ali N, et al. Percutaneous transmyocardial laser revascularisation for severe angina: the PACIFIC randomised trial. Lancet 2000; 356: 1705–10.

116. Soroff HS, Hui J, Giron F. Current status of external counterpulsation. Crit Care Clin 1986; 2: 277–95.

117. Kumar A, Aronow WS. Use of enhanced counterpulsation in the treatment of refractory angina pectoris and congestive heart failure. Compr Ther 2009; 35: 133–8.

118. Lawson WE, Hui JCK, Soroff HS, et al. Efficacy of enhanced external counterpulsation in the treatment of angina pectoris. Am J Cardiol 1992; 70: 859–62.

119. Arora R, Chou T, Jain D, et al. External Counter Pulsation (MUST-EECP): effect of EECP on exercise-induced myocardial ischemia and anginal episodes. J Am Coll Cardiol 1999; 33: 1833–40.

120. Kumar A, Aronow WS, Vadnerkar A, et al. Effect of enhanced external counterpulsation on clinical symptoms, quality of life, 6-minute walking distance, and echocardiographic measurements of left ventricular systolic and diastolic function after 35 days of treatment and at 1-year follow-up in 47 patients with chronic refractory angina pectoris. Am J Ther 2009; 16: 116–18.

121. Aronow WS, Frishman WH. Spinal cord stimulation for the treatment of angina pectoris. Curr Treat Options Cardiovasc Med 2004; 6: 79–83.

122. Aronow WS, Frishman WH. Spinal cord stimulation for the treatment of angina pectoris. In: Frishman WH, Weintraub WI, Micozzi MS, eds. Complementary and Integrative Therapies for Cardiovascular Disease. Philadelphia: Elsevier, 2005: 390–5.

123. Banai S, Muvhar SB, Parikh KH, et al. Coronary sinus reducer stent for the treatment of chronic refractory angina pectoris. A prospective, open-label, multicenter, feasibility first-in-man study. J Am Coll Cardiol 2007; 49: 1783–9.

10
Therapy of acute myocardial infarction

Michael W. Rich and Wilbert S. Aronow

SUMMARY

Acute myocardial infarction (MI) occurs at increasing frequency with advancing age, and older patients with acute MI are at increased risk for major complications, including HF, arrhythmias and conduction disturbances, myocardial rupture, cardiogenic shock, and death. Older patients thus comprise a large high-risk subgroup of the MI population who may derive substantial benefits from appropriately selected therapeutic interventions. At the same time, many interventions are associated with increased risk in the elderly, so that individualization of treatment is essential. Optimal therapy is thus based on a careful risk–benefit assessment of the available treatment options in conjunction with appropriate consideration of patient preferences and other relevant factors. Although many therapeutic trials in acute MI patients have either excluded elderly patients or enrolled too few older subjects to permit definitive conclusions, sufficient data are available to make specific recommendations in several areas. As shown in Table 10.1, aspirin, low-molecular-weight heparin, fibrinolytic agents, and primary percutaneous coronary intervention are of proven value during the acute phase of MI in selected elderly patients. Early initiation of β-blockers, angiotensin-converting enzyme (ACE) inhibitors, and statins is also likely to be beneficial. Following MI, aspirin, β-blockers, ACE inhibitors, and statins are of proven benefit and should be considered standard therapy in most patients. Selected patients may also benefit from clopidogrel, warfarin, percutaneous or surgical revascularization, or insertion of an implantable cardioverter defibrillator. Conversely, routine use of calcium channel blockers and antiarrhythmic agents is not recommended.

As the age of the population continues to increase, the number of older patients at risk for acute MI will rise commensurately. Although progressively more sophisticated interventions may result in sizable reductions in post-MI morbidity and mortality, it is apparent, given the high risk of adverse outcomes in the elderly population, that the best treatment is prevention. Thus, the greatest potential for the future, as well as the greatest challenge, will be to develop more effective strategies for preventing atherosclerosis and for conquering the epidemic of coronary heart disease in our aging population.

INTRODUCTION

In 2005, there were 683,000 hospital admissions in the USA with a first-listed diagnosis of acute myocardial infarction (MI) (1). Of these, 430,000 (63.0%) occurred in the 12.4% of the population aged 65 years or older, 40.1% occurred in the 6.1% of the population over the age of 75, and 16.1% occurred in the 1.6% of the population over the age of 85 (1). Moreover, approximately 85% of all deaths attributable to acute MI occur in patients over age 65, and 60% occur in patients over age 75 (1,2). In 2008 in the USA, 935,000 Americans

Table 10.1 Efficacy of Selected Treatments for Acute Myocardial Infarction in Elderly Patients

Effective	Probably Effective	Uncertain Efficacy	Ineffective
Acute phase			
Aspirin	Intravenous heparin[a]	Nitrates	
LMWH[a]	β-Blockers[a]		Calcium antagonists
Fibrinolysis[a]	ACE inhibitors[a]		Antiarrhythmic agents
Primary PCI[a]	Glycoprotein IIb/IIIa		Magnesium
	inhibitors[a]		Erythropoeitin
	Statins		
Chronic phase			
Aspirin	Clopidogrel,[a] prasugrel,[a]		Antiarrhythmic agents
	ticagrelor[a]		
β-Blockers[a]	Warfarin[a]		Calcium channel blockers
ACE inhibitors	PCI[a]		
Statins	Coronary surgery[a]		
	ICDs[a]		

[a]Selected subgroups; see text.
Abbreviations: ACE, angiotensin-converting enzyme; ICDs, implantable cardioverter-defibrillators; LMWH, low-molecular-weight heparin; PCI, percutaneous coronary intervention.

had a first or recurrent MI with the incidence of first MI being highest in persons aged 65–74 years (9.2% for white men, 10.2% for black men, 5.1% for white women, and 7.2% for black women) (3). In the National Registry of Myocardial Infarction, chest pain was not the presenting symptom in 32.7% of 159,603 men and 37.9% of 107,877 women aged 65–74 years and in 46.6% of 210,292 men and 50.4% of 265,405 women aged 75–84 years (4). In-hospital mortality was higher in older men and women who did not present with chest pain (4). In the Korea Acute Myocardial Infarction Registry (KAMIR) study of 7288 patients mean age 62 years with ST-elevation MI, painless MI was associated with higher in-hospital mortality (5.9% vs. 3.6% in patients with chest pain, $p = 0.026$) and with more major adverse cardiac events at 1-year follow-up (26% vs. 19% in patients with chest pain, $p = 0.002$) (5). Late detection may have contributed to total ischemic burden (5). The National Cardiovascular Data Registry (NCDR) Acute Coronary Treatment and Intervention Network Registry-Get With The Guidelines (ACTION-GWTG) database showed that in patients with ST-elevation MI, the in-hospital mortality was 4% in 24,070 patients younger than 75 years, 12% in 4273 patients aged 75–84 years, and 19% in 1845 patients aged 85 years and older (6). Thus, acute MI is exceedingly common in older adults, and the case fatality rate is disproportionately high. This chapter reviews the treatment of elderly patients with acute MI, including the management of selected complications.

GUIDING PRINCIPLES
Numerous studies have demonstrated that elderly patients with acute MI are at increased risk for a variety of complications, including atrial fibrillation, heart failure (HF), myocardial rupture, cardiogenic shock, and death (7–13). The risk of each of these complications is two- to fourfold higher in patients over age 65 than in younger patients. Older age thus defines a high-risk subgroup of MI patients who could potentially derive substantial benefit from aggressive therapeutic interventions. On the other hand, elderly patients are at increased risk for serious adverse consequences arising from aggressive treatments such as fibrinolytic therapy or early catheterization and percutaneous coronary intervention (PCI). In addition, the risk–benefit ratio may be modulated by the presence of comorbid

conditions (e.g., diabetes, renal insufficiency, and dementia), and the desirability of specific therapies may be further affected by social considerations and patient preferences. Therefore, the potential benefits and risks of each intervention must be carefully considered on an individualized basis.

While elderly MI patients clearly represent a high-risk subgroup, it is important to recognize that they also comprise an extremely heterogeneous subgroup, and this heterogeneity has important therapeutic implications. For example, an 80-year-old patient presenting with a large anterior MI complicated by HF and hypotension has an expected mortality of over 50%. As a result, the potential benefit to be derived from maximally aggressive therapy (e.g., immediate catheterization and PCI) is large, thereby justifying a moderate increase in procedural risk. In contrast, an 80-year-old individual presenting with a small inferior MI of more than 12 hours' duration who is hemodynamically stable and free of chest pain has a relatively favorable prognosis, and the risks associated with thrombolysis and PCI may not be justified. Thus, in considering the interventions described below, the clinician should keep in mind that the "sickest" patients often have the most to gain from aggressive treatment, while those with a more favorable prognosis often respond satisfactorily to conservative management.

GENERAL MEASURES

As in younger patients, the early management of older patients with acute MI should include measures designed to relieve the patient's discomfort and treat any hemodynamic disturbances, such as HF or hypotension (Table 10.2). Morphine sulfate in doses of 2–4 mg intravenously is the recommended agent for treating chest pain in patients with acute MI (14). Empiric administration of supplemental oxygen is appropriate if the baseline arterial saturation is less than 92%. Nitroglycerin is safe in the majority of patients with acute MI, and it is effective in reducing myocardial oxygen demand when administered sublingually, transdermally, or intravenously. Nitrates can occasionally result in a precipitous fall in blood pressure, especially when given sublingually to patients with inferior MI associated with right ventricular involvement (15). Intravenous β-blockers are also effective in relieving chest pain, and both metoprolol and atenolol have been approved for use in patients with acute MI (16,17). As discussed below, contraindications to β-blockers include marked bradycardia, hypotension, moderate or severe HF, advanced atrioventricular (AV) block, and significant bronchospastic lung disease. Recent data indicate that the optimal serum potassium level for survival in MI patients is 3.5–4.0 mEq/L (18).

HF and hypotension are common complications of acute MI in the elderly, and each is discussed in more detail later in this chapter. They are mentioned briefly here because they are often present when the patient arrives in the emergency room and empiric therapy may be necessary. In most cases, HF occurring in the early stages of acute MI can be effectively treated with a combination of diuretics, nitrates, and supplemental oxygen. In patients who do not respond to these measures, further investigation into the etiology of HF is appropriate. Urgent echocardiography is the most useful noninvasive test in this setting, since it allows assessment of left and right ventricular function, valvular structures, and the pericardium. Sympathomimetic agents such as dobutamine and dopamine are best avoided in the early hours of acute MI because they increase myocardial oxygen demand and may worsen ischemia, but patients with severe HF, particularly when accompanied by hypotension, may require inotropic therapy. In the absence of supraventricular tachyarrhythmias, digitalis has little value in the management of HF associated with acute MI.

Hypotension, particularly when accompanied by HF or impaired tissue perfusion, is a grave prognostic sign warranting prompt intervention. Hypotension without HF should be treated with IV fluids at a rate of 75–250 cc/hr until an adequate blood pressure has been

Table 10.2 General Measures for the Early Management of Elderly Patients with Acute Myocardial Infarction

Symptom or sign	Agent	Dose	Comment
Chest pain	Oxygen	2–5 L/min	Probably not helpful if O_2 saturation ≥92%
	Morphine	2–4 mg IV, q 5–15 min	Watch for respiratory depression
	Nitroglycerin	0.4 mg sublingually; 2% ointment, 1/2–2" transdermally; 10–200 μg/min IV	Watch for hypotension, especially in inferior myocardial infarction
	Metoprolol	2.5–5 mg IV, q 2–5 min, up to 15 mg	Watch for bradycardia, hypotension, heart, block, bronchospasm, worsening heart failure
	Atenolol	2.5–5 mg IV, q 10 min up to 10 mg	
Heart Failure	Oxygen	As needed to maintain arterial saturation ≥92%	
	Furosemide	20–80 mg IV	Watch for hypotension
	Bumetanide	0.5–2 mg IV	Watch for hypotension
	Nitroglycerin	2% ointment, 1/2–2" transdermally; 10–200 μg/min IV	Avoid hypotension
Hypotension	IV fluids	As needed to maintain adequate perfusion	Watch for worsening heart failure
	Dobutamine	2.5–10 μg/kg/min	Watch for worsening hypotension; may aggravate ischemia
	Dopamine	2–40 μg/kg/min	May worsen ischemia
	Norepinephrine	0.5–30 μg/min	May worsen ischemia

Abbreviation: IV, intravenous.

restored or until signs of HF develop. In patients with inferior MI, hypotension associated with bradycardia may be due to heightened vagal tone and may respond to 0.5–1 mg of subcutaneous or IV atropine. Further investigation is required if the blood pressure fails to respond to fluid resuscitation, and both noncardiac (e.g., sepsis, pulmonary embolism, and medications) and cardiac causes of hypotension should be considered. In patients with persistent unexplained hypotension, the use of an inotropic or vasopressor agent may be necessary, but the precautions noted above should be borne in mind.

REPERFUSION THERAPY

Prompt reperfusion of the infarct-related artery has been shown to reduce infarct size and peri-infarct complications, including death, in a broad range of patients with acute MI associated with ST-segment elevation (STEMI) or new left bundle branch block (LBBB), as well as in selected patients with non-ST-segment elevation (NSTEMI) acute coronary syndromes (ACS). Although early studies of reperfusion therapy focused on administration of fibrinolytic agents, in the past decade primary PCI has become the preferred reperfusion strategy if the procedure can be performed expeditiously, usually defined as within 60–90 minutes of the patient's arrival to the hospital. As discussed in more detail below, several studies have examined the role of reperfusion therapy in older patients. In one study, eligibility for reperfusion was present in 87% of patients younger than 75 years, 75% of patients aged 75–84 years, and 58% of patients aged 85 years and older. Although patients who received reperfusion had better outcomes than eligible patients who did not receive reperfusion, this was only significant for patients younger than 75 years (odds ratio = 0.58; 95% CI, 0.40–0.84) (6). In another study of 140 patients aged 80–100 years hospitalized with acute MI, an invasive strategy conferred a significant survival advantage during the first year after hospital discharge (multivariable, propensity-adjusted hazard ratio for death 0.30, $p = 0.01$) (19). Similarly, among 73 patients aged 85–94 years hospitalized for STEMI, primary PCI was the only independent predictor of survival at a median follow-up of 429 days (hazard ratio = 0.3, $p = 0.02$) (20).

FIBRINOLYTIC THERAPY

In the mid to late 1980s, a series of large randomized clinical trials demonstrated that IV administration of a fibrinolytic agent within 6–12 hours of symptom onset in patients with acute MI associated with ST-segment elevation or LBBB led to a significant reduction in short-term and long-term mortality (21–25). These studies ushered in the reperfusion era and revolutionized the approach to treatment of patients with ACS. However, despite the fact that more than 25 years have elapsed since the publication of the first, large trial of fibrinolytic therapy (22), the value of this treatment in patients over age 75 remains controversial.

In 1994, the Fibrinolytic Therapy Trialists' (FTT) Collaborative Group published a meta-analysis of all major trials, including a subgroup analysis by age (Fig. 10.1) (26). Although the greatest absolute benefit was seen in patients 65–74 years of age (26 fewer deaths per 1000 treated patients), the benefit was more modest in patients over age 75 years (10 fewer deaths per 1000 treated patients) and failed to achieve statistical significance. Reanalysis of the FTT data, limited to patients presenting within 12 hours of symptom onset with ST-segment elevation or LBBB, showed that among patients aged 75 years or older, mortality was reduced from 29.4% to 26.0% (34 fewer deaths per 1000 treated patients, $p = 0.03$) (27). Moreover, the absolute benefit was similar to that seen in other age groups, and greater than in patients younger than age 55.

In contrast to the FTT analysis, several observational studies have suggested that the use of fibrinolytic therapy in patients over 75 years of age may be associated with adverse outcomes (28–30). In one study, Thiemann et al. examined the outcomes in 7864 Medicare

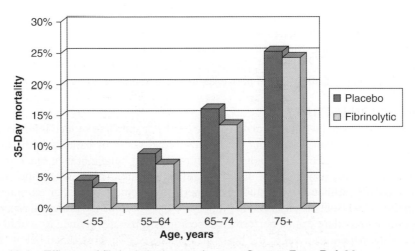

Figure 10.1   Efficacy of fibrinolytic therapy by age. *Source*: From Ref. 26.

patients with acute MI who were suitable candidates for fibrinolytic therapy (28). Among patients 65–75 years of age, administration of a fibrinolytic agent was associated with reduced mortality, consistent with the randomized trials. However, among patients aged 76–86, mortality was 38% higher in those who received a fibrinolytic drug. In another study, also based on the Medicare database, Berger et al. found that 30-day mortality tended to be higher among patients over 75 years of age receiving fibrinolytic therapy, although the 1-year mortality was lower (perhaps reflecting selection bias) (29). In another study, Soumerai et al. examined outcomes of fibrinolytic therapy at 37 Minnesota hospitals and found that fibrinolytic treatment was associated with a 40% higher mortality rate among patients 80 years of age or older (30). The findings of these studies are mitigated somewhat by a report from Stenestrand et al., who examined outcomes in 6891 patients aged 75 years or older hospitalized in Sweden with STEMI from 1995 to 1999 (31). Using propensity score analysis, these investigators found that patients who received fibrinolytic treatment had a 13% lower adjusted relative risk of death or nonfatal cerebral bleeding during a 1-year follow-up period ($p = 0.001$). Although the beneficial effects of fibrinolytic therapy were significant in patients 75–79 and 80–84 years of age, the absolute benefit was lower and no longer statistically significant among patients aged 85 years or older.

One plausible explanation for the apparent discrepancy between the clinical trials and some of the community-based analyses is that criteria for fibrinolysis were strictly regulated in clinical trials, thus ensuring an optimal risk–benefit ratio. Nonadherence to these criteria in clinical practice may have led to overutilization of fibrinolytic agents in patients who were less-than-ideal candidates for such therapy, resulting in diminished benefit and increased complications.

In summary, data from multiple randomized clinical trials demonstrate that fibrinolytic therapy is beneficial in appropriately selected elderly patients, including those over 75 years of age. However, observational studies indicate that caution is advised in the very elderly, and suggest that strict adherence to established criteria for use of fibrinolytic drugs is essential in patients over age 75 in order to maximize benefit and minimize risk (32).

One factor that limits utilization of fibrinolytic therapy in elderly patients is concern about increased risk of bleeding, particularly intracranial hemorrhage (ICH). In the FTT overview of nine large fibrinolytic trials, strokes occurred in 1.2% of patients receiving a fibrinolytic agent, compared to 0.8% in control group patients (absolute difference 0.4%; $p < 0.0001$) (27), and the excess in strokes attributable to fibrinolysis increased with age. Thus, in patients over 75 years of age, the stroke rate was 2.0% in patients receiving fibrinolytic therapy, as compared with 1.2% in controls. Other serious bleeding complications, defined as either life-threatening or requiring transfusion, were relatively uncommon, occurring in 1.1% of patients over 75 years of age receiving fibrinolytic treatment, as compared with 0.5% of control group patients. Notably, the excess in major bleeding complications attributable to fibrinolysis was similar in older and younger patients. Thus, the absolute excess risk for both strokes and major bleeding is less than 1%. Nonetheless, caution is advised when using fibrinolytic agents in elderly patients at increased risk for stroke (e.g., those with prior cerebrovascular disease, severe uncontrolled hypertension, or a markedly increased arterial pulse pressure), as well as in patients at increased risk for serious bleeding (33–35).

Several large trials have compared the effects of different fibrinolytic agents on clinical outcomes (36–39). In the Global Utilization of Streptokinase and tPA for Occluded Arteries (GUSTO)-I trial, which randomized over 40,000 acute MI patients to one of four fibrinolytic regimens, alteplase was associated with lower 30-day mortality than streptokinase in patients up to the age of 85 (39). However, the absolute benefit was small in patients over 75 years of age, and alteplase was associated with a significantly higher risk of ICH compared with streptokinase in this age group (2.1% vs. 1.2%; $p < 0.05$) (40). Subsequent studies with the newer fibrinolytic agents reteplase and tenecteplase failed to demonstrate a survival advantage of these agents compared with alteplase (41,42), and in the GUSTO-III trial, reteplase was associated with a higher rate of ICH than alteplase (2.5% vs. 1.7%) among patients over 75 years of age (41). Thus, currently available data indicate that the more fibrin-specific fibrinolytic agents (i.e., alteplase, reteplase, and tenecteplase) are associated with increased risk of ICH compared with streptokinase in patients over age 75, and the merits of these agents with respect to other clinical outcomes, including mortality, have not been convincingly established in the very elderly.

Streptokinase is administered in a dose of 1.5 million units intravenously over 1 hour, and no dosage adjustment is required for elderly patients. Alteplase should be administered as an initial bolus of 15 mg, followed by 0.75 mg/kg over 30 minutes (not to exceed 50 mg), and 0.5 mg/kg over the next 60 minutes (not to exceed 35 mg) (39). Reteplase is administered in two bolus doses of 10 units at an interval of 30 minutes (41). Tenecteplase is given as a single 30–50 mg bolus based on the weight of the patient (42). Aspirin 160–325 mg should be given to all patients receiving fibrinolytic therapy. Patients treated with alteplase, reteplase, or tenecteplase should also receive IV heparin to maintain the activated partial thromboplastin time (aPTT) in the range of 50–70 seconds for the first 24–48 hours (43,44). For patients treated with streptokinase, data from the GUSTO study indicate that IV heparin increases bleeding complications but does not improve survival relative to high dose subcutaneous heparin (12,500 U every 12 hours) (39).

PERCUTANEOUS CORONARY INTERVENTION

PCI has several potential applications in the acute MI setting: as a primary reperfusion strategy; as an adjunct to thrombolysis; as a "rescue" procedure for failed thrombolysis; and in the management of recurrent ischemia (45,46).

In several studies, PCI has been shown to be more effective than fibrinolytic therapy in recanalizing the infarct-related coronary artery, with reperfusion rates of over 90% in some series (46). In addition, three randomized trials suggest that PCI is associated with superior outcomes relative to fibrinolytic therapy in older patients with STEMI (47–49). deBoer et al. randomized 87 acute MI patients over 75 years of age to streptokinase or PCI. At 30-day follow-up, patients allocated to PCI had a reduced risk of death, reinfarction or stroke ($p = 0.01$), and this benefit persisted for at least 1 year (47). In another study involving 130 patients with STEMI 70 years of age or older receiving tissue plasminogen activator or PCI, treatment with PCI was an independent predictor of lower mortality, reinfarction, or revascularization for recurrent ischemia at 6-month follow-up (48). In the largest trial reported to date, Grimes et al. randomized 481 patients aged 70 years or older presenting within 12 hours of onset of STEMI to fibrinolytic therapy or PCI (49). In this study, PCI was associated with a 55% reduction in death, stroke, or reinfarction relative to fibrinolysis ($p = 0.05$). Of note, the benefit of PCI was limited to patients 70–79 years of age; among 131 patients aged 80 years or older, outcomes did not differ between reperfusion strategies.

The findings of these studies are also supported by subgroup analysis from a systematic overview of 22 randomized trials comparing PCI with fibrinolytic therapy in 6763 patients with acute MI (45). Overall, PCI was associated with a significant 37% reduction in 30-day mortality, and the absolute benefit was greater in patients over age 65 than in younger patients. Moreover, the absolute benefit of PCI increased progressively with age, from 1.0% in patients less than 65 years to 4.2%, 5.1%, and 6.9% in patients of ages 65–74, 75–84, and 85 or older, respectively (32). By comparison, among 1126 patients, mean age 80 years, who did not undergo reperfusion therapy, in-hospital and 1-year

Table 10.3 Class I and IIa Indications for Performing PCI in Patients with ST-Elevation Myocardial Infarction

1. Primary PCI should be performed within 12 hr of onset of MI (class I)
2. Prirmary PCI should be performed in patients presenting to a hospital with PCI capability within 90 min of first medical contact as a systems goal (class I)
3. Primary PCI should be performed in patients presenting to a hospital without PCI capability within 120 min of first medical contact as a systems goal (class I)
4. Primary PCI should be performed in patients with severe heart failure or cardiogenic shock who are suitable for revascularization irrespective of time delay (class I)
5. Primary PCI should be performed in patients with contraindications to fibrinolytic therapy and with ischemic symptoms for less than 12 hr (class I)
6. Primary PCI is reasonable if there is clinical and/or electrocardiographic evidence of ongoing ischemia between 12 and 24 hr after symptom onset (Class IIa)

Source: Adapted from Ref. 51.

mortality were 53% and 69%, respectively (50). Table 10.3 shows the 2011 American College of Cardiology Foundation/American Heart Association/Society for Cardiovascular Angiography and Interventions class I and class IIa indications for performing PCI in patients with STEMI (51).

In summary, current data suggest that PCI can be performed safely in elderly patients with acute MI and that it is associated with fewer hemorrhagic strokes and more favorable clinical outcomes compared to fibrinolysis (32). Although present data are insufficient to allow definitive conclusions on primary PCI versus fibrinolytic therapy in patients over 80 years of age, PCI is an effective therapeutic option in appropriately selected patients and should be strongly considered when fibrinolytic therapy is contraindicated (14,32). In particular, very high-risk elderly patients, such as those with large anterior MIs or severe hemodynamic disturbances, may be most likely to benefit from this approach (52).

The routine use of PCI following fibrinolysis was evaluated in several trials prior to the era of intracoronary stents and none of these studies demonstrated improved outcomes relative to conservative management (53–58). In contrast, two later trials reported favorable outcomes among patients who underwent routine stent implantation following fibrinolysis compared with conservative management (59,60). Both of these studies were relatively small and primarily involved younger patients with no subgroup analysis by age. Therefore, the role of routine PCI following successful fibrinolysis in older patients remains uncertain.

Patients who experience recurrent ischemic pain or marked ST-segment changes on a predischarge stress test are at high risk for recurrent ischemic events following hospital discharge. Coronary angiography and revascularization with either PCI or coronary bypass surgery is appropriate in these patients (61) and age per se is not a contraindication to these procedures (14,32,45). Patients with persistent ischemic pain following administration of a fibrinolytic agent, particularly when accompanied by hemodynamic instability (e.g., hypotension or marked HF), are also at high risk for adverse outcomes, and "rescue" PCI appears to improve prognosis in this subgroup (45,46,62,63). For example, a meta-analysis of 8 trials including 1177 patients demonstrated that rescue PCI was associated with improved clinical outcomes for patients with STEMI after failed fibrinolytic therapy (53). In contrast, repeat fibrinolysis was not associated with clinical improvement but was associated with increased minor bleeding (64). Thus, although cardiac catheterization and revascularization are not recommended as routine procedures for all older patients following acute STEMI, they should be strongly considered in patients with persistent chest pain, marked hemodynamic instability, or recurrent ischemia in the early post-MI period (14,32).

ANTITHROMBOTIC AGENTS
Aspirin

Aspirin is of proven benefit in patients with either unstable angina (65,66) or acute MI (24) and it should be considered standard therapy in all patients presenting with ACS in the absence of major contraindications. Evidence supporting the use of aspirin for acute MI derives from the second International Study of Infarct Survival (ISIS-2), in which 17,187 patients with suspected MI were randomized to receive either aspirin 162.5 mg or placebo, and either streptokinase 1.5 million units or placebo (23). Overall, patients receiving aspirin experienced a 23% reduction in the risk of vascular death within 35 days of hospitalization, and this effect was independent of whether or not the patient received streptokinase. In 3411 patients over 70 years of age, aspirin was associated with a 21% reduction in vascular deaths (17.6% vs. 22.3%; $p < 0.01$) (23). With respect to aspirin dosage, available evidence suggests that the minimum effective dose in patients with acute MI is 160 mg, and that doses in excess of 325 mg provide no additional benefit (67). Importantly, the initial dose of aspirin should be administered as soon as possible after presentation, and the nonenteric-coated form should be used to ensure rapid absorption. When possible, the first dose should be chewed rather than swallowed. Following MI, aspirin should be continued indefinitely at a dose of 75–325 mg daily or every other day (68,69).

Heparin

Subcutaneous heparin in a dose of 7500 U for every 12 hours reduces the risk of venous thromboembolic complications in patients hospitalized with acute MI (70). Since older patients are at increased risk for deep vein thrombosis and pulmonary embolism, prophylaxis against these events is appropriate in this age group.

At present, the value of routine IV heparin for all patients with acute ST-elevation MI remains unproven (71), but several subgroups do appear to benefit (14,72). Patients with large anterior MIs, acute or chronic atrial fibrillation, or severe left ventricular dysfunction with congestive HF are at increased risk for mural thrombus formation and embolization. Intravenous heparin at doses adjusted to maintain the a PTT at 1.5–2 times the control value appears to reduce arterial thromboembolism in patients with large anterior MIs (70,72,73), and routine heparinization is appropriate (14). Patients with atrial fibrillation should be anticoagulated with heparin, warfarin, or one of the newer agents (e.g., dabigatran, rivaroxaban, and apixaban), but the value of systemic anticoagulation in patients with severe left ventricular dysfunction is unproven, and its use in this situation should be individualized (14). Patients who experience recurrent ischemia during the first few days after MI are at increased risk for infarct extension, and IV heparin is recommended (14,70).

Low-Molecular-Weight Heparin

Compared with unfractionated IV heparin, low-molecular-weight heparins (LMWHs) offer several advantages: once or twice daily subcutaneous dosing, no need to monitor aPTTs, and fewer side effects (especially thrombocytopenia). In a meta-analysis of 14 trials involving 25,280 patients with ST-elevation MI receiving fibrinolytic therapy and aspirin, Eikelboom et al. reported that relative to placebo, LMWH reduced the risk of reinfarction by 28% and death by 10%, but increased the risk of major bleeding and intracranial bleeding (74). Compared with unfractionated heparin, LMWH reduced the risk of reinfarction by 45%, increased the risk of minor bleeding, and had no effect on mortality or major bleeding. Subgroup analyses by age were not reported. In addition, since all patients in these trials were treated with a fibrinolytic agent, the findings may not be applicable to patients receiving PCI or no reperfusion therapy. Further, careful attention to dosing of LMWH is required in older patients with decreased renal function, since excess dosing has been associated with an increased risk for major bleeding. (75). Based on available data, current guidelines recommend unfractionated heparin in preference to LMWH in patients with ST-elevation MI undergoing reperfusion therapy with either PCI or a fibrinolytic agent (14). In other patients for whom antithrombotic therapy is warranted, either unfractionated heparin or LMWH may be used.

Bivalirudin

The Harmonizing Outcomes with Revascularization and Stents in Acute Myocardial Infarction (HORIZONS-AMI) trial randomized 3602 patients, median age 60 years, undergoing primary PCI for STEMI to bivalirudin or heparin plus a glycoprotein (GP) IIb/IIIa inhibitor (76). At 1-year follow-up, the rate of net adverse clinical events, consisting of major bleeding or death, reinfarction, target vessel revascularization for ischemia, or stroke, was 17% lower (P = 0.022) in patients treated with bivalirudin (15.6% versus 18.3%) due to a lower rate of major bleeding in the bivalirudin group (5.8% vs. 9.2%, $p < 0.0001$). The rate of major adverse cardiovascular events was 11.9% in both groups (76). On the basis of these data, the 2009 American College of Cardiology/American Heart Association guidelines for the management of patients with ST-elevation MI recommended that it is reasonable to use bivalirudin in STEMI patients undergoing PCI who are at high risk for bleeding (class IIa) (77).

Glycoprotein IIb/IIIa Inhibitors

The GP IIb/IIIa inhibitors are potent antiplatelet agents that block the final common pathway leading to platelet aggregation. Three GP IIb/IIIa inhibitors—abciximab, eptifibatide, and tirofiban—have been shown to improve outcomes in patients with ACS, primarily in the setting of non-ST-elevation MI (NSTEMI) (78–82). However, although the benefits of GP IIb/IIIa inhibitors in patients up to the age of 75 years are similar to those in younger patients, the value of these agents in older patients is less clear. For example, in a trial involving over 10,000 patients, eptifibatide reduced the risk of death or nonfatal MI in patients up to the age of 79, but there was an increase in event rates among patients over 80 years of age receiving eptifibatide (82). In another study involving a smaller number of patients ($n = 1915$), tirofiban was associated with improved outcomes in patients younger or older than age 65, but outcomes for patients over 75 years were not reported (81). A retrospective analysis from the Intracoronary Stenting and Antithrombotic Regimen: Rapid Early Action for Coronary Treatment (ISAR-REACT) trial found that although abciximab reduced the risk of major coronary events by 43% in ACS patients under the age of 70 years undergoing PCI, there was no benefit in patients age 70 or older (83). Furthermore, meta-analysis of 7 randomized trials of 19,929 high-risk patients with an ACS undergoing an early invasive strategy showed that upstream administration of GP IIb/IIIa inhibitors does not improve clinical outcomes compared to downstream selective administration but is associated with an increased risk for major bleeding ($p = 0.0002$) (84). Nonetheless, on the basis of current evidence, the addition of abciximab to aspirin and heparin is recommended for patients with acute STEMI undergoing cardiac catheterization and PCI (8). In patients with STEMI not undergoing PCI, routine use of GP IIb/IIIa inhibitors is not recommended (14). Importantly, the risk of bleeding complications associated with these agents' increases with age, which may negate the clinical benefit of GP IIb/IIIa inhibitors in the very elderly.

Thienopyridines

Ticlopidine, clopidogrel, and prasugrel are thienopyridine derivatives that inhibit platelet aggregation through multiple mechanisms and are more effective antiplatelet agents than aspirin. Clopidogrel has been shown to be superior to ticlopidine with respect to both efficacy and safety (85). In addition, the combination of clopidogrel and aspirin reduces the risk of cardiovascular death, MI, or stroke by about 20% compared to aspirin alone during the 12-month period following hospitalization for unstable angina or NSTEMI, with similar absolute benefits in patients younger or older than age 65 (86).

In the Trial to Assess Improvement in Therapeutic Outcomes by Optimizing Platelet Inhibition with Prasugrel-Thrombolysis in Myocardial Infarction (TRITON-TIMI-38), 13,608 patients, median age 61 years, with moderate- to high-risk ACS and scheduled for PCI were randomized to prasugrel or to clopidogrel in addition to aspirin (87). After a median follow-up of 14.5 months, the primary endpoint of cardiovascular death, nonfatal MI, or nonfatal stroke was significantly lower in patients treated with aspirin plus prasugrel than in those treated with aspirin plus clopidogrel, 9.9% versus 12.1%, a relative risk reduction of 19% and an absolute risk reduction of 2.2%. Life-threatening bleeding was significantly increased from 0.9% in patients treated with aspirin plus clopidogrel to 1.4% in patients treated with aspirin plus prasugrel, a relative risk increase of 52% and an absolute risk increase of 0.5% (87). Among patients with a history of stroke or transient ischemic attack, ICH was significantly increased from 0% on clopidogrel to 2.3% on prasugrel. Patients aged 75 years and older and patients with a body weight less than 60 kg had a similar incidence of cardiovascular death, nonfatal MI, and nonfatal stroke if they were treated with prasugrel (16.1%) or clopidogrel (16.0%) (87). In the 3534 patients undergoing PCI for STEMI, the primary endpoint at 15 months was 10.0% in patients treated with prasugrel versus 12.4% in patients treated with clopidogrel, a relative risk reduction of 21% and an absolute risk reduction of 2.4% ($p = 0.022$) (88). TIMI major bleeding after coronary artery bypass graft surgery was significantly higher with prasugrel by a factor of 8.19 ($p = 0.0033$) (87).

The United States Food and Drug administration approved prasugrel with a black box warning stating that prasugrel should not be used in patients with a prior stroke or transient ischemic attack, in patients with active pathological bleeding, and in patients with an urgent need for surgery, including coronary artery bypass graft surgery. The 2012 American College of Cardiology Foundation/American Heart Association guidelines for the management of patients with unstable angina pectoris/non-STEMI (89) and the 2009 American College of Cardiology/American Heart Association guidelines for the management of patients with STEMI (77) recommend that prasugrel should not be used in patients with prior stroke or transient ischemic attack (class III indication). Clopidogrel should be used instead of prasugrel in patients with ACS who have had a prior ischemic stroke or transient ischemic attack, in patients aged 75 years and older, in patients with a body weight less than 60 kg, and in patients at high risk for bleeding. Thienopyridine therapy should be continued for at least 1–3 months following placement of a bare metal stent and for at least 9–12 months following placement of a drug-eluting stent. If feasible, these agents should be discontinued 5–7 days prior to coronary bypass surgery because of an increased risk for perioperative bleeding.

Ticagrelor

In the Study of Platelet Inhibition and Patient Outcomes (PLATO), 18,624 patients, median age 62 years, hospitalized with an ACS with or without ST-segment elevation were randomized in a double-blind trial to aspirin (98%) plus either ticagrelor or clopidogrel (90). At 12-month follow-up, the primary endpoint of cardiovascular death, nonfatal MI or nonfatal stroke was significantly lower in patients treated with ticagrelor than in those treated with clopidogrel, 9.8% versus 11.7%, a relative risk decrease of 16% and an absolute risk decrease of 1.9% (90). All-cause mortality was 5.9% in patients treated with clopidogrel compared to

4.5% in patients treated with ticagrelor, a significant relative risk decrease of 24% and an absolute risk decrease of 1.4%. No significant difference in major bleeding was found between groups. However, the incidence of major bleeding not related to coronary artery bypass graft surgery was significantly higher on ticagrelor (4.5%) than on clopidogrel (3.8%) ($p = 0.03$). Fatal intracranial bleeding occurred significantly more often in patients treated with ticagrelor (0.1%) than in patients treated with clopidogrel (0.01%) ($p = 0.02$) (90). In the USA, there was a non-significant 27% increase in the primary outcome in patients treated with ticagrelor versus clopidogrel (91). These findings were attributed to the use of higher dose aspirin in US patients (325 mg daily) compared to non-US patients (75 or 100 mg of aspirin daily). Ticagrelor was approved by the U.S. Food and Drug Administration for the treatment of patients with ACS with a recommended aspirin dose of 75–100 mg daily.

In the PLATO study, an invasive strategy was planned for 13,408 of the 18,624 patients (72%), median age 61 years, hospitalized for ACS (92). At 360-day follow-up of these patients, the primary endpoint of cardiovascular death, nonfatal MI, or nonfatal stroke was significantly lowered from 10.7% in patients treated with clopidogrel to 9.0% in patients treated with ticagrelor, a relative risk reduction of 16% and an absolute risk reduction of 1.7% with no significant difference in major bleeding or severe bleeding between groups (92).

Warfarin

Long-term anticoagulation with warfarin has been shown to reduce the risk of reinfarction and cardiac death in post-MI patients, including the elderly (93–95), and two studies indicate that warfarin, with or without aspirin, is superior to aspirin alone (96,97). However, the addition of warfarin to aspirin increases the risk of bleeding, and this risk is greater in elderly patients. Current indications for warfarin in the post-MI setting include allergy to aspirin, chronic or paroxysmal atrial fibrillation, the presence of a mechanical prosthetic heart valve, or active thromboembolic disease. Anticoagulation for a minimum of 3 months is also recommended for patients with apical akinesis or a left ventricular mural thrombus following acute MI (14). Warfarin may also be considered in other patients deemed to be at high risk for left ventricular thrombus or recurrent coronary events.

Bleeding Complications

An important consideration when using antithrombotic therapy in older patients is the increased bleeding risk accompanying the administration of multiple antithrombotic agents (e.g., aspirin, heparin, thienopyridine, and a GP IIb/IIIa inhibitor). Although there is no precise method to quantify this risk and to accurately assess the risk–benefit ratio of using multiple antithrombotic drugs in an individual patient, it is worth noting that in a study to evaluate the effects of LMWH and abciximab (a GP IIb/IIIa inhibitor) in patients receiving tenecteplase for acute MI, abciximab was associated with a marked increase in bleeding complications among patients over 75 years of age, resulting in overall worse outcomes in this age group (98). In addition, advanced age has been associated with increased risk for excessive dosing and major bleeding complications in patients with ACS treated with heparin, LMWH, or GP IIb/IIIa inhibitors (71). Thus, the benefits of aggressive antithrombotic therapy in reducing recurrent ischemic events must be carefully balanced against the risk of serious bleeding complications, particularly in the very elderly.

β-BLOCKADE

Most of the major trials evaluating β-blockers for the treatment of acute MI were conducted prior to the reperfusion era. However, since many elderly patients with acute MI do not undergo primary PCI or thrombolysis (99,100), the results of these earlier trials remain applicable.

Table 10.4 summarizes data from three large randomized trials of early IV β-blockade in patients with suspected MI (16,17,101). In the ISIS-1 study, administration of IV atenolol followed by oral therapy was associated with a 15% reduction in vascular deaths within the first 7 days (12). Among 5222 patients 65 years of age or older, there was a 23% mortality reduction ($p = 0.001$) (18). Similarly, in two trials using IV metoprolol, older patients benefited more than younger patients (17,101). In pooling the results of these three trials, mortality was reduced by 23% in older patients ($p = 0.005$), but by only 5% in younger patients (p = not significant). These data clearly indicate that older patients, who are at higher risk for adverse outcomes, derive proportionately greater benefit from early β-blocker therapy than younger patients. As a result, β-blockers should not be withheld on the basis of age.

The value of IV β-blockade in combination with fibrinolytic therapy was assessed in the second Thrombolysis in Myocardial Infarction trial (TIMI-II) (102,103). In this study, 1434 patients with acute MI were treated with alteplase and then randomized to receive IV metoprolol or placebo. Although there was no difference in hospital or 6-week mortality, patients receiving metoprolol experienced significantly fewer nonfatal ischemic events during follow-up. These findings provide support for the use of early β-blockade as an adjunct to fibrinolysis in patients with acute MI.

Subsequently, Wienbergen et al. examined the impact of early β-blocker therapy in 17,809 consecutive patients with STEMI enrolled in the German Maximal Individual Therapy of Acute Myocardial Infarction PLUS (MITRA PLUS) registry (104). After adjusting for covariates, early β-blocker treatment was associated with a 30% lower hospital mortality, and the greatest benefit was seen in high-risk patients, including those over age 65. In addition, in an analysis from the VALIANT registry, 55.2% of 306 patients with sustained ventricular tachycardia or ventricular fibrillation and HF were treated with intravenous or oral beta blockers in the first 24 hours (105). Use of beta blockers in these patients was associated with a 72% reduction in hospital mortality ($p = 0.013$) without worsening HF (105).

Despite these favorable results, findings from the Clopidogrel and Metoprolol in Myocardial Infarction Trial (COMMIT) have raised questions about the value of IV

Table 10.4 Mortality in Three Large Trials of Intravenous β-Blockade

		Mortality (%)				
	Number	Active	Control	Difference	% Change	*p* value
Atenolol						
ISIS-1 (18)	16,027					
<65 yr	10,805	2.5	2.6	−0.1	−4.0	NS
≥65 yr	5222	6.8	8.8	−2.0	−22.7	0.001
Metoprolol						
Goteborg (105)	1395					
<65 yr	917	4.5	5.7	−1.2	−21.1	NS
65–74 yr	478	8.1	14.8	−6.6	−45.0	0.03
MIAMI (19)	5778					
<60 yr	2965	1.9	1.8	+0.1	+3.1	NS
61–74 yr	2813	6.8	8.2	−1.5	−17.8	NS
Pooled totals	23,200					
Younger	14,687	2.5	2.6	−0.1	−5.0	NS
Older	8513	6.9	8.9	−2.1	−23.2	0.0005

Abbreviations: ISIS-1, First International Study of Infarct Survival; MIAMI, Metoprolol in Acute Myocardial Infarction; NS, not significant.

β-blockers in patients with acute MI (106). In this study, 45,852 patients with acute MI, 93% of whom had ST-elevation or LBBB, were randomized to IV metoprolol or placebo. Overall, metoprolol did not reduce the risk of death, reinfarction, or cardiac arrest, but the risk of cardiogenic shock was increased by 30% in patients randomized to metoprolol. Among 11,934 patients aged 70 years or older enrolled in the trial, hospital mortality was 13.6% with metoprolol compared with 13.3% in the placebo group.

Current guidelines recommend prompt administration of an oral β-blocker to all patients with acute MI in the absence of contraindications (14). Intravenous β-blocker therapy may be considered in stable patients with tachycardia or hypertension who have no contraindication to β-blocker therapy.

The long-term use of β-blockers for secondary prevention following acute MI has been extensively investigated, and Table 10.5 summarizes data from three of the largest and most frequently cited trials (101,107–111). Notably, reductions in mortality and reinfarction during long-term therapy were at least as great in the elderly as in younger patients. Carvedilol has also been associated with a 23% reduction in mortality relative to placebo in patients with a left ventricular ejection fraction less than or equal to 40% following acute MI (112). In addition, observational studies indicate that the survival benefits of β-blockers following MI appear to extend to patients over 75 years of age (113–115). In one study, covariate-adjusted 2-year mortality rates in patients prescribed β-blockers, relative to those who were not, were 50% lower among patients 65–74 years of age, 44% lower in patients age 75–84, and 28% lower in patients over age 85 (113). β-Blockers are also highly cost-effective in all age groups (116). Thus, β-blockers are recommended for all patients following acute MI in the absence of contraindications.

At the present time, only atenolol and metoprolol have been approved by the FDA for IV use in the acute MI setting. The recommended dose for intravenous atenolol is two 5 mg boluses at an interval of 10 minutes. Oral atenolol 50 mg every 12 hours should be initiated 10 minutes after the second IV dose. For metoprolol, the recommended IV dose is 15 mg

Table 10.5 Mortality in Three Large Trials of Long-term β-Blockade

		Mortality (%)				
	Number	Active	Control	Difference	% Change	p value
Propranolol						
BHAT (107,108)	3837					
30–59 yr	2588	6.0	7.4	−1.4	−18.7	NS
60–69 yr	1249	9.7	14.7	−5.0	−33.7	0.01
Timolol						
Norwegian						
(109–111)	1884					
<65 yr	1149	5.0	9.7	−4.7	−48.3	0.003
65–75 yr	735	8.0	15.3	−7.3	−47.8	0.003
Metoprolol						
Goteborg (112)	1395					
<65 yr	917	4.5	5.7	−1.2	−21.1	NS
65–74 yr	478	8.1	14.8	−6.6	−45.0	0.03
Pooled totals	7116					
Younger	4654	5.5	7.6	−2.2	−28.3	0.004
Older	2462	8.9	14.9	−6.0	−40.1	0.0001

Abbreviations: BHAT, β-Blocker Heart Attack Trial; NS, not significant.

(three 5 mg doses at 2 minute intervals). Oral metoprolol 25–50 mg every 6 hours should be started 15 minutes after the last IV dose, progressing to 100 mg twice daily in 24–48 hours. In very elderly patients, it may be advisable to reduce the dosages of both the agents.

Contraindications to the use of IV β-blockers include marked sinus bradycardia (heart rate < 45/min), systolic blood pressure less than 100 mmHg, marked first-degree AV block (PR interval ≥ 0.24 seconds) or higher levels of block, moderate or severe HF, active wheezing, or a history of significant bronchospastic pulmonary disease. Mild HF and chronic lung disease without bronchospasm are not contraindications to β-blocker therapy.

Propranolol, metoprolol, timolol, and carvedilol have all been approved for long-term use following MI. Recommended daily dosages for these agents are as follows: propranolol 180–240 mg, metoprolol 200 mg, timolol 20 mg, and carvedilol 50 mg. Elderly patients may require lower doses to avoid adverse effects, and there are data suggesting that lower doses may be as effective as higher ones for reducing mortality in older patients (117). Contraindications to oral β-blockers are similar to those listed for the IV drugs.

NITRATES

Nitrates are widely used in the treatment of acute MI (118), but two large studies (GISSI-3 and ISIS-4) failed to confirm a beneficial effect when nitrates were initiated within 24 hours of MI onset (119,120). However, among 5234 patients aged 70 years or older enrolled in GISSI-3, the combined endpoint of death or severe left ventricular dysfunction at 6-month follow-up was significantly reduced by nitroglycerin (odds ratio 0.88; $p = 0.04$) (121). This finding, coupled with the fact that both GISSI-3 and ISIS-4 demonstrated that nitrates can be administered safely to the majority of older patients, suggests that the continued use of nitrates for treating ischemic pain and peri-infarctional HF is appropriate. Routine use of nitrates in elderly patients without pain or pulmonary congestion is of unproven value. Nitrates are contraindicated in patients with right ventricular infarction or systolic blood pressure less than 90 mmHg in the setting of acute MI (14).

CALCIUM ANTAGONISTS

Calcium channel blockers have been widely studied in both the acute MI and post-MI settings (122,123). At present, there is no evidence that treatment with calcium antagonists is beneficial in patients with acute MI, and the use of short-acting calcium antagonists may be harmful (122). One relatively small study showed that diltiazem 60–90 mg administered every 6 hours beginning 24–72 hours after admission for non-STEMI reduced the rate of reinfarction during short-term follow-up, but there was no effect on mortality (124). In another study, long-term diltiazem administration following MI did not affect overall mortality, but a modest benefit was seen in the subgroup of patients with preserved left ventricular function and no HF (125). Similar results have been reported with long-term verapamil use in post-MI patients (126), although a later study failed to confirm these findings (127). Thus, calcium antagonists are not recommended for routine use in acute MI patients, but administration of diltiazem or verapamil is reasonable in patients with preserved ventricular function and no HF who are not candidates for β-blockade (14). Calcium channel blockers are contraindicated in patients with acute MI complicated by HF or left ventricular systolic dysfunction.

ANGIOTENSIN CONVERTING ENZYME INHIBITORS

Early administration of an ACE inhibitor to acute MI patients has been evaluated in several large trials. The first of these, the Cooperative New Scandinavian Enalapril Survival Study (CONSENSUS-2), was discontinued after 6000 patients were enrolled due to a higher frequency of adverse outcomes in patients receiving IV enalapril (128). Moreover, patients over 70 years of age experienced an increased incidence of serious hypotension. In contrast, the GISSI-3 and ISIS-4 trials reported small but statistically significant reductions in mortality in patients receiving oral captopril or lisinopril within 24 hours of MI onset (119,120). In addition, patients 70 years or older treated with lisinopril in GISSI-3 experienced a 14% reduction in the combined endpoint of death or severe left ventricular dysfunction at 6-month follow-up ($p = 0.01$) (121). Subsequently, the Survival of Myocardial Infarction Long-term Evaluation (SMILE) investigators randomized 1556 patients with anterior MI who were not candidates for fibrinolytic therapy to either the ACE inhibitor zofenopril or to placebo within the first 24 hours after symptom onset (129). The incidence of death or severe HF at 6-week follow-up was reduced 34% by zofenopril, and this benefit was maintained for 1 year. Moreover, the absolute benefit was threefold greater in individuals over 65 years of age compared with younger patients (129).

The applicability of the above findings to the general MI population is unclear, since the small benefit seen in the largest trials (absolute mortality reduction less than 1%) (119,120) may reflect a larger benefit in some patients (e.g., those with anterior MI or significant left ventricular dysfunction), but no benefit or even harm in other subgroups. At the present time, early administration of an oral ACE inhibitor is recommended in hemodynamically stable patients with anterior MIs, as well as in patients with HF or a left ventricular ejection fraction of less than 40% in the absence of hypotension (systolic blood pressure < 100 mmHg) or other contraindications (8). In other cases, early ACE inhibitor therapy is optional (14).

The value of ACE inhibitors in post-MI patients with significant left ventricular dysfunction (ejection fraction < 40%) or clinical HF has been well established by the Salvage and Ventricular Enlargement (SAVE) (130) and Acute Infarction Ramipril Efficacy (AIRE) trials (131,132). In SAVE, captopril reduced mortality and the occurrence of other cardiac events during an average follow-up of 42 months in asymptomatic or minimally symptomatic patients with left ventricular dysfunction after MI (ejection fraction < 40%) (130). In AIRE, ramipril produced similar effects in post-MI patients with clinical HF (131,132). Therapy was initiated 3–16 days after MI in SAVE (mean, 11 days), and 2–10 days after MI in AIRE (mean, 5 days). The maximum dose of captopril in SAVE was 50 mg thrice daily, while the target dose of ramipril in AIRE was 5 mg twice daily. Importantly, in both SAVE and AIRE, the beneficial effects of therapy were most pronounced in elderly patients (130,131). In 783 patients over 65 years of age enrolled in SAVE, mortality was reduced by 23% with captopril (27.9% vs. 36.1%; $p = 0.017$); by comparison, patients under the age of 65 experienced a statistically insignificant 9% mortality reduction (16.6% vs. 18.3%) (130). Similarly, ramipril significantly decreased mortality in patients over the age of 65 enrolled in AIRE, but not in younger patients (131). The Heart Outcomes Prevention Evaluation (HOPE) study also showed that the ACE inhibitor ramipril in a dose of 10 mg once daily reduced mortality and major vascular events in a broad spectrum of patients 55 years of age or older with established vascular disease (including chronic coronary artery disease) or diabetes (133). Similarly, the European trial on reduction of cardiac events with perindopril in stable coronary artery disease (EUROPA) randomized 13,655 patients with stable coronary artery disease, of whom 64% had prior MI, to perindopril or placebo (134). After a mean follow-up period of 4.2 years, perindopril was associated with a 20% reduction in cardiovascular death, MI, or cardiac arrest and the benefits were similar in younger and older patients. These findings are also supported by a retrospective analysis of 14,129 patients 65 years of age or older hospitalized with acute MI (135). In this study, patients discharged on an ACE inhibitor had a covariate-adjusted 1-year mortality rate that was 15% lower than in patients not receiving an ACE inhibitor, including a 27% lower mortality in patients over the age of 80.

In summary, ACE inhibitors are indicated for all patients following acute MI, including the elderly, in the absence of contraindications (14). The therapy should be initiated within the first few days in hemodynamically stable patients, but may be deferred in other cases. Dosages should be titrated to those proven to be effective in clinical trials, while monitoring blood pressure, renal function, and serum potassium levels at regular intervals.

ANGIOTENSIN RECEPTOR BLOCKERS

Angiotensin receptor blockers (ARBs) bind to the angiotensin-1 (AT1) receptor on the cell membrane, thereby inhibiting the effects of angiotensin II. ARBs are associated with less cough than ACE inhibitors, but the rates of hyperkalemia and worsening renal function are similar with both drug classes. Two large trials have evaluated ARBs in the post-MI setting. In the Optimal Trial in Myocardial Infarction with Angiotensin II Antagonist Losartan (OPTIMAAL), patients 50 years of age or older with acute MI accompanied by HF, anterior Q waves on ECG, or an ejection fraction less than 35% were randomized to losartan or captopril and followed for an average of 2.7 years (136). Mortality was non-significantly higher in the losartan group (18.2% vs. 16.4%, $p = 0.069$), with similar outcomes in older and younger subjects. In the Valsartan in Acute Myocardial Infarction Trial (VALIANT), 14,703 patients with acute MI were randomly assigned to receive captopril, valsartan, or both drugs and followed for a median of 25 months (137). Mortality was similar in all three arms, but side effects and withdrawals were more common in patients randomized to combination therapy. More than 50% of the patients in VALIANT were 65 years of age or older, 3160 patients were aged 75 years or older, and outcomes with respect to the three treatment groups were similar across age categories, including patients over age 85 (12).

On the basis of currently available evidence, ACE inhibitors remain the preferred agents in patients with recent acute MI, including the elderly (14). ARBs are indicated in patients with HF or left ventricular systolic dysfunction who are intolerant to ACE inhibitors. In addition, combination therapy with an ACE inhibitor and an ARB may be considered in patients with persistent symptomatic HF and an ejection fraction less than 40%.

ALDOSTERONE ANTAGONISTS

In the Eplerenone Post-acute myocardial infarction Heart Failure Efficacy and Survival Study (EPHESUS), the selective aldosterone antagonist eplerenone reduced mortality by 17% in patients with left ventricular dysfunction (ejection fraction < 40%) and HF after MI (138). However, the benefit of eplerenone was attenuated in patients 65 years of age or older, and there was no apparent benefit in patients aged 75 years or older. In addition, the risk of hyperkalemia was higher in older subjects. Therefore, the value of eplerenone in elderly patients following acute MI remains unproven (32).

MAGNESIUM

Although several relatively small studies suggested that selected patients with acute MI, including the elderly, might benefit from routine administration of magnesium (139,140), two large randomized trials failed to confirm a beneficial effect (120,141). Therefore, the routine use of IV magnesium in elderly patients with acute MI is not recommended (14).

ERYTHROPOETIN

Administration of intravenous erythropoeitin in patients with STEMI was associated with an increased rate of adverse cardiovascular events as well as concern about the potential for an increase in infarct size among older patients (142). Therefore, this agent is contraindicated in patients with acute MI.

ANTIARRHYTHMIC AGENTS AND DEVICES

The administration of prophylactic lidocaine to patients with acute MI was once a common practice. However, a meta-analysis suggested that lidocaine does not improve survival and may increase the incidence of asystolic cardiac arrest (143). Moreover, elderly patients hospitalized with acute MI appear to be at lower risk for primary ventricular fibrillation than younger patients (144), and toxicity from lidocaine is more common in the elderly. Thus, the routine use of lidocaine in elderly patients with acute MI is not recommended (14).

Intravenous amiodarone is more effective than lidocaine in the treatment of life-threatening ventricular arrhythmias in the setting of acute ischemic heart disease, and two trials have addressed the role of prophylactic oral amiodarone in the treatment of high-risk post-MI patients (145,146). In these studies, which involved a total of 2688 patients, amiodarone reduced the incidence of arrhythmic death by 35–38%, but there was no difference in total mortality. In one study, the absolute reduction in arrhythmic deaths was greatest in patients over 70 years of age (146). A subsequent meta-analysis, based on data from 13 amiodarone trials, found that amiodarone was associated with a 13% reduction in total mortality ($p = 0.03$) and a 29% reduction in arrhythmic deaths ($p = 0.0003$) (147). In patients over 65 years of age, amiodarone reduced arrhythmic deaths by 32%, but total mortality was reduced by only 8% (not significant) (147). In addition, use of amiodarone in 825 patients in VALIANT was associated with a significant 50% increase in mortality during days 1–16 ($p = 0.02$), and a significant 210% increase in mortality during days 17–45 ($p < 0.001$) after MI; amiodarone was also associated with increased mortality during late follow-up (148). Based on amiodarone's apparent lack of efficacy for reducing total mortality and the high side effect profile associated with this drug, prophylactic use of amiodarone in high-risk patients following acute MI is not recommended.

An implantable cardioverter-defibrillator (ICD) is indicated in patients who develop ventricular fibrillation or hemodynamically significant sustained ventricular tachycardia more than 48 hours after acute MI (14). The value of prophylactic ICD insertion in other post-MI patients is uncertain because of conflicting results from clinical trials (149–152). In a study, 898 high-risk post-MI patients were randomized to receive an ICD or no ICD 5–31 days after acute MI (152). Although ICD implantation reduced the risk of sudden cardiac death by 45%, there was no difference in total mortality during a mean follow-up period of 37 months. Thus, routine implantation of an ICD in post-MI patients is not warranted at the present time. Ongoing studies should clarify whether ICDs are beneficial in selected patients following MI, including the elderly.

STATINS

Statins have been shown to reduce long-term mortality and morbidity in patients up to 85 years of age with vascular disease (153,154). In addition, early administration of high-dose statin therapy within the first 96 hours of acute MI has been shown to reduce the risk of recurrent ischemic events during the 4-month period following hospital discharge, with similar effects in older and younger patients (155). The Pravastatin or Atorvastatin Evaluation and Infection Therapy (PROVE-IT) trial also demonstrated that high-dose atorvastatin was more effective than standard dose pravastatin in reducing the composite endpoint of death, MI, hospitalization for unstable angina, coronary revascularization, or stroke following acute MI (156). The benefit of high-dose atorvastatin appeared to be limited, however, to patients less than 65 years of age. In another trial, early initiation of simvastatin 40 mg with a subsequent increase to 80 mg did not significantly improve outcomes relative to deferred treatment with simvastatin 20 mg in 4497 patients hospitalized with ACS, and the results were similar in younger and older patients (157). In a recent study of 12,853 patients with acute MI, mean age 64 years, use of statin therapy reduced major adverse cardiac events at 1-year of follow-up (158). On the basis of the totality of evidence, prescription of statin therapy is recommended for all patients with acute MI regardless of age or baseline lipid profile (14,32).

MANAGEMENT OF COMPLICATIONS

Elderly patients are at increased risk for several major complications of acute MI, including HF, hypotension, supraventricular arrhythmias, conduction disturbances, myocardial rupture, and cardiogenic shock. In general, the management of these complications is similar in older and younger patients. In the following sections, the treatment of each of these complications is briefly reviewed, with special attention to the elderly.

Heart Failure

Several factors predispose the elderly patient with acute MI to the development of HF, including an increased incidence of prior MI, higher prevalence of multivessel disease, impaired diastolic relaxation, reduced contractile reserve, and an increased prevalence of comorbid illnesses, both cardiac (e.g., aortic stenosis) and noncardiac (e.g., renal insufficiency) (159). As a result, HF occurs in approximately 50% of older patients with acute MI (13), and HF is often the presenting manifestation of MI in the elderly (160).

The initial treatment of HF includes supplemental oxygen, diuretics, and nitrates. In more severe cases, morphine should also be given. Once therapy has been initiated, it is essential to determine the etiology of HF, which is frequently multifactorial in elderly patients. Commonly occurring factors that may contribute to HF in the elderly include persistent or recurrent ischemia, extensive myocardial damage, aortic or mitral valve disease (especially aortic stenosis or mitral regurgitation), arrhythmias (especially atrial fibrillation), uncontrolled hypertension, diastolic dysfunction due to left ventricular hypertrophy, inappropriate bradycardia, mechanical complications (e.g., papillary muscle rupture or ventricular septal perforation), severe renal insufficiency, and medications (e.g., β-blockers, calcium antagonists, and antiarrhythmic agents). In most cases, an echocardiogram with Dopplers, in conjunction with a careful review of the patient's medications and laboratory data, will be sufficient for determining the pathogenesis of HF (14). Infrequently, supplemental studies, such as pulmonary artery catheterization or left ventricular angiography, may be necessary (14).

Once the etiology has been established, an effort should be made to correct treatable disorders and to reduce the dose or discontinue offending medications. If HF persists despite aggressive diuresis, placement of a pulmonary artery catheter should be considered as an aid to diagnosis and therapy. When indicated, treatment with an inotropic agent and/ or an IV vasodilator should be instituted. Dobutamine is the most frequently used IV inotrope for treating severe left ventricular dysfunction, but dobutamine may be less effective in the elderly due to an age-related decline in β-adrenergic responsiveness (161,162). Phosphodiesterase inhibitors such as milrinone have theoretical advantages over sympathomimetic agents in coronary patients because they augment cardiac output without increasing myocardial oxygen demand (163). Nonetheless, in elderly patients with severe HF without recent MI, dobutamine appears to be at least as effective as a phosphodiesterase inhibitor (164).

Nitroglycerin, nitroprusside, and nesiritide are the most commonly used IV vasodilators, but nitroglycerin is the only one recommended for treatment of HF in the setting of acute MI (16). Intravenous nitroglycerin has a very short half-life, which allows rapid drug titration. Hypotension is the most common serious adverse effect, so blood pressure should be monitored closely. In patients with acute decompensated HF, nesiritide is more effective than nitroglycerin in relieving pulmonary congestion and reducing dyspnea (165), but data on the use of nesiritide in patients with acute MI are very limited, and there is concern that nesiritide may be associated with worsening renal function and increased short-term mortality (166,167). In addition, the Acute Study of Clinical Effectiveness of Nesiritide in Decompensated Heart Failure (ASCEND-HF) trial randomized 7141 patients, median age 67 years, with acute decompensated HF to nesiritide or placebo and found no significant effect on dyspnea at 6 or 24 hours and no significant effect on rehospitalization for HF or death within 30 days between groups; there was, however, a significant increase in hypotension in patients treated with nesiritide (26.6% for nesiritide vs. 15.3% for placebo, $p < 0.001$) (168). On the basis of these data, nesiritide should be avoided in patients with HF in the setting of acute MI. Intravenous enalaprilat is another alternative to nitroglycerin and may be useful in patients who are likely to require long-term ACE inhibition. However, enalaprilat may also induce hypotension and renal dysfunction, and it offers no clear advantage over conventional agents in the acute MI setting (169).

Patients who fail to respond to the above measures have refractory HF, and the prognosis is grave unless a correctable problem, such as a ventricular aneurysm, can be identified. Additional interventions that may help stabilize patients with refractory HF include endotracheal intubation with assisted ventilation and placement of an intra-aortic balloon pump. Such therapies are usually appropriate only in patients with potentially reversible pathology.

Hypotension

Hypotension in the setting of acute MI usually reflects a low cardiac output state arising from extensive myocardial damage, intravascular volume depletion, right ventricular infarction, valvular dysfunction (especially mitral regurgitation), pericardial effusion, or arrhythmias (both tachycardias and bradycardias). Other factors that may contribute to hypotension in elderly patients include pre-existing cardiac conditions such as aortic stenosis or cardiomyopathy, ventricular septal perforation, aortic dissection, sepsis, bleeding (e.g., from fibrinolytic therapy or catheterization), and medications. The cause of hypotension is frequently multifactorial, and it is incumbent upon the physician to consider all potential etiologies and to perform appropriate diagnostic investigations as indicated. If the history, physical examination, and laboratory data fail to provide an explanation, echocardiography should be performed promptly (14). If hypotension persists or if the etiology remains unexplained, pulmonary artery catheterization is indicated (14).

In the absence of HF, intravascular volume expansion is the appropriate initial treatment for hypotension. Subsequent therapy will depend on the response to fluid administration and the underlying etiology. Patients who fail to respond to IV fluids or who have coexistent HF may require pulmonary artery catheterization (14). On the basis of the hemodynamic findings and the severity of hypotension, treatment with sympathomimetic agents such as dobutamine, dopamine, or norepinephrine may be necessary to maintain organ perfusion. Other supportive measures include assisted ventilation and intra-aortic balloon counterpulsation (14). It is important to emphasize that all of these interventions are palliative, and unless the underlying etiology of hypotension can be corrected, the prognosis is grave.

Arrhythmias and Conduction Disturbances

Elderly patients with acute MI are at increased risk for supraventricular arrhythmias, particularly atrial fibrillation, and for conduction disturbances, including bundle branch block and high-degree AV block. The incidence of ventricular tachycardia is similar in older and younger patients, but primary ventricular fibrillation occurs less frequently in the elderly (144), possibly reflecting reduced β-adrenergic responsiveness in this age group.

New-onset atrial fibrillation following acute MI usually results from atrial distension due to an increase in ventricular diastolic pressure. Contributing factors may include mitral or tricuspid regurgitation, atrial infarction, pericarditis, electrolyte abnormalities (particularly hypokalemia), and medications (e.g., inotropic agents, bronchodilators). Because elderly patients frequently have pre-existing diastolic dysfunction and an increased reliance on atrial contraction to augment ventricular filling (the "atrial kick") (159), atrial fibrillation often precipitates HF or a low cardiac output state.

Treatment of atrial fibrillation includes correcting any reversible abnormalities (e.g., hypokalemia), controlling the ventricular rate, and restoring sinus rhythm. In patients who are hemodynamically stable, rate control with β-blockers or rate-lowering calcium channel blockers (i.e., diltiazem or verapamil) is appropriate. In most cases, heparinization to maintain the aPTT in the range of 50–70 seconds is also indicated. Although effective rate control often results in spontaneous conversion to sinus rhythm, if atrial fibrillation persists longer than 24 hours, pharmacological or electrical cardioversion should be considered. Antiarrhythmic agents commonly used in the cardioversion of recent-onset atrial fibrillation include amiodarone, sotalol, and ibutilide. All of these agents are negatively inotropic and should be used with caution in the presence of significant left ventricular dysfunction. In patients who exhibit hypotension, severe HF, or organ hypoperfusion attributable to atrial fibrillation, immediate direct current (DC) cardioversion is the treatment of choice (14). Patients should be sedated before cardioversion is attempted, and an initial energy level of 200 J is appropriate (14). Patients with persistent or chronic atrial fibrillation should receive long-term antithrombotic therapy (170). Warfarin, dabigatran, rivaroxaban, and apixaban have all been approved by the FDA for treatment of patients with atrial fibrillation. Aspirin is an acceptable, albeit less effective alternative in patients with major contraindications to systemic anticoagulation (170).

The treatment of peri-infarctional ventricular tachyarrhythmias is similar in older and younger patients and will not be reviewed here. In general, initial therapy should follow the Advanced Cardiac Life Support (ACLS) guidelines (171), and subsequent therapy should be individualized on the basis of symptoms, severity of arrhythmia, and other factors, such as left ventricular function. Similarly, the treatment of bradyarrhythmias and conduction disturbances does not differ in younger and older patients. In general, temporary pacing (transthoracic or transvenous) should be considered in patients with symptomatic or hemodynamically compromising bradyarrhythmias unresponsive to atropine, in patients with new bundle branch block, and in patients with second- or third-degree infranodal block complicating anterior MI. The ACLS guidelines should be followed in treating life-threatening bradyarrhythmias such as asystole (171).

Right Ventricular Infarction

Right ventricular infarction occurs in up to 50% of patients with inferior MI, with somewhat higher frequency in older than in younger patients (172). The pathophysiology, clinical features, and treatment of right ventricular infarction have previously been reviewed and will not be discussed in detail here (15). However, it is worth noting that the presence of right ventricular infarction, as evidenced by ST-segment elevation in the right precordial electrocardiographic leads, is associated with a marked increase in hospital mortality in both younger and older patients (172,173).

Myocardial Rupture

Myocardial rupture is an infrequent complication of acute MI, occurring in less than 5% of patients (174–176). However, when rupture does occur, the course is frequently catastrophic, with death ensuing in over 50% to almost 100% of cases, depending on location. There are three principal types of rupture: ventricular free wall rupture, papillary muscle rupture (PMR), and ventricular septal perforation (acute VSD). PMR almost always occurs following an inferoposterior or posterolateral MI, whereas septal rupture occurs somewhat more frequently following an anterior infarct. Free wall rupture can complicate an infarct of any location.

Although precise figures are unavailable, all forms of rupture appear to occur more frequently in patients over 65 years of age (175,176). Other risk factors for myocardial rupture include female gender and persistent peri-infarctional hypertension (176). Fibrinolytic therapy may also increase the risk of myocardial rupture within the first 24–48 hours after treatment, particularly in older patients undergoing delayed fibrinolysis (i.e., more than 6 hours after symptom onset) (174,176,177).

Impending myocardial rupture is occasionally heralded by persistent vague chest discomfort or unexplained hypotension, but sudden hemodynamic deterioration, new or worsening HF, or asystolic cardiac arrest may be the first indication of the rupture (178). The presence of a new systolic murmur, particularly in association with hemodynamic deterioration, strongly suggests the possibility of papillary muscle dysfunction or ventricular septal perforation, and prompt investigation is warranted. Urgent bedside Doppler echocardiography should be performed, since this will enable accurate diagnosis in the majority of cases (179,180). Pulmonary artery catheterization can provide definitive confirmation of a septal perforation by demonstrating an oxygen saturation step up of greater than 10% at the level of the shunt (usually the right ventricle). Similarly, the presence of an abnormally elevated V-wave in the pulmonary capillary wedge pressure waveform suggests acute mitral regurgitation. Cardiac catheterization is usually necessary to define coronary anatomy in elderly patients with cardiac rupture, and left ventriculography can provide diagnostic information on the severity of mitral regurgitation and on the presence and location of an acute VSD.

Once a diagnosis of acute VSD or PMR has been confirmed, supportive measures should be rapidly instituted, and urgent surgical consultation should be obtained (14). Diuretics, an IV inotropic agent, and after-load reduction with IV nitroglycerin or nitroprusside (blood pressure permitting) are appropriate therapy in most cases. Intra-aortic balloon counterpulsation is often effective in stabilizing the patient and should be strongly considered in all surgical candidates (8). Mechanical ventilation is indicated in patients with severe HF or persistent hemodynamic instability.

Surgery is recommended in almost all cases of acute VSD or PMR, since medical therapy is associated with mortality rates of more than 75% (174,181). Perioperative mortality rates range from 10% to 70%, with preoperative left ventricular function and the presence of cardiogenic shock being the most important factors influencing survival (181–183). The long-term prognosis following successful surgical repair of acute VSD or PMR is favorable (181–183).

Rupture of the left ventricular free wall usually progresses rapidly to pericardial tamponade, asystole, and death. Occasionally, however, the rupture will be locally contained as a result of pericardial adhesions or other factors, resulting in the formation of a pseudoaneurysm. Differentiation of a pseudoaneurysm from a true left ventricular aneurysm can be difficult, but echocardiography, magnetic resonance imaging, and left ventriculography are all useful in making this distinction. The hemodynamic effects of a pseudoaneurysm are variable, depending on its size and location, but there is a tendency for pseudoaneurysms to undergo further rupture, resulting in pericardial tamponade (184,185). Although conservative management may be associated with a favorable outcome in some cases (186), prompt surgical attention is usually recommended once a pseudoaneurysm has been identified (185,187).

Cardiogenic Shock

Cardiogenic shock is defined as the combination of markedly reduced cardiac output (cardiac index < 1.8 L/min/m^2), increased left ventricular diastolic pressure or pulmonary wedge pressure (≥ 22 mmHg), hypotension (systolic blood pressure < 80 mmHg), and tissue hypoperfusion (e.g., prerenal azotemia, impaired sensorium) (188,189). This syndrome occurs twice as frequently in elderly patients with acute MI as in younger subjects, and it accounts for most of the excess mortality associated with acute MI in the elderly (190). Moreover, despite major advances in the treatment of acute MI over the last 30 years, the case fatality rate from cardiogenic shock remains high (190–192).

The causes of cardiogenic shock complicating acute MI are similar to the causes of HF and hypotension. Since a minority of patients survive cardiogenic shock in the absence of a treatable underlying disorder, immediate evaluation for a potentially correctable problem is critical. Emergent Doppler echocardiography should be performed to assess overall left ventricular function and to rule out valvular lesions, pericardial disease, and septal perforation (16). Pulmonary artery catheterization is indicated both to facilitate diagnosis and for guiding therapy (14). Cardiac catheterization may be necessary in some cases if the diagnosis remains in doubt, or as a prelude to PCI or corrective surgery. Although emergent catheterization and coronary revascularization have been shown to improve outcomes in patients up to age 75 with cardiogenic shock complicating acute MI, patients over age 75 may not benefit from these interventions (193).

In patients with a potentially reversible cause of shock, maximally aggressive therapy is indicated to stabilize the patient. In most cases, this will include assisted ventilation, an intra-aortic balloon pump (194), and IV vasoactive therapy. However, when shock is due to irreversible myocardial damage or other untreatable disorder, invasive interventions are unlikely to influence survival and should generally be avoided. For example, in a recent study of 598 patients, median age 70 years, with cardiogenic shock complicating acute MI who were randomized to intra-aortic balloon support or to a control group, use of intra-aortic balloon counterpulsation did not reduce 30-day mortality (195).

NON-ST-ELEVATION ACUTE CORONARY SYNDROMES

Non-ST-elevation ACS, including NSTEMI and unstable angina, increase in frequency with advancing age, and NSTEMI accounts for over 50% of all MIs in patients over the age of 70 (11,13). The National Registry of Myocardial Infarction showed that among 1950, 561 patients hospitalized for acute MI from 1990 to 2006, the proportion of NSTEMIs increased from 14.2% to 59.1% ($p < 0.0001$). In addition, the mean age of all patients increased from 64.1 to 66.4 years ($p < 0.0001$) and the proportion of women increased from 32.4% to 37.0% ($p < 0.0001$) (196). This study also showed that hospital mortality decreased in patients with STEMI from 11.5% to 8.0% ($p < 0.0001$) and in patients with NSTEMI from 7.1% to 5.2% ($p < 0.0001$) (196). While STEMIs are almost always caused by total thrombotic occlusion of the infarct-related vessel (197), the pathogenesis of NSTEMI is more variable. In the elderly, NSTEMI may be precipitated by a sustained imbalance between myocardial oxygen supply and demand resulting from severe hypertension, marked hypoxemia due to HF or pulmonary embolus, atrial fibrillation with rapid ventricular response, or acute hypotension due to sepsis or other causes. Diffuse, multivessel coronary disease is often present, but total occlusion of the infarct artery is the exception rather than the rule (198,199).

The short-term prognosis following NSTEMI tends to be better than that following STEMI, since NSTEMIs are usually smaller and associated with greater preservation of ventricular function (200). However, patients with NSTEMI are at increased risk for recurrent ischemia and reinfarction, and long-term survival is similar to that of patients with

STEMI (200,201). In one series, over 60% of all deaths within the first year after hospitalization for acute MI occurred in patients over the age of 70 presenting with NSTEMIs (202).

As the clinical course following NSTEMI is distinct from that following STEMI, numerous studies have focused specifically on the management of this disorder. In general, the pharmacotherapy NSTEMI should include aspirin, LMWH or unfractionated heparin, and a β-blocker (203). Clopidogrel should also be initiated in most cases, especially if PCI is anticipated (13,14,86). A GP IIb/IIIa inhibitor should also be considered in patients likely to undergo early PCI (81,82,203). Nitrates should be administered for persistent or recurrent chest pain or if HF is present. In the absence of ST-elevation or LBBB, fibrinolytic therapy has not been shown to be efficacious and should be avoided (26).

Several studies have compared early cardiac catheterization and revascularization with conventional medical therapy in patients with unstable angina or NSTEMI (204–211). Although the results of these trials have been somewhat inconsistent, on balance the data suggest that early revascularization is beneficial in high-risk patients, including the elderly (15). Based on these studies, current ACCF/AHA/SCAI guidelines recommend that patients with NSTEMI or unstable angina who have refractory ischemia or hemodynamic or electrical instability should undergo cardiac catheterization with intent to revascularize ischemic myocardium in the absence of serious comorbidities or contraindications to such procedures (class I) (51).It should be noted, however, that in the Can Rapid Risk Stratification of Unstable Angina Patients Suppress Adverse Outcomes with Early Implementation of the ACC/AHA Guidelines (CRUSADE) quality improvement initiative, an early invasive management strategy did not reduce hospital mortality after adjusting for relevant covariates in a cohort of 5794 patients 75 years of age or older with non-ST-elevation ACS (212). Therefore, caution is warranted in the selection of very elderly patients with NSTEMI for early catheterization and revascularization (13).

RISK STRATIFICATION

In the past 30 years, the concept of risk stratification has been developed as a means for selecting subgroups of post-MI patients who are most likely to benefit from further diagnostic and therapeutic measures, and conversely, to identify those with a favorable prognosis who are unlikely to benefit from high-cost interventions (213). Factors associated with an increased risk for adverse outcomes include older age, anterior MI location, ischemia occurring either spontaneously or during a post-MI stress test, reduced left ventricular systolic function (especially an ejection fraction less than 40%), frequent premature ventricular contractions or higher grades of ventricular ectopy, reduced heart rate variability (214), increased fibrinogen (215), and elevated C-reactive protein (215,216). Although none of the major risk stratification studies have specifically targeted older patients, key factors identified in younger individuals, particularly left ventricular dysfunction and residual myocardial ischemia, almost certainly retain their prognostic significance in the elderly. In older patients who are suitable candidates for invasive treatment, further risk stratification seems appropriate, and should include an echocardiogram or other procedure to assess left ventricular function, and an exercise or pharmacological stress test (e.g., regadenoson sestamibi or dobutamine echocardiogram) to determine the extent of residual ischemia (217–219). On the basis of the results of these investigations, additional intervention may be appropriate, but further study is needed to define the optimal approach to managing high-risk elderly patients.

ETHICAL ISSUES

In general, the foregoing discussion has been predicated on the notion that a given patient is an "appropriate" or "suitable" candidate for each intervention under consideration. These terms, while vague, imply that not all patients should receive every intervention, and that multiple factors must be taken into consideration during the decision-making process. Among these are the wishes of the patient, as expressed either directly or through a prior communication such as a living will; the anticipated impact of the intervention on quality of life and long-term prognosis; the potential for the intervention itself to add to the patient's suffering; and the concerns of the patient's family and friends.

The physician's role in guiding these decisions is critically important, and a high level of compassion, honesty, and respect for the patient's autonomy is required. Thus, the physician must provide a balanced view of the available therapeutic options, including a realistic appraisal of the likelihood of various outcomes and adverse events. The physician should avoid creating an overly grim picture, but at the same time must avoid fostering unrealistic hopes. Finally, when the patient's condition is such that death seems inevitable, the physician must be able to provide appropriate counsel to forego or withdraw interventions that are unlikely to be helpful, and which will only serve to prolong the dying process. In addition, the physician must provide comfort and emotional support for the patient and family. In this regard, the importance of the nursing staff, members of the clergy, and other health professionals (e.g., palliative care) in helping the patient and family deal with emotional issues and other concerns cannot be overemphasized.

In summary, acute MI occurs at increasing frequency with advancing age, and older patients with acute MI are at increased risk for major complications, including HF, arrhythmias and conduction disturbances, myocardial rupture, cardiogenic shock, and death. Older patients thus comprise a large high-risk subgroup of the MI population who may derive substantial benefits from appropriately selected therapeutic interventions. At the same time, many interventions are associated with increased risk in the elderly, so that individualization of treatment is essential. Optimal therapy is thus based on a careful risk–benefit assessment of the available treatment options in conjunction with appropriate consideration of patient preferences and other relevant factors. Table 10.1 shows the efficacy of selected treatments for acute MI in elderly patients.

Although many therapeutic trials in acute MI patients have either excluded elderly patients or enrolled too few older subjects to permit definitive conclusions, sufficient data are available to make specific recommendations in several areas. As shown in Table 10.1, aspirin, LMWH, fibrinolytic agents, and primary PCI are of proven value during the acute phase of MI in selected elderly patients. Early initiation of β-blockers, ACE inhibitors, and statins is also likely to be beneficial. Following MI, aspirin, β-blockers, ACE inhibitors, and statins are of proven benefit and should be considered standard therapy in most patients. Selected patients may also benefit from clopidogrel, warfarin, percutaneous or surgical revascularization, or implantation of an ICD. Conversely, routine use of calcium channel blockers and antiarrhythmic agents is not recommended.

As the age of the population continues to increase, the number of older patients at risk for acute MI will rise commensurately. Although progressively more sophisticated interventions may result in sizable reductions in post-MI morbidity and mortality, it is apparent, given the high risk of adverse outcomes in the elderly population, that the best treatment is prevention. Thus, the greatest potential for the future, as well as the greatest challenge, will be to develop more effective strategies for preventing atherosclerosis and for conquering the epidemic of coronary heart disease in our aging population.

REFERENCES

1. DeFrances CJ, Cullen KA, Kozak LJ; National Center for Health Statistics. National Hospital Discharge Survey: 2005 annual summary with detailed diagnosis and procedure data. Vital Health Stat 13 2007:1–209.
2. Rosamond W, Flegal K, Friday G, et al. Heart disease and stroke statistics - 2007 update. Circulation 2007; 115: e69–e171.

3. Roger VL, Go AS, Lloyd-Jones DM, et al. Heart disease and stroke statistics-2012 update: a report from the American Heart Association. Circulation 2012; 125: e2–e220.

4. Canto JG, Rogers WJ, Goldberg RJ, et al. Association of age and sex with myocardial infarction symptom presentation and in-hospital mortality. JAMA 2012; 307: 813–22.

5. Cho JY, Jeong MH, Ahn YK, et al. Comparison of outcomes of patients with painless versus painful ST-segment elevation myocardial infarction undergoing percutaneous coronary intervention. Am J Cardiol 2012; 109: 337–43.

6. Forman DE, Chen AY, Wiviott SD, et al. Comparison of outcomes in patients aged <75, 75 to 84, and ≥85 years with ST-elevation myocardial infarction (from the ACTION Registry-GWTG). Am J Cardiol 2010; 106: 1382–8.

7. Mehta RH, Rathore SS, Radford MJ, et al. Acute myocardial infarction in the elderly: differences by age. J Am Coll Cardiol 2001; 38: 736–41.

8. Roger VL, Jacobsen SJ, Weston SA, et al. Trends in the incidence and survival of patients hospitalized with myocardial infarction, Olmsted County, Minnesota, 1979 to 1994. Ann Intern Med 2002; 136: 341–8.

9. Wu AH, Parsons L, Every NR, et al. Hospital outcomes in patients presenting with congestive heart failure complicating acute myocardial infarction: a report from the Second National Registry of Myocardial Infarction (NRMI-2). J Am Coll Cardiol 2002; 40: 1389–94.

10. Alexander KP, Roe MT, Chen AY, et al. Evolution in cardiovascular care for elderly patients with non-ST-segment elevation acute coronary syndromes: results from the CRUSADE National Quality Improvement Initiative. J Am Coll Cardiol 2005; 46: 1479–87.

11. Rich MW, Bosner MS, Chung MK, et al. Is age an independent predictor of early and late mortality in patients with acute myocardial infarction? Am J Med 1992; 92: 7–13.

12. White HD, Aylward PE, Huang Z, et al. Mortality and morbidity remain high despite captopril and/or valsartan therapy in elderly patients with left ventricular systolic dysfunction, heart failure, or both after acute myocardial infarction: results from the Valsartan in Acute Myocardial Infarction Trial (VALIANT). Circulation 2005; 112: 3391–9.

13. Alexander KP, Newby LK, Cannon CP, et al. Acute coronary care in the elderly, part I: Non-ST-segment-elevation acute coronary syndromes: a scientific statement for healthcare professionals from the American Heart Association Council on Clinical Cardiology: in collaboration with the Society of Geriatric Cardiology. Circulation 2007; 115: 2549–69.

14. Antman EM, Anbe DT, Armstrong PW, et al. ACC/AHA guidelines for the management of patients with ST-elevation myocardial infarction—executive summary. J Am Coll Cardiol 2004; 44: 671–719.

15. Haji SA, Movahed A. Right ventricular infarction—diagnosis and treatment. Clin Cardiol 2000; 23: 473–82.

16. ISIS-1 (First International Study of Infarct Survival) Collaborative Group. Randomised trial of intravenous atenolol among 16027 cases of suspected acute myocardial infarction: ISIS-1. Lancet 1986; 2: 57–66.

17. The MIAMI Trial Research Group. Metoprolol in acute myocardial infarction (MIAMI). A randomised placebo-controlled international trial. Eur Heart J 1985; 6: 199–226.

18. Goyal A, Spertus JA, Gosch K, et al. Serum potassium levels and mortality in acute myocardial infarction. JAMA 2012; 307: 157–64.

19. Schloss TW, Gage BF, Rich MW. An invasive strategy is associated with decreased mortality in patients 80 years and older with acute myocardial infarction. Am J Geriatr Cardiol 2007; 16: 83–91.

20. Shah P, Najafi AH, Panza JA, Cooper HA. Oucomes and quality of life in patients ≥85 years of age with ST-elevation myocardial infarction. Am J Cardiol 2009; 103: 170–4.

21. Gruppo Italiano Per Lo Studio Delia Streptochinasi Nell'Infarto Miocardico (GISSI). Effectiveness of intravenous thrombolytic treatment in acute myocardial infarction. Lancet 1986; 1: 397–402.

22. The ISAM Study Group. A prospective trial of intravenous streptokinase in acute myocardial infarction (ISAM). Mortality, morbidity, and infarct size at 21 days. N Engl J Med 1986; 314: 1465–71.

23. ISIS-2 (Second International Study of Infarct Survival) Collaborative Group. Randomised trial of intravenous streptokinase, oral aspirin, both, or neither among 17187 cases of suspected acute myocardial infarction: ISIS-2. Lancet 1988; 2: 349–60.

24. Wilcox RG, von der Lippe G, Olsson CG, et al. Trial of tissue plasminogen activator for mortality reduction in acute myocardial infarction. Anglo-Scandinavian Study of Early Thrombolysis (ASSET). Lancet 1988; 2: 525–30.

25. AIMS Trial Study Group. Effect of intravenous APSAC on mortality after acute myocardial infarction: preliminary report of a placebo-controlled clinical trial. Lancet 1988; 1: 545–9.

26. Fibrinolytic Therapy Trialists' (FTT) Collaborative Group. Indications for fibrinolytic therapy in suspected acute myocardial infarction: collaborative overview of early mortality and major morbidity results from all randomised trials of more than 1000 patients. Lancet 1994; 343: 311–22.

27. White HD. Thrombolytic therapy in the elderly. Lancet 2000; 356: 2028–30.

28. Thiemann DR, Coresh J, Schulman SP, et al. Lack of benefit for intravenous thrombolysis in patients with myocardial infarction who are older than 75 years. Circulation 2000; 101: 2239–46.

29. Berger AK, Radford MJ, Wang Y, et al. Thrombolytic therapy in older patients. J Am Coll Cardiol 2000; 36: 366–74.

30. Soumerai SB, McLaughlin TJ, Ross-Degnan D, et al. Effectiveness of thrombolytic therapy for acute myocardial infarction in the elderly: cause for concern in the old-old. Arch Intern Med 2002; 162: 561–8.

31. Stenestrand U, Wallentin L. Fibrinolytic therapy in patients 75 years and older with ST-segment-elevation myocardial infarction: one-year follow-up of a large prospective cohort. Arch Intern Med 2003; 163: 965–71.

32. Alexander KP, Newby LK, Armstrong PW, et al. Acute coronary care in the elderly, part II: ST-segment-elevation myocardial infarction: a scientific statement for healthcare professionals from the American Heart Association Council on Clinical Cardiology: in collaboration with the Society of Geriatric Cardiology. Circulation 2007; 115: 2570–89.

33. Anderson JL, Karagounis L, Allan A, et al. Older age and elevated blood pressure are risk factors for intracerebral hemorrhage after thrombolysis. Am J Cardiol 1991; 68: 166–70.

34. Brass LM, Lichtman JH, Wang Y, et al. Intracranial hemorrhage associated with thrombolytic therapy for elderly patients with acute myocardial infarction: results from the Cooperative Cardiovascular Project. Stroke 2000; 31: 1802–11.

35. Selker HP, Beshansky JR, Schmid CH, et al. Presenting pulse pressure predicts thrombolytic therapy-related intracranial hemorrhage. Thrombolytic Predictive Instrument (TPI) Project results. Circulation 1994; 90: 1657–61.

36. Gruppo Italiano Per Lo Studio Delia Sopravvivenza Nell'Infarto Miocardico: GISSI-2. A factorial randomised trial of alteplase versus streptokinase and heparin versus no heparin among 12490 patients with acute myocardial infarction. Lancet 1990; 336: 65–71.

37. The International Study Group. In-hospital mortality and clinical course of20891 patients with suspected acute myocardial infarction ramdomised between alteplase and streptokinase with or without heparin. Lancet 1990; 336: 71–5.

38. ISIS-3 (Third International Study of Infarct Survival) Collaborative Group. ISIS-3: a randomised comparison of streptokinase vs. tissue plasminogen activator vs. anistreplase and of aspirin plus heparin vs. aspirin alone among 41299 cases of suspected acute myocardial infarction. Lancet 1992; 339: 753–70.

39. The GUSTO Investigators. An international randomized trial comparing four thrombolytic strategies for acute myocardial infarction. N Engl J Med 1993; 329: 673–82.

40. White HD, Barbash GI, Califf RM, et al. Age and outcome with contemporary thrombolytic therapy. Results from the GUSTO-I Trial. Circulation 1996; 94: 1826–33.

41. The Global Use of Strategies to Open Occluded Coronary Arteries (GUSTO III) Investigators. A comparison of reteplase with alteplase for acute myocardial infarction. N Engl J Med 1997; 337: 1118–23.

42. Assessment of the Safety and Efficacy of a New Thrombolytic Investigators. Single-bolus tenecteplase compared with front-loaded alteplase in acute myocardial infarction: the ASSENT-2 double-blind randomised trial. Lancet 1999; 354: 716–22.

43. Hsia J, Hamilton WP, Kleiman N, et al. A comparison between heparin and low-dose aspirin as adjunctive therapy with tissue plasminogen activator for acute myocardial infarction. N Engl J Med 1990; 323: 1433–7.

44. Granger CB, Hirsch J, Califf RM, et al. Activated partial thromboplastin time and outcome after thrombolytic therapy for acute myocardial infarction. Results from the GUSTO-I trial. Circulation 1996; 93: 870–8.

45. Boersma E; The Primary Coronary Angioplasty vs. Thrombolysis Group. Does time matter? A pooled analysis of randomized clinical trials comparing primary percutaneous coronary intervention and in-hospital fibrinolysis in acute myocardial infarction patients. Eur Heart J 2006; 27: 779–88.

46. Simari RD, Berger PB, Bell MR, et al. Coronary angioplasty in acute myocardial infarction: primary, immediate adjunctive, rescue, or deferred adjunctive approach? Mayo Clin Proc 1994; 69: 346–58.

47. deBoer MJ, Ottervanger JP, van't Hof AW, et al. Reperfusion therapy in elderly patients with acute myocardial infarction: a randomized comparison of primary angioplasty and thrombolytic therapy. J Am Coll Cardiol 2002; 39: 1723–8.

48. Goldenberg I, Matetzky S, Halkin A, et al. Primary angioplasty with routine stenting compared with thrombolytic therapy in elderly patients with acute myocardial infarction. Am Heart J 2003; 145: 862–7.

49. Grines C. Senior PAMI: a prospective randomized trial of primary angioplasty and thrombolytic therapy in elderly patients with acute myocardial infarction. Presented at Transcatheter Cardiovascular Therapeutics, Washington DC, October 2005.

50. Wood FO, Leonowicz NA, Vanhecke TE, et al. Mortality in patients with ST-segment elevation myocardial infarction who do not undergo reperfusion. Am J Cardiol 2012; 110: 509–14.

51. Levine GN, Bates ER, Blankenship JC, et al. 2011 ACCF/AHA/SCAI guideline for percutaneous coronary intervention: executive summary. A report of the American College of Cardiology Foundation/American Heart association Task Force on Practice Guidelines and the Society for Cardiovascular Angiography and Interventions. J Am Coll Cardiol 2011; 58: 2550–83.

52. Dzavik V, Sleeper LA, Cocke TP, et al. Early revascularization is associated with improved survival in elderly patients with acute myocardial infarction complicated by cardiogenic shock: a report from the SHOCK Trial Registry. Eur Heart J 2003; 24: 828–37.

53. Barbash GI, Roth A, Hod H, et al. Randomized controlled trial of late-in-hospital angiography and angioplasty versus conservative management after treatment with recombinant tissue-type plasminogen activator in acute myocardial infarction. Am J Cardiol 1990; 66: 538–45.

54. Ellis SG, Mooney MR, George BS, et al. Randomized trial of late elective angioplasty versus conservative management for patients with residual stenoses after thrombolytic treatment of myocardial infarction. Circulation 1992; 86: 1400–6.

55. Simoons ML, Arnold AER, Betriu A, et al. Thrombolysis with tissue plasminogen activator in acute myocardial infarction: no additional benefit from immediate percutaneous coronary angioplasty. Lancet 1988; 1: 197–203.

56. SWIFT (Should We Intervene Following Thrombolysis?) Trial Research Group. SWIFT trial of delayed elective intervention vs. conservative treatment after thrombolysis with anistreplase in acute myocardial infarction. Br Med J 1991; 302: 555–60.

57. TIMI Research Group. Immediate vs. delayed catheterization and angioplasty following thrombolytic therapy for acute myocardial infarction. TIMI IIA results. JAMA 1988; 260: 2849.

58. Topol EJ, Califf RM, George BS, et al. A randomized trial of immediate versus delayed elective angioplasty after intravenous tissue plasminogen activator in acute myocardial infarction. N Engl J Med 1987; 317: 581–8.

59. Scheller B, Hennen B, Hammer B, et al. Beneficial effects of immediate stenting after thrombolysis in acute myocardial infarction. J Am Coll Cardiol 2003; 42: 634–41.

60. Fernandez-Aviles F, Alonso JJ, Castro-Beiras A, et al. Routine invasive strategy within 24 hours of thrombolysis versus ischaemia-guided conservative approach for acute myocardial infarction with ST-segment elevation (GRACIA-1): a randomised controlled trial. Lancet 2004; 364: 1045–53.

61. Madsen JK, Grande P, Saunamaki K, et al. Danish multicenter randomized study of invasive versus conservative treatment in patients with inducible ischemia after thrombolysis in acute myocardial infarction (DANAMI). Circulation 1997; 96: 748–55.

62. Gershlick AH, Stephens-Lloyd A, Hughes S, et al. Rescue angioplasty after failed thrombolytic therapy for acute myocardial infarction. N Engl J Med 2005; 353: 2758–68.

63. Patel TN, Bavry AA, Kumbhani DJ, et al. A meta-analysis of randomized trials of rescue percutaneous coronary intervention after failed fibrinolysis. Am J Cardiol 2006; 97: 1685–90.

64. Wijeysundera HC, Vijayaraghavan R, Nallamothu BK, et al. Rescue angioplasty or repeat fibrinolysis after failed fibrinolytic therapy for ST-segment myocardial infarction. A meta-analysis of randomized trials. J Am Coll Cardiol 2007; 49: 422–30.

65. Cairns JA, Gent M, Singer J, et al. Aspirin, sulfinpyrazone, or both in unstable angina. N Engl J Med 1985; 313: 1369–75.

66. Lewis HD, Davis JW, Archibald DG, et al. Protective effects of aspirin against acute myocardial infarction and death in men with unstable angina. N Engl J Med 1983; 309: 396–403.

67. Patrano C. Aspirin as an antiplatelet drug. N Engl J Med 1994; 330: 1287–94.

68. Antiplatelet Trialists' Collaboration. Collaborative overview of randomised trials of anti-platelet therapy. I Prevention of death, myocardial infarction, and stroke by prolonged antiplatelet treatment in various categories of patients. Br Med J 1994; 308: 81–106.

69. Antithrombotic Trialists' Collaboration. Collaborative meta-analysis of randomised trials of antiplatelet therapy for prevention of death, myocardial infarction, and stroke in high risk patients. BMJ 2002; 324: 71–86.

70. Stein B, Fuster V. Antithrombotic therapy in acute myocardial infarction: Prevention of venous, left ventricular and coronary artery thromboembolism. Am J Cardiol 1989; 64: 33B–40B.

71. Krumholz HM, Hennen J, Ridker PM, et al. Use and effectiveness of intravenous heparin therapy for treatment of acute myocardial infarction in the elderly. J Am Coll Cardiol 1998; 31: 973–9.

72. Collins R, Peto R, Baigent C, et al. Aspirin, heparin, and fibrinolytic therapy in suspected acute myocardial infarction. N Engl J Med 1997; 336: 847–60.

73. Vaitkus PT, Barnathen ES. Embolic potential, prevention and management of mural thrombus complicating anterior myocardial infarction: a meta-analysis. J Am Coll Cardiol 1993; 22: 1004–9.

74. Eikelboom JW, Quinlan DJ, Mehta SR, et al. Unfractionated and low-molecular-weight heparin as adjuncts to thrombolysis in aspirin-treated patients with ST-elevation acute myocardial infarction: a meta-analysis of the randomized trials. Circulation 2005; 112: 3855–67.

75. Alexander KP, Chen AY, Roe MT, et al. Excess dosing of antiplatelet and antithrombin agents in the treatment of non-ST-segment elevation acute coronary syndromes. JAMA 2005; 294: 3108–16.

76. Mehran R, Lansky AJ, Witzenbichler B, et al. Bivalirudin in patients undergoing primary angioplasty for acute myocardial infarction (HORIZONS-AMI): 1-year results of a randomised controlled trial. Lancet 2009; 374: 1149–59.

77. Kushner FG, Hand M, Smith SC Jr, et al. 2009 focused updates: ACC/AHA guidelines for the management of patients with ST-elevation myocardial infarction (updating the 2004 guideline and 2007 focused update) and ACC/AHA/SCAI guidelines on percutaneous coronary intervention (updating the 2005 guideline and 2007 focused update). A report of the American College of Cardiology Foundation/American Heart Association Task Force on Practice Guidelines. Circulation 2009; 120: 2271–306.

78. The EPIC Investigators. Use of a monoclonal antibody directed against the platelet glyco-protein IIb/IIIa receptor in high-risk coronary angioplasty. N Engl J Med 1994; 330: 956–61.

79. The EPILOG Investigators. Platelet glycoprotein IIb/IIIa receptor blockade and low-dose heparin during percutaneous coronary revascularization. N Engl J Med 1997; 336: 1689–96.

80. Platelet Receptor Inhibition in Ischemic Syndrome Management (PRISM) Study Investigators. A comparison of aspirin plus tirofiban with aspirin plus heparin for unstable angina. N Engl J Med 1998; 338: 1498–505.

81. Platelet Receptor Inhibition in Ischemic Syndrome Management in Patients Limited by Unstable Signs and Symptoms (PRISM-PLUS) Study Investigators. Inhibition of the platelet glycoprotein IIb/IIIa receptor with tirofiban in unstable angina and non-Q-wave myocardial infarction. N Engl J Med 1998; 338: 1488–97.

82. The PURSUIT Investigators. Inhibition of platelet glycoprotein IIb/IIIa with eptifibatide in patients with acute coronary syndromes. N Engl J Med 1998; 339: 436–43.

83. Ndrepepa G, Kastrati A, Mehilli J, et al. Age-dependent effect of abciximab in patients with acute coronary syndromes treated with percutaneous coronary interventions. Circulation 2006; 114: 2040–6.

84. De Luca G, Navarese EP, Cassetti E, et al. Meta-analysis of randomized trials of glycoprotein IIb/IIIa inhibitors in high-risk acute coronary syndromes patients undergoing invasive strategy. Am J Cardiol 2011; 107: 198–203.

85. Bertrand ME, Rupprecht HJ, Urban P, et al. Double-blind study of the safety of clopidogrel with and without a loading dose in combination with aspirin compared with ticlopidine in combination with aspirin after coronary stenting: the clopidogrel aspirin stent international cooperative study (CLASSICS). Circulation 2000; 102: 624–9.

86. The Clopidogrel in Unstable Angina to Prevent Recurrent Events Trial Investigators. Effects of clopidogrel in addition to aspirin in patients with acute coronary syndromes without ST-segment elevation. N Engl J Med 2001; 345: 494–502.

87. Wiviott SD, Braunwald E, McCabe CH, et al. Prasugrel versus clopidogrel in patients with acute coronary syndromes. N Engl J Med 2007; 357: 2001–15.

88. Montalescot G, Wiviott SD, Braunwald E, et al. Prasugrel compared with clopidogrel in patients undergoing percutaneous coronary intervention for ST-elevation myocardial infarction (TRITON-TIMI 38): double-blind, randomised controlled trial. Lancet 2009; 373: 723–31.

89. Jneid H, Anderson JL, Wright RS, et al. 2012 ACCF/AHA focused update of the guideline for the management of patients with unstable angina/non-ST-elevation myocardial infarction (updating the 2007 guideline and replacing the 2011 focused update). J am Coll Cardiol 2012; 60: 645–81.

90. Wallentin L, Becker RC, Budaj A, et al. Ticagrelor versus clopidogrel in patients with acute coronary syndromes. N Engl J Med 2009; 361: 1045–57.

91. Gaglia MA Jr, Waksman R. Overview of the 2010 Food and Drug administration Cardiovascular and renal Drugs Advisory Committee meeting regarding ticagrelor. Circulation 2011; 123: 451–6.

92. Cannon CP, Harrington RA, James S, et al. Comparison of ticagrelor with clopidogrel in patients with a planned invasive strategy for acute coronary syndromes (PLATO) : a randomised double-blind study. Lancet 2010; 375: 283–93.

93. Anticoagulants in the Secondary Prevention of Events in Coronary Thrombosis (ASPECT) Research Group. Effect of long-term oral anticoagulant treatment on mortality and cardiovascular morbidity after myocardial infarction. Lancet 1994; 343: 499–503.

94. Smith P, Arnesen H, Holme I. The effect of warfarin on mortality and reinfarction after myocardial infarction. N Engl J Med 1990; 323: 147–52.

95. The Sixty Plus Reinfarction Study Research Group. A double-blind trial to assess long-term oral anticoagulant therapy in elderly patients after myocardial infarction. Lancet 1980; 2: 989–94.

96. Hurlen M, Abdelnoor M, Smith P, et al. Warfarin, aspirin, or both after myocardial infarction. N Engl J Med 2002; 347: 969–74.

97. van Es RF, Jonker JJC, Verheugt FWA, et al. Aspirin and coumadin after acute coronary syndromes (the ASPECT-2 study): a randomised controlled trial. Lancet 2002; 360: 109–13.

98. The Assessment of the Safety and Efficacy of a New Thrombolytic Regimen (ASSENT)-3 Investigators. Efficacy and safety of tenecteplase in combination with enoxaparin, abciximab, or unfractionated heparin: the ASSENT-3 randomised trial in acute myocardial infarction. Lancet 2001; 358: 605–13.

99. Gurwitz JH, Gore JM, Goldberg RJ, et al. Recent age-related trends in the use of thrombolytic therapy in patients who have had acute myocardial infarction. Ann Intern Med 1996; 124: 283–91.

100. Krumholz HM, Murillo JE, Chen J, et al. Thrombolytic therapy for eligible patients with acute myocardial infarction. JAMA 1997; 277: 1683–8.

101. Hjalmarson A, Elmfeldt D, Herlitz J, et al. Effect on mortality of metoprolol in acute myocardial infarction. A double-blind randomised trial. Lancet 1981; 2: 823–7.

102. Roberts R, Rogers WJ, Mueller HS, et al. Immediate vs. deferred β-blockade following thrombolytic therapy in patients with acute myocardial infarction. Results of the Throm-bolysis in Myocardial Infarction (TIMI) II-B Study. Circulation 1991; 83: 422–37.

103. The TIMI Study Group. Comparison of invasive and conservative strategies after treatment with intravenous tissue plasminogen activator in acute myocardial infarction. Results of the Thrombolysis in Myocardial Infarction (TIMI) Phase II Trial. N Engl J Med 1989; 320: 618–27.

104. Wienbergen H, Zeymer U, Gitt AK, et al. Prognostic impact of acute beta-blocker therapy on top of aspirin and angiotensin-converting enzyme inhibitor therapy in consecutive patients with ST-elevation acute myocardial infarction. Am J Cardiol 2007; 99: 1208–11.

105. Piccini JP, Hranitzky PM, Kilaru R, et al. Relation of mortality to failure to prescribe beta blockers acutely in patients with sustained ventricular tachycardia and ventricular fibrillation following acute myocardial infarction (from the VALsartan In Acute myocardial iNfarcTion trial [VALIANT] registry). Am J Cardiol 2008; 102: 1427–32.

106. COMMIT (Clopidogrel and Metoprolol in Myocardial Infarction Trial) Collaborative Group. Early intravenous then oral metoprolol in 45,852 patients with acute myocardial infarction: randomised placebo-controlled trial. Lancet 2005; 366: 1622–32.

107. β-Blocker Heart Attack Trial Research Group. A randomized trial of propranolol in patients with acute myocardial infarction. I Mortality results. JAMA 1982; 247: 1707–14.

108. β-Blocker Heart Attack Trial Research Group. A randomized trial of propranolol in patients with acute myocardial infarction. II Morbidity results. JAMA 1983; 250: 2814–19.

109. The Norwegian Multicenter Study Group. Timolol-induced reduction in mortality and reinfarction in patients surviving acute myocardial infarction. N Engl J Med 1981; 304: 801–7.

110. Gundersen T, Abrahamsen AM, Kjekshus J, et al. Timolol-related reduction in mortality and reinfarction in patients ages 65-75 years surviving acute myocardial infarction. Circulation 1982; 66: 1179–84.

111. Pederson TR; Norwegian Multicenter Study Group. Six-year follow-up of the Norwegian Multicenter Study on timolol after myocardial infarction. N Engl J Med 1985; 313: 1055–8.

112. The CAPRICORN Investigators. Effect of carvedilol on outcome after myocardial infarction in patients with left-ventricular dysfunction: the CAPRICORN randomised trial. Lancet 2001; 357: 1385–90.

113. Soumerai SB, McLaughlin TJ, Spiegelman D, et al. Adverse outcomes of under use of β-blocker in elderly survivors of acute myocardial infarction. JAMA 1997; 277: 115–21.

114. Krumholz H, Radford MJ, Wang Y, et al. National use and effectiveness of β-blockers for the treatment of elderly patients after acute myocardial infarction. JAMA 1998; 280: 623–9.

115. Krumholz HM, Radford MJ, Wang Y, et al. Early β-blocker therapy for acute myocardial infarction in elderly patients. Ann Intern Med 1999; 131: 648–54.

116. Goldman L, Sia STB, Cook EF, et al. Costs and effectiveness of routine therapy with longterm beta-adrenergic antagonists after acute myocardial infarction. N Engl J Med 1988; 319: 152–7.

117. Rochon PA, Tu JV, Anderson GM, et al. Rate of heart failure and 1-year survival for older people receiving low-dose beta-blocker therapy after myocardial infarction. Lancet 2000; 356: 639–44.

118. Yusuf S, Collins R, MacMahon S, et al. Effect of intravenous nitrates on mortality in acute myocardial infarction: an overview of the randomised trials. Lancet 1988; 1: 1088–92.
119. Gruppo Italiano per lo Studio defla Sopravvivenza nell'Infarto Miocardico. GISSI-3: effects of lisinopril and transdermal glyceryl trinitrate singly and together on 6-week mortality and ventricular function after acute myocardial infarction. Lancet 1994; 343: 1115–22.
120. ISIS-4 (Fourth International Study of Infarct Survival) Collaborative Group. ISIS-4: a randomised factorial trial assessing early oral captopril, oral mononitrate and intravenous magnesium sulphate in 58,050 patients with suspected acute myocardial infarction. Lancet 1995; 345: 669–85.
121. Gruppo Italiano per lo Studio della Sopravvivenza nell'Infarto Miocardico. Six-month effects of early treatment with lisinopril and transdermal glyceryl trinitrate singly and together withdrawn six weeks after myocardial infarction: the GISSI-3 Trial. J Am Coll Cardiol 1996; 27: 337–44.
122. Yusuf S, Held P, Furberg C. Update of effects of calcium antagonists in myocardial infarction or angina in light of the Second Danish Verapamil Infarction Trial (DAVIT-II) and other recent studies. Am J Cardiol 1991; 67: 1296–8.
123. Hanse JF. Secondary prevention with calcium antagonists after a myocardial infarction. Arch Intern Med 1993; 153: 2281–2.
124. Gibson RS, Boden WE, Theroux P, et al. Diltiazem and reinfarction in patients with non-Q-wave myocardial infarction. Results of a double-blind, randomized, multicenter trial. N Engl J Med 1986; 315: 423–9.
125. The Multicenter Diltiazem Postinfarction Trial Research Group. The effect of diltiazem on mortality and reinfarction after myocardial infarction. N Engl J Med 1988; 319: 385–92.
126. The Danish Study Group on Verapamil in Myocardial Infarction. Effect of verapamil on mortality and major events after myocardial infarction (The Danish Verapamil Infarction Trial II-DAVIT II). Am J Cardiol 1990; 66: 779–85.
127. Rengo F, Carbonin P, Pahor M, et al. A controlled trial of verapamil in patients after acute myocardial infarction: results of the Calcium Antagonist Reinfarction Italian Study (CRIS). Am J Cardiol 1996; 77: 365–9.
128. Swedburg K, Held P, Kjekshus J, et al. Effects of early adminstration of enalapril on mortality in patients with acute myocardial infarction. Results of the Cooperative New Scandinavian Enalapril Survival Study II (CONSENSUS II). N Engl J Med 1992; 327: 678–84.
129. Ambrosioni E, Borghi C, Magnani B; Survival of Myocardial Infarction Long-Term Evaluation (SMILE) Study Investigators. The effect of the angiotensin-converting-enzyme inhibitor zofenopril on mortality and morbidity after anterior myocardial infarction. N Engl J Med 1995; 332: 80–5.
130. Pfeffer MA, Braunwald E, Moye L, et al. Effect of captopril on mortality and morbidity in patients with left ventricular dysfunction after myocardial infarction. Results of the Survival and Ventricular Enlargement Trial. N Engl J Med 1992; 327: 669–77.
131. The Acute Infarction Ramipril Efficacy (AIRE) Study Investigators. Effect of ramipril on mortality and morbidity of survivors of acute myocardial infarction with clinical evidence of heart failure. Lancet 1993; 342: 821–8.
132. Hall AS, Murray GD, Ball SG; AIREX Study Investigators. Follow-up study of patients randomly allocated ramipril or placebo for heart failure after acute myocardial infarction: AIRE Extension (AIREX) Study. Lancet 1997; 349: 1493–7.
133. Yusuf S, Sleight P, Pogue J, et al. Effects of an angiotensin-converting-enzyme inhibitor, ramipril, on cardiovascular events in high-risk patients. N Engl J Med 2000; 342: 145–53.
134. The EURopean trial on reduction of cardiac events with Perindopril in stable coronary Artery disease Investigators. Efficacy of perindopril in reduction of cardiovascular events among patients with stable coronary artery disease: randomised, double-blind, placebo-controlled, multicentre trial (the EUROPA study). Lancet 2003; 362: 782–8.
135. Krumholz HM, Chen YT, Wang Y, et al. Aspirin and angiotensin-converting enzyme inhibitors among elderly survivors of hospitalization for an acute myocardial infarction. Arch Intern Med 2001; 161: 538–44.
136. Dickstein K, Kjekshus J. Effects of losartan and captopril on mortality and morbidity in high-risk patients after acute myocardial infarction: the OPTIMAAL randomised trial. Lancet 2002; 360: 752–60.
137. Pfeffer MA, McMurray JJV, Velazquez EJ, et al. Valsartan, captopril, or both in myocardial infarction complicated by heart failure, left ventricular dysfunction, or both. N Engl J Med 2003; 349: 1893–906.
138. Pitt B, Remme W, Zannad F, et al. Eplerenone, a selective aldosterone blocker, in patients with left ventricular dysfunction after myocardial infarction. N Engl J Med 2003; 348: 1309–21.
139. Woods KL, Fletcher S, Roffe C, et al. Intravenous magnesium sulphate in suspected acute myocardial infarction: results of the second Leicester Intravenous Magnesium Intervention Trial (LIMIT-2). Lancet 1992; 339: 1553–8.

140. Schechter M, Hod H, Chouraqui P, et al. Magnesium therapy in acute myocardial infarction when patients are not candidates for thrombolytic therapy. Am J Cardiol 1995; 75: 321–3.

141. The MAGIC Trial Investigators. Early administration of intravenous magnesium to high-risk patients with acute myocardial infarction in the Magnesium in Coronaries (MAGIC) Trial: a randomised controlled trial. Lancet 2002; 360: 1189–96.

142. Najjar SS, Rao SV, Melloni C, et al. Intravenous erythropoeitin in patients with ST-segment elevation myocardial infarction REVEAL: a randomized controlled trial. JAMA 2011; 305: 1863–72.

143. Hine LK, Laird N, Hewitt P, et al. Meta-analytic evidence against prophylactic use of lidocaine in acute myocardial infarction. Arch Intern Med 1989; 149: 2694–8.

144. Volpi A, Maggioni A, Franzosi MG, et al. In-hospital prognosis of patients with acute myocardial infarction complicated by primary ventricular fibrillation. N Engl J Med 1987; 317: 257–61.

145. Julian DG, Camm AJ, Frangin G, et al. Randomised trial of effect of amiodarone on mortality in patients with left ventricular dysfunction after recent myocardial infarction: EMIAT. Lancet 1997; 349: 667–74.

146. Cairns JA, Connoly SJ, Roberts R, et al. Canaian Amiodarone Myocardial Infarction Arrhythmia Trial Investigators. Randomised trial of outcome after myocardial infarction in patients with frequent or repetitive ventricular premature depolarisations: CAMIAT. Lancet 1997; 349: 675–82.

147. Amiodarone Trials Meta-Analysis Investigators. Effect of prophylactic amiodarone on mortality after acute myocardial infarction and in congestive heart failure: meta-analysis of individual data from 6500 patients in randomised trials. Lancet 1997; 350: 1417–24.

148. Thomas KL, Al-Khatib SM, Lokhnygina Y, et al. Amiodarone use after acute myocardial infarction complicated by heart failure and/or left ventricular dysfunction may be associated with excess mortality. Am Heart J 2008; 155: 87–93.

149. Moss AJ, Hall WJ, Cannom DS, et al. Improved survival with an implanted defibrillator in patients with coronary disease at high risk for ventricular arrhythmia. Multicenter Automatic Defibrillator Implantation Trial Investigators. N Engl J Med 1996; 335: 1933–40.

150. Moss AJ, Zareba W, Hall WJ, et al. Prophylactic implantation of a defibrillator in patients with myocardial infarction and reduced ejection fraction. N Engl J Med 2002; 346: 877–83.

151. Hohnloser SH, Kuck KH, Dorian P, et al. Prophylactic use of an implantable cardioverter-defibrillator after acute myocardial infarction. N Engl J Med 2004; 351: 2481–8.

152. Steinbeck G, Andresen D, Seidi K, et al. Defibrillator implantation early after myocardial infarction. N Engl J Med 2009; 361: 1427–36.

153. Heart Protection Study Collaborative Group. MRC/BHF Heart Protection Study of cholesterol lowering with simvastatin in 20,536 high-risk individuals: a randomised placebo-controlled trial. Lancet 2002; 360: 7–22.

154. Shepherd J, Blauw GJ, Murphy MB, et al. Pravastatin in elderly individuals at risk of vascular disease (PROSPER): a randomised controlled trial. Lancet 2002; 360: 1623–30.

155. Schwartz GG, Olsson AG, Ezekowitz MD, et al. Effects of atorvastatin on early recurrent ischemic events in acute coronary syndromes: the MIRACL study: a randomized controlled trial. JAMA 2001; 285: 1711–18.

156. Cannon CP, Braunwald E, McCabe CH, et al. Intensive versus moderate lipid lowering with statins after acute coronary syndromes. N Engl J Med 2004; 350: 1495–504.

157. de Lemos JA, Blazing MA, Wiviott SD, et al. Early intensive vs. a delayed conservative simvastatin strategy in patients with acute coronary syndromes. Phase Z of the A to Z Trial. JAMA 2004; 292: 1307–16.

158. Lim SY, Bae EH, Choi JS, et al. Effect on short-and long-term major adverse cardiac events of statin treatment in patients with acute myocardial infarction and renal dysfunction. Am J Cardiol 2012; 109: 1425–30.

159. Rich MW. Epidemiology, pathophysiology, and etiology of congestive heart failure in older adults. J Am Geriatr Soc 1997; 45: 968–74.

160. Bayer AJ, Chadha JS, Farag RR, et al. Changing presentation of myocardial infarction with increasing age. J Am Geriatr Soc 1986; 34: 263–6.

161. Kyriakides ZS, Kelesides K, Melanidis J, et al. Systolic functional response of normal older and younger adult left ventricles to dobutamine. Am J Cardiol 1986; 58: 816–19.

162. Rich MW, Imburgia M. Inotropic response to dobutamine in elderly patients with decom-pensated heart failure. Am J Cardiol 1990; 65: 519–21.

163. Silke B, Verma SP, Midtbo KA, et al. Comparative haemodynamic dose-response effects of dobutamine and amrinone in left ventricular failure complicating acute myocardial infarction. J Cardiovasc Pharmacol 1987; 9: 19–25.

164. Rich MW, Woods WL, Davila-Roman VG, et al. A randomized comparison of intravenous amrinone versus dobutamine in older patients with decompensated congestive heart failure. J Am Geriatr Soc 1995; 43: 271–4.

165. Publication Committee for the VMAC Investigators. Intravenous nesiritide vs nitroglycerin for treatment of decompensated congestive heart failure: a randomized controlled trial. JAMA 2002; 287: 1531–40.
166. Sackner-Bernstein JD, Skopicki HA, Aaronson KD. Risk of worsening renal function with nesiritide in patients withacutely decompensated heart failure. Circulation 2005; 111: 1487–91.
167. Sackner-Bernstein JD, Kowalski M, Fox M, Aaronson K. Short-term risk of death after treatment with nesiritide for decompensated heart failure: a pooled analysis of randomized controlled trials. JAMA 2005; 293: 1900–5.
168. O'Connor CM, Starling RC, Hernandez PW, et al. Effect of nesiritide in patients with acute decompensated heart failure. N Engl J Med 2011; 365: 32–43.
169. Tohmo H, Karanko M, Korpilahti K, et al. Enalaprilat in acute intractable heart failure after myocardial infarction: a prospective, consecutive sample, before-after trial. Crit Care Med 1994; 22: 965–73.
170. Singer DE, Albers GW, Dalen JE, et al. Antithrombotic therapy in atrial fibrillation: the Seventh ACCP Conference on Antithrombotic and Thrombolytic Therapy. Chest 2004; 126: 429S–56S.
171. Neumar RW, Otto CW, Link MS, et al. Part 8: Adult advanced cardiovascular life support: 2010 American Heart Association guidelines for cardiopulmonary resuscitation and emergency cardiovascular care. Circulation 2010; 122: S729–67.
172. Bueno H, Lopez-Palop R, Bermejo J, et al. In-hospital outcome of elderly patients with acute inferior myocardial infarction and right ventricular involvement. Circulation 1997; 96: 436–41.
173. Zehender M, Kasper W, Kauder E, et al. Right ventricular infarction as an independent predictor of prognosis after acute inferior myocardial infarction. N Engl J Med 1993; 328: 981–8.
174. Becker RC, Gore JM, Lambrew C, et al. A composite view of cardiac rupture in the United States National Registry of Myocardial Infarction. J Am Coll Cardiol 1996; 27: 1321–6.
175. Becker RC, Hochman JS, Cannon CP, et al. Fatal cardiac rupture among patients treated with fibrinolytic agents and adjunctive thrombin antagonists: observations from the Thrombolysis and Thrombin Inhibition in Myocardial Infarction 9 Study. J Am Coll Cardiol 1999; 33: 479–87.
176. Solodky A, Behar S, Herz I, et al. Comparison of incidence of cardiac rupture among patients with acute myocardial infarction treated by thrombolysis versus percutaneous transluminal coronary angioplasty. Am J Cardiol 2001; 87: 1105–8.
177. Honan MB, Harrell FE, Reimer KA, et al. Cardiac rupture, mortality and the timing of fibrinolytic therapy: a meta-analysis. J Am Coll Cardiol 1990; 16: 359–67.
178. Oliva PB, Hammill SC, Edwards WD. Cardiac rupture, a clinically predictable complication of acute myocardial infarction: report of 70 cases with clinicopathologic correlations. J Am Coll Cardiol 1993; 22: 720–6.
179. Harrison MR, MacPhail B, Gurley JC, et al. Usefulness of color Doppler flow imaging to distinguish ventricular septal defect from acute mitral regurgitation complicating acute myocardial infarction. Am J Cardiol 1989; 64: 697–701.
180. Smyllie JH, Sutherland GR, Geuskens R, et al. Doppler color flow mapping in the diagnosis of ventricular septal rupture and acute mitral regurgitation after myocardial infarction. J Am Coll Cardiol 1990; 15: 1449–55.
181. Birnbaum Y, Fishbein MC, Blanche C, et al. Ventricular septal rupture after acute myocardial infarction. N Engl J Med 2002; 347: 1426–32.
182. Blanche C, Khan SS, Chaux A, et al. Postinfarction ventricular septal defect in the elderly: analysis and results. Ann Thorac Surg 1994; 57: 1244–7.
183. Clements SD, Story WE, Hurst JW, et al. Ruptured papillary muscle, a complication of myocardial infarction: clinical presentation, diagnosis, and treatment. Clin Cardiol 1985; 8: 93–103.
184. Vlodaver Z, Coe JI, Edwards JE. True and false left ventricular aneurysms. Propensity for the latter to rupture. Circulation 1975; 51: 567–72.
185. Frances C, Romero A, Grady D. Left ventricular pseudoaneurysm. J Am Coll Cardiol 1998; 32: 557–61.
186. Figueras J, Cortadellas J, Evangelista A, Soler-Soler J. Medical management of selected patients with left ventricular free wall rupture during acute myocardial infarction. J Am Coll Cardiol 1997; 29: 512–18.
187. Raitt MH, Kraft CD, Gardner CJ, et al. Subacute ventricular free wall rupture complicating myocardial infarction. Am Heart J 1993; 126: 946–55.
188. Califf RM, Bengtson JR. Cardiogenic shock. N Engl J Med 1994; 330: 1724–30.
189. Menon V, Hochman JS. Management of cardiogenic shock complicating acute myocardial infarction. Heart 2002; 88: 531–7.
190. Leor J, Goldbourt U, Reicher-Reiss H, et al. Cardiogenic shock complicating acute myocardial infarction in patients without heart failure on admission: incidence, risk factors, and outcome. Am J Med 1993; 94: 265–73.

191. Goldberg RJ, Gore JM, Alpert JS, et al. Cardiogenic shock after acute myocardial infarction. Incidence and mortality from a community-wide perspective, 1975 to 1988. N Engl J Med 1991; 325: 1117–22.

192. Berger AK, Radford MJ, Krumholz HM. Cardiogenic shock complicating acute myocardial infarction in elderly patients: does admission to a tertiary center improve survival? Am Heart J 2002; 143: 768–76.

193. Hochman JS, Sleeper LA, Webb JG, et al. Early revascularization in acute myocardial infarction complicated by cardiogenic shock. SHOCK Investigators. Should we emergently revascularize occluded coronaries for cardiogenic shock. N Engl J Med 1999; 341: 625–34.

194. Anderson RD, Ohman EM, Homes DR, et al. Use of intra-aortic balloon counterpulsation in patients presenting with Cardiogenic shock: observations from the GUSTO-I Study. J Am Coll Cardiol 1997; 30: 708–15.

195. Thiele H, Zeymer U, Neumann F-J, et al. Intraaortic balloon support for myocardial infarction with cardiogemic shock. N Engl J Med 2012; 367: 1287–96.

196. Rogers WJ, Frederick PD, Stoehr E, et al. Trends in presenting characteristics and hospital mortality among patients with ST elevation and non-ST elevation myocardial infarction in the National Registry of Myocardial Infarction from 1990 to 2006. Am Heart J 2008; 156: 1026–34.

197. DeWood MA, Spores J, Notske R, et al. Prevalence of total coronary occlusion during the early hours of transmural myocardial infarction. N Engl J Med 1980; 303: 897–902.

198. DeWood MA, Stifter WF, Simpson CS, et al. Coronary arteriographic findings soon after non-Q-wave myocardial infarction. N Engl J Med 1986; 315: 417–23.

199. Keen WD, Savage MP, Fischman DL, et al. Comparison of coronary angiographic findings during the first six hours of non-Q-wave and Q-wave myocardial infarction. Am J Cardiol 1994; 74: 324–8.

200. Berger CJ, Murabito JM, Evans JC, et al. Prognosis after first myocardial infarction. Comparison of Q-wave and non-Q-wave myocardial infarction in the Framingham Heart Study. JAMA 1992; 268: 1545–51.

201. Krone RJ, Friedman E, Thanavaro S, et al. Long-term prognosis after first Q-wave (trans-mural) or non-Q-wave (nontransmural) myocardial infarction: analysis of 593 patients. Am J Cardiol 1983; 52: 234–9.

202. Chung MK, Bosner MS, McKenzie JP, et al. Prognosis of patients is ≥70 years of age with. non-Q-wave acute myocardial infarction compared with younger patients with similar infarcts and with patients ≥70 years of age with Q-wave acute myocardial infarction. Am J Cardiol 1995; 75: 18–22.

203. Braunwald E, Antman EM, Beasley JW, et al. ACC/AHA guideline update for the management of patients with unstable angina and non-ST-segment elevation myocardial infarction-2002: summary article: a report of the American College of Cardiology/American Heart Association Task Force on Practice Guidelines. Circulation 2002; 106: 1893–900.

204. Fragmin and Fast Revascularization during Instability in Coronary artery disease Investigators. Invasive compared with non-invasive treatment in unstable coronary-artery disease: FRISC II prospective randomised multicentre study. Lancet 1999; 354: 708–15.

205. Wallentin L, Lagerqvist B, Husted S, et al. Outcome at 1 year after an invasive compared with a non-invasive strategy in unstable coronary-artery disease: the FRISC II invasive randomized trial. Lancet 2000; 356: 9–16.

206. Cannon CP, Weintraub WS, Demopoulos LA, et al. Comparison of early invasive and conservative strategies in patients with unstable coronary syndromes treated with the glycoprotein IIb/IIIa inhibitor tirofiban. N Engl J Med 2001; 344: 1879–87.

207. Fox KA, Poole-Wilson PA, Henderson RA, et al. Interventional versus conservative treatment for patients with unstable angina or non-ST-elevation myocardial infarction: the British Heart Foundation RITA 3 randomised trial. Randomized Intervention Trial of unstable Angina. Lancet 2002; 360: 743–51.

208. Spacek R, Widimsky P, Straka Z, et al. Value of first day angiography/angioplasty in evolving non-ST segment elevation myocardial infarction: an open multicenter randomized trial. The VINO Study. Eur Heart J 2002; 23: 230–8.

209. Bach RG, Cannon CP, Weintraub WS, et al. The effect of routine, early invasive management on outcome for elderly patients with non-ST-segment elevation acute coronary syndromes. Ann Intern Med 2004; 141: 186–95.

210. deWinter RJ, Windhausen F, Cornel JH, et al. Early invasive versus selectively invasive management for acute coronary syndromes. N Engl J Med 2005; 353: 1095–104.

211. Mehta SR, Cannon CP, Fox KA, et al. Routine vs. selective invasive strategies in aptients with acute coronary syndromes: a collaborative meta-analysis of randomized trials. JAMA 2005; 293: 2908–17.

212. Bhatt DL, Roe MT, Peterson ED, et al. Utilization of early invasive management strategies for high-risk patients with non-ST-segment elevation acute coronary syndromes: results from the CRUSADE Quality Improvement Initiative. JAMA 2004; 292: 2096–104.

213. Krone RJ. The role of risk stratification in the early management of a myocardial infarction. Ann Intern Med 1992; 116: 223–37.

214. Kleiger RE, Miller JP, Bigger JT, et al. Decreased heart rate variability and its association with increased mortality after acute myocardial infarction. Am J Cardiol 1987; 59: 256–62.

215. Toss H, Lindahl B, Siegbahn A, et al. Prognostic influence of increased fibrinogen and C-reactive protein levels in unstable coronary artery disease. Circulation 1997; 96: 4204–10.

216. Tommasi S, Carluccio E, Bentivoglio M, et al. C-reactive protein as a marker for cardiac ischemic events in the year after a first, uncomplicated myocardial infarction. Am J Cardiol 1999; 83: 1595–9.

217. Ciaroni S, Delonca J, Righetti A. Early exercise testing after acute myocardial infarction in the elderly: clinical evaluation and prognostic significance. Am Heart J 1993; 126: 304–11.

218. Jain S, Baird JB, Fischer KC, et al. Prognostic value of dipyridamole thallium imaging after acute myocardial infarction in older patients. J Am Geriatr Soc 1999; 47: 295–301.

219. de la Torre MM, San Roman JA, Bermejo J, et al. Prognostic power of dobutamine echocardiography after uncomplicated acute myocardial infarction in the elderly. Chest 2001; 120: 1200–5.

11

Management of the older patient after myocardial infarction

Wilbert S. Aronow

SUMMARY

After myocardial infarction, elderly patients should have their modifiable coronary risk factors intensively treated. Hypertension should be treated with β-blockers and angiotensin-converting-enzyme (ACE) inhibitors. The blood pressure should be reduced to 130–139/80–89 mm Hg in patients younger than 80 years and to a systolic blood pressure of 140–145 mm Hg if tolerated in patients aged 80 years and older. The serum low-density lipoprotein cholesterol should be reduced with statins to <70 mg/dL. Diabetics should have their hemoglobin A_{1c} reduced to <7.0%. Body mass index should be 18.5–24.9 kg/m^2. Regular aerobic exercise should be performed for 30 minutes daily, preferably seven times a week. Aspirin or clopidogrel, β-blockers, and ACE inhibitors should be administered indefinitely unless there are contraindications to their use. Long-acting nitrates are effective antianginal and anti-ischemic drugs. Patients at very high risk for sudden cardiac death should receive an implantable cardioverter-defibrillator. Hormonal replacement therapy should not be given to postmenopausal women. The two indications for coronary revascularization are prolongation of life and relief of unacceptable symptoms despite optimal medical management.

INTRODUCTION

Coronary artery disease (CAD) is the leading cause of death in older persons. Although persons older than 65 years comprise 12% of the population (1), approximately 60% of hospital admissions for acute myocardial infarction (MI) occur in persons older than 65 years of age, and persons older than 75 years of age account for nearly half of these admissions of patients with MI older than 65 years (2). Not only is the in-hospital mortality higher in older patients with MI than in younger patients with MI, but the postdischarge mortality rate is higher in older persons, with the 1-year cardiac mortality rate of 12% for patients aged 65–75 years and 17.6% for patients older than 75 years (3). Approximately two-thirds of these 1-year deaths were sudden or related to a new MI (3). This chapter discusses the management of the older patient after MI.

CONTROL OF CORONARY RISK FACTORS
Cigarette Smoking

The Chicago Stroke Study demonstrated that current cigarette smokers 65–74 years of age had a 52% higher mortality from CAD than nonsmokers, ex-smokers, and pipe and cigar smokers (4). Ex-smokers who had stopped smoking for 1–5 years had a similar mortality from CAD as did nonsmokers (4). The Systolic Hypertension in the Elderly Program pilot project showed that smoking was a predictor of first cardiovascular event and MI/sudden death (5). At 30-year follow-up of persons 65 years of age and older in the Framingham Study, cigarette smoking was not associated with the incidence of CAD in older men and women but was associated with mortality from CAD in older men and women (6).

At 12-year follow-up of men aged 65–74 years in the Honolulu Heart Program, cigarette smoking was an independent risk factor for nonfatal MI and fatal CAD (7). The absolute excess risk associated with cigarette smoking was 1.9 times higher in older men than in middle-aged men. At 5-year follow-up of 7178 persons 65 years of age or older in three communities, current cigarette smokers had a higher incidence of cardiovascular mortality than nonsmokers (relative risk = 2.0 for men and 1.6 for women) (8). The incidence of cardiovascular death in former smokers was similar to those who had never smoked (8). At 6-year follow-up of older men and women in the Coronary Artery Surgery Study registry, the relative risk of MI or death was 1.5 for persons aged 65–69 years and 2.9 for persons 70 years of age or older who continued smoking compared with quitters during the year before study enrollment (9).

At 40-month follow-up of 664 older men, mean age 80 years, and at 48-month follow-up of 1488 older women, mean age 82 years, current cigarette smoking increased the relative risk of new coronary events (nonfatal or fatal MI or sudden cardiac death) 2.2 times in older men and 2.0 times in older women (Table 11.1) (10). We have also observed that cigarette smoking aggravates angina pectoris and precipitates silent myocardial ischemia in older persons with CAD. At 6-month follow-up of 2231 patients a left ventricular ejection fraction (LVEF) ≤40% after MI, smoking cessation was associated with a significant

Table 11.1 Risk Factors for New Coronary Events in 664 Older Men and in 1488 Older Women

Risk Factor	Relative Risk of New Coronary Events	
	Men	Women
Age	1.04	1.03
Prior coronary artery disease	1.7	1.9
Cigarette smoking	2.2	2.0
Hypertension	2.0	1.6
Diabetes mellitus	1.9	1.8
Obesity	NS	NS
Serum total cholesterol	1.12[a]	1.12[a]
Serum HDL cholesterol	1.70[b]	1.95[c]
Serum triglycerides	NS	1.002

[a]1.12 times higher probability of developing new coronary events for an increment of 10 mg/dL of serum total cholesterol.
[b]1.70 times higher probability of developing new coronary events for a decrement of 10 mg/dL of serum HDL cholesterol.
[c]1.95 times higher probability of developing new coronary events for a decrement of 10 mg/dL of serum HDL cholesterol.
Abbreviations: HDL, high-density lipoprotein; NS, not significant by multivariate analysis.
Source: Adapted from Ref. 10.

reduction in all-cause mortality of 43%, in death or recurrent MI of 32%, and in death or heart failure hospitalization of 35% (11).

On the basis of the available data, older persons who smoke should be strongly encouraged to stop smoking because it will reduce cardiovascular mortality and all-cause mortality after MI. The American College of Cardiology Foundation (ACCF)/American Heart Association (AHA) 2011 guidelines recommend that patients should be asked about tobacco use at every office visit (12). A smoking cessation program should be recommended to smokers. Patients should be advised at every office visit to avoid exposure to environmental tobacco smoke at work, at home, and at public places (12).

Hypertension

Increased peripheral vascular resistance is the cause of systolic and diastolic hypertension in older persons. Systolic hypertension in older persons is diagnosed if the systolic blood pressure is 140 mm Hg or higher on three occasions (13–15). Diastolic hypertension in older persons is diagnosed if the diastolic blood pressure is 90 mm Hg or higher on three occasions (13–15). Isolated systolic hypertension in older persons is diagnosed if the systolic blood pressure is 140 mm Hg or higher on three occasions, and the diastolic blood pressure is normal (13–15). Isolated systolic hypertension occurred in 51% of 499 older persons with hypertension (14).

Isolated systolic hypertension and diastolic hypertension are both associated with increased cardiovascular morbidity and mortality in older persons (15,16). Increased systolic blood pressure is a greater risk factor for cardiovascular morbidity and mortality than is increased diastolic blood pressure (15,16). The higher the systolic or diastolic blood pressure, the greater the morbidity and mortality from CAD in older men and women.

At 30-year follow-up of persons aged 65 years and older in the Framingham Study, systolic hypertension correlated with the incidence of CAD in older men and women (6). Diastolic hypertension correlated with CAD in older men but not in older women (6). At 40-month follow-up of older men and 48-month follow-up of older women, systolic or diastolic hypertension increased the relative risk of new coronary events 2.0 times in men and 1.6 times in women (Table 11.1) (10).

Older persons with hypertension should be treated initially with salt restriction, weight reduction if necessary, cessation of drugs that increase blood pressure, avoidance of alcohol and tobacco, increase in physical activity, reduction of dietary saturated fat and cholesterol, and maintenance of adequate dietary potassium, calcium, and magnesium intake (15).

Antihypertensive drugs have been demonstrated to decrease new coronary events in older men and women with hypertension (Table 11.2) (17–22). Hypertension is present in 69% of patients with a first MI (23). A meta-analysis of 147 randomized trials including 464,000 persons with hypertension showed that β-blockers were the best drugs to use in patients after MI (24).

Persons with prior MI should be treated with β-blockers and angiotensin-converting-enzyme (ACE) inhibitors (13,15,24–32).. If a third drug is needed, aldosterone antagonists may be used based on the EPHESUS trial (33). Patients treated with aldosterone antagonists should not have significant renal dysfunction or hyperkalemia. In an observational prospective study of 1212 older men and women, mean age 80 years, with prior MI and hypertension treated with β-blockers, ACE inhibitors, diuretics, calcium channel blockers, or alpha-blockers, at 40-month follow-up, the incidence of new coronary events in persons treated with one antihypertensive drug was lowest in persons treated with β-blockers or ACE inhibitors (32). In older persons treated with two antihypertensive drugs, the incidence of new coronary events was lowest in persons treated with β-blockers plus ACE inhibitors (32).

Table 11.2   Decrease in New Coronary Events in Older Persons with Hypertension Treated with Antihypertensive Drugs Versus Placebo

Study	Follow-Up	Result
European Working Party on High Blood Pressure in the Elderly (17) (age 60–97 yr)	4.7 yr	Drug therapy caused a 60% reduction in fatal MIs and a 47% reduction in cardiac deaths
Swedish Trial in Old Patients with Hypertension (18) (age 70–84 yr)	25 mo	Drug therapy caused a 25% decrease in fatal MIs and a 67% decrease in sudden deaths
Medical Research Council (19) (age 65–74 yr)	5.8 yr	Drug therapy caused a 19% reduction in coronary events
Systolic Hypertension in the Elderly Program (20) (mean age 72 yr)	4.5 yr	Drug therapy caused a 27% decrease in nonfatal MIs plus coronary deaths
Systolic Hypertension in Europe (21) (mean age 70 yr)	2.0 yr	Drug therapy caused a 26% reduction in fatal and nonfatal cardiac events
Hypertension in the Very Elderly Trial (22) (mean age 83.6 yr)	1.8 yr	Drug therapy caused a 39% reduction in fatal stroke, a 21% reduction in all-cause mortality, and a 64% reduction in heart failure

Abbreviation: MIs, myocardial infarctions.

The benefit of β-blockers in reducing coronary events in older persons with prior MI is especially increased in persons with diabetes mellitus (28), symptomatic peripheral arterial disease (29), abnormal LVEF (27,34), complex ventricular arrhythmias with abnormal LVEF (35) or normal LVEF (36), and with congestive heart failure (CHF) with abnormal LVEF (37) or normal LVEF (38). B-blockers should also be used to treat older persons with hypertension who have angina pectoris (39), myocardial ischemia (40), supraventricular tachyarrhythmias such as atrial fibrillation with a rapid ventricular rate (41), hyperthyroidism (42), preoperative hypertension (13), migraine (13), or essential tremor (13).

In addition to β-blockers, older persons with hypertension and CHF should be treated with diuretics and ACE inhibitors or angiotensin receptor blockers (ARBs) and patients with persistent severe symptoms with aldosterone antagonists (13,33,43,44). ACE inhibitors or ARBs should also be administered to persons with diabetes mellitus, renal insufficiency, or proteinuria (13,15,45). After MI, the blood pressure should be lowered to 130–139/80–89 mm Hg in patients younger than 80 years and the systolic blood pressure to 140–145 mm Hg if tolerated in patients aged 80 years and older (15).

Dyslipidemia
Serum Total Cholesterol
In the Framingham Study, serum total cholesterol was an independent risk factor for CAD in older men and women (46). Among patients aged 65 years or older with prior MI in the Framingham Study, serum total cholesterol was most strongly related to death from CAD and to all-cause mortality (47). Many other studies have documented that a high serum total cholesterol is a risk factor for new coronary events in older men and women (5,10,48–50).

During 9-year follow-up of 350 men and women, mean age 79 years, in the Bronx Aging Study, a consistently increased serum low-density lipoprotein (LDL) cholesterol was associated with the development of MI in older women (51). In the Established Populations for Epidemiologic Studies of the Elderly study, serum total cholesterol was a risk factor for mortality from CAD in older women but not in older men (52). At 40-month follow-up of older men and 48-month follow-up of older women, an increment of 10 mg/dL of serum total cholesterol increased the relative risk of new coronary events 1.12 times in men and 1.12 times in women (Table 11.1) (10).

Serum High-Density Lipoprotein Cholesterol

A low serum high-density lipoprotein (HDL) cholesterol is a risk factor for new coronary events in older men and women (5,10,46,51–54). In the Framingham Study (46), in the Established Populations for Epidemiologic Studies of the Elderly Study (52), and in our study (10), a low serum HDL cholesterol was a more powerful predictor of new coronary events than was serum total cholesterol.

During 9-year follow-up of 350 men and women in the Bronx Aging Study, a consistently low serum HDL cholesterol level was independently associated with the development of MI, cardiovascular disease, or death in men (51). At 40-month follow-up of 664 older men and 48-month follow-up of 1488 older women, multivariate analysis showed that there was a 1.70 times higher probability of developing new coronary events in men and a 1.95 times higher probability of developing new coronary events in women for a decrement of 10 mg/dL of serum HDL cholesterol (Table 11.1) (10).

Serum Triglycerides

Hypertriglyceridemia has been reported to be a risk factor for new coronary events in older women but not in older men (10,46). At 40-month follow-up of older men and at 48-month follow-up of older women, multivariate analysis demonstrated that serum triglycerides was not a risk factor for new coronary events in older men and was a very weak risk factor for new coronary events in older women (Table 11.1) (10).

Drug Therapy of Hypercholesterolemia

At 5.4-year median follow-up of 4444 men and women (1021 aged 65–70 years) with CAD and hypercholesterolemia in the Scandinavian Simvastatin Survival Study, compared with placebo, simvastatin 20–40 mg daily significantly decreased in patients aged 65–70 years total mortality by 34%, CAD mortality by 43%, major coronary events by 34%, nonfatal MI by 33%, any acute CAD-related endpoint by 33%, any atherosclerosis-related endpoint by 34%, and coronary revascularization procedures by 41% (Table 11.3) (55). The absolute risk reduction for both all-cause mortality and CAD mortality was approximately twice as great in persons 65–70 years of age at study entry as in those younger than 65 years (55).

At 5-year follow-up of 4159 men and women (1283 aged 65–75 years) with MI and serum total cholesterol levels below 240 mg/dL but serum LDL cholesterol levels ≥115 mg/dL in the Cholesterol and Recurrent Events trial, compared with placebo, pravastatin 40 mg daily significantly reduced in patients aged 65–75 years CAD death by 45%, CAD death or nonfatal MI by 39%, major coronary events by 32%, coronary revascularization by 32%, and insignificantly reduced unstable angina pectoris by 8% and CHF by 23% (Table 11.3) (56). For every 1000 patients 65 years and older treated for 5 years with pravastatin, 225 cardiovascular hospitalizations would be prevented compared with prevention of 121 cardiovascular hospitalizations in 1000 patients younger than 65 years (56).

At 6.1-year mean follow-up of 9014 men and women (3514 of whom were aged 65–75 years) with MI (64%) or unstable angina pectoris (36%) and serum total cholesterol levels of 155–271 mg/dL in the Long-Term Intervention with Pravastatin in Ischaemic Disease Study, compared with placebo, pravastatin 40 mg daily significantly reduced

Table 11.3 Effects of Lowering Increased Serum Total Cholesterol and Low-Density Lipo-protein Cholesterol Levels by Simvastatin and Pravastatin Versus Placebo in Older Patients with Coronary Artery Disease

Study	Follow-Up (Years)	Results
Scandinavian Simvastatin Survival Study (55) (4444 men and women, 1021 aged 65–70 yr, with CAD and hypercholesterolemia)	5.4	In patients 65 yr and older, compared with placebo, simvastatin decreased all-cause mortality by 34%, CAD mortality by 43%, major coronary events by 34%, nonfatal MI by 33%, any acute CAD-related event by 33%, any atherosclerosis-related endpoint by 34%, and coronary revascularization procedures by 41%
Cholesterol and Recurrent Events trial (56) (4159 men and women, 1283 aged 65–75 yr, with MI and serum total cholesterol <240 mg/dL but serum LDL cholesterol ≥115 mg/dL)	5.0	Compared with placebo, pravastatin decreased CAD death by 45%, CAD death or nonfatal MI by 39%, major coronary events by 32%, coronary revascularization by 32%, stroke by 40%, and insignificantly decreased unstable angina by 8% and congestive heart failure by 23%
Long-Term Intervention with Pravastatin in Ischaemic Disease Study (57) (9014 men and women, 3514 aged 65–75 yr, with MI or unstable angina and mean serum total cholesterol 218 mg/dL)	6.1	Compared with placebo, pravastatin reduced all-cause mortality by 22%, death from CAD by 24%, fatal and nonfatal MI by 29%, death from cardiovascular disease by 25%, need for coronary artery surgery by 22%, need for coronary angioplasty by 19%, hospitalization for unstable angina by 12%, and stroke by 19%
Heart Protection Study (58) (20,536 men and women, 10,697 aged 65–85 yr, with CAD, occlusive arterial disease of noncoronary arteries, diabetes, or treated hypertension and no serum lipid requirement)	5.0	Compared with placebo, simvastatin reduced all-cause mortality by 13%, any vascular mortality by 17%, major coronary events by 27%, any stroke by 25%, any revascularization procedure by 24%, and any major vascular event by 24%

Abbreviations: CAD, coronary artery disease; LDL, low-density lipoprotein; MI, myocardial infarction.

all-cause mortality by 22%, death from CAD by 24%, fatal and nonfatal MI by 29%, death from cardiovascular disease by 25%, need for coronary artery bypass surgery by 22%, need for coronary angioplasty by 19%, hospitalization for unstable angina pectoris by 12%, and stroke by 19% (Table 11.3) (57). The absolute benefits of treatment with pravastatin were greater in groups of persons at higher absolute risk for a major coronary event such as older persons, those with a higher serum LDL cholesterol level, those with a lower serum HDL cholesterol level, and those with a history of diabetes mellitus or smoking (57).

At 5-year follow-up of 20,536 British men and women (10,697 of whom were aged 65–80 years) with either CAD, occlusive arterial disease of noncoronary arteries, diabetes mellitus, or treated hypertension and no serum lipid requirement in the Heart Protection Study, compared with placebo, simvastatin 40 mg daily significantly reduced all-cause mortality by 13%, any vascular mortality by 17%, major coronary events by 27%, any stroke by 25%, any revascularization procedure by 24%, and any major vascular event by 24% (Table 11.3) (58). In the 1263 persons aged 75–80 years at study entry and 80–85 years at follow-up, any major vascular event was significantly reduced 28% by simvastatin. Lowering serum LDL cholesterol from <116 mg/dL to <77 mg/dL by simvastatin caused a 25% significant reduction in vascular events (58).

In the Heart Protection Study, 3500 persons had initial serum LDL cholesterol levels less than 100 mg/dL (58). Decrease of serum LDL cholesterol from 97 mg/dL to 65 mg/dL by simvastatin in these persons caused a similar decrease in risk as did treating patients with higher serum LDL cholesterol levels. The Heart Protection Study Investigators recommended treating persons at high risk for cardiovascular events with statins, regardless of the initial levels of serum lipids, age, or gender (58). In the Study Assessing Goals in the Elderly (SAGE), 893 ambulatory patients with CAD were randomized to atorvastatin 80 mg daily or to pravastatin 40 mg daily (59). At 1-year follow-up, compared with pravastatin, atorvastatin significantly reduced serum LDL cholesterol and significantly reduced all-cause mortality by 67% (59).

On the basis of these data and other data (60–63), the ACCF/AHA guidelines (12) and the updated National Cholesterol Education Program III guidelines (64) state that in very high-risk persons, a serum LDL cholesterol level of <70 mg/dL is a reasonable clinical strategy. When a high-risk person has hypertriglyceridemia or low HDL cholesterol, consideration can be given to combining a fibrate with an LDL cholesterol-lowering drug. (12,64).

Diabetes Mellitus

Diabetes mellitus is a risk factor for new coronary events in older men and in older women (10,65). At 40-month follow-up of older men and 48-month follow-up of older women, diabetes mellitus was found by multivariate analysis to increase the relative risk of new coronary events 1.9 times in men and 1.8 times in women (Table 11.1) (10).

Diabetic patients are more often obese and have higher serum LDL cholesterol and triglycerides levels and lower serum HDL cholesterol levels than do nondiabetics. Diabetics also have a higher prevalence of hypertension and left ventricular hypertrophy than do nondiabetics. These risk factors contribute to the higher incidence of new coronary events in diabetics than in nondiabetics. Diabetics with microalbuminuria have more severe angiographic CAD than diabetics without microalbuminuria (66). Diabetics also have a significant increasing trend of hemoglobin A_{1c} levels over the increasing number of vessels with CAD (67).

Older diabetics after MI should be treated with dietary therapy, weight reduction if necessary, and appropriate drugs if needed to control hyperglycemia. Other coronary risk factors such as smoking, hypertension, dyslipidemia, obesity, and physical inactivity should be controlled. Hypertension should be treated with an ACE inhibitor or by an ARB (13,15,45,68). The serum LDL cholesterol level should be reduced to <70 mg/dL (12,64). Because there are data that show an increased incidence of coronary events and of mortality in diabetics with CAD treated with sulfonylureas (69–71), these drugs should be avoided if possible in postinfarction patients with diabetes mellitus. Metformin should be the initial drug to treat hyperglycemia in most patients (12,72). The hemoglobin A_{1c} level should be reduced to <7% in patients with diabetes mellitus (12). Hypoglycemia must be avoided in patients with CAD. In 10,251 high-risk diabetics in the Action to Control Cardiovascular Risk in Diabetes (ACCORD) Study, patients randomized to a hemoglobin A_{1c} of 6.4% rather than 7.5% had at 3.5-year follow-up a 22% increase in all-cause mortality from 4.0% to 5.9% (73).

Obesity

In the Framingham Study, obesity was an independent risk factor for new coronary events in older men and in older women (65). Disproportionate distribution of fat to the abdomen assessed by the waist-to-hip circumference ratio has also found to be a risk factor for cardiovascular disease, mortality from CAD, and total mortality in older men and women (74,75). At 40-month follow-up of older men and 48-month follow-up of older women, obesity was a risk factor for new coronary events in men and in women by univariate analysis but not by multivariate analysis (Table 11.1) (10).

Obese patients who have had a MI must undergo weight reduction (12). Weight reduction is also a first approach to controlling hyperglycemia, mild hypertension, and dyslipidemia before placing persons on long-term drug therapy. Regular aerobic exercise should be added to diet in treating obesity. The body mass index should be reduced to 18.5 from 24.9 kg/m² (12).

Physical Inactivity

Physical inactivity is associated with obesity, dyslipidemia, hyperglycemia, and hypertension. At 12-year follow-up in the Honolulu Heart Program, physically active men aged 65 years or older had a relative risk of 0.43 for CAD compared with inactive men (76). Exercise training programs are not only beneficial in preventing CAD (77) but also have been shown to improve endurance and functional capacity in older persons after MI (78,79). The goal to be achieved is at least 30 minutes of exercise daily for 7 days per week with a minimum of 5 days of physical exercise per week (12).

ASPIRIN

Aspirin decreases the aggregation of platelets exposed to thrombogenic stimuli by inhibiting the cyclooxygenase enzyme reaction within the platelet and thereby blocking synthesis of thromboxane A_2, a powerful stimulus to platelet aggregation and vasoconstriction (80).

Randomized trials involving 20,006 patients showed that aspirin and other antiplatelet drugs administered to patients after MI decreased the incidence of recurrent MI, stroke, or vascular death by 36 events per 1000 patients treated for 2 years (81). The benefit of aspirin in decreasing MI, stroke, or vascular death in patients after MI was irrespective of age, sex, blood pressure, and diabetes mellitus (81).

Data from the Multicenter Study of Myocardial Ischemia in 936 patients enrolled 1 to 6 months after an acute MI (70% of patients) or unstable angina pectoris (30% of patients) showed at 23-month follow-up that the cardiac mortality rate was 1.6% for aspirin users and 5.4% for nonusers of aspirin (82). Cardiac mortality was reduced 90% in aspirin users who underwent thrombolytic therapy compared with nonusers of aspirin who underwent thrombolytic therapy (82).

The Coumadin Aspirin Reinfarction Study (CARS) randomized 8803 low-risk patients after MI to aspirin 160 mg daily, aspirin 80 mg plus warfarin 1 mg daily, or to aspirin 80 mg plus warfarin 3 mg daily (83). At follow-up, the combined incidence of cardiovascular death, recurrent MI, and stroke was similar in the three treatment groups (74). The incidence of mortality was similar in the three treatment groups. However, the incidence of nonfatal stroke was reduced by aspirin 160 mg daily (83). Data from the Combination Hemotherapy and Mortality and Prevention Study showed in 5059 postinfarction patients that warfarin administered in a dose to achieve an INR of 1.8 combined with low-dose aspirin did not provide a clinical benefit beyond that achieved with aspirin alone (84).

Of 5490 survivors of acute MI aged ≥65 years with no contraindications to aspirin, 4149 patients (76%) received aspirin at the time of hospital discharge (85). At the 6-month follow-up evaluation, aspirin users had a significant 23% reduction in mortality (85).

In an observational prospective study of 1410 patients, mean age 81 years, with prior MI and a serum LDL cholesterol of 125 mg/dL or higher, 832 patients (59%) were treated with aspirin (86). At 3-year follow-up, use of aspirin caused a 52% significant independent reduction in new coronary events (95% CI, 0.41–0.55) (86). Use of statins caused a 54% significant independent reduction in the incidence of new coronary events (95% CI, 0.40–0.53) (86).

On the basis of the available data, all patients should receive aspirin in a dose of 160 mg to 325 mg daily on day 1 of an acute MI and continue aspirin in a dose of 75–162 mg daily for an indefinite period unless there is a specific contraindication to its use (12,87).

Clopidogrel is also an excellent antiplatelet drug which is effective in reducing MI, ischemic stroke, and vascular death in postinfarction patients (88). The ACC/AHA guidelines recommend the use of clopidogrel in postinfarction patients who cannot tolerate aspirin for an indefinite period unless there is a specific contraindication to its use (12,87).

ANTICOAGULANTS

The routine use of warfarin after MI is controversial (89). However, three well-controlled studies have shown a reduction in mortality and/or morbidity in patients receiving long-term oral anticoagulation therapy after MI (90–92). The Sixty Plus Reinfarction Study Group reported at 2-year follow-up after MI of patients, mean age 68 years, that compared with placebo, acenocoumarin or phenprocoumon caused a 26% nonsignificant decrease in mortality, a 55% significant reduction in recurrent MI, and a 40% nonsignificant decrease in stroke (90). The Warfarin Reinfarction Study Group showed at 37-month follow-up after MI of patients 75 years of age or younger that compared with placebo, warfarin caused significant reductions in mortality (24%), recurrent MI (34%), and stroke (55%) (91). The Anticoagulation in the Secondary Prevention of Events in Coronary Thrombosis Research Group reported at 37-month follow-up after MI of patients, mean age 61 years, that compared with placebo, nicoumalone or phenprocoumon caused a 10% nonsignificant decrease in mortality, a 53% significant reduction in recurrent MI, and a 42% significant decrease in stroke (92).

The ACCF/AHA guidelines recommend as Class I indications for long-term oral anticoagulant therapy after MI (*i*) secondary prevention of MI in post-MI patients unable to tolerate daily aspirin or clopidogrel; (*ii*) in post-MI patients with persistent atrial fibrillation; and (*iii*) post-MI patients with LV thrombus (12,87). Long-term warfarin should be administered in a dose to achieve an INR between 2.0 and 3.0 (12,87).

β-BLOCKERS

B-blockers are very effective antianginal and anti-ischemic agents and should be administered to all patients with angina pectoris or silent myocardial ischemia due to CAD unless there are specific contraindications to their use (39). Teo et al. (93) analyzed 55 randomized controlled trials comprising 53,268 patients that investigated the use of β-blockers after MI. B-blockers significantly decreased mortality by 19% in these studies (93). A randomized, double-blind, placebo-controlled study of propranolol in high-risk survivors of acute MI at 12 Norwegian hospitals showed a 52% reduction in sudden cardiac death in persons treated with propranolol for 1 year (94).

Table 11.4 shows that metoprolol (85), timolol (96,97), and propranolol (98) caused a greater decrease in mortality after MI in older persons than in younger persons. The reduction in mortality after MI in patients treated with β-blockers was due both to a reduction in sudden cardiac death and recurrent MI (96–98). In persons with an LVEF ≤40% after MI, compared with placebo, persons aged 25–90 years randomized to carvedilol had a 23% significant reduction in mortality at 1.3-year follow-up (99). A retrospective cohort study also showed that MI patients aged 60–89 years treated with metoprolol had an age-adjusted mortality decrease of 76% (100).

Table 11.4   Effect of β-Blockers on Mortality After Myocardial Infarction

Study	Follow-Up	Results
Goteborg Trial (95)	90 day	Compared with placebo, metoprolol caused a 21% nonsignificant decrease in mortality in patients <65 yr and a 45% significant decrease in mortality in patients 65–74 yr
Norwegian Multicenter Study (96)	17 mo (up to 33 mo)	Compared with placebo, timolol caused a 31% significant reduction in mortality in persons <65 yr and a 43% significant reduction in mortality in persons 65–74 yr
Norwegian Multicenter Study (97)	61 mo (up to 72 mo)	Compared with placebo, timolol caused a 13% nonsignificant decrease in mortality in persons <65 yr and a 19% significant decrease in mortality in persons 65–74 yr
β-Blocker Heart Attack Trial (98)	25 mo (up to 36 mo)	Compared with placebo, propranolol caused a 19% nonsignificant reduction in mortality in persons <60 yr and a 33% significant reduction in mortality in persons 60–69 yr
CAPRICORN Trial (99)	1.3 yr	In patients, mean age 63 yr (range 25–90 yr) with a left ventricular ejection fraction ≤40% after myocardial infarction, compared with placebo, carvedilol caused a 23% significant reduction in mortality

In the B-Blocker Heart Attack Trial, propranolol caused a 27% decrease in mortality in patients with a history of CHF and a 25% decrease in mortality in patients without CHF (101). In this study, propranolol caused a 47% reduction in sudden cardiac death in patients with a history of CHF and a 13% reduction in sudden cardiac death in patients without CHF (101).

In the B-Blocker Pooling Project, results from nine studies involving 3519 patients with CHF at the time of acute MI demonstrated that β-blockers caused a 25% decrease in mortality (102). In the Multicenter Diltiazem Postinfarction Trial, the 2.5-year risk of total mortality in patients with an LVEF <30% was 24% for patients receiving β-blockers (relative risk = 0.53) versus 45% for patients not receiving β-blockers (103). β-blockers have also been found to reduce mortality in patients with CAD and CHF associated with an LVEF ≤35% (37,104–106) or ≥40% (38,105).

An observational prospective study was performed in 477 patients, mean age 79 years, with prior MI and an LVEF <40% (mean LVEF 31%) (27). At 34-month follow-up, patients treated with β-blockers without ACE inhibitors had a 25% significant reduction in new coronary events and a 41% significant reduction in CHF (27). At 41-month follow-up, patients treated with both β-blockers and ACE inhibitors had a significant 37% reduction in new coronary events and a significant 60% reduction in CHF (27).

A retrospective analysis of the use of β-blockers after MI in a New Jersey Medicare population from 1987 to 1992 showed that only 21% of older persons after MI without contraindications to β-blockers were treated with β-blockers (107). Older patients who were treated with β-blockers after MI had a 43% decrease in 2-year mortality and a 22% decrease in 2-year cardiac hospital readmissions than older patients who were not treated with β-blockers (107). Use of a calcium channel blocker instead of a β-blocker after MI doubled the risk of mortality (107).

B-blockers have also been demonstrated to reduce mortality in older patients with complex ventricular arrhythmias after MI and an LVEF ≥40% (36) or ≤40% (35). The decrease in mortality in older patients with heart disease and complex ventricular arrhythmias caused by propranolol is due more to an anti-ischemic effect than to an antiarrhythmic effect (40). In these patients, propranolol also markedly decreased the circadian variation of ventricular arrhythmias (108), abolished the circadian variation of myocardial ischemia (109), and abolished the circadian variation of sudden cardiac death or fatal MI (110).

A meta-analysis of trials also showed that the use of β-blockers after non-Q-wave MI is likely to reduce mortality and recurrent MI by 25% (111). Therefore, older patients with Q-wave MI or non-Q-wave MI without contraindications to β-blockers should be treated with β-blockers for at least 6 years after MI. β-blockers with intrinsic sympathomimetic activity should not be used. The ACCF/AHA guidelines recommend that patients without a clear contraindication to β-blocker therapy should receive β-blockers within a few days of MI (if not initiated acutely) and continue them indefinitely (12,87). Carvedilol, metoprolol succinate, and bisoprolol are recommended (12).

NITRATES
Long-acting nitrates are effective antianginal and anti-ischemic drugs (112). These drugs should be administered along with β-blockers to patients after MI who have angina pectoris. The dose of oral isosorbide dinitrate prescribed should be gradually increased to a dose of 30–40 mg administered three times daily if tolerated. Isosorbide-5-mononitrate in a dose of 60 mg may also be administered once daily. To avoid nitrate tolerance, there should be a nitrate-free interval of 12 hours each day (113). B-blockers should be used to prevent angina pectoris and rebound myocardial ischemia during the nitrate-free interval.

ANGIOTENSIN-CONVERTING-ENZYME INHIBITORS
ACE inhibitors improve symptoms, quality of life, and exercise tolerance in patients with CHF and an abnormal LVEF (114) or a normal LVEF (115). An overview of 32 randomized trials comprising 7105 patients with CHF showed that ACE inhibitors reduced mortality by 23% and mortality or hospitalization for CHF by 35% (116). Patients who develop CHF after MI should be treated with ACE inhibitors unless there are specific contraindications to their use.

Table 11.5 shows that ACE inhibitors reduce mortality in patients after MI (26,117–121). In the Survival and Ventricular Enlargement Trial, asymptomatic patients with an LVEF ≤40% treated with captopril 3–16 days after MI had at 42-month follow-up compared with placebo, a 19% reduction in mortality, a 21% decrease in death from cardiovascular causes, a 37% reduction in development of severe CHF, a 22% decrease in development of CHF requiring hospitalization, and a 25% reduction in recurrent MI (117). Captopril decreased mortality independent of age, sex, blood pressure, LVEF, and use of thrombolytic therapy, aspirin, or β-blockers (117). In the Heart Outcomes Prevention Evaluation Study, 9217 patients aged ≥55 years (55% aged ≥65 years) with MI (53%), cardiovascular disease (88%), or diabetes mellitus (38%) but no CHF or abnormal LVEF were randomized to ramipril 10 mg daily or placebo (26). At 4.5-year follow-up, compared with placebo, ramipril significantly reduced the incidence of MI, stroke, and cardiovascular death by 22% (95% CI, 0.70–0.86) (26). At 4.2-year follow-up of

Table 11.5 Effect of Angiotensin-Converting-Enzyme Inhibitors on Mortality in Patients After Myocardial Infarction

Study	Follow-Up	Results
Survival and Ventricular Enlargement Trial (117)	42 mo (up to 60 mo)	In patients with MI and LVEF ≤40%, compared with placebo, captopril reduced mortality 8% in patients aged ≤55 yr, 13% in patients aged 56–64 yr, and 25% in patients aged ≥65 yr
Acute Infarction Ramipril Efficacy Study (118)	15 mo	In patients with MI and clinical evidence of CHF, compared with placebo, ramipril decreased mortality 2% in patients aged <65 yr and 36% in patients aged ≥65 yr
Survival of Myocardial Infarction Long-Term Evaluation Trial (119)	1 yr	In patients with anterior MI, compared with placebo, zofenopril reduced mortality or severe CHF 32% in patients aged <65 yr and 39% in patients aged ≥65 yr
Trandolapril Cardiac Evaluation Study (120)	24–50 mo	In patients, mean age 68 yr, with LVEF ≤35%, compared with placebo, trandolapril reduced mortality 33% in patients with anterior MI and 14% in patients without anterior MI
Heart Outcomes Prevention Evaluation Study (26)	4.5 yr (up to 6 yr)	In patients aged ≥55 yr with MI (53%), cardiovascular disease (88%), or diabetes (38%) but no CHF or abnormal LVEF, ramipril reduced MI, stroke, and cardiovascular death 22%
EUROPA study (121)	4.2 yr	In patients, mean age 60 yr, with prior MI, compared with placebo, perindopril significantly reduced cardiovascular death, MI, or cardiac arrest by 20%

Abbreviations: CHF, congestive heart failure; LVEF, left ventricular ejection fraction; MI, myocardial infarction.

13,655 patients with prior MI and stable CAD in the EUROPA trial, compared with placebo, patients randomized to perindopril had a 20% significant reduction in cardiovascular death, recurrent MI, or cardiac arrest (121).

On the basis of the available data, ACE inhibitors should be administered to all patients after MI unless there are specific contraindications to their use (12,87).

ALDOSTERONE ANTAGONISTS

At 16-month follow-up of 6632 patients after MI with an LVEF ≤40% and either CHF or diabetes mellitus treated with ACE inhibitors or ARBs and 75% with β-blockers, compared with placebo, patients randomized to eplerenone 50 mg daily had a significant 15% reduction in mortality and a 13% significant reduction in death from cardiovascular causes or hospitalization for cardiovascular events (122). The ACCF/AHA guidelines recommend an aldosterone antagonist in patients after MI treated with ACE inhibitors plus β-blockers if they have an LVEF ≤40% with either CHF or diabetes mellitus if they do not have significant renal dysfunction or hyperkalemia (12).

CALCIUM CHANNEL BLOCKERS

Teo et al. (93) analyzed randomized controlled trials comprising 20,342 patients that investigated the use of calcium channel blockers after MI. Mortality was insignificantly higher (relative risk = 1.04) in patients treated with calcium channel blockers (93). A meta-analysis of randomized, clinical trials of the use of calcium channel blockers in patients with MI, unstable angina pectoris, and stable angina pectoris showed that the relative risk for mortality in the trials using dihydropyridines such as nifedipine that increase heart rate was 1.16 (123). The calcium channel blockers diltiazem and verapamil which reduce heart rate had no effect on survival (123).

Furberg et al. (124) performed a meta-analysis of the effect of nifedipine on mortality in 16 randomized secondary prevention clinical trials in patients with CAD. In this study, the relative risk for mortality was 1.06 for patients treated with nifedipine 30 mg to 50 mg daily, 1.18 for patients treated with nifedipine 60 mg daily, and 2.83 for patients treated with nifedipine 80 mg daily (124).

The Multicenter Diltiazem Postinfarction Trial demonstrated at 25-month follow-up in patients after MI that compared with placebo, diltiazem caused no significant effect on mortality or recurrent MI (125). However, in patients with pulmonary congestion at baseline or an LVEF <40%, diltiazem caused a significant increase in new cardiac events (hazard ratios = 1.41 and 1.31, respectively) (125). In this study, diltiazem also increased the incidence of late-onset CHF in patients with an LVEF <40% (126). Use of a calcium channel blocker instead of a β-blocker after MI in a New Jersey Medicare population also doubled the risk of mortality (107).

Since no calcium channel blocker has been shown to improve survival after MI except for the subgroup of patients with normal LVEF treated with verapamil in the Danish Verapamil Infarction Trial II (127), calcium channel blockers should not be used in the treatment of patients after MI. However, if patients after MI have persistent angina pectoris despite treatment with β-blockers and nitrates, a nondihydropyridine calcium channel blocker such as verapamil or diltiazem should be added to the therapeutic regimen if the LVEF is normal. If the LVEF is abnormal, amlodipine or felodipine should be added to the therapeutic regimen. The ACC/AHA guidelines state that there are no Class I indications for the use of calcium channel blockers after MI (87).

ANTIARRHYTHMIC THERAPY
Class I Drugs

A meta-analysis of 59 randomized controlled trials comprising 23,229 patients that investigated the use of quinidine, procainamide, disopyramide, imipramine, moricizine, lidocaine, tocainide, phenytoin, mexiletine, aprindine, encainide, and flecainide after MI demonstrated that mortality was significantly higher in patients receiving class I antiarrhythmic drugs than in patients receiving no antiarrhythmic drugs (odds ratio = 1.14) (93). None of the 59 studies showed a decrease in mortality by class I antiarrhythmic drugs (93).

In the Cardiac Arrhythmia Suppression Trials I and II, older age also increased the likelihood of adverse effects including death in patients after MI receiving encainide, flecainide, or moricizine (128). Compared with no antiarrhthmic drug, quinidine or procainamide did not decrease mortality in older patients with CAD, normal or abnormal LVEF, and presence versus absence of ventricular tachycardia (129). On the basis of the available data, patients after MI should not receive class I antiarrhythmic drugs.

d, l-Sotalol and d-Sotalol

Studies comparing the effect of d, l-sotalol with placebo on mortality in patients with complex ventricular arrhythmias have not been performed. Compared with placebo, d, l-sotalol did not reduce mortality in post-MI patients followed for 1 year (130). In the Survival with Oral d-Sotalol (SWORD) trial, 3121 survivors of MI with an LVEF ≤40% were randomized to d-sotalol or placebo (131). Mortality was significantly higher at 148-day follow-up in patients treated with d-sotalol (5.0%) than in patients treated with placebo (3.1%) (131). On the basis of the available data, d, l-sotalol and d-sotalol, should not be used to treat patients after MI.

Amiodarone

In the European Myocardial Infarction Amiodarone Trial, 1486 survivors of MI with an LVEF ≤40% were randomized to amiodarone (743 patients) or to placebo (743 patients) (132). At 2-year follow-up, 103 patients treated with amiodarone and 102 patients treated with placebo had died (132). In the Canadian Amiodarone Myocardial Infarction Arrhythmia Trial, 1202 survivors of MI with nonsustained ventricular tachycardia or complex ventricular arrhythmias were randomized to amiodarone or to placebo (133). Amiodarone was very effective in suppressing ventricular tachycardia and complex ventricular arrhythmias. However, the mortality rate at 1.8-year follow-up was not significantly different in the patients treated with amiodarone or placebo (133). In addition, early permanent discontinuation of drug for reasons other than outcome events occurred in 36% of patients taking amiodarone (133).

In the Sudden Cardiac Death in Heart Failure Trial (SCD-HEFT), 2521 patients, mean age 60 years, with Class II or III CHF, an LVEF of ≤35%, and a mean QRS duration on the resting ECG of 120 ms, were randomized to placebo, amiodarone or an automatic implantable cardioverter-defibrillator (AICD) (134). At 46-month median follow-up, compared with placebo, amiodarone insignificantly increased mortality by 6% (134). At 46-month median follow-up, compared with placebo, ICD therapy significantly reduced all-cause mortality by 23% (134).

In the Cardiac Arrest in Seattle: Conventional Versus Amiodarone Drug Evaluation Study, the incidence of pulmonary toxicity was 10% at 2 years in patients receiving amiodarone in a mean dose of 158 mg daily (135). The incidence of adverse effects for amiodarone also approaches 90% after 5 years of therapy (136). On the basis of the available data, amiodarone should not be used in the treatment of patients after MI.

β-Blockers

However, β-blockers have been demonstrated to reduce mortality in patients with nonsustained ventricular tachycardia or complex ventricular arrhythmias after MI in patients with normal or abnormal LVEF (35,36,137,138). On the basis of the available data, β-blockers should be used in the treatment of older patients after MI, especially if nonsustained ventricular tachycardia or complex ventricular arrhythmias are present, unless there are specific contraindications to their use.

Automatic Implantable Cardioverter-Defibrillator

In the Antiarrhythmics Versus Implantable Defibrillators (AVID) trial, 1016 patients, mean age 65 years, with a history of ventricular fibrillation or serious sustained ventricular tachycardia were randomized to an AICD or to drug therapy with amiodarone or d, l-sotalol (139). Patients treated with an AICD had a 39% reduction in mortality at 1 year, a 27% decrease in mortality at 2 years, and a 31% reduction in mortality at three years (139). If patients after MI have life-threatening ventricular tachycardia or ventricular fibrillation, an AICD should be inserted. The efficacy of the AICD implanted for ventricular fibrillation or recurrent sustained ventricular tachycardia on survival is similar in older and younger patients (140).

The Multicenter Automatic Defibrillator Implantation Trial (MADIT) randomized 196 patients with prior MI, an LVEF ≤35%, a documented episode of asymptomatic non-sustained ventricular tachycardia, and inducible ventricular tachycardia or ventricular fibrillation not suppressed by intravenous procainamide or an equivalent drug at electro-physiologic study to conventional medical therapy or implantation of an AICD (141). At 27-month follow-up, patients treated with an AICD had a 54% reduction in mortality (132). These data favor the prophylactic implantation of an AICD in post-MI patients at very high risk for sudden cardiac death.

MADIT II randomized 1232 patients, mean age 64 years, with a prior MI and an LVEF of ≤30% to an AICD or to conventional medical therapy (142). At 20-month follow-up, compared with conventional medical therapy, the AICD significantly reduced all-cause mortality from 19.8% to 14.2% (hazard ratio = 0.69; 95% CI, 0.51–0.93) (142). The effect of AICD therapy in improving survival was similar in patients stratified according to age, sex, LVEF, New York Heart Association class, and QRS interval (142).

In MADIT II, the reduction in sudden cardiac death in patients treated with an AICD was significantly reduced by 68% in 574 patients aged <65 years ($p = 0.02$), by 65% in 455 patients aged 65–74 years ($p = 0.005$), and by 68% in 204 patients aged ≥75 years ($p = 0.05$) (143). The median survival in 348 octogenarians treated with AICD therapy was >4 years (144). These data favor considering the prophylactic implantation of an AICD in postinfarction patients with an LVEF of ≤30%.

HORMONE REPLACEMENT THERAPY

The Heart Estrogen/Progestin Replacement Study (HERS) investigated in 2763 women with documented CAD the effect of hormonal replacement therapy versus double-blind placebo on coronary events (145). At 4.1-year follow-up, there were no significant differences between hormonal replacement therapy and placebo in the primary outcome (nonfatal MI or CAD death) or in any of the secondary cardiovascular outcomes. However, there was a 52% significantly higher incidence of nonfatal MI or death from CAD in the first year in patients treated with hormonal replacement therapy (relative hazard = 1.52; 95% CI, 1.01–2.29) than in patients treated with placebo (145). Women on hormonal replacement herapy had a significantly higher incidence of venous thromboembolic events (relative hazard = 2.89, 95% CI, 1.50–5.58) and a significantly higher incidence of gallbladder disease requiring surgery (relative hazard = 1.38, 95% CI, 1.00–1.92) than women on placebo.

The Estrogen Replacement and Atherosclerosis trial randomized 309 postmenopausal women, mean age 66 years, with coronary angiographic evidence of significant CAD to estrogen plus progestin, estrogen alone, or double-blind placebo (146). At 3.2-year follow-up, quantitative coronary angiography showed no between-group differences in progression of coronary atherosclerosis (146).

At 6.8-year follow-up in the HERS trial, hormonal replacement therapy did not reduce the risk of cardiovascular events in women with CAD (147). The investigators concluded that hormonal replacement therapy should not be used to reduce the risk of coronary events in women with CAD (147). At 6.8-year follow-up in the HERS trial, all-cause mortality was insignificantly increased 10% by hormonal replacement therapy (relative hazard = 1.10; 95% CI, 0.92–1.31) (147). The overall incidence of venous thromboembolism at 6.8-year follow-up was significantly increased 208% by hormonal replacement therapy (relative hazard = 2.08; 95% CI, 1.28–3.40) (148). At 6.8-year follow-up, the overall incidence of biliary tract surgery was significantly increased 48% (relative hazard = 1.48; 95% CI, 1.12–1.95), the overall incidence for any cancer was insignificantly increased 19% (relative hazard = 1.19; 95% CI, 0.95–1.50), and the overall incidence for any fracture was insignificantly increased 4% (relative hazard = 1.04; 95% CI, 0.92–1.31) (148).

The estrogen plus progestin component of the Women's Health Initiative (WHI) study included 16,608 healthy postmenopausal women aged 50–79 years with an intact uterus who were randomized to estrogen plus progestin or to placebo (149). At 5.2-year follow-up, this component of the WHI study was prematurely discontinued because the excess risk of events included in the global index was 19 per 10,000 person-years (149). Absolute excess risks per 10,000 person-years included seven more coronary events, eight more strokes, eight more episodes of pulmonary embolism, and eight more invasive breast cancers, while absolute risk reductions per 10,000 person-years were six fewer colorectal cancers and five fewer hip fractures (149).

On the basis of the available data, hormonal replacement therapy should not be used in postmenopausal women with CAD (87).

INFLUENZA VACCINATION

Evidence from cohort studies and a randomized clinical trial indicate that annual vaccination against seasonal influenza prevents cardiovascular morbidity and mortality in patients with cardiovascular disease (150). The ACCF/AHA guidelines recommend influenza immunization with inactivated vaccine administered intramuscularly as part of secondary prevention in persons with CAD or other atherosclerotic vascular disease with a Class I indication (12,150).

CORONARY REVASCULARIZATION

Medical therapy alone is the preferred treatment in older patients after MI. The two indications for coronary revascularization in older patients after MI are prolongation of life and relief of unacceptable symptoms despite optimal medical management (151). In a prospective study of 305 patients aged ≥75 years with chest pain refractory to at least two antianginal drugs, 150 patients were randomized to optimal medical therapy and 155 patients to invasive therapy (152,153). In the invasive group, 74% had coronary revascularization (54% coronary angioplasty and 20% coronary artery bypass graft surgery). During the 6-month follow-up, one-third of the medically treated group needed coronary revascularization for uncontrollable symptoms. At 6-month follow-up, death, nonfatal MI, or hospital admission for an acute coronary syndrome was significantly higher in the medically treated group (49%) than in the invasive group (19%) (152,153). However, a randomized trial of 2287 patients with stable CAD and myocardial ischemia treated with optimal medical therapy alone or optimal medical therapy plus percutaneous coronary intervention showed at 4.6-year follow-up no significant difference in death, MI, or other major cardiovascular events (154). Revascularization by percutaneous coronary intervention (chap. 13) or by coronary artery bypass graft surgery (chap. 12) is extensively discussed elsewhere. If coronary revascularization is performed, aggressive medical therapy must be continued.

REFERENCES

1. Stenson WB, Sanders CA, Smith HC. Cardiovascular care of the elderly: economic considerations. J Am Coll Cardiol 1987; 10:18A–21A.
2. Weaver WD, Litwin PE, Martin JS, et al. Effect of age on the use of thrombolytic therapy and mortality in acute myocardial infarction. J Am Coll Cardiol 1991; 18: 657–62.
3. Smith SC Jr, Gilpin E, Ahnve S, et al. Outlook after acute myocardial infarction in the very elderly compared with that in patients aged 65 to 75 years. J Am Coll Cardiol 1990; 16: 784–92.
4. Jajich CL, Ostfield AM, Freeman DH Jr. Smoking and coronary heart disease mortality in the elderly. JAMA 1984; 252: 2831–4.
5. Siegel D, Kuller L, Lazarus NB, et al. Predictors of cardiovascular events and mortality in the Systolic Hypertension in the Elderly Program pilot project. Am J Epidemiol 1987; 126: 385–99.
6. Kannel WB, Vokonas PS. Primary risk factors for coronary heart disease in the elderly: The Framingham Study. In: Wenger NK, Furberg CD, Pitt B, eds. Coronary Heart Disease in the Elderly. New York: Elsevier Science Publishing Co, Inc, 1986: 60–92.

7. Benfante R, Reed D, Frank J. Does cigarette smoking have an independent effect on coronary heart disease incidence in the elderly? Am J Public Health 1991; 81: 897–9.
8. LaCroix AZ, Lang J, Scherr P, et al. Smoking and mortality among older men and women in three communities. N Engl J Med 1991; 324: 1619–25.
9. Hermanson B, Omenn GS, Kronmal RA, Gersh BJ. Beneficial six-year outcome of smoking cessation in older men and women with coronary artery disease. Results from the CASS registry. N Engl J Med 1988; 319: 1365–9.
10. Aronow WS, Ahn C. Risk factors for new coronary events in a large cohort of very elderly patients with and without coronary artery disease. Am J Cardiol 1996; 77: 864–6.
11. Shah AM, Pfeffer MA, Hartley LH, et al. Risk of all-cause mortality, recurrent myocardial infarction, and heart failure hospitalization associated with smoking status following myocardial infarction with left ventricular dysfunction. Am J Cardiol 2010; 106: 911–16.
12. Smith SC Jr, Benjamin EJ, Bonow RO, et al. AHA/ACCF secondary prevention and risk reduction therapy for patients with coronary and other atherosclerotic vascular disease: 2011 update. A guideline from the American Heart Association and American College of Cardiology Foundation. Endorsed by the World Heart Federation and the Preventive Cardiovascular Nurses Association. J Am Coll Cardiol 2011; 58: 2432–46.
13. 2003 Joint National Committee. The Seventh Report of the Joint National Committee on the Detection, Evaluation, and Treatment of High Blood Pressure (JNC VII). JAMA 2003; 289: 2560–72.
14. Aronow WS, Ahn C, Kronzon I, Koenigsberg M. Congestive heart failure, coronary events and atherothrombotic brain infarction in elderly blacks and whites with systemic hypertension and with and without echocardiographic and electrocardiographic evidence of left ventricular hypertrophy. Am J Cardiol 1991; 67: 295–9.
15. Aronow WS, Fleg JL, Pepine CJ, et al. ACCF/AHA 2011 expert consensus document on hypertension in the elderly: a report of the American College of Cardiology Foundation Task Force on Clinical Expert Consensus Documents. Developed in collaboration with the American Academy of Neurology, American Geriatrics Society, American Society for Preventive Cardiology, American Society of Hypertension, Association of Black Cardiologists, and European Society of Hypertension. J Am Coll Cardiol 2011; 57: 2037–114.
16. Applegate WB, Rutan GH. Advances in management of hypertension in older persons. J Am Geriatr Soc 1992; 40: 1164–74.
17. Amery A, Birkenhager W, Brixko P, et al. Mortality and morbidity results from the European Working Party on Hypertension in Elderly Trial. Lancet 1985; 1: 1349–54.
18. Dahlof B, Lindholm LH, Hansson L, et al. Morbidity and mortality in the Swedish Trial in Old Patients with Hypertension (STOP Hypertension). Lancet 1991; 338: 1281–5.
19. MRC Working Party. Medical Research Council Trial of treatment of hypertension in older adults: principal results. Brit Med J 1992; 304: 405–12.
20. SHEP Cooperative Research Group. Prevention of stroke by antihypertensive drug treatment in older persons with isolated systolic hypertension: final results of the Systolic Hypertension in the Elderly Program (SHEP). JAMA 1991; 265: 3255–64.
21. Staessen JA, Fagard R, Thijs L, et al. Randomised double-blind comparison of placebo and active treatment for older patients with isolated systolic hypertension. Lancet 1997; 350: 757–64.
22. Beckett NS, Peters R, Fletcher AE, et al. HYVET Study Group. Treatment of hypertension in patients 80 years of age or older. N Engl J Med 2008; 358: 1887–98.
23. Lloyd –Jones D, Adams R, Carnethon M, et al. Heart disease and stroke statistics—2009 update: a report from the American Heart association Statistics Committee and Stroke Statistics Stroke Subcommittee. Circulation 2009; 119: e21–e181.
24. Law MR, Morris JK, Wald NJ. Use of blood pressure lowering drugs in the prevention of cardiovascular disease: meta-analysis of 147 randomised trials in the context of expectations from prospective epidemiological studies. Brit Med J 2009; 339: b1665.
25. Smith SC Jr, Allen J, Blair SN, et al. ACC/AHA guidelines for secondary prevention for patients with coronary and other atherosclerotic vascular disease: 2006 update: endorsed by the National Heart, Lung, and Blood Institute. Circulation 2006; 113: 2363–72.
26. HOPE (Heart Outcomes Prevention Evaluation) Study Investigators. Effects of an angiotensin-converting-enzyme inhibitor, ramipril, on cardiovascular events in high-risk patients. N Engl J Med 2000; 342: 145–53.
27. Aronow WS, Ahn C, Kronzon I. Effect of beta blockers alone, of angiotensin-converting enzyme inhibitors alone, and of beta blockers plus angiotensin-converting enzyme inhibitors on new coronary events and on congestive heart failure in older persons with healed myocardial infarcts and asymptomatic left ventricular systolic dysfunction. Am J Cardiol 2001; 88: 1298–300.

28. Aronow WS, Ahn C. Effect of beta blockers on incidence of new coronary events in older persons with prior myocardial infarction and diabetes mellitus. Am J Cardiology 2001; 87: 780–1.

29. Aronow WS, Ahn C. Effect of beta blockers on incidence of new coronary events in older persons with prior myocardial infarction and symptomatic peripheral arterial disease. Am J Cardiol 2001; 87: 1284–6.

30. Pahor M, Psaty BM, Alderman MH, et al. Health outcomes associated with calcium antagonists compared with other first-line antihypertensive therapies: a meta-analysis of randomised controlled trials. Lancet 2000; 356: 1949–54.

31. ALLHAT Officers and Coordinators for the ALLHAT Collaborative Research Group. Major cardiovascular events in hypertensive patients randomized to doxazosin vs chlorthalidone. The Antihypertensive and Lipid-Lowering Treatment to Prevent Heart Attack Trial (ALLHAT). JAMA 2000; 283: 1967–75.

32. Aronow WS, Ahn C. Incidence of new coronary events in older persons with prior myocardial infarction and systemic hypertension treated with beta blockers, angiotensin-converting enzyme inhibitors, diuretics, calcium antagonists, and alpha blockers. Am J Cardiol 2002; 89: 1207–9.

33. Pitt B, White H, Nicolau J, et al. Eplerenone reduces mortality 30 days after randomization following acute myocardial infarction in patients with left ventricular systolic dysfunction and heart failure. J Am Coll Cardiol 2005; 46: 425–31.

34. Furberg CD, Hawkins CM, Lichstein E; For the Beta-Blocker Heart Attack Trial Study Group. Effect of propranolol in postinfarction patients with mechanical or electrical complications. Circulation 1984; 69: 761–5.

35. Kennedy HL, Brooks MM, Barker AH, et al. Beta-blocker therapy in the Cardiac Arrhythmia Suppression Trial. Am J Cardiol 1994; 74: 674–80.

36. Aronow WS, Ahn C, Mercando AD, et al. Effect of propranolol versus no antiarrhythmic drug on sudden cardiac death, total cardiac death, and total death in patients ≥62 years of age with heart disease, complex ventricular arrhythmias, and left ventricular ejection fraction ≥40%. Am J Cardiol 1994; 74: 267–70.

37. MERIT-HF Study Group. Effect of metoprolol CR/XL in chronic heart failure: metoprolol CR/XL Randomised Intervention Trial in Congestive Heart Failure (MERIT-HF). Lancet 1999; 353: 2001–7.

38. Aronow WS, Ahn C, Kronzon I. Effect of propranolol versus no propranolol on total mortality plus nonfatal myocardial infarction in older patients with prior myocardial infarction, congestive heart failure, and left ventricular ejection fraction ≥40% treated with diuretics plus angiotensin-converting-enzyme inhibitors. Am J Cardiol 1997; 80: 207–9.

39. Aronow WS, Frishman WH. Angina in the elderly. In: Aronow WS, Fleg J, Rich MW, eds. Cardiovascular Disease in the Elderly, 4th edn. New York: Informa Healthcare, 2008: 269–92.

40. Aronow WS, Ahn C, Mercando AD, et al. Decrease of mortality by propranolol in patients with heart disease and complex ventricular arrhythmias is more an anti-ischemic than an antiarrhythmic effect. Am J Cardiol 1994; 74: 613–15.

41. Aronow WS. Management of the older person with atrial fibrillation. J Gerontol Med Sci 2002; 57A: M352–63.

42. Aronow WS. The heart and thyroid disease. In: Gambert SR, ed. Clinics in Geriatric Medicine. Thyroid Disease. Philadelphia: W. B. Saunders Co, 1995: 219–29.

43. Jessup M, Abraham WT, Casey DE, et al. 2009 focused update: ACCF/AHA guidelines for the diagnosis and management of heart failure in adults: a report of the American College of Cardiology Foundation/American Heart Association Task Force on Practice Guidelines: developed in collaboration with the International Society for Heart and Lung Transplantation. Circulation 2009; 119: 1977–2016.

44. Aronow WS. Epidemiology, pathophysiology, prognosis, and treatment of systolic and diastolic heart failure. Cardiol Rev 2006; 14: 108–24.

45. American Diabetes Association. Treatment of hypertension of adults with diabetes. Diabetes Care 2003; 26: 580–2.

46. Castelli WP, Wilson PWF, Levy D, Anderson K. Cardiovascular disease in the elderly. Am J Cardiol 1989; 63: 12H–9H.

47. Wong ND, Wilson PWF, Kannel WB. Serum cholesterol as a prognostic factor after myocardial infarction: the Framingham Study. Ann Intern Med 1991; 115: 687–93.

48. Benfante R, Reed D. Is elevated serum cholesterol level a factor for coronary heart disease in the elderly? JAMA 1990; 263: 393–6.

49. Barrett-Connor E, Suarez L, Khaw K-T, et al. Ischemic heart disease risk factors after age 50. J Chron Dis 1984; 37: 903–8.

50. Rubin SM, Sidney S, Black DM, et al. High blood cholesterol in elderly men and the excess risk for coronary heart disease. Ann Intern Med 1990; 113: 916–20.

51. Zimetbaum P, Frishman WH, Ooi WL, et al. Plasma lipids and lipoproteins and the incidence of cardiovascular disease in the very elderly. The Bronx Aging Study. Arterioscler Thromb 1992; 12: 416–23.
52. Corti M-C, Guralnik JM, Salive ME, et al. HDL cholesterol predicts coronary heart disease mortality in older persons. JAMA 1995; 274: 539–44.
53. Aronow WS, Ahn C. Correlation of serum lipids with the presence or absence of coronary artery disease in 1,793 men and women aged ≥62 years. Am J Cardiol 1994; 73: 702–3.
54. Lavie CJ, Milani RV. National Cholesterol Education Program's recommendations, and implications of "missing" high-density lipoprotein cholesterol in cardiac rehabilitation programs. Am J Cardiol 1991; 68: 1087.
55. Miettinen TA, Pyorala K, Olsson AG, et al. Cholesterol-lowering therapy in women and elderly patients with myocardial infarction or angina pectoris. Findings from the Scandinavian Simvastatin Survival Study (4S). Circulation 1997; 96: 4211–18.
56. Lewis SJ, Moye LA, Sacks FM, et al. Effect of pravastatin on cardiovascular events in older patients with myocardial infarction and cholesterol levels in the average range. Results of the Cholesterol and Recurrent Events (CARE) trial. Ann Intern Med 1998; 129: 681–9.
57. The Long-Term Intervention with Pravastatin in Ischaemic Disease (LIPID) Study Group. Prevention of cardiovascular events and death with pravastatin in patients with coronary heart disease and a broad range of initial cholesterol levels. N Engl J Med 1998; 339: 1349–57.
58. Heart Protection Study Collaborative Group. MRC/BHF Heart Protection Study of cholesterol lowering with simvastatin in 20,536 high-risk individuals: a randomised placebo-controlled trial. Lancet 2002; 360: 7–22.
59. Deedwania P, Stone PH, Merz CNB, et al. Effects of intensive versus moderate lipid-lowering therapy on myocardial ischemia in older patients with coronary heart disease. Results of the Study Assessing Goals in the Elderly (SAGE). Circulation 2007; 115: 700–7.
60. Cannon CP, Braunwald E, McCabe CH, et al. Comparison of intensive and moderate lipid lowering with statins after acute coronary syndromes. N Engl J Med 2004; 350: 1495–504.
61. LaRosa JC, Grundy SM, Waters DD, et al. Intensive lipid lowering with atorvastatin in patients with stable coronary disease. N Eng J Med 2005; 352: 1425–35.
62. Aronow WS, Ahn C. Incidence of new coronary events in older persons with prior myocardial infarction and serum low-density lipoprotein cholesterol ≥125 mg/dL treated with statins versus no lipid-lowering drug. Am J Cardiol 2002; 89: 67–9.
63. Nissen SE, Tuzcu EM, Schoenhagen P, et al. Effect of intensive compared with moderate lipid-lowering therapy on progression of coronary atherosclerosis. A randomized controlled trial. JAMA 2004; 291: 1071–80.
64. Grundy SM, Cleeman JI, Merz CN, et al. Implications of recent clinical trials for the National Cholesterol Education Program Adult Treatment Panel III guidelines. Circulation 2004; 110: 227–39.
65. Gregoratos G, Leung G. Diabetes mellitus and cardiovascular disease in the elderly. In: Aronow WS, Fleg JL, eds. Cardiovascular Disease in the Elderly, 3rd edn. revised and expanded. New York: Marcel Dekker, 2004: 163–88.
66. Sukhija R, Aronow WS, Kakar P, et al. Relation of microalbuminuria and coronary artery disease in patients with and without diabetes mellitus. Am J Cardiol 2006; 98: 279–81.
67. Ravipati G, Aronow WS, Ahn C, et al. Association of hemoglobin A1c level with the severity of coronary artery disease in patients with diabetes mellitus. Am J Cardiol 2006; 97: 968–9.
68. Brenner BM, Cooper ME, de Zeeuw D, et al. Effects of losartan on renal and cardiovascular outcomes in patients with type 2 diabetes and nephropathy. N Engl J Med 2001; 345: 861–9.
69. Garratt KN, Brady PA, Hassinger NL, et al. Sulfonylurea drugs increase early mortality in patients with diabetes mellitus after direct angioplasty for acute myocardial infarction. J Am Coll Cardiol 1999; 33: 119–24.
70. O'Keefe JH, Blackstone EH, Sergeant P, McCallister BD. The optimal mode of coronary revascularization for diabetics. Eur Heart J 1998; 19: 1696–703.
71. Aronow WS, Ahn C. Incidence of new coronary events in older persons with diabetes mellitus and prior myocardial infarction treated with sulfonylureas, insulin, metformin, and diet alone. Am J Cardiol 2001; 88: 556–7.
72. Qaseem A, Humphrey LL, Sweet DE, et al. Oral pharmacologic treatment of type 2 diabetes mellitus: a clinical practice guideline from the American College of Physicians. Ann Intern Med 2012; 156: 218–31.
73. The Action to Control Cardiovascular Risk in Diabetes Study Group. Effects of intensive glucose lowering in type 2 diabetes. N Engl J Med 2008; 358: 2545–59.
74. Kannel WB, Cupples LA, Ramaswami R, et al. Regional obesity and risk of cardiovascular disease. J Clin Epidemiol 1991; 44: 183–90.

75. Folsom AR, Kaye SA, Sellers TA, et al. Body fat distribution and 5-year risk of death in older women. JAMA 1993; 269: 483–7.

76. Donahue RP, Abbott RD, Reed DM, Yano K. Physical activity and coronary heart disease in middle-aged and elderly men: the Honolulu Heart Program. Am J Public Health 1988; 78: 683–5.

77. Wenger NK. Physical inactivity as a risk factor for coronary heart disease in the elderly. Cardiol Elderly 1994; 2: 375–9.

78. Williams MA, Maresh CM, Aronow WS, et al. The value of early out-patient cardiac exercise programmes for the elderly in comparison with other selected age groups. Eur Heart J 1984; 5:113–15.

79. Aronow WS. Exercise therapy for older persons with cardiovascular disease. Am J Geriatr Cardiol 2001; 10: 245–52.

80. Cairns JA, Theroux P, Lewis HD Jr, et al. Antithrombotic agents in coronary artery disease. Chest 1998; 114(Suppl): 611S–33S.

81. Antithrombotic Trialists' Collaboration. Collaborative meta-analysis of randomised trials of antiplatelet therapy for prevention of death, myocardial infarction, and stroke in high risk patients. Br Med J 2002; 324: 71–86.

82. Goldstein RE, Andrews M, Hall WJ, et al. Marked reduction in long-term cardiac deaths with aspirin after a coronary event. J Am Coll Cardiol 1996; 28: 326–30.

83. Coumadin Aspirin Reinfarction Study (CARS) Investigators. Randomised double-blind trial of fixed low-dose warfarin with aspirin after myocardial infarction. Lancet 1997; 350: 389–96.

84. Fiore LD, Ezekowitz MD, Brophy MT, et al. Combination Hemotherapy and Mortality Prevention (CHAMP) Study Group. Department of Veterans Affairs Cooperative Studies Program Clinical Trial comparing combined warfarin and aspirin with aspirin alone in survivors of acute myocardial infarction: primary results of the CHAMPs study. Circulation 2002; 105: 557–63.

85. Krumholz HM, Radford MJ, Ellerbeck EJ, et al. Aspirin for secondary prevention after acute myocardial infarction in the elderly: prescribed use and outcome. Ann Intern Med 1996; 124: 292–8.

86. Aronow WS, Ahn C. Reduction of coronary events with aspirin in older patients with prior myocardial infarction treated with and without statins. Heart Dis 2002; 4: 159–61.

87. Smith SC Jr, Blair SN, Bonow RO, et al. AHA/ACC guidelines for preventing heart attack and death in patients with atherosclerotic cardiovascular disease: 2001 update. A statement for healthcare professionals from the American Heart Association and the American College of Cardiology. J Am Coll Cardiol 2001; 38: 1581–3.

88. CAPRIE Steering Committee. A randomised, blinded, trial of clopidogrel versus aspirin in patients at risk of ischaemic events (CAPRIE). Lancet 1996; 348: 1329–39.

89. Chalmers TC, Matta RJ, Smith H Jr, Kunzler A-M. Evidence favoring the use of anticoagulants in the hospital phase of acute myocardial infarction. N Engl J Med 1977; 297: 1091–6.

90. The Sixty Plus Reinfarction Study Group. A double-blind trial to assess long-term oral anticoagulant therapy in elderly patients after myocardial infarction. Lancet 1980; 2: 989–94.

91. Smith P, Arnesen H, Holme I. Effect of warfarin on mortality and reinfarction after myocardial infarction. N Engl J Med 1990; 323: 147–52.

92. Anticoagulants in the Secondary Prevention of Events in Coronary Thrombosis (ASPECT) Research Group. Effects of long-term oral anticoagulant treatment on mortality and cardiovascular morbidity after myocardial infarction. Lancet 1994; 343: 499–503.

93. Teo KK, Yusuf S, Furberg CD. Effects of prophylactic antiarrhythmic drug therapy in acute myocardial infarction. An overview of results from randomized controlled trials. JAMA 1993; 270: 1589–95.

94. Hansteen V. Beta blockade after myocardial infarction: the Norwegian Propranolol Study in high-risk patients. Circulation 1983; 67: I-57–60.

95. Hjalmarson A, Elmfeldt D, Herlitz J, et al. Effect on mortality of metoprolol in acute myocardial infarction. Lancet 1981; 2: 823–7.

96. Gundersen T, Abrahamsen AM, Kjekshus J, et al. Timolol-related reduction in mortality and reinfarction in patients ages 65-75 years surviving acute myocardial infarction. Circulation 1982; 66: 179–1184.

97. Pedersen TR for the Norwegian Multicentre Study Group. Six-year follow-up of the Norwegian Multicentre Study on Timolol after acute myocardial infarction. N Engl J Med 1985; 313: 1055–8.

98. Beta-Blocker Heart Attack Trial Research Group. A randomized trial of propranolol in patients with acute myocardial infarction. JAMA 1982; 247: 1707–14.

99. The CAPRICORN Investigators. Effect of carvedilol on outcome after myocardial infarction in patients with left-ventricular dysfunction: the CAPRICORN randomised trial. Lancet 2001; 357: 1385–90.

100. Park KC, Forman DE, Wei JY. Utility of beta-blockade treatment for older postinfarction patients. J Am Geriatr Soc 1995; 43: 751–5.

101. Chadda K, Goldstein S, Byington R, Curb JD. Effect of propranolol after acute myocardial infarction in patients with congestive heart failure. Circulation 1986; 73: 503–10.

102. The Beta-Blocker Pooling Project Research Group. The Beta-Blocker Pooling Project (BBPP): subgroup findings from randomised trials in post-infarction patients. Eur Heart J 1988; 9: 8–16.

103. Lichstein E, Hager WD, Gregory JJ, et al. Relation between beta-adrenergic blocker use, various correlates of left ventricular function and the chance of developing congestive heart failure. J Am Coll Cardiol 1990; 16: 1327–32.

104. CIBIS-II Investigators and Committees. The Cardiac Insufficiency Bisoprolol Study II (CIBIS-II): a randomised trial. Lancet 1999; 353: 9–13.

105. Packer M, Coats AJS, Fowler MB, et al. Effect of carvedilol on survival in chronic heart failure. N Engl J Med 2001; 344: 651–8.

106. Flather MD, Shibata MC, Coats AJS, et al. Randomized trial to determine the effect of nevibolol on mortality and cardiovascular hospital admission in elderly patients with heart failure (SENIORS). Eur Heart J 2005; 26: 215–25.

107. Soumerai SB, McLaughlin TJ, Spiegelman D, et al. Adverse outcomes of underuse of beta-blockers in elderly survivors of acute myocardial infarction. JAMA 1997; 277: 115–21.

108. Aronow WS, Ahn C, Mercando AD, Epstein S. Effect of propranolol on circadian variation of ventricular arrhythmias in elderly patients with heart disease and complex ventricular arrhythmias. Am J Cardiol 1995; 75: 514–16.

109. Aronow WS, Ahn C, Mercando AD, Epstein S. Effect of propranolol on circadian variation of myocardial ischemia in elderly patients with heart disease and complex ventricular arrhythmias. Am J Cardiol 1995; 75: 837–9.

110. Aronow WS, Ahn C, Mercando AD, Epstein S. Circadian variation of sudden cardiac death or fatal myocardial infarction is abolished by propranolol in patients with heart disease and complex ventricular arrhythmias. Am J Cardiol 1994; 74: 819–21.

111. Yusuf S, Wittes J, Probstfield J. Evaluating effects of treatment subgroups of patients within a clinical trial: the case of non-Q-wave myocardial infarction and beta blockers. Am J Cardiol 1990; 60: 220–2.

112. Danahy DT, Aronow WS. Hemodynamics and antianginal effects of high dose oral isorbide dinitrate after chronic use. Circulation 1977; 56: 205–12.

113. Parker JO, Farrell B, Lahey KA, Moe G. Effect of interval between doses on the development of tolerance to isosorbide dinitrate. N Engl J Med 1987; 316: 1440–4.

114. Cohn J, Johnson G, Ziesche S, et al. A comparison of enalapril with hydralazine-isosorbide dinitrate in the treatment of chronic congestive heart failure. N Engl J Med 1991; 325: 303–10.

115. Aronow WS, Kronzon I. Effect of enalapril on congestive heart failure treated with diuretics in elderly patients with prior myocardial infarction and normal left ventricular ejection fraction. Am J Cardiol 1993; 71: 602–4.

116. Garg R, Yusuf S; For the Collaborative Group on ACE Inhibitor Trials. Overview of randomized trials of angiotensin-converting enzyme inhibitors on mortality and morbidity in patients with heart failure. JAMA 1995; 273: 1450–6.

117. Pfeffer MA, Braunwald E, Moye LA, et al. Effect of captopril on mortality and morbidity in patients with left ventricular dysfunction after myocardial infarction. Results of the Survival and Ventricular Enlargement Trial. N Engl J Med 1992; 327: 669–77.

118. The Acute Infarction Ramipril Efficacy (AIRE) Study Investigators. Effect of ramipril on mortality and morbidity of survivors of acute myocardial infarction with clinical evidence of heart failure. Lancet 1993; 342: 821–8.

119. Ambrosioni E, Borghi C, Magnani B; For the Survival of Myocardial Infarction Long-Term Evaluation (SMILE) Study Investigators. The effect of the angiotensin-converting-enzyme inhibitor zofenopril on mortality and morbidity after anterior myocardial infarction. N Engl J Med 1995; 332: 80–5.

120. Kober L, Torp-Pedersen C, Carlsen JE, et al. A clinical trial of the angiotensin-converting-enzyme inhibitor trandolapril in patients with left ventricular dysfunction after myocardial infarction. N Engl J Med 1995; 333: 1670–6.

121. The European trial on reduction of cardiac events with perindopril in stable coronary artery disease investigators. Efficacy of perindopril in reduction of cardiovascular events among patients with stable coronary artery disease: randomised, double-blind, placebo-controlled, multicentre trial (the EUROPA study). Lancet 2003; 362: 782–8.

122. Pitt B, Remme W, Zannad F, et al. Eplerenone, a selective aldosterone blocker, in patients with left ventricular dysfunction after myocardial infarction. N Engl J Med 2003; 348: 1309–21.

123. Yusuf S, Held P, Furberg C. Update of effects of calcium antagonists in myocardial infarction or angina in light of the second Danish Verapamil Infarction Trial (DAVIT-II) and other recent studies. Am J Cardiol 1991; 67: 1295–7.

124. Furberg CD, Psaty BM, Meyer JV. Nifedipine: dose-related increase in mortality in patients with coronary heart disease. Circulation 1995; 92: 1326–1.

125. The Multicenter Diltiazem Postinfarction Trial Research Group. The effect of diltiazem on mortality and reinfarction after myocardial infarction. N Engl J Med 1988; 319: 385–92.

126. Goldstein RE, Boccuzzi SJ, Cruess D, et al. Diltiazem increases late-onset congestive heart failure in postinfarction patients with early reduction in ejection fraction. Circulation 1991; 83: 52–60.

127. Danish Study Group on Verapamil in Myocardial Infarction. Trial II-DAVIT II. Effect of verapamil on mortality and major events after acute myocardial infarction. Am J Cardiol 1990; 66: 779–85.

128. Akiyama T, Pawitan Y, Campbell WB, et al. Effects of advancing age on the efficacy and side effects of antiarrhythmic drugs in post-myocardial infarction patients with ventricular arrhythmias. J Am Geriatr Soc 1992; 40: 666–72.

129. Aronow WS, Mercando AD, Epstein S, Kronzon I. Effect of quinidine or procainamide versus no antiarrhythmic drug on sudden cardiac death, total cardiac death, and total death in elderly patients with heart disease and complex ventricular arrhythmias. Am J. Cardiol 1990; 66: 423–8.

130. Julian DJ, Prescott RJ, Jackson FS, Szekely P. Controlled trial of sotalol for one year after myocardial infarction. Lancet 1982; 1: 1142–7.

131. Waldo AL, Camm AJ, deRuyter H, et al. Effect of d-sotalol on mortality in patients with left ventricular dysfunction after recent and remote myocardial infarction. Lancet 1996; 348: 7–12.

132. Julian DG, Camm AJ, Frangin G, et al. Randomised trial of effect of amiodarone on mortality in patients with left-ventricular dysfunction after recent myocardial infarction: EMIAT. Lancet 1997; 349: 667–74.

133. Cairns JA, Connolly SJ, Roberts R, et al. Randomised trial of outcome after myocardial infarction in patients with frequent or repetitive ventricular premature depolarisations: CAMIAT. Lancet 1997; 349: 675–82.

134. Bardy GH, Lee KL, Mark DB, et al. Amiodarone or an implantable cardioverter-defibrillator for congestive heart failure. N Eng J Med 2005; 352: 225–37.

135. Greene HL; For the CASCADE Investigators. The CASCADE study. Randomized antiarrhythmic drug therapy in survivors of cardiac arrest in Seattle. Am J Cardiol 1993; 72: 70F–4F.

136. Herre J, Sauve M, Malone P, et al. Long-term results of amiodarone therapy in patients with recurrent sustained ventricular tachycardia or ventricular fibrillation. J Am Coll Cardiol 1989; 13: 442–9.

137. Friedman LM, Byington RP, Capone RJ, et al. Effect of propranolol in patients with myocardial infarction and ventricular arrhythmia. J Am Coll Cardiol 1986; 7: 8.

138. Norris RM, Barnaby PF, Brown MA, et al. Prevention of ventricular fibrillation during acute myocardial infarction by intravenous propranolol. Lancet 1984; 2: 883–6.

139. The Antiarrhythmics Versus Implantable Defibrillators (AVID) Investigators. A comparison of antiarrhythmic-drug therapy with implantable defibrillators in patients resuscitated from near-fatal ventricular arrhythmias. N Engl J Med 1997; 337: 1576–83.

140. Tresch DD, Troup PJ, Thakur RK, et al. Comparison of efficacy of automatic implantable cardioverter defibrillator in patients older and younger than 65 years of age. Am J Med 1991; 90: 717–24.

141. Moss AJ, Hall WJ, Cannom DS, et al. Improved survival with an implanted defibrillator in patients with coronary disease at high risk for ventricular arrhythmia. N Engl J Med 1996; 335: 1933–40.

142. Moss AJ, Zareba W, Hall WJ, et al. Prophylactic implantation of a defibrillator in patients with myocardial infarction and reduced ejection fraction. N Engl J Med 2002; 346: 877–83.

143. Goldenberg I, Moss AJ. Treatment of arrhythmias and use of implantable cardioverter-defibrillators to improve survival in elderly patients with cardiac disease. In: Aronow WS, ed. Clinics in Geriatric Medicine on Heart Failure. Philadelphia: Elsevier, 2007; 23: 205–19.

144. Koplan BA, Epstein LM, Albert CM, Stevenson WG. Survival in octogenarians receiving implantable defibrillators. Am Heart J 2006; 152: 714–19.

145. Hulley S, Grady D, Bush T, et al. Randomized trial of estrogen plus progestin for secondary prevention of coronary heart disease in postmenopausal women. JAMA 1998; 280: 605–13.

146. Herrington DM, Reboussin DM, Brosnihan B, et al. Effects of estrogen replacement on the progression of coronary-artery atherosclerosis. N Engl J Med 2000; 343: 522–9.

147. Grady D, Herrington D, Bittner V, et al. Cardiovascular disease outcomes during 6.8 years of hormone therapy. Heart and Estrogen/Progestin Replacement Study Follow-up (HERS II). JAMA 2002; 288: 49–57.

148. Hulley S, Furberg C, Barrett-Connor E, et al. Noncardiovascular disease outcomes during 6.8 years of hormone therapy. Heart and Estrogen/Progestin Replacement Study Follow-up (HERS II). JAMA 2002; 288: 58–66.

149. Writing Group for the Women's Health Initiative Investigators. Risks and benefits of estrogen plus progestin in healthy postmenopausal women. Principal results from the Women's Health Initiative randomized controlled trial. JAMA 2002; 288: 321.

150. Davis MM, Taubert K, Benin AL, et al. Influenza vaccination as secondary prevention for cardiovascular disease: a science advisory from the American Heart Association/American College of Cardiology. J Am Coll Cardiol 2006; 48: 1498–502.
151. Stemmer EA, Aronow WS. Surgical management of coronary artery disease in the elderly. In: Aronow WS, Fleg J, Rich MW, eds. Cardiovascular Disease in the Elderly, 4th edn. New York: Informa Healthcare, 2008: 351–85.
152. The TIME Investigators. Trial of invasive versus medical therapy in elderly patients with chronic symptomatic coronary-artery disease (TIME): a randomised trial. Lancet 2001; 358: 951–7.
153. Aronow WS; Commentary. Approach to symptomatic coronary disease in the elderly: TIME to change? Lancet 2001; 358: 945–6.
154. Boden WE, O'Rourke RA, Teo KK, et al. Optimal medical therapy with or without PCI for stable coronary disease. N Engl J Med 2007; 356: 1503–16.

12

Surgical management of coronary artery disease

Melissa M. Anastacio and Jennifer S. Lawton

SUMMARY

The prevalence of coronary artery disease (CAD) increases with age, and older patients tend to have more severe CAD, including multi-vessel disease and left main disease, compared to younger patients. In addition, as the population ages, the number of older adults with clinically significant CAD will continue to rise. Over the past 20 years, morbidity and mortality associated with coronary artery bypass grafting (CABG) in older adults, including those over 80 years of age, have declined progressively due to improved surgical techniques and perioperative care. Moreover, among older adults with severe CAD, CABG provides equivalent or, in many situations, superior long-term outcomes compared to percutaneous coronary intervention or optimal medical therapy. Conversely, the rate of non-fatal peri-operative complications, including stroke, cognitive dysfunction, renal insufficiency, and pulmonary disorders, is higher in elderly patients undergoing CABG compared to younger patients. Very elderly patients with severe left ventricular dysfunction, poor functional status, frailty, dementia, or multiple comorbid conditions may not be suitable candidates for CABG. Thus, the treatment for CAD in older patients must be individualized, but CABG remains a highly effective therapy for improving quality of life and extending functional survival and should be offered to appropriately selected elderly patients with advanced CAD.

EPIDEMIOLOGY OF AGING

According to the US Census Bureau, there were 304,280,000 persons living in the USA in 2010 (1). Over 38.6 million were over the age of 65 years, accounting for 13% of the total population (1).

Older adults are the fastest growing segment of the population. People are living longer and the projected life expectancies are 77.1 years for men and 81.9 years for women in 2020 (2). Baby boomers, born between 1946 and 1964, started turning 65 years in 2011 (3). By 2050, it is estimated that there will be 108 million elderly in the USA (Figs. 12.1–12.3) (4). Women will comprise over 50% of the elderly population (4). The increasing proportion of elderly is evident across all racial groups, a reflection of the overall demographic changes in the USA (3).

The same trend has been observed in the rest of the world. It is expected that the worldwide population of persons over the age of 65 years will increase in developed and developing countries alike (5).

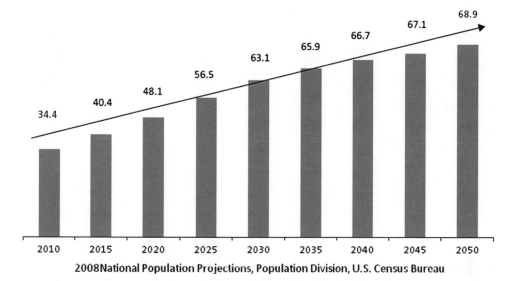

2008National Population Projections, Population Division, U.S. Census Bureau

Figure 12.1 Projected population aged 65–84 years in the United States through 2050. Projected population between the age of 65 and 84 years (in millions) based on the 2008 National Population Projections from the US Census Bureau.

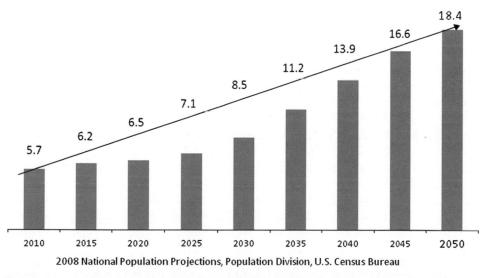
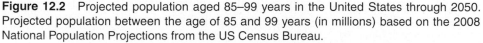

2008 National Population Projections, Population Division, U.S. Census Bureau

Figure 12.2 Projected population aged 85–99 years in the United States through 2050. Projected population between the age of 85 and 99 years (in millions) based on the 2008 National Population Projections from the US Census Bureau.

Prevalence of Coronary Artery Disease in the Elderly

The prevalence of coronary artery disease (CAD), as with most other forms of cardiovascular disease (CVD), increases with age. From 2005 to 2008, an estimated 72% of men and women between the ages of 60 and 79 years had some form of cardiovascular disease (6). There are 16.3 million persons in the USA who carry the diagnosis of CAD (7). By 2030, 40.5% of the US population is projected to have some form of CVD with CAD accounting for 9.3%, an increase of 16.6% from 2010 (8).

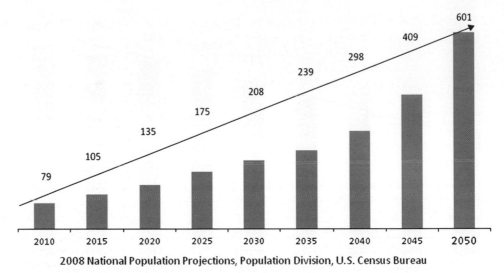

2008 National Population Projections, Population Division, U.S. Census Bureau

Figure 12.3   Projected population aged >100 years in the United States through 2050. Projected population for 100 years and older (in thousands) based on the 2008 National Population Projections from the US Census Bureau.

With the exception of tobacco use, the prevalence of risk factors associated with CAD (including hypertension, hyperlipidemia, diabetes mellitus, obesity, and physical inactivity) also increases with age. The elderly typically present with more of these risk factors and their associated sequelae (9–12). The elderly are also more likely to have severe CAD, left ventricular systolic dysfunction, concomitant valvular disease, previous percutaneous coronary intervention (PCI) or sternotomy, and they are on more cardiovascular medications (9,11,13). Women also represent a greater proportion of these patients.

Morbidity and Mortality of Cardiovascular Disease in the Elderly Population
According to the US Census Bureau, over 14 million elderly persons lived with a disability (hearing, vision, cognitive, ambulatory, self-care, or independent living deficits) in 2009 (14). Approximately 5.3 million were between the ages of 65 and 74 years and 8.9 million were over the age of 75 years. CAD, stroke, and hypertension are among the 15 leading conditions associated with disabilities in an estimated 45 million people with functional disabilities in the USA (6). It is expected that these figures will increase as the elderly population continues to grow.

Cardiovascular disease continues to be the number one cause of all deaths in the USA and CAD is the number one cause of death attributable to CVD (7,15). This is true regardless of gender and regardless of race. Approximately 81% of people who die of CAD are 65 years of age or older (6). Nearly 40% of octogenarians have symptomatic cardiovascular disease, which accounts for more than 50% of the mortality in this age group (16).

Economic Impact of Coronary Artery Disease in the Elderly
CAD imposes a significant economic impact in the elderly. In 2009, CAD accounted for over 14 million ambulatory care visits and 1,537,000 hospital admissions (6). Hospitalization rates increased with age with the highest rates for those over the age of 85 years, among whom women accounted for the majority (6). In 2009, an estimated 416,000 inpatient bypass procedures, 1.1 million PCI procedures, and 1 million diagnostic cardiac catheterizations were performed in the USA (6). The estimated direct and indirect cost of heart

disease in 2008 was $190.3 billion, and from 2010 to 2030, real total direct medical costs of cardiovascular disease are projected to triple from $273 billion to $818 billion (6,8).

The prevalence of CAD in persons over the age of 65 years and its associated morbidity and mortality will continue to grow as the size of the elderly population increases. In addition, older adults increasingly desire longer life with preserved functional capacity and independence. As a result, the role of coronary revascularization, both percutaneous and surgical, as a means to improve quality of life and reduce mortality, is expanding. It is against this backdrop that we will discuss the surgical treatment of CAD in the elderly.

INDICATIONS FOR CORONARY ARTERY BYPASS GRAFTING

Medical therapy and lifestyle modification form the foundation of CAD management regardless of disease severity. Surgical revascularization in the form of coronary artery bypass grafting (CABG) is often required for patients presenting with significant or complex coronary disease and/or symptoms.

The American Heart Association and American College of Cardiology have established guidelines for CABG and PCI (12). Patients with significant stenosis (≥50% diameter) of the left main coronary artery (LMCA) or significant stenosis (≥70%) involving the left anterior descending artery (LAD) and one other major coronary artery or 2- or 3-vessel involvement (≥70%) with or without involvement of the LAD benefit from surgical revascularization (12). Patients with these anatomic lesions involving large viable areas of myocardium or extensive ischemia, decreased left ventricular function (ejection fraction 35–50%), and/or symptoms unrelieved by optimal medical therapy may also benefit from CABG. In addition, CABG is the preferred revascularization strategy in patients with diabetes and multivessel CAD (12,17).

Surgical revascularization in the elderly is associated with several benefits (Table 12.1). Relief of angina has been documented in the elderly in retrospective reviews where 84% of patients following CABG were free of angina (18) as well as in randomized trials when compared to medical management (19) and PCI (20). The elderly also benefit from improved quality of life (19–22), with mid-term quality of life following CABG, which approaches that of the general population (23). Reduced major adverse cardiac events at 6-month follow-up were noted with revascularization (PCI or CABG) in a randomized trial of medical therapy versus invasive treatment (19). Although there have been no randomized trials to document increased survival in the elderly following CABG compared to PCI (24), retrospective reviews have reported improved long-term survival in patients following CABG versus PCI (25) and versus medical therapy (26). In addition, CABG has been demonstrated to provide equivalent long-term survival in patients ≥80 years compared to the age matched general population (23). The same authors reported enhanced survival in women following CABG (6.7 years vs. 5.2 years in men), although only 41% of patients had a left internal mammary artery (LIMA) graft used in this study (24).

Table 12.1 Benefits of CABG in Older Patients

- Relief of angina
- Improved quality of life
- Prevent myocardial infarction
- Improve survival/Prolong life

Abbreviation: CABG, coronary artery bypass grafting.

Notably, elderly patients may not consider survival as the most important factor when considering a revascularization strategy. Higher emphasis may be placed on quality of life, need for transitional care in a nursing home following surgery, the re-intervention rate, and the potential for neurological injury (19,24).

CABG Versus Medical Therapy in the Elderly

The earliest randomized controlled trials, Veteran's Administration Cooperative Study, Coronary Artery Surgery Study (CASS), and European Coronary Surgery Study (ECSS), which evaluated the effectiveness of CABG compared to standard medical therapy consistently demonstrated superiority of CABG in providing symptom relief and survival advantage in high-risk patients (those with 2- or 3-vessel involvement, with or without depressed left ventricular function) (27–32). However, most of these studies excluded patients over the age of 65 years and it is uncertain whether these findings are applicable to the elderly population.

Retrospective studies have documented cost benefit and survival benefit compared to medical therapy in elderly patients undergoing CABG (22,26). In a retrospective review of patients stratified by age (<70 years, 70–79 years, and ≥80 years), Graham and colleagues demonstrated significantly improved adjusted survival in each age group following CABG compared to medical therapy (Fig. 12.4) (26). Interestingly, they also found that the largest risk reduction with invasive revascularization compared to medical therapy was noted in the oldest patients (Fig. 12.4C).

Similarly, in a subgroup analysis of patients over the age of 65 years with 2- or 3-vessel disease from the CASS Registry, CABG provided a survival benefit and improvement in functional status both overall and within each age category (age 65–69 years, 70–74 years, and over 75 years) at 6-year follow-up (33). In a randomized trial with 6-month follow-up comparing medical treatment versus invasive treatment (CABG or PCI) in patients ≥75 years, the TIME Investigators reported that invasive treatment was associated with better relief of angina and improved quality of life versus medical treatment (19). This was similarly observed in MASS II, which included patients over the age of 65 years with 3-vessel disease (≥70% stenosis), ejection fraction (EF) >40%, and documented ischemia who were randomized to CABG or PCI or medical therapy (34). CABG patients had significantly fewer anginal symptoms and lower rates of postoperative myocardial infarction (MI) at 1 year, as well as a survival advantage at 5 years (35). Others have noted that patients (mean age of 62.3 ± 9.8 years) with significant LMCA stenosis (≥50%) and depressed left ventricular function (EF < 45%), who underwent CABG had significantly fewer anginal symptoms and decreased mortality compared to medical therapy or PCI (mean age of 65 ± 10.7 years) (36).

In summary, CABG in the elderly bestows a survival advantage and improvement in functional status over medical therapy in patients with LMCA disease, multi-vessel disease, and those with left ventricular dysfunction.

CABG Versus PCI in the Elderly

The elderly have been excluded from most randomized trials comparing PCI and CABG in the past (27–32). Therefore, much of the available data are from retrospective reviews. Contemporary randomized and observational studies have shown no overall mortality difference between patients who underwent CABG versus PCI (with or without stenting), but there were higher rates of repeat revascularization and decreased improvement in angina symptoms in patients who underwent PCI (37–41). Although these studies included patients who were 65 years and older, they did not have an adequate representation of the elderly, especially those over the age of 70 years.

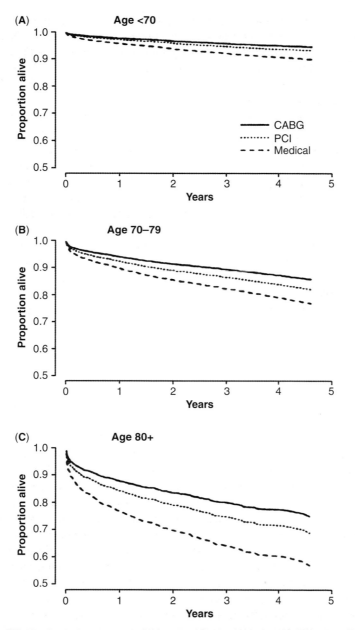

Figure 12.4   Risk-adjusted 5-year survival curves for 3 age groups (<70 years, 70–79 years, >80 years) of patients who underwent revascularization (coronary artery bypass grafting or percutaneous coronary intervention) or medical therapy. There was a statistically significant survival advantage to revascularization compared to medical therapy in all 3 age groups. *Source*: From Ref. 26.

A retrospective study of patients aged 80–89 years undergoing first time CABG with 2- or 3-vessel CAD reported lower in-hospital mortality for PCI versus CABG (3.0% vs. 5.9%) as well as better survival at 6 months following PCI but significantly better survival after 6 months and up to 8 years in CABG patients (25).

A meta-analysis of 66 studies in 65,376 patients over 80 years of age undergoing PCI or CABG reported similar 30 day mortality, as well as1-, 3-, and 5-year survival rates

(7.3%, 86%, 78%, and 68% for CABG and 5.4%, 87%, 78%, and 62% for PCI, respectively) (24). The authors stressed that it remains unknown if octogenarians derive the same survival advantage following CABG as younger patients compared to PCI as older patients have been excluded from large randomized trials designed to answer this question.

The SYNTAX trial, the largest, prospective randomized controlled trial, compared CABG to PCI (with drug-eluting stents) in patients with untreated left main or 3-vessel CAD (mean age 65 years ± 9.7 years) (42). At 1 year, PCI was associated with higher rates of major adverse cardiac or cerebrovascular events (MACCE) (17.8% PCI vs. 12.4% CABG, $p = 0.002$) and higher rates of repeat revascularization (13.5% PCI vs. 5.9% CABG, $p < 0.001$), but CABG was associated with higher rates of stroke. Further subgroup analysis revealed that rates of MACCE (37.3% PCI vs. 21.2% CABG, $p = 0.003$) and rates of repeat revascularization (27.2% PCI vs. 9.2% CABG, $p < 0.001$) were higher in those with SYNTAX scores greater than 33 who underwent PCI. There was no difference in rates of MACCE in patients with low or intermediate SYNTAX scores. For patients with 3-vessel disease, 3-year follow-up revealed continued survival advantage with lower mortality (5.7% vs. 9.5%, $p = 0.002$), lower MACCE rates (20.2% vs. 28%, $p < 0.001$), lower MI rates (3.6% vs. 7.1%, $p = 0.002$), and less need for repeat revascularization (10.7% vs. 19.7%, $p < 0.001$) in the CABG versus PCI group (43). Stroke was no longer significantly different between the two groups. Unlike 3-vessel disease, CABG for LMCA stenosis showed no mortality benefit or difference in MACCE compared to PCI. However, CABG patients had lower rates of repeat revascularization and PCI patients had fewer strokes.

Boudriot and colleagues also showed that 1-year rates of death and MI were similar for patients who underwent PCI or CABG for >50% LMCA stenosis with or without involvement of other coronary arteries (44). Symptom relief was comparable although there were higher rates of revascularization in the PCI group and higher rates of stroke in the CABG group.

Additionally, Weintraub and colleagues analyzed data from the Society of Thoracic Surgeons (STS) Adult Cardiac database and the CathPCI registry linked to data from the Centers for Medicare and Medicaid Services from 2004 to 2008 to compare outcomes for CABG versus PCI (78% received drug eluting stents, 16% had bare metal stents) in patients greater than 65 years of age who underwent elective or urgent revascularization for 2–3-vessel disease without an acute myocardial infarction (<7 days prior to intervention) (45). Although mortality at 1 year was similar between the two treatment groups, there was a survival advantage at 4 years among those who underwent isolated CABG. This benefit was observed in patients regardless of age, race, gender, body mass index, ejection fraction, number of diseased vessels, and presence or absence of diabetes, chronic lung disease, peripheral vascular disease, or renal failure (45).

In summary, multiple studies demonstrate that CABG in the elderly offers a survival advantage, lower incidence of MACCE, and lower repeat revascularization rates in patients with increasing disease severity and complexity.

CABG Outcomes in Older Patients

In an analysis of data from the National Inpatient Sample designed to assess in-hospital outcomes after CABG from 1988 to 2004, the adjusted rate for all CABG-related mortality steadily decreased from 300.3 per 100,000 in 1988 to a rate of 104.69 per 100,000 in 2004 (46). Total mortality also declined from 5.5% to 3.06% irrespective of the presence of heart failure, type 2 diabetes mellitus, or acute myocardial infarction. Improvements in short-term outcomes have been attributed to advances in medical therapy, surgical technique, and postoperative care.

In a review of the STS database, 30-day operative mortality associated with first time isolated CABG was 1.6%, down from 2.1% in 2000 (13). The overall rate of major morbidity or operative mortality in the 2008 STS Report for patients undergoing isolated on-pump CABG was 16.9% (risk adjusted rate 13.6%) (47). The incidence of stroke has also declined to 1.1% from 1.6% in 2000. Rates of reoperation for bleeding, sternal wound infections, and new-onset renal failure have also declined. The STS 2008 Report observed rate of deep sternal wound infection to be 0.4% (risk adjusted 0.3%), respiratory failure manifesting as prolonged intubation was 11.6% (risk adjusted 8.8%), and renal failure 3.7% (risk adjusted 3.2%) (postoperative creatinine >2 mg/dL or doubling of preoperative creatinine) (47). Postoperative atrial fibrillation is the most common cause of morbidity following isolated CABG, occurring in up to 40% of patients (48,49).

Postoperative in hospital morbidity rates in a study of 1062 patients ≥80 years of age who underwent isolated CABG between 1989 and 2001 with mean follow-up of 3.4 years and late follow-up for survival of 5.6 years included: renal insufficiency 9.8%, stroke 3.2%, bleeding 3.2%, MI 1.5%, and deep sternal wound infection 1.5% (50). Overall hospital mortality was 9.7% and declined to 2.2% in past few years. Notably, only 41% of patients received a LIMA graft. Variables that correlated with in hospital mortality using a logistic regression model included: date of surgery, arrhythmia, abnormal EF, renal insufficiency, non-elective surgery, no IMA, and longer cardiopulmonary bypass (CPB) time. Others have found predictors of operative mortality in octogenarians to be chronic renal failure, urgent or emergent CABG, and incomplete revascularization (51).

Alexander and colleagues retrospectively reviewed 4306 patients ≥80 years of age that underwent isolated CABG at 22 centers and compared outcomes to younger patients (52). The octogenarians had higher 30-day mortality (8.1% vs. 3.0%) compared to the younger patients, but in the absence of comorbidities, the mortality rate was similar in octogenarians (4.2%) to younger patients. Predictors of operative mortality included age, emergent surgery, and prior CABG. The incidence of renal failure in octogenarians was 6.9% and the incidence of stroke was 3.9%. In addition, octogenarians had a median postoperative length of hospital stay that was 1 day longer than younger patients. The authors concluded that in-hospital mortality, postoperative neurologic events, and renal failure increased with advancing age with the greatest risk after the age of 75 years (Fig. 12.5) (52).

Older patients undergoing CABG are at increased risk for postoperative cognitive impairment and delirium (53). Risk factors for postoperative cognitive dysfunction include preoperative cognitive impairment, which is present in 20–46% of older patients referred for CABG, older age, prior stroke or cerebrovascular disease, and the presence of multiple co-existing conditions (53). The mechanisms of postoperative cognitive decline are unclear, but are likely multifactorial, including microemboli, activation of a systemic inflammatory response to CPB, pain, sleep disturbances, and medications (especially pain medications and sedatives, e.g., benzodiazepines). In most patients with postoperative cognitive impairment, cognitive function returns to baseline within 1–3 months. In a minority of cases, cognitive dysfunction persists, but it is not clear whether this is due to CABG or progression of underlying impaired cognition (53). Although some studies have suggested that off-pump CABG may be associated with less cognitive dysfunction than on-pump CABG, others have not confirmed this observation (53,54).

Early and late outcomes following CABG in the elderly have continued to improve. Although the elderly incur more postoperative complications, have longer hospital stays, and have higher short-term mortality, isolated CABG for the elderly is associated with acceptable mortality (23,55). CABG also leads to improved functional status and overall quality of life (20,23).

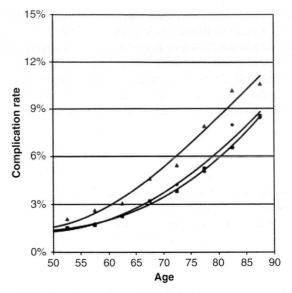

Figure 12.5   In-hospital mortality and morbidity following coronary artery bypass grafting increases with age. Diamond = mortality; square = renal failure; triangle = neurologic events. *Source*: From Ref. 52.

In a retrospective review, patients over the age of 80 years, who underwent isolated CABG incurred higher costs during the initial hospitalization compared to those who underwent medical management (22). However, the rate of subsequent hospitalizations over the following 3 years for cardiac-related illnesses was 2.2 per patient managed medically and 1.6 per patient managed surgically. The cost per quality-adjusted life year (QALY) gained was not significantly different between the two groups.

More recently, SYNTAX investigators analyzed the economic impact of CABG versus PCI with drug eluting stents (56). The total cost of the index revascularization procedure was higher for PCI ($14,407 vs. $8100, $p < 0.01$) attributable to the cost of equipment associated with PCI. However, associated hospital costs including physician services and ancillary/operating room costs were higher with CABG. Therefore, the total costs were higher for those who underwent CABG (average of $5693 higher per patient). At 1-year follow-up, CABG patients still incurred higher total costs. In subgroup analysis based on the SYNTAX score, there was an economic advantage to PCI for those with scores less than 23 or between 23 and 32. However, for those with SYNTAX scores greater than 32, CABG was associated with a favorable cost-effectiveness ratio of $43,000/QALY gained (56).

Cardiac rehabilitation has been shown to be beneficial in patients who have sustained an acute myocardial infarction or have had PCI or CABG. In a meta-analysis of randomized controlled trials exploring the benefit of exercise-based cardiac rehabilitation, there was a 13% reduction in all-cause mortality, 26% reduction in cardiovascular mortality, and 31% reduction in hospital admissions in those who received cardiac rehabilitation (57). Similarly, a survival benefit of cardiac rehabilitation was observed at 1- and 5-years post event (hospitalization for acute myocardial infarction or PCI or CABG) (56). Overall, cardiac rehabilitation users were less likely to have died than non-cardiac rehabilitation users (2.2% vs. 5.3% at 1 year, 16.3% vs. 24.6% at 5 years with relative risk reduction of 58% at 1 year and 34% at 5 years ($p < 0.001$) (58). There was an additional survival benefit in those who utilized cardiac rehabilitation more frequently (1.1% vs. 2.6% at 1 year, 14% vs. 17.2% at 5 years) compared to those who did not. Compared to patients who did not participate in cardiac rehabilitation, those who did experienced significant mortality reductions regardless of age ($p < 0.001$ for 65–74 years, $p < 0.001$ for 75–84 years, and $p < 0.013$ for 85 years or older) or gender.

Despite the proven benefits of cardiac rehabilitation in quality of life and survival, there remains an underutilization of cardiac rehabilitation. Participation rates remain low nationally, averaging 10–30% (59). In a review of Medicare claims in 1997 for outpatient cardiac rehabilitation utilization after hospitalization for either an acute myocardial infarction or CABG in individuals over the age of 65 years, there was a low utilization of outpatient rehabilitation overall (13.9% and 31%, after myocardial infarction and CABG, respectively) (59). Cardiac rehabilitation was used less frequently by women, non-whites, and older patients, as well as those with lower mean incomes, less education, more comorbid conditions, and more associated disabilities (60). There was also a correlation between utilization and distance from the nearest outpatient cardiac rehabilitation facility.

In summary, CABG provides important benefits to the elderly when compared to medical therapy and PCI and it should be offered as a revascularization strategy in patients with a reasonable life expectancy and acceptable operative risk. Outcomes following CABG in the elderly have improved over time due to improved medical and surgical perioperative care.

Patient Selection and Risk Assessment

Traditionally, retrospective reviews summarizing results in the elderly have been hampered by the fact that only those deemed to be "fit for surgery" were likely offered surgical revascularization. Patients offered CABG may have less comorbidity and may be physiologically younger than patients who were not offered surgical revascularization. Older patients typically have more comorbidities, concomitant valvular pathology, depressed left ventricular function, previous cardiac procedures, and have an increased incidence of atherosclerotic disease of the aorta. They also have a slower recovery or regeneration phase following surgery. The estimated risk of CABG using the STS score increases with age, however, this is often difficult to quantify. The surgeon must weigh the risks and benefits of surgical revascularization with the elderly patient and determine if the benefits warrant taking the increased short-term risk. In this regard, recent data suggest that gait speed, an easily performed objective measure, and indices of frailty and disability provide incremental information for assessing perioperative risk in older patients being considered for CABG (61,62).

In addition to well established risk assessment algorithms (STS or Euroscore), surgeons typically have individualized algorithms for assessing risk for coronary revascularization surgery. The assessment begins with a complete history and physical exam. This leads to an individualized risk and benefit assessment for each patient. Depending upon the physical status of the patient and other comorbidities, factors associated with excessive risk must be considered. *Relative contraindications* for surgical coronary revascularization may include poor LV ejection fraction (<30%) with lack of myocardial viability in corresponding ischemic anatomic territories, poor coronary artery targets (small in size, extensive calcium, or multiple stents), lack of available conduit for bypass (previous vein stripping or lower extremity bypass), unacceptable pulmonary function (home oxygen therapy, poor FEV1 on pulmonary function testing), porcelain aorta, history of mediastinal radiation, severe dementia, bleeding dyscrasias, liver dysfunction or cirrhosis, life expectancy significantly limited by other disease (metastatic cancer), advanced age (>90+ years), and poor physical status (sedentary lifestyle, wheelchair bound, excessive frailty).

After having performed a careful physical assessment, most surgeons would recommend a less aggressive option in the frail, debilitated, sedentary patient with multiple comorbidities compared to the active elderly patient with fewer comorbidities.

Table 12.2   Intraoperative Strategies for
Older Patients Undergoing CABG

- Maintain high mean arterial pressure
- Reduce aortic manipulation
- Utilize LIMA graft
- Consider off pump or beating heart techniques
- Provide complete revascularization

Abbreviations: CABG, coronary artery bypass grafting;
LIMA, left internal mammary artery.

SURGICAL TECHNIQUE
Technical Considerations
Specific technical considerations should be given to the elderly undergoing CABG to improve outcomes and survival (Table 12.2). To improve cerebral perfusion and reduce postoperative delirium, a higher mean arterial pressure should be maintained on CPB (63). Due to the increase in aortic atherosclerotic plaques with age, reduced aortic manipulation should be stressed including: off pump no-touch aortic techniques, consideration of less aortic manipulation with beating heart techniques, the use of epi-aortic ultrasound prior to aortic cannulation, and avoidance of femoral cannulation for CPB.

Older Adults Benefit from Off-Pump CABG
Several studies (propensity adjusted retrospective, randomized trials, and meta-analysis) have documented acceptable quality of life, in-hospital mortality, and reduced morbidity in octogenarians undergoing off-pump CABG, indicating that off-pump CABG provides benefit to the elderly patient and should be considered as a potential operative choice (21,64,65).

Completeness of Revascularization
Similar to observations in younger patients, octogenarians have a significant reduction in long-term survival following incomplete revascularization (i.e., residual ungrafted ischemic regions at the time of CABG) compared to patients with complete revascularization (51).

Use of Arterial Grafts
The use of arterial grafts is associated with prolonged survival in patients following CABG. This creates a dilemma in elderly patients who may have a perceived risk of increased perioperative complications or added technical difficulty associated with the use of arterial grafting by some surgeons without a long-term survival benefit due to advanced age. Surgeons may thus incorrectly conclude that the patient's life expectancy may limit the net benefit of a more aggressive operative strategy.

Although there is no doubt that the use of the LIMA increases long-term survival (66), the LIMA has been underused in the elderly (estimated to be 10–15% less than that of the younger STS population) (67). Ferguson and colleagues reported that the LIMA was utilized in 99,942 patients ≥75 years included in the US STS database between 1996 and1999 (67). These patients had improved acute (30-day) mortality without an associated increased risk in perioperative complications related to use of the LIMA graft. In addition, the use of LIMA graft in the elderly conveyed an early survival advantage across all levels of preoperative risk. Use of the LIMA in 100% of CABG operations is presently a Medicare national quality measure in the USA for patients of ALL ages.

In addition, reports have documented safety with the use of radial artery, skeletonized IMA, and bilateral IMA grafts in the elderly (68–72). A survival advantage was found

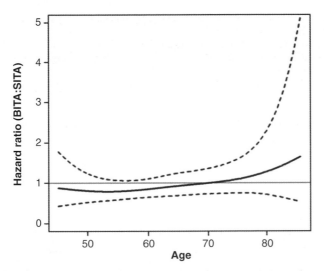

Figure 12.6 Relationship of hazard ratio for bilateral internal thoracic artery related to single internal thoracic artery across age in patients undergoing coronary artery bypass grafting. The solid line is the hazard ratio and the dotted lines are the 95% confidence interval around the hazard ratio. A hazard ratio of less than 1 suggests decreased mortality with bilateral internal thoracic artery grafting relative to single internal thoracic artery grafting up to 70 years. *Source*: From Ref. 74.

with the use of bilateral IMA grafting versus single IMA grafting in elderly (>75 years) patients in a propensity matched comparison (50) and also in a prior retrospective study (73). The benefits of using bilateral IMA grafts were documented to outweigh the risks up to the age of 74 years in one study (68) and up to age 70 in another (Fig. 12.6) (74).

CONCLUSIONS
CABG continues to offer superior coronary revascularization in cases of complex or high risk disease (LMCA disease, LMCA equivalent, complex multi-vessel disease, 2–3-vessel CAD with proximal LAD involvement) when compared to medical therapy and PCI. These disease characteristics often describe patients who are of advanced age and who have multiple comorbid conditions. Although age is an important risk factor, patients of advanced age have been shown to benefit from the more invasive revascularization technique (CABG), and CABG is associated with acceptable operative mortality and survival up to 5 years in octogenarians (24). As the population ages, the number of older adults with CAD will continue to rise. As medical therapy and percutaneous technology continue to improve, so too will surgical coronary revascularization. Continued improvements in care (both intraoperatively and postoperatively), increased use of internal mammary artery grafts, and increased use of intraoperative strategies (Table 12.2) have led to better outcomes in the elderly. Elderly patients who are appropriate candidates with reasonable life expectancy should be offered CABG when indicated.

REFERENCES
1. Current Population Survey. Annual Social and Economic Supplement, 2010. U.S. Census Bureau Internet Release Date 2011: 1–365.
2. US Census Bureau "2008 National Population Projections" released August 2008. [Available From http://www.census.gov/population/www/projections/2008projections.html]
3. He W, Sengupta M, Velkoff VA, et al. 65+ in the United States: 2005. Current Population Reports. U.S. Department of Health and Human Services National Institutes of Health and U.S. Department of Commerce Economics and Statistics Administration U.S. Census Bureau, 2005: 23–209.

4. Projections of the Population by Selected Age Groups and Sex for the United States: 2010-2050. U.S. Census Bureau: Population Division, 2008.

5. World Population Ageing: 1950-2050. Department of Economic and Social Affairs Population Division, United Nations, 2002. [Available From http://www.un.org/esa/population/publications/worldageing19502050]

6. Roger VL, Go AS, Lloyd-Jones DM, et al. Writing Group Members of American Heart Association. Heart disease and stroke statistics-2012 update: a report from the American Heart Association. Circulation 2012; 125: e2–e220.

7. National Health and Nutrition Examination Survey 2005-2008. National Center for Health Statistics and National Heart, Lung, and Blood Institute 2008. National Heart, Lung, and Blood Institute 2011 Fact Book.

8. Heidenreich PA, Trogdon JG, Khavjou OA, et al. Forecasting the future of cardiovascular disease in the United States: a policy statement from the American Heart Association. Circulation 2011; 123: 933–44.

9. Bridges CR, Edwards FH, Peterson ED, et al. Cardiac surgery in nonagenarians and centenarians. J Am Coll Surg 2003; 197: 347–57.

10. Maganti M, Rao V, Brister S, et al. Decreasing mortality for coronary artery bypass surgery in octogenarians. Can J Cardiol 2009; 25: e32–5.

11. Saito A, Motomura N, Miyata H, et al. Age-specific risk stratification in 13,488 isolated coronary artery bypass grafting procedures. J Thorac Cardiovasc Surg 2011; 12: 575–81.

12. Hillis LD, Smith PK, Anderson JL, et al. 2011 ACCF/AHA guideline for coronary artery bypass graft surgery: a report of the American College of Cardiology Foundation/American Heart Association task force on practice guidelines. Circulation 2011; 124: e652–735.

13. ElBardissi AW, Aranki SF, Sheng S, et al. Trends in isolated coronary artery bypass grafting: an analysis of the Society of Thoracic Surgeons Adult Cardiac Surgery Database. J Thorac Cardiovasc Surg 2012; 143: 273–81.

14. US Census Bureau, 2008 American community survey. B18101 "Sex by age by disability status", B18102 "Sex by age by hearing difficulty", B18103 "Sex by age by vision difficulty", B18104 "Sex by age by cognitive difficulty", B18105 "Sex by age by ambulatory difficulty", B18106 "Sex by age by self care difficulty", B18107 "Sex by age by independent living difficulty". [Available From http://factfinder.census.gov/]

15. Murphy SL, Xu J, Kochanek KD. Deaths: preliminary data for 2010. National Vital Statistics Reports 2012; 60:1–69.

16. National Center for Health Statistics. National Health Interview Survey 1983-1985. Hyattsville, MD: National Center for Health Statistics, 1986.

17. Farkouh ME, Domanski M, Sleeper LA, et al. Strategies for multivessel revascularization in patients with diabetes. N Engl J Med 2012; 367: 2375–84.

18. Kozower BD, Moon MR, Barner HB, et al. Impact of complete revascularization on long–term survival after coronary artery bypass grafting in octogenarians. Ann Thorac Surg 2005; 80: 112–17.

19. TIME Investigators. Trial of invasive versus medical therapy in elderly patients with chronic symptomatic coronary – artery disease (TIME): a randomized trial. Lancet 2001; 358: 951–7.

20. Cohen DJ, Van Hout B, Serruys PW, et al. Quality of life after PCI with drug-eluting stents or coronary artery bypass surgery. N Engl J Med 2011; 364: 1016–26.

21. Houlind K, Kjeldsen J, Madsen SN, DOORS Study Group. Mortality in coronary artery bypass grafting. What's next? Circulation 2012; 125: 2431–9.

22. Sollano JA, Rose EA, Williams DL, et al. Cost–effectiveness of coronary artery bypass surgery in octogenarians. Ann Surg 1998; 228: 297–306.

23. Kurlansky PA, Williams DB, Traad EA, et al. Eighteen–year follow-up demonstrates prolonged survival and enhanced quality of life for octogenarians after coronary artery bypass grafting. J Thorac Cardiovasc Surg 2011; 141: 394–9.

24. McKellar SH, Brown ML, Frye RL, et al. Comparison of coronary revascularization procedures in octogenarians: a systematic review and meta–analysis. Nature Clin Pract Cardio 2008; 5: 738–46.

25. Dacey LJ, Likosky DS, Ryan TJ, et al. Northern New England Cardiovascular Disease Study Group. Long–term survival after surgery versus percutaneous intervention in octogenarians with multi-vessel coronary disease. Ann Thorac Surg 2007; 84: 1904–11.

26. Graham MM, Ghali WA, Faris PD, et al. APPROACH Investigators. Survival after coronary revascularization in the elderly. Circulation 2002; 105: 2378–84.

27. Peduzzi P, Hultgren HN. Effect of medical vs surgical treatment on symptoms in stable angina pectoris. The Veterans Administration cooperative study of surgery for coronary arterial occlusive disease. Circulation 1979; 60: 888–900.

28. The Veterans Administration Coronary Artery Bypass Surgery Cooperative Study Group. Eleven-year survival in the Veterans Administration randomized trial of coronary artery bypass surgery for stable angina. N Engl J Med 1984; 311: 1333–9.
29. CASS Principal Investigators and Their Associates. Coronary Artery Surgery Study (CASS): a randomized trial of coronary artery bypass surgery. Survival data. Circulation 1983; 68: 939–50.
30. Alderman EL, Bourassa MG, Cohen LS, et al. Ten-year follow-up of survival and myocardial infarction in the randomized coronary artery surgery study. Circulation 1990; 82: 1629–46.
31. European Coronary Surgery Study Group. Long-term results of prospective randomized study of coronary artery bypass surgery in stable angina pectoris. Lancet 1982; 2: 1173–80.
32. Varnauskas E; The European Coronary Surgery Study Group. Twelve-year follow-up of survival in the randomized European Coronary Surgery Study. N Engl J Med 1988; 319: 332–7.
33. Passamani E, Davis KB, Gillespie MJ, et al. CASS Principal Investigators and Their Associates. A randomized trial of coronary artery bypass surgery. Survival of patients with a low ejection fraction. N Engl J Med 1985; 312: 1665–71.
34. Hueb W, Soares PR, Gersh BJ, et al. The medicine, angioplasty, or surgery study (MASS-II): a randomized, controlled clinical trial of three therapeutic strategies for multi-vessel coronary artery disease. One year results. J Am Coll Cardiol 2004; 43: 1743–51.
35. Hueb W, Lopes NH, Gersh BJ, et al. Five year follow-up of the medicine, angioplasty, or surgery study (MASS II): a randomized controlled clinical trial of 3 therapeutic strategies for multi-vessel coronary artery disease. Circulation 2007; 115: 1082–9.
36. De Lorenzo A, Tura B, Bassan F, et al. Outcomes of patients with left main coronary artery disease undergoing medical or surgical treatment: a propensity matched analysis. Coron Artery Dis 2011; 22: 585–9.
37. Rodriguez A, Bernard V, Navia J, et al. Argentine randomized study: coronary angioplasty with stenting versus coronary artery bypass surgery in patients with multi-vessel disease (ERACI II): 30-day and one-year follow up results. J Am Coll Cardiol 2001; 37: 51–8.
38. Serruys PW, Unger F, Sousa JE, et al. Comparison of coronary artery bypass surgery and stenting for the treatment of multi-vessel disease. New Engl J Med 2001; 344: 1117–24.
39. The SoS Investigators. Coronary artery bypass surgery versus percutaneous coronary intervention with stent implantation in patients with multi-vessel coronary artery disease (the stent or surgery trial): a randomized controlled trial. Lancet 2002; 360: 965–70.
40. Hlatky MA, Boothroyd DB, Bravata DM, et al. Coronary artery bypass surgery compared with percutaneous coronary interventions for multi-vessel disease: a collaborative analysis of individual patient data from ten randomized trials. Lancet 2009; 373: 1190–7.
41. Takagi H, Kawai N, Umemoto T. Meta-analysis of four randomized controlled trials on long-term outcomes of coronary artery bypass grafting versus percutaneous coronary intervention with stenting for mult-ivessel coronary artery disease. Am J Cardiol 2008; 101: 1259–62.
42. Serruys PW, Morice MC, Kappetein AP, et al. Percutaneous coronary intervention versus coronary artery bypass grafting for severe coronary artery disease. N Engl J Med 2009; 360: 961–72.
43. Kappetein AP, Feldman TE, Mack MJ, et al. Comparison of coronary bypass surgery with drug-eluting stenting for the treatment of left main and/or three-vessel disease: three-year follow-up of the SYNTAX trial. Eur Heart J 2011; 32: 2125–34.
44. Boudriot E, Thiele H, Walther T, et al. Randomized comparison of percutaneous coronary intervention with sirolimus-eluting stents versus coronary artery bypass grafting in unprotected left main stem stenosis. J Am Coll Cardiol 2011; 57: 538–45.
45. Weintraub WS, Grau-Sepulveda MV, Weiss JM, et al. Comparative effectiveness of revascularization strategies. New Engl J Med 2012; 366: 1467–76.
46. Movahed MR, Ramaraj R, Khoynezhad A, et al. Declining in-hospital mortality in patients undergoing coronary bypass surgery in the United States irrespective of presence of type 2 diabetes or congestive heart failure. Clin Cardiol 2012; 35: 297–300.
47. Society of Thoracic Surgeons. [Available from: www.sts.org]
48. Almassi GH, Schowalter T, Nicolosi AC, et al. Atrial fibrillation after cardiac surgery: a major morbid event? Ann Surg 1997; 226: 501–11.
49. Creswell LL, Alexander JC, Ferguson TB, et al. American College of Chest Physicians. Intraoperative interventions: American College of Chest Physicians guidelines for the prevention and management of postoperative atrial fibrillation after cardiac surgery. Chest 2005; 128: 28S–35S.
50. Kurlansky PA, Traad EA, Dorman MJ, et al. Thirty-year follow-up defines survival benefit for second internal mammary artery in propensity-matched groups. Ann Thorac Surg 2010; 90: 101–8.
51. Aziz A, Lee AM, Pasque MK, et al. Evaluation of revascularization subtypes in octogenarians undergoing coronary artery bypass grafting. Circulation 2009; 120: S65–9.

52. Alexander KP, Anstrom KJ, Muhlbaier LH, et al. Outcomes of cardiac surgery in patients age ≥ 80 years: results from the National Cardiovascular Network. J Am Coll Cardiol 2000; 35: 731–8.

53. Selnes OA, Gottesman RF, Grega MA, et al. Cognitive and neurologic outcomes after coronary-artery bypass surgery. N Engl J Med 2012; 366: 250–7.

54. Stroobant N, Van Nooten G, De Bacquer D, Van Belleghem Y, Vingerhoets G. Neuropsychological functioning 3-5 years after coronary artery bypass grafting: does the pump make a difference? Eur J Cardiothorac Surg 2008; 34: 396–401.

55. Saxema A, Dinh DT, Yap CH, et al. Critical analysis of early and late outcomes after isolated coronary artery bypass surgery in elderly patients. Ann Thorac Surg 2011; 92: 1703–11.

56. Cohen DJ, Lavelle TA, Van Hout B, et al. Economic outcomes of percutaneous coronary intervention with drug-eluting stents versus bypass surgery for patients with left main or three vessel coronary artery disease: one year results from the SYNTAX trial. Catheter Cardiovasc Intervent 2012; 9: 198–209.

57. Heran BS, Chen JM, Ebrahim S, et al. Exercise-based cardiac rehabilitation for coronary heart disease. Cochrane Database Systemic Review 2007; 7: CD001800. doi:10.1002/14651858.CD001800.pub2.

58. Suaya JA, Stason WB, Ades PA, et al. Cardiac rehabilitation and survival in older coronary patients. J Amer Coll Cardiol 2009; 54: 25–33.

59. Suaya JA, Shepard DS, Norman SL, et al. Use of cardiac rehabilitation by medicare beneficiaries after myocardial infarction or coronary bypass surgery. Circulation 2007; 116: 1653–62.

60. Balady GJ, Ades PA, Bittner VA, et al. Referral, enrollment, and delivery of cardiac rehabilitation/secondary prevention programs at clinical centers and beyond: a presidential ad56. Advisory from the American Heart Association. Circulation 2011; 124: 2951–60.

61. Afilalo J, Eisenberg MJ, Morin JF, et al. Gait speed as an incremental predictor of mortality and major morbidity in elderly patients undergoing cardiac surgery. J Amer Coll Cardiol 2010; 56:1668–76.

62. Afilalo J, Mottillo B, Eisenberg MJ, et al. Addition of frailty and disability to cardiac surgical risk scores identifying elderly patients at high risk of mortality and major morbidity. Circ Cardiovasc Qual Outcomes 2012; 5: 222-228.

63. Siepe M, Pfeiffer T, Gieringer A, et al. Increased systemic perfusion pressure during cardiopulmonary bypass is associated with less early postoperative cognitive dysfunction and delirium. Eur J Cardiothorac Surg 2011; 40: 200–2007.

64. Sarin EL, Kayatta MO, Kilgo P, et al. Short- and long–term outcomes in octogenarian patients undergoing off–pump coronary artery bypass grafting. Innovations 2011; 6: 110–15.

65. Pawlaczyk R, Swietlik D, Lango R, Rogowski J. Off–pump coronary surgery may reduce stroke, respiratory failure, and mortality in octogenarians. Ann Thorac Surg 2012; 94: 29–37.

66. Loop FD, Lytle BW, Cosgrove DM, et al. Influence of internal mammary artery graft on 10-year survival and other cardiac events. N Engl J Med 1986; 314: 6.

67. Ferguson TB, Coombs LP, Peterson ED. Internal throacic artery grafting in the elderly patient undergoing coronary artery bypass grafting: room for process improvement? J Thorac Cardiovasc Surg 2002; 123: 869–80.

68. Song SW, Sul SY, Lee HJ, et al. Comparison of the radial artery and saphenous vein as composite grafts in off–pump coronary artery bypass grafting in elderly patients: a randomized controlled trial. Korean Circ J 2012; 42: 107–12.

69. Olivera Sa MP, Santos CA, Figueiredo OJ, et al. Skeletonized internal thoracic artery is associated with lower rates of mediastinitis in elderly undergoing coronary artery bypass grafting surgery. Rev Bras Cir Cardiovasc 2011; 26: 617–23.

70. Elmistekawy EM, Gawad N, Bourke M, et al. Is bilateral internal thoracic artery use safe in the elderly? J Card Surg 2012; 27: 1–5.

71. Kinoshita T, Asai T, Suzuki T, et al. Off-pump bilateral skeletonized internal thoracic artery grafting in elderly patients. Ann Thorac Surg 2012; 93: 531–6.

72. Hirotani T, Nakamichi T, Munakata M, et al. Extended use of bilateral internal thoracic arteries for coronary artery bypass grafting in the elderly. Jpn J Thorac Cardiovasc Surg 2003; 51: 488–95.

73. Lytle BW, Blackstone EH, Loop FD, et al. Two internal thoracic artery grafts are better than one. J Thorac Cardiovasc Surg 1999; 117: 855–72.

74. Kieser TM, Lewin AM, Graham MM, et al. APPROACH Investigators. Outcomes associated with bilateral internal thoracic artery grafting: The importance of age. Ann Thorac Surg 2011; 92: 1269–76.

13

Percutaneous coronary intervention in the elderly

Andrew Cassar and David R. Holmes Jr.

SUMMARY

With a growing elderly population, over 50% of percutaneous coronary interventions (PCI) are now performed in patients ≥65 years of age. Due to more frequent and more severe medical comorbidities, frailty, as well as poorer success and higher complication rates with PCI in the elderly, the decision to perform coronary revascularization is often challenging. However, the elderly also have more extensive CAD and ischemic burden, and therefore may derive great benefit from revascularization. With the rapid evolution of PCI techniques and improvement in outcomes in the elderly, one must continually reevaluate PCI's applicability in the setting of older, sicker patients so as to better advise its relative benefit versus alternative treatment strategies.

Cardiovascular disease is the leading cause of morbidity and mortality among the elderly (1). The numbers of old (≥65 years) and older (≥75 years) patients with coronary artery disease (CAD) are increasing in our society at a tremendous rate. Indeed, there has been unsurpassed 15% growth in the elderly population between the years 2000 and 2010 (2). In the 2010 US census, one-sixth of the population, representing 40 million people, were 65 years or older with one-third of these being 75 years or older (2). The elderly have a high prevalence (about 60%) of significant atherosclerotic CAD in at least one coronary vessel, with many becoming symptomatic enough to require definitive treatment (3). The increase in prevalence of CAD with increasing age is seen irrespective of gender status (Fig. 13.1) (1). In current practice, over 50% of percutaneous coronary interventions (PCIs) are performed in patients ≥65 years, almost 25% in patients ≥75 years, and 12% in patients ≥80 years old (4–8).

Unfortunately, many studies of revascularization for symptomatic CAD in the past have either excluded patients over the age of 70–75 or have included insufficient numbers to draw effective conclusions (9). This is possibly due to more frequent and more severe medical comorbidities, frailty, and poorer success rates leading to higher complication/death rates in the elderly, both with PCI (4,8,10,11) (Fig. 13.2) as well as with coronary artery bypass surgery (CABG) (12). These factors make the decision to perform coronary revascularization challenging. However, the elderly also have more extensive CAD (11) and ischemic burden, and therefore may derive great benefit from revascularization. With the rapid evolution of PCI techniques, one must continually reevaluate PCI's applicability in the setting of older, sicker patients so as to better advise its relative benefit versus alternative treatment strategies.

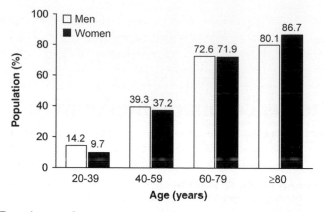

Figure 13.1   Prevalence of coronary artery disease in adults by age and sex. *Source*: From Ref. 1.

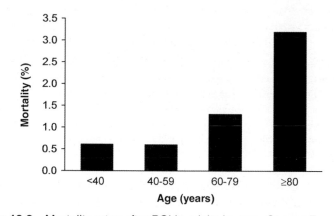

Figure 13.2   Mortality rates after PCI in adults by age. *Source*: From Ref. 4.

BASIS FOR INTERVENTION IN THE ELDERLY

Previous studies have shown that elderly patients with symptomatic CAD have poorer long-term and event-free survival with medical therapy alone compared with revascularization (13,14). The large observational Alberta Provincial Project for Outcomes Assessment in Coronary Heart Disease (APPROACH) study, set in the mid-1990s (6000 patients with CAD over the age of 70 years and about 1000 patients over the age of 80 years) noted age-related differences in adjusted 4-year survival in the elderly with medical treatment (MED) compared with PCI and CABG as follows: aged <70 MED = 90.5%, PCI = 93.8%, CABG = 95.0%; aged 70–79 MED = 79.1%, PCI = 83.9%, CABG = 87.3%; aged >80 MED = 60.3%, PCI = 71.6%, CABG = 77.4% (13). Elderly patients in general did poorer with medical therapy, and this trend seemed to worsen with increasing patient age. Graham et al. and others (13,15) have shown that benefits of revascularization in carefully selected elderly patients are more pronounced. In addition to frequent symptoms, some 50% of medically treated patients will be admitted with an acute coronary event, a trend that can be favorably impacted with timely revascularization therapy (14).

Other factors in the elderly limit some of the pharmacologic options for treatment of CAD. Although it is still essential to try to optimize medical therapy, there are challenges in this regard in older patients because of their more extensive disease and ischemic burden and thereby often refractory symptoms. The use of multiple medications can be problematic because of multiple adverse drug–drug interactions (14,16). Elderly patients often have a substantial degree of medication intolerance (due to peptic ulcer disease among others) as well as cognitive impairment that can lead to poorer compliance with medications than younger patients (9,17,18). Undoubtedly, for a multitude of reasons, older patients tend to downplay their symptoms and delay seeking care; when they do present with active coronary ischemia, they are more likely to do so late, with signs of severe congestive heart failure (CHF), acute myocardial infarction (MI), and/or cardiogenic shock (10,11). It is these very subsets of elderly who are shown to carry a poorer prognosis with medical therapy in the absence of revascularization (19,20). Together with a high prevalence of chronic symptomatic ischemia, a high burden of atherosclerosis, and many medical comorbidities, active CAD can be a tremendously disabling problem in the elderly, one that often prompts patients to consider the more definitive benefits offered by revascularization therapy.

The TIME trial (14) randomized 301 elderly patients ≥75 years of age to either coronary angiography and revascularization or to further optimization of medical therapy. At baseline, three-quarters of the patients had CCS Class III or IV angina pectoris despite using an average of 2.5 antianginal drugs. The primary endpoint was quality of life assessed at 6 months. Although angina severity decreased and quality of life improved in both groups, these improvements were significantly greater in the group of patients treated with revascularization. In the invasive group, 19% had a major adverse cardiac event at 6 months versus 49% in the medical group ($p < 0.0001$). Pfisterer et al. reported the 1-year follow-up of the TIME trial in 282 elderly patients with Canadian Cardiac Society Class II or higher angina who survived for the first 6 months after enrollment. The mean age was 80 years; and at 1 year, there was no statistically significant difference in death [11.1% for invasive versus 8.1% for medical therapy hazard ratio (HR) 1.51, 95% CI 0.72–3.16 $p = 0.28$] or the combined endpoint of death or non fatal infarction (17% for the invasive group versus 19.6% for the medical therapy group [HR 0.90, 95% CI 0.51–1.53, $p = 0.71$]). There was however a marked difference in subsequent revascularization. Patients randomized to medical therapy had almost a 50% chance of later hospitalization and revascularization (46% for medical therapy versus 10% for an invasive approach [HR 0.17, 95% CI 0.11–0.32, $p < 0.001$]) (21). After 4 years, the patient survival was 70.6% in the invasive group versus 73% in the medically treated group (NS, nonsignificant). Survival rates were better, however, if patients were revascularized within the first year of study entry. At 4 years, freedom from major adverse cardiac event rate remained significantly higher (39% vs. 20%) in the invasive group (22).

Quality of life has also been compared after invasive versus medical therapy (23). Graham evaluated 4-year health status in elderly patients using the Seattle Angina Questionnaire. At 4 years of follow-up, health status was better in those patients who had undergone revascularization at the index procedure compared with medical therapy. Finally, cost effectiveness has also been studied in the setting of the TIME trial. Costs were determined by resource utilization at 1 year. The two strategies had different cost profiles, with invasive treated patients having higher initial costs, but medically treated patients had higher later costs. Accordingly, at 1 year, patients treated with an invasive strategy had improved clinical outcomes at only marginally higher costs (24).

CHARACTERISTICS OF THE ELDERLY PCI POPULATION

Elderly subjects undergoing PCI are generally sicker than younger ones due to a higher prevalence of comorbid medical conditions (8,25). Patients over the age of 65 years frequently have hypertension and diabetes leading to more advanced CAD, peripheral vascular disease, and cerebrovascular disease (7,8,25). In addition, older patients have a greater burden of coronary atherosclerosis associated with a relatively high percentage of prior MI, prior history of PCIs and/or CABG, and resultant lower left ventricular ejection fraction (LVEF) (7,16,26,27). Based on a multicenter registry study, CHF is common in the elderly and comparatively rare in younger patients undergoing PCI: only 4% of patients younger than 65 years have had CHF versus some 9% over 65 years and 17% over 75 years (16). In addition, there is a higher percentage of women undergoing PCI over the age of 75 years (40—50%) compared with those younger than 65 (21%), a factor that alone predisposes toward a higher need for subsequent revascularization procedures (25).

The presence of many adverse risk predictors in the elderly has a major impact on the coronary lesion's suitability for PCI and is inherent in their higher procedural risk. There is a high incidence of multivessel CAD in patients with lower LVEFs. One study noted that 50% of patients over the age of 75 years versus 33% of younger patients have multivessel disease, with some 13% of those over the age of 80 years having left main coronary disease (28). Furthermore, age is a significant predictor of both coronary calcification (29) as well as tortuous vessels, which are associated with increased risk of coronary and vascular access complications with PCI. Thus, in the early balloon era, only 31% of patients in their 80s were considered suitable candidates for angioplasty, due to diffuse extensive CAD (28,30). With the rise of improved PCI techniques such as stenting, interventions for many of these advanced "type C" lesions are now routine, but the modified AHA/ACC character-istics still predict poorer overall short-and long-term success in this setting (31).

As a consequence of more extensive disease, elderly patients are often more unstable upon presentation for intervention than younger patients, not uncommonly having had prior silent infarctions (32). They have a higher frequency of class III/IV angina, which is present during intervention in as many as 70% of patients over 65 and in an even higher number of those over age 80, compared with less than 50% of younger patients (7,16,24–26,33).

OUTCOMES OF BALLOON ANGIOPLASTY IN THE ELDERLY

Initial results in elderly patients undergoing coronary angioplasty in the early 1980s showed relatively low acute success rates, higher procedural complications, and higher mortality than in younger patients (16,24). The results have been age-dependent, with those over the age 75 years having poorer outcomes than younger patients (16,24–27,34,35). Elderly patients who underwent angioplasty at the Mayo Clinic between 1980 and 1989 showed procedural mortality of 1.2% for patients below the age of 75 years but 6.7% for those over the age of 75 years (7). This is in keeping with data from other large centers during the same period (36). In a large Medicare database of some 20,000 patients, Jollis et al. reported in-hospital mortality rates of 7% in patients over age 80 of age with angioplasty (37). With lower profile balloons, in-lab monitoring of anticoagulation status, increasing operator experience and stenting, angioplasty success had significantly improved by the early 1990s to an acceptable level of 88% to 93% (38) in elderly patients with single-vessel disease, but was still lower in the oldest subjects.

From 1990 to 1992 (compared to the 1980s), results of angioplasties performed at Mayo Clinic showed a 50% drop in hospital mortality to 0.8% in patients aged 65–74 and to 3% in those over 75 years of age (38). The rate of complications had also fallen during this time period, with procedural infarction rates in those over age 65 falling to 2.2% (vs. 3.9% previously) and emergency bypass rates of 0.65% (vs. 5.5%).

Feldman et al. (39) evaluated the effect of age on outcome in the New York State Registry using data from 2000/2001. In this series, 10,964 patients had undergone emer-gency PCI, and 71,176 patients elective PCI. Patients were divided into three age groups, <60 years, 60–80 years, and >80 years. In both elective and emergency PCI, elderly patients had more comorbidities. Age was strongly predictive of in-hospital mortality for both elective and emergency cases. In the elective cases, mortality was 0.1, 0.4, and 1.1% respectively ($p < 0.05$); in the emergency cases, mortality was 1.0, 4.1, and 11.5% respectively ($p < 0.05$).

Other medical complications post procedure have also been a particular concern in the elderly. After angioplasty, Maiello and colleagues (40) described a 1.1% rate of renal insufficiency and a 5.4% rate of need for transfusion in patients over 70 years of age. As a result, the elderly tend to have longer hospital stays, although this may be favorably altered by careful attention to the amount of contrast dye used, better preprocedural hydration, less aggressive anticoagulant dosing, and the use of smaller caliber equipment. Of interest, longer hospital stays are associated with higher mortality, presumably reflecting complications which necessitate an extended hospitalization.

PCI with the radial approach significantly reduces rates of vascular complications in high-risk patients aged 80 years and older. In one study (41), patients aged 80–97 years during 2003–2007 undergoing elective PCI were divided into two groups by femoral ($n = 156$) or radial approach ($n = 112$). Rates of access site bleeding (2.7% vs. 9.6%, $p = 0.004$), hematoma (4.5% vs. 10.9%, $P = 0.006$), or any vascular complication (7.1% vs. 23.7%, $p < 0.001$) were significantly reduced with the radial approach as opposed to femoral. Also ambulation time (5 ± 2 hours vs. 20 ± 4 hours, $p < 0.001$) was improved. The radial approach was associated with longer cannulation, fluoroscopy time (23 ± 15 minutes vs. 19 ± 12 minutes, $P = 0.03$), and higher rate of crossover to an alternative access site (9.8% vs. 3.8%, $p = 0.02$) compared with the femoral approach. These findings were confirmed in another study (42) in which the incidence of vascular complications was found to be significantly less in the radial group (1.6% vs. 6.5%, $p = 0.03$), without any decrease in the efficacy of PCI and only a slight increase in procedure duration for coronary angiography. The most recent RIFLE_STEACS study (43) randomized 1001 patients (mean age 65 years) with ST-elevation MI to radial versus femoral access; the primary endpoint of 30-day net adverse clinical events (composite of cardiac death, stroke, MI, target lesion revascularization, and bleeding) occurred in 13.6% in the radial arm and 21.0% in the femoral arm ($p = 0.003$). In particular, compared with femoral access, radial access was associated with significantly lower rates of cardiac mortality (5.2% vs. 9.2%, $p = 0.020$), bleeding (7.8% vs. 12.2%, $p = 0.026$), and shorter hospital stay [5 days (IQR 4–7 days) vs. 6 days (IQR 5–8 days); $p = 0.03$].

PREDICTORS OF POOR EARLY OUTCOME WITH PCI IN THE ELDERLY

The strongest predictor of hospital death in the elderly is the presence of extensive or multiple-vessel coronary disease (44). In patients over the age of 75 years, Maiello and colleagues showed a high success rate, approaching 100% in single-vessel angioplasty versus a success rate in multiple-vessel treatment of only 52% (45). The overall procedural success rate depends on the additive number of vessels treated. Calcified coronary artery lesions have definitely been predictors of failed angioplasty procedures in the past and, even in contemporary practice with stenting, are associated with poorer long-term event-free survival (31,46) due to a higher need for repeat revascularization procedures.

LONG-TERM OUTCOMES IN THE ELDERLY FOLLOWING PCI

The long-term results after a successful angioplasty in the elderly have shown consistent improvement. By the early 1990s, Buffet (34) and Thompson (7) had shown 4-year survivals of 83% and 86%, respectively. The overall long-term survival rates were not significantly different between those over and those under 75 years of age. However, there was less satisfactory event-free survival in patients over 75 years in these series (34,38) that was probably due less to restenosis than to continued untreated advanced CAD or its progression. Restenosis rates after angioplasty have been quite similar, in the range of 31–44%, in patients over 80 years, patients between 65 and 79, and in younger patients (26,47–50)

The strongest predictor of event-free survival in the elderly post-PCI is the extent of CAD. DeJaegere (51) reported an 81% event-free survival post-angioplasty in patients over the age of 70 years with single-vessel disease versus 45% in patients with multivessel disease. The extent of disease also was a multivariate risk predictor in a prior review of the Mayo Clinic angioplasty experience in the elderly (44). Other predictors of long-term event-free survival were the left ventricular systolic function, the presence of unstable angina, and the number of noncardiac medical problems (37,38,44,48–52).

Clearly, there is a wide variation in risk in PCI patients: this is most true in the elderly. The number of adverse risk factors present greatly impacts the long-term risk of death or MI. In a Mayo Clinic series with stratification by the number of risk predictors, we noted that elderly patients undergoing angioplasty with three-vessel CAD, recent CHF, and two other concomitant medical problems had a 3-year survival rate free of MI of only 66%, while in the absence of these factors, it was 96% (44).

RESULTS OF CORONARY STENTING IN THE ELDERLY

Coronary stenting has become the dominant revascularization mode in the elderly in those with one- and two-vessel CAD and, occasionally, in those with three-vessel CAD with a low risk SYNTAX score or those felt to be too high risk for CABG. In the early stenting era, Yokoi et al. (53) reported initial successful stent results to be lower in those over 75 years compared with younger patients for the initial Palmaz-Schatz stent (86% vs. 95%) with associated higher hospital mortality (4.1% vs. 1.2%). By the mid-1990s, the procedural success rate with lower profile, more deliverable stents had improved to 90.8% and 90.2% in two series by Chevalier and Batchelor (54,55) of 142 and 7472 octogenarians, respectively, but with poorer results compared to younger patients' success rates of 95.5%. Overall in-hospital mortality was still around 3.5% and combined death/infarction and stroke risks were 5.2%; stenting was associated with better procedural success rates, lower need for repeat revascularization but higher vascular complication rates compared to balloon angioplasty (54). Overall procedural success with stenting has increased compared with results from the early series and now ranges between 90% and 97% success rates at major medical centers (56–58).

The National Heart, Lung and Blood Institutes (NHLBI) Dynamic Registry study of PCIs from 1997 to 1999 (59) compared 307 patients over 80 years of age (oldest), 1776 patients aged 65–79 years (older), and 2537 patients under 65 years (youngest). Successful procedural treatment of all lesions attempted was lower in those 80 years and over versus those under age 80 (84% vs. 92–93%) despite similar IIB/IIIA receptor inhibitor use (26–29%), similar stent rates (72–73%) and similar rates of rotational atherectomy (5.2–7.2%). Accounting for the lower success in the oldest patients was a higher burden of CAD with more vessels (two or more in 15% vs. 9.4% vs. 9.4%), more lesions (2 or more in 39.1 % vs. 34.2% vs. 29.0%), and more graft vessels (8.5% vs. 8.3% vs. 3.9%) treated. Complication rates included higher stroke rates in those 80 years and over (1.0% vs. 0.5% vs. 0.2%), higher in-hospital mortality (4.6% vs. 2.2% vs. 0.6%) and more nonfatal MIs (6.2% vs. 3.1% vs. 2.2%). One-year survival, although lower with increasing age, was identical to the age-expected mortality rates of the general population, suggesting that successful revascularization in the elderly is beneficial (59).

Registry studies from the Mayo Clinic and nationally have shown encouraging improvement in outcomes in elderly patients undergoing PCI. Nonagenarians at the Mayo Clinic presented with acute coronary syndrome 91% of the time, and PCI technical success

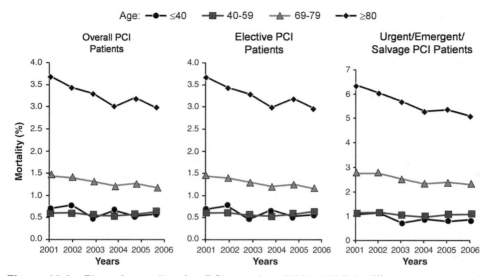

Figure 13.3   Plots of mortality after PCI over time (2001–2006) in different age groups in the National Cardiovascular Disease Registry. *Source*: From Ref. 4.

rate was 91% with an in-hospital death rate of 9.4% but a long-term survival which was not significantly different than that of age- and gender-matched persons in the community. The in-hospital mortality decreased markedly over time when the cohort was divided into pre-2000 and the 2000–2006 groups: 22% to 6% ($p = 0.006$) (60). In the National Cardiovascular Data Registry (4), in-hospital mortality after PCI in 1,410,069 patients admitted from January 1, 2001 to December 31, 2006 was age stratified into 4 groups: group 1 (age <40, $n = 25,679$), group 2 (40–59, $n = 496,204$), group 3 (60–79, $n = 732,574$), and group 4 ($\geq$80, $n = 155,612$). In-hospital mortality was 0.60%, 0.59%, 1.26%, and 3.16% in groups 1–4, respectively, $p < 0.0001$ (Fig. 13.2). Overall temporal improvement per calendar year in the adjusted in-hospital mortality after PCI was noted in most groups; however, this finding was significant only in the 2 older age groups, group 3 (odds ratio (OR) 0.94, 95% CI 0.92–0.96) and group 4 (OR, 0.95, 95% CI 0.92–0.97). The absolute mortality reduction was greatest in the group $\geq$80 years (Fig. 13.3).

LONG-TERM RESULTS OF STENTING IN THE ELDERLY

The earliest study that included a large number of elderly patients undergoing stenting with first-generation stents reported increased angiographic restenosis rates in 137 patients aged 75 years and older compared with 2551 younger individuals (47% vs. 28%) (58). The presence of more advanced coronary disease in those over versus those under the age of 75 years was evidenced by higher rates of stenting in multiple vessels (44% vs. 27%), left main (7.4% vs. 1.5%), ostial lesions (15.5% vs. 7%), and more frequent use of rotational atherectomy for debulking of calcified lesions in the elderly (notably, all factors in restenosis). Other studies by Chauhan et al. (56) in 300 octogenarians, Abizaid et al. (57) in over 700 patients over the age of 70 years, and Alfonso et al. (61) in 378 patients over the age of 65 years have all shown similar clinical restenosis rates when compared to younger patients, but higher in-hospital mortality rates (1.3–3.0% in those over the age of 80 years vs. 0.2–0.7% in younger patients), higher procedural infarction rates (7–10% vs. 2%), higher bleeding and vascular complications (5% vs. 1.0%), and higher subsequent 1-year mortality (5–9% vs. 1–2%). Many studies with coronary interventions in the past have shown that late events are related mostly to repeat revascularization; despite similar restenosis rates, patients over the age of 75 years are less likely to undergo repeat revascularization, possibly due to less aggressive late treatment (62).

Drug-eluting stents (DES) have come to dominate interventional cardiology on the basis of multiple randomized clinical trials which document marked reduction in both angiographic and clinical restenosis compared with conventional bare metal stents (BMS). There is limited information on the effect of age on outcome in this setting. Observational data from Groeneveld et al. (63) from a national sample of >70,000 patients undergoing PCI with a mean age of 75 years found that those receiving DES had a lower mortality (HR 0.83, 95% CI 0.81–0.86) than those receiving BMS as well as having less likelihood for revascularization within 2 years or hospitalizations for MI. A Medicare observational study (64) of >260,000 patients with a mean age of 73 years showed lower risk for patients treated with DES versus BMS with regard to adjusted mortality (HR 0.75, 95% CI 0.72–0.79) and MI (HR 0.77, 95% CI 0.72–0.81). Caution is required when interpreting these observational data, and randomized clinical trials would be beneficial. Until then, it seems safe and possibly beneficial to use DES in elderly patients.

Vlaar et al. (65) analyzed 2453 patients who received DES at Mayo Clinic to evaluate the effect of age. They classified patients into two groups: <80 and ≥80 years old. Procedural success in the older group was 97%, nonsignificantly less than in the younger patients (98%, $p = 0.10$). In-hospital mortality in patients ≥80 years was 1.9% versus 0.6% in those patients <80 years old ($p = 0.011$). At 12 months of follow-up, target lesion revascularization rates were similar at 4.9% and 4.5% in the ≥80- and <80-year-old groups respectively ($p = 0.38$). There were, however, significantly higher MACE rates and higher mortality rates at 16.1% vs. 9.4% and 8.9% vs. 3.0% respectively (both $p < 0.001$). Despite this increase in overall mortality, the life expectancy of octogenarians undergoing DES treatment was similar to that of the general Minnesota population of the same age and gender (65).

Hassani et al. (66) also evaluated the outcome of DES placement in patients ≥80 years of age compared with younger patients. There were 339 octogenarians and 2827 younger patients. As expected, octogenarians had more adverse characteristics including more chronic renal failure, CHF, more extensive CAD, and lower LVEF. Multivariate analysis identified age >80 years at the index procedure, cardiogenic shock, Q-wave MI, and length of hospital stay to be independent predictors of mortality.

PREDICTORS OF STENTING OUTCOME IN THE ELDERLY

In a landmark study reflecting relatively current practice in PCI, Klein (67) examined 8828 octogenarians undergoing intervention with predominant stenting (75%) in the 100,000 patient ACC-National Cardiovascular Data Registry from 1998 to 2000. The most important factor identified as a predictor of in-hospital death in the elderly was the presence of an acute MI within 6 hours of PCI. For those over the age of 80 years, treated in a nonemergency fashion, the overall mortality was only 1.4% (vs. 13.8% for intervention in the setting of acute infarction), with low stroke rates (0.34%) and infrequent renal failure (1.5%), though a notable degree of vascular complications (3.0%). The overall success rate was 93%, with slightly lower success in those with acute infarctions (91% vs. 94%). Other predictors of increased procedural mortality in octogenarians, if present (vs. if not present), included decreased LVEF, acute renal failure (29% vs. 3.2%), peripheral vascular disease with vascular complications (8.2% vs. 3.3%), procedural Q-wave infarction (17.4% vs. 3.7%), and stroke (17% vs. 3.3%). Predictors of higher mortality were two to three times as frequent with acute MI.

Other studies have identified the presence of multivessel disease, CHF, left main disease, thrombus, vein graft treatment, cardiogenic shock, chronic renal failure, prior MI, prior CABG as additive predictors of poor outcome in PCI in the elderly in the stent era

Table 13.1 Factors Predicting Adverse Outcome and/or Mortality with Percutaneous Coronary Revascularization in the Elderly

Baseline Characteristics	Procedural Issues
Age over 80 years	Decreased LVEF
Numerous comorbid illnesses	Respiratory failure/intubation
Frailty	Multivessel disease
Prior CABG	Left main coronary disease
Prior myocardial infarction	Intracoronary thrombus
Cardiogenic shock	Saphenous vein graft disease
Acute myocardial infarction	Acute renal failure post-PCI
Chronic renal failure	Q-wave infarction post-PCI
Peripheral vascular disease	Stroke post-PCI
Congestive heart failure	Vascular access complication

Abbreviations: CABG, coronary artery bypass surgery; LVEF, left ventricular ejection fraction; PCI, percutaneous coronary intervention.

(8,10). The SYNTAX score, defined by the sum of the points assigned to each individual lesion identified in the 16 segments of the coronary tree with >50% diameter narrowing in vessels >1.5 mm diameter, can also help predict mortality at 30 days in patients undergoing primary PCI for acute coronary syndrome (37.1% for high SYNTAX score vs. 5.1% for low/intermediate SYNTAX score; $p < 0.0001$). The clinical SYNTAX score also predicted 1-year MACE rates (12.1% for high clinical SYNTAX score vs. 3.1% for low/intermediate clinical SYNTAX score, $p = 0.03$) (68).

In past few years, there has been an increasing interest in studying the impact of frailty on the success of PCI in the elderly. Frailty, the clinical syndrome of physical functional decline, decreased nutrition, and reduced cognitive and physical resistance to stressors, occurs in about 10% of 75–85 year olds and >25% of patients >85 years old. Frail elderly patients undergoing PCI had an increased 3-year mortality rate of 28% (vs. 6% for nonfrail patients) and increased 3-year rates of death or MI of 41% (vs. 17% for nonfrail patients). The hazard ratio of frailty for mortality in patients undergoing PCI was 4.2 [CI 1.85, 9.51] (69). The factors associated with adverse procedural outcome with PCI are listed in Table 13.1.

PCI FOR ACUTE CORONARY SYNDROMES IN THE ELDERLY
The elderly have been underrepresented in many clinical trials, including those of PCI for acute coronary syndrome. This relates to the atypical presentation of acute coronary syndrome in the elderly (less likely to present with chest pain, longer prehospital delay and higher prevalence of left bundle branch block) and as well as more frequent comorbidities, including CHF (70), and higher rates of adverse outcomes, including bleeding and mortality (11), in this group (71,72).

ST-Elevation Myocardial Infarction
Approximately 60–65% of ST-elevation myocardial infarctions (STEMIs) occur in patients ≥65 years of age, and up to 33% occur in patients ≥75 years of age (73). Furthermore, up to 80% of deaths due to STEMI occur in patients ≥65 years of age. Reperfusion therapy has become the standard of care in STEMI. The GUSTO-I trial was one of the first to recognize the survival advantage of rapid restoration of normal coronary blood flow in the infarct-related artery. Reperfusion therapy was introduced with thrombolytic agents, but it became

apparent that in the elderly, particularly those over the age of 75, thrombolysis resulted in worrisome levels of disabling and/or fatal strokes, negating some of the survival benefits of opened arteries (74,75). The stroke risk appeared to be higher with tissue plasminogen activator (tPA) therapy than with streptokinase. As angioplasty and stenting techniques became accepted therapy in chronic stable angina, their use as primary therapy in acute infarction in the elderly was studied.

Gottlieb et al. (76) studied trends in management of acute MI in 1475 patients ≥75 years of age in Israel. Over the 10 years from 1992–2002, there was a significant increase in reperfusion therapy (27–48%), PCI (3% to 33%), medical therapy including aspirin (53–88%), beta-blockers (18 65%), and ACE inhibitors (26–63%). During the same decade, there was a 42% reduction in the 30-day mortality (27–16% OR 0.57, 95% CI 0.36–0.93) and a 20% reduction in 1-year mortality (37–29%).

Marked regional differences in care have been documented in older coronary patients. Ko et al. (77) compared procedural and medication use and 30-day risk standardized mortality in 38,886 US fee-for-service Medicare beneficiaries versus 5634 similarly aged Canadian patients and found significant differences. Overall, the use of invasive procedures was higher in the USA (38.5% vs. 16.8% ($p < 0.001$)). Despite this, the standardized 30-day mortality was not different. This finding has not been universal. Harpaz et al. (78) studied 1009 patients ≥75 years of age in all coronary care units in Israel. Those patients who underwent coronary angiography were on average 2.2 years younger, had a higher systolic pressure, better Killip class, and were more likely to have NSTEMI. Of the patients who underwent coronary angiography, 67% underwent revascularization either with PCI or with surgery. These authors found that both the crude and adjusted 1-year mortality rates were lower in patients who underwent angiography (21% vs. 37%, $p < 0.0001$).

There are several potential reasons for the worse outcome in the elderly versus younger patients with acute coronary syndrome. Popitean et al. (79) evaluated the French regional survey data. They found that with increasing age, there are increased prehospital delays. In addition, once in hospital, the time to recognition is increased in elderly patients in part because of atypical symptom presentations. The elderly are also more likely to have heart failure (70) and are less likely to receive guideline-based medication regimens (80,81).

These and other data have moved the practice of reperfusion in elderly patients with acute coronary syndrome toward an invasive strategy. Sakai et al. (82) evaluated 1087 patients treated by primary angioplasty and subdivided them by age ≥75 years and those <75 years of age. They found that the mortality in the older patients was higher (8.1% vs. 4.0%, $p = 0.0057$). Successful reperfusion was achieved in 91.6% and 92.9% of patients respectively. When reperfusion was successful, cardiac mortality in older patients was not statistically significantly higher (4.6% vs. 2.8%, $p = 0.14$). Guagliumi et al. (83) analyzed the outcome of elderly patients in the Controlled Abciximab and Device Investigation to Lower Late Angioplasty Complications (CADILLAC) trial of PCI in acute MI. They found that 1-year mortality increased for each decile of age. In those patients <55 years, 1-year mortality was 1.6% but increased to 11.1% for patients >75 years ($p < 0.0001$). In addition, elderly patients had increased rates of stroke and major bleeding. Among patients ≥65 years, 1-year rates of ischemic target revascularization (7.0% vs. 17.6%, $p < 0.0001$) and subacute or late thrombosis (0% vs. 2.2%, $p = 0.005$) were reduced with stenting compared with balloon angioplasty. Routine abciximab administration, although safe, was not of definite benefit in elderly patients.

In a Medicare analysis from the Cooperative Cardiovascular Project, the 2.5% of elderly patients who underwent primary PCI, when compared to the 23% treated with fibrinolytic therapy, had significant reductions in mortality at 30 days and 1 year (8.7% vs. 11.9% and 14.4% vs. 17.6%, respectively). After adjusting for baseline cardiac risk factors and admission and hospital characteristics, primary PCI was associated with improved 30-day (hazard ratio [HR] of death 0.74, 95% confidence interval [CI] 0.63–0.88) and 1-year (HR 0.88, 95% CI 0.73–0.94) survival (84).

Two randomized trials of reperfusion therapy for acute infarction specifically in the elderly have been reported. Boer et al. (85) randomized 87 patients over the age of 75 years PCI (46 patients) versus streptokinase therapy (41 patients). Of the 41 patients who actually received PCI (21 receiving stents), 90% had a successful procedure. The results were dramatic, with in-hospital mortality (7% vs. 20%), 30-day mortality (7% vs. 22%), 1-year mortality (13% vs. 41%), stroke (1% vs. 7%) and reinfarction rates (2% vs. 15%) showing significant advantages of PCI over thrombolysis. Goldenberg et al. (86) randomized 130 consecutive patients ≥70 years with STEMI to alteplase or primary angioplasty with routine stenting. At 6 months, patients treated with primary angioplasty, compared with those treated with thrombolytic therapy, had a lower incidence of reinfarction (2% vs. 14%, $p = 0.05$) and revascularization for recurrent ischemia (9% vs. 61%, $p < 0.001$) and a significant reduction in the prespecified combined end point of death, reinfarction, or revascularization for recurrent ischemia (29% vs. 93%, $p < 0.01$). Major bleeding complications were also significantly reduced in the primary angioplasty group (0% vs. 17%, $p = 0.03$). A meta-analysis (87) of 22 randomized trials comparing primary PCI with fibrinolysis showed mortality reduction as well as MI and stroke reduction with PCI in all age strata.

Non-ST-Segment Elevation Myocardial Infarction

Elderly patients with NSTEMI generally have more adverse baseline clinical characteristics than STEMI patients and are more likely to present with a TIMI risk score of ≥3 than younger patients (91% vs. 63%). In the TACTICS-TIMI 18 substudy, an early invasive strategy compared to a conservative strategy significantly reduced the incidence of death or MI at 30 days (5.7% vs. 9.8%) and 6 months (8.8% vs.13.6%) in patients ≥65 years of age. Among patients >75 years of age, the advantage of an early invasive strategy in reducing the incidence of death or MI at 6 months was even more marked (10.8% vs. 21.6%) at the expense of increased frequency of major bleeding (16.6% vs. 6.5%) (88). Unfortunately, patients with major comorbidities such as previous stroke or heart failure were excluded from this analysis.

Despite this scientific data, the elderly are often treated differently than younger patients. Yan et al. (89) stratified 4627 patients admitted with an acute coronary syndrome in the Canadian Acute Coronary Syndrome Registry into three groups (<65, 65–74, and ≥75 years of age). Across a broad spectrum, the elderly patients were at higher risk but were less likely to receive evidence-based medical therapy or to undergo revascularization. Another registry confirmed a lower use of coronary angiography (35% vs. 73%) and PCI (9% vs. 31%) in patients ≥75 years old compared to those <65 years of age for non-STEMI acute coronary syndromes (90). In another large survey from Europe, Rosengren et al. (91) analyzed 10,253 patients with acute coronary syndrome from 25 countries. There was a significant inverse association between age and the likelihood of presenting with a STEMI, and once again, elderly patients were investigated less intensively and were more apt to be seen by a general medical physician rather than a cardiologist.

Substantial variability in care of the elderly with acute coronary syndrome has also been documented. Alexander et al. (92) used data from the SYMPHONY trials to compare 1794 patients ≥75 years of age versus 14,043 <75 years of age. Elderly patients presented with higher risk and underwent catheterization less frequently than younger patients [53% vs. 63%; adjusted OR 0.53 (0.46, 0.60)]. Absolute catheterization rates varied from 27% (non-US cohort) to 77% (US cohort). Revascularization of elderly who underwent cardiac catheterization was also higher in US than non-US cohorts (71.3% vs. 53.6%). Of interest in this study, performance of cardiac catheterization was not an independent predictor of 90-day death and the combined endpoint of death or MI.

Finally, Avezum et al. (93) evaluated the effect of age on treatment in the GRACE Registry of 24,165 acute coronary syndrome patients from 14 countries. Aspirin, beta-blockers, thrombolytic therapy, statins, and IIb/IIIa glycoprotein inhibitors were all used less frequently with increasing age. In addition, performance of coronary angiography and PCI was also less frequent in the older patients. The CRUSADE study showed that in-hospital mortality and complication rates in acute coronary syndrome increased with advancing age, but those patients receiving more recommended therapies had lower mortality, even after adjustment for other covariates, than those who did not (94).

ACUTE INTERVENTION IN CARDIOGENIC SHOCK COMPLICATING MI IN THE ELDERLY

The SHould we emergently revascularize Occluded Coronaries for Cardiogenic ShocK? (SHOCK) Trial suggested a survival advantage with rapid revascularization for younger patients with cardiogenic shock complicating acute MI (95). However, there was a trend toward poorer outcome in those over the age of 75 years who were revascularized versus those receiving aggressive MED, which included use of an intra-aortic balloon pump (75% vs. 53% 30-day morality). A portion of this trial occurred during an era of lower stent use and also may not be reflective of contemporary use of glycoprotein IIb/IIIa receptor inhibitors. On the other hand, the SHOCK registry (96) showed that the relative risk for in-hospital mortality was significantly reduced with early revascularization compared to initial medical therapy with or without late revascularization in both older (relative risk 0.46) and younger patients (relative risk 0.76).

The observational studies of acute intervention in the elderly for cardiogenic shock complicating acute MI have suggested significant survival advantages with stenting. The large Global Registry of Acute Coronary Events (GRACE) Investigation of 583 patients (April 1999 to June 2001), of which 40% were ≥75 years, showed an overall mortality rate of 59%, with a rate of only 35% in those treated with stenting as compared to 74% in those who had no cardiac catheterization (20).Revascularization was used in only 33% of patients ≥75 years compared with 50% of nonelderly patients with shock ($p < 0.001$). On multivariate analysis, PCI with stenting was the most powerful positive predictor of hospital survival (OR 3.99, 95% CI 2.41–6.62) and older age the most powerful negative predictor of hospital survival (OR 0.70, 95% CI 0.60–0.83 for every 10-year increase). Two smaller studies have shown similar benefits, but have attributed much of the effect to synergy between use of stents and the use of abciximab. In 96 and 113 patients, respectively (mean age 66 years in both studies), Chan (97) and Giri (98) noted angiographic success rates (TIMI-3 flow) of 85% in the abciximab-stenting patients versus lower rates (64–67%) with stenting alone, angioplasty plus abciximab and angioplasty alone. Mortality in the abciximab-stenting groups was 13% to 22% (vs. 36–38% in both angioplasty groups and 36%–52% mortality in the stent only groups), indicating significant benefit in these high-risk patients. Prasad et al. (99) evaluated the outcome of elderly patients with shock at Mayo Clinic who underwent PCI. They found in 61 patients with a mean age of 79.5 years that in hospital mortality occurred in 44%. However, the 1 year survival after hospital discharge was 75%. Although the momentum is building toward a preferred role for acute interventions in elderly patients with acute cardiogenic shock after acute MI, one must await randomized multicenter trials to make firm recommendations. In an elderly patient with minimal prior comorbidities, PCI with stenting in acute cardiogenic shock may be a consideration, whereas it may not be appropriate in a frail patient with numerous health concerns.

DRUGS FOR PCI IN THE ELDERLY

Medication choice and dosing is challenging in the elderly due to age-related changes in drug distribution and metabolism. The elderly have ~20% less adipose-free mass, reduced hepatic metabolism and higher likelihood of renal insufficiency. Pharmacotherapy must be tailored with these age-associated physiological changes in mind so as to prevent increased morbidity.

Clopidogrel dosing in the elderly is not different from non-elderly patients and is usually given orally prior to PCI as 600 mg to achieve a maximal antiplatelet effect in 2 hours or as 300 mg to achieve a maximal antiplatelet effect in 6 hours, followed by 75 mg daily. Subgroup analysis from PCI-CURE revealed an almost significant trend toward benefit in acute coronary syndrome in patients ≥65 years of age (relative risk 0.79 compared to placebo, 95% CI 0.57–1.08) (100). Age remains a significant predictor of bleeding in patients ≥75 years with a hazard ratio of 2.4 (95% CI 1.97–2.91, $p < 0.0001$) in the CHARISMA trial (101).

Prasugrel was evaluated in the TRITON-TIMI 38 study (102) of primary PCI in patients with acute coronary syndrome. Prasugrel at a loading dose of 60 mg followed by 10 mg daily resulted in a 19% reduction in major cardiac adverse events compared to clopidogrel, but this risk reduction decreased with increasing age from 25% in <65 year olds to 14% in 65–74 year olds and to 6% in patients age ≥75 years. This benefit came at the cost of increased major bleeding (HR 1.32, 95% CI 1.03–1.68). Patients 75 years of age or older had no net benefit from prasugrel (HR 0.99, 95% CI 0.81–1.21, $p = 0.92$), and its use in the elderly is thus not recommended. Similarly, patients weighing less than 60 kg had no net benefit from prasugrel (HR 1.03, 95% CI 0.69–1.53, $p = 0.89$), and patients who had a previous stroke or transient ischemic attack had net harm from prasugrel (HR 1.54, 95% CI 1.02–2.32, $p = 0.04$).

The antiplatelet option for patients undergoing PCI is ticagrelor—an oral, reversible, direct-acting inhibitor of the adenosine diphosphate receptor P2Y12 that has a more rapid onset and more pronounced platelet inhibition than clopidogrel. In the multicenter PLATO study (103), ticagrelor (180 mg loading dose, 90 mg twice daily thereafter) was compared to clopidogrel for the prevention of cardiovascular events in 18,624 patients admitted to the hospital with an acute coronary syndrome, with or without ST-segment elevation. At 12 months, the primary end point—a composite of death from vascular causes, MI, or stroke—had occurred in 9.8% of patients receiving ticagrelor as compared with 11.7% of those receiving clopidogrel (HR 0.84, 95% CI 0.77–0.92, $p < 0.001$). This included lower rates of MI alone (5.8% in the ticagrelor group vs. 6.9% in the clopidogrel group, $p = 0.005$) and death from vascular causes (4.0% vs. 5.1%, $p = 0.001$) but not stroke alone (1.5% vs. 1.3%, $p = 0.22$). The rate of death from any cause was also reduced with ticagrelor (4.5% vs. 5.9% with clopidogrel; $p < 0.001$). There was no significant difference in the rates of major bleeding between the ticagrelor and clopidogrel groups (11.6% and 11.2%, respectively; $p = 0.43$), but ticagrelor was associated with a higher rate of major bleeding not related to coronary-artery bypass grafting (4.5% vs. 3.8%, $p = 0.03$), including more instances of fatal intracranial bleeding and fewer of fatal bleeding of other types. Subgroup analysis showed no interaction of age for either the primary endpoint or major bleeding, making ticagrelor an important option in the elderly undergoing PCI.

Use of GP IIb/IIIa inhibitors in the elderly has both significant anti-ischemic benefits as well as possible increased risk of bleeding. Limited data from a subgroup analysis of the ADMIRAL trial (104) found that the benefit with GP IIb/IIIa inhibitors was greater in STEMI patients ≥65 years of age than in younger patients (RR 0.35 (0.12–0.98)) with the composite endpoint of death, MI or revascularization at 6 months being 7.6% with abciximab versus 21.7% without. In NSTEMI, age was not a significant determinant of the benefit of GP IIb/IIIa inhibitors in one meta-analysis (105). In the ESPRIT study (106), patients undergoing PCI for acute or chronic coronary disease with eptifibatide had a lower composite risk of death, MI, urgent target-vessel revascularization or thrombotic use of GP IIb/IIIa inhibitors versus placebo, and this was predominantly in the subgroup of patients ≥65 years of age (RR 0.47, 95% CI 0.31–0.72) rather than in younger patients (RR 0.84, 95% CI 0.56–1.25).

The greatest concern of use of GP IIb/IIIa inhibitors in the elderly is the increased risk of bleeding, both at the access site (26% vs. 20%) and non-access site (5.2% vs. 2.5%), but without increased intracranial hemorrhage or increased need for blood transfusion (107). Most of this excess bleeding risk could be decreased with careful dosing since an evaluation of the CRUSADE registry showed a remarkable 64.5% overdoing of GP IIb/IIIa inhibitors in patients aged ≥75 years compared to only 8.5% in patients <65 years old. Overdosing GP IIb/IIIa inhibitors was associated with increased risk of bleeding (OR 1.38, 95% CI 1.12–1.70). Abciximab is given at a dose of 0.25 mg/kg IV bolus, then 0.125 mcg/kg/min IV (max 10 mcg/min), and no adjustment is needed for renal clearance. However, dose adjustment is required for eptifibatide and tirofiban. With normal renal function, eptifibatide is given as 180 mcg/kg IV bolus x2, 10 min apart (max 22.6 mg each bolus) and then an infusion of 2 mcg/kg/min (max 15 mg/hr) after first bolus. For patients with a creatinine clearance of < 50 ml/min, the infusion should be decreased to 1 mcg/kg/min (max 7.5 mg/hr). It is contraindicated in dialysis patients.

No dose adjustment is needed for unfractionated heparin, but low molecular weight heparin should be avoided in patients with a creatinine clearance ≤30 ml/min or on dialysis. The direct thrombin inhibitor bivalirudin has been shown to have similar outcomes compared to heparin and GP IIb/IIIa inhibitors with regard to death, MI or revascularization in the REPLACE 2 trial (108), but better composite outcome in patients >75 years old (OR 0.51, 95% CI 0.26–0.98). Similarly in the ACUITY trial, the risk of bleeding in acute coronary syndrome patients undergoing PCI was decreased most in patients ≥75 years (NNT of 16 vs. 38 in patients <55 years). If bivalirudin is used, the bolus dose is 0.75 mg/kg IV followed by infusion of 1.75 mg/kg/hr IV, which should be decreased to 1 mg/kg/hr in patients with a creatinine clearance of 10–29 ml/min and to 0.25 mg/kg/hr in hemodialysis patients.

OPTIONS FOR REVASCULARIZATION IN THE ELDERLY

From early in the revascularization era, a definite role for CABG has emerged in higher risk patient groups based on its consistent beneficial effect on long-term survival and in reducing anginal symptoms (13,109–113). The success of CABG versus PCI in the elderly has been attributed mostly to CABG's greater efficacy at achieving complete revascularization of all or most affected vessel territories in the setting of multivessel CAD, left main CAD, advanced AHA/ACC lesion class, and/or lower LVEF (11,48,99,110–112,114–120). Whereas balloon angioplasty in the 1980s and early 1990s was an accepted therapy for single-vessel disease (121), the frequent problem of restenosis, as demonstrated by 5-year revascularization rates exceeding 50% in BARI, has limited its widespread application in multivessel disease, particularly in the presence of diabetes (109,122). Past studies with PCI, even with stenting, have shown frequent recurrent angina leading to repeat PCIs and ultimate need for CABG in up to 20% of patients (55–57,109,115,117,122,123).

Unfortunately, CABG surgery in the elderly is not entirely a benign procedure. The overall mortality rate of CABG in a 1990 Medicare database of nearly 24,500 patients over age 80 was higher compared with patients aged 65–70, with higher in-hospital mortality (11.5% vs. 4.4%), 1-year mortality (19.3% vs. 7.9%), and 3-year mortality (28.8% vs. 13.1%) rates (124). Many elderly patients are also at substantial risk of perioperative MI, pneumonia, renal failure, prolonged mechanical ventilation, and neurological events, with rates between 2% and 10% (122,125). Given these risks, in addition to cognitive impairments seen in 60% short-term and 20% long-term post-CABG in the elderly (125–127), many patients will not regain their previous level of function and, thus, suffer a loss in their quality of life. Some elderly patients, particularly those who have extensive CAD, a recent or prior MI, prior revascularization, or additional comorbidities, will have even higher potential morbidity and mortality with CABG.

The search for a viable alternative to CABG has continued to make steady progress. The PCI studies with predominant stent use demonstrate comparable or slightly better survival with PCI versus CABG, but have still failed to avoid the subsequent need for additional revascularization in the PCI group, especially in the setting of diabetes (98,99,114–117,123). A systematic review and meta-analysis (128) of 66 studies of coronary revascularization in patients aged over 80 years comparing CABG and PCI showed similar pooled estimated 30 day mortality rates (7.3% for CABG vs. 5.4% for PCI) and 1-year survival rates (86% for CABG vs. 87% for PCI). The question, when deciding upon the most suitable revascularization modality, is whether the higher procedural morbidity/mortality with CABG is justified by the 20% lower 5-year need for repeat revascularization compared with PCI. In the setting of numerous comorbidities or frailty, elderly patients may be better served with moderate-duration symptomatic improvement offered by PCI. Indeed, one issue many studies fail to recognize when reporting poorer long-term survival in the elderly after either CABG or PCI is that the long-term survival with a successful revascularization modality is not very different compared to others of similar age (10,124). Factors favoring preferential attempts at PCI with stenting compared to those favoring CABG in the elderly are listed in Table 13.2.

Table 13.2 Factors Favoring Better Revascularization Results with Either Percutaneous Coronary Intervention or Coronary Artery Bypass Surgery in the Elderly

Patient Characteristics	
Percutaneous Intervention Better	**Coronary Bypass Better**
Age over 80	Diabetes (extensive disease)
Numerous comorbid illnesses	No major comorbid illnesses
Frail health/limited life expectancy	Active lifestyle/expect longevity
Major depression	Dedicated to lifestyle changes
Poor motivation to rehabilitate	Great motivation to rehabilitate
Morbid obesity/severe COPD	Thin, athletic in past
Angiographic Characteristics	
Percutaneous Intervention Better	**Coronary Bypass Better**
Focal/limited 1- or 2-vessel CAD	3-vessel CAD/left main CAD
3-vessel CAD—low SYNTAX score	3-vessel CAD—intermediate/high SYNTAX score
Good left ventricular function	Poor left ventricular function
AHA/ACC Type A, B1 lesion	AHA/ACC Type B2, C lesion
Bifurcation: risk to small branch	Bifurcation: risk to large branch
Crossable total occlusion	Uncrossable occlusion/large area of "jeopardized" tissue
Acute MI/cardiogenic shock	Stable CAD
Procedure goal: symptom relief	Goal: survival/symptom relief

Abbreviations: CAD, coronary artery disease; COPD, chronic obstructive pulmonary disease.

ELDERLY PATIENTS WITH MULTIVESSEL DISEASE: PCI VERSUS SURGERY

Some authors have suggested that the reduced event-free survival with PCI seen in the elderly may relate to the frequency of incomplete revascularization with PCI, but others believe it indirectly reflects the greater extent of active coronary disease in this population (44,51,52), associated with more coronary risk factors. Nonetheless, the relative lack of complete and durable revascularization achieved with PCI for multivessel disease in the elderly is a prime reason why many elderly patients will ultimately require surgery (129).

This was one of the major findings in the elderly subset of the largest randomized multivessel coronary angioplasty versus bypass study, the BARI (Bypass Angioplasty Revascularization Investigation) trial, which enrolled patients from 1988 to 1991 (122). No significant difference in 30-day mortality (1.7% in each arm) was noted in the 709 patients aged 65–80 who were randomized, although many patients with angioplasty required repeat revascularization and some ultimately had CABG. Only the subset with diabetes showed higher long-term mortality with angioplasty versus bypass surgery in all age groups, and this is definitely a consideration in elderly patients undergoing angioplasty in lieu of CABG (109). The rate of strokes with CABG was significantly higher in the elderly than with angioplasty (122). Given the prohibitively high repeat revascularization rates with balloon angioplasty seen in the overall population in BARI (52% vs. 6% with CABG at 5 years), stenting has become the preferred therapy. Importantly, even in the present era, not all lesions are suitable for stenting, and some may still be better treated with balloon angioplasty; hence these results are still clinically relevant in as many as 25–30% of PCI involving the elderly, particularly in small vessels, branch vessels, or those with heavy calcification.

With the advent of BMS in 1995 (130) and subsequently DES since 2003 (131), better techniques/devices to address higher risk ACC/AHA Type C lesions, and the greater use of antiplatelet therapies, outcomes with PCI have improved in general (114,132), primarily evidenced by decreased rates of restenosis requiring revascularization. Thus, PCI has become an attractive, if not preferred, alternative to CABG, especially in candidates not favorable for or desiring CABG. The questions are whether it is appropriate to perform multivessel stenting in the elderly and what are its benefits/problems versus CABG?

A number of contemporary trials of multivessel stenting compared with CABG for extensive disease have been reported. The ARTS (Arterial Revascularization Therapy Study) trial randomly assigned 1205 patients (600 to PCI vs. 605 to CABG) (115). The results in the nondiabetics showed low 1-year mortality in both assigned therapies (1.6% PCI vs. 2.8% CABG), with an overall 76% event-free survival at 12 months with stents compared to 88% with CABG ($p < 0.001$). Some 11.7% of PCI-assigned patients (vs. 2.9% CABG patients, $p < 0.001$) required subsequent PCI while 3.9% later underwent CABG (vs. 0.6% CABG patients, $p < 0.001$). Although CABG showed significantly better symptom-free survival, the stenting results were much more favorable than those at a similar follow-up stage in the BARI angioplasty subset (109), despite 70% of patients having complex type B2/C lesions. Results in the 208 randomized diabetic patients were not as attractive with PCI as with CABG (63% vs. 84% event-free survival at 18 months, $p < 0.001$), possibly related to the low 3.5% rate of abciximab use in this high-risk subset. Increasing age was not an independent predictor of worse outcome in the PCI group but was in the CABG group (OR 1.06/yr) in the ARTS trial.

In contrast to ARTS, multivessel stenting showed a better 18-month survival rate than CABG (96.9% vs. 92.5%; $p < 0.02$) in the ERACI-2 trial (Argentine Randomized Study) of multivessel therapy options (116), possibly related to the 28% use of abciximab and the higher procedural CABG mortality (5.7% vs. 0.9%). In the 225-patient PCI arm versus a similar-sized CABG arm, there was also a lower long-term rate of infarction (2.3% vs. 6.6%; $p < 0.02$), but the rate of repeat revascularization with PCI versus CABG patients was 16.8% compared to 4.8%. Age was not an independent predictor of MACE in the overall ERACI-2 population, but age ≥ 65 years was predictive of worse outcome in males (OR 2.22, 95%CI 1.00–4.95, $p < 0.05$). The randomized Stent or Surgery (SoS) trial, with 500 CABG patients and 488 multivessel PCI patients, also showed a high rate of 2-year repeat procedures of 21% in the PCI group versus 6% in the CABG patients (117). In patients aged 65 or older who were randomized to PCI, 19.5% required repeat revascularization versus 3.4% of patients treated with CABG ($p < 0.001$). In the older patients, 1 year health status, which included physical limitations, frequency of angina, and quality of life, was similar irrespective of whether the initial treatment was PCI or CABG (133). The low surgical mortality rate of 2% was in keeping with some 50% of patients having stable angina; the mortality rate in patients with unstable angina in the ERACI-2 trial was 7.9% (134).

Perhaps one of the most relevant trials to date in the elderly and in high-risk patients is the AWESOME trial (Angina With Serious Operative Mortality Evaluation). It enrolled 454 medically refractory veterans from 1995 to 2000 with one or more high-risk characteristics: age over 70 years, cardiac shock needing intra-aortic balloon pumping, LVEF <35%, prior CABG, and recent infarction (118). With 222 patients receiving multivessel stenting and 232 receiving CABG and at least 50% over age 67, it showed low 30-day (5% vs. 3%), 6-month (10% vs. 6%), and similar 3-year mortalities (21% vs. 20%) with CABG versus PCI, respectively. Thus, elderly patients who are high risk due to one or more of the above risk factors may be able to avoid the longer recovery of CABG and live just as long with multivessel stenting.

The SYNTAX trial (135) randomly assigned patients with previously untreated left main stem or three-vessel disease to undergo state-of-the-art CABG or PCI with DES. Despite not being a study specifically of the elderly, the mean age in both groups was 65 years. At 36-months follow-up, there was no difference between the two groups in the composite endpoint of death, MI, and stroke (PCI 14.1% vs. CABG 12.0%, $p = 0.21$), but the patients in the PCI group needed repeat revascularization more often than the CABG group (19.7% vs. 10.7%, $p < 0.001$). The rate of MI was also higher in the PCI group over 3 years (7.1% vs. 3.6%, $p = 0.002$), most likely due to the fact that PCI targets culprit lesions while CABG bypasses whole segments and thus possibly future culprit lesions. The rate of stroke was higher in the CABG group in the first year (2.2% vs. 0.6%, $p = 0.003$), possibly due to the lesser utilization of anti-platelet agents in this group, but this was no longer significant after 3 years (2.0% vs. 3.4%, $p = 0.07$). Furthermore, the investigators used an angiographic grading tool (the SYNTAX score) to determine the complexity of CAD. The SYNTAX score may help identify patients at low risk who may be appropriately treated with PCI with at least equivalent outcomes as CABG. On the other hand, intermediate- and high-risk patients by SYNTAX score were shown to have decreased major adverse cardiac and cerebrovascular events when assigned to CABG rather than PCI after 3 years (135).

GOALS OF REVASCULARIZATION IN THE ELDERLY

One drawback of comparing results of angioplasty and PCI in the elderly versus younger patients is that there is often a different emphasis on the goals of the procedure. More often, elderly patients are poor surgical candidates, with the palliative goal of reducing symptoms whereas younger patients are freer to consider the options: either the most effective procedure that will avoid the need for future procedures versus the one that will interfere the least with their active lifestyle. The options in the elderly are often less applicable or consist of picking the "better" of two "unappealing" therapy alternatives.

Choice of revascularization method depends on angiographic characteristics and likelihood of technical success with PCI, left ventricular function, presence of diabetes and other comorbidities, thrombotic and bleeding risk, risk of death, quality-of-life expectations, and patient preference. Improvement of interventional methods and medications has made PCI a preferred revascularization option in the oldest and/or sickest patients or in patients with a low SYNTAX score. Hybrid revascularization with combined surgical (left internal mammary artery graft to the left anterior descending artery) and percutaneous (DES to other lesions) treatment has some promise of combining the best of both worlds and is being actively studied (136). Hopefully, clinical trialists will continue to address revascularization issues in the elderly, recognizing their unique needs.

REFERENCES

1. Roger VL, Go AS, Lloyd-Jones DM, et al. Heart disease and stroke statistics--2012 update: a report from the American Heart Association. Circulation 2012; 125: e2–e220.
2. U.S. Census Bureau The Older Population. 2010. [Available From http://www.census.gov/prod/cen2010/briefs/c2010br-09.pdf] [accessed 21 06 2012].
3. Elveback L, Lie JT. Continued high incidence of coronary artery disease at autopsy in Olmsted County, Minnesota, 1950 to 1979. Circulation 1984; 70: 345–9.
4. Singh M, Peterson ED, Roe MT, et al. Trends in the association between age and in-hospital mortality after percutaneous coronary intervention: National Cardiovascular Data Registry experience. Circ Cardiovasc Interv 2009; 2: 20–6.
5. Feinleib M, Havlik RJ, Gillum RF, et al. Coronary heart disease and related procedures. National Hospital Discharge Survey data. Circulation 1989; 79: I13–18.
6. Lytle BW, Cosgrove D, Loop FD. Future implications of current trends in bypass surgery. Cardiovasc Clin 1991; 21: 265–78.
7. Thompson RC, Holmes DR Jr, Gersh BJ, Mock MB, Bailey KR. Percutaneous transluminal coronary angioplasty in the elderly: early and long-term results. J Am Coll Cardiol 1991; 17: 1245–50.
8. Singh M, Lennon RJ, Holmes DR Jr, Bell MR, Rihal CS. Correlates of procedural complications and a simple integer risk score for percutaneous coronary intervention. J Am Coll Cardiol 2002; 40: 387–93.
9. Gurwitz JH, Col NF, Avorn J. The exclusion of the elderly and women from clinical trials in acute myocardial infarction. JAMA 1992; 268: 1417–22.
10. Holmes DR Jr, Berger PB, Garratt KN, et al. Application of the New York State PTCA mortality model in patients undergoing stent implantation. Circulation 2000; 102: 517–22.
11. Singh M, Mathew V, Garratt KN, et al. Effect of age on the outcome of angioplasty for acute myocardial infarction among patients treated at the Mayo Clinic. Am J Med 2000; 108: 187–92.
12. Gersh BJ, Kronmal RA, Frye RL, et al. Coronary arteriography and coronary artery bypass surgery: morbidity and mortality in patients ages 65 years or older. A report from the Coronary Artery Surgery Study. Circulation 1983; 67: 483–91.
13. Graham MM, Ghali WA, Faris PD, et al. Survival after coronary revascularization in the elderly. Circulation 2002; 105: 2378–84.
14. TIME Investigators. Trial of invasive versus medical therapy in elderly patients with chronic symptomatic coronary-artery disease (TIME): a randomised trial. Lancet 2001; 358: 951–7.
15. Bell MR, Gersh BJ, Schaff HV, et al. Effect of completeness of revascularization on long-term outcome of patients with three-vessel disease undergoing coronary artery bypass surgery. A report from the Coronary Artery Surgery Study (CASS) Registry. Circulation 1992; 86: 446–57.
16. Kelsey SF, Miller DP, Holubkov R, et al. Results of percutaneous transluminal coronary angioplasty in patients greater than or equal to 65 years of age (from the 1985 to 1986 National Heart, Lung, and Blood Institute's Coronary Angioplasty Registry). Am J cardiol 1990; 66: 1033–8.
17. Backes RJ, Gersh BJ. The treatment of coronary artery disease in the elderly. Cardiovasc Drugs Ther 1991; 5: 449–55.
18. Nolan L, O'Malley K. Prescribing for the elderly. Part I: sensitivity of the elderly to adverse drug reactions. J Am Geriatr Soc 1988; 36: 142–9.
19. Dauerman HL, Goldberg RJ, Malinski M, et al. Outcomes and early revascularization for patients > or = 65 years of age with cardiogenic shock. Am J Cardiol 2001; 87: 844–8.
20. Dauerman HL, Goldberg RJ, White K, et al. Revascularization, stenting, and outcomes of patients with acute myocardial infarction complicated by cardiogenic shock. Am J Cardiol 2002; 90: 838–42.

21. Pfisterer M, Buser P, Osswald S, et al. Outcome of elderly patients with chronic symptomatic coronary artery disease with an invasive vs optimized medical treatment strategy: one-year results of the randomized TIME trial. JAMA 2003; 289: 1117–23.

22. Pfisterer M. Long-term outcome in elderly patients with chronic angina managed invasively versus by optimized medical therapy: four-year follow-up of the randomized Trial of Invasive versus Medical therapy in Elderly patients (TIME). Circulation 2004; 110: 1213–18.

23. Graham MM, Norris CM, Galbraith PD, Knudtson ML, Ghali WA. Quality of life after coronary revascularization in the elderly. Eur Heart J 2006; 27: 1690–8.

24. Claude J, Schindler C, Kuster GM, et al. Cost-effectiveness of invasive versus medical management of elderly patients with chronic symptomatic coronary artery disease. Findings of the randomized trial of invasive versus medical therapy in elderly patients with chronic angina (TIME). Eur Heart J 2004; 25: 2195–203.

25. Macaya C, Alfonso F, Iniguez A, Zarco P. Long-term clinical and angiographic follow-up of percutaneous transluminal coronary angioplasty in patients greater than or equal to 65 years of age. Am J Cardiol 1990; 66: 1513–15.

26. ten Berg JM, Bal ET, Gin TJ, et al. Initial and long-term results of percutaneous transluminal coronary angioplasty in patients 75 years of age and older. Cathet Cardiovasc Diagn 1992; 26: 165–70.

27. Voudris V, Antonellis J, Salachas A, et al. Coronary angioplasty in the elderly: immediate and long-term results. Angiology 1993; 44: 933–7.

28. Kowalchuk GJ, Siu SC, Lewis SM. Coronary artery disease in the octogenarian: angiographic spectrum and suitability for revascularization. Am J Cardiol 1990; 66: 1319–23.

29. Newman AB, Naydeck BL, Sutton-Tyrrell K, et al. Coronary artery calcification in older adults to age 99: prevalence and risk factors. Circulation 2001; 104: 2679–84.

30. Botas J, Stadius ML, Bourassa MG, et al. Angiographic correlates of lesion relevance and suitability for percutaneous transluminal coronary angioplasty and coronary artery bypass grafting in the Bypass Angioplasty Revascularization Investigation study (BARI). Am J Cardiol 1996; 77: 805–14.

31. Kastrati A, Schomig A, Elezi S, et al. Prognostic value of the modified american college of Cardiology/American heart association stenosis morphology classification for long-term angiographic and clinical outcome after coronary stent placement. Circulation 1999; 100: 1285–90.

32. Margolis JR, Kannel WS, Feinleib M, Dawber TR, McNamara PM. Clinical features of unrecognized myocardial infarction--silent and symptomatic. Eighteen year follow-up: the Framingham study. Am J Cardiol 1973; 32: 1–7.

33. Lindsay J Jr, Reddy VM, Pinnow EE, Little T, Pichard AD. Morbidity and mortality rates in elderly patients undergoing percutaneous coronary transluminal angioplasty. Am Heart J 1994; 128: 697–702.

34. Buffet P, Danchin N, Juilliere Y, et al. Percutaneous transluminal coronary angioplasty in patients more than 75 years old: early and long-term results. Int J Cardiol 1992; 37: 33–9.

35. Imburgia M, King TR, Soffer AD, et al. Early results and long-term outcome of percutaneous transluminal coronary angioplasty in patients age 75 years or older. Am J Cardiol 1989; 63: 1127–9.

36. Bedotto JB, Rutherford BD, McConahay DR, et al. Results of multivessel percutaneous transluminal coronary angioplasty in persons aged 65 years and older. Am J Cardiol 1991; 67: 1051–5.

37. Jollis JG, Peterson ED, Bebchuk JD, et al. Coronary angioplasty in 20,006 patients over age 80 in the United States. J Am Coll Cardiol 1995; 25: 47A.

38. Thompson RC, Holmes DR Jr, Grill DE, Mock MB, Bailey KR. Changing outcome of angioplasty in the elderly. J Am Coll Cardiol 1996; 27: 8–14.

39. Feldman DN, Gade CL, Slotwiner AJ, et al. Comparison of outcomes of percutaneous coronary interventions in patients of three age groups (<60, 60 to 80, and >80 years) (from the New York State Angioplasty Registry). Am J Cardiol 2006; 98: 1334–9.

40. Maiello L, Colombo A, Gianrossi R, Thomas J, Finci L. Percutaneous transluminal coronary angioplasty in patients aged 70 years and older: immediate and long-term results. Int J Cardiol 1992; 36: 1–8.

41. Hu F, Yang Y, Qiao S, et al. Comparison between radial and femoral approach for percutaneous coronary intervention in patients 80 years or older. J Interv Cardiol 2012; 25:513–17.

42. Louvard Y, Benamer H, Garot P, et al. Comparison of transradial and transfemoral approaches for coronary angiography and angioplasty in octogenarians (the OCTOPLUS study). Am J Cardiol 2004; 94: 1177–80.

43. Romagnoli E, Biondi-Zoccai G, Sciahbasi A, et al. Radial versus femoral randomized investigation in ST-segment elevation acute coronary syndrome: the RIFLE-STEACS (Radial Versus Femoral Randomized Investigation in ST-Elevation Acute Coronary Syndrome) study. J Am Coll Cardiol 2012; 60:2481–9.

44. Thompson RC, Holmes DR Jr, Gersh BJ, Bailey KR. Predicting early and intermediate-term outcome of coronary angioplasty in the elderly. Circulation 1993; 88: 1579–87.

45. Maiello L, Colombo A, Gianrossi R, Thomas J, Finci L. Results of coronary angioplasty in patients aged 75 years and older. Chest 1992; 102: 375–9.

46. Ellis SG, Vandormael MG, Cowley MJ, et al. Coronary morphologic and clinical determinants of procedural outcome with angioplasty for multivessel coronary disease. Implications for patient selection. Multivessel Angioplasty Prognosis Study Group. Circulation 1990; 82: 1193–202.

47. Jackman JD Jr, Navetta FI, Smith JE, et al. Percutaneous transluminal coronary angioplasty in octogenarians as an effective therapy for angina pectoris. Am J Cardiol 1991; 68: 116–19.

48. Bourassa MG, Lesperance J, Eastwood C, et al. Clinical, physiologic, anatomic and procedural factors predictive of restenosis after percutaneous transluminal coronary angioplasty. J Am Coll Cardiol 1991; 18: 368–76.

49. Hirshfeld JW Jr, Schwartz JS, Jugo R, et al. Restenosis after coronary angioplasty: a multivariate statistical model to relate lesion and procedure variables to restenosis. The M-HEART Investigators. J Am Coll Cardiol 1991; 18: 647–56.

50. Holmes DR Jr, Vlietstra RE, Smith HC, et al. Restenosis after percutaneous transluminal coronary angioplasty (PTCA): a report from the PTCA Registry of the National Heart, Lung, and Blood Institute. Am J Cardiol 1984; 53: 77C–81C.

51. de Jaegere P, de Feyter P, van Domburg R, et al. Immediate and long term results of percutaneous coronary angioplasty in patients aged 70 and over. Br Heart J 1992; 67: 138–43.

52. O'Keefe JH Jr, Sutton MB, McCallister BD, et al. Coronary angioplasty versus bypass surgery in patients >70 years old matched for ventricular function. J Am Coll Cardiol 1994; 24: 425–30.

53. Yokoi H, Kimaura T, Sawada, Y. Efficacy and safety of Palmatz-Schatz stent in the elderly (>75 years old) patients: early and follow-up results [abstr]. J Am Coll Cardiol 1995; 25: 47.

54. Chevalier B, Guyon P, Glatt B. Coronary angioplasty in the elderly in the stenting era. J Am Coll Cardiol 1998; 31: 234.

55. Batchelor WB, Anstrom KJ, Muhlbaier LH, et al. Contemporary outcome trends in the elderly undergoing percutaneous coronary interventions: results in 7,472 octogenarians. National Cardiovascular Network Collaboration. J Am Coll Cardiol 2000; 36: 723–30.

56. Chauhan MS, Kuntz RE, Ho KL, et al. Coronary artery stenting in the aged. J Am Coll Cardiol 2001; 37: 856–62.

57. Abizaid AS, Mintz GS, Abizaid A, et al. Influence of patient age on acute and late clinical outcomes following Palmaz-Schatz coronary stent implantation. Am J Cardiol 2000; 85: 338–43.

58. De Gregorio J, Kobayashi Y, Albiero R, et al. Coronary artery stenting in the elderly: short-term outcome and long-term angiographic and clinical follow-up. J Am Coll Cardiol 1998; 32: 577–83.

59. Cohen HA, Williams DO, Holmes DR Jr, et al. Impact of age on procedural and 1-year outcome in percutaneous transluminal coronary angioplasty: a report from the NHLBI Dynamic Registry. Am Heart J 2003; 146: 513–19.

60. From AM, Rihal CS, Lennon RJ, Holmes DR Jr, Prasad A. Temporal trends and improved outcomes of percutaneous coronary revascularization in nonagenarians. JACC Cardiovasc Interv 2008; 1: 692–8.

61. Alfonso F, Azcona L, Perez-Vizcayno MJ, et al. Initial results and long-term clinical and angiographic implications of coronary stenting in elderly patients. Am J Cardiol 1999; 83: 1483–7; A7.

62. Munoz JC, Alonso JJ, Duran JM, et al. Coronary stent implantation in patients older than 75 years of age: clinical profile and initial and long-term (3 years) outcome. Am Heart J 2002; 143: 620–6.

63. Groeneveld PW, Matta MA, Greenhut AP, Yang F. Drug-eluting compared with bare-metal coronary stents among elderly patients. J Am Coll Cardiol 2008; 51: 2017–24.

64. Douglas PS, Brennan JM, Anstrom KJ, et al. Clinical effectiveness of coronary stents in elderly persons: results from 262,700 Medicare patients in the American College of Cardiology-National Cardiovascular Data Registry. J Am Coll Cardiol 2009; 53: 1629–41.

65. Vlaar PJ, Lennon RJ, Rihal CS, et al. Drug-eluting stents in octogenarians: early and intermediate outcome. Am Heart J 2008; 155: 680–6.

66. Hassani SE, Wolfram RM, Kuchulakanti PK, et al. Percutaneous coronary intervention with drug-eluting stents in octogenarians: characteristics, clinical presentation, and outcomes. Catheter Cardiovasc Interv 2006; 68: 36–43.

67. Klein LW, Block P, Brindis RG, et al. Percutaneous coronary interventions in octogenarians in the American College of Cardiology-National Cardiovascular Data Registry: Development of a nomogram predictive of in-hospital mortality. J Am Coll Cardiol 2002; 40: 394–402.

68. Scherff F, Vassalli G, Surder D, et al. The SYNTAX score predicts early mortality risk in the elderly with acute coronary syndrome having primary PCI. J Invasive Cardiol 2011; 23: 505–10.

69. Singh M, Rihal CS, Lennon RJ, et al. Influence of frailty and health status on outcomes in patients with coronary disease undergoing percutaneous revascularization. Circ Cardiovasc Qual Outcomes 2011; 4: 496–502.

70. Mehta RH, Rathore SS, Radford MJ, et al. Acute myocardial infarction in the elderly: differences by age. J Am Coll Cardiol 2001; 38: 736–41.

71. Alexander KP, Newby LK, Cannon CP, et al. Acute coronary care in the elderly, part I: Non-ST-segment-elevation acute coronary syndromes: a scientific statement for healthcare professionals from the American Heart Association Council on Clinical Cardiology: in collaboration with the Society of Geriatric Cardiology. Circulation 2007; 115: 2549–69.

72. Alexander KP, Newby LK, Armstrong PW, et al. Acute coronary care in the elderly, part II: ST-segment-elevation myocardial infarction: a scientific statement for healthcare professionals from the American Heart Association Council on Clinical Cardiology: in collaboration with the Society of Geriatric Cardiology. Circulation 2007; 115: 2570–89.

73. Goldberg RJ, McCormick D, Gurwitz JH, et al. Age-related trends in short- and long-term survival after acute myocardial infarction: a 20-year population-based perspective (1975-1995). Am J Cardiol 1998; 82: 1311–17.

74. White HD, Barbash GI, Califf RM, et al. Age and outcome with contemporary thrombolytic therapy. Results from the GUSTO-I trial. Global Utilization of Streptokinase and TPA for Occluded coronary arteries trial. Circulation 1996; 94: 1826–33.

75. Holmes DR Jr, White HD, Pieper KS, et al. Effect of age on outcome with primary angioplasty versus thrombolysis. J Am Coll Cardiol 1999; 33: 412–19.

76. Gottlieb S, Behar S, Hod H, et al. Trends in management, hospital and long-term outcomes of elderly patients with acute myocardial infarction. Am J Med 2007; 120: 90–7.

77. Ko DT, Krumholz HM, Wang Y, et al. Regional differences in process of care and outcomes for older acute myocardial infarction patients in the United States and Ontario, Canada. Circulation 2007; 115: 196–203.

78. Harpaz D, Rozenman Y, Behar S, et al. Coronary angiography in the elderly with acute myocardial infarction. Int J Cardiol 2007; 116: 249–56.

79. Popitean L, Barthez O, Rioufol G, et al. Factors affecting the management of outcome in elderly patients with acute myocardial infarction particularly with regard to reperfusion. Data from the French regional RICO survey. Gerontology 2005; 51: 409–15.

80. Magid DJ, Masoudi FA, Vinson DR, et al. Older emergency department patients with acute myocardial infarction receive lower quality of care than younger patients. Ann Emerg Med 2005; 46: 14–21.

81. Lee DC, Pancu DM, Rudolph GS, Sama AE. Age-associated time delays in the treatment of acute myocardial infarction with primary percutaneous transluminal coronary angioplasty. Am J Emerg Med 2005; 23: 20–3.

82. Sakai K, Nakagawa Y, Soga Y, et al. Comparison of 30-day outcomes in patients <75 years of age versus >or=75 years of age with acute myocardial infarction treated by primary coronary angioplasty. Am J Cardiol 2006; 98: 1018–21.

83. Guagliumi G, Stone GW, Cox DA, et al. Outcome in elderly patients undergoing primary coronary intervention for acute myocardial infarction: Results from the Controlled Abciximab and Device Investigation to Lower Late Angioplasty Complications (CADILLAC) trial. Circulation 2004; 110: 1598–604.

84. Berger AK, Schulman KA, Gersh BJ, et al. Primary coronary angioplasty vs thrombolysis for the management of acute myocardial infarction in elderly patients. JAMA 1999; 282: 341–8.

85. de Boer MJ, Ottervanger JP, van 't Hof AW, et al. Reperfusion therapy in elderly patients with acute myocardial infarction: a randomized comparison of primary angioplasty and thrombolytic therapy. J Am Coll Cardiol 2002; 39: 1723–8.

86. Goldenberg I, Matetzky S, Halkin A, et al. Primary angioplasty with routine stenting compared with thrombolytic therapy in elderly patients with acute myocardial infarction. Am Heart J 2003; 145: 862–7.

87. de Boer SP, Westerhout CM, Simes RJ, et al. Mortality and morbidity reduction by primary percutaneous coronary intervention is independent of the patient's age. JACC Cardiovasc Interv 2010; 3: 324–31.

88. Bach RG, Cannon CP, Weintraub WS, et al. The effect of routine, early invasive management on outcome for elderly patients with non-ST-segment elevation acute coronary syndromes. Ann Intern Med 2004; 141: 186–95.

89. Yan RT, Yan AT, Tan M, et al. Age-related differences in the management and outcome of patients with acute coronary syndromes. Am Heart J 2006; 151: 352–9.

90. Paul SD, O'Gara PT, Mahjoub ZA, et al. Geriatric patients with acute myocardial infarction: cardiac risk factor profiles, presentation, thrombolysis, coronary interventions, and prognosis. Am Heart J 1996; 131: 710–15.

91. Rosengren A, Wallentin L, Simoons M, et al. Age, clinical presentation, and outcome of acute coronary syndromes in the Euroheart acute coronary syndrome survey. Eur Heart J 2006; 27: 789–95.

92. Alexander KP, Newby LK, Bhapkar MV, et al. International variation in invasive care of the elderly with acute coronary syndromes. Eur Heart J 2006; 27: 1558–64.

93. Avezum A, Makdisse M, Spencer F, et al. Impact of age on management and outcome of acute coronary syndrome: observations from the Global Registry of Acute Coronary Events (GRACE). Am Heart J 2005; 149: 67–73.

94. Alexander KP, Roe MT, Chen AY, et al. Evolution in cardiovascular care for elderly patients with non-ST-segment elevation acute coronary syndromes: results from the CRUSADE National Quality Improvement Initiative. J Am Coll Cardiol 2005; 46: 1479–87.

95. Hochman JS, Sleeper LA, Webb JG, et al. Early revascularization in acute myocardial infarction complicated by cardiogenic shock. SHOCK Investigators. Should We Emergently Revascularize Occluded Coronaries for Cardiogenic Shock. N Engl J Med 1999; 341: 625–34.

96. Dzavik V, Sleeper LA, Cocke TP, et al. Early revascularization is associated with improved survival in elderly patients with acute myocardial infarction complicated by cardiogenic shock: a report from the SHOCK Trial Registry. Eur Heart J 2003; 24: 828–37.

97. Chan AW, Chew DP, Bhatt DL, et al. Long-term mortality benefit with the combination of stents and abciximab for cardiogenic shock complicating acute myocardial infarction. Am J Cardiol 2002; 89: 132–6.

98. Giri S, Mitchel J, Azar RR, et al. Results of primary percutaneous transluminal coronary angioplasty plus abciximab with or without stenting for acute myocardial infarction complicated by cardiogenic shock. Am J Cardiol 2002; 89: 126–31.

99. Prasad A, Lennon RJ, Rihal CS, Berger PB, Holmes DR Jr. Outcomes of elderly patients with cardiogenic shock treated with early percutaneous revascularization. Am Heart J 2004; 147: 1066–70.

100. Mehta SR, Yusuf S, Peters RJ, et al. Effects of pretreatment with clopidogrel and aspirin followed by long-term therapy in patients undergoing percutaneous coronary intervention: the PCI-CURE study. Lancet 2001; 358: 527–33.

101. Berger PB, Bhatt DL, Fuster V, et al. Bleeding complications with dual antiplatelet therapy among patients with stable vascular disease or risk factors for vascular disease: results from the Clopidogrel for High Atherothrombotic Risk and Ischemic Stabilization, Management, and Avoidance (CHARISMA) trial. Circulation 2010; 121: 2575–83.

102. Wiviott SD, Braunwald E, McCabe CH, et al. Prasugrel versus clopidogrel in patients with acute coronary syndromes. N Engl J Med 2007; 357: 2001–15.

103. Wallentin L, Becker RC, Budaj A, et al. Ticagrelor versus clopidogrel in patients with acute coronary syndromes. N Engl J Med 2009; 361: 1045–57.

104. Montalescot G, Barragan P, Wittenberg O, et al. Platelet glycoprotein IIb/IIIa inhibition with coronary stenting for acute myocardial infarction. N Engl J Med 2001; 344: 1895–903.

105. Boersma E, Harrington RA, Moliterno DJ, et al. Platelet glycoprotein IIb/IIIa inhibitors in acute coronary syndromes: a meta-analysis of all major randomised clinical trials. Lancet 2002; 359: 189–98.

106. ESPRIT Investigators. Enhanced Suppression of the Platelet IIb/IIIa Receptor with Integrilin Therapy. Novel dosing regimen of eptifibatide in planned coronary stent implantation (ESPRIT): a randomised, placebo-controlled trial. Lancet 2000; 356: 2037–44.

107. Sadeghi HM, Grines CL, Chandra HR, et al. Percutaneous coronary interventions in octogenarians. glycoprotein IIb/IIIa receptor inhibitors' safety profile. J Am Coll Cardiol 2003; 42: 428–32.

108. Lincoff AM, Kleiman NS, Kereiakes DJ, et al. Long-term efficacy of bivalirudin and provisional glycoprotein IIb/IIIa blockade vs heparin and planned glycoprotein IIb/IIIa blockade during percutaneous coronary revascularization: REPLACE-2 randomized trial. JAMA 2004; 292: 696–703.

109. Influence of diabetes on 5-year mortality and morbidity in a randomized trial comparing CABG and PTCA in patients with multivessel disease: the Bypass Angioplasty Revascularization Investigation (BARI). Circulation 1997; 96: 1761 9.

110. Murphy ML, Hultgren HN, Detre K, Thomsen J, Takaro T. Treatment of chronic stable angina. A preliminary report of survival data of the randomized Veterans Administration cooperative study. N Engl J Med 1977; 297: 621–7.

111. European Coronary Surgery Study Group. Long-term results of prospective randomised study of coronary artery bypass surgery in stable angina pectoris. Lancet 1982; 2: 1173–80.

112. Coronary artery surgery study (CASS): a randomized trial of coronary artery bypass surgery. Survival data. Circulation 1983; 68: 939–50.

113. Wilson MF, Baig MK, Ashraf H. Quality of life in octagenarians after coronary artery bypass grafting. Am J Cardiol 2005; 95: 761–4.

114. Srinivas VS, Brooks MM, Detre KM, et al. Contemporary percutaneous coronary intervention versus balloon angioplasty for multivessel coronary artery disease: a comparison of the National Heart, Lung and Blood Institute Dynamic Registry and the Bypass Angioplasty Revascularization Investigation (BARI) study. Circulation 2002; 106: 1627–33.

115. Abizaid A, Costa MA, Centemero M, et al. Clinical and economic impact of diabetes mellitus on percutaneous and surgical treatment of multivessel coronary disease patients: insights from the Arterial Revascularization Therapy Study (ARTS) trial. Circulation 2001; 104: 533–8.

116. Rodriguez A, Bernardi V, Navia J, et al. Argentine Randomized Study: Coronary Angioplasty with Stenting versus Coronary Bypass Surgery in patients with Multiple-Vessel Disease (ERACI II): 30-day and one-year follow-up results. ERACI II Investigators. J Am Coll Cardiol 2001; 37: 51–8.

117. SoS Investigators. Coronary artery bypass surgery versus percutaneous coronary intervention with stent implantation in patients with multivessel coronary artery disease (the Stent or Surgery trial): a randomised controlled trial. Lancet 2002; 360: 965–70.

118. Morrison DA, Sethi G, Sacks J, et al. Percutaneous coronary intervention versus coronary artery bypass graft surgery for patients with medically refractory myocardial ischemia and risk factors for adverse outcomes with bypass: a multicenter, randomized trial. Investigators of the Department of Veterans Affairs Cooperative Study #385, the Angina With Extremely Serious Operative Mortality Evaluation (AWESOME). J Am Coll Cardiol 2001; 38: 143–9.

119. Whitlow PL, Dimas AP, Bashore TM, et al. Relationship of extent of revascularization with angina at one year in the Bypass Angioplasty Revascularization Investigation (BARI). J Am Coll Cardiol 1999; 34: 1750–9.

120. Passamani E, Davis KB, Gillespie MJ, Killip T. A randomized trial of coronary artery bypass surgery. Survival of patients with a low ejection fraction. N Engl J Med 1985; 312: 1665–71.

121. Ryan TJ, Bauman WB, Kennedy JW, et al. Guidelines for percutaneous transluminal coronary angioplasty. A report of the American Heart Association/American College of Cardiology Task Force on Assessment of Diagnostic and Therapeutic Cardiovascular Procedures (Committee on Percutaneous Transluminal Coronary Angioplasty). Circulation 1993; 88: 2987–3007.

122. Mullany CJ, Mock MB, Brooks MM, et al. Effect of age in the Bypass Angioplasty Revascularization Investigation (BARI) randomized trial. Ann Thorac Surg 1999; 67: 396–403.

123. Morrison DA, Sethi G, Sacks J, et al. Percutaneous coronary intervention versus coronary bypass graft surgery for patients with medically refractory myocardial ischemia and risk factors for adverse outcomes with bypass: The VA AWESOME multicenter registry: Comparison with the randomized clinical trial. J Am Coll Cardiol 2002; 39: 266–73.

124. Peterson ED, Cowper PA, Jollis JG, et al. Outcomes of coronary artery bypass graft surgery in 24,461 patients aged 80 years or older. Circulation 1995; 92: II85–91.

125. Shaw PJ, Bates D, Cartlidge NE, et al. Long-term intellectual dysfunction following coronary artery bypass graft surgery: A six month follow-up study. Q J Med 1987; 62: 259–68.

126. Smith PL, Treasure T, Newman SP, et al. Cerebral consequences of cardiopulmonary bypass. Lancet 1986; 1: 823–5.

127. Sotaniemi KA, Mononen H, Hokkanen TE. Long-term cerebral outcome after open-heart surgery. A five-year neuropsychological follow-up study. Stroke 1986; 17: 410–16.

128. McKellar SH, Brown ML, Frye RL, Schaff HV, Sundt TM III. Comparison of coronary revascularization procedures in octogenarians: a systematic review and meta-analysis. Nature clinical practice. Cardiovasc Med 2008; 5: 738–46.

129. van den Brand MJ, Rensing BJ, Morel MA, et al. The effect of completeness of revascularization on event-free survival at one year in the ARTS trial. J Am Coll Cardiol 2002; 39: 559–64.

130. Brophy JM, Belisle P, Joseph L. Evidence for use of coronary stents. A hierarchical bayesian meta-analysis. Ann Intern Med 2003; 138: 777–86.

131. Kastrati A, Mehilli J, Pache J, et al. Analysis of 14 trials comparing sirolimus-eluting stents with bare-metal stents. N Engl J Med 2007; 356: 1030–9.

132. Trikalinos TA, Alsheikh-Ali AA, Tatsioni A, Nallamothu BK, Kent DM. Percutaneous coronary interventions for non-acute coronary artery disease: a quantitative 20-year synopsis and a network meta-analysis. Lancet 2009; 373: 911–18.

133. Zhang Z, Mahoney EM, Spertus JA, et al. The impact of age on outcomes after coronary artery bypass surgery versus stent-assisted percutaneous coronary intervention: one-year results from the Stent or Surgery (SoS) trial. Am Heart J 2006; 152: 1153–60.

134. Rodriguez AE, Baldi J, Fernandez Pereira C, et al. Five-year follow-up of the Argentine randomized trial of coronary angioplasty with stenting versus coronary bypass surgery in patients with multiple vessel disease (ERACI II). J Am Coll Cardiol 2005; 46: 582–8.

135. Serruys PW, Morice MC, Kappetein AP, et al. Percutaneous coronary intervention versus coronary-artery bypass grafting for severe coronary artery disease. N Engl J Med 2009; 360: 961–72.

136. Shannon J, Colombo A, Alfieri O. Do hybrid procedures have proven clinical utility and are they the wave of the future? : hybrid procedures have proven clinical utility and are the wave of the future. Circulation 2012; 125: 2492–503.

14

Exercise training and cardiac rehabilitation in older cardiac patients

Philip A. Ades

SUMMARY

Older coronary patients are characterized by high rates of disability but are quite heterogeneous in overall physical functioning and disease severity. Cardiac rehabilitation training programs have been demonstrated to be safe and to improve aerobic fitness capacity, muscular strength, mental depression, and cardiac risk factors for older individuals. Additionally, cardiac rehabilitation increases survival in older coronary patients and may reverse and prevent cardiac disability. Yet, cardiac rehabilitation participation is quite low in the clinical setting due largely to low referral rates despite available third party coverage.

The goals of cardiac rehabilitation in older coronary populations are to decrease cardiac disability, cardiac-related symptoms, and to extend disability-free survival. Compared with younger patients with coronary heart disease (CHD), older patients have higher rates of disability and mobility limitations, and a diminished exercise capacity (1–3). Coronary artery disease (CAD) in the elderly is also characterized by a greater severity of angiographic disease (4), more severe and more diffuse left ventricular systolic dysfunction (5), and increased levels of peripheral vascular and left ventricular stiffness also termed "diastolic dysfunction", compared with younger cardiac patients (6). The higher rate of diastolic dysfunction results in the fact that dyspnea is a more common symptom than chest pain in many older patients suffering a myocardial infarction (7,8). Compared with older men, older women with CHD have a higher prevalence of chronic heart failure (CHF), a greater prevalence of coronary risk factors, a more complex clinical course, and higher rates of physical disability (1,9). Despite the fact that primary prevention has resulted in a lower prevalence of CAD in the elderly, the rapidly increasing size of the older population is such that the absolute number of older patients with CHD is increasing (10,11). Cardiac rehabilitation exercise training designed to decrease disability and overall coronary risk in older CHD patients should come to play an increasingly important role as the size of the older CHD population continues to grow.

CARDIAC DISABILITY

The Social Security Administration has no guidelines or definitions for cardiac disability for patients over the age of 65 years, because at this age disability pensions are simply converted to "old-age" pensions (12). In practice, disability in older CHD patients is defined by limitations in physical activity, mobility, and ability to perform activities of daily living with an underlying psychological component. Data from the Framingham Disability Study provides insight into the effects of various CHD manifestations on disability and mobility in older populations (1). The Framingham Disability Study included 2576 participants and yielded a quantitative assessment of levels of physical and social disability in older adults, based upon self-reported information. The measures of disability were primarily based upon three questions: "Are you able to walk up and down stairs to the second floor without help?" "Are you able to walk a half mile without help?" and "Are you able to do heavy work around the house, like shoveling snow or washing windows, walls, or floors without help?" The presence of any negative responses determined a component of physical disability.

At a given age, women were more likely to report disability than men, and the presence of CHD was a major predictor of activity limitations in both men and women (Table 14.1). In the 55–69-year age group, 49% of men and 67% of women with CHD were disabled as compared with 9% of men and 25% of women without CHD. In coronary patients over the age of 70 years with symptoms of angina pectoris or CHF, disability was reported by over 80% of women and 55% of men. The presence of CHD in the "older-old" was particularly powerful, with estimated disability rates of up to 76% in men 75 years of age and older.

Other studies on this topic are complementary to the Framingham study. In the Medical Outcomes Study, angina was related to the total physical activity score in older patients, although past myocardial infarction was not (13). Chirikos and Nickel studied 976 men and women hospitalized for acute coronary syndromes (myocardial infarction or unstable angina). By multivariate analysis, they found that the presence of cardiac disease, in particular angina pectoris, was predictive of disability at 6, 18, and 24 months of follow-up (14). In a subsequent analysis, they found that angina was more disabling in older women than older men, supporting the findings of the Framingham study (2).

Data from our laboratory provides further insight into the determinants of physical functional capacity in older coronary patients (15). A group of 51 men and women over the age of 65 years with established chronic CHD underwent comprehensive evaluations with exercise echocardiography, measurement of peak aerobic capacity, strength, and body composition along with detailed clinical histories, and self-reported measures of

Table 14.1 Framingham Disability Study by Age and Coronary Disease Status

	Percentage with Disability (Age 55–69 yr)	Percentage with Disability (Age 70–88 yr)
No CAD or CHF		
Women	25	49
Men	9	27
Coronary heart disease		
Women	67	79
Men	49	49
Angina pectoris		
Women	67	84
Men	57	56
Chronic heart failure		
Women	80	88
Men	43	57

Abbreviations: CHF, chronic heart failure; CAD, coronary artery disease.
Source: From Ref. 1.

physical function and mental depression. Univariate predictors of physical function score included peak aerobic capacity, depression score, handgrip strength, gender, and comorbidity score (16). By multivariate analysis, the only independent predictors of physical function score were peak aerobic capacity and depression score. Left ventricular systolic function, which varies inversely with infarct size, was not related to the physical function score (15).

In summary, the presence of clinical CHD is a powerful predictor of disability and mobility limitations in the elderly. Disability rates are highest in women, the older-old, and in the presence of angina pectoris, CHF, and mental depression.

AEROBIC TRAINING

The goals of cardiac rehabilitation exercise training in older coronary populations are, above all, to decrease cardiac disability and to extend disability-free survival. These goals are accomplished by programs that will increase aerobic capacity, muscle strength, and flexibility and which will provide associated psychosocial and cardiac risk factor benefits. Exercise training programs in the elderly also need to take into account commonly associated comorbidities that can alter the modalities and intensities of the exercise stimulus that is required. These include, but are not limited to, CHF, arthritis, chronic lung disease, diabetes, osteoporosis, and peripheral and cerebrovascular disease. In middle-aged coronary patients and in patients with CHF, reduced cardiovascular fitness [peak oxygen uptake (VO_2)] is a primary clinical predictor of impaired physical function and of clinical survival (17,18). Furthermore, favorable training-induced changes in peak aerobic capacity are associated with a lower mortality for patients with the greatest training effect (19). Meta-analyses of randomized trials of cardiac rehabilitation, including over 4000 patients, document a 25% decreased mortality over an average follow-up of 3 years after cardiac rehabilitation (20,21). These studies are limited, however, by the inclusion of few patients over the age of 65, and the fact that over 80% of the subjects were male. Most of these studies antedated current thrombolytic and interventional approaches to acute myocardial infarction as well as the many interventions available for secondary prevention, such as lipid lowering, antiplatelet therapy, β-adrenergic blockade, and angiotensin-converting-enzyme inhibitors. The Cochrane Database systematic review of cardiac rehabilitation in 2001 extends these findings to contemporary populations, although these remain primarily middle-aged patients (22).

Data from an analysis of over 600,000 US Medicare beneficiaries hospitalized with either acute myocardial infarction or coronary bypass surgery assessed the effect of cardiac rehabilitation on 5-year mortality rates (23). Using three statistical techniques a 5-year survival benefit was found ranging from 21% to 34% reduction in mortality. Mortality reductions extended to all demographic and diagnostic sub-groups including patients with acute myocardial infarction, patients after coronary bypass grafting, and patients who experienced congestive heart failure. A second analysis of Medicare data assessed the relationship between the number of sessions of cardiac completed and 4-year risk of death or myocardial infarction (24). Patients who attended 36 sessions had a 14% lower risk of death and a 12% lower risk of MI than those who attended 24 sessions and a 47% lower risk of death and a 31% lower risk of MI than those who attended just 1 session; thus, a strong dose–response relationship existed. Finally, a large observational study, the British Regional Heart Study of almost 6000 men with established CHD, found that regular light-to-moderate physical activity was associated with a lower 5-year all-cause mortality (25).

The goals of cardiac rehabilitation in the elderly include both extending disability-free survival and on improving physical functioning. Secondarily, exercise rehabilitation plays an important role in coordination of coronary risk factor therapy, including management of hypertension, lipid abnormalities, insulin resistance, and obesity (26).

The cardiac rehabilitation literature supports the safety and efficacy of exercise training regimens in older coronary patients (3,27–30). Compared with younger coronary patients, older patients are significantly less fit at entry into a rehabilitation program 1–3 months after suffering a major coronary event, such as myocardial infarction or coronary bypass surgery (3,31) (Fig. 14.1). In a cross-sectional analysis of cardiac patients, peak aerobic capacity decreased by 40% in men and 33% in women from age 40 to 80 (31). In addition, it is notable that older patients after coronary artery bypass grafting surgery are significantly less fit compared with patients after myocardial infarction or a percutaneous coronary intervention (31). However, after 3 months of aerobic conditioning, older coronary patients derive a similar relative training benefit as younger patients, with peak VO_2 increasing from 16% to 20%, effectively distancing themselves from mobility limitations and disability (Fig. 14.2). Training programs have been extended to a year and longer with long-term maintenance of exercise-related benefits (29,32).

The effects of aerobic exercise training programs on submaximal exercise response in older coronary patients are more relevant to the performance of daily activities than the maximal exercise response. In a study of 45 older coronary patients, mean age 69 ± 6 years, subjected to a 3-month aerobic conditioning program, submaximal indices of exercise performance were closely studied (33). Training effects were assessed during an exhaustive submaximal exercise protocol, with patients exercising at a steady intensity of 80% of a previously measured peak aerobic capacity. Outcome measures included endurance time, serum lactate, perceived exertion, heart rate, blood pressure, and expired ventilatory measures. Exhaustive endurance time increased by more than 40% after conditioning, with associated decreases in serum lactate, perceived exertion, minute ventilation, heart rate, and systolic blood pressure during relatively steady state exercise. Respiratory exchange ratio during steady state exercise, an indicator of substrate utilization, decreased, indicating a shift toward greater use of free fatty acids as a more efficient metabolic fuel. Activities that were exhaustive before training became sustainable for extended periods of time at a lower perceived exertion.

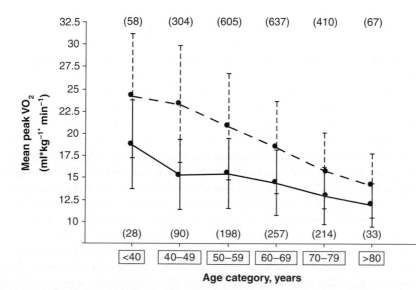

Figure 14.1 Peak aerobic capacity (peak VO_2) by age and gender entering cardiac rehabilitation. Upper graph *(hatched lines)* are women. Lower graph *(solid lines)* are men. *Abbreviation*: VO_2, oxygen uptake. *Source*: From Ref. 31.

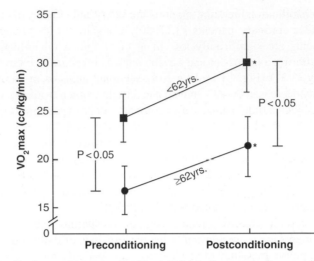

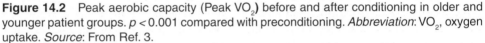

Figure 14.2   Peak aerobic capacity (Peak VO_2) before and after conditioning in older and younger patient groups. $p < 0.001$ compared with preconditioning. *Abbreviation*: VO_2, oxygen uptake. *Source*: From Ref. 3.

   The mechanisms of physiological adaptations to aerobic exercise conditioning in the elderly may differ somewhat from those seen in younger (i.e., middle-aged) coronary patients. In younger patients, physiological responses to training include both peripheral adaptations (skeletal muscle and vascular) that result in a widened arteriovenous oxygen difference at maximal exercise (34,35), and cardiac adaptations, which include increases in cardiac dimensions, stroke work, cardiac output, and afterload-corrected indices of left ventricular function (36–40). In older coronary patients, coronary and peripheral vascular diseases are superimposed on "age-related" increases in left ventricular and arterial wall thickness and stiffness (6,8,41) that may reduce their adaptability to remodeling. We found that after 3 months of intensive aerobic conditioning in 60 older coronary patients (mean age 68 ± 5 years, range 62–82 years), conditioning-induced adaptations were localized almost exclusively to the periphery (42). Peak exercise cardiac output, hyperemic calf blood flow, and vascular conductance were unaffected by the conditioning program. In contrast, at 3 and 12 months, arteriovenous oxygen difference at peak exercise was increased in intervention subjects but not in age-matched controls that explains the 16% increase in peak aerobic capacity. Histological analysis of skeletal muscle documented a 34% increase in capillary density and a 23% increase in oxidative enzyme capacity after 3 months. After 12 months, an increase in individual fiber area was seen compared with baseline measures. Thus, even after 12 months of aerobic exercise, in contrast with middle-aged coronary patients, we saw no discernible improvements in cardiac output or calf blood flow. It is acknowledged; however, that the absolute amount of exercise performed by older coronary patients is less than that performed by younger patients, and this may potentially confound comparisons of physiological response to training by age group.

   Practical issues related to the implementation of exercise training programs in older coronary patients include the frequent need for training regimens to be adjusted to accommodate the presence of comorbidities such as arthritis, diabetes, and peripheral vascular disease (Table 14.2). The least fit individuals are often unable to sustain exercise for extended periods and do well with repeated intermittent brief bouts of exercise (often termed "interval training") that are gradually extended. Some authors recommend long-term exercise programs for the elderly, partly related to their low baseline functional

Table 14.2   Implementing Exercise in Older Coronary Patients

- Optimally performed in the cardiac rehabilitation setting
- Intensity of exercise generally based on an exercise tolerance test
- In severely disabled patients, forego exercise test and begin with
  low level interval training on treadmill and/or cycle
- Resistance training based on single-repetition maximal testing
- Advance intensity actively
- Long-term goals and follow-up

capacity (32). It should however, be noted, that even patients who use canes and walkers can perform an exercise test and can train on a treadmill with surround bars or on a cycle ergometer.

Patients entering cardiac rehabilitation are becoming progressively older and more overweight. From 1996 to 2006, the mean age of participants has increased from 60.6 to 63.4 years and the mean body weight has increased from 84.7 to 88.5 kg (43). For many individuals the accomplishment of weight reduction will significantly lower the burden of coronary risk factors. An exercise program in cardiac rehabilitation that emphasizes daily longer distance walking to maximize caloric expenditure, associated with behavioral weight loss dietary counseling has been shown to accomplish significant weight reduction associated with a comprehensive reduction of coronary risk factors. (44). This approach was found to be associated with an improved quality of life in older, overweight cardiac patients (45).

Despite the documented value of exercise regimens in older patients and the low baseline measures of functional capacity, older coronary patients are far less likely than younger patients to participate in cardiac rehabilitation (46). Our data documented a 21% participation rate in cardiac rehabilitation for patients over the age of 62 years, who recently suffered a coronary event and who lived within 1 hour driving time of the rehabilitation center, compared with a 42% participation rate in younger patients (46). By far, the most powerful predictor of cardiac rehabilitation participation in the clinical setting was the strength of the primary physician's recommendation for participation as described by the patient. The physician's recommendation was scored from 1 to 5, ranging from no encouragement to participate (a score of 1) to a strong encouragement to participate (a score of 5). When the recommendation was weak (a score of 1–3), a 2% participation rate was noted, compared with a rate of 66% when it was strong (a score of 4–5). Older women had a lower participation rate than men (15% vs. 25%; $p = 0.06$); this difference was primarily related to lower physician recommendation scores for women than men (47). Other factors weighing against participation for women include more comorbid conditions, greater difficulty with transportation, lower likelihood of being married, and higher likelihood of having a dependent spouse at home. Data from the American Heart Association's "Get with the Guidelines" program affirms these results with older patients less likely to be referred to cardiac rehabilitation than younger patients (48). As noted above, older cardiac patients perceive greater barriers to cardiac rehabilitation participation than do younger patients (49). Finally, with increasing utilization of electronic medical records, computerized "automatic" referral of appropriate patients to cardiac rehabilitation at hospital discharge is showing great promise as a means to increase cardiac rehabilitation referral and participation (50).

RESISTANCE TRAINING

Resistance training has been advocated as a particularly useful intervention in older coronary patients for several reasons (51–53). First and foremost, even "normal" aging is associated with a significant loss of muscle mass and strength, related both to diminished activity profiles and to decreased rates of muscle protein synthesis (51,54–56). Furthermore, in older populations ranging from healthy community living elders to institutionalized octogenarians, resistance training has been demonstrated to improve walking endurance, muscle mass, and strength (57,58). In coronary patients, aging-related musculoskeletal abnormalities are superimposed upon activity restrictions related to chronic disease (59), and diminished muscle mass and strength, termed "sarcopenia", is even more severe.

In a study that focused upon resistance training in older CAD patients who had recently suffered a myocardial infarction, relative increases in strength were found to be similar to increases seen in younger CAD patients (52). In older women with chronic CHD, where the negative effects of age, gender, and chronic disease all conspire to result in a severe loss of strength and function (15), the effects of strength training have been studied (60). Brochu et al. assessed the effects of 6 months of resistance training on strength, endurance, and on a physical performance test designed to assess physical function during practical household activities in 30 older women, mean age 71 ± 5 years (61). Compared with patients randomized to a control group, strength-trained women increased strength, endurance, and capacity to perform a wide range of household activities such as carrying groceries, doing household activities, and climbing stairs. The increase in strength after resistance training correlated with improvements in the overall physical function score (Fig. 14.3).

Strength training should also be considered for stable patients with CHF due to the well described skeletal muscle abnormalities (fiber atrophy, diminished oxidative capacity) (62). Pu et al. found that 10 weeks of strength training in women with CHF led to increased strength, and 6-minute walk distance and was supported by increases in skeletal muscle fiber area and oxidative capacity (63).

From a practical point of view, the onset of upper body resistance training should be delayed until 3 months after coronary bypass surgery to allow for full sternal healing, while it can commence as soon as 1 month of postmyocardial infarction after performance of a satisfactory baseline exercise tolerance test. The resistance training program should include

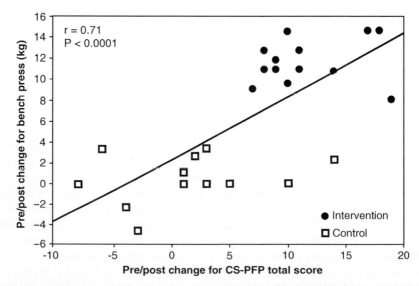

Figure 14.3 Association between percent changes in total CS-PFP and percent changes in maximal strength on the bench press before and after strength training in older women with coronary heart disease. *Abbreviation*: CS-PFP, continuous scale physical functional performance test score. *Source*: From Ref. 60.

training of the leg extensor muscles to assist with walking, stair climbing and fall prevention, and upper body training to aid in the lifting and pushing required for the performance of daily household activities. Training is based upon the performance of a single-repetition maximal (1-RM) lift supplemented by a Borg scale for perceived exertion (64). Patients begin their resistance training with 8–10 repetitions of each exercise at 40–50% of their 1-RM for a given exercise and gradually increase exercise intensity, as tolerated, to 50–80% of updated 1-RMs.

EXERCISE TRAINING FOR CHRONIC HEART FAILURE

The syndrome of CHF is particularly common in the elderly and its prevalence is increasing both in the USA and around the world (65). Over 75% of CHF patients are aged 65 years or greater. These patients are at a particularly high risk of disability and have an exercise capacity that is 25–70% below normal levels (66). Systematic reviews and meta-analyses of studies of exercise training for stable patients with CHF have demonstrated reductions in cardiac mortality and hospitalizations whereas single individual trials have been less conclusive (67–69). The single largest trial of exercise training in CHF; HF-ACTION (Heart Failure: A Controlled Trial Investigating Outcomes of Exercise Training) found a trend towards a lower combined endpoint of total mortality and hospitalizations (reduced by 7%; $p = 0.13$) and when results were adjusted by pre-specified predictors of mortality, the combined endpoint of mortality and hospitalizations was reduced by 11% ($p < 0.05$) (69). This same study found a significantly improved quality of life versus control subjects and virtually all studies have found an improved exercise capacity in intervention patients versus controls. Optimally, patients with CHF should begin their exercise training process in the supervised confines of a cardiac rehabilitation program whereas it has also been demonstrated that in well screened patients, exercise in the home setting is safe (69).

SCREENING AND IMPLEMENTATION

Optimally, older coronary patients begin exercise training only after a careful screening process, which should include an electrocardiographically monitored exercise tolerance test, strength measures, and a clinical review, including an analysis of disease severity and questionnaire or interview-derived data regarding physical and psychosocial function. Diagnostic categories appropriate for consideration of cardiac rehabilitation exercise training in older cardiac patients include myocardial infarction, stable angina pectoris, coronary bypass surgery, percutaneous coronary revascularization (angioplasty, or stenting), heart valve replacement, and CHF.

Exercise modalities should include options for aerobic, resistance, and flexibility exercise. Aerobic choices include treadmills, a walking course, cycles, airdynes, and rowers. Aerobic exercise is often guided by an exercise heart rate range and/or scales of perceived exertion such as the Borg scale. A gradual increment of exercise heart rate from 60% to 65% of maximal attained heart rate to higher levels of up to 85% is balanced against the greater risk of injury at higher levels and past demonstration of measurable benefits even with low levels of exercise (70). It has been observed that older coronary patients are less likely to exercise to a physiological maximum at their baseline exercise test than younger patients; therefore, strict adherence to an exercise heart rate range is often inappropriate (3). Duration of the exercise stimulus can begin with very brief, intermittent bouts of exercise, gradually increasing to 20–25 minutes or longer. Special considerations in the elderly include that training regimens often need to be adjusted to accommodate the presence of comorbidities. For example, patients with hip or knee arthritis may do better with cycling or rowing exercises to avoid the weight bearing of treadmill walking. However, walking is generally a preferred modality because of its direct relevance to daily activities. Finally, it should be noted that for many elders, flexibility, or lack thereof, can be an exercise-limiting factor. Flexibility exercises can be as simple as 5–10 minutes of stretching per day to more complex protocols of yoga and tai chi.

Gender Issues

Healthy older women have lower levels of habitual physical activity and physical functioning than older men, explained, in part, by lower strength and muscle mass (71–73). Older women with CAD further curtail their activities because of apprehension regarding the safety of specific physical activities that compounds their deconditioning. Following a coronary event, women have lower fitness levels than men (31), yet are less likely to be referred to an exercise-based rehabilitation program by their physicians (46). This distinction may relate, in part, to the older age of women after infarction, compared with men, or to higher rates of angina pectoris, but is most likely related to the physician misunderstanding regarding the benefits of rehabilitation in the most severely debilitated patients. Women make similar improvements in aerobic fitness and in muscular strength compared with men in rehabilitation programs (51,52). The current model of cardiac rehabilitation was developed primarily in middle-aged male coronary patients in the 1960s and 1970s. The differing clinical profile of women in cardiac rehabilitation may require a different model relevant to their older age, increased prevalence of comorbid conditions, more prominent cardiac risk factor profiles, higher rates of depression, higher risk of recurrent coronary events, and differing personal preferences (74–77).

Supervised versus Home Exercise

Roughly, only 15% of eligible patients in the USA receive cardiac rehabilitation services, with the lowest participation rates noted in older patients (26,46). In many cases, cardiac rehabilitation programs are not geographically available (78), whereas in other cases, patients are unable to travel, or the primary physician does not recommended formal rehabilitation. While cardiac rehabilitation services have classically been delivered on-site at an established exercise training facility, a need to expand preventive cardiology services to include the majority of eligible patients in a cost-effective manner necessitates a redefinition of this classical model.

The development of alternate approaches to the delivery of cardiac rehabilitation services is an ongoing process, with a goal of expanding the base of patients who receive services at the lowest possible healthcare costs. Older patients tend to require a more "hands on" approach early in the rehabilitative process, but often can transition to a home program with appropriate follow-up. Case management, that is, evaluation and management of the exercise program and risk factors for the individual patient by a nurse "case manager" allows for the individualization of preventive care in health-care delivery systems that focus on efficiency and outcomes. Exercise programs can be individualized, with moderate- and high-risk patients referred to a rehabilitation program for closer supervision and monitoring.

CARDIAC REHABILITATION ON CORONARY RISK FACTORS

Exercise plays an important adjunctive role in the management of blood lipid levels, obesity, blood pressure, and psychological factors such as social isolation and mental depression. In older coronary populations, exercise rehabilitation has well-defined metabolic benefits that include improved blood lipid values, decreased body fat, improved glucose tolerance, and lower blood pressure (30,79,80). In addition, cardiac rehabilitation in the elderly has been shown to have important effects on mental health that include decreased measures of depression, anxiety, and hostility (Table 14.3) (81–84). These measures, in

Table 14.3 Noncardiac Benefits of Exercise Rehabilitation in Older Coronary Patients

Effect	Refs.
Increased HDL cholesterol (+8% to 10%)	(30,79)
Decreased triglycerides (−10% to 25%)	
Decreased body fat (−1% to 2%)	(30,79)
Improved glucose tolerance	(80)
Lowered blood pressure (−5 mmHg to 7 mmHg systolic)	(81)
Diminished depression, anxiety, and hostility	(30,82–84)

Abbreviation: HDL, high-density lipoprotein.

summary, constitute important outcome measures for older CHD patients engaging in therapeutic exercise.

Cardiac rehabilitation programs have been termed as "secondary prevention centers" and thus should function as a location to systematically measure and treat coronary risk factors with both lifestyle approaches (exercise and nutrition) and pharmacological therapy. For example, a systematic approach to measuring lipid profiles in all patients entering cardiac rehabilitation, with an active stance towards pharmacological therapy, resulted in a tripling of the number of patients that attain nationally recognized therapeutic lipid goals (85). Similarly, blood-pressure monitoring and treatment, and obesity assessment and treatment should be coordinated in the cardiac rehabilitation setting (86).

The magnitude of exercise-related effects on blood lipid measures depends, in part, on whether or not there is associated weight loss. In a study of cardiac rehabilitation without weight loss, lipid effects were relatively modest with high density lipoprotein (HDL)-cholesterol increasing by 8%, but no significant effects on low density lipoprotein (LDL)-cholesterol, triglyceride levels, or glucose levels (79). On the other hand, when exercise was associated with 10 lbs of exercise-induced weight loss, favorable effects were noted on serum triglycerides (−24%), HDL-cholesterol (+7%), on the atherogenic ratio [total cholesterol/HDL-cholesterol (−14%)], and fasting serum insulin levels (−22%) (87). Exercise rehabilitation has also been shown to be associated with a decrease in the high-sensitive C-reactive protein, a predictor of prognosis after myocardial infarction (88). The benefits in older coronary patients of lipid-lowering, smoking-cessation, angiotensin-converting-enzyme inhibition, antiplatelet agents, and β-adrenergic blockade have all been demonstrated in appropriately selected populations (89,90).

FUTURE DIRECTIONS

As the older cardiac population continues to grow in size and complexity, the role of cardiac rehabilitation in the elderly should proportionately expand. The effects of aerobic and resistance-training protocols on measures of physical functioning need to be better studied in older coronary populations, with the inclusion of patients disabled by angina or CHF. Whether training regimens can improve physical functioning in the most severely disabled patients is of particular importance, although preventing disability in the less severely affected "younger-old" is also a priority. Effects of exercise regimens on other important outcomes, including lipid levels, blood pressure measures, insulin levels, body composition, and body fat distribution need to be further studied to better define expected benefits of rehabilitation. Finally, whether training regimens can affect the economics of health care is crucial, especially if costly hospitalizations and/or home-care services can be minimized.

In summary, the older coronary population is a highly disabled group, yet quite heterogeneous as to physical functioning and disease severity. Cardiac rehabilitation training programs have been demonstrated to be safe and to improve aerobic fitness capacity, muscular strength, and cardiac risk factors for older individuals yet it is recommended far too infrequently in the clinical setting. Exercise training may, in fact, reverse and prevent cardiac disability. Thus, cardiac rehabilitation can pay great medical, social, and economic dividends in the older coronary population.

REFERENCES

1. Pinsky JL, Jette AM, Branch LG, et al. The Framingham Disability Study: relationship of various coronary heart disease manifestations to disability in older persons living in the community. Am J Public Health 1990; 80: 1363–8.
2. Nickel JT, Chirikos TN. Functional disability of elderly patients with long-term coronary heart disease: a sex-stratified analysis. J Gerontol 1990; 45: 560–8.
3. Ades PA, Grunvald MH. Cardiopulmonary exercise testing before and after conditioning in older coronary patients. Am Heart J 1990; 120: 585–9.
4. Sugiura M, Hiraoka K, Ohkawa S. Severity of coronary sclerosis in the aged: a pathological study of 968 consecutive autopsy cases. Jpn Heart J 1976; 17: 471–8.
5. Hochman J, Boland J, Sleeper L. Current spectrum of cardiogenic shock and effect of early revascularization on mortality: results of an international registry. Circulation 1995; 91: 873–81.
6. Rockman HA, Lew W. Left ventricular remodeling and diastolic dysfunction in chronic ischemic heart disease. In: Gaasch WH, LeWinter MM, eds. Left Ventricular Diastolic Dysfunction and Heart Failure. Philadelphia, PA: Lea and Febiger, 1994.
7. Bayer A, Chadha J, Farad R, et al. Changing presentation of myocardial infarction with increasing old age. J Am Geriatr Soc 1986; 34: 263–6.
8. Solomon C, Lee T, Cook E, et al. Comparison of clinical presentation of acute myocardial infarction in patients older than 65 years of age to younger patients: the multicenter chest pain study experience. Am J Cardiol 1989; 63: 772–6.
9. Malacrida R, Genoni M, Maggioni A, et al. A comparison of the early outcome of acute myocardial infarction in women and men. N Engl J Med 1998; 338: 8–14.
10. Weinstein W, Coxson P, Williams L, et al. Forecasting coronary heart disease incidence, mortality and cost: the Coronary Heart Disease Policy Model. Am J Public Health 1987; 77: 1417–26.
11. Salomaa V, Rosamond W, Mahonen M. Decreasing mortality from acute myocardial infarction: effect of incidence and prognosis. J Cardiovasc Risk 1999; 6: 69–75.
12. Social Security Administration. Disability Evaluation Under Social Security. Washington, DC: U.S. Department of Health and Human Services, 1992; Report no.: ICN 468 600.
13. Stewart AL, Hays RD, Ware JE. The MOS short-form general health survey. Reliability and validity in a patient population. Med Care 1988; 26: 724–35.
14. Chirikos T, Nickel J. Socioeconomic determinants of disablement from chronic disease episodes. Soc Sci Med 1986; 22: 1329–35.
15. Ades P, Savage P, Tischler M, et al. Determinants of disability in older coronary patients. Am Heart J 2002; 143: 151–6.
16. Yesavage JA, Brink TL, Rose TL. Development and validation of a geriatric depression screening scale: A preliminary report. J Psychiatr Res 1983; 17: 37–49.
17. McNeer J, Margolis J, Lee K, et al. The role of the exercise test in the evaluation of patients for ischemic heart disease. Circulation 1978; 57: 64–70.
18. Mancini D, Eisen H, Kussmaul W, et al. Value of peak oxygen consumption for optimal timing of cardiac transplantation in ambulatory patients with heart failure. Circulation 1991; 83: 778–86.
19. Vanhees L, Fagard R, Thijs L, et al. Prognostic value of training-induced change in peak exercise capacity in patients with myocardial infarcts and patients with coronary bypass surgery. Am J Cardiol 1995; 76: 1014–19.
20. O'Connor GT, Buring JE, Yusuf S, et al. An overview of randomized trials of rehabilitation with exercise after myocardial infarction. Circulation 1989; 80: 234–44.
21. Oldridge NB, Guyatt GH, Fischer ME, et al. Cardiac rehabilitation after myocardial infarction: combined experience of randomized clinical trials. JAMA 1988; 260: 945–50.
22. Jolliffe J, Rees K, Taylor R, et al. Exercise-based rehabilitation for coronary heart disease. Cochrane Database Syst Rev 2001: CD001800.

23. Suaya JA, Stason WB, Ades PA, et al. Cardiac rehabilitation and survival in older coronary patients. J Am Coll Cardiol 2009; 54: 25–33.
24. Hammill BG, Curtis LH, Schulman KA, Whellan DJ. Relationship between cardiac rehabilitation and long-term risks of death and myocardial infarction among elderly medicare beneficiaries. Circulation 2010; 121: 63–70.
25. Wannamethee SG, Shaper AG, Walker M. Physical activity and mortality in older men with diagnosed coronary heart disease. Circulation 2000; 102: 1358–63.
26. Wenger NK, Froehlicher ES, Smith LK, et al. Cardiac rehabilitation as secondary prevention. Agency for Health Care Policy and Research and the National Heart, Lung and Blood Institute. 1995:1–23.
27. Williams MA, Maresh CM, Esterbrooks DJ, et al. Early exercise training in patients older than age 65 years compared with that in younger patients after acute myocardial infarction of coronary bypass grafting. Am J Cardiol 1985; 55: 263–6.
28. Ades PA, Hanson JS, Gunther PG, et al. Exercise conditioning in the elderly coronary patient. J Am Geriatr Soc 1987; 35: 121–4.
29. Ades PA, Waldmann ML, Gillespie C. A controlled trial of exercise training in older coronary patients. J Gerontol 1995; 50: M7–M11.
30. Lavie CJ, Milani RV, Littman AB. Benefits of cardiac rehabilitation and exercise training in secondary coronary prevention in the elderly. J Am Coll Cardiol 1993; 22: 678–83.
31. Ades PA, Savage PD, Brawner CA, et al. Aerobic capacity in patients entering cardiac rehabilitation. Circulation 2006; 113: 2706–12.
32. Williams M, Maresh C, Esterbrooks D, et al. Characteristics of exercise responses following short and long term aerobic training in elderly cardiac patients. J Am Geriatr Soc 1987; 35: 904–9.
33. Ades PA, Waldmann ML, Poehlman ET, et al. Exercise conditioning in older coronary patients: submaximal lactate response and endurance capacity. Circulation 1993; 88: 572–7.
34. Detry JMR, Rousseau M, Vandenbroecke O, et al. Increased arteriovenous oxygen difference after physical training in coronary heart disease. Circulation 1971; 44: 109–18.
35. Clausen JP. Circulatory adjustments to dynamic exercise and effect of physical training in normal subjects and in patients with coronary artery disease. Prog Cardiovasc Dis 1976; 18: 459–95.
36. Ehsani A, Martin WH, Heath GW, et al. Cardiac effects of prolonged intense exercise training in patients with coronary artery disease. Am J Cardiol 1982; 50: 246–54.
37. Hagberg JM, Ehsani AA, Holloszy JO. Effects of 12 months of intense exercise training on stroke volume in patients with coronary artery disease. Circulation 1983; 67: 1194–9.
38. Ehsani AA, Biello DR, Schultz J, et al. Improvement of left ventricular contractile function by exercise training in patients with coronary artery disease. Circulation 1986; 74: 350–8.
39. Hagberg JM. Physiologic adaptations to prolonged high-intensity exercise training in patients with coronary artery disease. Med Sci Sports 1991; 23: 661–7.
40. Lakatta E, Mitchell J, Pomerance A, et al. Human aging: changes in cardiac structure and function. J Am Coll Cardiol 1987; 10: 42A–7A.
41. Vaitkevicius P, Fleg J, Engel J, et al. Effects of age and aerobic capacity on arterial stiffness in healthy adults. Circulation 1993; 88: 1456–62.
42. Ades P, Waldmann ML, Meyer WL, et al. Skeletal muscle and cardiovascular adaptations to exercise conditioning in older coronary patients. Circulation 1996; 94: 323–30.
43. Audelin MC, Savage PD, Ades PA. Changing clinical profile of patients entering cardiac rehabilitation/secondary prevention programs: 1996 to 2006. J Cardiopulm Rehabil Prev 2008; 299–306.
44. Ades PA, Savage PD, Toth MJ, et al. High-Caloric expenditure exercise: a new approach to cardiac rehabilitation for overweight coronary patients. Circulation 2009; 119: 2671–8.
45. Pope E, Harvey-Berino J, Savage PD, et al. The impact of high-calorie-expenditure exercise and behavioral weight loss on quality of life and exercise enjoyment in older adults with coronary heart disease. J Aging Phys Act 2011; 19: 99–116.
46. Ades PA, Waldmann ML, McCann W, et al. Predictors of cardiac rehabilitation participation in older coronary patients. Arch Intern Med 1992; 152: 1033–5.
47. Ades PA, Waldmann ML, Polk D, et al. Referral patterns and exercise response in the rehabilitation of female coronary patients aged ≥ 62 years. Am J Cardiol 1992; 69: 1422–5.
48. Brown TM, Hernandez AF, Bittner V, et al. Predictors of cardiac rehabilitation referral in coronary artery disease patients: findings from the American Heart Association's Get With The Guidelines Program. J Am Coll Cardiol 2009; 54: 515–21.
49. Grace SL, Shanmugasegaram S, Gravely-Witte S, et al. Barriers to cardiac rehabilitation: does age make a difference? J Cardiopulm Rehabil Prev 2009; 29: 183–7.

50. Grace SL, Russell KL, Reid RD, et al. Effect of cardiac rehabilitation referral strategies on utilization rates: a prospective, controlled study. Arch Intern Med 2011; 171: 235–41.

51. Brechue W, Pollack M. Exercise training for coronary artery disease in the elderly. Clin Geriatr Med 1996; 1: 207–29.

52. Fragnoli-Munn K, Savage P, Ades P. Combined resistive-aerobic training in older coronary patients early after myocardial infarction. J Cardiopulm Rehabil 1998; 18: 416–20.

53. Squires RW, Muri AJ, Amderson LJ, et al. Weight training during phase II (early outpatient) cardiac rehabilitation: heart rate and blood pressure responses. J Cardiopulm Rehabil 1991; 11: 360–4.

54. Frontera W, Meredith CN, O'Reilly KP, et al. Strength conditioning in older men: skeletal muscle hypertrophy and improved function. J Appl Physiol 1988; 64: 1038–44.

55. Frontera WR, Meridith CN, O'Reilly KP, et al. Strength training and determinants of VO2 max. J Appl Physiol 1990; 68: 329–33.

56. Balagopal P, Rooyackers O, Adey D, et al. Effects of aging on in-vivo synthesis of skeletal muscle myosin heavy chain and sarcoplasmic protein in humans. Am J Physiol 1997; 273: E790–800.

57. Ades PA, Ballor DL, Ashikaga T, et al. Weight training improves walking endurance in the healthy elderly. Ann Intern Med 1996; 124: 568–72.

58. Fiatorone MA, Marks EC, Ryan ND, et al. High intensity strength training in nonagenarians: effects of skeletal muscle. JAMA 1990; 263: 3029–34.

59. Neill WA, Branch LG, DeJong G. Cardiac disability: the impact of coronary disease on patients' daily activities. Arch Intern Med 1981; 145: 1642–7.

60. Brochu M, Savage P, Lee N, et al. Effects of resistance training on physical function in older disabled women with coronary heart disease. J Appl Physiol 2002; 92: 672–8.

61. Cress ME, Buchner DM, Questad KA, et al. Continuous-scale physical functional performance in a broad range of older adults: a validation study. Arch Phys Med Rehabil 1996; 7: 1243–50.

62. Middlekauff HR. Making the case for skeletal myopathy as the major limitation of exercise capacity in heart failure. Circ Heart Fail 2010; 3: 537–46.

63. Pu CT, Johnson MT, Forman DE, et al. Randomized trial of progressive resistance training to counteract the myopathy of chronic heart failure. J Appl Physiol 2001; 90: 2341–50.

64. Borg GA. Perceived exertion: a note on history and methods. Med Sci Sports 1973; 5: 90–3.

65. Roger VL, Go AS, Lloyd-Jones DM, et al. Heart disease and stroke statistics--2012 update: a report from the American Heart Association. Circulation 2012; 125: e2–e220.

66. Kitzman DW, Little WC, Brubaker PH, et al. Pathophysiological characterization of isolated diastolic heart failure in comparison to systolic heart failure. JAMA 2002; 288: 2144–50.

67. Piepoli MF, Davos C, Francis DP, Coats AJ. ExTraMATCH Collaborative. Exercise training meta-analysis of trials in patients with chronic heart failure (ExTraMATCH). BMJ 2004; 328: 189.

68. Davies EJ, Moxham T, Rees K, et al. Exercise based rehabilitation for heart failure. Cochrane Database Syst Rev 2010: CD003331.

69. O'Connor CM, Whellan DJ, Lee KL, et al. Efficacy and safety of exercise training in patients with chronic heart failure: HF-ACTION randomized controlled trial. JAMA 2009; 301: 1439–50.

70. Lee JY, Jensen BE, Oberman A, et al. Adherence in the training levels comparison trial. Med Sci Sports Exerc 1996; 28: 47–52.

71. Reaven PD, McPhillips JB, Barrett-Connor EL, et al. Leisure time exercise and lipid and lipoprotein levels in an older population. J Am Geriatr Soc 1990; 38: 847–54.

72. Cress M. Quantifying physical functional performance in older adults. Muscle Nerve 1997; 5: S17–20.

73. Wells CL, Plowman SA. Sexual differences in athletic performance: biological or behavioral? Phys Sportsmed 1983; 11: 52–63.

74. Bueno H. Influence of sex on the short-term outcome of elderly patients with a first acute myocardial infarction. Circulation 1995; 92: 1133–40.

75. Cannistra LB, Balady GJ, O'Malley CJ, et al. Comparison of the clinical profile and outcome of women and men in cardiac rehabilitation. Am J Cardiol 1992; 69: 1274–9.

76. Rich MW, Bosner MS, Chung MK, et al. Is age an independent predictor of early and late mortality in patients with acute myocardial infarction? Am J Med 1992; 92: 7–13.

77. Moore SM, Kramer FM. Women's and men's preferences for cardiac rehabilitation program features. J Cardiopulm Rehabil 1996; 16: 163–8.

78. Curnier D, Savage PD, Ades PA. Geographic distribution of cardiac rehabilitation programs in the U.S. J Cardiopulm Rehabil 2005; 25: 80–4.

79. Brochu M, Poehlman ET, Savage P, et al. Modest effects of exercise training alone on coronary risk factors and body composition in coronary patients. J Cardiopulm Rehabil 2000; 20: 180–8.

80. Dylewicz P, Bienkowska S, Szczesniak S, et al. Beneficial effect of short-term endurance training on glucose metabolism during rehabilitation after coronary bypass surgery. Chest 2000; 117: 47–51.

81. Kokkinos PF, Papademetriou V. Exercise and hypertension. Coron Artery Dis 2000; 11: 99–102.
82. Ades PA, Maloney AE, Savage P, et al. Determinants of physical function in coronary patients: response to cardiac rehabilitation. Arch Intern Med 1999; 159: 2357–60.
83. Milani RV, Lavie CJ. Prevalence and effects of cardiac rehabilitation on depression in the elderly with coronary heart disease. Am J Cardiol 1998; 81: 1233–6.
84. Lavie CV, Milani RV. Impact of aging on hostility in coronary patients and effects of cardiac rehabilitation and exercise training in elderly persons. Am J Geriatr Cardiol 2004; 13: 125–30.
85. Ades PA, Savage PD, Poehlman ET, et al. Lipid lowering in the cardiac rehabilitation setting. J Cardiopulm Rehabil 1999; 19: 255–60.
86. Savage PD, Ades PA. The obesity epidemic in the United States: role of cardiac rehabilitation Cor Art Dis. 2006; 17: 227–31.
87. Savage P, Brochu M, Poehlman E, et al. Reduction in obesity and coronary risk factors after high caloric exercise training in overweight coronary patients. Am Heart J 2003; 146: 317–23.
88. Milani RV, Lavie CJ, Mehra MR. Reduction in C-reactive protein through cardiac rehabilitation and exercise training. J Am Coll Cardiol 2004; 43: 1056–61.
89. Williams MA, Fleg JL, Ades PA, et al. Secondary prevention of coronary heart disease in the elderly (with emphasis on patients ≥ years of age). Circulation 2002; 105: 1735–43.
90. Smith SC Jr. Secondary prevention in the elderly. Coron Artery Dis 1998; 9: 715–18.

15

Aortic valve disease in the elderly

Wilbert S. Aronow

SUMMARY

Elderly patients with aortic stenosis (AS) have an increased prevalence of coronary risk factors, of coronary artery disease (CAD), and of other atherosclerotic vascular diseases. Angina pectoris, syncope or near syncope, and congestive heart failure are the three classic manifestations of severe AS. Prolonged duration and late peaking of an aortic systolic ejection murmur best differentiate severe AS from mild AS on physical examination. The severity of aortic regurgitation (AR) correlates with the duration of the diastolic murmur. Doppler echocardiography is used to diagnose the severity of AS and AR. Indications for aortic valve replacement (AVR), for use of warfarin after AVR in patients with mechanical prostheses and for use of aspirin or warfarin after AVR in patients with bioprostheses, are discussed. Transcatheter aortic valve implantation (TAVI) should be performed in nonoperable patients with symptomatic severe AS to improve survival and quality of life compared with medical management.

AORTIC STENOSIS
Etiology and Prevalence

Valvular AS in elderly patients is usually due to stiffening, scarring, and calcification of the aortic valve leaflets. The commissures are not fused as in rheumatic AS. Calcific deposits in the aortic valve are common in elderly patients and may lead to valvular AS (1–7). Aortic cuspal calcium was present in 295 of 752 men (36%), mean age 80 years, and in 672 of 1663 women (40%), mean age 82 years (6). Of 2358 patients, mean age 81 years, 378 (16%) of them had valvular AS, 981 (42%) had valvular aortic sclerosis (thickening of or calcific deposits on the aortic valve cusps with a peak flow velocity across the aortic valve ≤1.5 m/s), and 999 (42%) had no valvular AS or aortic sclerosis (7). Calcific deposits in the aortic valve were present in 22 of 40 necropsy patients (55%) aged 90–103 years (2). Calcium of the aortic valve and mitral annulus may coexist (1–3,8,9).

In the Helsinki Aging Study, calcification of the aortic valve was diagnosed by Doppler echocardiography in 28% of 76 patients aged 55–71 years, in 48% of 197 patients aged 75–76 years, in 55% of 155 patients aged 80–81 years, and in 75% of 124 patients aged 85–86 years (5). Aortic valve calcification, aortic sclerosis, and mitral annular calcium (MAC) are degenerative processes (1,2,10–12), accounting for their high prevalence in an elderly population.

Otto et al. (11) demonstrated that the early lesion of degenerative AS is an active inflammatory process with some similarities to atherosclerosis, including lipid deposition, macrophage and T-cell infiltration, and basement membrane disruption. In a prospective study of 571 unselected patients, mean age 82 years, 292 patients (51%) had calcified or thickened aortic cusps or root (13). A serum total cholesterol ≥200 mg/dL, a history of hypertension, diabetes mellitus, and a serum high-density lipoprotein cholesterol <35 mg/dL were more prevalent in elderly patients with calcified or thickened aortic cusps or root than in elderly patients with normal aortic cusps and root (13).

In the Helsinki Aging Study, age, hypertension, and a low body mass index were independent predictors of aortic valve calcification (14). In 5201 patients older than 65 years of age in the Cardiovascular Health Study, independent clinical factors associated with degenerative aortic valve disease included age, male gender, smoking, history of hypertension, height, and high lipoprotein(a) and low-density lipoprotein cholesterol levels (12). In 1275 elderly patients, mean age 81 years, AS was present in 52 of 202 patients (26%) with 40–100% extracranial carotid arterial disease (ECAD) and in 162 of 1073 patients (15%) with 0–39% ECAD (15). In 2987 elderly patients, mean age 81 years, symptomatic peripheral arterial disease was present in 193 of 462 patients (42%) with AS and in 639 of 2525 patients (25%) without AS (16).

In 290 patients, mean age 79 years, with valvular AS who had follow-up Doppler echocardiograms, elderly patients with MAC had a greater reduction in aortic valve area/ year than elderly patients without MAC (17). Significant independent risk factors for progression of valvular AS in 102 patients, mean age 76 years, who had follow-up Doppler echocardiograms were cigarette smoking and hypercholesterolemia (18). Palta et al. (19) also found that cigarette smoking and hypercholesterolemia accelerate the progression of AS. These and other data suggest that aortic valve calcium, MAC, and coronary atherosclerosis in elderly patients have similar predisposing factors (11–21).

A retrospective analysis of 180 elderly patients with mild AS who had follow-up Doppler echocardiograms at ≥2 years showed that significant independent predictors of the progression of AS were male gender, cigarette smoking, hypertension, diabetes mellitus, a serum low-density lipoprotein cholesterol ≥125 mg/dL at follow-up, a serum high-density lipoprotein cholesterol <35 mg/dL at follow-up, and use of statins (inverse association) (22). Novaro et al. (23) reported in a retrospective analysis of 174 patients, mean age 68 years, with mild-to-moderate AS that statin therapy reduced the progression of AS.

In a retrospective study of 156 patients, mean age 77 years, with AS, at 3.7-year follow-up, statin therapy reduced the progression of AS by 54% (24). However, a randomized, double-blind trial in which 1873 patients with mild-to-moderate AS randomized to simvastatin 40 mg plus ezetimibe 10 mg daily versus placebo showed at 52-month follow-up that the primary outcome of cardiovascular death, aortic valve replacement (AVR), nonfatal myocardial infarction, hospitalization for unstable angina pectoris, coronary artery bypass graft surgery (CABGS), percutaneous coronary intervention, or nonhemorrhagic stroke was 35.3% in the simvastatin–ezetimibe group versus 38.2% in the placebo group (p not significant) (25).

The frequency of AS increases with age. Valvular AS diagnosed by Doppler echocardiography was present in 141 of 924 men (15%), mean age 80 years, and in 322 of 1881 women (17%), mean age 81 years (26). Severe valvular AS (peak gradient across aortic valve of ≥50 mm Hg or aortic valve area <0.75 cm^2) was diagnosed in 62 of 2805 elderly patients (2%) (26). Moderate valvular AS (peak gradient across aortic valve of 26–49 mm Hg or aortic valve area of 0.75–1.49 cm^2) was present in 149 of 2805 elderly patients (5%) (26). Mild valvular AS (peak gradient across aortic valve of 10–25 mm Hg or aortic valve area ≥1.50 cm^2) occurred in 25 of 2805 elderly patients (9%) (26). In 924 elderly men, mean age 80 years, AS was present in 36 of 236 African-Americans (15%), in 19 of 135 Hispanics (14%), and in 86 of 553 whites (16%) (25). In 1881 elderly women, mean age 81 years, AS was present in 84 of 494 African-Americans (17%), in 33 of 188

Hispanics (18%), and in 205 of 1199 white women (17%) (26). In 501 unselected patients aged 75–86 years in the Helsinki Aging Study, critical AS was present in 3% and moderate-to-severe AS in 5% of the 501 elderly patients (5).

Pathophysiology

In valvular AS, there is resistance to ejection of blood from the left ventricle (LV) into the aorta, with a pressure gradient across the aortic valve during systole and an increase in LV systolic pressure. The pressure overload on the LV leads to concentric LV hypertrophy, with an increase in LV wall thickness and mass, normalizing systolic wall stress, and maintenance of normal LV ejection fraction and cardiac output (27,28). A compensated hyperdynamic response is common in elderly women (29). Elderly patients with a comparable degree of AS have more impairment of LV diastolic function than do younger patients (30). Coronary vasodilator reserve is more severely impaired in the subendocardium in patients with LV hypertrophy caused by severe AS (31).

The compensatory concentric LV hypertrophy leads to abnormal LV compliance, LV diastolic dysfunction with reduced LV diastolic filling, and increased LV end-diastolic pressure, further increased by left atrial systole. Left atrial enlargement develops. Atrial systole plays an important role in diastolic filling of the LV in patients with AS (32). Loss of effective atrial contraction may cause immediate clinical deterioration in patients with severe AS.

Sustained LV hypertrophy eventually leads to LV chamber dilatation with decreased LV ejection fraction and, ultimately, congestive heart failure (CHF). The stroke volume and cardiac output decrease, the mean left atrial and pulmonary capillary pressures increase, and pulmonary hypertension occurs. Elderly patients with both obstructive and nonobstructive coronary artery disease (CAD) have an increased incidence of LV enlargement and LV systolic dysfunction (33). In a percentage of elderly patients with AS, the LV ejection fraction will remain normal and LV diastolic dysfunction will be the main problem.

In 48 elderly patients with CHF associated with unoperated severe valvular AS, the LV ejection fraction was normal in 30 patients (63%) (34). The prognosis of patients with AS and LV diastolic dysfunction is usually better than that of patients with AS and LV systolic dysfunction, but is worse than that of patients without LV diastolic dysfunction (34,35).

Symptoms

Angina pectoris, syncope or near syncope, and CHF are the three classic manifestations of severe AS. Angina pectoris is the most common symptom associated with AS in elderly patients. Coexistent CAD is frequently present in these patients. However, angina pectoris may occur in the absence of CAD as a result of an increase in myocardial oxygen demand with a reduction in myocardial oxygen supply at the subendocardial level. Myocardial ischemia in patients with severe AS and normal coronary arteries is due to inadequate LV hypertrophy with increased LV systolic and diastolic wall stresses causing decreased coronary flow reserve (36).

Syncope in patients with AS may be caused by reduced cerebral perfusion following exertion when arterial pressure drops because of systemic vasodilatation in the presence of a fixed cardiac output. LV failure with a decrease in cardiac output may also cause syncope. In addition, syncope at rest may be caused by a marked reduction in cardiac output secondary to transient ventricular fibrillation or transient atrial fibrillation (AF) or transient atrioventricular block related to extension of the valve calcification into the conduction system. Coexistent cerebrovascular disease with transient cerebral ischemia may contribute to syncope in elderly patients with AS.

Exertional dyspnea, paroxysmal nocturnal dyspnea, orthopnea, and pulmonary edema may be caused by pulmonary venous hypertension associated with AS. Coexistent CAD and hypertension may contribute to CHF in elderly patients with AS. AF may also precipitate CHF in these patients.

CHF, syncope, or angina pectoris was present in 36 of 40 elderly patients (90%) with severe AS, in 66 of 96 elderly patients (69%) with moderate valvular AS, and in 45 of 165 elderly patients (27%) with mild valvular AS (37).

Sudden death occurs mainly in symptomatic valvular AS patients (34,37–40). It may also occur in 3–5% of asymptomatic patients with AS (38,40). Marked fatigue and peripheral cyanosis in patients with AS may be caused by a low cardiac output. Cerebral emboli causing stroke or transient cerebral ischemic attack, bacterial endocarditis, and gastrointestinal bleeding may also occur in elderly patients with AS.

Signs

A systolic ejection murmur heard in the second right intercostal space, down the left sternal border toward the apex, or at the apex is classified as an aortic systolic ejection murmur (ASEM) (3,4,41,42). An ASEM is commonly heard in elderly patients (1,3,41), occurring in 265 of 565 unselected elderly patients (47%) (3). Of 220 elderly patients with an ASEM and technically adequate M-mode and two-dimensional echocardiograms of the aortic valve, 207 (94%) had aortic cuspal or root calcification or thickening (3). Of 75 elderly patients with an ASEM, valvular AS was diagnosed by continuous-wave Doppler echocardiography in 42 patients (56%) (42).

Table 15.1 shows that an ASEM was heard in 100% of 19 elderly patients with severe AS, in 100% of 49 elderly patients with moderate AS, and in 95% of 74 elderly patients with mild AS (4). However, the ASEM may become softer or absent in patients with CHF associated with severe AS because of a low cardiac output. The intensity and maximal location of the ASEM and transmission of the ASEM to the right carotid artery do not differentiate among mild, moderate, and severe AS (3,4,42). The ASEM may be heard only at the apex in some elderly patients with AS. The apical systolic ejection murmur may also be louder and more musical than the basal systolic ejection murmur in some elderly patients with AS. The intensity of the ASEM in valvular AS increases with squatting and by inhalation of amyl nitrite and decreases during the Valsalva maneuver.

Prolonged duration of the ASEM and late peaking of the ASEM best differentiate severe AS from mild AS (3,4,42). However, the physical signs do not distinguish between severe and moderate AS (Table 15.1) (4,42).

Table 15.1 Correlation of Physical Signs of Valvular Aortic Stenosis with the Severity of Aortic Stenosis in Elderly Patients

Physical sign	Severity of aortic stenosis		
	Mild ($n = 74$)%	Moderate ($n = 49$)%	Severe ($n = 19$)%
ASEM	95	100	100
Prolonged duration ASEM	3	63	84
Late-peaking ASEM	3	63	84
Prolonged carotid upstroke time	3	33	53
A_2 absent	0	10	16
A_2 decreased or absent	5	49	74

Abbreviations: ASEM, aortic systolic ejection murmur; A_2, aortic component of second heart sound.
Source: Adapted from Ref. 4.

A prolonged carotid upstroke time does not differentiate between severe and moderate AS in elderly patients (4). A prolonged carotid upstroke time was palpable in 3% of elderly patients with mild AS, in 33% of elderly patients with moderate AS, and in 53% of elderly patients with severe AS (Table 15.1) (4). Stiff noncompliant arteries may mask a prolonged carotid upstroke time in elderly patients with severe AS. The pulse pressure may also be normal or wide rather than narrow in elderly patients with severe AS because of loss of vascular elasticity. An aortic ejection click is rare in elderly patients with severe AS because of loss of vascular elasticity. An aortic ejection click is rare in elderly patients with AS because the valve cusps are immobile (4,42).

An absent or decreased A_2 occurs more frequently in elderly patients with severe or moderate AS than in patients with mild AS (Table 15.1) (4,42). However, an absent or decreased A_2 does not differentiate between severe and moderate AS (4,41). The presence of AF, reversed splitting of S_2, or an audible fourth heart sound at the apex also does not differentiate between severe and moderate AS in elderly patients (42). The presence of a third heart sound in elderly patients with AS usually indicates the presence of LV systolic dysfunction and elevated LV filling pressure (43).

Electrocardiography and Chest Roentgenography

Table 15.2 shows that echocardiography is more sensitive than electrocardiography in detecting LV hypertrophy in elderly person with AS (4). Rounding of the LV border and apex may occur as a result of concentric LV hypertrophy. Poststenotic dilatation of the ascending aorta is commonly seen. Calcification of the aortic valve is best seen by echocardiography or fluoroscopy.

In the Simvastatin and Ezetimibe in Aortic Stenosis study of 1533 patients with asymptomatic AS, electrocardiographic LVH was associated at 4.3-year follow-up with a 5.8 times increase in heart failure, with a 2.0 times increase in AVR, and with a 2.5 times increase in myocardial infarction, heart failure, or cardiovascular death (44). LV strain was associated with a 3.1 times increase in myocardial infarction (44).

Involvement of the conduction system by calcific deposits may occur in elderly patients with AS. In a study of 51 elderly patients with AS who underwent aortic valve replacement, conduction defects occurred in 58% of 31 patients with MAC and in 25% of 20 patients without MAC (9). In another study of 77 elderly patients with AS, first-degree atrioventricular block occurred in 18% of patients, left bundle branch block in 10% of patients, intraventricular conduction defect in 6% of patients, right bundle branch block in 4% of patients, and left axis deviation in 17% of patients (45).

Complex ventricular arrhythmias may be detected by 24-hour ambulatory electrocardiograms in patients with AS. Elderly patients with complex ventricular arrhythmias associated with AS have a higher incidence of new coronary events than elderly patients with AS and no complex ventricular arrhythmias (46).

Table 15.2 Prevalence of Electrocardiographic and Echocardiographic Left Ventricular Hypertrophy in Elderly Patients with Mild, Moderate, and Severe Valvular Aortic Stenosis

	Severity of valvular aortic stenosis		
	Mild ($n = 74$)%	Moderate ($n = 49$)%	Severe ($n = 19$)%
Electrocardiographic LVH	11	31	58
Echocardiographic LVH	74	96	100

Abbreviation: LVH, left ventricular hypertrophy.
Source: Adapted from Ref. 4.

Echocardiography and Doppler Echocardiography

M-mode and 2-dimensional echocardiography and Doppler echocardiography are very useful in the diagnosis of AS. Of 83 patients with CHF or angina pectoris and a systolic precordial murmur in whom severe AS was diagnosed by Doppler echocardiography, AS was not clinically diagnosed in 28 patients (34%) (47). Echocardiography can detect thickening, calcification, and reduced excursion of aortic valve leaflets (3). LV hypertrophy is best diagnosed by echocardiography (4). Chamber dimensions and measurements of LV end-systolic and end-diastolic volumes, LV ejection fraction, and assessment of global and regional LV wall motion give important information on LV systolic function.

Doppler echocardiography is used to measure peak and mean transvalvular gradients across the aortic valve and to identify associated valve lesions. Aortic valve area can be calculated by the continuity equation using pulsed Doppler echocardiography to measure LV outflow tract velocity, continuous-wave Doppler echocardiography to measure transvalvular flow velocity, and two-dimensional long-axis view to measure LV outflow tract area (48,49). Aortic valve area can be detected reliably by the continuity equation in elderly patients with AS (47). Figures 15.1–15.5 illustrate two-dimensional echocardiographic findings (Figs. 15.1 and 15.3), continuous-wave Doppler echocardiographic findings (Figs. 15.2 and 15.4), and simultaneous LV and femoral arterial pressure tracings (Fig. 15.5) in elderly patients with severe valvular AS.

Shah and Graham (50) reported that the agreement in quantitation of the severity of AS between Doppler echocardiography and cardiac catheterization was greater than 95%. Patients with a peak jet velocity ≥4.5 m/s had critical AS, and those with a peak jet velocity

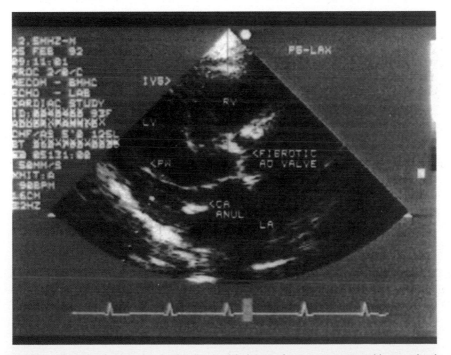

Figure 15.1   Two-dimensional echocardiographic image from a parasternal long-axis view of a 93-year-old female with aortic stenosis and moderately depressed left ventricular function showing a fibrotic aortic valve and mitral annular calcification. *Abbreviations*: PS-LAX, parasternal long-axis view; RV, right ventricular cavity; LV, left ventricular cavity; IVS, interventricular septum; PW, posterior wall; CA ANUL, mitral annulus calcification; LA, left atrium; AO, aorta.

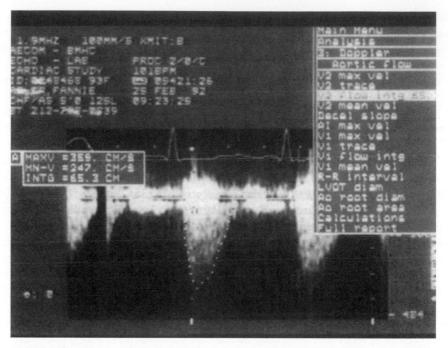

Figure 15.2   Continuous-wave Doppler recording of the velocity profile across the aortic valve in the same patient shown in Figure 15.1. A 52 mm Hg gradient across the aortic valve is measured using the Bernoulli equation. Indexed aortic valve area measured by the continuity equation using Doppler data = 0.5 cm^2/m^2.

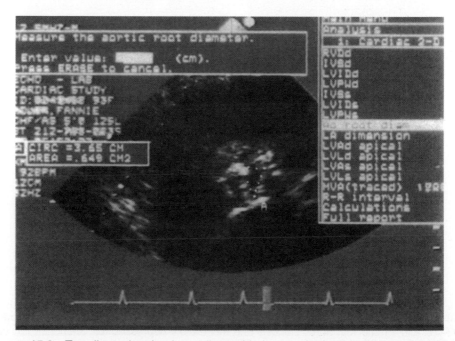

Figure 15.3   Two-dimensional echocardiographic image obtained in the same patient in Figures 15.1 and 15.2 from a short-axis parasternal view in which the aortic valve orifice is mapped, yielding an indexed area of 0.4 cm^2/m^2.

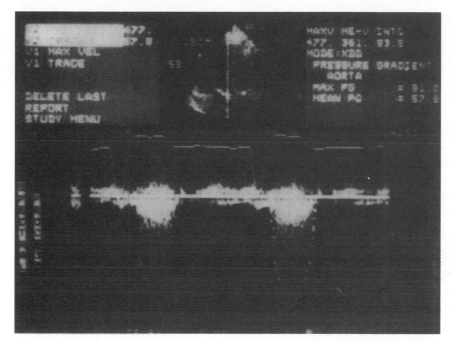

Figure 15.4 Continuous-wave Doppler recording of the velocity profile across the aortic valve in an elderly patient with aortic stenosis and normal left ventricular systolic function. The indexed aortic valve area is 0.5 cm²/m² by both Gorlin's formula and the Doppler continuity equation. The peak gradient across the aortic valve by Bernoulli's equation is 81 mm Hg, a value higher than that recorded in Figure 15.2 for the same indexed aortic valve area.

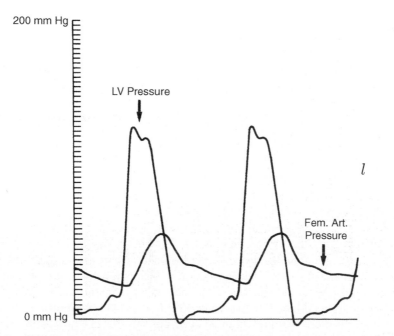

Figure 15.5 Simultaneous left ventricular and femoral artery pressure recordings obtained in the same patient in Figure 15.4 confirming a large gradient across the aortic valve with a maximum value of 81 mm Hg (instantaneous pressure). *Abbreviations*: Fem. Art., femoral artery pressure tracing; LV, left ventricular pressure tracing.

<3.0 m/s had noncritical AS. Slater et al. (51) demonstrated a concordance between Doppler echocardiography and cardiac catheterization in the decision to operate or not to operate in 61 of 73 patients (84%) with valvular AS. In 75 patients, mean age 76 years, with valvular AS, the Bland–Altman plot showed that four of the 75 patients (5%) had disagreement between cardiac catheterization and Doppler echocardiography that was outside the 95% confidence limits (52).

Cardiac catheterization was performed in 105 patients in which Doppler echocardiography demonstrated an aortic valve area ≤0.75 cm^2 or a peak jet velocity ≥4.5 m/s, consistent with critical AS (53). Doppler echocardiography was 97% accurate in this subgroup. Cardiac catheterization was performed in this study in 133 patients with noncritical AS. Doppler echocardiography was 95% accurate in this subgroup. Although most elderly patients do not require cardiac catheterization before aortic valve surgery, they require selective coronary arteriography before aortic valve surgery. Patients in whom Doppler echocardiography shows a peak jet velocity between 3.6 and 4.4 m/s and an aortic valve area >0.8 cm^2 should undergo cardiac catheterization if they have cardiac symptoms attributable to AS (49). Patients with a peak jet velocity between 3.0 and 3.5 m/s and an LV ejection fraction <50% may have severe AS, requiring aortic valve replacement, and should undergo cardiac catheterization (50). Patients with a peak jet velocity between 3.0 and 3.5 m/s and an LV ejection fraction >50% probably do not need aortic valve replacement but should undergo cardiac catheterization if they have symptoms of severe AS (50).

Natural History

Ross and Braunwald (38) found that the average survival rate was 3 years after the onset of angina pectoris in patients with severe AS. Ross and Braunwald (38) reported that the average survival rate after the onset of syncope in patients with severe AS was 3 years. Ross and Braunwald (38) demonstrated that the average survival rate after the onset of CHF in patients with severe AS was 1.5–2 years.

Patients with symptomatic severe valvular AS have a poor prognosis (37–40,54). At the National Institutes of Health, 52% of patients with symptomatic severe valvular AS not operated on were dead at 5 years (39,40). At 10-year follow-up, 90% of these patients were dead.

At 4-year follow-up of patients aged 75–86 years in the Helsinki Aging Study, the incidence of cardiovascular mortality was 62% in patients with severe AS and 35% in patients with moderate AS (55). At 4-year follow-up the incidence of total mortality was 76% in patients with severe AS and 50% in patients with moderate AS (55).

In a prospective study, at 19-month follow-up (range 2–36 months), 90% of 30 patients with CHF associated with unoperated severe AS and a normal LV ejection fraction were dead (34). At 13-month follow-up (range 2–24 months), 100% of 18 patients with CHF associated with unoperated severe AS and an abnormal LV ejection fraction were dead (34).

Table 15.3 shows the incidence of new coronary events in elderly patients with no, mild, moderate, and severe AS. Independent risk factors for new coronary events in this study were prior myocardial infarction, AS, male gender, and increasing age (37). In this prospective study, at 20-month follow-up of 40 elderly patients with severe AS, CHF, syncope, or angina pectoris was present in 36 of 37 patients (97%) who developed new coronary events and in none of three patients (0%) without new coronary events (37). At 32-month follow-up of 96 elderly patients with moderate valvular AS, CHF, syncope, or angina pectoris was present in 65 of 77 patients (84%) who developed new coronary events and in 1 of 19 patients (5%) without new coronary events (37). At 52-month follow-up of

Table 15.3 Incidence of New Coronary Events in Older Persons with No, Mild, Moderate, and Severe Valvular Aortic Stenosis

	No AS (*n* = 1496)	Mild AS (*n* = 165)	Moderate AS (*n* = 96)	Severe AS (*n* = 40)
Age (yr)	81	84	85	85
Follow-up (mo)	49	52	32	20
New coronary events (%)	41	62	80	93

Abbreviation: AS, aortic stenosis.
Source: Adapted from Ref. 37.

165 elderly patients with mild AS, CHF, syncope, or angina pectoris was present in 40 of 103 patients (39%) who developed new coronary events and in 5 of 62 patients (8%) without new coronary events (37).

In a prospective study of 981 patients, mean age 82 years, with aortic sclerosis and of 999 patients, mean age 80 years, without valvular aortic sclerosis, elderly patients with aortic sclerosis had at 46-month follow-up a 1.8 times higher chance of developing a new coronary event than those without valvular aortic sclerosis (7). Otto et al. (56) also reported in 5621 men and women ≥65 years of age that AS and aortic sclerosis increased cardiovascular morbidity and mortality.

Kennedy et al. (57) followed 66 patients with moderate AS diagnosed by cardiac catheterization (aortic valve area 0.7–1.2 cm²). In 38 patients with symptomatic moderate AS and 28 patients with minimally symptomatic moderate AS, the probabilities of avoiding death from AS were 0.86 for patients and 1.0 for patients with minimally symptomatic moderate AS at 1-year follow-up, 0.77 for patients with symptomatic AS and 1.0 for patients with minimally symptomatic AS at 2 years, 0.77 for patients with symptomatic AS and 0.96 for patients with minimally symptomatic AS at 3 years, and 0.70 for patients with symptomatic AS and 0.90 for patients with minimally symptomatic AS at 4 years (57). During 35-month mean follow-up in this study, 21 patients underwent aortic valve replacement.

Hammermeister et al. (58) followed 106 patients with unoperated AS in the Veterans Administration Cooperative Study on Valvular Heart Disease for 5 years. During follow-up, 60 of 106 patients (57%) died. Multivariate analysis demonstrated that measures of the severity of the AS, the presence of CAD, and the presence of CHF were the important predictors of survival in unoperated patients.

Studies have demonstrated that patients with asymptomatic severe AS are at low risk for death and can be followed until symptoms develop (57–60). Turina et al. (59) followed 17 patients with asymptomatic or mildly symptomatic AS. During the first 2 years, none died or had aortic valve surgery. At 5-year follow-up, 94% were alive and 75% were free of cardiac events. Kelly et al. (60) followed 51 asymptomatic patients with severe AS. During 17-month follow-up, 21 (41%) of the patients became symptomatic. Only 2 of the 51 patients (4%) died of cardiac causes. In both patients, death was preceded by the development of angina pectoris or CHF. Pellikka et al. (61) observed that 113 of 143 patients (79%), mean age 72 years, with asymptomatic severe AS were not initially referred for AVR or percutaneous aortic balloon valvuloplasty. During 20-month follow-up, 37 of 113 patients (33%) became symptomatic. The actuarial probability of remaining free of cardiac events associated with AS, including cardiac death and aortic valve surgery, was 95% at 6 months, 93% at 1 year, and 74% at 2 years. No asymptomatic person with severe AS developed sudden death while asymptomatic.

Rosenheck et al. (62) followed 126 patients with asymptomatic severe AS for 22 months. Eight patients died and 59 patients developed symptoms necessitating AVR. Event-free survival was 67% at 1 year, 56% at 2 years, and 33% at 4 years. Five of the six deaths from cardiac disease were preceded by symptoms. Of the patients with moderately or severely calcified aortic valves whose aortic jet velocity increased by 0.3 m/s or more within 1 year, 79% underwent AVR or died within 2 years of the observed increase.

When patients with low gradient AS due to abnormal LV ejection fraction are considered for AVR, failure to respond to dobutamine and large preoperative LV end-systolic and end diastolic volumes are poor prognostic signs (63–65). The American College of Cardiology (ACC)/American Heart Association (AHA) guidelines state that dobutamine stress echocardiography is reasonable to evaluate patients with low-flow/low-gradient AS and abnormal LV ejection fraction (66).

Medical Management

Prophylactic antibiotics are not recommended to prevent bacterial endocarditis in patients with AS regardless of severity according to updated ACC/AHA guidelines (67). Patients with CHF, exertional syncope, or angina pectoris associated with moderate or severe AS should undergo AVR promptly. Valvular surgery is the only definitive therapy in these elderly patients (66,68). Medical therapy does not relieve the mechanical obstruction to LV outflow and does not relieve symptoms or progression of the disorder. Patients with asymptomatic AS should report the development of symptoms possibly related to AS immediately to the physician. If significant AS is present in asymptomatic elderly patients, clinical examination and an electrocardiogram and Doppler echocardiogram should be performed at 6-month intervals. Nitrates should be used with caution in patients with angina pectoris and AS to prevent the occurrence of orthostatic hypotension and syncope. Diuretics should be used with caution in patients with CHF to prevent a decrease in cardiac output and hypotension. Vasodilators should be avoided. Digitalis should not be used in patients with CHF and a normal LV ejection fraction unless needed to control a rapid ventricular rate associated with AF.

Aortic Valve Replacement

Table 15.4 lists four Class I indications and one Class II_a indication for performing AVR in elderly patients with AS (66). AVR is the procedure of choice for symptomatic elderly patients with severe AS. Other Class I indications for AVR in elderly patients with severe AS include patients undergoing CABGS, undergoing surgery on the aorta or other heart valves, and patients with an LV ejection fraction <50% (66). Patients with moderate AS undergoing CABGS or surgery on the aorta or other heart valves have a Class II_a indication for AVR (66).

Although the ACC/AHA guidelines do not recommend AVR in patients with asymptomatic severe AS and normal LV ejection fraction, there are data suggesting otherwise. (69–73). Pai et al. (69) found in their database that 99 of 338 patients (29%), mean age 71 years, with asymptomatic severe AS had AVR during 3.5-year follow-up. Survival at 1, 2, and 5 years was 67%, 56%, and 38%, respectively, for nonoperated patients and 94%, 93%, and 90%, respectively, for those who had AVR (69). In the unoperated group, beta-blocker use significantly reduced mortality by 48%, and statin use significantly reduced mortality by 48% (69).

Severe asymptomatic AS was present in 622 patients, mean age 72 years, at the Mayo Clinic (70). Of the 622 patients, 166 (27%) developed symptoms and had AVR. Another 97 patients (16%) had AVR in the absence of symptoms. At 3-year follow-up, 52% of the 622

Table 15.4 American College of Cardiology/American Heart Association Class I Indications for Aortic Valve Replacement in Persons with Severe Aortic Stenosis

1. Patients with symptomatic severe AS
2. Patients with severe AS undergoing coronary artery bypass surgery
3. Patients with severe AS undergoing surgery on the aorta or other heart valves
4. Patients with severe AS and a left ventricular ejection fraction <50%
5. Patients with moderate AS undergoing coronary artery bypass surgery or surgery on the aorta or other heart valves (Class II$_a$ indication)

Abbreviation: AS, aortic stenosis.
Source: Adapted from Ref. 66.

patients had had symptoms develop, undergone AVR, or died. The most important risk factor for 10-year mortality was absence of AVR (hazard ratio = 3.53, p <0.001) (70).

Of 197 consecutive patients with asymptomatic severe AS, early AVR was performed in 102 patients (52%) (71). The estimated actuarial 6-year all-cause mortality rates were 2% for AVR and 32% for the conventional treatment group (p<0.001) (71).

Despite being asymptomatic, patients with very severe AS have a poor prognosis. (72). Early elective AVR should be considered in these patients (72).

Of 73 patients with severe AS who did not undergo AVR, 15 (14%) died at 15-month follow-up (73). Of these 73 patients, symptoms were thought to be unrelated to the AS in 31 patients. Exercise stress tests for symptoms were performed in only 4% of the 42 asymptomatic patients (73).

Asymptomatic patients with low-gradient severe AS and normal LV ejection fraction with reduced stroke volume index had at 46-month follow-up aortic valve events similar to those with normal stroke volume index (74). Of 248 patients with severe AS and a normal LV ejection fraction, 94 had a low-gradient (<30 mm Hg mean gradient) (group 1), 87 had a moderate gradient (30–40 mm Hg mean gradient) (group 2), and 67 had a severe gradient (>40 mm Hg mean gradient) (group 3) (75). Symptoms were present in 49% of group 1 patients, in 55% of group 2 patients, and in 60% of group 3 patients (p not significant). At 45–60-month follow-up, the incidence of AVR or death was 71% for group 1, 77% for group 2, and 76% for group 3 (p not significant). Kaplan–Meier survival curves for time to death in all 3 groups were significantly better for patients with AVR versus no AVR (75). E/E$^1_{lateral}$ was an independent predictor of time to death in patients who did not receive AVR (76).

Echocardiography is recommended in asymptomatic patients with AS every 1 year for severe AS, every 1–2 years for moderate AS, and every 3–5 years for mild AS (66) Echocardiography should be repeated more frequently if there are changes in symptoms or LV function.

The bioprosthesis has less structural failure in elderly patients than in younger patients and may be preferable to the mechanical prosthetic valve for AS replacement in the elderly due to the anticoagulation issue (77–80). Patients with mechanical prostheses need anticoagulant therapy indefinitely. Patients with porcine bioprostheses may be treated with aspirin in a dose of 75–100 mg daily unless the patient has AF, abnormal LV ejection fraction, previous thromboembolism, or a hypercoagulable condition (66,80). Table 15.5 lists four Class I indications and two Class II$_a$ indications for antithrombotic therapy in patients with AVR (66).

Arom et al. (81) performed AVR in 273 patients aged 70–89 years (mean age 75 years), 162 with aortic valve replacement alone, and 111 with aortic valve replacement plus CABGS. Operative mortality was 5%. Late mortality at 33-month follow-up was 18%.

Table 15.5   Class I Indications for Antithrombotic Therapy in Patients with Aortic Valve Replacement

1. After AVR with bileaflet mechanical or Medtronic Hall prostheses, in patients with no risk factors, administer warfarin to maintain INR between 2.0 and 3.0; if risk factors are present, the INR should be maintained between 2.5 and 3.5
2. After AVR with Starr–Edwards valves or mechanical disc valves (other than Medtronic Hall prostheses), in patients with no risk factors, warfarin should be administered to maintain INR between 2.5 and 3.5
3. After AVR with a bioprosthesis and no risk factors, administer aspirin in a dose of 75–100 mg daily
4. After AVR with a bioprosthesis and risk factors, administer warfarin to maintain an INR between 2.0 and 3.0
5. During the first 3 mo after AVR with a mechanical prosthesis, it is reasonable to give warfarin to maintain an INR between 2.5 and 3.5 (Class II$_a$ indication)
6. During the first 3 mo after AVR with a bioprosthesis in patients with no risk factors, it is reasonable to give warfarin to maintain an INR between 2.0 and 3.0 (Class II$_a$ indication)

Risk factors include atrial fibrillation, prior thromboembolism, left ventricular systolic dysfunction, and hypercoagulable condition. *Abbreviations*: AVR, aortic valve replacement; INR, international normalized ratio. *Source*: Adapted from Ref. 66.

Actuarial analysis showed at 5-year follow-up that overall survival was 66% for patients with AVR alone, 76% for patients with AVR plus CABGS, and 74% for a similar age group in the general population.

A UK heart valve registry observed in 1100 patients aged ≥80 years (56% women) who underwent AVR that the 30-day mortality was 6.6% (82). The actuarial survival was 89% at 1 year, 79% at 3 years, 69% at 5 years, and 46% at 8 years. The survival of patients with severe AS, an LV ejection fraction <35%, and a low transvalvular gradient at one year and at 4 years was 82% and 78% respectively in 39 patients, mean age 73 years, who underwent AVR versus 41% and 15% respectively in 56 patients, mean age 75 years, in a control group (83). In 242 patients, mean age 83 years, with AS who had AVR, actuarial survival was 92% at 1 year and 66% at 5 years (84). Concomitant CABGS did not affect late survival (84).

Paroxysmal or chronic AF is a risk factor for mortality in patients with severe AS and an LV ejection fraction ≤ 35% undergoing AVR (85). Of 83 patients, mean age 70 years, with severe AS and an LV ejection fraction ≤ 35%, 29 (35%) had paroxysmal or chronic AF (85). The perioperative mortality was 24% in the AF group versus 5.5% in the non-AF group (p = 0.03) (85).

AVR is associated with a reduction in LV mass and in improvement of LV diastolic filling (86–88). Hoffman and Burckhardt (89) performed a prospective study in 100 patients who had AVR. At 41-month follow-up, the yearly cardiac mortality rate was 8% in patients with electrocardiographic LV hypertrophy and repetitive ventricular premature complexes ≥2 couplets per 24 hours during 24-hour ambulatory monitoring and 0.6% in patients without either of these findings (89).

If LV systolic dysfunction in patients with severe AS is associated with critical narrowing of the aortic valve rather than myocardial fibrosis, it often improves after successful aortic valve replacement (90). In 154 patients, mean age 73 years, with AS and an LV ejection fraction ≤35% who underwent AVR, the 30-day mortality was 9%. The 5-year survival was 69% in patients without significant CAD and 39% in patients with significant CAD. NYHA functional class III or IV was present in 58% of patients before surgery versus 7% of patients after surgery. Postoperative LV ejection fraction was measured in

76% of survivors at a mean of 14 months after surgery. Improvement in LV ejection fraction was found in 76% of patients (90).

Balloon Aortic Valvuloplasty

AVR is the procedure of choice for symptomatic elderly patients with severe AS. In a Mayo Clinic study, the actuarial survival of 50 elderly patients, mean age 77 years, with symptomatic severe AS in whom aortic valve replacement was refused (45 patients) or deferred (5 patients) was 57% at 1 year, 37% at 2 years, and 25% at 3 years (91). Because of the poor survival in this group of patients, balloon aortic valvuloplasty should be considered when operative intervention is refused or deferred. On the basis of the available data, balloon aortic valvuloplasty should be considered for elderly patients with symptomatic severe AS who are not candidates for aortic valve surgery and possibly for patients with severe LV dysfunction as a bridge to subsequent valve surgery (92–94).

Percutaneous Transcatheter Implantation of Aortic Valve Prostheses

Percutaneous heart valve implantation may be performed in nonsurgical patients with end-stage calcific AS (95,96). Eighteen high-risk patients, mean age 76 years, with severe AS and moderate CAD amenable to percutaneous coronary intervention (PCI) had combined PCI followed by minimally invasive AVR (97). One of 18 patients (6%) died postoperatively with no late mortality after a mean follow-up of 19 months (97). This hybrid strategy may be a new therapeutic approach for elderly high-risk patients with combined CAD and severe AS.

The UK Transcatheter Aortic Valve Implantation (TAVI) Registry followed prospectively 870 high-risk patients, mean age 82 years, with severe AS undergoing 877 TAVI procedures (98). Survival was 92.9% at 30 days, 78.6% at 1 year, and 73.7% at 2 years (98).

Of 442 patients with severe AS at increased surgical risk, mean age 82 years, 78 were treated with medical management, 107 with AVR, and 257 with TAVI (99). At 30-month follow-up, adjusted mortality was 49% significantly lower for AVR compared with medical treatment and 62% significantly lower for TAVI compared with medical treatment. At 1-year, 92.3% of AVR patients, 93.2% of TAVI patients, and 70.8% of medically treated patients were NYHA functional class I or II (99).

In the Placement of Aortic Transcatheter Valves (PARTNER) trial, 699 high-risk patients with severe AS, mean age 84 years, were randomized to AVR or TAVI (100). All-cause mortality was 3.4% for the TAVI group versus 6.5% for the AVR group at 30 days (p not significant) and 24.2% for the TAVI group versus 26.8% for the AVR group at 1 year (p not significant). Major stroke was 3.8% for the TAVI group versus 2.1% for the AVR group at 30 days (p not significant) and 5.1% for the TAVI group versus 2.4% for the AVR group at 1 year (p not significant). Major vascular complications at 30 days were 11.0% for the TAVI group versus 3.2% for the AVR group ($p<0.001$). At 1-year, there were similar improvements in cardiac symptoms for both groups (99). In the PARTNER trial, among inoperable patients with severe AS, compared with standard care, TAVI caused significant improvements in health-related quality of life maintained for at least 1 year (101).

One-third of 270 patients undergoing a CoreValve TAVI needed a permanent pacemaker implanted within 30 days (102). In 138 patients undergoing TAVI, mean age 79 years, with no prior history of AF, new-onset AF developed in 44 patients (32%) at a median time of 48 hours after TAVI (103). A modified procedure of transapical TAVI with a balloon-expandable prosthesis was associated with a low incidence of relevant prosthetic regurgitation (104).

On the basis of the available data, AVR should be performed in operable patients with severe AS. However, TAVI should be performed in nonoperable patients with symptomatic severe AS to improve survival and quality of life compared with medical management.

After TAVI, treatment with clopidogrel for 3 months in addition to aspirin is widely practiced. However, a small study of 161 patients randomized to clopidogrel for 3 months (a loading dose of 300 mg on the day before TAVI followed by 75 mg daily) plus aspirin 100 mg daily or aspirin 100 mg daily alone showed no significant difference in major adverse cardiac and cerebrovascular events at 30 days and at 6 months (105). These data need confirmation by a larger study.

AORTIC REGURGITATION
Etiology and Prevalence
Acute AR in elderly patients may be due to infective endocarditis, rheumatic fever, aortic dissection, trauma following prosthetic valve surgery, or rupture of the sinus of Valsalva, and causes sudden severe LV failure. Chronic AR in elderly patients may be caused by valve leaflet disease (secondary to any cause of AS, infective endocarditis, rheumatic fever, congenital heart disease, rheumatoid arthritis, ankylosing spondylitis, following prosthetic valve surgery, or myxomatous degeneration of the valve) or by aortic root disease. Examples of aortic root disease causing chronic AR in elderly patients include association with systemic hypertension, syphilitic aortitis, cystic medial necrosis of the aorta, ankylosing spondylitis, rheumatoid arthritis, Reiter's disease, systemic lupus erythematosus, Ehler–Danlos syndrome, and pseudoxanthoma elasticum. Mild or moderate AR was also diagnosed by Doppler echocardiography in 9 of 29 patients (31%) with hypertrophic cardiomyopathy (106). Margonato et al. (107) linked the increased prevalence of AR with age to aortic valve thickening.

The prevalence of AR increases with age (107–109). In a prospective study of 450 unselected patients, mean age 82 years, AR was diagnosed by pulsed Doppler echocardiography in 39 of 114 men (34%) and in 92 of 336 women (27%) (109). Severe or moderate AR was diagnosed in 74 of 450 elderly patients (16%). Mild AR was diagnosed in 57 of 450 elderly patients (13%). In a prospective study of 924 men, mean age 80 years, and 1,881 women, mean age 82 years, valvular AR was diagnosed by pulsed Doppler recordings of the aortic valve in 282 of 924 men (31%) and in 542 of 1881 women (29%) (26).

Pathophysiology
The primary determinants of AR volume are the regurgitant orifice area, the transvalvular pressure gradient, and the duration of diastole (110). Chronic AR increases LV ventricular end-diastolic volume. The largest LV end-diastolic volumes are seen in patients with chronic severe AR. LV stroke volume increases to maintain the forward stroke volume. The increased preload causes an increase in LV diastolic stress and the addition of sarcomeres in series. This results in an increase in the ratio of the LV chamber size to wall thickness. This pattern of LV hypertrophy is called eccentric LV hypertrophy.

Primary myocardial abnormalities or ischemia due to coexistent CAD depress the contractile state. LV diastolic compliance decreases, LV end-systolic volume increases, LV end-diastolic pressure rises, left atrial pressure increases, and pulmonary venous hypertension results. When the LV end-diastolic radius-to-wall thickness ratio rises, LV systolic wall stress increases abnormally because of the preload and afterload mismatch (28,111). Additional stress then decreases the LV ejection fraction response to exercise (112). Eventually, the LV ejection fraction, forward stroke volume, and effective cardiac output are decreased at rest. We demonstrated that an abnormal resting LV ejection fraction occurred in 8 of 25 elderly patients (32%) with CHF associated with chronic severe AR (113).

In patients with acute severe AR, the LV cannot adapt to the increased volume over-load. Forward stroke volume falls, LV end-diastolic pressure increases rapidly to high lev-els, (114), and pulmonary hypertension and pulmonary edema result. The rapid rise of the LV end-diastolic pressure to exceed the left atrial pressure in early diastole causes prema-ture closure of the mitral valve (115). This prevents backward transmission of the elevated LV end-diastolic pressure to the pulmonary venous bed.

Symptoms

Patients with acute AR develop symptoms due to the sudden onset of CHF, with marked dyspnea and weakness. Patients with chronic AR may remain asymptomatic for many years. Mild dyspnea on exertion and palpitations, especially on lying down, may occur. Exertional dyspnea, orthopnea, paroxysmal nocturnal dyspnea, fatigue, and edema are common clinical symptoms when LV failure occurs. Syncope is rare. Angina pectoris occurs less often in patients with AR than in patients with AS and may be due to coexistent CAD. However, nocturnal angina pectoris, often accompanied by flushing, diaphoresis, and palpitations, may develop when the heart rate slows and the arterial diastolic pressure falls to very low levels. Most patients with severe AR who do not have surgery die within 2 years after CHF develops (116).

Signs

The AR murmur is typically a high-pitched blowing diastolic murmur that begins immedi-ately after A_2. The diastolic murmur is best heard along the left sternal border in the third and fourth intercostal spaces when AR is due to valvular disease. The murmur is best heard along the right sternal border when AR is due to dilatation of the ascending aorta. The diastolic murmur is best heard with the diaphragm of the stethoscope with the person sit-ting up, leaning forward, and holding the breath in deep expiration. The severity of AR correlates with the duration of the diastolic murmur, not with the intensity of the murmur.

Grayburn et al. (117) heard an AR murmur in 73% of 82 patients with AR and in 8% of 24 patients without AR. Saal et al. (118) heard an AR murmur in 80% of 35 patients with AR and in 10% of 10 patients without AR. Meyers et al. (119) heard an AR murmur in 73% of 66 patients with AR and in 22% of nine patients without AR. Table 15.6 shows that an AR murmur was heard in 95% of 74 elderly patients with severe or moderate AR diagnosed by pulsed Doppler echocardiography, in 61% of 57 elderly patients with mild AR, and in 3% of 319 elderly patients with no AR (109).

In patients with chronic severe AR, the LV apical impulse is diffuse, hyperdynamic, and displaced laterally and inferiorly. A rumbling diastolic murmur (Austin Flint) may be heard at the apex, with its intensity decreased by inhalation of amyl nitrite. A short basal systolic ejection murmur is heard. A palpable LV rapid filling wave and an audible S_3 at the

Table 15.6 Correlation of Aortic Regurgitation Murmur with Severity of Aortic Regurgitation in Elderly Patients with Chronic Aortic Regurgitation

	AR murmur (%)
Severe or moderate AR ($n = 74$)	95
Mild AR ($n = 57$)	61
No AR ($n = 319$)	3

Abbreviation: AR, aortic regurgitation.
Source: Adapted from Ref. 109.

apex are usually found. Physical findings due to a large LV stroke volume and a rapid diastolic runoff in patients with severe AR include a wide pulse pressure with an increased systolic arterial pressure and an abnormally low diastolic arterial pressure, an arterial pulse that abruptly rises and collapses, a bisferiens pulse, bobbing of the head with each heart beat, booming systolic and diastolic sounds heard over the femoral artery, capillary pulsations, and systolic and diastolic murmurs heard over the femoral artery when compressing it proximally and distally.

Electrocardiography and Chest Roentgenography

The electrocardiogram may initially be normal in patients with acute severe AR. Roberts and Day (120) showed in 30 necropsy patients with chronic severe AR that the electrocardiogram did not accurately predict the severity of AR or cardiac weight. Using various electrocardiographic criteria, the prevalence of LV hypertrophy varied from 30% (RV_6>RV_5) to 90% (total 12-lead QRS voltage >175 mm). The P–R interval was prolonged in 28% of patients, and the QRS duration was ≥0.12 seconds in 20% of patients (120).

The chest X ray in patients with acute severe AR may show a normal heart size and pulmonary edema. The chest X ray in patients with chronic severe AR usually shows a dilated LV, with elongation of the apex inferiorly and posteriorly and a dilated aorta. Aneurysmal dilatation of the aorta suggests that aortic root disease is causing the AR. Linear calcifications in the wall of the ascending aorta are seen in syphilitic AR and in degenerative disease.

Echocardiography and Doppler Echocardiography

M-mode and two-dimensional echocardiography and Doppler echocardiography are very useful in the diagnosis of AR. Two-dimensional echocardiography can provide information showing the etiology of the AR and measurements of LV function. Eccentric LV hypertrophy is diagnosed by echocardiography if the LV mass index is increased with a relative wall thickness <0.45 (121–123). Echocardiographic measurements reported to predict an unfavorable response to aortic valve replacement in patients with chronic AR include an LV end-systolic dimension >55 mm (124), an LV shortening fraction <25% (124), an LV diastolic radius-to-wall thickness ratio >3.8 (125), an LV end-diastolic dimension index >38 mm/m^2 (2,125), and an LV ventricular end-systolic dimension index >26 mm/m^2 (2,125).

Grayburn et al. (117) showed that pulsed Doppler echocardiography correctly identified the presence of AR in 57 of 57 patients (100%) with ≥2+ AR and in 22 of 25 patients (88%) with 1+ AR. Saal et al. (118) demonstrated that pulsed Doppler echocardiography identified the presence of AR in 34 of 35 patients (97%) with documented AR. Continuous-wave Doppler echocardiography has also been shown to be very useful in diagnosing and quantitating AR (126,127). AR is best assessed by color flow Doppler imaging (128). Figure 15.6 illustrates two-dimensional echocardiographic and color Doppler findings in an elderly patient with chronic severe AR. Figure 15.7 illustrates continuous-wave Doppler findings in the elderly patient with chronic severe AR shown in Figure 15.6.

Natural History

The natural history of chronic AR is significantly different than the natural history of acute AR. Patients with acute AR should have immediate aortic valve replacement because death may occur within hours to days. In one study of patients with hemodynamically significant chronic AR treated medically, 75% were alive at 5 years after diagnosis (52,111). Of patients with moderate-to-severe chronic AR, 50% were alive at 10 years after diagnosis (54,129). The 10-year survival rate for patients with mild-to-moderate chronic AR was 85–95% (54,130).

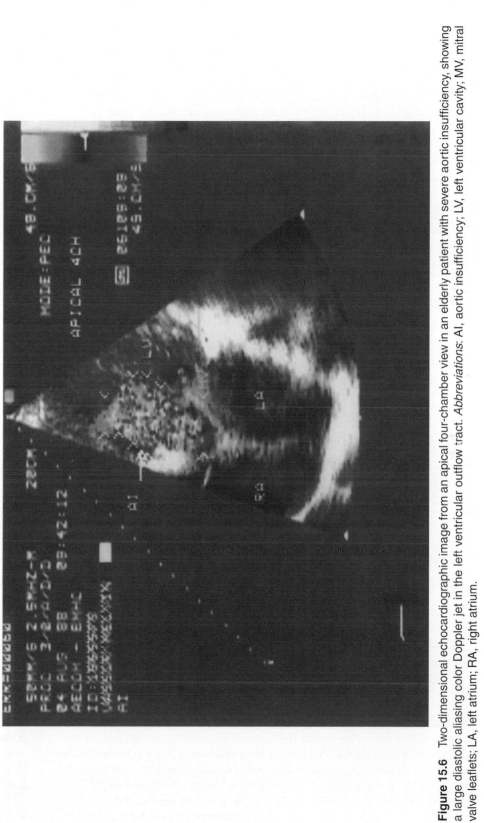

Figure 15.6 Two-dimensional echocardiographic image from an apical four-chamber view in an elderly patient with severe aortic insufficiency, showing a large diastolic aliasing color Doppler jet in the left ventricular outflow tract. *Abbreviations*: AI, aortic insufficiency; LV, left ventricular cavity; MV, mitral valve leaflets; LA, left atrium; RA, right atrium.

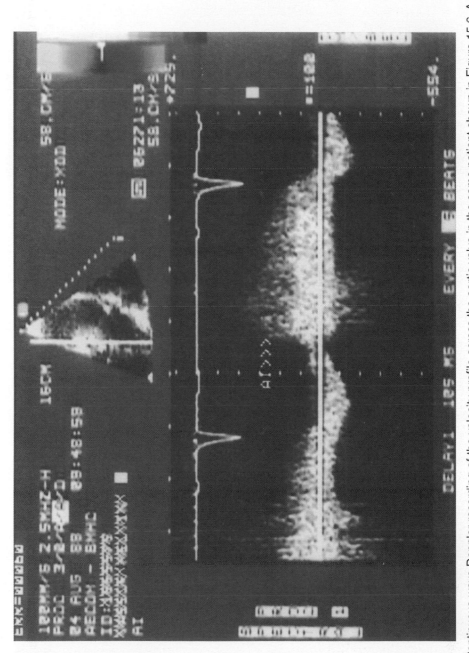

Figure 15.7 Continuous-wave Doppler recording of the velocity profile across the aortic valve in the same patient shown in Figure 15.6. A holosystolic decrescendo high-velocity profile is recorded from the left ventricular outflow tract, characteristic of aortic insufficiency. *Abbreviation:* AI, aortic insufficiency.

In another study of 14 patients with chronic severe AR who did not have surgery, 13 (93%) died within 2 years of developing CHF (116). The mean survival time after the onset of angina pectoris is 5 years (129).

During 8-year follow-up of 104 asymptomatic patients with chronic severe AR and normal LV ejection fraction, 2 patients (2%) died suddenly, and 23 patients (22%) had aortic valve replacement (131). Of the 104 patients, 19 (18%) had aortic valve replacement because of cardiac symptoms and four patients (4%) had aortic valve replacement because of the development of LV systolic dysfunction in the absence of cardiac symptoms. Multivariate analysis showed that age, initial end-systolic dimension, and rate of change in end-systolic dimension and resting LV ejection fraction during serial studies predicted the outcome.

In a prospective study, at 24-month follow-up (range 7–55 months) of 17 patients, mean age 83 years, with CHF associated with unoperated severe chronic AR and a normal LV ejection fraction, 15 patients (88%) were dead (113). At 15-month follow-up (range 8–21 months) of 8 patients, mean age 85 years, with CHF associated with unoperated severe chronic AR and an abnormal LV ejection fraction, 8 patients (100%) were dead (113).

The overall 15-year mortality for AR in 1156 patients was 74% and increased 1.94 times in patients with moderate or greater pulmonary artery systolic hypertension (132).

Medical and Surgical Management

Asymptomatic patients with mild or moderate AR do not require therapy. Prophylactic antibiotics are not recommended to prevent bacterial endocarditis in patients with AR according to updated ACC/AHA guidelines (67). Echocardiographic evaluation of LV end-systolic dimension should be performed yearly if the measurement is less than 50 mm but every 3–6 months if the LV end-systolic dimension is 50–54 mm. AVR should also be considered when the LV ejection fraction approaches 50% before the decompensated state (110).

Patients with asymptomatic, chronic severe AR have been treated with hydralazine (133), nifedipine (134), or angiotensin-converting-enzyme therapy (135) to decrease the LV volume overload. Vasodilator therapy is indicated for chronic therapy in patients with severe AR who have symptoms or an abnormal LV ejection fraction when AVR is not recommended because of additional cardiac or noncardiac factors (Class I indication) and for short-term therapy to improve the hemodynamic profile of patients with severe CHF symptoms and severe LV systolic dysfunction before proceeding with AVR (Class II$_a$ indication) (66). Long-term vasodilator therapy with enalapril or nifedipine did not reduce or delay the need for AVR in patients with asymptomatic severe AR and normal LV ejection fraction (136).

Infections should be treated promptly. Systemic hypertension increases the regurgitant flow and should be treated. Drugs that depress LV function should not be used. Arrhythmias should be treated. Patients with AR due to syphilitic aortitis should receive a course of penicillin therapy. Prophylactic resection should be considered in patients with Marfan's syndrome when the aortic root diameter exceeds 55 mm (137).

Bacterial endocarditis should be treated with intravenous antibiotics. Indications for AVR in patients with AR due to bacterial endocarditis are CHF, uncontrolled infection, myocardial or valvular ring abscess, prosthetic valve dysfunction or dehiscence, and multiple embolic episodes (138–140).

CHF should be treated with sodium restriction, diuretics, digoxin if the LV ejection fraction is abnormal, vasodilator therapy, and AVR. Angina pectoris should be treated with nitrates.

Table 15.7 American College of Cardiology/American Heart Association Class I Indications for Aortic Valve Replacement in Persons with Chronic Severe Aortic Regurgitation

---

1. Symptomatic patients with severe AR and normal or abnormal left ventricular ejection fraction
2. Asymptomatic patients with severe AR and LV ejection fraction ≤50% at rest
3. Patients with severe AR undergoing coronary artery bypass surgery or surgery on the aorta or other heart valves
4. Asymptomatic patients with severe AR with LV ejection fraction >50% but an LV end-diastolic dimension >75 mm or an LV end-systolic dimension >55 mm (Class II$_a$ indication)

Abbreviations: AR, aortic regurgitation; LV, left ventricular.
Source: Adapted from Ref. 66.

Patients with acute severe AR should undergo AVR immediately. Patients with chronic severe AR should have AVR if they develop symptoms of CHF, angina pectoris or syncope (66,131). AVR should also be performed in asymptomatic patients with chronic severe AR if their LV ejection fraction is ≤ 50% at rest (66,131). Table 15.7 shows three Class I and one Class II$_a$ ACC/AHA indications for AVR in patients with chronic severe AR (66). The Class I indications for AVR include symptoms with an abnormal or normal LV ejection fraction, no symptoms but an LV ejection fraction ≤50% at rest, and asymptomatic patients undergoing CABGS or surgery on the aorta or other heart valves (66). The Class II$_a$ indication for AVR is asymptomatic patients with severe AR with an LV ejection fraction >50% but an LV end-diastolic dimension >75 mm or an LV end-systolic dimension >55 mm (66).

Elderly patients undergoing AVR for severe AR have an excellent postoperative survival if the preoperative LV ejection fraction is normal (141–143). If LV systolic dysfunction was present for less than 1 year, patients also did well postoperatively. However, if the person with severe AR has an abnormal LV ejection fraction and impaired exercise tolerance and/or the presence of LV systolic dysfunction for longer than 1 year, the postoperative survival is poor (141–143). However, the Cleveland Clinic has reported that for the patient with AR and severe LV dysfunction, AVR is the preferred treatment and can be performed with acceptable risk and late survival (144). After AVR, women exhibit an excess late mortality, suggesting that surgical correction of severe chronic AR should be considered at an earlier stage in women (145).

The operative mortality for AVR in elderly patients with severe AR is similar to that in elderly patients with AVR for valvular AS. The mortality rate is slightly increased in patients with infective endocarditis and in those patients needing replacement of the ascending aorta plus aortic valve replacement.

Of 450 patients with severe AR, 273 (61%) had an LV ejection fraction ≥ 50%, 134 (30%) had an LV ejection fraction of 35–50%, and 43 patients (10%) had an LV ejection fraction <35% (146). The operative mortality was 3.7% for patients with a normal LV ejection fraction, 6.7% for patients with an LV ejection fraction of 35–50%, and 14% for patients with an LV ejection fraction <35% (146). At 10-year follow-up, survival rates were 70% for patients with a normal LV ejection fraction, 56% for patients with an LV ejection fraction of 35–50%, and 41% for patients with an LV ejection fraction <35% (146).

The bioprosthesis is preferable to the mechanical prosthetic valve for AVR in elderly patients with severe AR as in elderly patients with valvular AS (77–80). Patients with porcine bioprostheses may be treated with antiplatelet therapy alone unless they have AF, abnormal LV ejection fraction, previous thromboembolism, or a hypercoagulable state (66).

In a prospective study, AVR in 38 patients with severe AR normalized LV chamber size and mass in two-thirds of patients undergoing surgery (147). At 9-month follow-up after AVR, 58% of patients had a normal LV end-diastolic dimension, and 50% of patients had a normal LV mass. During further follow-up (18–56 months postoperatively) 66% of patients had a normal LV end-diastolic dimension and 68% of patients had a normal LV mass. The LV end-diastolic dimension normalized in 86% of patients with a preoperative LV end-systolic dimension ≤55 mm. A preoperative LV end-systolic dimension >55 mm was present in 81% of patients with postoperative persistent LV dilatation (147).

In 56 patients undergoing AVR for chronic severe AR, the best predictor of LV remodeling and of outcomes at 3 years was a preoperative stroke volume of ≥97 mL (148). In 171 patients undergoing AVR for severe chronic AR, preoperative indexed LV end-systolic and end-diastolic dimensions were independent predictors of restored LV systolic function (149). Of 690 patients, mean age 81 years, with severe AS treated with TAVI, 119 patients (17.2%) developed ≥2+ AR (150). In this study, ≥2+ AR was an independent predictor of in-hospital death with an adjusted odds ratio of 2.4 (150).

REFERENCES

1. Roberts WC, Perloff JK, Costantino T. Severe valvular aortic stenosis in patients over 65 years of age. Am J Cardiol 1971; 27: 497–506.
2. Waller BF, Roberts WC. Cardiovascular disease in the very elderly. An analysis of 40 necropsy patients aged 90 years or over. Am J Cardiol 1983; 51: 403–21.
3. Aronow WS, Schwartz KS, Koenigsberg M. Correlation of aortic cuspal and aortic root disease with aortic systolic ejection murmurs and with mitral anular calcium in persons older than 62 years in a long-term health care facility. Am J Cardiol 1986; 58: 651–2.
4. Aronow WS, Kronzon I. Prevalence and severity of valvular aortic stenosis determined by Doppler echocardiography and its association with echocardiographic and electrocardiographic left ventricular hypertrophy and physical signs of aortic stenosis in elderly patients. Am J Cardiol 1991; 67: 776–7.
5. Lindroos M, Kupari M, Heikkila J, Tilvis R. Prevalence of aortic valve abnormalities in the elderly: an echocardiographic study of a random population sample. J Am Coll Cardiol 1993; 21: 1220–5.
6. Aronow WS, Ahn C, Kronzon I. Association of mitral annular calcium and of aortic cuspal calcium with coronary artery disease in older patients. Am J Cardiol 1999; 84: 1084–5.
7. Aronow WS, Ahn C, Shirani J, Kronzon I. Comparison of frequency of new coronary events in older subjects with and without valvular aortic sclerosis. Am J Cardiol 1999; 83: 599–600.
8. Roberts WC, Perloff JK. Mitral valvular disease. A clinicopathologic survey of the conditions causing the mitral valve to function normally. Ann Intern Med 1972; 77: 939–75.
9. Nair CK, Aronow WS, Stokke K, et al. Cardiac conduction defects in patients older than 60 years with aortic stenosis with and without mitral anular calcium. Am J Cardiol 1984; 53: 169–72.
10. Sell S, Scully RE. Aging changes in the aortic and mitral valves. Am J Pathol 1965; 46: 345–65.
11. Otto CM, Kuusisto J, Reichenbach DD, et al. Characterization of the early lesion of 'degenerative' valvular aortic stenosis. Circulation 1994; 90: 844–53.
12. Stewart BF, Siscovick D, Lind BK, et al. Clinical factors associated with calcific aortic valve disease. J Am Coll Cardiol 1997; 29: 630–4.
13. Aronow WS, Schwartz KS, Koenigsberg M. Correlation of serum lipids, calcium, and phosphorus, diabetes mellitus and history of systemic hypertension with presence or absence of calcified or thickened aortic cusps or root in elderly patients. Am J Cardiol 1987; 59: 998–9.
14. Lindroos M, Kupari M, Valvanne J, et al. Factors associated with calcific aortic valve degeneration in the elderly. Eur Heart J 1994; 15: 865–70.
15. Aronow WS, Kronzon I, Schoenfeld MR. Prevalence of extracranial carotid arterial disease and of valvular aortic stenosis and their association in the elderly. Am J Cardiol 1995; 75: 304–5.
16. Aronow WS, Ahn C, Kronzon I. Association of valvular aortic stenosis with symptomatic peripheral arterial disease in older persons. Am J Cardiol 2001; 88: 1046–7.
17. Nassimiha D, Aronow WS, Ahn C, Goldman ME. Rate of progression of valvular aortic stenosis in persons ≥60 years. Am J Cardiol 2001; 87: 807–9.
18. Nassimiha D, Aronow WS, Ahn C, Goldman ME. Association of coronary risk factors with progression of valvular aortic stenosis in older persons. Am J Cardiol 2001; 87: 1313–14.
19. Palta S, Pai AM, Gill KS, Pai RG. New insights into the progression of aortic stenosis. Implications for secondary prevention. Circulation 2000; 101: 3497–2502.

20. Roberts WC. The senile cardiac calcification syndrome. Am J Cardiol 1986; 58: 572–4.
21. Aronow WS, Schwartz KS, Koenigsberg M. Correlation of serum lipids, calcium and phosphorus, diabetes mellitus, aortic valve stenosis and history of systemic hypertension with presence or absence of mitral anular calcium in persons older than 62 years in a long-term health care facility. Am J Cardiol 1987; 59: 381–2.
22. Aronow WS, Ahn C, Kronzon I, Goldman ME. Association of coronary risk factors and use of statins with progression of mild valvular aortic stenosis in older persons. Am J Cardiol 2001; 88: 693–5.
23. Novaro GM, Tiong IY, Pearce GL, et al. Effect of hydroxymethylglutaryl coenzyme A reductase inhibitors on the progression of calcific aortic stenosis. Circulation 2001; 104: 2205–9.
24. Bellamy MF, Pellikka PA, Klarich KW, et al. Association of cholesterol levels, hydroxymethylglutaryl coenzyme-A reductase inhibitor treatment, and progression of aortic stenosis in the community J Am Coll Cardiol 2002; 40: 1723–30.
25. Rossebo AB, Pedersen TR, Boman K, et al. Intensive lipid lowering with simvastatin and ezetimibe in aortic stenosis. N Engl J Med 2008; 359: 1343–56.
26. Aronow WS, Ahn C, Kronzon I. Comparison of echocardiographic abnormalities in African-American, Hispanic, and white men and women aged >60 years. Am J Cardiol 2001; 87: 1131–3.
27. Kennedy JW, Twiss RD, Blackmon JR, Dodge HT. Quantitative angiocardiography. III. Relationships of left ventricular pressure, volume and mass in aortic valve disease. Circulation 1968; 38: 838–45.
28. Hood WP Jr, Rackley CE, Rolett EL. Wall stress in the normal and hypertrophied human left ventricle. Am J Cardiol 1968; 22: 550–8.
29. Carroll JD, Carroll EP, Feldman T, et al. Sex-associated differences in left ventricular function in aortic stenosis of the elderly. Circulation 1992; 86: 1099–107.
30. Villari B, Vassalli G, Schneider J, et al. Age dependency of left ventricular diastolic function in pressure overload hypertrophy. J Am Coll Cardiol 1997; 29: 181–6.
31. Rajappan K, Rimoldi OE, Dutka DP, et al. Mechanisms of coronary microcirculatory dysfunction in patients with aortic stenosis and angiographically normal coronary arteries. Circulation 2002; 105: 470–6.
32. Stott DK, Marpole DG, Bristow JD, et al. The role of left atrial transport in aortic and mitral stenosis. Circulation 1970; 41: 1031–41.
33. Vekshtein VI, Alexander RW, Yeung AC, et al. Coronary atherosclerosis is associated with left ventricular dysfunction and dilatation in aortic stenosis. Circulation 1990; 82: 2068–74.
34. Aronow WS, Ahn C, Kronzon I, Nanna M. Prognosis of congestive heart failure in patients aged ≥62 years with unoperated severe valvular aortic stenosis. Am J Cardiol 1993; 72: 846–8.
35. Hess OM, Villari B, Krayenbuehl HP. Diastolic dysfunction in aortic stenosis. Circulation 1993; 87:73–6.
36. Julius BK, Spillmann M, Vassalli G, et al. Angina pectoris in patients with aortic stenosis and normal coronary arteries. Mechanisms and pathophysiological concepts. Circulation 1997; 95: 892–8.
37. Aronow WS, Ahn C, Shirani J, Kronzon I. Comparison of frequency of new coronary events in older persons with mild, moderate, and severe valvular aortic stenosis with those without aortic stenosis. Am J Cardiol 1998; 81: 647–9.
38. Ross J Jr, Braunwald E. Aortic stenosis. Circulation 1968; 37:61–7.
39. Frank S, Johnson A, Ross J Jr. Natural history of valvular aortic stenosis. Br Heart J 1973; 35: 41–56.
40. Braunwald E. On the natural history of severe aortic stenosis. J Am Coll Cardiol 1990; 15: 1018–20.
41. Bruns DL, Van Der Hauwaert LG. The aortic systolic murmur developing with increased age. Br Heart J 1958; 20: 370–8.
42. Aronow WS, Kronzon I. Correlation of prevalence and severity of valvular aortic stenosis determined by continuous-wave Doppler echocardiography with physical signs of aortic stenosis in patients aged 62 to 100 years with aortic systolic ejection murmurs. Am J Cardiol 1987; 60: 399–401.
43. Folland ED, Kriegel BJ, Henderson WG, et al. Implications of third heart sounds in patients with valvular heart disease. N Engl J Med 1992; 327: 458–62.
44. Greve AM, Boman K, Gohlke-Baerwolf C, et al. Clinical implications of electrocardiographic left ventricular strain and hypertrophy in asymptomatic patients with aortic stenosis. The Simvastatin and Ezetimibe in Aortic Stenosis study. Circulation 2012; 125: 346–53.
45. Finegan RE, Gianelly RE, Harrison DC. Aortic stenosis in the elderly. Relevance of age to diagnosis and treatment. N Engl J Med 1969; 281: 1261–4.
46. Aronow WS, Epstein S, Koenigsberg M, Schwartz KS. Usefulness of echocardiographic abnormal left ventricular ejection fraction, paroxysmal ventricular tachycardia and complex ventricular arrhythmias in predicting new coronary events in patients over 62 years of age. Am J Cardiol 1988; 61: 1349–51.
47. Rispler S, Rinkevich D, Markiewicz W, Reisner SA. Missed diagnosis of severe symptomatic aortic stenosis. Am J Cardiol 1995; 76: 728–30.

48. Teirstein P, Yeager M, Yock PG, Popp RL. Doppler echocardiographic measurements of aortic valve area in aortic stenosis: a noninvasive application of the Gorlin formula. J Am Coll Cardiol 1986; 8: 1059–65.
49. Come PC, Riley MF, McKay RG, Safian R. Echocardiographic assessment of aortic valve area in elderly patients with aortic stenosis and of changes of valve area after percutaneous balloon valvuloplasty. J Am Coll Cardiol 1987; 10: 115–24.
50. Shah PM, Graham BM. Management of aortic stenosis: is cardiac catheterization necessary? Am J Cardiol 1991; 67: 1031–2.
51. Slater J, Gindea AJ, Freedberg RS, et al. Comparison of cardiac catheterization and Doppler echocardiography in the decision to operate in aortic and mitral valve disease. J Am Coll Cardiol 1991; 67: 1007–12.
52. Nassimiha D, Aronow WS, Ahn C, Goldman ME. Comparison of aortic valve area determined by Doppler echocardiography and cardiac catheterization in 75 older patients with valvular aortic stenosis. Cardiovasc Rev and Reports 2000; 21: 507–9.
53. Galan A, Zoghbi WA, Quinones MA. Determination of severity of valvular aortic stenosis by Doppler echocardiography and relation of findings to clinical outcome and agreement with hemodynamic measurements determined at cardiac catheterization. Am J Cardiol 1991; 67: 1007–12.
54. Rapaport E. Natural History of aortic and mitral valve disease. Am J Cardiol 1975; 35: 221–7.
55. Livanainen AM, Lindroos M, Tilvis R, et al. Natural history of aortic valve stenosis of varying severity in the elderly. Am J Cardiol 1996; 78: 97–101.
56. Otto CM, Lind BK, Kitzman DW, et al. Association of aortic-valve sclerosis with cardiovascular mortality and morbidity in the elderly. N Engl J Med 1999; 341: 142–7.
57. Kennedy KD, Nishimura RA, Holmes DR Jr, Bailey KR. Natural history of moderate aortic stenosis. J Am Coll Cardiol 1991; 17: 313–19.
58. Hammermeister KE, Cantor AB, Burchfield CM, et al. Clinical haemodynamic and angiographic predictors of survival in unoperated patients with aortic stenosis. Eur Heart J 1988; 9:65–9.
59. Turina J, Hess O, Sepulcri F, Krayenbuehl HP. Spontaneous course of aortic valve disease. Eur Heart J 1987; 8: 471–83.
60. Kelly TA, Rothbart RM, Cooper CM, et al. Comparison of outcome of asymptomatic to symptomatic patients older than 20 years of age with valvular aortic stenosis. Am J Cardiol 1988; 61: 123–30.
61. Pellikka PA, Nishimura RA, Bailey KR, Tajik AJ. The natural history of adults with asymptomatic hemodynamically significant aortic stenosis. J Am Coll Cardiol 1990; 15: 1012–17.
62. Rosenhek R, Binder T, Porenta G, et al. Predictors of outcome in severe, asymptomatic aortic stenosis. N Engl J Med 2000; 343: 611–17.
63. Smith RL, Larsen D, Crawford MH, Shively BK. Echocardiographic predictors of survival in low gradient aortic stenosis. Am J Cardiol 2000; 86: 804–7.
64. Monin J-L, Monchi M, Gest V, et al. Aortic stenosis with severe left ventricular dysfunction and low transvalvular pressure gradients. Risk stratification by low-dose dobutamine echocardiography. J Am Coll Cardiol 2001; 37: 2101–7.
65. Monin J-L, Quere J-P, Monchi M, et al. Low-gradient aortic stenosis. Operative risk stratification and predictors for long-term outcome: a multicenter study using dobutamine stress hemodynamics. Circulation 2003; 108: 319–24.
66. Bonow RO, Carabello BA, Chatterjee K, et al. ACC/AHA 2006 practice guidelines for the management of patients with valvular heart disease. Executive Summary. A Report of the American College of Cardiology/American Heart Association task force on Practice Guidelines (Writing Committee to Revise the 1988 Guidelines for the Management of Patients With Valvular Heart Disease). Developed in collaboration with the Society of Cardiovascular Anesthesiologists. Endorsed by the Society for Cardiovascular Angiography and Interventions and the Society of Thoracic Surgeons. J Am coll Cardiol 2006; 48: 598–675.
67. Nishimura RA, Carabello BA, Faxon DP, et al. ACC/AHA 2008 guideline update on valvular heart disease: focused update on infective endocarditis. A Report of the American College of Cardiology/American Heart Association Task Force on Practice Guidelines. Endorsed by the Society of Cardiovascular Anesthesiologists, Society for Cardiovascular Angiography and Interventions, and Society of Thoracic Surgeons. J Am Coll Cardiol 2008; 52: 676–85.
68. Tresch DD, Knickelbine T. Aortic valvular stenosis in the elderly: a disorder with a favorable outcome if correctly diagnosed and treated. Cardiovasc Rev Rep 1994; 15:35–8.
69. Pai RG, Kapoor N, Bansal RC, Varadarajan P. Malignant natural history of asymptomatic severe aortic stenosis: benefit of aortic valve replacement. Ann Thorac Surg 2006; 82: 2116–22.
70. Brown ML, Pellikka PA, Schaff HV, et al. The benefits of early valve replacement in asymptomatic patients with severe aortic stenosis. J Thorac Cardiovasc Surg 2008; 135: 308–15.

71. Kang D-H, Park S-J, Rim JH, et al. Early surgery versus conventional treatment in asymptomatic very severe aortic stenosis. Circulation 2010; 121: 1502–9.
72. Rosenhek R, Zilberszac R, Schemper M, et al. Natural history of very severe aortic stenosis. Circulation 2010; 121: 151–6.
73. Freed BH, Sugeng L, Furlong K, et al. Reasons for nonadherence to guidelines for aortic valve replacement in patients with very severe aortic stenosis and potential solutions. Am J Cardiol 2010; 105: 1339–42.
74. Jander N, Minners J, Holme I, et al. Outcome of patients with low-gradient "severe" aortic stenosis and preserved ejection fraction. Circulation 2011; 123: 887–95.
75. Belkin RN, Khalique O, Aronow WS, et al. Outcomes and survival with aortic valve replacement compared with medical therapy in patients with low-, moderate-, and severe-gradient severe aortic stenosis and normal left ventricular ejection fraction. Echocardiography 2011; 28: 378–87.
76. Khalique O, Belkin RN, Li Y-W, et al. Diastolic function and survival in patients with severe aortic stenosis and normal left ventricular ejection fraction (abstract). J Am coll cardiol 2012; 59: E1363.
77. Hammermeister K, Sethi GK, Henderson WG, et al. Outcomes 15 years after valve replacement with a mechanical versus a bioprosthetic valve: final report of the Veterans Affairs Randomized Trial. J Am Coll Cardiol 2000; 36: 1152–8.
78. Borkon AM, Soule LM, Baughman KL, et al. Aortic valve selection in the elderly patient. Ann Thorac Surg 1988; 46: 270–7.
79. Culliford AT, Galloway AC, Colvin SB, et al. Aortic valve replacement for aortic stenosis in persons aged 80 years and older. Am J Cardiol 1991; 67: 1256–60.
80. Huang G, Rahimtoola SH. Prosthetic heart valve. Circulation 2011; 123: 2602–5.
81. Arom K, Nicoloff D, Lindsay W, et al. Aortic valve replacement in the elderly: operative risks and long-term results (abstract). J Am Coll Cardiol 1990; 15: 96A.
82. Asimakopoulos G, Edwards M-B, Taylor KM. Aortic valve replacement in patients 80 years of age and older. Survival and cause of death based on 1100 cases: collective results from the UK Heart Valve Registry. Circulation 1997; 96: 3403–8.
83. Pereira JJ, Lauer MS, Bashir M, et al. Survival after aortic valve replacement for severe aortic stenosis with low transvalvular gradients and severe left ventricular dysfunction. J Am Coll Cardiol 2002; 39: 1356–63.
84. Unic D, Leacche M, Paul S, et al. Early and late results of isolated and combined heart valve surgery in patients ≥ 80 years of age. Am J Cardiol 2005; 95: 1500–3.
85. Levy F, Garayalde E, Quere JP, et al. Prognostic value of preoperative atrial fibrillation in patients with aortic stenosis and low ejection fraction having aortic valve replacement. Am J Cardiol 2006; 98: 809–11.
86. Gilchrist IC, Waxman HL, Kurnik PB. Improvement in early diastolic filling dynamics after aortic valve replacement. Am J Cardiol 1990; 66: 1124–9.
87. Villari B, Vassalli G, Monrad ES, et al. Normalization of diastolic dysfunction in aortic stenosis late after valve replacement. Circulation 1995; 91: 2353–8.
88. Kuhl HP, Franke A, Puschmann D, et al. Regression of left ventricular mass one year after aortic valve replacement for pure severe aortic stenosis. Am J Cardiol 2002; 89: 408–13.
89. Hoffman A, Burckhardt D. Patients at risk for cardiac death late after aortic valve replacement. Am Heart J 1990; 120: 1142–7.
90. Connolly HM, Oh JK, Orszulak TA, et al. Aortic valve replacement for aortic stenosis with severe left ventricular dysfunction. Prognostic indicators. Circulation 1997; 95: 2395–400.
91. O'Keefe JH Jr, Vlietstra RE, Bailey KR, Holmes DR Jr. Natural history of candidates for balloon aortic valvuloplasty. Mayo Clin Proc 1987; 62: 986–91.
92. Kuntz RE, Tosteson ANA, Berman AD, et al. Predictors of event free survival after balloon aortic valvuloplasty. N Engl J Med 1991; 325: 17–23.
93. Cheitlin MD. Severe aortic stenosis in the sick octogenarian. A clear indicator for balloon valvuloplasty as the initial procedure. Circulation 1989; 80: 1906–8.
94. Rahimtoola SH. Catheter balloon valvuloplasty for severe calcific aortic stenosis: a limited role. J Am Coll Cardiol 1994; 23: 1076–8.
95. Cribier A, Eltchaninoff H, Tron C, et al. Early experience with percutaneous transcatheter implantation of heart valve prosthesis for the treatment of end-stage inoperable patients with calcific aortic stenosis. J Am Coll Cardiol 2004; 43: 698–703.
96. Feldman T, Herrmann HC, Goar FS. Percutaneous treatment of valvular heart disease: catheter-based aortic valve replacement and mitral valve repair therapies. Am J Geriatr Cardiol 2006; 15: 291–301.
97. Brinster DR, Byrne M, Rogers CD, et al. Effectiveness of same day percutaneous coronary intervention followed by minimally invasive aortic valve replacement for aortic stenosis and moderate coronary disease ("hybrid approach"). Am J Cardiol 2006; 98: 1501–3.

98. Moat NE, Ludman P, de Belder MA, et al. Long-term outcomes after transcather aortic valve implantation in high-risk patients with severe aortic stenosis. The U.K. TAVI (United Kingdom Transcatheter Aortic Valve Implantation) Registry. J Am Coll Cardiol 2011; 58: 2130–8.

99. Wenaweser P, Pilgrim T, Kadner A, et al. Clinical outcomes of patients with severe aortic stenosis at increased surgical risk according to treatment modality. J Am Coll Cardiol 2011; 58: 2151–62.

100. Smith CR, Leon MB, Mack MJ, et al. Transcatheter versus surgical aortic-valve replacement in high-risk patients. N Engl J Med 2011; 364: 2187–98.

101. Reynolds MR, Magnuson EA, Lei Y, et al. Health-related quality of life after transcatheter aortic valve replacement in inoperable patients with severe aortic stenosis. Circulation 2011; 124: 1964–72.

102. Khawaja MZ, Rajani R, Cook A, et al. Permanent pacemaker insertion after CoreValve transcatheter aortic valve implantation. Incidence and contributing factors (the UK CoreValve Collaborative). Circulation 2011; 123: 951–60.

103. Amat-Santos IJ, Rodes-Cabau J, Urena M, et al. Incidence, predictive factors, and prognostic value of new-onset atrial fibrillation following transcatheter aortic valve implantation. J Am Coll Cardiol 2012; 59: 178–88.

104. Unbehaun A, Pasic M, Dreysse S, et al. Transapical aortic valve implantation. Incidence and predictors of paravalvular leakage and transvalvular regurgitation in a series of 358 patients. J Am coll Cardiol 2012; 59: 211–21.

105. Ussia GP, Scarabelli M, Mule M, et al. Dual antiplatelet therapy versus aspirin alone in patients undergoing transcatheter aortic valve implantation. Am J Cardiol 2011; 108: 1772–6.

106. Theard MA, Bhatia SJS, Plappert T, St. John Sutton MG. Doppler echocardiographic study of the frequency and severity of aortic regurgitation in hypertrophic cardiomyopathy. Am J Cardiol 1987; 60: 1143–7.

107. Margonato A, Cianflone D, Carlino M, et al. Frequency and significance of aortic valve thickening in older asymptomatic patients and its relation to aortic regurgitation. Am J Cardiol 1989; 64: 1061–2.

108. Akasaka T, Yoshikawa J, Yoshida K, et al. Age-related valvular regurgitation: a study by pulsed Doppler echocardiography. Circulation 1987; 76: 262–5.

109. Aronow WS, Kronzon I. Correlation of prevalence and severity of aortic regurgitation detected by pulsed Doppler echocardiography with the murmur of aortic regurgitation in elderly patients in a long-term health care facility. Am J Cardiol 1989; 63: 128–9.

110. Gaasch WH, Sundaram M, Meyer TE. Managing asymptomatic patients with chronic aortic regurgitation. Chest 1997; 111: 1702–9.

111. Ross J Jr. Afterload mismatch and preload reserve: a conceptual framework for the analysis of ventricular function. Prog Cardiovasc Dis 1976; 18: 256–64.

112. Greenberg B, Massie B, Thomas D, et al. Association between the exercise ejection fraction response and systolic wall stress in patients with chronic aortic insufficiency. Circulation 1985; 71: 458–65.

113. Aronow WS, Ahn C, Kronzon I, Nanna M. Prognosis of patients with heart failure and unoperated severe aortic valvular regurgitation and relation to ejection fraction. Am J Cardiol 1994; 74: 286–8.

114. Welch GH Jr, Braunwald E, Sarnoff SJ. Hemodynamic effects of quantitatively varied experimental aortic regurgitation. Circ Res 1957; 5: 546–51.

115. Mann T, McLaurin LP, Grossman W, Craige E. Assessing the hemodynamic severity of acute aortic regurgitation due to infective endocarditis. N Engl J Med 1975; 293: 108–13.

116. Massell BF, Amezcua FJ, Czoniczer G. Prognosis of patients with pure or predominant aortic regurgitation in the absence of surgery (abstract). Circulation 1966; 34:164.

117. Grayburn PA, Smith MD, Handshoe R, et al. Detection of aortic insufficiency by standard echocardiography, pulsed Doppler echocardiography, and auscultation. A comparison of accuracies. Ann Intern Med 1986; 104: 599–605.

118. Saal AK, Gross BW, Franklin DW, Pearlman AS. Noninvasive detection of aortic insufficiency in patients with mitral stenosis by pulsed Doppler echocardiography. J Am Coll Cardiol 1985; 5: 176–81.

119. Meyers DG, Sagar KB, Ingram RF, et al. Diagnosis of aortic insufficiency: comparison of auscultation and M-mode echocardiography to angiography. South Med J 1982; 75: 1192–4.

120. Roberts WC, Day PJ. Electrocardiographic observations in clinically isolated, pure, chronic, severe aortic regurgitation: analysis of 30 necropsy patients aged 19 to 65 years. Am J Cardiol 1985; 55: 431–8.

121. Savage DD, Garrison RJ, Kannel WB, et al. The spectrum of left ventricular hypertrophy in a general population sample: the Framingham Study. Circulation 1987; 75:26–33.

122. Aronow WS, Ahn C, Kronzon I, Koenigsberg M. Congestive heart failure, coronary events, and atherothrombotic brain infarction in elderly blacks and whites with systemic hypertension and with and without echocardiographic and electrocardiographic evidence of left ventricular hypertrophy. Am J Cardiol 1991; 67: 295–9.

123. Koren MJ, Devereux RB, Casale PN, et al. Relation of left ventricular mass and geometry to morbidity and mortality in uncomplicated essential hypertension. Ann Intern Med 1991; 114: 345–52.

124. Henry WL, Bonow RO, Borer JS, et al. Observations on the optimum time for operative intervention for aortic regurgitation. I. Evaluation of the results of aortic valve replacement in symptomatic patients. Circulation 1980; 61: 471–83.

125. Gaasch WH, Carroll JD, Levine HJ, Criscitiello MG. Chronic aortic regurgitation: prognostic value of left ventricular end-systolic dimension and end-diastolic radius/thickness ratio. J Am Coll Cardiol 1983; 1: 775–82.

126. Grayburn PA, Handshoe R, Smith MD, et al. Quantitative assessment of the hemodynamic consequences of aortic regurgitation by means of continuous wave Doppler recordings. J Am Coll Cardiol 1987; 10: 135–41.

127. Beyer RW, Ramirez M, Joscphson MA, Shah PM. Correlation of continuous-wave assessment of chronic aortic regurgitation with hemodynamics and angiography. Am J Cardiol 1987; 60: 852–6.

128. Perry GJ, Helmcke F, Nanda NC, et al. Evaluation of aortic insufficiency by Doppler color flow mapping. J Am Coll Cardiol 1987; 9: 952–9.

129. Dexter L. Evaluation of the results of cardiac surgery. In: Jones AM, ed. Modern Trends in Cardiology. Vol. 2 New York: Appleton-Century-Crofts, 1969: 311–33.

130. Hegglin R, Scheu H, Rothlin M. Aortic insufficiency. Circulation 1968; 38:77–92.

131. Bonow RO, Lakatos E, Maron BJ, Epstein SE. Serial long-term assessment of the natural history of asymptomatic patients with chronic aortic regurgitation and normal left ventricular systolic function. Circulation 1991; 84: 1625–35.

132. Parker MVV, Mittleman MA, Waksmonski CA, et al. Pulmonary hypertension and long-term mortality in aortic and mitral regurgitation. Am J Med 2010; 123: 1043–8.

133. Greenberg B, Massie B, Bristow JD, et al. Long-term vasodilator therapy of chronic aortic insufficiency: a randomized double-blind, placebo-controlled clinical trial. Circulation 1988; 78: 92–103.

134. Scognamiglio R, Rahimtoola SH, Fasoli G, et al. Nifedipine in asymptomatic patients with severe aortic regurgitation and normal left ventricular function. N Engl J Med 1994; 331: 689–94.

135. Lin M, Chiang H-T, Lin S-L, et al. Vasodilator therapy in chronic asymptomatic aortic regurgitation: enalapril versus hydralazine therapy. J Am Coll Cardiol 1994; 24: 1046–53.

136. Evangelista A, Tornos P, Sambola A, et al. Long-term vasodilator therapy in patients with severe aortic regurgitation. N Engl J Med 2005; 353: 1342–9.

137. McDonald GR, Schaff HV, Pyeritz RE, et al. Surgical management of patients with the Marfan syndrome and dilatation of the ascending aorta. J Thorac Cardiovasc Surg 1981; 81: 180–6.

138. Alsip SG, Blackstone EH, Kirklin JW, Cobbs CG. Indications for cardiac surgery in patients with active infective endocarditis. Am J Med 1985; 78:138–48.

139. Karp RB. Role of surgery in infective endocarditis. Cardiovasc Clin 1987; 17:141–62.

140. Cobbs CG, Gnann JW. Indications for surgery. In: Sande MA, Kaye D, Root RK, eds. Endocarditis. New York: Churchill Livingstone, 1984: 201–12.

141. Bonow RO, Picone AL, McIntosh CL, et al. Survival and functional results after valve replacement for aortic regurgitation from 1976 to 1983: impact of preoperative left ventricular function. Circulation 1985; 72: 1244–56.

142. Bonow RO. Noninvasive evaluation: prognosis and timing of operation in symptomatic and asymptomatic patients with chronic aortic regurgitation. In: Cohn LH, DiSesa VJ, eds. Aortic Regurgitation: Medical and Surgical Management. New York: Marcel Dekker, 1986: 55–86.

143. Turina J, Milincic J, Seifert B, Turina M. Valve replacement in chronic aortic regurgitation. True predictors of survival after extended follow-up. Circulation 1998; 98: II-100–7.

144. Bhudia SK, McCarthy PM, Kumpati GS, et al. Improved outcomes after aortic valve surgery for chronic aortic regurgitation with severe left ventricular dysfunction. J Am Coll Cardiol 2007; 49: 1465–71.

145. Klodas E, Enriquez-Sarano M, Tajik AJ, et al. Surgery for aortic regurgitation in women. Contrasting indications and outcomes compared with men. Circulation 1996; 94: 2472–8.

146. Chaliki HP, Mohty D, Avierinos JF, et al. Outcomes after aortic valve replacement in patients with severe aortic regurgitation and markedly reduced left ventricular function. Circulation 2002; 106: 2687–93.

147. Roman MJ, Klein L, Devereux RB, et al. Reversal of left ventricular dilatation, hypertrophy, and dysfunction by valve replacement in aortic regurgitation. Am Heart J 1989; 118: 553–63.

148. Senechal M, Bernier M, Dagenais F, et al. Usefulness of preoperative stroke volume as strong predictor of left ventricular remodeling and outcomes after aortic valve replacement in patioents with severe pure aortic regurgitation. Am J cardiol 2011; 108: 1008–13.

149. Cho SH, Byun CS, Kim KW, et al. Preoperative indexed left ventricular dimensions to predict early recovery of left ventricular function after aortic valve replacement for chronic aortic regurgitation. Circ J 2010; 74: 2340–5.
150. Abdel-Wahab M, Zahn R, Horack M, et al. Aortic regurgitation after transcatheter aortic valve implantation: incidence and early outcome. Results from the German transcatheter aortic valve interventions registry. Heart 2011; 97: 899–906.

16

Mitral regurgitation, mitral stenosis, and mitral annular calcification in the elderly

Melvin D. Cheitlin and Wilbert S. Aronow

SUMMARY

Mitral valve disease in the elderly differs from that in the younger patients in several ways. Since rheumatic fever is now uncommon in North America and Western Europe, most rheumatic heart disease is seen in younger patients not born in the USA or in older patients. In patients born in North America or Western Europe, mitral stenosis (MS) is predominantly seen in patients over age of 50–60 years, many of whom have had one or more surgical or balloon valuloplasties. At present, balloon valvuloplasty is the procedure of choice, even in the elderly and even in patients who have had previously valvulotomy and are who now have mitral restenosis. Mitral regurgitation (MR) has many etiologies, the commonest of which are degenerative or mitral valve prolapse, functional MR due to ischemia or cardiomyopathy. In patients with grade I or II ischemic MR, revascularization alone can reduce or eliminate the MR. With grade III or IV ischemic MR revascularization and concomitant annuloplasty or valve replacement can markedly reduce the degree of MR and result in better outcomes. With mitral valve disease, atrial fibrillation (AF) is a common complication and if valve surgery is indicated, consideration should be given to a concomitant Maze procedure or ablation for AF. Mitral annular calcification (MAC) is most frequently seen in the elderly patient and is probably a marker for vascular atherosclerosis and an independent predictor of adverse cardiovascular events such as myocardial infarction and stroke. The American Heart Association recommendations for antibiotic prophylaxis for valvular disease has been markedly altered so that now prophylaxis is no longer recommended for valvular regurgitation. However, many physicians still prescribe antibiotic prophylaxis for their patients with valve disease.

ETIOLOGY
Mitral Stenosis

The etiology of mitral stenosis (MS) in the elderly as in the young patient is chronic rheumatic heart disease. There is a small incidence of mitral annular calcification (MAC) with exuberant atherosclerotic encroachment from the annulus into the base of the left ventricle such that the mitral orifice is decreased, producing some degree of MS, most often not severe. Reduced anterior leaflet mobility seems to be necessary to produce obstruction sufficient for a gradient of greater than 5 mmHg (1,2).

With the marked decrease in the incidence of acute rheumatic fever in the USA over the last half century, the prevalence of MS in those people under the age of 40 years, born and raised in the USA with chronic rheumatic heart disease and MS or mitral regurgitation

Table 16.1 Etiologies of MR

1. Rheumatic heart disease
2. Mitral valve prolapse (myxomatousdegeneration)[a]
3. Infective endocarditis[a]
4. Left ventricular dilatation (left ventricular failure)
5. Idiopathic rupture of chordae tendinae[a]
6. Trauma, penetrating and nonpenetrating[a]
7. Coronary artery disease
   a. Transient ischemia[a]
   b. Myocardial infarction
   c. Ruptured papillary muscle[a]
8. Connective tissue diseases (lupus erythematosus, Marfan disease)
9. Mitral annular calcification
10. Postmitralvalvotomy[a]
11. Valve dehiscence[a]
12. Paraprosthetic MR
13. Degeneration of a bioprosthetic valve
14. Drug associated valvulopathy (fenfluoramine, pergolide)
15. Hypertrophic cardiomyopathy

[a]Etiologies where clinical picture may be that of acute MR.
Abbreviation: MR, mitral regurgitation.

(MR) has markedly decreased, so that MS in this population is seen predominantly in the elderly patient, frequently the older patient who has had earlier mitral valve surgery. Since rheumatic fever is still very common in eastern Europe, Asia, Latin and South America, and Africa, most of the younger patients with MS in the USA were born and raised in these countries.

Mitral Regurgitation

In the elderly patient mitral valve disease, especially MR, is more frequently seen than aortic valve disease, although aortic stenosis is much more often the reason for valve surgery in this age group (3). MR has numerous etiologies (Table 16.1) (4). The most frequent etiologies in elderly patients are myxomatous degeneration (mitral valve prolapse), functional MR due to left ventricular dilatation, coronary artery disease, rheumatic heart disease, and MAC. Since MAC is seen predominantly in the elderly patient and poses problems beyond those related to volume overload, a detailed discussion of this topic will be presented separately at the end of this chapter.

Anorexogenic drugs (fenfluoramine, benfluorex that was withdrawn in France in 2009 (5)) possibly related to serotonergic medications that are agonists at the 5-hydroxytryptamine 2B (5-HT 2B) receptor. Have been shown to produce valvulopathy similar to that seen in carcinoid valve disease (6). Ergot-derived dopamine receptor agonists (pergolide, cabergoline) often used in Parkinson's disease have been associated with increased risk of valvular regurgitation (7).

PATHOPHYSIOLOGY
Mitral Stenosis

The major pathology is that of commissural fusion and fusion and shortening of the chordae tendinae. Later, there is increasing fibrosis and calcification of the valve leaflets. Therefore, the obstruction to diastolic flow across the mitral valve can be due to the narrowed mitral orifice caused by commissural fusion and to the thickening and calcification of the leaflets, so that they do not open without a pressure gradient in spite of open commissures, or to obstruction due to a subvalvular component caused by fused, shortened chordae tendinae. In these latter two instances, commissurotomy will not relieve the obstruction and valve replacement is necessary.

The normal mitral valve orifice is approximately 5.0 cm². With a normal stroke volume there is no obstruction to diastolic flow until the valve area is reduced to approximately 2.0 cm². When the valve area reaches about 1.0 cm², there is sufficient obstruction at resting flow rates to result in a diastolic gradient across the mitral valve, so the left atrial pressure as well as pulmonary venous and pulmonary capillary pressures rise enough to cause pulmonary congestive symptoms (8).

The obstruction and pressure gradient between the left atrium and left ventricle in diastole accelerates the blood through the narrowed orifice, causing the turbulence and vortex formation that generates the characteristic low-frequency diastolic murmur. The loudness of the murmur is related to the magnitude of the pressure gradient and to the volume of blood accelerated across the obstructed valve as well as to the nearness of the chamber in which the murmur is generated (here the left ventricle) to the ear. Since the left ventricular apex pushes the chest wall in systole creating the point of maximal impulse (PMI), this is where the murmur is best heard. In the elderly, the antero-posterior (AP) diameter of the chest may be increased, so that the left ventricular apex no longer contacts the chest wall and the low pitched murmur of MS may be inaudible.

As left atrial pressure rises, pulmonary capillary pressure rises and overcomes the colloid osmotic pressure in the pulmonary capillary bed, leading to increasing congestion in the interstitial areas of the lung and finally to pulmonary edema. As left atrial pressure rises, there is a *pari passu* rise in right ventricular systolic pressure, increasing afterload on the right ventricle, right ventricular hypertrophy, finally resulting in right ventricular failure. In 10–15% of cases, there is a marked increase in pulmonary artery pressure and pulmonary vascular resistance due to edema pressure on the interstitial small arteries and vasoconstriction probably mediated by pulmonary artery endothelial release of vasoconstrictive amines such as endothelin. Eventually, with right ventricular failure, there is a decrease in cardiac output, and signs of right ventricular failure with increased central venous pressure, edema, and even ascites (8).

As left atrial pressure rises, the left atrium enlarges resulting in atrial fibrillation (AF), which may occur relatively early in the course of MS. With AF, stasis of blood, especially in the left atrial appendage, as well as endocardial changes (9) that promote platelet activation and release of thrombogenic substances result in atrial clotting and form the basis for the high incidence of systemic thromboemboli, the most important of which is embolic stroke that is so common in MS (10).

Hemoptysis occurs in these patients as pulmonary venous pressure increases, opening collaterals for run-off to the bronchial veins. These protrude into the lumen of the bronchi and, when rupture occurs, cause hemoptysis (8). Ortner's syndrome (paralysis of the left vocal cord) can occur with the recurrent laryngeal nerve, which hooks around the ligamentum arteriosus being stretched by the enlarging left pulmonary artery and left atrium (11).

Mitral Regurgitation
Mechanism of Regurgitant Orifice Formation
The development of MR depends on the formation during systole of a regurgitant orifice. There are a number of mechanisms by which this can occur. Dilatation of the left ventricular OS (including the mitral annulus) is seen in any cause of ventricular failure with left

ventricular dilatation. The valve itself remains normal, but the area of the mitral opening is too great to be closed by coaptation of the leaflets. There is also displacement of the papillary muscles and more lateral tension in systole on the leaflet edges, thus restricting leaflet motion (12). A similar problem occurs with ischemia and myocardial fibrosis where the mural leaflet is held from coapting with the anterior leaflet. Other mechanisms of regurgitant orifice formation are loss of leaflet tissue and fibrosis, retraction of leaflet tissue as is seen in rheumatic heart disease, or tearing of the leaflet as in infective endocarditis, seen also in penetrating and non-penetrating trauma. With hypertrophic obstructive cardiomyopathy, a regurgitant orifice is formed by the displacement of the anterior leaflet to the septum during systole. Finally, there can be loss of infravalvular support as seen in chordal and papillary muscle rupture.

With myxomatous leaflets, mitral valve prolapse occurs where there may be coaptation of the leaflets early in systole, but as the left ventricle empties and becomes smaller, the redundant leaflet is displaced back above the mitral annulus into the left atrium, and at some point a regurgitant orifice is created (13). With myocardial infarction and fibrosis of the papillary muscle and its origin from the left ventricular wall, as systole progresses, the mitral valve leaflets prolapse toward the left atrium and a regurgitant orifice forms. With annular calcification, the OS of the left ventricle is prevented from constricting during systole and the mural leaflet can be immobilized, preventing it from coapting with the anterior leaflet.

Pathophysiology Causing Symptoms
Acute Mitral Regurgitation

The pathophysiology of MR depends on the severity of the leak (regurgitant volume) and the rapidity with which the MR occurred. With sudden chordal or leaflet rupture or valve dehiscence, a sudden low-resistance runoff in systole from the left ventricle develops. If the regurgitant orifice is large, the regurgitant volume will be large. The total left ventricular stroke volume is now divided into the stroke volume going out of the aorta (effective forward stroke volume) and the blood regurgitating back into the left atrium (regurgitant volume). The left ventricle in this situation empties rapidly during systole. Since much of the regurgitant volume goes into the left atrium against low resistance, the left ventricle faces a decreased afterload early in systole, permitting it to empty more easily and achieving a smaller end-systolic volume and a higher ejection fraction (EF) (8).

The increased blood coming into the left atrium during systole results in a higher "V" wave. With the next diastole, the blood coming from the pulmonary veins adds to the regurgitant blood thus increasing the left ventricular end-diastolic volume (LVEDV). The Frank–Starling mechanism increases the next left ventricular stroke volume so that the regurgitant volume can be maintained as well as the effective forward stroke volume. In acute MR, the sudden increase in LVEDV, resisted by the unprepared left ventricle and unstretched pericardium, results in a marked rise in left ventricular filling pressure. With the increased filling pressure the left atrial and pulmonary capillary pressure is increased causing pulmonary congestion and pulmonary edema. With the rise in left atrial pressure there is a sudden increase in afterload on the right ventricle, which may dilate and rapidly fail (8).

Chronic Mitral Regurgitation

With gradually increasing regurgitant volume, there is stimulus and time for remodeling of the left ventricle and eccentric hypertrophy to occur. As the ventricle dilates, left ventricular hypertrophy (LVH) occurs so that the wall does not become thinner, preventing an increase in left ventricular wall tension. The ventricle remains compliant and the pericardium stretches to keep the left ventricular filling pressure and the left atrial pressure normal. The dilated more compliant left atrium limits the height of the "V" wave to 30–35 mmHg. The left ventricular filling pressure remains normal until the left ventricle fails, at which time the filling pressure rises.

Since the left ventricle is contracting against a lower afterload, the EF remains normal or even higher than normal. As the left ventricular end-diastolic diameter increases, eventually the wall tension and afterload increases and the EF begins to fall (14). At this stage, even with the EF still "within normal limits", there is a decrease in myocardial contractility. When the left atrial mean pressure rises, there is increased afterload on the right ventricle, which eventually leads to right ventricular failure. Here, right ventricular failure is very late in the course of the natural history.

Age Modifies the Pathophysiology of Mitral Regurgitation

In the elderly there is decreased compliance of the left ventricle (15) as well as LVH, which leads to a further, more rapid increase in left ventricular filling pressure given the volume load present in MR. With the increased aortic stiffness present in the elderly (16), there is increased left ventricular impedance to ejection and increased left ventricular afterload leading to earlier decompensation of the left ventricle in MR.

CLINICAL PICTURE
Mitral Stenosis
Symptoms

For many years, the patient may remain asymptomatic. In the elderly, many patients have had a previous intervention, either surgical or balloon valvotomy. In elderly patients, pulmonary congestion almost always results in progressive dyspnea on exertion and eventually orthopnea and paroxysmal nocturnal dyspnea (PND). Wall tension and enlargement of the left atrium lead to the development of AF and the increased danger of systemic emboli, especially stroke (8). Frequently the first symptoms occur with the onset of AF or, in the young patient, during the course of pregnancy, secondary to the increased cardiac output and diastolic flow across the mitral valve, usually in the late second or third trimester (8). With decreasing right ventricular function, the patient may have fewer symptoms and signs of pulmonary congestion and more problems with decreased exercise tolerance. Eventually, the clinical picture is dominated by the signs and symptoms of right heart failure, pedal edema, engorged neck veins, and finally ascites and the stasis cyanosis of low cardiac output.

Signs

The murmur of MS is a characteristic low-pitched, rumbling diastolic murmur best heard at the apex. With flexible valve leaflets, the first heart sound is loud and even palpable and there is an opening snap after the S_2 in early diastole. The second heart sound may be increased and even palpable if the pulmonary artery pressure is elevated. With severe pulmonary hypertension, a diastolic blowing murmur of pulmonic insufficiency may be heard along the left-sternal border, indistinguishable from the murmur of aortic regurgitation (Graham–Steele murmur). With right ventricular hypertrophy, there may be a precordial lift. With right heart failure, a systolic murmur along the left sternal border of tricuspid regurgitation may be present, as well as an elevated central venous pressure, hepatomegaly, edema, and even ascites (8).

Age Modifies Signs and Symptoms of Mitral Stenosis

In the elderly, symptoms of MS may be far advanced before the patient recognizes them. Elderly patients may accept shortness of breath and decreased exercise tolerance as an inevitable consequence of "getting older". In addition, accompanying comorbidities, such as chronic obstructive pulmonary disease, may be accepted as the cause of the increasing symptoms. In the elderly patient, the AP diameter of the chest is frequently increased so that the left ventricle no longer contacts the chest wall. Also, dilatation of the right ventricle may move the left ventricle posteriorly away from contact with the chest wall. Since the low-frequency murmur does not conduct well through the blood of the right ventricle, the murmur may be inaudible (8). Sometimes, rolling the patient into the left lateral position can bring the left ventricle into contact with the chest wall and make the murmur detectable with the bell of the stethoscope over the PMI. In addition, increasing the heart rate and cardiac output with exercise increases the diastolic gradient across the mitral valve and makes the murmur louder.

Since the elderly are more likely to have a fibrotic, calcified valve, the first heart sound may not be loud and the opening snap may be absent. In these patients, the MS may be truly silent and the patient simply looks like a patient with heart failure.

Laboratory Findings and Diagnosis

The classic findings on a chest X-ray are those of right ventricular dilatation, prominence of the pulmonary artery and pulmonary veins, especially with redistribution to the upper lung fields. There is also a double density behind the right cardiac silhouette protruding beyond the right heart border of left atrial enlargement, and a filling in below the main pulmonary artery segment in the PA view of the left atrial appendage. In the lateral film, at times, calcification of the mitral valve can be seen, but can be observed better on fluoroscopy.

The classic findings on electrocardiogram (ECG) are left atrial abnormality and right ventricular hypertrophy. In the elderly, AF is common.

The restricted opening of the mitral valve can be seen in the 2-D echocardiogram and the mitral orifice can be planimetered. The diastolic area of the open mitral valve can be accurately measured using magnetic resonance imaging (MRI) (17). The increased diastolic velocity across the mitral valve is measured by Doppler echocardiography and the diastolic gradient is calculated by the formula (18):

$$\text{Gradient} = 4V^2$$

The severity of the MS can be calculated from the diastolic half-time (19) and the mitral orifice area from the continuity equation (20):

$$\text{Mitral valve area} = \text{LV outflow tract area} \times \text{Velocity/Velocity across mitral valve}$$

or by the proximal isovelocity surface area (PISA) method (21)

$$\text{Mitral area} = \text{Flow } (2\pi r^2)/\text{Velocity across mitral valve}$$

where r is determined from the Nyquist limit.

There are several echocardiographic scores (22,23), which by looking at the thickness and mobility of the leaflets, the degree of leaflet and commissural calcification, and subvalvular chordal fusion, can reliably identify those patients who will benefit from balloon or surgical valvotomy and those who should have valve replacement. Other imaging techniques such as MRI and computed angiographic tomography (CAT) scanning can demonstrate the pathophysiologic abnormalities in MS but generally do not contribute significantly to the more common laboratory studies and therefore are not generally indicated.

Mitral Regurgitation
Symptoms
Acute Mitral Regurgitation
With sudden development of severe MR, there is no time for compensatory eccentric hypertrophy or enlargement of the left atrium, so the patient frequently develops severe shortness of breath, orthopnea, PND, early pulmonary edema, and even right heart failure. Since the left atrium is not dilated, it is unusual for the patient to be in AF (24).

Chronic Mitral Regurgitation
The patient may remain asymptomatic for years. Eventually the earliest symptom may be a decrease in exercise tolerance rather than dyspnea on exertion since with left ventricular dysfunction the forward stroke volume may decrease with exercise. Later, shortness of breath, orthopnea, PND, and left heart failure occur. Finally, right heart failure is very late in the course of the disease (25).

The elderly patient may deny symptoms thinking that decreased exercise tolerance is due to aging and shortness of breath is due to pulmonary disease. In addition, with a gradual decrease in the patient's ability to exercise, symptoms may be avoided by decreasing the level of activity so that the patient may have very severe MR and still deny symptoms.

Signs
Acute Mitral Regurgitation
With acute MR the PMI may not be displaced but is hyperactive, especially compared with the radial pulse, and may be rapid rising and abbreviated. If the regurgitant orifice is very large, pressure in the left atrium and left ventricle may approach equality, in which case the murmur may be short or even absent. These patients are usually extremely dyspneic or in pulmonary edema (24). With posterior leaflet prolapse, the regurgitant jet may be directed anteriorly and superiorly so that the murmur may be heard well at the base as well as at the apex. With anterior leaflet prolapse, the jet is directed posteriorly and is well heard in the back.

The murmur of acute MR may be confused with that of aortic stenosis but with a premature ventricular contraction, the postextrasystolic beat results in a murmur that does not get louder, unlike that of the postextrasystolic beat in aortic stenosis.

Chronic Mitral Regurgitation
With chronic MR, the left ventricle is dilated and the PMI is displaced laterally and sustained. With the PMI and carotid pulse felt simultaneously, instead of the PMI collapsing before the carotid pulse, with LVH the PMI collapses after the carotid pulse. The pansystolic murmur of MR, best heard at the apex, is flat throughout systole.

Since the regurgitation continues throughout all of left ventricular systole, there are no isovolumic contraction or relaxation phases and the murmur classically buries the first and second heart sounds (25). In patients where the regurgitant orifice does not form until the ventricle is ejecting, such as in mitral valve prolapse, nonejection click or clicks may be present as the leaflet prolapses and is suddenly stopped in its motion. Since the regurgitant orifice continues to enlarge as the ventricle empties, the murmur starts after the click, crescendos in loudness, and incorporates the second sound (13). With the marked increase in diastolic blood flow across the mitral valve, there may be a short diastolic rumble and an S_3 sound. AF is common in the elderly patient with significant MR.

Other signs and symptoms may be related to the etiology of the MR. For instance, with MR secondary to a dilated left ventricle, the findings of cardiomyopathy may be present with an S_3 and S_4 gallop. Fever and immunoembolic signs may be present in patients with infective endocarditis, physical signs of connective tissue diseases such as Marfan disease, or a history of trauma, angina, or acute myocardial infarction.

Laboratory Findings and Diagnosis
Chest X-Ray
Since there is no time for atrial or ventricular remodeling, in acute MR the heart may not be enlarged on the chest X-ray. Pulmonary congestion and edema are commonly seen. With chronic severe MR, the left atrium and ventricle are dilated and appear enlarged on the chest X-ray. With chronic MR, occasionally the left atrium can become extremely dilated so that it touches the right lateral chest wall compressing the right lower lung.

Electrocardiogram
With acute MR, the ECG may be normal, except for sinus tachycardia, or have only non-specific ST–T-wave changes. With chronic MR, LVH, left atrial abnormality, and AF are common.

Echocardiography
The regurgitant volume and size of the regurgitant orifice can be estimated by Doppler echocardiography. The effect of the MR on the size and function of the cardiac chambers can also be evaluated. With acute severe MR, there is frequently pulmonary hypertension that can be estimated by identifying a tricuspid regurgitant jet, which allows estimation of the pulmonary artery systolic pressure (26). The direction of the MR regurgitant jet as well as multiple views on transesophageal echocardiogram (TEE) can reliably show which scallops of the mitral leaflets are prolapsing and define the anatomical and functional mechanism causing the MR; and it is necessary for planning the surgical procedure (27).

The severity of MR is more difficult to quantitate than the severity of MS. By Doppler echocardiography, the regurgitant jet by color-flow mapping is composed of a roughly hemispherical area of flow convergence resulting from serial aliasing (PISA), the regurgitant orifice and the fully developed regurgitant jet. Multiple measurements have been used to quantitate the magnitude of MR. The jet area in proportion to the left atrial area, the width of the jet at the regurgitant oriface, the calculated regurgitant volume, the intensity of the continuous-wave MR signal, the mitral inflow/pulmonary vein Doppler signs have all been used. Using PISA, it is possible to calculate the regurgitant volume and the effective oriface area. This measurement should be the best estimate of regurgitant severity, although the accuracy of the flow rate depends on many variables such as the shape of the PISA, the oriface geometry, aliasing velocity and others (28). All methods of measuring the severity of MR have limitations and should be used with other signs and measurements of regurgitant severity such as LV chamber size and pulmonary venous flow patterns (29).

Thomas and colleagues (30) developed an MR index using six echo-Doppler findings, three related to the regurgitant volume and three to the effect on the cardiac chambers. The index correlated well with regurgitant fraction and other measures of MR severity and identified patients with severe MR with a 90% sensitivity, a 88% specificity, and a 79% positive predictive value.

As in the case of MS, the imaging techniques of MRI and CAT scanning can demonstrate similar pathophysiologic abnormalities, but are generally not used clinically.

NATURAL HISTORY OF MITRAL STENOSIS AND MR IN THE ELDERLY
Mitral Stenosis
A patient over the age of 65 years with MS who has not already had a commissurotomy will have had mild MS for many years, or may have progressed to moderate MS. Others

have progressed to severe MS by valvular fibrosis and calcification. Many have had MS diagnosed at an early age and, if symptomatic, had a valvotomy or valve replacement.

Once MS becomes symptomatic, the course usually is to become progressively more symptomatic, going through the pulmonary congestive phase, then the right heart failure phase, and finally the low-cardiac-output stage leading to death (8). Since valvotomy or valve replacement has been available for over half a century, it is unusual to see an elderly person with severe MS who has not had at least one attempt at valvotomy. Mainly in newly arrived patients in the USA do we see the elderly with previously unrecognized severe MS.

Mitral Regurgitation

The natural history of patients with MR depends on the acuteness of onset, severity, and etiology of MR. The presence of echocardiographic MR early after acute myocardial infarction is predictive of decreased survival (31,32). The prevalence of MR increases with age, diabetes, hypertension, and previous revascularization. However, mild or moderate MR may not be an independent prognostic predictor (30). In patients who have decreased ventricular function or heart failure after an acute myocardial infarction, increased MR at baseline was associated with larger LVEDV and left ventricular end-systolic volume, increased sphericity index, and reduced EF. Moderate to severe MR is an independent predictor of total mortality, cardiovascular mortality, and hospitalization for heart failure on follow-up. If the severity of the MR progresses during the first post-myocardial infarction month, patients are likely to die or develop heart failure (33). With MR caused by ischemia or myocardial infarction, the prognosis is poor unless there is minimal myocardial damage and the ischemic muscle can be revascularized and the valve made competent (34). In patients with MR at the time of revascularization, there is conflicting evidence that repair of the mitral valve alters long-term functional status or survival (35). In addition, there is good evidence that after coronary bypass surgery, the preoperative MR will decrease. In one study (36), 66% of 131 patients preoperatively had mild, 31% had moderate, and 3% had severe ischemic MR. On follow-up after coronary bypass surgery, 52% had no or mild, 27% had moderate and 6% had severe MR. With endocarditis the cause of the MR, the course depends on the infecting organism and the complications seen with infective endocarditis. If trauma is the etiology, the damage to the heart and other organs determines the course.

Acute Mitral Regurgitation

How large the regurgitant volume is when the acute MR occurs will determine the symptomatic state of the patient. In the elderly patient, the stiffer left ventricle results in a higher filling pressure for a given volume overload. With a single chord rupture, there may be minimal to moderate regurgitation and the patient may not exhibit the clinical picture of acute MR. With the rupture of several primary chords or of the papillary muscle tip, the patient exhibits the classic clinical picture of acute MR and frequently presents with pulmonary edema, culminating in early demise (24).

With the decrease in afterload, the ventricle empties in systole to a greater extent than normal and the EF increases. With myocardial dysfunction, the left ventricular end-diastolic and end-systolic volumes increase and the EF begins to fall, at times into the normal range (14). The decrease in EF in this case still identifies myocardial dysfunction that has a negative effect on prognosis even after surgical correction of the MR (37). Although in one study a relatively high incidence of sudden death has been reported in patients with acute MR due to flail leaflets (38), it has not been confirmed because in that study coronary artery disease could not be ruled out as the etiology (39).

After a period of time, remodeling of the left atrium and left ventricle allows the filling pressure to fall and the effective forward stroke volume to be maintained. The patient may become less symptomatic and the clinical picture may become that of chronic MR.

Chronic Mitral Regurgitation

Patients with chronic MR can remain asymptomatic for many years with good exercise tolerance (40). At some point, the volume load on the left ventricle combined with increasing afterload due to the ventricle becoming more spherical and increasing its radius results in myocardial dysfunction. The course becomes that of increasing symptoms and death, usually from congestive heart failure (25).

TREATMENT OF MITRAL STENOSIS AND MITRAL REGURGITATION IN THE ELDERLY

Mitral Stenosis

Balloon Valvotomy for Mitral Stenosis

In elderly patients with mild-to-moderate MS who have good or acceptable exercise tolerance consistent with their age and not interfering with their life, controlling volume overload, the ventricular rate if in AF, and anticoagulation with warfarin because of the high risk of systemic embolization is the best approach. If the patient develops symptoms that do not respond to gentle diuresis and rate control with β blockers or calcium channel blockers, valvotomy should be considered. If the valve is flexible, with minimal calcification, no left atrial thrombus, and no more than mild (grade 2 or less) MR, the patient is a candidate for valvotomy (41,42). Commissural calcification has an adverse effect on the results of balloon valvotomy with smaller increases in mitral valve area as calcification increases and a smaller reduction in functional class after balloon mitral valvotomy (43). In evaluating 848 consecutive patients with MS in normal sinus rhythm by both TTE and TEE, the prevalence of atrial thrombus was 6.6%. TEE is warranted when the individual is over the age of 44 years, the left atrial inferior-superior diameter is >6.9 cm or the mean diastolic gradient is >18 mmHg. When spontaneous echo contrast is absent on TEE, thrombus is unlikely (44). At the present time with experienced operators, balloon valvotomy is the treatment of choice rather than open commissurotomy (42,45). With balloon valvotomy, the success rate of increasing the valve area to 1.5 cm^2 or greater, effectively doubling the valve area, is high—about 90%, even in valves with a high echo score (46). Pre-existing MR is a risk factor predicting poor outcome (46,47). The presence of commissural calcium is related to the development of MR after balloon valvotomy, and with calcification of the valve there is less chance that the valve can be opened to greater than or equal to 1.5 cm^2 and less improvement in symptoms.

Iung and colleagues (48) reported results of balloon valvotomy in 1514 patients, 45 ± 15 years of age. Twenty-five percent had calcified valves. A good result, defined as opening the mitral valve to 1.5 cm^2 or more without creating 2+ or greater MR, was obtained in 1348 (89%) patients. Important predictors of a good result were younger age, echo score less than or equal to 8, and relatively large predilation valve area. Palacios and colleagues (45) reported 327 patients with balloon valvotomy. There were seven in-hospital deaths. The follow-up period was 26 ± 12 months. The echo score, which evaluates the anatomical suitability for valvotomy using the Wilkins scoring system (22), was determined. Patients with an echo score greater than eight compared with those less than or equal to eight were older (64 ± 11 years vs. 48 ± 14 years) had more AF (65% vs. 40%), more valve calcification (81% vs. 29%) and more previous surgical commissurotomy (30% vs. 16%). Event-free survival was 79 ± 10% for those with echo score less than 8 versus 39 ± 18% with echo score greater than or equal to 8.

Fawzy reported the results of mitral valvuloplasty in 547 consecutive patients, mean age 31.5 years, followed for 1.5–19 years after valvotomy. Valve area increased from 0.92 cm^2 to 1.95 cm^2. Restenosis occurred in 169 (31%) patients; it was less common in those with echocardiographic scores of ≤8. Event-free survival at 10, 15, and 19 years was 89%, 60%, and 28%, respectively. Multivariate analysis identified an echocardiographic score of ≤8 and post procedure valve area ≤1.8 cm^2 as predictors of restenosis. The long-term outcome can be predicted from the baseline characteristics of the mitral valve (49).

There is limited experience with valvotomy in patients over ages 60–70. Remadi and colleagues (50) reported the immediate and late outcomes of balloon mitral valvotomy in 745 patients, 45 of whom were aged 60 years or older. They compared the immediate and late outcomes with those below 60 years. The baseline hemodynamic parameters were comparable in the two groups as was the degree of mitral valve opening and favorable hemodynamic response. Complication rates, including the development of grade I and II MR, were also similar. After a mean of 43 months of follow-up, a good result was maintained in 60% of patients, even though some degree of restenosis occurred in 40% of the older patients, compared to 25% of the younger patients. Le Feuvre and colleagues (51) reported 234 patients who had a balloon valvotomy, only 28 (10%) aged 70 years or older. Compared to younger patients, the 70 years and older patients had a higher percentage of New York Heart Association (NYHA) class III and IV (84% vs. 67%), and higher echo scores (9.3 ± 2.1 vs. 8.0 ± 1.6), meaning they were less suitable for valvotomy. They also had more AF (61% vs. 36%), more complications (27% vs. 9%), and a higher 30-day mortality (12% vs. 0.8%). The success rate in opening the valve was similar in both groups.

Long-term survival without cardiac events (death, cerebrovascular accidents, another intervention) depends on the patient's age as well as comorbidity. In general, the older the patient and the more the comorbidity, the shorter the survival.

Meneveau and colleagues (52) reported 532 patients after balloon valvotomy (Table 16.2). The event-free survival was age dependent. The anatomical form of the mitral valve was the second important factor in event-free survival. Given the fact that a calcified valve is unfavorable for valvotomy, in those very symptomatic patients with calcified valves believed to be too great a risk for surgery, balloon valvotomy can be palliative, achieving a moderate increase in valve area at low procedural risk and with improvement of symptoms in the majority of patients (53). Patients with echo scores that make them unsuitable for balloon valvotomy and rejected for surgery because of frailty or comorbidity can benefit from balloon valvotomy. Sutaria and colleagues (54) reported 80 patients over 70 years of age. Fifty-five were considered unsuitable for surgery. There was a 95% success rate in opening the valve. One year later, 28 of the 55 unsuitable patients (51%) had

Table 16.2   Long-Term Follow-Up of 532 Patients with Balloon Valvotomy

Event-free survival	**3 yr**	**5 yr**	**7.5 yr**
Entire group	84%	74%	52%
Age ≤65	80%	70%	45%
Age >65	52%	38%	17%
The anatomic form of the mitral valve was the second important factor in event-free survival			
	3 yr	**5 yr**	**7.5 yr**
Favorable anatomy (echo score of 1)	92%	84%	70%
Intermediate anatomy	86%	73%	34%

Source: From Ref. 52.

improved at least one NYHA class and 14 (25%) at 5 years. Of the 25 with suitable valves, 16 (64%) had achieved this outcome at 1 year and 9 (36%) at 5 years. Shaw and colleagues (55) reported similar results in 20 patients 70 years of age and older. The absence of commissural calcification is a significant predictor of the frequency of achieving a mitral valve opening of 1.5 cm^2 without creating severe MR. Sutaria and colleagues (56) reported that calcification of one or more commissures predicts a less than 50% chance of achieving a valve area of greater than or equal to 1.5 cm^2. Its influence is greatest in valves with an echo score of less than or equal to 8. Those with commissural calcification grade of 0/1 had a significantly larger number of patients with improvement in symptoms and achieving a valve area of 1.5 cm^2 (67%) than those with a grade of 3/4 (46%) (56). If the echo score is greater than 8, the degree of commissural calcification is less important.

Complications of balloon valvotomy reported in the literature are a mortality of 0.5–1%, development of MR requiring surgery of 1.3–3%, and cerebrovascular accident 0.5–1%. These complications compare favorably with those reported after surgical commissurotomy. Restenosis after balloon valvotomy ranges from 4% to 70% depending on patient selection, morphology of the valve and length of follow-up (57).

In patients age 80 and older, there is limited experience of balloon valvotomy. Sutaria and colleagues (58) reported 20 octogenarians (age range 80–89) with balloon valvuloplasty, all functional classes II–IV, and 14 among them were unfit for surgery. The mitral valve area was increased by 106% from 0.81 ± 0.3 cm^2 to 1.67 ± 0.8 cm^2. Eight patients attained a valve area of greater than or equal to 1.5 cm^2 and 16 an area greater than or equal to 1.2 cm^2. Eighty percent improved at least one NYHA functional class.

Since many elderly patients with MS have had a previous surgical commissurotomy, the question arises whether balloon valvotomy could be successful if restenosis occurs. Iung and colleagues (59) reported the results of balloon valvotomy in 232 patients, mean age 47 ± 14 years, who had undergone a surgical commissurotomy 16 ± 8 years before. Eighty-one of these patients had valve calcification and bilateral commissural fusion. One patient died (0.4%), MR > 2/4 developed in 4% and 82% achieved an immediate valve area of greater than or equal to 1.5 cm^2 without significant MR. Predictors of a poor result were age ($p < 0.001$), smaller initial valve area ($p = 0.01$), and use of a double-balloon technique ($p = 0.015$), indicating that results in the elderly would not be as good. In the 175 patients with follow-up, 8-year survival without operation and in NYHA class I and II was 48 ± 5% and in those with good immediate results, 58 ± 6%.

Aslanabadi and colleagues (60) reported 47 post-balloon valvotomy restenosis patients with unfavorable valve characteristics assigned either to repeat balloon valvotomy (25) or to mitral valve replacement (22). The mean follow-up was 41 months for the repeat valvotomy patients and 63 months for the mitral valve replacement patients. The 10 year survival was higher in the re-balloon patients than in the surgical patients, 96% versus 73%, respectively ($p < 0.05$), but the event-free survival was similar (52% vs. 50%) due to a high re-intervention rate in the re-balloon group (48% vs. 18%) ($p = 0.02$). Others have had similar results with re-balloon valvotomy in patients with restenosis and found that independent predictors of event-free survival were an echo score of <7 and absence of prior surgical commissurotomy (61).

The question of whether balloon valvotomy in the patient with MS or in the patient in normal sinus rhythm will prevent the later development of AF addresses the argument that early commissurotomy is necessary to avoid his complication. Eid Fawzy and colleagues (62) reported a retrospective analysis of 382 consecutive patients with severe MS in sinus rhythm who had successful balloon valvotomy and were followed for a mean of 5.6 years. Thirty-four (8.9%) patients developed AF compared with 348 (91.1%) who remained in sinus rhythm at follow-up. They compared these results with a reported series in the literature of patients with MS where AF occurred in 29% of patients with similar baseline characteristics who did not have an intervention. The baseline characteristics that were predictive of the late postvalvotomy development of AF were older age, larger left atrium, and a smaller mitral valve area at follow-up.

These findings differ from an earlier report by Krasuski and colleagues (63) of a prospective cohort of patients with MS and no history of atrial arrhythmias, who showed no decrease in AF after successful versus unsuccessful balloon valvotomy. Advanced age and left atrial dimension were the best predictors of AF at follow-up, whereas procedural success at balloon valvotomy and left trial pressure reduction did not have an impact on the incidence of late AF.

Surgical Management of Mitral Valve Disease

The surgical management of mitral valve disease in the 65–75 age groups is not much different than in younger patients, except that older patients have more comorbidity, which increases the mortality and morbidity of surgery. Over the age of 75 years, there is a marked increase in surgical mortality and morbidity related to limited cardiac, renal, and pulmonary reserves. Since prolongation of life is not as likely in this age group, other therapeutic goals must justify surgery, such as improvement in quality of life (QOL) and return to independent lifestyle (64). Surgery in an unacceptably symptomatic patient should not be denied on the basis of age alone, and a patient who is symptomatically doing well should not be subjected to surgery with its higher mortality and morbidity.

Mitral Stenosis

Open commissurotomy should be considered when the valve is flexible enough to open when the commissures are released, there is minimal MR, but the subvalvular apparatus is obstructive, when there is thrombus in the left atrium, especially in the body of the left atrium, that remains after 2–3 months of anticoagulation, which would make balloon valvotomy hazardous (41). At surgery, the subvalvular structures can be separated, the commissures opened, and the valve preserved. If not, the valve can be replaced.

Cotrufo and colleagues (65) reported 540 consecutive MS patients, 340 with mitral commissurotomy and 240 with a bileaflet valve replacement. The majority of patients were less than 65 years of age at the time of surgery. Hospital mortality was 2% in each group (Table 16.3). With a 15-year follow-up, late mortality was lower in the open commissurotomy group (1%) than in the valve replacement group (3%). With the exception of a greater incidence of reoperation, long-term results were better in the open commissurotomy group. This observation is consistent with many other studies that found that mitral valve repair is preferable to replacement (66).

With balloon valvotomy available for most patients with MS, the incidence of open commissurotomy has decreased. With the operative technique of preserving the papillary muscle-chordal apparatus in mitral valve replacement, the long-term outcome has

Table 16.3   Mitral Commissurotomy Vs. Mitral Valve Replacement

	Commissurotomy	**Valve Replacement**
10-yr survival rate	98.7 ± 1%	93.7 ± 3%
Freedom from reop	88.1 ± 2%	97.7 ± 1%
Freedom from emboli	93.7 ± 2%	83.9 ± 7%
Freedom from hemorrhage	99.3 ± 0.5%	98.4 ± 1%

Source: From Ref. 65.

approached that of valve commissurotomy. Ismeno and colleagues (67) report 313 patients with isolated MS who received either balloon valvulotomy, open commissur-otomy, or valve replacement. (Table 16.4). There was no difference in operative mortality or 7-year actuarial survival. Freedom from reoperation was significantly better in those with mitral valve replacement and the mean functional class at the end of the follow-up period was lowest in those with open commissurotomy. At present, conservative techniques are the best, especially in the elderly. With the latest operative techniques, the late outcome after mitral valve replacement has markedly improved. Similar results have been reported in other studies (68).

Mitral Regurgitation

With the present techniques, most patients with MR (except those with extensive loss of flexible leaflet tissue) can have the valve repaired successfully, but the selection of patients and the expertise of the surgeon are critical factors for success (66,69,70) MR due to rheumatic heart disease is characterized by fibrosis and retraction of the leaflet edges as well as chordal shortening and fusion (71). Repair is least successful in this group and selection of the proper patients for repair is essential (71,72). Most MR in the elderly is caused by myxomatous redundant leaflets, and these are ideal candidates for valve repair (69). With ischemic MR or a dilated left ventricle and left ventricular OS, annuloplasty, with or without an annular ring, is frequently sufficient to create a competent valve (72–74). However, restricted leaflet motion can make the repair less predictable.

Contraindications for repair are loss of leaflet area, extreme leaflet thickening, or calcification of leaflets or commissures (71). Some surgeons have suggested that calcification of the annulus or leaflets does not preclude successful valve repair (75). Grossi and colleagues (76) reported the results of mitral valve repair in 558 patients. Debridement of calcification in annulus and/or leaflets was necessary in 64 (11.5%) patients. Freedom from reoperation at 10 years was 88.1% for debrided patients and 82.6% for those not needing debridement. When good annulus and leaflet mobility can be achieved in calcified valves, calcium debridement allows durable valve repair.

Patients with a small mitral annulus or multiple leaflet defects have a small probability of being successfully repaired. Patients with small left ventricular cavities, most often seen in elderly women, have a high incidence of postoperative systolic anterior motion and left ventricular outflow tract obstruction (66). Patients with mitral valve prolapse involving the posterior leaflet have the most success with repair. However, although less successful than repair with mural leaflet prolapse, there have been reports of successful repair of anterior leaflet prolapse (77,78). For the best results, patient needs a careful evaluation by TEE and an experienced surgeon.

Table 16.4 Outcome of MS Intervention

	BV	OC	VR
Number	111	82	120
7-yr survival (%)	95.4	95.1	92.8 (p = NS)
Freedom from emboli (%)	95.8	98.8	92.5 (p > 0.05)
Freedom from reop (%)	84.4	96.4	97.7 (p > 0.05)
NYHA class at follow-up	1.39	1.14	1.41 (p = 0.001)

Abbreviations: BV, balloon valvulotomy; OC, open commissurotomy; VR, valve replacement; NS, not significant.
Source: From Ref. 67.

Because the expected lifespan after surgery is shorter for the elderly patient at the time of surgery, there is an advantage of bioprosthetic valves over mechanical valves in older patients since anticoagulation is not necessary in the absence of AF. The frequency of AF in elderly patients with moderate-to-severe chronic MR lessens the advantage because these patients require anticoagulants to prevent systemic emboli (41). There is evidence that valve degeneration occurs much more slowly in the elderly than in younger patients. In one study, the rate of primary structural deterioration in patients over the age of 65 years was 0.95% per patient–year (79). For this reason, in patients over 65 years of age, the prevailing opinion is that the preferred valve is a bioprosthetic one.

Chikwe and colleagues (80) reported 322 consecutive octogenarian patients with MR, mean age 82.6 years, 70% undergoing mitral valve repair and 30% replacement. A propensity-adjusted analysis showed that elective mitral valve repair can be performed with low operative mortality and good long-term outcomes in patients with degenerative MR. In octagenarians with mitral valve prolapse, repair is associated with better survival than with replacement, although this is more questionable in patients with non-degenerative MR.

Dalrymple-Hay and colleagues (81) reported 329 patients with MR due to myxomatous degeneration, mean age of 65.5 years with valve repair in 169 and valve replacement in 160 patients. Operative mortality occurred in four (1.2%), all in those with valve replacement. Actuarial survival at 1, 5, and 10 years was $94 \pm 1.4\%$, $77 \pm 2.9\%$, and $41 \pm 5.8\%$, respectively, with survival in patients with repair significantly better ($p < 0.05$) than with valve replacement. Reoperation was required in 10 (6%) of those with valve repair and in 13 (8%) of those with valve replacement. Increased age, worse left ventricular function, the type of operation (repair vs. replacement), and left ventricular size all were significantly associated with poorer survival.

Gogbashian and colleagues (82) reported a 10-year experience of mitral valve repair versus replacement in 292 patients aged 70 years and over for MR due to mitral valve prolapse, including patients with concomitant revascularization. Comparing repair to replacement, in-hospital mortality was higher (0.7% vs. 13.9%), length of hospital stay longer (8.7 vs. 9.6 days), and with greater 5-year survival (81% vs. 63%). The 10-year freedom from valve reoperation in the patients with repair was 93.9% and for repair plus coronary bypass surgery 98.2%. They concluded that the preferred option for elderly patients was mitral valve repair.

A report by Daneshmand and colleagues (83) from Duke University of 2064 patients with mitral valve surgery with and without coronary bypass surgery, followed for a median of 5 years, maximal follow-up was 20 years. Mitral valve repair had a better survival across all ages than mitral valve replacement. If replacement was required, mechanical valves achieved better outcomes than tissue valves, even in the elderly. The recommendation from this study was that in patients needing valve replacement, tissue valves should be reserved for those where anticoagulation is contraindicated.

Lee and colleagues (84) reported 614 patients with valve surgery for severe MR 190, aged 70 and older and 424 under age 70. In the older patients, there was significantly more myxomatous disease, coronary disease, worse left ventricular function, and worse NYHA class III–IV symptoms. Operative mortality in both young and old patients was low (3.5% vs. 3.7%). In the older patients, 7-year survival was lower than in the young ($49 \pm 6\%$ vs. $72 \pm 3\%$) as were overt heart failure ($74 \pm 3\%$ vs. $44 \pm 7\%$) and complication-related deaths ($78 \pm 3\%$ vs. $57 \pm 7\%$). However, both young and old patients who were NYHA class I with an EF greater than 40% had the same freedom from complication-related death ($93 \pm 3\%$ in the younger vs. $90 \pm 7\%$ in the elderly). These findings support the approach to early surgery once symptoms occur and before the EF begins to fall, especially if valve repair is possible.

There is good evidence that valve repair or replacement for MR improves the QOL (64). Goldsmith and colleagues (85), in a prospective study of 61 consecutive patients with severe MR, mean age 64 ± 12 years, who had mitral valve repair (40) or replacement (21) obtained QOL scores using the short form 36-questionnaire before and 3 months after surgery. There was significant improvement in seven out of eight QOL parameters in those with repair and in three out of eight in those with valve replacement. Patients with EF greater than or equal to 50% improved in seven out of eight parameters. Those with impaired function or end-systolic dimensions of greater than or equal to 45 mm showed no improvement in any of the parameters. These findings support the importance of early surgery before a decline in left ventricular function.

Grossi and colleagues (86) studied 278 patients with mitral valve repair aged 70 and older (mean age 75.2 years). Concomitant procedures were done in 72.3%, with over half having coronary revascularization. Mortality was lower in those with isolated mitral valve repair than in those with concomitant revascularization (6.5% vs. 17%). With an additional valve procedure, the mortality was 13.2%. Long-term survival was excellent with freedom from cardiac death in 100% of those with isolated mitral valve repair, lower in those with a concomitant procedure (79.7%; $p = 0.006$), and freedom from reoperation in 91.2% patients.

Surgery for MR in octogenarians is usually reserved for patients who are very symptomatic despite optimal medical management. There is evidence of improvement in the results of surgery for MR in these elderly patients. DeTaint and colleagues (87) reported the results of surgery for MR performed from 1980 to 1995 in patients greater than or equal to 75 years of age (group 1), 65–75 (group 2), and less than 65 (group 3). Preoperatively, group 1 patients had a higher prevalence of Functional Class III–IV symptoms, more AF and coronary disease, increased creatinine, and higher comorbidity index. The temporal trend of operative mortality showed a decrease in each age group from 27% to 5% in group 1, 21% to 4% in group 2, and 7% to 2% in group 3. Over time, the feasibility of valve repair also increased, in all groups from 30% to 54%, and in those with degernerative MR (mitral valve prolapse) from 31% to 93%. Multivariate analysis of relative survival showed no difference in restoration of life expectancy compared with younger patients (Table 16.5).

There are several reports of valve surgery in patients over the age of 75 years including reports in octagenarians that conclude that surgery can be performed with acceptable mortality and good long-term outcomes including good QOL. All stress the importance of risk evaluation, avoidance of non-elective surgery whenever possible, and early surgery before moderate-to-severe symptoms develop (3,88,89).

Present guidelines (41) recommend that surgery may be postponed safely in asymptomatic patients with severe MR, even if repair is possible, until the patient develops symptoms or AF, evidence of left ventricular dysfunction with EF falling below 60%, or LVESD increases to 45 mm, or pulmonary hypertension becomes greater than 50 mmHg at rest or greater than 60 mmHg with exercise. Rosenheek and colleagues (40) reported 132 such

Table 16.5 Long-Term Survival After Surgery For MR

	Gr 1	Gr 2	Gr 3
Number	284	504	556
5-yr survival	$57 \pm 3\%$	$73 \pm 2\%$	$85 \pm 2\%$ ($p < 0.001$)
Rate of observed/expected survival (for age)	83%	85%	88% ($p = $ NS)

Abbreviations: MR, mitral regurgitation; NS, not significant.
Source: From Ref. 87.

patients, 55 ± 15 years of age with severe MR due to mitral valve prolapse or flail leaflet. They underwent serial clinical and echocardiographic monitoring and were followed prospectively for 62 ± 26 months. They were referred for surgery for the above criteria. Only 30% of patients needed surgery by 5 years and fewer than half by 8 years. Symptoms were the commonest indication for surgery. There was no operative mortality and the postoperative outcome was good with regards to survival, symptomatic status and late left ventricular function.

The question of the timing of surgery in asymptomatic or mildly symptomatic patients with degenerative MR is addressed in the ACC/AHA guidelines (41) with the recommendation that surgery be done with the onset of symptoms or in asymptomatic patients, with EF < 60%, or left ventricular systolic diameter > 40 mm. Supporting these recommendations are the studies of Suri and colleagues (90) who report 204 patients with mitral valve prolapse and less than severe MR followed for a mean of 8.6 years. Over half the patients developed left ventricular dysfunction or worsening MR. Despite optimal medical management, left ventricular dysfunction can develop in the absence of MR progression. Gillinov and colleagues (91) reviewed 4586 patients with surgery for degenerative mitral valve disease with repair in 93%. Thirty percent of the patients were asymptomatic and even the development of mild symptoms by the time of surgery was associated with deleterious changes in cardiac structure and function. Finally, in a cohort of 481 patients with severe degenerative mitral valve disease and one ACC/AHA indication for surgery, 168 patients were grouped into those with early surgery (<2 months from the development of the surgical indication), 94 who had late surgery (>2 months), and 219 who were managed medically. Follow-up time was 5.6 years. Those selected for early surgery had a hazard ratio of 0.54 compared to those with late surgery (92). These studies support the guidelines for early referral for surgery in patients with severe MR and the development of symptoms, enlarged left ventricular dimensions, or decreased EF, providing that repair is possible and the surgical mortality is low (≤1%). Optimal timing of surgery in asymptomatic patients with MR is crucial to avoid excess morbidity and mortality. In asymptomatic patients with severe MR, both elevation of brain-type natriuretic peptide (BNP) on serial measurements and pulmonary hypertension have been shown by multivariate analysis to independently predict early deterioration of left ventricular function or the onset of symptoms (93). The presence of pulmonary hypertension in the resting patient and the development of systolic pulmonary artery pressure ≥56 mm Hg on exercise has been shown to be a good predictor of symptom development in asymptomatic patients with degenerative MR (94).

Valve replacement is performed in more elderly patients for aortic valve than for mitral valve disease, most often calcific aortic stenosis, and operative mortality is lower than with mitral valve replacement (95). Helft and colleagues (79) reported 110 patients, 65 and older (mean 73.4 years), with bioprosthetic valve replacement, 71 with aortic, 32 with mitral, and 7 with both. Follow-up was 8.5 years. At 5 years the actuarial survival was 79.6% and at 10 years 62.4%. Of the 44 patients who died, over half (52.3%) died from non-valve-related causes. Reoperation was needed in 13 patients (11.8%), 10 for structural deterioration, with one death (7.7%). Anticoagulation for AF was needed in 26%, with 6.4% developing severe bleeding (2.9% per patient–year). Similar results have been reported in octogenarians (96,97). In examining the reasons for a higher mortality in octogenarians with MR surgery compared to aortic valve surgery, it is probable that the higher mortality is related more to the patients' preoperative clinical state and comorbidities than to the type of surgery (96).

Ischemic MR results from ventricular remodeling related to the position and extent of the ischemic or infarcted left ventricular myocardium (98). With MR due to ischemia, operative and late mortality is higher than with MR due to myxomatous degeneration (30).

Table 16.6 Surgery for Ischemic MR

			Op Mort With EF		Actuarial Survival Rate		
Type of operation	*n*	Op mort	10–30%	>30%	2 yr	5 yr	7 yr
Valve repair	140	12.1%	33.3%	8.4%	75.4%	66.8%	61.7%
Valve replace	197	14.2%	30.3%	11.0%	78.6%	73.4%	67.2%
When MR reduced to grade 0–1 patient survival best					81.0%	78.4%	77.2%

Abbreviations: Op mort, Operative mortality; EF, ejection fraction.
Source: From Ref. 34.

Operative mortality is also higher when the EF is 30% or lower. Hausmann and colleagues (34) reported 337 patients with ischemic MR and mitral valve repair or replacement (Table 16.6). The goal of surgery in patients with ischemic MR is to reduce the MR to no more than grade 1. Schurr and colleagues (99) compared 196 patients with coronary bypass surgery alone with 102 patients with bypass surgery and mitral valve repair or replacement. Perioperative mortality was double in the patients with bypass surgery and mitral valve surgery (10.8% vs. 5.1%) ($p < 0.05$). In patients with moderate to severe MR, postoperative echocardiography showed improvement in MR in 95% in those with bypass and mitral valve surgery and in 64% of only bypass surgery patients. With lesser degrees of MR, improvement rates were similar (74% vs. 69%, respectively). Significant predictors of postoperative mortality were renal insufficiency, older age and NYHA Class III–IV.

A frequent problem with ischemia and 1 to 3+ MR is whether to simply revascularize the patient or also make the mitral valve more competent, usually with an annuloplasty. Kang and colleagues (100) reported an observational study of 185 consecutive patients, age 63 ± 9 years, with significant ischemic MR. Sixty-six had percutaneous angioplasty (PCI) and 119 coronary bypass surgery. Of those with surgical revascariztion, 68 had concomitant mitral annuloplasty. In a median of 54 months of follow-up, survival and crdiac mortality rates were similar between the two groups. For the 45 propensity score-matched pairs, the risk of cardiac events was significantly lower in the operative group[hazard ratio 0.499 (95% CI 0.251–0.990, $p = 0.043$). Compared to those with bypass surgery alone, patients with concomitant annuloplasty had a significantly higher event-free survival rate. Grossi and colleagues (101) in evaluating the impact of moderate MR in patients undergoing isolated coronary surgery followed 2242 consecutive patients with no to moderate MR. They found that independent of ventricular function, that mild to moderate MR is associated with significantly decreased survival.

Tolis and colleagues (102) had 49 patients, mean age 66.3 years with advanced ischemic heart disease, 1 to 3+ MR (62% had 2 to 3+ MR), and an EF of 10–30% (mean 22.4%). In-hospital mortality was 2% and the mean degree of MR went from 1.73 down to 0.54 ($p < 0.05$). The NYHA class decreased from 3.3 to 1.8 ($p < 0.05$) and the EF rose from 22% to 31.5% ($p < 0.05$). The 1-, 3-, and 5-year survivals were 88%, 65%, and 50%, respectively. They concluded that in such patients revascularization was sufficient and that improvement in MR and EF occur from improved left ventricular function and size after revascularization.

Aklog and colleagues (73) reported 136 patients, mean age 70.5 years with ischemic heart disease and more severe 3+ MR with a mean EF of 38.1% who had isolated coronary bypass surgery. Operative mortality was 2.9%. They found the intraoperative TEE underestimated the degree of MR and the postoperative TTE revealed that 40% of the patients still had 3+ MR, 51% improved to 2+ MR, and only 9% had 0 to 1+ MR. They concluded that ischemic MR required more than just revascularization, usually concomitant annuloplasty. Campwala and colleagues (103) reported the fate of MR following surgical revascularization in 523 patients, 92 of whom had 3 to 4+ MR on preoperative echocardio-gram. Post surgery, residual 3 to 4+ MR was present in 43 (47%) patients and was associ-ated with a trend to increased mortality ($p = 0.3$) over a mean follow-up of 3.9 years. Other studies have reported benefit in terms of symptoms and improved survival in patients with severe left ventricular dysfunction and MR, not only due to coronary artery disease but also in patients with cardiomyopathy and chronic valvular regurgitation (104,105).

AF is common in patients with mitral valve disease, both MS and MR. At the time of surgery, consideration should be given to performing a Cox–Maze procedure with particu-lar attention to isolating the entrance of the pulmonary veins. Saint and colleagues (106) reported 101 patients with the Cox–Maze IV procedure for lone AF and 99 concomitantly with mitral valve operations. Operative mortality was similar in both groups and at 1-year freedom from AF and antiarrhythmic drugs was also similar in both groups (76% vs. 77%). In patients with mitral valve replacement and AF, the addition of the Maze procedure was associated with a reduction in thromboembolic events and better long-term event-free sur-vival in patients with AF undergoing mechanical mitral valve replacement (107). Other studies including radiofrequency ablation for AF in conjunction with mitral valve surgery was equally effective in restoring normal sinus rhythm (108,109).

Finally, there are constant innovations in cardiac surgery that should make surgery easier on the patient and possibly safer for elderly patients with multiple comorbidities. These include minimally invasive surgery compared to standard thoracotomy (110,111), and robotic surgery (112,113). Catheter interventions have also shown promise in rela-tively non-invasively repaired MR. Whitlow and colleagues reported the acute and 1-year results of the Endovascular Valve Edge-to-Edge Repair (EVEREST II) study where the mitral valve is converted into a double orifice by clipping the edges of the two leaflets together using a percutaneous catheter (MitraClip device). Seventy-eight patients, mean age 77 years old, with 3-to-4+ MR who were high risk for surgery had the procedure. At 1 year the patients had improvement in clinical symptoms and significant left ventricular reverse remodeling (114). Another innovative technique for performing a mitral annulo-plasty by transcatheter implantation of a coronary sinus device has been developed. The 1-year results in 59 patients with MR grade ≥2 has been reported with a reduction in MR by ≥1 grade. However, there was coronary compression in 15 patients where the great car-diac vein passes over a coronary artery, so strategies for avoiding this occurrence must be developed before this becomes a useful technique (115).

MITRAL ANNULAR CALCIFICATION

MAC is a chronic degenerative process that is common in elderly persons, especially women. The amount of calcium may vary from a few spicules to a large mass behind the posterior cusp, often extending to form a ridge or ring encircling the mitral leaflets, occa-sionally lifting the leaflets toward the left atrium and protruding into the left ventricular cavity below the mural leaflet of the mitral valve. Sphincter function loss of the mitral annulus and mechanical stretching of the mitral leaflets can cause improper coaptation of the leaflets during systole, resulting in MR (78). Although the calcific mass may immobilize the mitral valve, actual calcification of the leaflets is rare. In persons with severe MAC, the calcification may extend inward to involve the underside of the leaflets. MS may result from severe calcific deposits within the mitral annulus protruding into the orifice (1), but the obstruction is rarely severe (116). Calcific deposits may extend from the mitral annulus into the membranous portions of the ventricular septum, involving the conduction system and causing rhythm and conduction disturbances (117). Although the annular calcium is cov-ered with a layer of endothelium, ulceration of this lining can expose the underlying calcific deposits, which may serve as a nidus for platelet-fibrin aggregation and subsequent thromboembolic episodes (118). Rodriguez and colleagues (119) reported a substudy of the Cardiovascular Health Study involving 2680 subjects without a history of stroke or transient ischemic attacks who had an MRI head scan. The mean age was 74.5 years. They found an increased prevalence of covert brain infarcts in those with MAC, aortic annular or valve calcification or aortic valve sclerosis. After adjusted analysis for known risk factors, the risk ratio was 1.24 and the severity of valvular calcification was directly related to the covert brain MRI findings. In patients with endocarditis associated with MAC, the avascular nature of the mitral annulus predisposes to periannular and myocardial abscesses (120,121).

Prevalence

MAC is a degenerative process that increases with age and occurs more frequently in women than in men (122). In an unselected multi-ethnic population of 6814 men and women ages 45–84-years old, MAC was present by CT in 9%, highest in Caucasians (12%) and lowest in Chinese (5%) (123). In a prospective study of 1797 unselected elderly persons in a long-term health-care facility, mean age 81 ± 8 years (range 60–103 years), with technically adequate M-mode and two-dimensional echocardiograms of the mitral valve, MAC was present in 665 of 1243 women (53%) and in 194 of 554 men (35%) (124). Table 16.7 shows the prevalence of MAC with increasing age in elderly men and elderly women (125).

Predisposing Factors

Because calcific deposits in the mitral annulus, in the aortic valve cusps, and in the epicardial coronary arteries are commonly associated in elderly persons and have similar predisposing factors, Roberts (126) suggested that MAC and aortic cuspal calcium are a form of atherosclerosis. MAC and aortic cuspal calcium may coexist (117,122,126,127). Breakdown of lipid deposits on the ventricular surface of the posterior mitral leaflet at or below the mitral annulus and on the aortic surfaces of the aortic valve cusps is probably responsible for the calcification (117). Increased left ventricular systolic pressure due to aortic valve stenosis increases stress on the mitral apparatus and may accelerate development of MAC (117,128). Tricuspid annular calcium and MAC may also coexist and have similar predisposing factors (129). MAC has been suggested as a time-averaged marker of atherosclerosis and is associated with coronary artery disease, stroke, and increased mortality (119,130,131). Consistent with this is the association of coronary risk factors including age, hypertension, diabetes and smoking (123,132). In a 27-year follow-up, the Framingham Offspring study demonstrated that exposure to multiple atherosclerotic risk factors in early to mid adulthood is associated with aortic and mitral valve calcification (132).

Table 16.7   Prevalence of MAC with Increasing Age in Elderly Men and Elderly Women

| Age (yr) | MAC | | | |
| | Men | | Women | |
	n	%	*n*	%
62–70	4/22	18	7/35	20
71–80	13/42	31	40/116	34
81–90	44/75	59	146/226	65
91–100	19/22	86	56/63	89
101–103	—	—	3/3	100

Abbreviation: MAC, Mitral Annular Calcium.
Source: Adapted from Ref. 125.

Systemic hypertension increases with age and predisposes to MAC (117,120,122,124). Persons with diabetes mellitus also have a higher prevalence of MAC than nondiabetic persons (117,133). MAC occurs in the teens with serum total cholesterol levels greater than 500 mg/dL (134). Waller and Roberts (135) suggested that hypercholesterolemia predisposes to MAC. The prevalence of hypercholesterolemia with serum total cholesterol greater than 200 mg/dL was higher in elderly persons with MAC than in elderly persons without MAC (133). Yetkin and colleagues (136) reported 484 consecutive patients, mean age 60 ± 10 years, undergoing coronary arteriography for suspected coronary artery disease. Twenty percent of them had MAC. There were no statistically significant differences between those with and without MAC with respect to body mass index, diabetes mellitus, hypercholesterolemia, or the presence of coronary artery disease.

Roberts and Waller (137) found that chronic hypercalcemia predisposes to MAC. Patients undergoing dialysis for chronic renal insufficiency have an increased prevalence of MAC (137,138). MAC has also been found to be a marker of left ventricular dilatation and decreased left ventricular systolic function in patients with end-stage renal disease on peritoneal dialysis (139). Fox and colleagues (140) studying 3047 participants in the Framingham study of patients with chronic kidney disease, defined by a glomerular filtration rate less than 60 ml/min/1.73 m², found that the odds of having MAC was increased by 60% in those with chronic kidney disease. Nair and colleagues (141) demonstrated a similar mean serum calcium, a higher mean serum phosphorus, and a higher mean product of serum calcium and phosphorus in patients younger than 60 years with MAC than in a control group. However, Aronow and colleagues (133) observed no significant difference in mean serum calcium, serum phosphorus, or product of serum calcium and phosphorus between elderly persons with and without MAC. By accelerating the rate of rise of left ventricular systolic pressure, hypertrophic cardiomyopathy predisposes to MAC (117). Kronzon and Glassman (142) diagnosed MAC in 12 of 18 patients (67%) older than 55 years with hypertrophic cardiomyopathy and in 4 of 28 patients (14%) younger than 55 years with hypertrophic cardiomyopathy. Motamed and Roberts (143) demonstrated MAC in 30 of 100 autopsy patients (30%) with hypertrophic cardiomyopathy older than 40 years and in none of 100 autopsy patients (0%) younger than 40 years with hypertrophic cardiomyopathy. Aronow and Kronzon (144) diagnosed MAC in 13 of 17 older persons (76%) with hypertrophic cardiomyopathy and in 176 of 362 older persons (49%) without hypertrophic cardiomyopathy.

Elderly men and women with MAC have a higher prevalence of coronary artery disease (145,146), of peripheral arterial disease (146,147), of extracranial carotic arterial disease (ECAD) (146,148) and of aortic atherosclerotic disease (146) than elderly men and women without MAC. MAC has also been shown to be associated with thoracic aorta calcium in patients with systemic hypertension (149).

Diagnosis

Calcific deposits in the mitral annulus are J-, C-, U-, or O-shaped and are visualized in the posterior third of the heart shadow (150,151). MAC may be diagnosed by chest X-ray films or by fluoroscopy (151) and by computed tomography (132,152). However, the procedures of choice for diagnosing MAC are M-mode and two-dimensional echocardiography.

Posterior MAC (Fig. 16.1) is diagnosed by M-mode echocardiography when a band of dense echoes is recorded anterior to the left ventricular posterior wall and moving parallel with it (153). These echoes end at the atrioventricular junction and merge with the left ventricular posterior wall on echocardiographic sweep from the aortic root to the left ventricular apex.

Anterior MAC (Fig. 16.1) is diagnosed by M-mode echocardiography when a continuous band of dense echoes is observed at the level of the anterior mitral leaflet in both systole and diastole (153). These echoes are contiguous with the posterior wall of the aortic root. Calcification may extend from the mitral annulus throughout the base of the heart and into the mitral and aortic valves.

Figures 16.2 and 16.3 are two-dimensional echocardiograms showing increased echogenicity and brightness of the mitral annulus characteristic of MAC. Using multiple

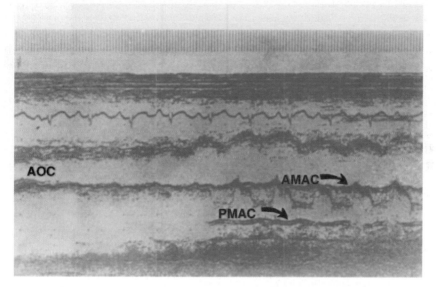

Figure 16.1 M-mode echocardiogram with scan from the aortic root to the left ventricular apex in a patient with both anterior and posterior mitral annular calcium. *Abbreviations*: AOC, aortic calcium; AMAC, anterior mitral annular calcium; PMAC, posterior mitral annular calcium.

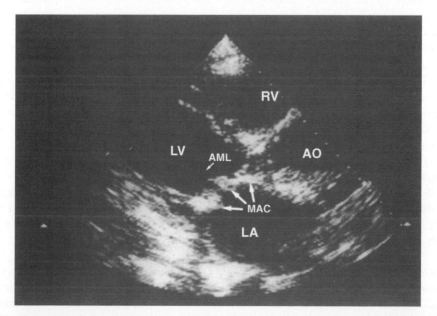

Figure 16.2 Two-dimensional echocardiogram long-axis view depicting MAC. *Abbreviations*: LA, left atrium; LV, left ventricle; RV, right ventricle; AO, aorta; AML, anterior mitral leaflet; MAC, mitral annular calcium.

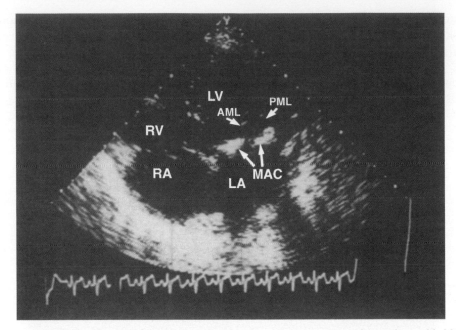

Figure 16.3 Two-dimensional echocardiogram four-chamber view of a patient with MAC. *Abbreviations*: LA, left atrium; RA, right atrium; RV, right ventricle; LV, left ventricle; AML, anterior mitral leaflet; PML, posterior mitral leaflet; MAC, mitral annular calcium.

echocardographic views, MAC may be classified as mild, moderate, or severe (154). The echo densities in mild MAC involve less than one-third of the annular circumference (<3 mm in width) and are usually restricted to the angle between the posterior leaflet of the mitral valve and the left ventricular posterior wall. The echo densities in moderate MAC involve less than two-thirds of the annular circumference (3–5 mm in width). The echo densities in severe MAC involve more than two-thirds of the annular circumference (>5 mm in width), usually extending beneath the entire posterior mitral leaflet with or without making a complete circle.

In a blinded prospective study, MAC was diagnosed by M-mode and two-dimensional echocardiography in 55% of 604 unselected elderly patients in a long-term healthcare facility (151). The diagnosis of MAC by chest X-ray films using a lateral chest X-ray in addition to the posterior-anterior or anterior posterior chest X-ray had a sensitivity of 12%, a specificity of 99%, a positive predictive value of 95%, and a negative predictive value of 47%. Patients with radiographic MAC were more likely than patients without radiographic MAC to have a more severe form of the disease, with significant MR, functional MS, or conduction defects. However, patients with echocardiographically severe MAC and significant MR, functional MS, or conduction defects may have no evidence of MAC on chest X-ray films. Figure 16.4 shows C-shaped calcification of the mitral annulus. Figure 16.5 illustrates J-shaped calcification of the mitral annulus.

Chamber Size
Patients with MAC have a higher prevalence of left atrial enlargement (117,122,124,125,138,154) and left ventricular enlargement (122,138,154) than patients without MAC. In a prospective study of 976 elderly patients (526 with MAC and 450 without MAC), left atrial enlargement was 2.4 times more prevalent in patients with MAC than in the group without MAC (120).

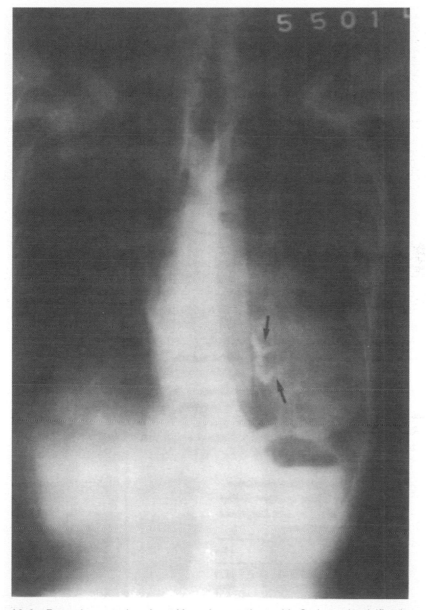

Figure 16.4   Posterior-anterior chest X-ray in a patient with C-shaped calcification of the mitral annulus (arrows).

Atrial Fibrillation

Patients with MAC also have a higher prevalence of AF than patients without MAC (120,122,125,154,155) Table 16.8 shows that the prevalence of AF was increased 12, 5, and 2.8 times in patients with MAC than in patients without MAC (122,138,155).

Conduction Defects

Because of the close proximity of the mitral annulus to the atrioventricular node and the bundle of His, patients with MAC have a higher prevalence of conduction defects, such as sinoatrial disease, atrioventricular block, bundle branch block, left anterior fascicular

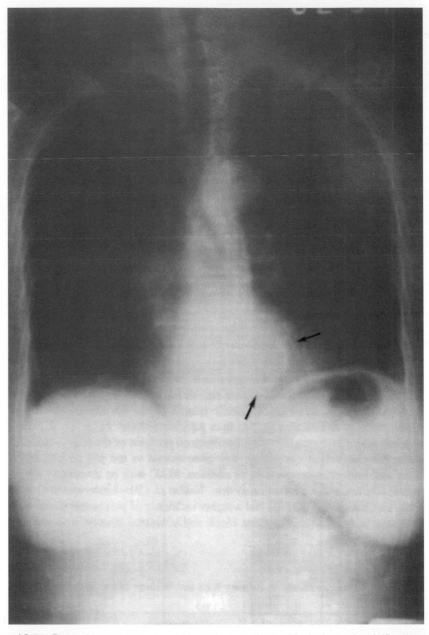

Figure 16.5 Posterior-anterior chest X-ray in a patient with J-shaped calcification of the mitral annulus (arrow).

block, and intraventricular conduction defect, than patients without MAC (118,128,154) The calcific deposits may also extend into the membranous portions of the interventricular septum involving the conduction system, or may even extend to the left atrium, interrupting interatrial and intra-atrial conduction. In addition, MAC may be associated with a sclerodegenerative process in the conduction system. Nair et al. (154) showed in their prospective study that patients with MAC had a higher incidence of permanent pacemaker implantation because of both atrioventricular block and sinoatrial disease than patients without MAC.

Mitral Regurgitation

MAC is thought to generate systolic murmurs by the sphincter action loss of the annulus and the mechanical stretching of the mitral leaflets causing MR and from vibration of the calcified ring or vortex formation around the annulus. Table 16.9 shows that the prevalence of apical systolic murmurs of MR in patients with MAC ranged from 12% to 100% in different studies (122,138,156–159). Table 16.10 states the prevalence of MR diagnosed by Doppler echocardiography in patients with MAC (155,159–161). The prevalence of MR associated with MAC ranged from 54% to 97% in the Doppler echocardiographic studies (159–161). Figure 16.6 illustrates severe MR due to MAC diagnosed by color Doppler echocardiography.

Table 16.8 Prevalence of Atrial Fibrillation in Patients With and Without MAC

	Atrial Fibrillation				
	MAC		No MAC		
	n	%	*n*	%	Relative Risk
Framingham study (122)	20/162	12	53/5532	1	12
Patients younger than 61 yr (138)	11/107	10	2/107	2	5
Patients older than 60 yr (mean age 81 + 8 yr) (155)	225/1028	22	85/1120	8	2.8

Abbreviation: MAC, mitral annular calcium.

Table 16.9 Prevalence of Apical Systolic Murmurs of MR in Patients with MAC

	Prevalence of MR Murmur	
	n	%
Korn et al. (156)	14/14	100
Schott et al. (157)	10/14	71[a]
Savage et al. (122)	26/132	12
Nair et al. (138)	17/104	16
Aronow et al. (158)	129/293	44
Aronow et al. (159)	43/100	43

[a]MAC due to noninflammatory calcific disease.
Abbreviations: MR, mitral regurgitation; MAC, mitral annular calcium.

Table 16.10 Prevalence of MR Diagnosed by Doppler Echocardiography in Patients with MAC

	MR		Moderate-to-Severe MR	
	n	%	*N*	%
Labovitz et al. (161)	28/51	55	17/51	33
Aronow et al. (159)	54/100	54	18/100	18
Kaul et al. (160)	28/29	97[a]	—	
Aronow et al. (155)	—	—	24/1028	22

[a]Severe MR in 2 of 29 patients (7%).
Abbreviations: MR, mitral regurgitation; MAC, mitral annular calcium.

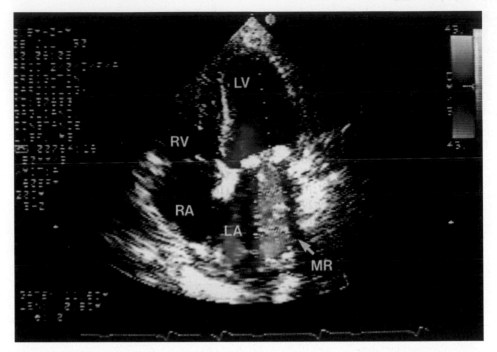

Figure 16.6   Color Doppler echocardiographic findings in a patient with mitral annular calcium and severe MR. *Abbreviations*: LA, left atrium; RA, right atrium; RV, right ventricle; LV, left ventricle; MR, mitral regurgitation.

The greater the severity of MAC, the greater is the severity of MR associated with MAC. Moderate-to-severe MR was diagnosed by Doppler echocardiography in 33% of 51 patients with MAC by Labovitz and colleagues (161) and in 22% of 1028 patients with MAC by Aronow and colleagues (155). Kaul and colleagues (160) diagnosed severe MR in 7% of their 29 patients with MAC, and concluded that MR in patients with MAC is caused by a reduced sphincteric action of the mitral annulus, with MAC preventing the posterior annulus from contracting and assuming a flatter shape during systole.

Mitral Stenosis
An apical diastolic murmur may be heard in patients with MAC as a result of turbulent flow across the calcified and narrowed annulus (annular stenosis). Table 16.11 shows that the prevalence of apical diastolic murmurs of MS in patients with MAC ranged from 0% to 25% in different studies (122,154–159,161). Table 16.11 also indicates that MS associated with MAC was diagnosed by Doppler echocardiography in 8% of 51 patients by Labovitz and colleagues (161), in 6% of 100 patients by Aronow and Kronzon (159), and in 8% of 1028 patients by Aronow et al. (155). Figure 16.7 illustrates MS due to MAC diagnosed by Doppler echocardiography.

The reduction of mitral valve orifice in patients with MAC is due to the annular calcium and to decreased mitral excursion and mobility secondary to calcium at the base of the leaflets (159). The commissures are fused in rheumatic MS but are not fused in MS associated with MAC. The mitral leaflet margins in MAC may be thin and mobile, and the posterior mitral leaflet may move normally during diastole. However, Doppler echocardiographic recordings show increased transvalvular flow velocity and prolonged pressure halftime and, therefore, smaller mitral valve orifice in patients with MS, regardless of the etiology. Pressman and colleagues (2) followed 32 patients with severe MAC (>5 mm) with

Table 16.11   Prevalence of Apical Diastolic Murmurs of MS and of MS in Patients with MAC

	Prevalence of MS Murmur		Prevalence of MS by Doppler Echocardiography	
	n	%	*n*	%
Korn et al. (156)	3/14	21	—	—
Schott et al. (157)	2/14	14[a]	—	—
Savage et al. (122)	2/132	2	—	—
Nair et al. (154)	7/104	7	—	—
Aronow et al. (158)	28/293	10	—	—
Labovitz et al. (161)	0/51	0	4/51	8
Aronow et al. (159)	6/100	6	6/100	6
Aronow et al. (155)	—	—	83/1028	8

[a]MAC due to noninflammatory calcific disease.
Abbreviations: MS, mitral stenosis; MAC, mitral annular calcium.

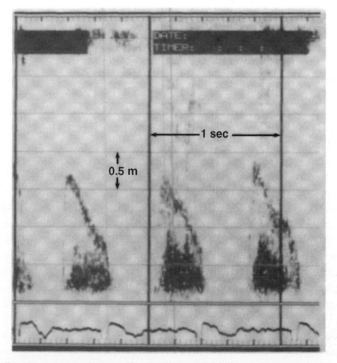

Figure 16.7   Continuous-wave Doppler tracing across a stenotic mitral valve orifice due to mitral annular calcium. Peak diastolic gradient = 12 mmHg. Pressure halftime = 200 ms. Mitral valve area = 1.1 cm².

echocardiography for 2.6 ± 1.6 years and found that increase in the diastolic gradient occurred in 50% with several subjects progressing at 9 mmHg/year.

Bacterial Endocarditis

Bacterial endocarditis, with a high incidence of *Staphylococcus aureus* endocarditis, may complicate MAC (120,129). Patients with MAC associated with chronic renal failure are especially at increased risk for developing bacterial endocarditis (157). The calcific mass erodes the endothelium under the mitral valve that is exposed to transient bacteremia. The avascular nature of the mitral annulus interferes with antibiotics reaching a nidus of bacteria, predisposing to periannular and myocardial abscesses and, consequently, to a poor prognosis (162). Therefore, Burnside and DeSanctis (162) recommended prophylactic antibiotics to prevent bacterial endocarditis in patients with MAC. Nair and colleagues (154) observed at 4.4-year mean follow-up with no significant difference in incidence of bacterial endocarditis in 99 patients younger than 61 years with MAC compared to a control group of 101 patients. However, Aronow and colleagues (120) demonstrated at 39-month mean follow-up a 3% incidence of bacterial endocarditis in 526 elderly patients with MAC and a 1% incidence of bacterial endocarditis in 450 elderly patients without MAC. Until 2007, prophylactic antibiotics were recommended to prevent bacterial endocarditis in patients with MAC, according to American Heart Association guidelines (163). At that time, after reevaluating the evidence in the literature, the consensus was that the vast majority of cases of infective endocarditis were the result of bacteremias which occur extremely frequently as a result of daily activities such as vigorous chewing, brushing the teeth, and flossing and not from dental manipulations. Therefore, the present American Hear Association's recommendation is that antibiotic prophylaxis should be reserved for high-risk patients such as those with prosthetic valves, cyanotic and other high-risk congenital heart disease, patients with a previous episode of infective endocarditis, and cardiac transplant patients with valvulopathy (164). Despite the American Heart Association recommendations, many physicians still prescribe antibiotic prophylaxis for their patients with valvular disease.

Cardiac Events

The presence of MAC, a marker of atherosclerosis, is associated with an increase in cardiovascular events, including myocardial infarction, stroke and death. Utsunomiya and colleagues (131) in 322 patients referred for 64-multidetector computed tomography showed that the combination of aortic valve calcification and MAC were highly associated with the presence, extent and vulnerability characteristics of coronary artery plaques. Gondrie and colleagues (127), using a case-cohort design evaluated 10,410 subjects undergoing chest CT, excluding patients referred for cardiovascular disease. The mean follow-up was 17 months and there were 515 cardioivascular events in 1285 subjects. Patients with MAC compared to those without valve calcification had a risk ratio of 1.53 (95% CI 1.13–2.00). Potpara and colleagues (130) in the Belgrade Atrial Fibrillation Study followed for a mean of 9.9 years, 1056 patients with AF, 33 (3.1%) of whom had MAC. The age of the population was 52.7 ± 12.2 years. In multivariate analysis MAC was independently related to all-cause death, cardiovascular death, and new cardiac morbidity (hazard ratio of 4.3, 3.5, and 2.4, respectively).

In a prospective study of 107 patients (eight lost to follow-up) younger than 61 years with MAC and 107 (six lost to follow-up) age- and sex-matched control subjects, Nair and colleagues (154) demonstrated at 4.4-year mean follow-up that patients with MAC had a higher incidence of new cardiac events than control subjects (Table 16.12). In a prospective study of 526 elderly patients with MAC and 450 elderly patients without MAC, Aronow and colleagues (120) found at 39-month mean follow-up that the incidence of new cardiac events (myocardial infarction, primary ventricular fibrillation, or sudden cardiac death) was also higher in elderly patients with MAC than in elderly patients without MAC.

Table 16.12   Incidence of New Cardiac Events in Patients With and Without MAC

| | | Cardiac Events | | | | |
| | | MAC | | No MAC | | |
	Follow-Up	n	%	n	%	Relative risk
Nair et al. (154)	4.4 yr	31/99	31	2/101	2	15.5
Total cardiac death		12/99	12	1/101	1	12.0
Sudden cardiac death		41/99	41	6/101	6	6.8
Congestive heart failure Mitral or aortic valve replacement		9/99	9	0/101	0	—
Aronow et al. (120) cardiac events[a] if:	39 mo					
Atrial fibrillation		62/90	69	22/41	54	1.3
Sinus rhythm		157/436	36	106/409	26	1.4
All patients		219/526	42	128/450	28	1.5

[a]Myocardial infarction, primary ventricular fibrillation, or sudden cardiac death.
Abbreviation: MAC, mitral annular calcium.

Mitral Valve Replacement

Nair and colleagues (165) reported that mitral valve replacement could be accomplished in patients with MAC with morbidity and mortality similar to that in patients without MAC. Following mitral valve replacement, subsequent morbidity and mortality during 4.4-year mean follow-up were also similar in patients with and without MAC.

Cerebrovascular Events

Although the increased prevalence of AF, MS, MR, left atrial enlargement and congestive heart failure predisposes patients with MAC to thromboembolic stroke, some investigators consider MAC a marker of other vascular disease causing stroke rather the primary embolic source (166). Others believe that MAC with ulcerated endothelium and platelet agglutination is responsible for clinically silent brain infarcts. Rodriguez and colleagues (119) reported cerebral MRIs in 2680 Cardiovascular Health Study subjects without a clinical history of strokes or transient ischemic attacks. The mean age of the population was 7.5 ± 4.8 years. The presence of any left sided valvular or annular calcification was associated with covert brain infarcts with a risk ratio compared to those with no calcification of 1.24 (95% CI 1.05–1.47) and the severity of calcification was directly related to the presence of MRI findings. In a retrospective study of 110 elderly patients with chronic AF, 44 (40%) had documented thromboembolic stroke (167). In this study, the prevalence of MAC was not significantly different in elderly patients with thromboembolic stroke (80%) or without thromboembolic stroke (65%) (relative risk = 1.2). However, six prospective studies have demonstrated an increased incidence of new cerebrovascular events in patients with MAC than in patients without MAC (Tables 16.13–16.15) (120,154,155,168–170) ranging from a relative risk of 1.5 up to 5.0.

Aronow and colleagues studied the incidence of new thromboembolic stroke at 44-month mean follow-up in 310 unselected elderly patients with chronic AF in a long-term health-care facility (155) (Table 16.14). MS and the severity of MR were diagnosed by Doppler echocardiography in this study (155). In elderly persons with chronic AF, MAC increased the incidence of new thromboembolic stroke 2.1 times if MS was associated with MAC, 1.7 times if 2–4+ MR was associated with MAC, and 1.4 times if 0–1+ MR was present. Table 16.15 shows the incidence of new thromboembolic stroke at 44-month mean follow-up in 1838 unselected older persons, mean age 81 years, with sinus rhythm, in a

Table 16.13   Incidence of New Cerebrovascular Events in Patients With and Without MAC

| | | Cerebrovascular Events | | | | |
| | | MAC | | No MAC | | |
	Follow-Up	n	%	n	%	Relative Risk
Nair et al. (154)	4.4 yr	10/99	10	2/101	2	5.0
TE cardiovascular events						
Benjamin et al. (167)	8 yr	22/160	14	51/999	5	2.7
stroke						
Aronow et al. (120)	39 mo					
TE stroke if:						
Atrial fibrillation		45/90	50	14/41	34	1.5
Sinus rhythm		59/436	14	38/409	9	1.6
All patients		104/526	20	52/450	12	1.7
Boston Area Anticoagulation	2.2 yr	10/129	8	5/291	2	4.0
Trial for Atrial Fibrillation (169)						
ischemia stroke						
Aronow et al. (170)	45 mo					
TE stroke if:						
40–100% ECD		52/101	51	16/49	33	1.5
0–39% ECD		88/365	24	47/413	11	2.2
TIA if:						
40–100% ECD		8/101	8	3/49	6	1.3
0–39% ECD		11/365	3	3/413	1	3.0

Abbreviations: MAC, mitral annular calcium; TE, thromboembolic; ECD, extracranial carotid arterial disease; TIA, cerebral transient ischemic attack.

Table 16.14   Incidence of New Thromboembolic Stroke at 44-Month Mean Follow-Up in Elderly Patients with Chronic Atrial Fibrillation

	Thromboembolic Stroke (%)
Atrial fibrillation, no MAC (n = 85)	35
Atrial fibrillation with MS due to MAC (n = 42)	74
Atrial fibrillation with MAC and 2–4+ MR (n = 90)	59
Atrial fibrillation with MAC and 0–1+ MR (n = 93)	48

Abbreviation: MAC, mitral annular calcium.
Source: From Ref. 155.

long-term health-care facility (155). In elderly persons with sinus rhythm, MAC increased the incidence of new thromboembolic stroke 3.6 times if MS was associated with MAC, 3.1 times if 2–4+ MR was associated with MAC, and 2.7 times if 0–1+ MR was present. Using the multivariate Cox regression model, independent risk factors for new thromboembolic stroke in this study were prior stroke (risk ratio = 2.4), MAC (risk ratio = 2.6), AF (risk ratio = 3.0), and male gender (risk ratio = 1.6).

There was a higher prevalence of MAC in elderly patients with 40–100% ECAD (67% of 150 patients) than in elderly patients with 0–39% ECAD (47% of 778 patients) (170). The increased prevalence of significant ECAD contributes to a higher stroke rate. Thrombi of the mitral annulus also contribute to thromboembolic stroke in elderly patients

Table 16.15 Incidence of New Thromboembolic Stroke at 44-Month Mean Follow-Up in Elderly Patients with Sinus Rhythm

	Thromboembolic Stroke (%)
Sinus rhythm, no MAC ($n = 1035$)	9
Sinus rhythm with MS due to MAC ($n = 41$)	32
Sinus rhythm with MAC and 2–4+ MR ($n = 134$)	28
Sinus rhythm with MAC and 0–1+ MR ($n = 625$)	24

Abbreviations: MR, mitral regurgitation; MAC, mitral annular calcium.
Source: From Ref. 155.

with MAC (171). In addition, MAC is associated with aortic atheromatous disease (146), complex intra-aortic debris (172), and thoracic aorta calcium (149)that could contribute to thromboembolic stroke. Some patients with MAC who experienced thromboembolic events also had a mobile component that was associated with the thromboembolic events (173). There was no significant difference in the association of MAC with prior stroke between elderly whites and elderly African-Americans, between elderly whites and elderly Hispanics, and between elderly African-Americans and elderly Hispanics (174).

Kizer and colleagues (175) from the Strong Heart Study, followed 2723 American-Indians without clinical cardiovascular disease and with baseline echocardiograms for 7 years. Eighty-six strokes occurred. The presence of MAC but not aortic valve sclerosis was a strong risk factor for incident stroke after extensive adjustment for other predictors. Since patients with MAC and AF or sinus rhythm have a higher incidence of thromboembolic stroke than patients without MAC, antithrombotic therapy should be considered in patients with MAC and no contraindications to antithrombotic therapy. In the Boston Area Anticoagulation Trial for Atrial Fibrillation study, warfarin reduced the incidence of thrombembolic stroke in patients with MAC by about 90% (176,177).

Until data from prospective, randomized studies evaluating the efficacy and risk of antithrombotic therapy in patients with MAC are available, patients with MAC associated with either AF, MS, or moderate-to-severe MR should be considered for treatment with warfarin if they have no contraindications to anticoagulant therapy. The international normalised ratio should be maintained between 2.0 and 3.0. The efficacy of antiplatelet therapy in patients with MAC is unknown.

REFERENCES

1. Muddassir SM, Pressman GS. Mitral annular calcification as a cause of mitral valve gradients. Int J Cardiol 2007; 123: 58–62.
2. Pressman GS, Agarwal A, Braitman LE, et al. Mitral annular calcium causing mitral stenosis. Am J Cardiol 2010; 105: 389–91.
3. Speziale G, Nasso G, Barattoni MC, et al. Short-term and long-term results of cardiac surgery in elderly and very elderly patients. J Thorac Cardiovasc Surg 2011; 141: 725–31.
4. Cheitlin MD. Management of valve disease in the elderly. Am J Geriatr Cardiol 1996; 5: 65–7.
5. Weill A, Païta M, Tuppin P, et al. Benfluorex and valvular heart disease: a cohort study of a million people with diabetes mellitus. Pharmacoepidemiol Drug Saf 2010; 19: 1256–62.
6. Rothman RB, Baumann MH, Savage JE, et al. Evidence for possible involvement of 5-HT(2B) receptors in the cardiac valvulopathy associated with fenfluramine and other serotonergic medications. Circulation 2000; 102: 2836–41.
7. Zanettini R, Antonini A, Gatto G, et al. Valvular heart disease and the use of dopamine agonists for Parkinson's disease. N Engl J Med 2007; 356: 39–46.
8. Cheitlin MD. The timing of surgery in mitral and aortic valve disease. Curr Probl Cardiol 1987; 12: 69–149.

9. Goldsmith I, Kumar P, Carter P, et al. Atrial endocardial changes in mitral valve disease: a scanning electron microscopy study. Am Heart J 2000; 140: 777–84.

10. Chiang CW, Lo SK, Kuo CT, et al. Noninvasive predictors of systemic embolism in mitral stenosis. An echocardiographic and clinical study of 500 patients. Chest 1994; 106: 396–9.

11. Subramaniam V, Herle A, Mohammed N, et al. Ortner's syndrome: case series and literature review. Braz J Otorhinolaryngol 2011; 77: 559–62.

12. Otsuji Y, Handschumacher MD, Liel-Cohen N, et al. Mechanism of ischemic mitral regurgitation with segmental left ventricular dysfunction: three-dimensional echocardio-graphic studies in models of acute and chronic progressive regurgitation. J Am Coll Cardiol 2001; 37: 641–8.

13. Cheitlin MD, Byrd RC. Prolapsed mitral valve: the commonest valve disease? Curr Prob Cardiol 1984; 8: 1–54.

14. Carabello BA. Progress in mitral and aortic regurgitation. Prog Cardiovasc Dis 2001; 43: 457–75.

15. Swinne CJ, Shapiro EP, Lima SD, et al. Age-associated changes in left ventricular diastolic performance during isometric exercise in normal subjects. Am J Cardiol 1992; 69: 823–6.

16. Vaitkevicius PV, Fleg JL, Engel JH, et al. Effects of age and aerobic capacity on arterial stiffness in healthy adults. Circulation 1993; 88: 1456–62.

17. Lanjewar C, Ephrem B, Mishra N, et al. Planimetry of mitral valve stenosis in rheumatic heart disease by magnetic resonance imaging. J Heart Valve Dis 2010; 19: 357–63.

18. Handshoe R, DeMaria AN. Doppler assessment of intracardiac pressures. Echocardiogr Rev Cardiovasc Ultrasound 1985; 2: 127–39.

19. Fredman CS, Pearson AC, Labovitz AJ, et al. Comparison of hemodynamic pressure half-time method and Gorlin formula with Doppler and echocardiographic determinations of mitral valve area in patients with combined mitral stenosis and regurgitation. Am Heart J 1990; 119: 121–9.

20. Taylor R. Evolution of the continuity equation in the Doppler echocardiographic assessment of the severity of valvular aortic stenosis. J Am Soc Echocardiogr 1990; 3: 326–30.

21. Shiota T, Jones M, Teien DE, et al. Evaluation of mitral regurgitation using a digitally determined color Doppler flow convergence 'centerline' acceleration method. Studies in an animal model with quantified mitral regurgitation. Circulation 1994; 89: 2879–87.

22. Abascal VM, Wilkins GT, O'Shea JP, et al. Prediction of successful outcome in 130 patients undergoing percutaneous balloon mitral valvotomy. Circulation 1990; 82: 448–56.

23. Padial LR, Freitas N, Sagie A, et al. Echocardiography can predict which patients will develop severe mitral regurgitation after percutaneous mitral valvulotomy. J Am Coll Cardiol 1996; 27: 1225–31.

24. Cheitlin MD, Ardehali A. Acute valvular regurgitation. In: Chatterjee K, Parmley WW, Cheitlin MD, et al. eds. Cardiology: An Illustrated Text/Reference. Vol. 1 2nd edn. Philadelphia, PA: Lippincott, 1991: 1–13.

25. Cheitlin MD, Byrd RC. Acquired mitral valve disease. In: Greenberg BH, Murphy E, eds. Valvular Heart Disease. Littleton, MA: PSG, 1987: 92–122.

26. Tramarin R, Torbicki A, Marchandise B, et al. Doppler echocardiographic evaluation of pulmonary artery pressure in chronic obstructive pulmonary disease. A European multicentre study. Eur Heart J 1991; 12: 103–11.

27. Grewal KS, Malkowski MJ, Kramer CM, et al. Multiplane transesophageal echocardiographic identification of the involved scallop in patients with flail mitral valve leaflet: intraoperative correlation. J Am Soc Echocardiogr 1998; 11: 966–71.

28. Pai RG, Shah PM. Echocardiographic and other noninvasive measurements of cardiac hemodynamics and ventricular function. Curr Probl Cardiol 1995; 20: 681–770.

29. Grayburn PA, Bhella P. Grading severity of mitral regurgitation by echocardiography: science or art? JACC 2010; 3: 244–6.

30. Thomas L, Foster E, Hoffman JI, Schiller NB. Prospective validation of an echocardiographic index for determining the severity of chronic mitral regurgitation. Am J Cardiol 2002; 90: 607–12.

31. Zamorano J, Perez de Isla L, Oliveros L, et al. Prognostic influence of mitral regurgitation prior to a first myocardial infarction. Eur Heart J 2005; 26: 343–9.

32. Lamas GA, Mitchell GF, Flacker GC, et al. Clinical significance of mitral regurgitation after myocardial infarction. Circulation 1997; 96: 827–33.

33. Amigoni M, Meris A, Thune JJ, et al. Mitral regurgitation in myocardial infarction complicated by heart failure, left ventricular dysfunction, or both: prognostic significance and relation to ventricular size and function. Eur Heart J 2007; 28: 326–33.

34. Hausmann H, Siniawski H, Hetzer R. Mitral valve reconstruction and replacement for ischemic mitral insufficiency: seven years' follow up. J Heart Valve Dis 1999; 8: 536–42.

35. Mihaljevic T, Lam B-U, Rajeswaran J, et al. Impact of mitral valve annuloplasty combined with revascularization in patients with functional ischemic mitral regurgitation. J Am Coll Cardiol 2007; 49: 2191–201.

36. Mustonen J, Suurmunne H, Kouri J, et al. Impact of coronary artery bypass surgery on ischemic mitral regurgitation. Scand J Surg 2011; 100: 114–19.
37. Ling LH, Enriquez-Sarano M, Seward JB, et al. Clinical outcome of mitral regurgitation due to flail leaflet. N Engl J Med 1996; 335: 1417–23.
38. Grigioni F, Enriquez-Sarano M, Ling LH, et al. Sudden death in mitral regurgitation due to flail leaflet. J Am Coll Cardiol 1999; 34: 2078–85.
39. Carabello BA. Sudden death in mitral regurgitation: why was I so surprised? J Am Coll Cardiol 1999; 34: 2086–7.
40. Rosenhek R, Rader F, Klaar U, et al. Outcome of watchful waiting in asymptomatic severe mitral regurgitation. Circulation 2006; 113: 2238–44.
41. Bonow RO, Carabello B, Chatterjee K, et al. ACC/AHA 2006 guidelines for the management of patients with valvular heart disease. a report of the American College of Cardiology/American Heart Association Task Force on Practice Guidelines (writing Committee to Revise the 1998 guidelines on the management of patients with valvular heart disease): developed in collaboration with the Society of Cardiovascular Anestheiologists: endorsed by the Society for Cardiovascular Angiography and Interventions. Circulation 2006; 114: e84–e231.
42. Nobuyoshi M, Arita T, Shirai S, et al. Percutaneous balloon mitral valvuloplasty: a review. Circulation 2009; 119: e211–19.
43. Wei T, Zeng C, Chen F, et al. Influence of commissural calcification on the immediate outcomes of percutaneous balloon mitral valvuloplasty. Acta Cardiol 2003; 58: 411–H5.
44. Manjunath CN, Srinivasa KH, Panneerselvam A, et al. Incidence and predictors of left atrial thrombus in patients with rheumatic mitral stenosis and sinus rhythm: a transesophageal echocardiographic study. Echocardiography 2011; 28: 457–60.
45. Palacios IF, Tuzcu ME, Weyman AE, et al. Clinical follow-up of patients undergoing percutaneous mitral balloon valvotomy. Circulation 1995; 91: 671–6.
46. Iung B, Garbarz E, Doutrelant L, et al. Late results of percutaneous mitral commissurotomy for calcific mitral stenosis. Am J Cardiol 2000; 85: 1308–14.
47. Zhang HP, Yen GS, Allen JW, et al. Comparison of late results of balloon valvotomy in mitral stenosis with versus without mitral regurgitation. Am J Cardiol 1998; 81: 51–5.
48. Iung B, Cormier B, Ducimetiere P, et al. Immediate results of percutaneous mitral commissurotomy. A predictive model on a series of 1514 patients. Circulation 1996; 94: 2124–30.
49. Fawzy ME. Long-term results up to 19 years of mitral balloon valvuloplasty. Asian Cardiovasc Thorac Ann 2009; 17: 627–33.
50. Remadi F, Boughzala E, Neffati E, et al. Percutaneous mitral commisurotomy in patients aged 60 years and more. Ann Cardiol Angeiol 2006; 55: 149–52.
51. Le Feuvre C, Bonan R, Lachurie ML, et al. Balloon mitral commissurotomy in patients aged > or = 70 years. Am J Cardiol 1993; 71: 233–6.
52. Meneveau N, Schiele F, Seronde MF, et al. Predictors of event-free survival after percutaneous mitral commissurotomy. Heart 1998; 80: 359–64.
53. Hildick-Smith DJ, Taylor GJ, Shapiro LM. Inoue balloon mitral valvuloplasty: long-term clinical and echocardiographic follow-up of a predominantly unfavourable population. Eur Heart J 2000; 21: 1690–7.
54. Sutaria N, Elder AT, Shaw TR. Long term outcome of percutaneous mitral balloon valvotomy in patients aged 70 and over. Heart 2000; 83: 433–8.
55. Shaw TR, Elder AT, Flapan AD, et al. Mitral balloon valvuloplasty for patients aged over 70 years: an alternative to surgical treatment. Age Ageing 1991; 20: 299–303.
56. Sutaria N, Northridge DB, Shaw TR. Significance of commissural calcification on outcome of mitral balloon valvotomy. Heart 2000; 84: 398–402.
57. Fawzy ME. Percutaneous mitral balloon valvotomy. Catheter Cardiovasc Interv 2007; 69: 313–21.
58. Sutaria N, Elder AT, Shaw TR. Mitral balloon valvotomy for the treatment of mitral stenosis in octogenarians. J Am Geriatr Soc 2000; 48: 971–4.
59. Iung B, Garbarz E, Michaud P, et al. Percutaneous mitral commissurotomy for restenosis after surgical commissurotomy: late efficacy and implications for patient selection. J Am Coll Cardiol 2000; 35: 1295–302.
60. Aslanabadi N, Golmohammadi A, Sohrabi B, et al. Repeat percutaneous balloon mitral valvotomy vs. mitral valve replacement in patients with restenosis after previous balloon mitral valvotomy and unfavorable valve characteristics. Clin Cardiol 2011; 34: 401–6.
61. Chmielak Z, Klopotowski M, Kruk M, et al. Repeat percutaneous mitral balloon valvuloplasty for patients with mitral valve restenosis. Catheter Cardiovasc Interv 2010; 76: 986–92.
62. Eid Fawzy M, Shoukri M, Al Sergani H, et al. Favorable effect of balloon mitral valvuloplasty on the incidence of atrial fibrillation in patients with severe mitral stenosis. Catheter Cardiovasc Interv 2006; 68: 536–41.

63. Krasuski RA, Assar MD, Wang A, et al. Usefulness of percutaneous balloon mitral commissurotomy in preventing the development of atrial fibrillation in patients with mitral stenosis. Am J Cardiol 2004; 93: 936–9.

64. Rumsfeld JS. Valve Surgery in the elderly. A question of quality (of Life)? J Amer Coll Cardiol 2003; 42: 1215–17.

65. Cotrufo M, Renzulli A, Vitale N, et al. Long-term follow-up of open commissurotomy versus bileaflet valve replacement for rheumatic mitral stenosis. Eur J Cardiothorac Surg 1997; 12: 335–9.

66. Lawrie GM. Mitral valve repair vs. replacement. Current recommendations and long-term results. Cardiol Clin 1998; 16: 437–48.

67. Ismeno G, Renzulli A, De Feo M, et al. Surgery of rheumatic mitral stenosis: comparison of different techniques. Acta Cardiol 2001; 56: 155–61.

68. Ben Farhat M, Ayari M, Maatouk F, et al. Percutaneous balloon versus surgical closed and open mitral commissurotomy seven-year follow-up results of a randomized trial. Circulation 1998; 97: 245–50.

69. Nardi P, Pellegrino A, Scafuri A, et al. Survival and durability of mitral valve repair surgery for degenerative mitral valve disease. J Card Surg 2011; 26: 360–6.

70. Zhou YX, Leobon B, Berthoumieu P, et al. Long-term outcomes following repair or replacement in degenerative mitral valve disease. Thorac Cardiovasc Surg 2010; 58: 415–21.

71. Cheitlin MD, Sokolow M, McIlroy MB. Valvular heart disease; mitral valve disease. In: Sokolow M, McIlroy MB, eds. Clinical Cardiology, 6th edn. New York, NY: Appleton & Lange, 1997: 407–37.

72. Fedakar A, Sasmazel A, Bugra O, et al. Results of mitral valve repair in rheumatic mitral lesions. Heart Surg Forum 2010; 13: E86–90.

73. Aklog L, Filsoufi F, Flores KQ, et al. Does coronary artery bypass grafting alone correct moderate ischemic mitral regurgitation? Circulation 2001; 104: 168–75.

74. Grossi EA, Woo YJ, Patel N, et al. Outcomes of coronary artery bypass grafting and reduction annuloplasty for functional ischemic mitral regurgitation: a prospective multicenter study (Randomized Evaluation of a Surgical Treatment for Off-Pump Repair of the Mitral Valve). J Thorac Cardiovasc Surg 2011; 141: 91–7.

75. Skoularigis J, Sinovich V, Joubert G, et al. Evaluation of the long-term results of mitral valve repair in 254 young patients with rheumatic mitral regurgitation. Circulation 1994; 90: II167–74.

76. Grossi EA, Galloway AC, Steinberg BM, et al. Severe calcification does not affect long-term outcome of mitral valve repair. Ann Thorac Surg 1994; 58: 685–7.

77. El Khoury G, Noirhomme P, Verhelst R, et al. Surgical repair of the prolapsing anterior leaflet in degenerative mitral valve disease. J Heart Valve Dis 2000; 9: 75–80.

78. Galloway AC, Grossi EA, Bizekis CS, et al. Evolving techniques for mitral valve reconstruction. Ann Surg 2002; 236: 288–93.

79. Helft G, Tabone X, Georges JL, et al. Late results with bioprosthetic valves in the elderly. J Card Surg 1999; 14: 252–8.

80. Chikwe J, Goldstone AB, Passage J, et al. A propensity score-adjusted retrospective comparison of early and mid-term results of mitral valve repair versus replacement in octogenarians. Eur Heart J 2011; 32: 618–26.

81. Dalrymple-Hay MJ, Bryant M, Jones RA, et al. Degenerative mitral regurgitation: when should we operate? Ann Thorac Surg 1998; 66: 1579–84.

82. Gogbashian A, Sepic J, Soltesz EG, et al. Operative and long-term survival of elderly is significantly improved by mitral valve repair. Am Heart J 2006; 151: 1325–33.

83. Daneshmand MA, Milano CA, Rankin JS, et al. Influence of patient age on procedural selection in mitral valve surgery. Ann Thorac Surg 2010; 90: 1479–85.

84. Lee EM, Porter JN, Shapiro LM, et al. Mitral valve surgery in the elderly. J Heart Valve Dis 1997; 6: 22–31.

85. Goldsmith IR, Lip GY, Patel RL. A prospective study of changes in the quality of life of patients following mitral valve repair and replacement. Eur J Cardiothorac Surg 2001; 20: 949–55.

86. Grossi EA, Zakow PK, Sussman M, et al. Late results of mitral valve reconstruction in the elderly. Ann Thorac Surg 2000; 70: 1224–6.

87. Detaint D, Sundt TM, Nkomo VT, et al. Surgical correction of mitral regurgitation in the elderly: outcomes and recent improvements. Circulation 2006; 114: 265–72.

88. Aoyagi S, Fukunaga S, Arinaga K, et al. Heart valve surgery in octogenarians: operative and long-term results. Heart Vessels 2010; 25: 522–8.

89. Rizzoli G, Bejko J, Bottio T, et al. Valve surgery in octogenarians: does it prolong life? Eur J Cardiothorac Surg 2010; 37: 1047–55.

90. Suri RM, Aviernos JF, Dearani JA, et al. Management of less-than-severe mitral regurgitation: should guidelines recommend earlier surgical intervention? Eur J Cardiothorac Surg 2011; 40: 496–502.

91. Gillinov AM, Mihaljevic T, Blackstone EH, et al. Should patients with severe degenerative mitral regurgitation delay surgery until symptoms develop? Ann Thorac Surg 2010; 90: 481–8.

92. Samad Z, Kaul P, Shaw LK, et al. Impact of early surgery on survival of patients with severe mitral regurgitation. Heart 2011; 97: 221–4.

93. Klaar U, Gabriel H, Bergler-Klein J, et al. Prognostic value of serial B-type natriuretic peptide measurement in asymptomatic organic mitral regurgitation. Eur J Heart Fail 2011; 13: 163–9.

94. Magne J, Lancellotti P, Piérard LA. Exercise pulmonary hypertension in asymptomatic degenerative mitral regurgitation. Circulation 2010; 122: 33–41.

95. Ralph-Edwards AC, Robinson AG, Gordon RS, et al. Valve surgery in octogenarians. Can J Cardiol 1999; 15: 1113–19.

96. Bossone E, Di Benedetto G, Frigiola A, et al. Valve surgery in octogenarians: in-hospital and long-term outcomes. Can J Cardiol 2007; 23: 223–7.

97. Cheitlin MD. Significant valve disease in the octogenarian: when is intervention warranted? Am J Geriartr Cardiol 2000; 9: 33–9.

98. Fattouch K, Sampognaro R, Speziale G, et al. Impact of moderate ischemic mitral regurgitation after isolated coronary artery bypass grafting. Ann Thorac Surg 2010; 90: 1187–94.

99. Schurr P, Boeken U, Limathe J, et al. Impact of mitral valve repair in patients with mitral regurgitation undergoing coronary artery bypass grafting. Acta Cardiol 2010; 65: 441–7.

100. Kang DH, Sun BJ, Kim DH, et al. Percutaneous versus surgical revascularization in patients with ischemic mitral regurgitation. Circulation 2011; 124:S156–62.

101. Grossi EA, Crooke GA, DiGiorgi PL, et al. Impact of moderate functional mitral insufficiency in patients undergoing surgical revascularization. Circulation 2006; 114:I573–6.

102. Tolis GA Jr, Korkolis DP, Kopf GS, et al. Revascularization alone (without mitral valve repair) suffices in patients with advanced ischemic cardiomyopathy and mild-to-moderate mitral regurgitation. Ann Thorac Surg 2002; 74: 1476–80.

103. Campwala SZ, Bansal RC, Wang N, et al. Factors affecting regression of mitral regurgitation following isolated coronary artery bypass surgery. Eur J Cardiothorac Surg 2005; 28: 783–7.

104. Bishay ES, McCarthy PM, Cosgrove DM, et al. Mitral valve surgery in patients with severe left ventricular dysfunction. Eur J Cardiothorac Surg 2000; 17: 213–21.

105. De Bonis M, Lapenna E, La Canna G, et al. Mitral valve repair for functional mitral regurgitation in end-stage dilated cardiomyopathy: role of the "edge-to-edge" technique. Circulation 2005; 112: I402–8.

106. Saint LL, Bailey MS, Prasad S, et al. Cox-Maze IV results for patients with lone atrial fibrillation versus concomitant mitral disease. Ann Thorac Surg 2012; 93: 789–94.

107. Kim JB, Ju MH, Yun SC, et al. Mitral valve replacement with or without a concomitant Maze procedure in patients with atrial fibrillation. Heart 2010; 96: 1126–31.

108. Tekumit H, Uzun K, Cenal AR, et al. Midterm results of left atrial bipolar radiofrequency ablation combined with a mitral valve procedure in persistent atrial fibrillation. Cardiovasc J Afr 2010; 21: 137–41.

109. Wu M, Zhang S, Dong A, et al. Long-term outcomes of maze procedure plus valve replacement in treating rheumatic valve disease resulting in atrial fibrillation. Ann Thorac Surg 2010; 89: 1942–9.

110. Lamelas J, Sarria A, Santana O, et al. Outcomes of minimally invasive valve surgery versus median sternotomy in patients age 75 years or greater. Ann Thorac Surg 2011; 91: 79–84.

111. Holzhey DM, Shi W, Borger MA, et al. Minimally invasive versus sternotomy approach for mitral valve surgery in patients greater than 70 years old: a propensity-matched comparison. Ann Thorac Surg 2011; 91: 401–5.

112. Mihaljevic T, Jarrett CM, Gillinov AM, et al. Robotic repair of posterior mitral valve prolapse versus conventional approaches: potential realized. J Thorac Cardiovasc Surg 2011; 141: 72–80.

113. Suri RM, Burkhart HM, Daly RC, et al. Robotic mitral valve repair for all prolapse subsets using techniques identical to open valvuloplasty: establishing the benchmark against which percutaneous interventions should be judged. J Thorac Cardiovasc Surg 2011; 142: 970–9.

114. Whitlow PL, Feldman T, Pedersen WR, et al. Acute and 12-month results with catheter-based mitral valve leaflet repair: the EVEREST II (Endovascular Valve Edge-to-Edge Repair) High Risk Study. J Am Coll Cardiol 2012; 59: 130–9.

115. Harnek J, Webb JG, Kuck KH, et al. Transcatheter implantation of the MONARC coronary sinus device for mitral regurgitation: 1-year results from the EVOLUTION phase I study (Clinical Evaluation of the Edwards Lifesciences Percutaneous Mitral Annuloplasty System for the Treatment of Mitral Regurgitation). JACC Cardiovasc Interv 2011; 4: 115–22.

116. Pressman GS, Agarwal A, Braitman LE, et al. Mitral annular calcium causing mitral stenosis. Am J Cardiol 2010; 105: 389–91.

117. Roberts WC, Perloff JK. Mitral valvular disease. A clinicopathologic survey of the conditions causing the mitral valve to function normally. Ann Intern Med 1972; 77: 939–75.
118. Nair CK, Sketch MH, Desai R, et al. High prevalence of symptomatic bradyarrhythmias due to atrio-ventricular node-fascicular and sinus node- atrial disease in patients with mitral anular calcification. Am Heart J 1982; 103: 226–9.
119. Rodriguez CJ, Bartz TM, Longstreth WT Jr, et al. Association of annular calcification and aortic valve sclerosis with brain findings on magnetic resonance imaging in community dwelling older adults: the cardiovascular health study. J Am Coll Cardiol 2011; 57: 2172–80.
120. Aronow WS, Koenigsberg M, Kronzon I, et al. Association of mitral anular calcium with new thromboembolic stroke and cardiac events at 39- month follow-up in elderly patients. Am J Cardiol 1990; 65: 1511–12.
121. Mambo NC, Silver MD, Brunsdon DF. Bacterial endocarditis of the mitral valve associated with annular calcification. Can Med Assoc J 1978; 119: 323–6.
122. Savage DD, Garrison RJ, Castelli WP, et al. Prevalence of submitral (anular) calcium and its correlates in a general population-based sample (the Framingham Study). Am J Cardiol 1983; 51: 1375–8.
123. Kanjanauthai S, Nasir K, Katz R, et al. Relationships of mitral annular calcification to cardiovascular risk factors: the Multi-Ethnic Study of Atherosclerosis (MESA). Atherosclerosis 2010; 213: 558–62.
124. Aronow WS, Ahn C, Kronzon I. Prevalence of echocardiographic findings in 554 men and in 1,243 women aged >60 years in a long-term health care facility. Am J Cardiol 1997; 79: 379–80.
125. Aronow WS, Schwartz KS, Koenigsberg M. Correlation of atrial fibrillation with presence or absence of mitral anular calcium in 604 persons older than 60 years. Am J Cardiol 1987; 59: 1213–14.
126. Roberts WC. The senile cardiac calcification syndrome. Am J Cardiol 1986; 58: 572–4.
127. Gondrie MJ, van der Graaf Y, Jacobs PC, et al. The association of incidentally detected heart valve calcification with future cardiovascular events. Eur Radiol 2011; 21: 963–73.
128. Nair CK, Sketch MH, Ahmed I, et al. Calcific valvular aortic stenosis with and without mitral anular calcium. Am J Cardiol 1987; 60: 865–70.
129. Aronow WS, Schwartz KS, Koenigsberg M. Prevalence of tricuspid anular calcium diagnosed by echocardiography in elderly patients. Am J Noninvas Cardiol 1987; 1: 275–7.
130. Potpara TS, Vasiljevic ZM, Vujisic-Tesic BD, et al. Mitral annular calcification predicts cardiovascular morbidity and mortality in middle-aged patients with atrial fibrillation: The Belgrade Atrial Fibrillation Study. Chest 2011; 140: 902–10.
131. Utsunomiya H, Yamamoto H, Kunita E, et al. Combined presence of aortic valve calcification and mitral annular calcification as a marker of the extent and vulnerable characteristics of coronary artery plaque assessed by 64-multidetector computed tomography. Atherosclerosis 2010; 213: 166–72.
132. Thanassoulis G, Massaro JM, Cury R, et al. Associations of long-term and early adult atherosclerosis risk factors with aortic and mitral valve calcium. J Am Coll Cardiol 2010; 55: 2491–8.
133. Aronow WS, Schwartz KS, Koenigsberg M. Correlation of serum lipids, calcium and phosphorus, diabetes mellitus, aortic valve stenosis and history of systemic hypertension with presence or absence of mitral anular calcium in persons older than 62 years in a long-term health care facility. Am J Cardiol 1987; 59: 381–2.
134. Sprecher DL, Schaefer EJ, Kent KM, et al. Cardiovascular features of homozygous familial hypercholesterolemia: analysis of 16 patients. Am J Cardiol 1984; 54: 20–30.
135. Waller BF, Roberts WC. Cardiovascular disease in the very elderly. An analysis of 40 necropsy patients aged 90 years or over. Am J Cardiol 1983; 51: 403–21.
136. Yetkin E, Yagmur C, Yagmur J, et al. Evaluation of cardiovascular risk factors and bone mineral density in patients undergoing coronary angiography and relation of findings to mitral annular calcium. Am J Cardiol 2007; 99: 159–62.
137. Roberts WC, Waller BF. Effect of chronic hypercalcemia on the heart: an analysis of 18 necropsy patients. Am J Med 1981; 71: 371–84.
138. Aronow WS, Kronzon I. Prevalence of aortic valve calcium and mitral annular calcium in older persons with and without chronic renal insufficiency. Cardiovasc Rev Rep 2000; 21: 623–4.
139. Huting J. Mitral valve calcification as an index of left ventricular dysfunction in patients with end-stage renal disease on peritoneal dialysis. Chest 1994; 105: 383–8.
140. Fox CS, Larson MG, Vasan RS, et al. Cross-sectional association of kidney function with valvular and annular calcification: the Framingham heart study. J Am Soc Nephrol 2006; 17: 521–7.
141. Nair CK, Sudhakaran C, Aronow WS, et al. Clinical characteristics of patients younger than 60 years with mitral anular calcium: comparison with age- and sex-matched control subjects. Am J Cardiol 1984; 54: 1286–7.
142. Kronzon I, Glassman E. Mitral ring calcification in idiopathic hypertrophic subaortic stenosis. Am J Cardiol 1978; 42: 60–6.

143. Motamed HE, Roberts WC. Frequency and significance of mitral anular calcium in hypertrophic cardiomyopathy: analysis of 200 necropsy patients. Am J Cardiol 1987; 60: 877–84.

144. Aronow WS, Kronzon I. Prevalence of hypertrophic cardiomyopathy and its association with mitral anular calcium in elderly patients. Chest 1988; 94: 1295–6.

145. Aronow WS, Ahm C, Kronzon I. Association of mitral annular calcium and of aortic cuspal calcium with coronary artery disease in older patients. Am J Cardiol 1999; 84: 1084–5.

146. Tolstrup K, Roldan CA, Qualls CR, et al. Aortic valve sclerosis, mitral annular calcium, and aortic root sclerosis as markers of atherosclerosis in men. Am J Cardiol 2002; 89: 1030–4.

147. Aronow WS, Ahn C, Kronzon I. Association of mitral annular calcium with symptomatic peripheral arterial disease in older persons. Am J Cardiol 2001; 88: 333–4.

148. Seo Y, Ishimitsu T, Ishizu T, et al. Relationship between mitral annular calcification and severity of carotid atherosclerosis in patients. J Cardiol 2005; 46: 17–24.

149. Adler Y, Motro M, Shemesh J, et al. Association of mitral annular calcium on spiral computed tomography (dual-slice mode) with thoracic aorta calcium in patients with systemic hypertension. Am J Cardiol 2002; 89: 1420–2.

150. Roberts WC, Waller BF. Mitral valve 'anular' calcium forming a complete circle or 'O' configuration: clinical and necropsy observations. Am Heart J 1981; 101: 619–21.

151. Aronow WS, Schwartz KS, Koenigsberg M. Sensitivity, specificity, positive predictive value, and negative predictive value of mitral anular calcium detected by chest roentgenograms correlated with mitral anular calcium diagnosed by echocardiography in elderly patients. Am J Noninvas Cardiol 1987; 1: 252–3.

152. Hamirani YS, Nasir K, Blumenthal RS, et al. Relation of mitral annular calcium and coronary calcium (from the Multi-Ethnic Study of Atherosclerosis [MESA]). Am J Cardiol 2011; 107: 1291–4.

153. Nair CK, Aronow WS, Sketch MH, et al. Clinical and echocardiographic characteristics of patients with mitral anular calcification. Comparison with age- and sex-matched control subjects. Am J Cardiol 1983; 51: 992–5.

154. Nair CK, Thomson W, Ryschon K, et al. Long-term follow-up of patients with echocardiographically detected mitral anular calcium and comparison with age- and sex-matched control subjects. Am J Cardiol 1989; 63: 465–70.

155. Aronow WS, Ahn C, Kronzon I, et al. Association of mitral annular calcium with new thromboembolic stroke at 44-month follow-up of 2,148 persons, mean age 81 years. Am J Cardiol 1998; 81: 105–6.

156. Korn D, DeSanctis RW, Sell S. Massive calcification of the mitral annulus: a clinicopathologic study of fourteen cases. N Engl J Med 1962; 267: 900–9.

157. Schott CR, Kotler MN, Parry WR, et al. Mitral annular calcification: clinical and echocardiography correlations. Arch Intern Med 1977; 137: 1143–50.

158. Aronow WS, Schwartz KS, Koenigsberg M. Correlation of murmurs of mitral stenosis and mitral regurgitation with presence or absence of mitral anular calcium in persons older than 62 years in a long-term health care facility. Am J Cardiol 1987; 59: 181–2.

159. Aronow WS, Kronzon I. Correlation of prevalence and severity of mitral regurgitation and mitral stenosis determined by Doppler echocardiography with physical signs of mitral regurgitation and mitral stenosis in 100 patients aged 62 to 100 years with mitral anular calcium. Am J Cardiol 1997; 60: 1189–90.

160. Kaul S, Pearlman JD, Touchstone DA, et al. Prevalence and mechanisms of mitral regurgitation in the absence of intrinsic abnormalities of the mitral leaflets. Am Heart J 1989; 118: 963–72.

161. Labovitz AJ, Nelson JG, Windhorst DM, et al. Frequency of mitral valve dysfunction from mitral anular calcium as detected by Doppler echocardiography. Am J Cardiol 1985; 55: 133–7.

162. Burnside JW, DeSanctis RW. Bacterial endocarditis on calcification of the mitral anulus fibrosus. Ann Intern Med 1972; 76: 615–18.

163. Dajani AS, Taubert KA, Wilson W, et al. Prevention of bacterial endocarditis. Recommendations by the American Heart Association. Circulation 1997; 96: 358–66.

164. Wilson W, Taubert KA, Gewitz M, et al. Prevention of infective endocarditis: guidelines from the American Heart Association: a guideline from the American Heart Association Rheumatic Fever, Endocarditis, and Kawasaki Disease Committee, Council on Cardiovascular Disease in the Young, and the Council on Clinical Cardiology, Council on Cardiovascular Surgery and Anesthesia, and the Quality of Care Outcomes Research Interdisciplinary Working Group. Circulation 2007; 116: 1736–54.

165. Nair CK, Biddle P, Kaneshige A, et al. Mitral valve replacement in patients with mitral anular calcium (abstract). Chest 1991; l00(Suppl): S109.

166. Sherman DG, Dyken ML, Fisher M, et al. Cerebral embolism. Chest 1986; 89: S82–98.

167. Aronow WS, Gutstein H, Hsieh FY. Risk factors for thromboembolic stroke in elderly patients with chronic atrial fibrillation. Am J Cardiol 1989; 63: 366–7.

168. Benjamin EJ, Plehn JF, D'Agostino RB, et al. Mitral annular calcification and the risk of stroke in an elderly cohort. N Engl J Med 1992; 327: 374–9.

169. Boston Area Anticoagulation Trial for Atrial Fibrillation Investigators. The effect of low-dose warfarin on the risk of stroke in patients with nonrhemnatic atrial fibrillation. N Engl J Med 1990; 323: 1505–11.

170. Aronow WS, Schoenfeld MR, Gutstein H. Frequency of thromboembolic stroke in persons ≥60 years of age with extracranial carotid arterial disease and/or mitral annular calcium. Am J Cardiol 1992; 70: 123–4.

171. Eicher JC, Soto FX, DeNadai L, et al. Possible association of thrombotic, nonbacterial vegetations of the mitral ring-mitral annular calcium and stroke. Am J Cardiol 1997; 79: 1712–15.

172. Rubin DC, Hawke MW, Plotnick GD. Relation between mitral annular calcium and complex intraaortic debris. Am J Cardiol 1993; 71: 1251–2.

173. Shohat-Zabarski R, Paz R, Adler Y, et al. Mitral annulus calcification with a mobile component as a possible source of embolism. Am J Geriatr Cardiol 2001; 10: 196–8.

174. Aronow WS, Ahn C, Kronzon I, et al. Association of mitral annular calcium with prior thromboembolic stroke in older white, African American, and Hispanic men and women. Am J Cardiol 2000; 85: 672–3.

175. Kizer JR, Wiebers DO, Whisnant JP, et al. Mitral annular calcification, aortic valve sclerosis, and incident stroke in adults free of clinical cardiovascular disease: the Strong Heart Study. Stroke 2005; 36: 2533–7.

176. Aronow WS. The effect of low-dose warfarin on the risk of non-rheumatic atrial fibrillation. Letter to the Editor. N Engl J Med 1991; 325: 130.

177. Singer DE, Hughes RA, Gress DR, et al. The effect of low-dose warfarin on the risk of stroke in patients with nonrheumatic atrial fibrillation. N Engl J Med 1991; 325: 131.

17

Infective endocarditis in older adults

Hendren Bajillan and Kevin P. High

SUMMARY

Age is a strong risk factor for infective endocarditis (IE). The annual incidence of IE is 145 cases per million in patients aged 70–80 years. IE in seniors is associated with a poor prognosis and high rate of complications due to insidious initial symptoms, delayed diagnosis, multimorbidity and a higher incidence of aggressive pathogens. Mitral and aortic valves are affected in the majority of IE in seniors. Recently, there has been a trend toward higher incidence of cardiovascular implantable electronic device-associated IE in older adults. Diagnosis of IE is frequently delayed in seniors due to atypical clinical presentations and difficulty interpreting echocardiographic findings, therefore it is recommended to pursue early transesophageal echocardiography in most patients with suspected IE. Seniors have a wider spectrum of causative microbiology compared to younger adults, thus broad spectrum empiric intravenous antibiotics should be initialed with narrowing of coverage after the etiologic organism and sensitivities have been confirmed. Consultation with an infectious diseases specialist can be helpful in evaluating antibiotic choices and long-term management that typically involves prolonged intravenous therapy.

DEFINITION

In 1835 Jean-Baptiste Bouillaud coined the term endocardium and described inflammation of this membranous tissue calling it "endocarditis" (1). He also noted that this lesion was frequently associated with acute inflammatory rheumatism (i.e., rheumatic fever). Rudolf Virchow described "small granules" under microscopic descriptions of these lesions, but it was not until 1869 when Emanuel Winge presented the findings of a patient with endocarditis in which he noted short rod-shaped bodies "similar to *Leptothrix*" on microscopy leading him to theorize that "parasitic organisms" may have entered the patient's body through a foot wound and later colonized the heart valve, thus providing the first description of infective endocarditis.

Infective endocarditis is a term that now refers to microbial infection of the endocardial surface of native heart valves (2), but it is also widely used to indicate infection of prosthetic material that crosses heart valves (e.g., pacemaker wires) and is embedded within endocardial tissues (e.g., ICD wires), as well as artificial or bioprosthetic heart valves. These important distinctions have great impact on classification, diagnosis, and treatment in older adults as addressed in this chapter.

CLASSIFICATION

IE is classified either based on acuity level—acute, subacute or chronic; localization (left-sided, right-sided, or valve involved); or valve type—native versus prosthetic valve

Table 17.1   Microbiology of prosthetic valve endocarditis

Pathogen	Early PVE (%)	Late PVE (%)
Methicillin-susceptible *Staphylococcus aureus*	15–29	13–22
Methicillin-resistant *S. aureus*	18–24	2–4
Coagulase-negative staphylococci	17–38	10–20
Viridans group streptococci	0–2	14–17
Enterococci	5–24	8–20
Gram-negative bacilli	2–15	1–7
Culture-negative	3–17	3–19
Polymicrobial	2–7	2–7
Fungi	5–15	2–3

Abbreviation: PVE, prosthetic valve endocarditis.
Source: Adapted from Refs. 2,29–32.

endocarditis (PVE). PVE is further divided into early PVE—usually defined as occurring within 12 months after implantation—versus late PVE which occurs more than 12 months after surgery. This distinction is important since the causative agents vary substantially by PVE subclass (see below). Most early PVE is due to acquisition of a pathogen during the index hospitalization either through surgical contamination or nosocomial bacteremia often from intravenous lines. Thus, coagulase-negative staphylococci, *Staphylococcus aureus* [including methicillin-resistant *S. aureus* (MRSA)] and hospital-acquired gram-negative rods are more common in early PVE than in late PVE or native valve IE. In contrast, late PVE endocarditis is felt to primarily result from community-acquired bacteremia with seeding of the valve and thus the microbiology more close resembles native valve disease (2) (Table 17.1).

Finally, in some studies, IE may be classified according to the mode of acquisition into community-acquired, hospital-acquired, or intravenous drug abuse-associated IE (3).

AGE, EPIDEMIOLOGIC FEATURES, RISK FACTORS, AND PROGNOSIS OF IE

Age is a strong risk factor for IE. The incidence of community acquired, native valve IE ranges from 1.7 to 6.2 cases per 100,000 person-years (2), with peak incidence of 14.5 episodes per 100,000 person-years in patients between 70 and 80 years of age (3). In a French population survey, the annual incidence of IE was 31 cases per million population, but the incidence increased dramatically in patients older than 50 years and peaked at 145 cases per million in men between 70 and 80 years (4). The male to female ratio of IE is 2–8:1 in patients older than 60 years (5,6).

For PVE, the risk of early PVE ranges from 1% to 3.1% at 12 months versus 2% to 5.7% for late PVE by 60 months post surgery (2).

Previous data show that IE has evolved from a typically subacute or chronic disease affecting young individuals with rheumatic heart disease to one normally afflicting older adults who often have underlying degenerative valve disease or a previously placed prosthetic valve or device (7).

The mean age of patients with IE has increased from about 30 years of age in the 1950s, 50 years in the 1980s, and 55–60 years in the 1990s (8). Prior to the 1940s less than 10% of IE patients were over 60 years of age. In the 1940s and 1950s about 20% of IE patients were over 60 years, increasing to 40% during the 1960s and to 55% in the 1970s and 1980s (9).

Most reports suggest that IE in the elderly is associated with a poor prognosis and high rate of complications attributed to insidious initial symptoms, delayed diagnosis, multimorbidity, and a higher incidence of more aggressive pathogens than occurs in young adults (3). Older age, PVE and cerebral embolism are risk factors for in-hospital mortality in those with IE (10). However, many studies that identified age as a risk factor did not adequately control for comorbid illnesses. Elderly IE patients are more likely to have diabetes mellitus, a gastrointestinal or genitourinary cancer, or another chronic illness (11), and these comorbid illnesses influence the causative micro-organisms (see below) as well as prognosis. Among IE patients > 70 years of age, 19–50% have a gastrointestinal and 13% have a urinary portal of entry (8,10).

Age also influences the anatomic location of IE. In one study the mitral valve was affected in 20 of 44 patients (45%), and the aortic valve was affected in 14 of 44 patients (32%) (12). Another study demonstrated mitral valve involvement in 52% of IE in seniors (13). Significantly more mitral and less aortic and tricuspid vegetations were found in elderly patients (50%, 41%, and 7%, respectively), as compared with 45%, 44%, and 17% for those valves in young adults (11). A higher frequency of pacemaker lead-associated IE has also been noted in elderly patients (14). Intracardiac device infection represents a sizable subset of IE in elderly patients (10% vs. 3% in young adults (11).

MICROBIOLOGY
Native Valve IE
The primary causative organisms for IE in the general population are Streptococcus species (spp.) 30–45%, *S. aureus* 25–30%, *Enterococcus* spp. 14–17%, coagulase-negative staphylococci 3–5%, gram-negative bacilli 5%, HACEK (*Haemophilus parainfluenzae, Haemophilus aphrophilus, Actinobacillus actinomycetemcomitans, Cardiobacterium hominis, Eikenella corrodens,* and *Kingella kingae*) organisms 5%, polymicrobial 1–3% and Fungi 1–2% (2).

Older adults have a significantly different spectrum of microbiology than that seen in the general population, and there is evidence that the spectrum is evolving. In a study from the 1990s, the majority of IE cases in seniors were due to *Streptococcus* spp. (43%) and *Staphylococcus* spp. (36%); a minority of cases were due to gram-negative rods (9%) and *Enterococcus faecalis* (7%) (12). However, another study published a few years later found that *Enterococcus* spp. were more common in seniors 32.2% versus 13.1%, $p = 0.001$ for young adults (15). In a study, the leading causative organism was *S. aureus*, with a higher rate of methicillin resistance; coagulase-negative staphylococci, enterococci, and *Streptococcus bovis* were also significantly more prevalent than in younger adults (11).

The incidence of blood culture-negative IE ranges from 5% to 21% (8,10–12,14–16) (also see the Section "Emerging and Special Pathogens"). In a study comparing characteristics of culture-negative versus culture-positive IE, no significant differences were found with regard to clinical or echocardiographic findings, predisposing factors, valve location, need for surgery, long-term prognosis, or overall mortality (16).

Prosthetic Valve IE
As noted above, the microbiology of PVE differs markedly from that of native valve disease by timing of disease onset. Staphylococci [*S. aureus* and coagulase-negative staphylococci (CoNS)] are the major causative organisms in both early and late PVE, but the relative distribution among staphylococci and involvement of other organisms varies markedly by time since implantation (Table 17.1). In general, early PVE is primarily caused by hospital-acquired organisms or skin/surgical contaminants, primarily CoNS. Late PVE more closely resembles native valve IE with regard to causative agents with the exception that staphylococci are more common in late PVE than native valve IE.

Prosthetic Devices—Pacemakers, Implantable Defibrillators

The microbiology of IE associated with intracardiac devices mirrors that of early PVE (17,18). CoNS account for more than 40% with *S. aureus* accounting for another 30%. The remaining cases are caused primarily by other gram-positive cocci and gram-negative bacilli with about 7% being culture negative and only 2% due to fungi.

Emerging and Special Pathogens

Several pathogens deserve further comment due to their increasing frequency, diagnostic requirements or therapeutic implications. *S. lugdunensis* is a coagulase-negative staphylococcus recognized with increasing frequency in IE including device-associated IE (19,20). Although this is a CoNS, it should never be dismissed as a contaminant. The organism is often aggressive causing valve destruction or abscess and surgical intervention/device removal is frequently required; in retrospective analyses medical treatment alone is associated with increased mortality (19). Unlike many other CoNS, the vast majority of *S. lugdunensis* are susceptible to β-lactams, with > 80% susceptible to penicillin in a series of IE cases (19).

Culture-negative (CN) endocarditis has always been a vexing clinical problem and is often caused by previous antibiotic exposure or difficult to grow organisms such as the HACEK group. New culture techniques and media support the growth of HACEK organisms, so that this group is now a relatively rare cause of culture-negative IE. When culture-negative IE is encountered in the absence of prior antibiotics, specific pathogens should be suspected that often require special diagnostic studies.

The most likely causes of culture-negative IE include *Coxiella burnetii*, *Bartonella* spp., and *Tropheryma whipplei*. *C. burnetii*, the causative agent of Q fever, is associated with animal contact. Patients with endocarditis often present with a flu-like illness. *Bartonella* spp. have been implicated as a cause of "culture-negative" endocarditis for several decades, primarily affecting younger adults particularly the homeless since the major *Bartonella* spp. that causes IE, *B. quintana*, is louse-borne. Other *Bartonella* spp. are carried by fleas/other vectors or can be transmitted by cat scratches/bites and have been also reported as a cause of IE (21). Recent reports of IE due to *Bartonella* spp. have emerged in older patients with prosthetic valve and device-associated IE (21,22). *T. whipplei*, the causative agent of Whipple's disease, is also well recognized as a cause of culture-negative endocarditis, and in a recent study of such patients the organism was the fourth most common pathogen identified by PCR of surgical valve material (causing 6% of cases) (23). Of the 16 patients in that series, the aortic valve was affected in 13, the mitral valve in 3. Also, 12 patients were age 60 years and older; 6 were older than age 70, and only 2 had GI symptoms. Thus, *T. whipplei* may be a relatively common cause of CN IE in seniors and appears to rarely present with classic signs of Whipple's disease.

A key point with all three of these pathogens is that the diagnosis is suggested by serologic studies but confirmed by polymerase chain reaction (PCR) of either blood or valvular material. Thus, high suspicion is needed to make the diagnosis. There are also important therapeutic implications in that treatment of *C. burnetii*, *Bartonella* spp., and *T. whipplei* requires very specific and prolonged therapy quite different from typical IE treatment, and enlisting an infectious diseases specialist is encouraged to assist with management.

CLINICAL AND LABORATORY MANIFESTATIONS

The clinical manifestations of IE in the elderly are frequently insidious and nonspecific (24) but the range of symptoms does not differ dramatically by age. However, the frequency of specific symptoms does vary by age complicating diagnosis and delaying treatment. For example, fever and chills appear to be less frequent in seniors according to some studies (9,12,14,15,) but not others (8,10,11,13). Constitutional symptoms like fatigue, anorexia, weight loss or malaise, myalgias/arthralgias are often present, but may be ignored as typical symptoms of aging by both patients and providers. Complicated end organ manifestations may also be present, such as pneumonia, septic pulmonary emboli, pleural effusion, empyema, meningitis, heart failure, acute/subacute renal failure, septic arthritis, and visceral abscesses.

Heart murmurs are relatively common in older adults due to degenerative valve disease and calcification so IE in seniors may not present with a new or changing murmur (9). Vascular and immune-mediated phenomena, such as embolic events, splenomegaly, Osler nodes, Roth spots, Janeway lesions, and conjunctival hemorrhages are all observed less commonly in elderly IE patients than in young adults (11,24). Heart failure, renal insufficiency and malignancy more commonly complicate IE in older versus young adults (12,13,15). Central nervous system manifestations are associated with increased long-term mortality (12,24,25).

Leukocytosis with left shift is commonly present (6), but less often in seniors than in young adults (11). Anemia appears to be more common in the elderly population (3), and elevation of the erythrocyte sedimentation rate occurs in 90% of cases (24,6). Microscopic examination of the urine sediment is recommended to detect proteinuria and microscopic hematuria, red blood cell casts, and bacteriuria. Up to 50% of cases have a positive rheumatoid factor. Reduced complement levels and increased circulating immune complexes may be noted (6,24).

Blood cultures are more likely to grow bacteria in elderly IE patients when compared to young adults (11). At least 3 sets of blood cultures (aerobic and anaerobic bottles) from different sites 1 hour apart are recommended to increase the yield up to 99% (24).

A chest X ray or a computed tomography scan of the chest may reveal pneumonia, septic pulmonary emboli, pleural effusion, and/or empyema, but age-specific data on the frequency of these findings are not available. Electrocardiography should be performed and may reveal conduction defects due to intramyocardial abscess formation (6).

DIAGNOSIS

The diagnosis of IE in older adults is frequently delayed due to atypical clinical presentations and difficulty interpreting echocardiographic findings. In one study, time to diagnosis was 7.2 ± 6.2 days in elderly patients versus 3.2 ± 3.5 days in younger patients ($p < 0.001$) (15). Delays in diagnosis may be a major cause for the poorer prognosis of older adults compared to younger patients (6).

The presence of calcified valvular lesions and prosthetic valves makes echocardiographic findings difficult to interpret in seniors limiting the utility of transthoracic echocardiography (6). The rate of detection for valvular vegetations by transthoracic echocardiography is lower, 45%, in elderly patients compared to 75% in younger patients. Importantly, the rate of detection using transesophageal echocardiography increases to 90% in both age groups. Vegetations are generally smaller in elderly patients compared to younger patients (14). Seniors with IE also have fewer vegetations but a higher rate of intracardiac abscess and prosthetic perivalvular complications (11). Therefore, it is recommended that a lower threshold for obtaining transesophageal echocardiography be employed in elderly patients suspected of having IE versus that in young adults.

The diagnosis of IE is generally established based on the modified Duke criteria (Table 17.2). The Duke criteria categorize patients as having definite, probable, or possible IE. Gagliardi et al. found the sensitivity of the Duke criteria to be 69% for classifying seniors (>64 years of age) as definite IE, and 100% for classifying patients as definite or probable IE. The Duke criteria appear more sensitive for identifying seniors with IE than other classification systems (e.g., Beth Israel criteria) (12).

Table 17.2 Modified Duke criteria for diagnosis of IE

Definitive IE
Pathological criteria
1. Microorganism demonstrated by culture or histological examination of a vegetation
2. Vegetation or intracardiac abscess confirmed by histological examination showing IE
Clinical criteria
1. 2 major criteria; or
2. 1 major and three minor criteria; or
3. 5 minor criteria

Possible IE
1. 1 major and one minor criterion; or
2. 3 minor criteria

Rejected IE
1. Firm alternative diagnosis; or
2. Resolution of IE syndrome with antibiotic therapy for ≤4 days; or
3. No pathological evidence of IE at surgery or autopsy, with antibiotic therapy for ≤4 days; or
4. Does not meet criteria for possible IE

Major criteria
Blood culture positive for IE
1. Typical microorganisms consistent with IE from two separate blood cultures:
   a. *Viridans streptococci, Streptococcus bovis, Staphylococcus aureus*, HACEK group; or
   b. Community-acquired enterococci, in the absence of a primary focus; or
2. Microorganisms consistent with IE from persistently positive blood cultures, defined as follows:
   a. At least two positive cultures of blood samples drawn 12 h apart; or
   b. All of the three or majority of ≥4 separate cultures of blood (with first and last sample drawn at least 1 h apart)
3. Single positive blood culture for *Coxiella burnetii* or antiphase I IgG antibody titer > 1:800
Evidence of endocardial involvement
Echocardiogram-positive for IE, defined as follows:
1. Oscillating intracardiac mass on valve or supporting structures, in the path of regurgitant jets, or on implanted material in the absence of an alternative anatomical explanation; or
2. Abscess; or
3. New partial dehiscence of prosthetic valve
New valvular regurgitation (worsening or changing of pre-existing murmur not sufficient)

Minor criteria
Predisposing heart condition or IDU
Fever, temperature > 38°C
Vascular phenomena: major arterial emboli, septic pulmonary infarcts, mycotic aneurysm, intracranial hemorrhage, conjunctival hemorrhage, Janeway lesion
Immunologic phenomena: glomerulonephritis, Osler's nodes, Roth's spots, rheumatoid factor
Microbiological evidence: positive blood cultures but does not meet a major criterion or serological evidence of active infection with organism consistent with IE

Abbreviations: HACEK, *Haemophilus parainfluenzae, Haemophilus aphrophilus, Actinobacillus actinomycetemcomitans, Cardiobacterium hominis, Eikenella corrodens, and Kingella kingae*; IDU, intravenous drug use; IE, infective endocarditis; IgG, immunoglobulin G.
Source: Adapted from Ref. 33.

TREATMENT

Broad spectrum empiric intravenous antibiotics should be initiated promptly *after* obtaining blood cultures. Antibiotics should then be adjusted based on microbiological data and whether native valve or prosthetic valve endocarditis is being treated (Table 17.3). Blood cultures should be repeated every 24–48 hours until clearance of bacteremia is documented. The first day of negative blood cultures "starts the clock" for the planned duration of antibiotic therapy.

Although an option for abbreviated courses of antibiotics with combination therapy of β-lactams and an aminoglycoside can be used in young adults for relatively penicillin-resistant viridians streptococci, this strategy is not favored in elderly patients due to the higher risk of renal dysfunction and ototoxicity in seniors (6).

When aminoglycosides are necessary (e.g., for treatment of enterococcal IE) close attention to renal function and therapeutic drug level measurements should be obtained in order to minimize toxicities. Some authors recommend audiometry at baseline and weekly to monitor for ototoxicity for all patients anticipated to receive aminoglycoside therapy for more than 2 weeks. Serum levels of aminoglycosides that are lower than levels generally considered "therapeutic" (i.e., peaks of 3–4) are adequate for synergy when administered with cell wall-active agents (6), and are associated with reduced risk of toxicity.

SURGICAL THERAPY

According to the AHA guidelines, surgery is recommended in patients with IE and congestive heart failure unresponsive to medical therapy, and in prosthetic valve endocarditis, particularly early PVE (<12 months after valve replacement). Other clinical situations for which surgery should be considered include fungal endocarditis; endocarditis with an aggressive antibiotic-resistant bacteria or bacteria that respond poorly to antibiotics; left-sided endocarditis caused by gram-negative bacteria; persistent infection with positive blood cultures after 1 week of effective antibiotic therapy; more than one embolic event during the first 2 weeks of antimicrobial therapy; persistent vegetation after systemic embolization; anterior mitral leaflet vegetations >10 mm; an increase in vegetation size despite appropriate antibiotic therapy; valve dehiscence, perforation, rupture, or fistula; large perivalvular abscess; and new heart block. The AHA guidelines recommend that decisions concerning surgical interventions should be individualized (26).

Early surgery is a reasonable treatment option in selected elderly patients with IE and may lead to better survival compared to medical treatment alone (27). In two studies, surgical management was an independent predictor of a favorable prognosis and lower in-hospital mortality in multivariate analyses (10,27). This was true despite data suggesting elderly patients had fewer vegetations or valve perforations at the time of surgery (11). Nonetheless, age older than 65 years is a significant independent predictor of reduced likelihood of surgical intervention (11), suggesting a reluctance to operate in this group.

Older adults with IE are more prone to complications after valve surgery, including prosthetic valve dysfunction, pericardial tamponade, renal insufficiency, rhythm disturbances, and the need for a second intervention (13). Although mortality is higher in older adults than in younger patients, selected elderly patients who undergo surgery have very good outcomes, similar to those of younger patients (10).

COMPLICATIONS

The length of hospitalization is longer for elderly patients with IE compared to young adults (12). There is increased use of antiplatelet and anticoagulant drugs in seniors, in addition to a less robust acute phase response, therefore; one study in elderly patients with IE actually showed lower rates than young adults of some complications such as septic

Table 17.3   Antimicrobial therapy for common causes of IE

Pathogen	Native Valve Endocarditis	Prosthetic Valve Endocarditis	Comments
Empiric initial regimen prior to pathogen identification	Vancomycin plus gentamicin	Vancomycin plus cefepime plus gentamicin (early) Vancomycin plus ceftriaxone plus gentamicin (late)	
Highly penicillin susceptible *Viridans streptococci, Streptococcus bovis*, and other streptococci with penicillin MIC ≤ 0.1 μg/mL	penicillin G or ceftriaxone for 4 wk	penicillin G or ceftriaxone for 6 wk	Vancomycin for patients unable to tolerate β-lactams
relative penicillin resistant *V. streptococci* and *S.bovis* with penicillin MIC > 0.12 μg/mL	penicillin G or ceftriaxone for 4 wk and gentamicin for 2 wk	penicillin G or ceftriaxone for 6 wk and gentamicin for 4 wk	Vancomycin for patients unable to tolerate β-lactams
Methicillin susceptible staphylococci	Nafcillin or oxacillin or cefazolin for 6 wk Optional gentamicin for the first 3–5 day of therapy	Nafcillin or oxacillin or cefazolin with rifampin for 6 wk and gentamicin for 2 wk	Vancomycin for patients unable to tolerate β-lactams
Methicillin-resistant staphylococci	Vancomycin for 6 wk	Vancomycin with rifampin for 6 wk and gentamicin for 2 wk	
Enterococci susceptible to penicillin	Ampicillin for 4–6 wk	Ampicillin for 4–6 wk	
Enterococci resistant to penicillin but susceptible to gentamicin and vancomycin	Ampicillin–sulbactam plus gentamicin or vancomycin plus gentamicin for 6 wk	Ampicillin–sulbactam plus gentamicin or vancomycin plus gentamicin for 6 wk	
E. faecium resistant to penicillin, gentamicin, and vancomycin	Linezolid or quinupristin–dalfopristin for ≥8 wk	Linezolid or quinupristin–dalfopristin for ≥8 wk	
E. faecalis resistant to penicillin, gentamicin, and vancomycin	Imipenem–cilastatin plus ampicillin or ceftriaxone plus ampicillin for ≥8 wk	Imipenem–cilastatin plus ampicillin or ceftriaxone plus ampicillin for ≥8 wk	
HACEK group organisms	Ceftriaxone or ampicillin–sulbactam for 4 wk	Ceftriaxone or ampicillin–sulbactam for 6 wk	
Culture-negative	Ampicillin–sulbactam plus getamicin or vancomycin plus gentamicin for 4–6 wk	Vancomycin plus gentamicin (for 2 wk) plus cefepime plus rifampin for 6 wk	Consultation with an infectious diseases specialist should be sought

Abbreviations: HACEK. *Haemophilus parainfluenzae, Haemophilus aphrophilus, Actinobacillus actinomycetemcomitans, Cardiobacterium hominis, Eikenella corrodens, and Kingella kingae;* IE, infective endocarditis.
Source: Adapted from Refs 2,3,26.

pulmonary infarcts, intracranial hemorrhages, and mycotic aneurysms (11). However, the in-hospital mortality rate of IE in elderly ranges from 16% to 30% (8–15,27). Comorbidity index, severe sepsis, valvular prosthesis, and major neurological events are factors that are associated with overall increased mortality in elderly IE patients (27). Among IE patients treated with medical therapy only, mortality is higher in patients older than 70 years compared to younger patients, 57% versus 21%. Conversely, mortality is similar in older and younger patients treated with combined medical and surgical therapy (11% vs. 8%) (10,14).

PREVENTION

Based on the revised AHA guidelines, all elderly patients with high risk cardiac conditions (prosthetic heart valves, previous endocarditis, unrepaired cyanotic congenital heart disease, repaired congenital heart defects with prosthetic materials or device, and cardiac transplantation recipients with valvulopathy) who are undergoing high risk dental procedures (procedures that involve manipulation of gingival tissue or the periapical region of the teeth or perforation or oral mucosa) should receive chemoprophylaxis (28). Antibiotic prophylaxis is NOT recommended for minor valvular pathology (e.g., mitral valve prolapse even with murmur), coronary stents, or implanted devices other than prosthetic valves (e.g., pacemakers, implantable defibrillators) (18,28).

Amoxicillin 2 g orally 30–60 min prior to dental procedures is the most common regimen for prophylaxis. For patients unable to take oral medications, either ampicillin 2 g IV or IM, or cefazolin or ceftriaxone 1 g IV or IM, is recommended. For patients who are allergic to penicillin or ampicillin either oral cephalexin 2 g, clindamycin 600 mg, azithromycin, or clarithromycin 500 mg can be used. Parenteral alternatives for penicillin allergic patients include clindamycin 600 mg IV or IM, and cefazolin or ceftriaxone 1 g IV or IM.

CONCLUSION

IE affects seniors at a much higher rate than young adults, primarily due to higher prevalence of degenerative valve disease and wider use of prosthetic devices in the older population among several other factors including an increased number of procedures that may predispose to bacteremia; poor dentition; higher incidence of other infections (especially urinary tract infection and pneumonia); diminished immune function due to immunosenescence; comorbid illnesses (e.g., cancer); nutritional deficits; and certain medications (e.g., prednisone and other immunosuppressants).

Key differences between IE in older adults versus IE in young adults include the following:

- Nonspecific clinical presentations with lower rates of fever, chills, embolic events, and leukocytosis, being factors that lead to delayed diagnosis of IE in seniors
- Higher rates of renal failure and heart failure on presentation, and a much higher burden of chronic disease/comorbidities that likely underlies age-associated increases in mortality
- More likely to have blood culture positivity with the causative agent more likely to be staphylococci, GU, or GI pathogens
- Poor sensitivity of TTE, but nearly equivalent sensitivity of TEE that should prompt more frequent use of TEE in older adults with suspected IE
- Empiric therapy directed broadly until culture-directed therapy can be used; careful use of nephrotoxic agents particularly aminoglycosides with monitoring of audiometry and renal function if use of aminoglycosides is necessary

REFERENCES

1. Contrepois A. Notes on the early history of infective endocarditis and the development of an experimental model. Clin Infect Dis 1995; 20: 461–6.
2. Mylonakis E, Calderwood SB. Infective endocarditis in adults. N Engl J Med 2001; 345: 1318–30.
3. Habib G, Hoen B, Tornos P, et al. ESC Committee for Practice Guidelines. Guidelines on the prevention, diagnosis, and treatment of infective endocarditis (new version 2009): the Task Force on the Prevention, Diagnosis, and Treatment of Infective Endocarditis of the European Society of Cardiology (ESC). Endorsed by the European Society of Clinical Microbiology and Infectious Diseases (ESC-MID) and the International Society of Chemotherapy (ISC) for Infection and Cancer. Eur Heart J 2009; 30: 2369–413.
4. Hoen B, Alla F, Selton-Suty C, et al. Changing profile of infective endocarditis: results of a 1-year survey in France. JAMA 2002; 288: 75–81.
5. Cunha BA, Gill MV, Lazar JM. Acute infective endocarditis. Diagnostic and therapeutic approach. Infect Dis Clin North Am 1996; 10: 811–34.
6. Dhawan VK. Infective endocarditis in elderly patients. Clin Infect Dis 2002; 34: 806–12.
7. Murdoch DR, Corey GR, Hoen B, et al. International Collaboration on Endocarditis-Prospective Cohort Study (ICE-PCS) Investigators. Clinical presentation, etiology, and outcome of infective endocarditis in the 21st century: the International Collaboration on Endocarditis-Prospective Cohort Study. Arch Intern Med 2009; 169: 463–73.
8. Selton-Suty C, Hoen B, Grentzinger A, et al. Clinical and bacteriological characteristics of infective endocarditis in the elderly. Heart 1997; 77: 260–3.
9. Terpenning MS, Buggy BP, Kauffman CA. Infective endocarditis: clinical features in young and elderly patients. Am J Med 1987; 83: 626–34.
10. Di Salvo G, Thuny F, Rosenberg V, et al. Endocarditis in the elderly: clinical, echocardiographic, and prognostic features. Eur Heart J 2003; 24: 1576–83.
11. Durante-Mangoni E, Bradley S, Selton-Suty C, et al. Current features of infective endocarditis in elderly patients: results of the International Collaboration on Endocarditis Prospective Cohort Study. Arch Intern Med 2008; 168: 2095–103.
12. Gagliardi JP, Nettles RE, McCarty DE, et al. Native valve infective endocarditis in elderly and younger adult patients: comparison of clinical features and outcomes with use of the Duke criteria and the Duke Endocarditis Database. Clin Infect Dis 1998; 26: 1165–8.
13. Netzer RO, Zollinger E, Seiler C, et al. Native valve infective endocarditis in elderly and younger adult patients: comparison of clinical features and outcomes with use of the Duke criteria. Clin Infect Dis 1999; 28: 933–5.
14. Werner GS, Schulz R, Fuchs JB, et al. Infective endocarditis in the elderly in the era of transesophageal echocardiography: clinical features and prognosis compared with younger patients. Am J Med 1996; 100: 90–7.
15. Zamorano J, Sanz J, Moreno R, et al. Better prognosis of elderly patients with infectious endocarditis in the era of routine echocardiography and nonrestrictive indications for valve surgery. J Am Soc Echocardiogr 2002; 15: 702–7.
16. Pérez de Isla L, Zamorano J, Lennie V, et al. Negative blood culture infective endocarditis in the elderly: long-term follow-up. Gerontology 2007; 53: 245–9.
17. Sohail MR, Uslan DZ, Khan AH, et al. Management and outcome of permanent pacemaker and implantable cardioverter-defibrillator infections. J Am Coll Cardiol 2007; 49: 1851–9.
18. Baddour LM, Epstein AE, Erickson CC, et al. Update on cardiovascular implantable electronic device infections and their management: a scientific statement from the American Heart Association. Circulation 2010; 121: 458–77.
19. Liu PY, Huang YF, Tang CW, et al. Staphylococcus lugdunensis infective endocarditis: a literature review and analysis of risk factors. J Microbiol Immunol Infect 2010; 43: 478–84.
20. Tsao YT, Wang WJ, Lee SW, et al. Characterization of Staphylococcus lugdunensis endocarditis in patients with cardiac implantable electronic devices. Int J Infect Dis 2012; 16: e464–7.
21. Chaloner GL, Harrison TG, Birtles RJ, et al. Bartonella species as a cause of infective endocarditis in the UK. Epidemiol Infect 2013; 141: 841–6.
22. Hajj-Chahine J, Houmaida H, Plouzeau C, et al. Bartonella as a cause of mechanical prosthetic aortic root endocarditis. Ann Thorac Surg 2012; 93: e93–5.
23. Geissdörfer W, Moos V, Moter A, et al. High frequency of Tropheryma whipplei in culture-negative endocarditis. J Clin Microbiol 2012; 50: 216–22.
24. Gregoratos G. Infective endocarditis in the elderly: diagnosis and management. Am J Geriatr Cardiol 2003; 12: 183–9.

25. Robbins N, DeMaria A, Miller MH. Infective endocarditis in the elderly. South Med J 1980; 73: 1335–8.
26. P, Baddour LM, Wilson WR, Bayer AS, et al. Infective endocarditis: diagnosis, antimicrobial therapy, and management of complications: a statement for healthcare professionals from the Committee on Rheumatic Fever, Endocarditis, and Kawasaki Disease, Council on Cardiovascular Disease in the Young, and the Councils on Clinical Cardiology, Stroke, and Cardiovascular Surgery and Anesthesia, American Heart Association: endorsed by the Infectious Diseases Society of America. Circulation 2005; 111: e394–434.
27. Remadi JP, Nadji G, Goissen T, et al. Infective endocarditis in elderly patients: clinical characteristics and outcome. Eur J Cardiothorac Surg 2009; 35: 123–9.
28. Wilson W, Taubert KA, Gewitz M, et al. Prevention of infective endocarditis: guidelines from the American Heart Association: a guideline from the American Heart Association Rheumatic Fever, Endocarditis, and Kawasaki Disease Committee, Council on Cardiovascular Disease in the Young, and the Council on Clinical Cardiology, Council on Cardiovascular Surgery and Anesthesia, and the Quality of Care and Outcomes Research Interdisciplinary Working Group. Circulation 2007; 116: 1736–54.
29. Rivas P, Alonso J, Moya J, et al. The impact of hospital-acquired infections on the microbial etiology and prognosis of late-onset prosthetic valve endocarditis. Chest 2005; 128: 764–71.
30. Wang A, Athan E, Pappas PA, et al. Contemporary clinical profile and outcome of prosthetic valve endocarditis. JAMA 2007; 297: 1354–61.
31. Hill EE, Herregods MC, Vanderschueren S, et al. Management of prosthetic valve infective endocarditis. Am J Cardiol 2008; 101: 1174–8.
32. López J, Revilla A, Vilacosta I, et al. Definition, clinical profile, microbiological spectrum, and prognostic factors of early-onset prosthetic valve endocarditis. Eur Heart J 2007; 28: 760–5.
33. Li JS, Sexton DJ, Mick N, et al. Proposed modifications to the Duke criteria for the diagnosis of infective endocarditis. Clin Infect Dis 2000; 30: 633–8.

18

Cardiomyopathies in the elderly

John Arthur McClung and Wilbert S. Aronow

SUMMARY

This chapter focuses on the nonischemic causes for cardiomyopathy encountered commonly in the elderly. The various presenting features as well as prevalence of the various types of nonischemic cardiomyopathy in older patients differ in a number of respects from those of younger patients. Heart failure with normal ejection fraction, hypertrophic cardiomyopathy, and dilated cardiomyopathy are reviewed with emphasis placed on the unique pathophysiology, presentation, and treatment of these entities in this age group.

PREVALENCE

The true prevalence of cardiomyopathy in the elderly may be underestimated because of the low sensitivity of the clinical criteria, particularly in milder cases. Data from the Framingham study demonstrate that the incidence of heart failure is 10% in patients older than 80 years of age as compared with only 1% in patients who are in their sixth decade (1). Approximately one-third of those identified expire within 2 years of diagnosis. The annual incidence in men aged 85–95 years was noted to be 4.4%, with a doubling of incidence noted with each 10 years of age, making heart failure the leading primary diagnosis in hospitalized elderly patients (1,2).

DIASTOLIC DYSFUNCTION

Diastolic dysfunction is especially prevalent in the elderly and accounts for a very high morbidity and mortality (3,4). Of patients identified as having congestive failure by the Framingham study, more than 50% had a left ventricular (LV) ejection fraction greater than 50% (5). Mortality, although lower than that noted for patients with diminished ejection fraction, remained four times greater than that of age- and sex-matched controls. Women appear to present with preserved ejection heart failure more frequently than men (6). A 15-year study of 4596 elderly patients performed at the Mayo Clinic demonstrated that the prevalence of heart failure with a preserved ejection fraction increased significantly between 1986 and 2002 (7). An analysis of 83 patients with clinical heart failure and LV ejection fractions greater than or equal to 45% participating in the Vasodilator-Heart Failure Trial (V-HeFT) has previously demonstrated that exercise tolerance in this population was only slightly better than that for patients with lower ejection fractions (8). In patients with comorbid conditions, hypoalbuminemia has been demonstrated to significantly exacerbate both the frequency and severity of heart failure episodes (9).

The pathophysiology of diastolic dysfunction combines delayed relaxation, impairment of LV filling, and decreased compliance of the ventricle (10). Delayed relaxation, or more properly prolonged systolic contraction, can be induced by any substance that will increase the pressure or volume load to the ventricle, such as angiotensin II or antidiuretic hormone. While, delayed relaxation represents a compensatory adjustment to loading phenomena, impaired relaxation with secondary reduction in ventricular filling constitutes active diastolic pathology that relates to a specific underlying cause. It is important to recognize that diastolic dysfunction is, to some extent, a function of aging per se, perhaps related to an increase in cellular apoptosis over time (11,12). This tendency toward diastolic dysfunction with aging has been demonstrated to be reversible with exercise in an animal model (13). Studies in humans have also demonstrated that patients presenting with heart failure and preserved ejection fraction manifest ventricular systolic and arterial stiffening in excess of that associated with aging or hypertension (14). As a result, the clinician must be able to differentiate between what could be a result of normal sedentary aging and abnormal deterioration in ventricular compliance.

Specific therapies that have been investigated in a preliminary fashion for patients with heart failure and preserved LV systolic function include AT_1 receptor blockade, statin therapy, and aldosterone antagonism (15–17). Although the SOLVD data base suggested that enalapril therapy might modestly improve diastolic function in patients with reduced ejection fraction, the use of AT_1 blockade has been demonstrated to be ineffective at reducing either mortality or prespecified morbidity endpoints in patients aged 60 or greater years with preserved ejection fraction and clinical heart failure (18,19). Spironolactone has been studied in a small cohort of 30 patients with isolated diastolic dysfunction over the age of 60 years and has been found to improve echocardiographic indices of diastolic function (20). No long-term hard endpoint trials have been reported to date. Pathologically, diastolic dysfunction with normal LV systolic dysfunction is associated with coronary artery disease (see Chaps. 8–14), restrictive cardiomyopathy, and both primary and secondary hypertrophic cardiomyopathy. In one trial, as many as 60% of elderly patients presenting with clinically significant diastolic dysfunction died of cardiovascular causes with sudden cardiac death and heart failure being the most common cause, however the overall prevalence of these modes of death remained lower in patients with diastolic dysfunction than in those with reduced ejection fraction (21).

RESTRICTIVE CARDIOMYOPATHY

Restrictive cardiomyopathy results from increased stiffness of the LV myocardium, generally as a result of infiltrative disease (22). As the infiltrative disorder is often biventricular, right-sided signs often predominate. Disturbances in conduction as well as dysrhythmia can also be common (23–26). Clinical findings are often similar to pericardial constriction, and care is required in order to establish the correct diagnosis (27).

Etiology

In contrast to younger patients, idiopathic restrictive myopathy is not only rare in the elderly, but also carries a better prognosis (28). Similarly, Loeffler's endocarditis is extremely rare in older populations (29). Amyloidosis constitutes the most common etiology in the elderly, followed by other infiltrative processes such as cardiac sarcoid, carcinoid, hemochromatosis, and systemic sclerosis (11,30). The broader use of both chest radiotherapy and anthracyclines in elderly patients with cancer leaves these patients at the risk of developing restrictive cardiomyopathy secondary to endomyocardial fibrosis (31).

Amyloid infiltration of the atria is extremely common in the elderly and has been documented in 91% of subjects of advanced age in a histological study (32). Primary

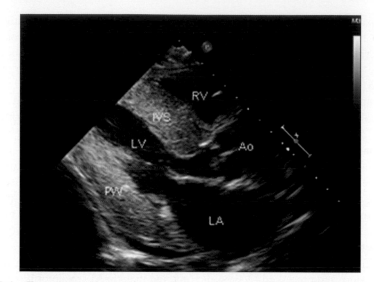

Figure 18.1 Two-dimensional echocardiogram from a parasternal long-axis view in an elderly patient with cardiac amyloidosis shows a hypertrophic interventricular septum and posterior wall with the characteristic "sparkling" appearance of myocardium. *Abbreviations*: RV, right ventricle; IVS, interventricular septum; AO, aorta; LA, left atrium; LV, left ventricle; PW, posterior wall.

amyloidosis, manifesting as a clinical syndrome with cardiac involvement, however, is considerably less common. The incidence of primary amyloidosis has been estimated to be between 6.1 and 10.5 per million person–years with the median age of presentation to medical attention being roughly 74 years (33). Diastolic dysfunction associated with primary amyloidosis may result directly from the presence of monoclonal immunoglobulins rather than requiring the presence of the amyloid deposit itself. Diastolic dysfunction similar to that observed in patients with cardiac involvement can be replicated in mice simply by the systemic infusion of light chains isolated from patients with cardiac amyloidosis (34).

The ventricular cavities are generally normal or small in size; however, mild dilatation can be noted (Fig. 18.1). The atria are characteristically dilated and in some cases may present with thrombi in the appendages (31). Only 25% of patients with primary amyloidosis present with congestive heart failure, while about one-sixth present with orthostatic hypotension (30). Median survival in patients presenting with congestive heart failure is 6 months. One of the key prognostic variables is LV wall thickness. Median survival is 2.4 years for patients presenting with normal ventricular dimensions and falls to 0.4 years for those with significant LV hypertrophy (LVH) (35,36). Prognosis is also reduced in patients presenting with shortened deceleration time and an increase in the E/A ratio as measured by Doppler echocardiography with a corresponding increase in the E/e' ratio on interrogation with tissue Doppler imaging. (Figs. 18.2,18.3) (37). Dysrhythmia associated with amyloidosis ranges from node dysfunction and bundle branch blocks to life-threatening ventricular dysrhythmia and is also related to the severity of the disease process as demonstrated by the above indices (38).

Familial amyloidosis, although responsible for only 10% of cases, also presents in the elderly. This autosomal dominant disorder is indistinguishable from primary amyloidosis by clinical criteria and requires identification of the variant protein by immunochemical modalities. Accurate diagnosis is important primarily because of the more favorable prognosis for survival, which is roughly twice that of primary amyloidosis (39).

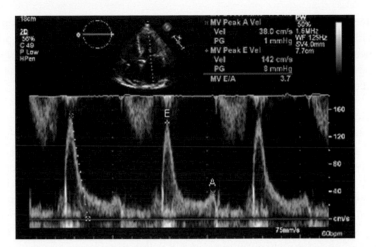

Figure 18.2 LV mitral inflow diastolic waveforms obtained with pulsed Doppler echocardiography in an elderly patient with cardiac amyloidosis show a sibstantial increase in the flow velocity of the early peak (E) and decreased maximal velocity of the late peak (A) that is characteristic of a marked increase in atrial pressure.

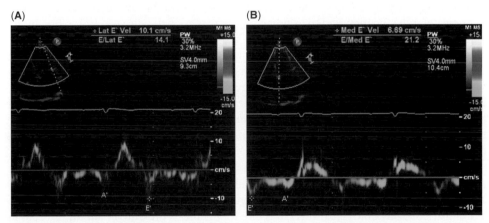

Figure 18.3 Tissue Doppler wave forms from the same patient as Figure 18.2. Tracings are from the lateral (**A**) and medial (**B**) portions of the mitral annulus obtained from the apical four chamber view, both of which demonstrate a marked increase in the E/e' ratio that is characteristic of severe diastolic dysfunction.

Cardiac sarcoidosis is associated with interstitial inflammation resulting in abnormal diastolic function (40). Incidence and prevalence of cardiac involvement remains largely unknown with only a minority of patients presenting in their elderly. Cardiac involvement can apparently be frequently subclinical with studies demonstrating between five and eight times as many patients presenting with cardiac infiltration at necropsy as had been previously diagnosed clinically (41,42). As many as half the patients presenting with sarcoidosis can have electrocardiographic abnormalities; however, the precise significance of these findings is unknown (43). Sudden death is the most common cause of mortality in patients presenting with cardiac sarcoid as a result of either complete heart block or malignant tachyarrhythmia (44).

The mean age of patients presenting with carcinoid syndrome has been reported to be 64 years with a range extending upto 83 years (45). Up to half of the cases present with carcinoid heart disease as a late complication (46). The majority of cases present with tricuspid regurgitation with additional fibrotic involvement of the pulmonic valve and the right ventricular endocardium.

Presentation and Diagnosis

Restrictive myopathies often present with generalized findings of fatigue, peripheral edema, paroxysmal nocturnal dyspnea, orthopnea, dyspnea, and occasionally, ascites. Chest pain can occur in patients presenting with amyloidosis (47). Similar clinical presentations require that this diagnosis be differentiated from pericardial constriction. This task is accomplished largely by a combination of clinical history with echocardiographic and Doppler findings, cardiac magnetic resonance imaging, and hemodynamic observations. Similar to pericardial constriction, restrictive myopathy often presents with a prominently descent in the jugular venous pulse, a positive Kussmaul's sign, an enlarged and pulsatile liver, ascites, and pedal edema. The presence of a third heart sound can serve to help differentiate restriction from constriction, which classically presents with a pericardial knock. The presence of pulmonary alveolar congestion on chest radiography favors restriction over constriction.

The classic echocardiographic presentation of amyloid heart disease includes LVH with characteristic sparkling of the myocardium (48). Mitral inflow velocities in patients with diastolic dysfunction vary depending on the extent of the disease. E/A ratios in the elderly customarily become less than one in most normal individuals. The first sign of diastolic dysfunction is often pseudonormalization of the Doppler spectral display in which the E/A ratio once again becomes greater than one associated with increasing prominence of the diastolic filling velocity in the pulmonary vein (49,50). Active restrictive physiology results in a very steep, high-velocity mitral E-wave with a short deceleration time, followed by a very small or absent A-wave (31). B-natriuretic peptide assay has been used to enhance the diagnosis of diastolic dysfunction in patients who present with normal systolic function on echocardiography (51).

Thickening of the pericardium, which is common in pericardial constriction, is absent in patients with restrictive cardiomyopathy on cardiac magnetic resonance imaging. At cardiac catheterization, the end-diastolic pressures can be equalized in both restrictive and constrictive physiology; however, it is rare for the pre-A pressure to fall toward zero in patients with restriction. In some patients, endomyocardial biopsy may be necessary for diagnosis (52).

Treatment

Specific therapy for patients with restrictive myopathy is poorly understood (53). Drug therapy has been primarily aimed at the presumed cause of the disorder (10). In patients in whom tachycardia appears to play a major role, the use of β-blockade, some calcium channel blockers, and occasionally digoxin has been advocated. Angiotensin-converting-enzyme (ACE) inhibitors have been used to reduce both pressure and volume load as well as assist in ventricular remodeling at the microstructural level (10). Diuretics reduce preload and improve exercise tolerance (54). Nitrates similarly decrease preload as well as potentially abbreviate systole, which could assist in the augmentation of diastolic filling (55,56). Warfarin may be indicated in those patients who present with atrial appendage thrombus on transesophageal echocardiography. Drugs such as amiodarone may be necessary to maintain sinus rhythm and enhance cardiac output in patients who develop atrial fibrillation (31). Pacing may be a requisite for patients who develop conduction system disease (57).

HYPERTROPHIC CARDIOMYOPATHY

Hypertrophic cardiomyopathies are common in the elderly. In some series, more than 80% of patients presenting to the hospital with newly diagnosed hypertrophic obstructive cardiomyopathy (HOCM) were older than 50 years of age and as many as 70% were at least 60 years of age (58–60). Hypertensive hypertrophic cardiomyopathy (HHC) is characteristically found in older populations. Whereas older males and females demonstrate generally equal prevalence of obstructive cardiomyopathy, HHC appears to predominate in females (59,61). Some of the hypertrophic cardiomyopathy seen in older patients has been recognized as a genetic disorder, as some late onset cases demonstrate sarcomere protein gene mutations with mutations in the cardiac myosin-binding protein C gene being the most common (62–64).

Hypertrophic cardiomyopathy in older adults needs to be differentiated from the septal bulge or "sigmoid septum" commonly seen in older patients without any other evidence of myocardial hypertrophy (65). The bulge is caused by an increased angulation of the interventricular septum, which can result in as much as a twofold increase in LV outflow tract velocity following amyl nitrate. Although demonstrating an increase in fractional shortening comparable to a patient with hypertrophic cardiomyopathy, subjects with septal bulge appear to have no decrease in end-diastolic dimension, no evidence of anterior malposition, and normal wall thickness apart from the basal septum, suggesting that this constitutes a separate physiological entity (66). Similarly, these patients tend to present with no evidence for myosin-binding protein C gene mutations (67).

HYPERTROPHIC OBSTRUCTIVE CARDIOMYOPATHY

HOCM has an autosomal dominant inheritance pattern with many different mutations, some of which are specific to phenotypic expression at an older age (62,68,69). Although disease severity can vary depending upon the type of mutation, phenotypic expression varies to such a degree as to render the type of mutation a poor indicator of prognosis on a case-by-case basis (70,71). The histological pattern of HOCM has been demonstrated to be distinctly different from the hypertrophy associated with hypertension (72).

Elderly patients diagnosed with HOCM present with an increased severity of symptoms compared to younger individuals; however, the progression of the disease appears to be slower with as many as 23% of elderly patients achieving a normal life expectancy (59,73–75). The annual mortality for the elderly patient with HOCM has been reported to be only 2.6% compared with 5.9% in younger patients, and does not appear to be demonstrably different from that of age- and sex-matched controls (61,76). A significant increase in baseline LV mass measured by either echocardiography or electrocardiography has been associated with a decrease in ejection fraction over time in a cohort of elderly patients (77).

The predominant symptom noted by multiple authors is dyspnea with between one-third and one-half of elderly patients presenting with chest pain (59,74,78,79). Presentation in New York Heart Association Class III or IV heart failure has been noted to increase the annual mortality rate to 36% (61). Between 20% and 30% of patients complain of syncope or presyncope, while some authors report palpitations in as many as half (61,74,76). Classic physical findings include the presence of carotid pulsus bisferiens, a fourth heart sound, and a systolic ejection murmur at the left sternal margin that becomes more prominent with the Valsalva maneuver and less audible with isometric exercise (80,81). The bisferiens pulse may be less noticeable in older patients as a result of increased atherosclerosis in the peripheral vasculature (74,82). Both atrial fibrillation and hypertension have been reported to be more commonly associated with the diagnosis in the elderly, and are also associated with decreased survival (76,83). Patients with obstructive hypertrophic cardiomyopathy and atrial fibrillation have an overall mortality risk ratio of 2.2 compared to HCM patients without obstruction (84). Electrocardiographic presentation in the older adult includes the presence of atrial abnormality, LVH, and bundle branch block; however, the anterior Q waves that are typical of HOCM in the young are only rarely seen (76,85).

Echocardiographic findings in the older patient with HOCM, similar to younger patients, include LVH, systolic anterior motion (SAM) of the anterior leaflet of the mitral valve, and increased LV outflow tract velocity (Figs. 18.4–18.7) (82). LV cavity shape in the elderly appears to be more oval than that of younger patients with HOCM (74). In addition,

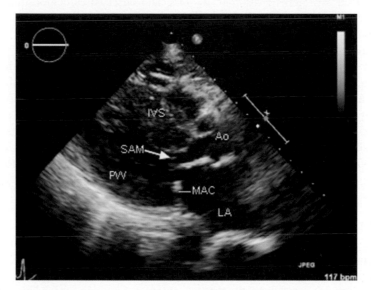

Figure 18.4 Early systolic frame from a two-dimensional parasternal long axis view in a 75-year-old female with HOCM showing a prominent septal bulge and systolic anterior motion of the mitral valve. *Abbreviations*: IVS, interventricular septum; Ao, aortic root; LA, left atrium; PW, posterior wall; MAC, mitral annulur calcification; SAM, systolic anterior motion of the mitral valve leaflets.

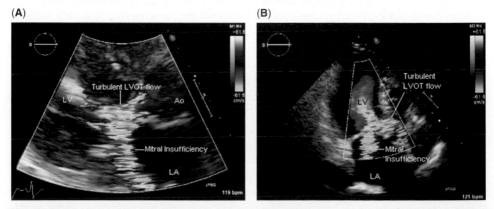

Figure 18.5 Color Doppler flow display superimposed on the same systolic frame from a parasternal long axis view (**A**) and a three chamber view (**B**) in the same patient shown in Figure 18.4, demonstrating significant eccentric mitral regurgitation and turbulent LVOT flow. *Abbreviations*: IVS, interventricular septum; LA, left atrium; LV, left ventricle; LVOT, left ventricular outflow tract.

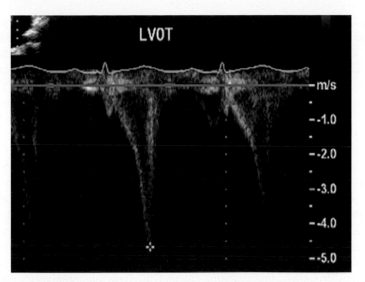

Figure 18.6 High PRF Doppler obtained from interrogation of the LVOT flow in the same patient shown in Figure 18.4, demonstrating a large increase of LVOT velocity (maximum = 5 m/sec) and a Bernoulli-derived gradient of 87 mmHg. The wave form demonstrates the dagger shape that is characteristic of HOCM with a late systolic peak. *Abbreviation*: LVOT, left ventricular outflow tract.

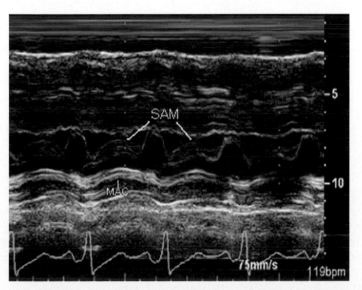

Figure 18.7 M-mode echocardiogram at the mitral valve level in the same patient illustrated in Figure 18.4. During midsystole, a smooth anterior motion at the mitral valve is noted. The mitral valve assumes a flattened curve appearance as it approaches the septum, and the contact with the septum is facilitated by the posterior motion of the septum. Mitral annular calcification is present behind the posterior leaflet. *Abbreviations*: SAM, systolic anterior motion of the mitral valve leaflets; MAC, mitral annular calcification.

mitral annular calcification is much more common in older patients presenting with HOCM, with prevalence rates reported to be anywhere between 30% and 100% (86–89). As a result, the mechanism for outflow tract obstruction may depend more on the posterior displacement of the septum and less on the anterior displacement of the mitral apparatus than it does in younger patients.

β-Adrenergic blocking agents and non-dihydropyridine calcium channel blockers, particularly verapamil, have been shown to reduce symptoms in patients with HOCM; however, no clear effect on mortality has been documented (80,90). As in patients with coronary disease, hypersensitivity to β-adrenergic stimulation accompanied by precipitous clinical deterioration occurs in patients who are abruptly withdrawn from β-blockers (91). Patients who do not respond to β-blockade can have a salutary response to large doses of verapamil (92). Controlled release disopyramide in doses of 150–900 mg daily has also been demonstrated to decrease symptoms in as many as 66% of patients, with a reduction in subaortic gradient of approximately 50% over 3 years (93). All of these agents are relatively contraindicated in patients with conduction system disease in the absence of cardiac pacing. Positive inotropic agents such as digoxin and load-reducing agents such as nitrates, diuretics, and dihydropyridine calcium channel blockers are relatively contraindicated because of their ability to increase the gradient across the LV outflow tract (59,84,89).

Dysrhythmia requires special attention in this patient population. Atrial fibrillation is associated with a diminished long-term prognosis and requires anticoagulation (94). Ventricular dysrhythmia poses a more vexing problem. One trial has demonstrated that ventricular tachycardia or fibrillation appears to be the primary mechanism for sudden death in patients carrying a diagnosis of hypertrophic cardiomyopathy (95). In these cases, implantable defibrillators were found to be efficacious in the treatment of these rhythms and the prevention of sudden death. Mean age in this patient population, however, was 40 ± 16 years with more than half the sample size younger than 41 years. In addition, it is not clear how many of these subjects presented with HOCM and how many had HHC, although the mean age suggests that HOCM might have been the prevailing diagnosis. A subsequent trial demonstrated that LV wall thickness is directly related to the risk of sudden death and may, therefore, be an indicator of the need for automatic implantable cardioverter-defibrillator placement (96).

Once again, however, the mean age was only 47 years with the mean age being youngest (31 years) for the patients with the thickest walls. As a result, it remains unclear at this time how much prescriptive relevance these data have for the older patient with obstructive myopathy. These findings in combination with other observations (vide infra), however, suggest that the appearance of complex ventricular dysrhythmia in the elderly patient with hypertrophic cardiomyopathy does, in fact, suggest a negative prognosis in comparison to patients in whom they do not appear, and these patients should be considered for cardioverter defibrillator placement.

Dual-chamber pacing for patients with HOCM who have not responded to medical therapy has been associated with variable results (97–99). Maron et al. demonstrated a significant reduction in outflow tract velocity in all subjects; however, this finding did not translate into improved functional capacity for any subgroup except for elderly patients, who are older than 65 years (100). As such, pacing may be of some benefit to older adults with HOCM who do not respond well to medical therapy.

In patients who continue to demonstrate Class III or IV symptoms, despite medication and pacing, surgery or transcatheter septal ablation must be considered. Older studies have described symptomatic improvement in as many as 80–90% of patients older than 65 years undergoing surgical myectomy (37,74). Operative mortality, however, has been observed to more than triple in patients older than 65 years when myectomy is combined with coronary artery bypass surgery (101). The concurrent presence of severe mitral annu-lar calcification may require mitral valve surgery as well (88). Data from a six-patient subset of patients with HOCM and mitral annular calcification undergoing myectomy (mean age 61 years) suggests that the myectomy alone may significantly reduce the amount of mitral regurgitation such that mitral surgery may be unnecessary (102). Initially, 1-year follow-up of patients with HOCM as old as 83 years undergoing transcatheter septal abla-tion with ethanol has been favorable (103). Therefore, this procedure may be an acceptable alternative to surgical intervention in selected cases.

Hypertensive Hypertrophic Cardiomyopathy of the Elderly

Topol and colleagues, who reported on 21 elderly patients in 1985, first described HHC (104). There has been significant concern as to whether or not this description represents a genu-inely different pathophysiological entity from other hypertrophic myopathies (105). One study has suggested that the cell cycle is actively deranged in patients (mean age 61 years) with non-HHC compared to patients with hypertensive LVH (106). Similarly, therapy with captopril was associated with regression of ventricular hypertrophy in hypertensive patients, but not in non-hypertensive patients with hypertrophic cardiomyopathy. As such, the pathophysiology of the two groups of patients appears to be different. Patients with HHC may represent a hybrid of pathology that superimposes aspects of hypertensive LVH on a genetic predisposition to primary hypertrophic cardiomyopathy (107). In contradis-tinction to HOCM, sudden death in this patient population appears to be rare, while prog-nosis for survival in general appears to be better (104).

Patients with HHC classically present with flash pulmonary edema in the absence of prior symptoms (59). Although frequently presenting with a chronic history of hyperten-sion, the extent of the blood pressure elevation often does not correlate with the severity of the ventricular hypertrophy (104). The findings on physical examination are somewhat similar to HOCM and feature the absence of neck vein distension, a palpable S4, a LV heave, and a systolic ejection murmur (108). The echocardiogram demonstrates severe LVH with hyperdynamic contractility and cavity obliteration, left atrial dilatation, and delayed opening of the mitral valve. Concentric LVH is more commonly seen than asymmetric sep-tal hypertrophy, and SAM is present in less than one-third of cases (59,104,106).

Medical therapy for patients with HHC is similar to that of patients with HOCM, with the exception that the need for diuretic therapy may be somewhat greater as a result of recurrent episodes of pulmonary edema.

DILATED CARDIOMYOPATHY

Idiopathic dilated cardiomyopathy is primarily a disease of ventricular muscle, with increased LV or biventricular volumes, without an appropriate increase in ventricular septal or free wall thickness, and with depression of LV systolic function (109). Other etiological factors that can cause diffuse LV systolic dysfunction must be excluded (53). Multiple cases of hypocalcemia induced dilated myopathy have been reported in the pediatric age group, however, a 76-year-old female patient has also been described with a reversible dilated myopathy induced by hypocalcemia (110,111). In a large cohort of 554 unselected men and 1243 women aged older than 60 years in a long-term healthcare facility, the preva-lence of idiopathic dilated cardiomyopathy was 1% for both sexes (112). In the same cohort, the prevalence of abnormal LV ejection fraction (<50%) was 29% in men and 21% in women. Approximately 10% of patients with dilated cardiomyopathy are older than 65 years of age (113–116). The diagnosis of dilated cardiomyopathy can be confirmed by echocardiography (Figs. 18.8–18.10) in elderly patients. Coronary angiography should be considered in patients with dilated cardiomyopathy and chest pain. Transthoracic coronary

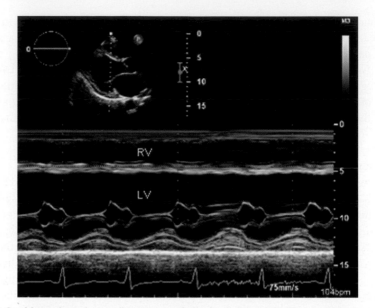

Figure 18.8   M-mode echocardiogram at the mitral valve level in an elderly patient with dilated cardiomyopathy shows thinning of the interventricular septum, a markedly dilated LV cavity (LV), and increased E point septal separation. *Abbreviations*: LV, left ventricle; RV, right ventricle.

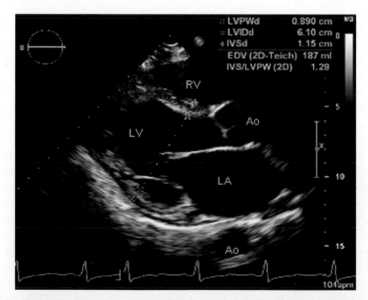

Figure 18.9   Diastolic frame of a two-dimensional echocardiogram from a parasternal long-axis view in an elderly patient with dilated cardiomyopathy shows thinning of the interventricular septum (IVS) and a large LV cavity (LV) with secondary enlargement of the left atrium (LA) and right ventricle (RV). *Abbreviations*: LV, left ventricle; RV, right ventricle; AO, aorta; PW, posterior wall; LA, left atrium.

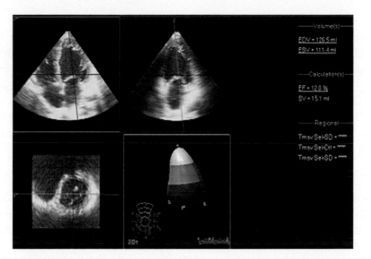

Figure 18.10 Three dimensional imaging of the same patient described in Figures 18.8 and 18.9 demonstrating a three-dimensional reconstruction of the ventricle in diastole with a calculated ejection fraction of only 12% and a stroke volume of only 15cc. *Abbreviations*: EDV, end diastolic volume; ESV, end systolic volume.

echocardiography has been proposed as a useful method for distinguishing between ischemic and non-ischemic dilated cardiomyopathy (117).

Symptoms

Symptoms due to dilated cardiomyopathy include fatigue and weakness resulting from decreased cardiac output, exercise intolerance, dyspnea due to pulmonary congestion, chest pain, and syncope. Symptoms due to systemic or pulmonary emboli may also occur. Physical examination reveals moderate-to-severe cardiomegaly and audible third and fourth heart sounds. Signs of LV or biventricular failure may be present.

Fuster et al. reported 104 patients at the Mayo Clinic with idiopathic dilated cardiomyopathy followed for 6–20 years (115). Of these 104 patients, 73% had congestive heart failure at the time of diagnosis, and 96% had congestive heart failure at follow-up. Systemic emboli were present in 4% of the patients at the time of diagnosis and in 18% of the patients at follow-up. Systemic thromboembolism developed in 8 of 24 patients (33%) with atrial fibrillation and in 11 of 80 patients (14%) with sinus rhythm (p = NS). Systemic thromboembolism developed in 18% of patients who did not receive anticoagulant therapy and in none of those who did (p = 0.05). Of 104 patients, 80 (77%) had died at follow-up, two-thirds of the deaths having occurred within 2 years.

Roberts et al. reported that 148 of 152 necropsy patients (97%) with idiopathic dilated cardiomyopathy had clinical evidence of chronic congestive heart failure (116). Sudden death was the initial manifestation in 114 of 152 patients (75%), and in most patients, ventricular dysrhythmia became intractable and caused death. The mean duration from the onset of chronic congestive heart failure to known death in 120 patients was 54 months. The cause of death was chronic congestive heart failure in 58% of patients, sudden death in 27% of patients, pulmonary emboli in 9% of patients, and other in 6% of patients. Clinical evidence of pulmonary emboli was present in 39% of patients. Clinical evidence of systemic emboli was present in 20% of patients. Of 131 patients, 79 (60%) had either clinical or necropsy evidence, or both, of pulmonary or systemic emboli.

Falk et al., studying 25 patients with non-ischemic dilated cardiomyopathy who were not receiving anticoagulant therapy, demonstrated that a LV thrombus was present on initial echocardiogram in 11 patients (44%), developed during 21.5 months of follow-up in an additional four patients (16%), and disappeared in two patients (8%) during follow-up (118). Systemic thromboembolism developed in 5 of 25 patients (20%) during follow-up. Of the five thromboembolic events, four occurred in patients with echocardiographic evidence of a LV thrombus. These five patients with thromboembolic events were treated with warfarin. No further embolic events occurred in these patients at 15 months of follow-up.

Therapy

The past two decades have witnessed a significant improvement in the prognosis for elderly patients presenting with dilated cardiomyopathy (119). Congestive heart failure in these patients should be treated with salt restriction, diuretics, and ACE inhibitor therapy. Of interest is the observation that elderly hypertensive patients enrolled in the Antihypertensive and Lipid-Lowering Treatment to Prevent Heart Attack Trial (ALLHAT) who were treated with a thiazide diuretic were less likely to develop heart failure than patients treated with an ACE inhibitor (120). Digoxin has been demonstrated to reduce the number of hospital admissions due to heart failure; however, its effect on total mortality appears to be neutral (121). An analysis of a combination of data from both the Randomized Assessment of Digoxin and Inhibitors of Angiotensin-Converting Enzyme (RADIANCE) and the Prospective Randomized Study of Ventricular Failure and Efficacy of Digoxin (PROVED) databases found that the effect of digoxin on clinical outcome was identical even at low serum digoxin levels (0.5–0.9 ng/mL) (122). A subsequent post hoc analysis of data from the Digitalis Investigation Group trial has suggested that there may be a survival benefit conferred on patients with serum digoxin levels less than 1 ng/mL (123). A second post hoc analysis of the same data also suggested an increase in mortality in women with congestive failure taking digoxin; however, a subsequent independent analysis demonstrated no increase in mortality in women with digoxin levels less than 1 ng/mL (124,125). An analysis of the effect of increasing age on patients in the Digitalis Investigation Group database specifically found that advanced age per se was not associated with an increased risk for digoxin intoxication (126).

β-Blockade has now been shown unequivocally to be associated with improvement in symptoms, quality of life, exercise capacity, ejection fraction, and survival (127–131). Multivariate analysis has demonstrated that shorter duration of congestive symptoms and the use of β-blockers are independently associated with reverse remodeling in patients older than 70 years of age with non-ischemic cardiomyopathy (132). This observation has been attributed to an increase in $β_1$-adrenergic receptor density, prolongation of the action potential with secondary increase in calcium influx, and induction of changes in gene expression (133). β-blockade also enhances calcium release channel function as well as increases plasma B-type natriuretic peptides in patients with heart failure (134,135). In addition, β-blockers have been demonstrated to improve contractile dyssynchrony in patients with heart failure who have narrow QRS complexes (136).

Beneficial effects have also been observed in patients with heart failure treated with spironolactone, allopurinol, and AT_1-blockade (131,137,138). The role of anticoagulants in the patient population presenting with sinus rhythm and LV dysfunction is unclear, with some sources suggesting this for severe LV dysfunction (vide supra).

There is no evidence that antiarrhythmic drugs prolong life or prevent sudden cardiac death in patients with dilated cardiomyopathy; however, there is clearly increased survival associated with automatic implantable cardioverter-defibrillator therapy in patients with dilated cardiomyopathy and a low ejection fraction (139). Cardiac resynchronization therapy with biventricular pacing has been shown to be of value in reducing symptoms, improving exercise capacity, reducing complications, and reducing mortality in patients with advanced heart failure, a wide QRS complex, and evidence of contraction dyssynchrony (140). There is also some evidence that biventricular pacing also improves symptoms and reverses remodeling in patients with heart failure, evidence of LV dyssynchrony on echocardiography, and narrow QRS complexes (141). Resynchronization therapy in concert with a cardioverter-defibrillator decreases the risk of clinical heart failure in patients presenting with a low ejection fraction, a wide QRS complex, and no significant pre-existent symptoms of heart failure (142).

The use of natriuretic peptides for the treatment of decompensated heart failure has been controversial. Although in-hospital mortality is apparently reduced in patients with decompensated heart failure at a mean hospitalization of 7.9 days with the use of the natriuretic peptide, nesiritide, when compared to therapy with positive inotropes, a meta-analysis of three trials suggests that mortality at 30 days is increased in patients treated with nesiritide (143,144). A meta-analysis of five trials has also demonstrated a decrease in renal function associated with the use of nesiritide (145).

Additional potential therapies for dilated cardiomyopathy include enhanced external counterpulsation, the use of vasopressin antagonists, and the intriguing possibility of H_2 receptor blockade. Enhanced external counterpulsation has been shown to improve exercise tolerance and New York Heart Association functional classification in patients with dilated cardiomyopathy as well as patients with ischemic disease (146). Tolvaptan, a vasopressin antagonist, has been shown to improve volume loss as well as sodium levels in patients hospitalized with heart failure (147). The H_2 receptor blocker famotidine has been demonstrated to improve symptoms and ventricular remodeling at 24 weeks in a relatively small series of patients, nearly half of which presented with dilated cardiomyopathy (148). Further investigation will be requisite before long-term efficacy and safety can be assessed.

Finally, it has been observed that mobility disability and dementia are independently associated with an increase in short- and long-term mortality in elderly patients with decreased ejection fractions that are admitted with heart failure (149,150). Whether or not active efforts to reverse these geriatric conditions can result in a decrease in overall mortality in elderly patients with heart failure remains to be determined.

REFERENCES

1. Kannel WB, Belanger AJ. Epidemiology of heart failure. Am Heart J 1991; 121: 951–7.
2. Haldeman GA, Croft JB, Giles WH, et al. Hospitalization of patients with heart failure: National Hospital Discharge Survey, 1985 to 1995. Am Heart J 1999; 137: 352–60.
3. Mandinov L. Diastolic heart failure. Cardiovasc Res 2000; 45: 813–25.
4. Gottdiener JS, McClelland RL, Marshall R, et al. Outcome of congestive heart failure in elderly persons: influence of left ventricular systolic function. Ann Intern Med 2002; 137: 631–9.
5. Vasan RS, Larson MG, Benjamin EJ, et al. Defining diastolic heart failure: a call for standardized diagnostic criteria. Circulation 2000; 101: 2118.
6. Bhatia RS, Tu JV, Lee DS, et al. Outcome of heart failure with preserved ejection fraction in a population based study. N Engl J Med 2006; 355: 260–9.
7. Owan TE, Hodge DO, Herges RM, et al. Trends in prevalence and outcome of heart failure with preserved ejection fraction. N Engl J Med 2006; 355: 251–9.
8. Cohn JN, Johnson G. Heart failure with normal ejection fraction. Circulation 1990; 81: 48–53.
9. Arques S, Ambrosi P, Gelisse R, et al. Hypoalbuminemia in elderly patients with acute diastolic heart failure. J Am Coll Cardiol 2003; 42: 712–16.
10. Brutsaert DL, Sys SU, Gillebert TC. Diastolic failure: pathophysiology and therapeutic implications. J Am Coll Cardiol 1993; 22: 318–25.
11. Backes RJ, Gersh BJ. Cardiomyopathies in the elderly. Cardiovasc Clin 1992; 22: 105–25.

12. Kajstura J, Cheng W, Sarangarajan R, et al. Necrotic and apoptotic myocyte cell death in the aging heart of Fischer 344 rats. Am J Physiol 1996; 217: H1215–28.

13. Brenner DA, Apstein CS, Saupe KW. Exercise training attenuates age-associated diastolic dysfunction in rats. Circulation 2001; 104: 221–6.

14. Kawaguchi M, Hay I, Fetics B, et al. Combined ventricular systolic and arterial stiffening in patients with heart failure and preserved ejection fraction: implications for systolic and diastolic reserve limitations. Circulation 2003; 107: 714–20.

15. Kasama S, Toyama T, Kumakura H, et al. Effects of candesartan on cardiac sympathetic nerve activity in patients with congestive heart failure and preserved left ventricular ejection fraction. J Am Coll Cardiol 2005; 45: 661–7.

16. Fukuta H, Sane DC, Brucks S, et al. Statin therapy may be associated with lower mortality in patients with diastolic heart failure: a preliminary report. Circulation 2005; 112: 357–63.

17. Mottram PM, Haluska B, Leano R, et al. Effect of aldosterone antagonism on myocardial dysfunction in hypertensive patients with diastolic heart failure. Circulation 2004; 110: 558–65.

18. Hayashida W, Van Eyll C, Rousseau MF, et al. Regional remodeling and nonuniform changes in diastolic function in patients with left ventricular dysfunction: modification by long-term enalapril treatment. J Am Coll Cardiol 1993; 22: 1403–10.

19. Massie BM, Carson PE, McMurray JJ, et al. Irbesartan in patientws with heart failure and preserved ejection fraction. N Engl J Med 2008; 359: 2456–67.

20. Roongsritong C, Sutthiwan P, Bradley J, et al. Spironolactone improves diastolic function in the elderly. Clin Cardiol 2005; 28: 484–7.

21. Zile MR, Gaasch WH, Anand IS, et al. Mode of death in patients with heart failure and a preserved ejection fraction: results from the Irbesartan in Heart Failure with Preserved Ejection Fraction Study (I-Preserve) trial. Circulation 2010; 121: 1393–405.

22. Zieman SJ, Fortuin NJ. Hypertrophic and restrictive cardiomyopathies in the elderly. Cardiol Clin 1999; 17: 159–72.

23. Eriksson P, Boman K, Jacobsson B, et al. Cardiac arrhythmias in familial amyloid polyneuropathy during anaesthesia. Acta Anaesthesiol Scand 1986; 30: 317–20.

24. Child JS, Perloff JK. The restrictive cardiomyopathies. Cardiol Clin 1988; 6: 289–316.

25. Winters SL, Cohen M, Greenberg S, et al. Sustained ventricular tachycardia associated with sarcoidosis: assessment of the underlying cardiac anatomy and the prospective utility of programmed ventricular stimulation, drug therapy and an implantable antitachycardia device. J Am Coll Cardiol 1991; 18: 937–43.

26. Nakata T, Shimamoto K, Yonekura S, et al. Cardiac sympathetic denervation in transthyretin-related familial amyloidotic polyneuropathy: detection with iodine-123-MIBG. J Nucl Med 1995; 36: 1040–2.

27. Schoenfeld MH. The differentiation of restrictive cardiomyopathy from constrictive pericarditis. Cardiol Clin 1990; 8: 663–71.

28. Tresch DD, McGough MF. Heart failure with normal systolic function: a common disorder in older people. J Am Geriatr Soc 1995; 43: 1035–42.

29. Fauci AS, Harley JB, Roberts WC, et al. The idiopathic hypereosinophilic syndrome: clinical pathophysiologic and therapeutic considerations. Ann Intern Med 1982; 97: 78–92.

30. Falk RH, Comenzo RL, Skinner M. The systemic amyloidoses. N Engl J Med 1997; 337: 898–909.

31. Kushwaha SS, Fallen JT, Fuster V. Restrictive cardiomyopathy. N Engl J Med 1997; 336: 267–76.

32. Kawamura S, Takahashi M, Ishihara T, et al. Incidence and distribution of isolated atrial amyloid: histologic and immunohistochemical studies of 100 aging hearts. Pathol Int 1995; 45: 335–42.

33. Kyle RA, Linos A, Beard CM, et al. Incidence and natural history of primary systemic amyloidosis in Olmsted County Minnesota 1950 through 1989. Blood 1992; 79: 1817–22.

34. Liao R, Jain M, Teller P, et al. Infusion of light chains from patients with cardiac amyloidosis causes diastolic dysfunction in isolated mouse hearts. Circulation 2001; 104: 1594–7.

35. Cueto-Garcia L, Reeder GS, Kyle RA, et al. Echocardiographic findings in systemic amyloidosis: spectrum of cardiac involvement and relation to survival. J Am Coll Cardiol 1985; 45: 335–43.

36. Katritsis D, Wilmshurst PT, Wendon JA, et al. Primary restrictive cardiomyopathy: clinical and pathologic characteristics. J Am Coll Cardiol 1991; 18: 1230–5.

37. Klein AL, Hatle LK, Taliercio CP, et al. Prognostic significance of Doppler measures of diastolic function in cardiac amyloidosis: a Doppler echocardiography study. Circulation 1991; 83: 808–16.

38. Falk RH, Rubinow A, Cohen AS. Cardiac arrhythmias in systemic amyloidosis: correlation with echocardiographic abnormalities. J Am Coll Cardiol 1984; 3: 107–13.

39. Dubrey SW, Cha K, Skinner M, et al. Familial and primary (AL) amyloidosis: echocardiographically similar diseases with distinctly different clinical outcomes. Heart 1997; 78: 74–82.

40. Angomachalelis N, Hourzamanis A, Vamvalis C, et al. Doppler echocardiographic evaluation of left ventricular diastolic function in patients with systemic sarcoidosis. Postgrad Med J 1992; 68: S52–6.
41. Matsui Y, Iwai K, Tachihana T, et al. Clinico-pathological study on fatal myocardial sarcoidosis. Ann N Y Acad Sci 1976; 278: 445–69.
42. Roberts WC, McAllister HA, Ferrans VJ. Sarcoidosis of the heart. Am J Med 1977; 63: 86–108.
43. Stein E, ladder I, Stimmel B, et al. Asymptomatic electrocardiographic alterations in sarcoidosis. Am Heart J 1973; 86: 474–7.
44. Mitchell DN, duBois RM, Oldershaw PJ. Cardiac sarcoidosis: a potentially fatal condition that needs expert assessment. Br Med J 1997; 314: 320–1.
45. Ballantyne GH, Savoca PE, Flannery JT, et al. Incidence and mortality of carcinoids of the colon: data from the Connecticut tumor registry. Cancer 1992; 69: 2400–5.
46. Pellikka PA, Tajik AJ, Khandheria BK, et al. Carcinoid heart disease: clinical and echocardiographic spectrum in 74 patients. Circulation 1993; 87: 1188–96.
47. Hesse A, Altland K, Linke RP, et al. Cardiac amyloidosis: a review and report of a new transthyretin (prealbumin) variant. Br Heart J 1993; 70: 111–15.
48. Falk RH, Plehn JF, Deering Sensitivity and specificity of the echocardiographic features of cardiac amyloidosis. Am J Cardiol 1987; 59: 418–22.
49. Pai RG, Shah PM. Echo-Doppler evaluation of left ventricular diastolic function. Am Coll Cardiol Curr J Rev 1994; 3: 30–3.
50. Vasan RS, Benjamin EJ, Levy D. Congestive heart failure with normal left ventricular systolic function. Arch Intern Med 1996; 156: 146–57.
51. Lubien E, DeMaria A, Krishnaswamy P, et al. Utility of B-natriuretic peptide in detecting diastolic dysfunction: comparison with Doppler velocity recordings. Circulation 2002; 105: 595–601.
52. Mason JW, O'Connell JB. Clinical merit of endomyocardial biopsy. Circulation 1989; 79: 971–9.
53. Shah PM, Abelmann WH, Gersh BJ. Cardiomyopathy in the elderly. J Am Coll Cardiol 1987; 10: 77A–9A.
54. Wilson JR, Reichek N, Dunkman WB, et al. Effect of diuresis on the performance of the failing left ventricle in man. Am J Med 1981; 70: 234–9.
55. Packer M. Abnormalities of diastolic function as a potential cause of exercise intolerance in chronic heart failure. Circulation 1990; 81: 78–86.
56. Shah AM, Lewis MJ, Henderson AH. Effects of 8-bromo-cyclic GMP on contraction and on inotropic response of ferret cardiac muscle. J Mol Cell Cardiol 1991; 23: 55–64.
57. McDougall NI, Purvis JA, Wilson CM, et al. Asystolic arrest as a presentation of sarcoidosis. Int J Cardiol 1994; 47: 165–7.
58. Petrin TJ, Tavel ME. Idiopathic hypertrophic subaortic stenosis as observed in a large community hospital: relation to age and history of hypertension. J Am Geriatr Soc 1979; 27: 43–6.
59. Cannan CR, Reeder GS, Bailey KR, et al. Natural history of hypertrophic cardiomyopathy: a population-based study, 1976 through 1990. Circulation 1995; 92: 2488–95.
60. Kubo T, Kitaoka H, Okawa M, Nishinaga M, Doi YL. Hypertrophic cardiomyopathy in the elderly. Geriatr Gerontol Int 2010; 10: 9–16.
61. Fay WP, Taliercio CP, Ilstrup DM, et al. Natural history of hypertrophic cardiomyopathy in the elderly. J Am Coll Cardiol 1990; 16: 821–6.
62. Niimura H, Bachinski LL, Sangwatanaroj S, et al. Mutations in the gene for cardiac myosin-binding protein C and late-onset familial hypertrophic cardiomyopathy. N Engl J Med 1998; 338: 1248–57.
63. Niimura H, Patton KK, McKenna WJ, et al. Sarcomere protein gene mutations in hypertrophic cardiomyopathy of the elderly. Circulation 2002; 105: 446–51.
64. Wang L, Seidman JG, Seidman CE. Narrative review: harnessing molecular genetics for the diagnosis and management of hypertrophic cardiomyopathy. Ann Intern Med 2010; 152: 5134–520.
65. Goor D, Lillehei CW, Edwards JE. The "sigmoid septum": variation in the contour of the left ventricular outlet. Arch Pathol 1969; 107: 366–76.
66. Krasnow N. Subaortic septal bulge simulates hypertrophic cardiomyopathy by angulation of the septum with age, independent of focal hypertrophy: an echocardiographic study. J Am Soc Echocardiogr 1997; 10: 545–55.
67. Binder J, Ommen SR, Gersh BJ, et al. Echocardiography guided genetic testing in hypertrophic cardiomyopathy: septal morphological features predict the presence of myofilament mutations. Mayo Clin Proc 2006; 81: 459–67.
68. Watkins H. Multiple disease genes cause hypertrophic cardiomyopathy. Br Heart J 1994; 72(Suppl): S4–9.

69. Konno T, Shimizu M, Ino H, et al. A novel missense mutation in the myosin binding protein-C gene is responsible for hypertrophic cardiomyopathy with left ventricular dysfunction and dilation in elderly patients. J Am Coll Cardiol 2003; 41: 781–6.

70. Seidman JG, Seidman C. The genetic basis for cardiomyopathy: from mutation identification to mechanistic paradigms. Cell 2001; 104: 557–67.

71. Ackerman MJ, VanDriest SL, Ommen SR, et al. Prevalence and age-dependence of malignant mutations in the beta-myosin heavy chain and troponin T genes in hypertrophic cardiomyopathy. J Am Coll Cardiol 2002; 39: 2042–8.

72. Davies MJ, McKenna WJ. Hypertrophic cardiomyopathy: an introduction to pathology and pathogenesis. Br Heart J 1994; 72: S2–3.

73. Spirito P, Maron BJ. Absence of progression of left ventricular hypertrophy in adult patients with hypertrophic cardiomyopathy. J Am Coll Cardiol 1987; 9: 1013–17.

74. Lewis JF, Maron BJ. Clinical and morphological expression of hypertrophic cardiomyopathy in patients ≥65 years of age. J Am Coll Cardiol 1994; 73: 1105–11.

75. Maron BJ, Casey S, Hauser RG, et al. Clinical course of hypertrophic cardiomyopathy with survival to advanced age. J Am Coll Cardiol 2003; 42: 882–8.

76. McKenna W, Deanfield J, Faruqui A, et al. Prognosis in hypertrophic cardiomyopathy: role of age and clinical, electrocardiographic and hemodynamic features. Am J Cardiol 1981; 47: 532–8.

77. Drazner MH, Rame JE, Marino EK, et al. Increased left ventricular mass is a risk factor for the development of a depressed left ventricular ejection fraction within five years. J Am Coll Cardiol 2004; 43: 2207–15.

78. Lever HM, Karam RF, Currie PJ, et al. Hypertrophic cardiomyopathy in the elderly: distinctions from the young based on cardiac shape. Circulation 1989; 79: 580–9.

79. Agaston AS, Polakoff R, Hippogoankar R, et al. The significance of increased left ventricular outflow tract velocities in the elderly measured by continuous wave Doppler. Am Heart J 1989; 117: 1320–6.

80. Wigle ED, Rakowski H, Kimball BP, et al. Hypertrophic cardiomyopathy: clinical spectrum and treatment. Circulation 1995; 92: 1680–92.

81. Cassidy J, Aronow WS, Prakash R. The effect of isometric exercise on the systolic murmur of patients with idiopathic hypertrophic subaortic stenosis. Chest 1975; 67: 395–7.

82. Shenoy MM, Khanna A, Nejat M, et al. Hypertrophic cardiomyopathy in the elderly: a frequently misdiagnosed disease. Arch Intern med 1986; 146: 658–61.

83. Chikamori T, Doi YL, Dickie S, et al. Comparison of clinical features in patients >60 years of age to those ≤40 years of age with hypertrophic cardiomyopathy. Am J Cardiol 1990; 66: 875–8.

84. Hamby RI, Aintablian A. Hypertrophic subaortic stenosis is not rare in the eighth decade. Geriatrics 1976; 31: 71–4.

85. Olivotto I, Cecchi F, Casey SA, et al. Impact of atrial fibrillation on the clinical course of hypertrophic cardiomyopathy. Circulation 2001; 104: 2517–24.

86. Kronzon I, Glassman E. Mitral ring calcification in Idiopathic hypertrophic subaortic stenosis. Am J Cardiol 1978; 4: 60–6.

87. Motamed HE, Roberts WC. Frequency and significance of mitral annular calcium in hypertrophic cardiomyopathy: analysis of 200 necropsy patients. Am J Cardiol 1987; 60: 877–84.

88. Aronow WS, Kronzon I. Prevalence of hypertrophic cardiomyopathy and its association with mitral annular calcium in elderly patients. Chest 1988; 94: 1295–6.

89. Lewis JF, Maron BJ. Elderly patients with hypertrophic cardiomyopathy: a subset with distinctive left ventricular morphology and progressive clinical course late in life. J Am Coll Cardiol 1989; 13: 36–45.

90. Seiler C, Hess OM, Schoenbeck M, et al. Long-term follow-up of medical versus surgical therapy for hypertrophic cardiomyopathy: a retrospective study. J Am Coll Cardiol 1991; 17: 634–42.

91. Gilligan DM, Chan WL, Stewart R, et al. Adrenergic hypersensitivity after beta-blocker withdrawal in hypertrophic cardiomyopathy. Am J Cardiol 1991; 68: 766–72.

92. Rosing DR, Idanpaan-Heikkila U, Maron BJ, et al. Use of calcium-channel blocking drugs in hypertrophic cardiomyopathy. Am J Cardiol 1985; 55: 185B–95B.

93. Sherrid MV, Barac I, McKenna WJ, et al. Multicenter study of the efficacy and safety of disopyramide in obstructive hypertrophic cardiomyopathy. J Am Coll Cardiol 2005; 45: 1251.

94. Maron BJ, Bonow RO, Cannon RO, et al. Hypertrophic cardiomyopathy: interrelations of clinical manifestations, pathophysiology, and therapy (second of two parts). N Engl J Med 1987; 316: 844–52.

95. Maron BJ, Shen W, Link MS, et al. Efficacy of implantable cardioverter-defibrillators for the prevention of sudden death in patients with hypertrophic cardiomyopathy. N Engl J Med 2000; 342: 365–73.

96. Spirito P, Bellone P, Harris KM, et al. Magnitude of left ventricular hypertrophy and the risk of sudden death in hypertrophic cardiomyopathy. N Engl J Med 2000; 342: 1778–85.

97. Betocchi S, Losi MA, Piscione F, et al. Effects of dual chamber pacing in hypertrophic cardiomyopathy on left ventricular outflow tract obstruction and on diastolic function. Am J Cardiol 1996; 77: 498–502.

98. Nishimura RA, Trusty JM, Hayes DL, et al. Dual-chamber pacing for hypertrophic obstructive cardiomyopathy: a randomized, double-blind crossover trial. J Am Coll Cardiol 1997; 29: 435–41.

99. Linde C, Gadler F, Kappenberger L, et al. Placebo effect of pacemaker implantation in obstructive hypertrophic cardiomyopathy. Am J Cardiol 1999; 83: 903–7.

100. Maron BJ, Nishimura RA, McKenna WJ, et al. Assessment of permanent dual-chamber pacing as a treatment for drug-refractory symptomatic patients with obstructive hypertrophic cardiomyopathy. Circulation 1999; 99: 2927–33.

101. Cooper MM, McIntosh CL, Tucker E, et al. Operation for hypertrophic subaortic stenosis in the aged. Ann Thorac Surg 1987; 44: 370–8.

102. Yu EHC, Omran AS, Wigle D, et al. Mitral regurgitation in hypertrophic obstructive cardiomyopathy: relationship to obstruction and relief with myectomy. J Am Coll Cardiol 2000; 36: 2219–25.

103. Lakkis NM, Nagueh SF, Dunn JK, et al. Nonsurgical septal reduction therapy for hypertrophic obstructive cardiomyopathy: one-year follow-up. J Am Coll Cardiol 2000; 36: 852–8.

104. Topol EJ, Traill TA, Fortuin NJ. Hypertensive hypertrophic cardiomyopathy of the elderly. N Engl J Med 1985; 312: 277–83.

105. Karam R, Lever HM, Healy BP. Hypertensive hypertrophic cardiomyopathy or hypertrophic cardiomyopathy with hypertension? A study of 78 patients. J Am Coll Cardiol 1988; 12: 989–95.

106. Takeda A, Takeda N. Different pathophysiology of cardiac hypertrophy in hypertension and hypertrophic cardiomyopathy. J Mol Cell Cardiol 1997; 29: 2961–5.

107. Shapiro LM. Hypertrophic cardiomyopathy in the elderly. Br Heart J 1990; 63: 265–6.

108. Williams B, Isaacson JH, Lauer MS. An 81-year-old woman with dyspnea on exertion. Cleve Clin J Med 1996; 63: 209–12.

109. Stevenson LW, Perloff JK. The dilated cardiomyopathies: clinical aspects. Cardiol Clin 1988; 6: 197–218.

110. Brown J, Nunez S, Russell M, Spurney C. Hypocalcemic rickets and dilated cardiomyopathy: case reports and review of literature. Pediatr Cardiol 2009; 30: 818–23.

111. Behagel A, Donal E. Hypocalcemia-induced dilated cardiomyopathy in elderly: a case report. Eur J Echocardiogr 2011; 12: E38.

112. Aronow WS, Ahn C, Kronzon I. Prevalence of echocardiographic findings in 554 men and in 1243 women aged >60 years in a long term health care facility. Am J Cardiol 1997; 79: 379–80.

113. Torp A. Incidence of congestive cardiomyopathy. Postgrad Med J 1978; 54: 435–9.

114. Segal JP, Stapleton JF, McClellan JR, et al. Idiopathic cardiomyopathy: clinical features, prognosis and therapy. Curr Probl Cardiol 1978; 3: 1–48.

115. Fuster V, Gersh BJ, Giuliani ER, et al. The natural history of idiopathic dilated cardiomyopathy. Am J Cardiol 1981; 47: 525–31.

116. Roberts WC, Siegel RJ, McManus BM. Idiopathic dilated cardiomyopathy: analysis of 152 necropsy patients. Am J Cardiol 1987; 60: 1340–55.

117. Sawada SG, Ryan T, Segar D, et al. Distinguishing ischemic cardiomyopathy from nonischemic dilated cardiomyopathy with coronary echocardiography. J Am Coll Cardiol 1992; 19: 1223–8.

118. Falk RH, Foster E, Coats MH. Ventricular thrombi and thromboembolism in dilated cardiomyopathy: a prospective follow up study. Am Heart J 1992; 123: 136–42.

119. Kubo T, Matsumura Y, Okawa M, et al. Improvement in prognosis of dilated cardiomyopathy in the elderly over the past 20 years. J Cardiol 2008; 52: 111–17.

120. Davis BR, Piller LB, Cutler JA, et al. Role of diuretics in the prevention of heart failure: the antihypertensive and lipid-lowering treatment to prevent heart attack trial. Circulation 2006; 113: 2201–10.

121. Van Veldhuisen DJ, de Graeff PA, Remme WJ, et al. Value of digoxin in heart failure and sinus rhythm: new features of an old drug. J Am Coll Cardiol 1996; 28: 813–19.

122. Adams KF, Gheorghiade M, Uretsky BF, et al. Clinical benefits of low serum digoxin concentrations in heart failure. J Am Coll Cardiol 2002; 39: 946–53.

123. Ahmed A, Rich MW, Love TE, et al. Digoxin and reduction in mortality and hospitalization in heart failure: a comprehensive post hoc analysis of the DIG trail. Eur Heart J 2006; 27: 178–86.

124. Rathore SS, Wang Y, Krumholz HM. Sex-based differences in the effect of digoxin for the treatment of heart failure. N Engl J Med 2002; 347: 1403–11.

125. Adams KF, Patterson JH, Gattis WA, et al. Relationship of serum digoxin concentration to mortality and morbidity in women in the digitalis investigation group trial: a retrospective analysis. J Am Coll Cardiol 2005; 46: 497–504.

126. Rich MW, McSherry F, Williford WO, et al. Effect of age on mortality, hospitalizations and response to digoxin in patients with heart failure: the DIG study. J Am Coll Cardiol 2001; 38: 806–13.

127. Packer M, Bristow M, Cohn J, et al. The effect of carvedilol on morbidity and mortality in patients with chronic heart failure. N Engl J Med 1996; 334: 1349–55.

128. Macdonald PS, Keogh AM, Aboyoun CL, et al. Tolerability and efficacy of carvedilol in patients with New York Heart Association class IV heart failure. J Am Coll Cardiol 1999; 33: 924–31.

129. Sanderson JE, Chan SKW, Yip G, et al. Beta-blockade in heart failure: a comparison of carvedilol with metoprolol. J Am Coll Cardiol 1999; 33: 1522–8.

130. MERIT-HF Study Group. Effect of metoprolol CR/XL in chronic heart failure: metoprolol CR/XL randomised intervention trial in congestive heart failure (MERIT-HF). Lancet 1999; 353: 2001–7.

131. Pitt B, Zannad F, Remme WJ, et al. The effect of spironolactone on morbidity and mortality in patients with severe heart failure. N Engl J Med 1999; 341: 709–17.

132. Cioffi G, Tarantini L, DeFeo S, et al. Pharmacological left ventricular reverse remodeling in elderly patients receiving optimal therapy for chronic heart failure. Eur J Heart Fail 2005; 7: 1040–8.

133. Barry WH, Gilbert EM. How do β-blockers improve ventricular function in patients with congestive heart failure? Circulation 2003; 107: 2395–97.

134. Reiken S, Wehrens XHT, Vest JA, et al. β-Blockers restore calcium release channel function and improve cardiac muscle performance in human heart failure. Circulation 2003; 107: 2459–66.

135. Davis ME, Richards AM, Nicholls G, et al. Introduction of metoprolol increases plasma B-type cardiac natriuretic peptides in mild, stable heart failure. Circulation 2006; 113: 977–85.

136. Takemoto Y, Hozumi T, Sugioka K, et al. Beta-blocker therapy induces ventricular resynchronization in dilated cardiomyopathy with narrow QRS complex. J Am Coll Cardiol 2007; 49: 778–83.

137. Cappola TP, Kass DA, Nelson GS, et al. Allopurinol improves myocardial efficiency in patients with idiopathic dilated cardiomyopathy. Circulation 2001; 104: 2407–11.

138. Cohn JN, Tognoni G. A randomized trial of the angiotensin-receptor blocker valsartan in chronic heart failure. N Engl J Med 2001; 345: 1667–75.

139. Goldberger Z, Lampert R. Implantable cardioverter-defibrillators: expanding indications and technologies. JAMA 2006; 295: 809–18.

140. Cleland JGF, Daubert J-C, Erdmann E, et al. The effect of cardiac resynchronization on morbidity and mortality in heart failure. N Engl J Med 2005; 352: 1539–49.

141. Bleeker GB, Holman ER, Steendijk P, et al. Cardiac resynchronization therapy in patients with a narrow QRS complex. J Am Coll Cardiol 2006; 48: 2243–50.

142. Moss AJ, Hall WJ, Cannom DS, et al. Cardiac-resynchronization therapy for the prevention of heart-failure events. N Engl J Med 2009; 361: 1329–38.

143. Abraham WT, Adams KF, Fonarow GC, et al. In-hospital mortality in patients with acute decompensated heart failure requiring intravenous vasoactive medications. J Am Coll Cardiol 2005; 46: 57–64.

144. Sackner-Bernstein JD, Kowalski M, Fox M, et al. Short-term risk of death after treatment with nesiritide for decompensated heart failure: a pooled analysis of randomized controlled trials. JAMA 2005; 293: 1900–5.

145. Sackner-Bernstein JD, Skopicki HA, Aaronson KD. Risk of worsening renal function with nesiritide in patients with acutely decompensated heart failure. Circulation 2005; 111: 1487–91.

146. Feldman AM, Silver MA, Francis GS, et al. Enhanced external counterpulsation improves exercise tolerance in patients with chronic heart failure. J Am Coll Cardiol 2006; 48: 1198–205.

147. Gheorghiade M, Gattis WA, O'Connor CM, et al. Effects of tolvaptan, a vasopressin antagonist, in patients hospitalized with worsening heart failure: a randomized controlled trial. JAMA 2004; 291: 1963–71.

148. Kim J, Ogai A, Nakatani S, et al. Impact of blockade of histamine H2 receptors on chronic heart failure revealed by retrospective and prospective randomized studies. J Am Coll Cardiol 2006; 48: 1378–84.

149. Chaudhry SI, Wang Y, Gill TM, Krumholz HM. Geriatric conditions and subsequent mortality in older patients with heart failure. J Am Coll Cardiol 2010; 55: 309–16.

150. Venkitachalam L, Spertus JA. Stepping outside of the heart: using nontraditional patient characteristics to understand and improve outcomes. J Am Coll Cardiol 2010l; 55: 317–19.

19
Thyroid heart disease in the elderly

Myron Miller and Steven R. Gambert

SUMMARY

Thyroid hormones have multiple effects on cardiac tissue, vasculature, and lipid metabolism. Thyroid disorders are common, especially in older persons, both as overt hyperthyroidism and hypothyroidism and as their subclinical forms. Consequent alterations in thyroid hormone production can have significant effects on cardiac and vascular function and are associated with increased risk of cardiovascular disorders, morbidity, and mortality. Recognition and effective management of altered thyroid function has the potential to correct the adverse effects of thyroid disease on the cardiovascular system and on altered lipid metabolism. Amiodarone, a drug commonly used in the management of cardiac arrhythmias, is associated with a high prevalence of alterations in thyroid function and with development of both hyperthyroidism and hypothyroidism. Careful monitoring of thyroid function will allow prompt recognition and effective management of these disorders.

INTRODUCTION

Thyroid dysfunction may be accompanied by a number of cardiovascular manifestations. In some circumstances, the presence of a cardiovascular disorder may lead to the clinical diagnosis of thyroid dysfunction. The effects of severe thyroid disease have been increasingly researched and expanded upon since the early nineteenth century and numerous studies have increased our understanding of the molecular and cellular basis for the cardiovascular changes occurring in thyroid disease. The hemodynamic changes associated with both hyper- and hypothyroidism have been measured and continue to be an area of research effort. The effects of subclinical stages of thyroid disease on the cardiovascular system and the potential benefits of treatment at this early disease stage are reported with increasing frequency in the literature. This review will address recent progress in defining the mechanism of thyroid hormone action on the heart as well as the hemodynamic changes, clinical consequences, and treatment options associated with both overt and subclinical disorders of thyroid function.

MECHANISMS OF THYROID HORMONE ACTION

Through the action of the hypothalamic releasing hormone (TRH), thyrotropin or thyroid-stimulating hormone (TSH) is released from the anterior pituitary and stimulates the release of thyroxine (T4) and triiodothyronine (T3) from the thyroid gland. T3 is the more active cellular form of thyroid hormone and has both genomic and nongenomic actions to influence cardiac function by effects on stimulation of transcriptional processes and cellular membrane activity. The genomic actions of T3 are mediated predominately by binding of T3 to nuclear receptors of the same super family as those for steroid hormones. This mechanism has been reviewed (1). In brief, T4 and T3 rapidly cross membranes because of their lipophilic nature and possibly through specific transport proteins located in the cell membrane of cardiac myocytes. Thyroid hormone enters the nucleus and binds with high affinity to thyroid hormone receptors. These are activated either as a homodimer or bind a second hormone receptor and become activated as a heterodimer (2,3). These in turn bind to the DNA of target genes' thyroid response elements in various configurations leading to either stimulation or inhibition of gene activity and transcriptional activity (4–7). The multiple hemodynamic changes reported in hyperthyroidism may be explained by the transcriptional changes of several genes. Thyroid hormone-responsive target genes include both regulatory and structural genes. These include transcriptional modulation of myosin heavy chain alpha, myosin heavy chain beta, making up the thick filament of cardiac myocytes, sarcoplasmic reticulum calcium-ATPase, Na,K-ATPase, phospholamban, voltage-gated potassium channels, adenylyl cyclase types V and VI, and the Na, Ca exchanger (8–14). The activation of the myosin heavy chain alpha gene results in an increase in muscle fiber velocity and theoretically in increased myocardial contractility. The dominant component in human myofibril proteins is myosin heavy chain beta, which is repressed (7,8) making the exact contribution of these structural proteins to human cardiovascular manifestations of thyroid disease less certain. Another indirect genomic action of thyroid hormone is the alteration in function of the sarcoplasmic reticulum, including sarcoplasmic reticulum calcium-ATPase and phospholamban. In hyperthyroid heart disease, the release of calcium and subsequent reuptake by the sarcoplasmic reticulum, which determines systolic contractile function as well as diastolic relaxation, is altered. This process favors an increase in myocardial contractility (inotropy) and an improvement in diastolic relaxation. Upregulation of sarcoplasmic reticulum calcium-ATPase and changes in the phosphorylation of phospholamban can increase contractility as well as diastolic relaxation and may account for the hemodynamic changes in thyroid disease (10–12).

Although thyroid hormone has a direct effect on the cardiovascular system by modulating the rate of transcription of multiple genes, T3 also exerts nongenomic effects on the cellular membrane. Thyroid hormone was first shown to exert a direct effect on myocardial tissue when T4 was incubated with fragments of cardiac tissues from chicken embryos resulting in an increased rate of contraction. Several studies using cardiac muscle, specifically cat papillary muscles, demonstrated an increase in heart rate, isometric tension, and velocity of muscle shortening in the presence of thyroid hormone, in the absence of adrenergic tissue, and in the presence of depletion or blockage of catecholamines (15,16). The rapid increase in cardiac output following an intravenous infusion of T3 supports a direct effect of T3 on cellular membranes (17). Extranuclear effects include alterations of various membrane channels and subsequent changes in calcium, sodium, and potassium as mediated through the ATPase system, notably Na, K-ATPase. This increase in concentration leads to short-term increases in both inotropy and chronotropy (18–23). The increase in myocyte contractile function in the presence of T3 is due to alterations of multiple cell membrane enzyme systems including a direct effect on myocyte sarcolemmal transduction (20). Not only are there alterations in solute transport (calcium and sodium), but there is also a modulation of mitochondrial respiration, changes in several kinases that may promote signal transduction pathways, and several relevant thyroid hormone-binding sites distinct from nuclear binding sites (22). In autoimmune-mediated hyperthyroidism, myocardial tissue pathology reveals fibroblast infiltration and degenerative changes. Patients with resulting cardiomyopathy have been found to have antibody receptor binding to TSH receptors in the human heart (4). The results of these studies support a role for a nongenomic or direct effect of the thyroid hormone on cardiovascular function. Because several of the membrane channel proteins are upregulated at a nuclear level by thyroid hormone, the boundaries of the genomic and nongenomic actions of thyroid hormone are not clear.

The manifestations of hyperthyroidism resemble an increased adrenergic state. For this reason, an increased sensitivity to adrenergic stimulation in hyperthyroidism has been proposed. Although hyperthyroidism does affect various components of the adrenergic system and a synergistic effect has been reported between thyroid hormone and epinephrine, other data have not supported the role of an increased sensitivity to catecholamines as the sole cause of the cardiovascular manifestations of hyperthyroidism. Early studies have suggested an adrenergic contribution secondary to the observation that sympathetic blockade could relieve thyroid storm and alterations in cardiovascular function (24,25). Also, sympatholytic agents, specifically β-adrenergic blockers, have been and continue to be effective in reducing many of the cardiovascular manifestations of hyperthyroidism (26–29). Several mechanisms have been proposed to explain the synergism between catecholamines and thyroid hormone including an increase in the number of adrenergic receptor sites, an increase in the sensitivity of adrenergic receptors, an increase in tissue levels of free catecholamines, and thyroid stimulation of adrenergic nerve terminals (30,31). Data support a positive or upregulation of β1-adrenergic receptors in hyperthyroidism, whereas several other components of the adrenergic-receptor complex are negatively or downregulated, so that the net effect on the sensitivity of the heart to adrenergic stimulation in hyperthyroidism remains normal (32–34). Despite an apparent increase in adrenergic activity in hyperthyroid patients, catecholamine concentrations in thyrotoxic patients are normal to low in the serum, and normal rates of epinephrine and norepinephrine secretion by the adrenal have been demonstrated (35–38). The physiologic basis for the effect of hyperthyroidism on the heart seems to be shifting away from the sympathetic system to the direct cellular mechanisms and transcriptional actions of thyroid hormone.

HYPERTHYROIDISM
Clinical Findings

Classical findings of hyperthyroidism include heat intolerance, irritability, emotional lability, nervousness, muscle weakness, menstrual abnormalities, loss of weight, increased appetite, tremor, hyperactive reflexes, excessive sweating, and fatigue (39). In one prospective study, atrial fibrillation and anorexia were the only findings more commonly noted in an elderly population as compared with a younger population (39). The majority of hyperthyroid elderly persons, however, present most frequently with one or more of the symptoms of tachycardia, fatigue, dyspnea, and weight loss. In a study of 3049 patients with hyperthyroidism, 54% of the 732 who were over the age of 61 years had 0–2 symptoms with the most common being weight loss and dyspnea. Atrial fibrillation was present in 13% of the over 61 years age group as compared to <3% in those under the age of 60 years (40).

Hemodynamic alterations include an increased resting heart rate, blood volume, left ventricular mass, stroke volume, ejection fraction, and cardiac output. Subsequent clinical manifestations involving the cardiovascular system may include palpitations, tachycardia, elevated systolic blood pressure, decreased peripheral vascular resistance, widened pulse pressure, atrial fibrillation, congestive heart failure (CHF), and angina. These latter problems are more common in the elderly and result from the increase in oxygen demand placed on the aged heart by excessive amounts of the thyroid hormones T4 and T3 and subsequent increased metabolic demands by both the heart and other body organs.

Thyroid Hormone Excess and Cardiovascular Function
Hemodynamic Changes
The pathophysiology of the changes in cardiac function associated with hyperthyroidism are multifactorial. The associated hemodynamic changes of increased heart rate, blood volume, left ventricular stroke volume, ejection fraction and cardiac output, and decreased systemic vascular resistance have been well defined (5,41). It is currently believed that the high cardiac output state associated with hyperthyroidism results from peripheral hemodynamic changes as well as direct changes in myocardial contractility. Cardiac contractility is also increased secondarily because of an increase in peripheral oxygen consumption and metabolic demands associated with excess thyroid hormone.

Tachycardia is frequently present in hyperthyroidism. Initially, this was felt to be associated with an altered responsiveness to adrenergic input. Other data support a direct effect of thyroid hormone on pacemaker activity through the sinoatrial (SA) node (42). An increased venous return, secondary to a decreased systemic vascular resistance, activated renin–angiotensin–aldosterone system, and subsequently increased blood volume contribute to the increase in preload reported in hyperthyroid states (5,6,41,43–45). Although these findings contribute to the augmented cardiac output associated with hyperthyroidism, cardiac contractility is increased in cardiac myocytes removed from peripheral effects (15,16). Systemic vascular resistance is decreased directly by thyroid hormone's action on vascular smooth muscle cells as evidenced by invasive measurement after coronary artery bypass surgery (17). This may be mediated through thyroid hormone-stimulated increased activity of adrenomedullin—a potent vasodilatory peptide (7). Afterload is reduced in hyperthyroid patients as a result of direct arterial smooth muscle relaxation, which leads to an improvement in stroke volume and subsequently cardiac output. A comprehensive review evaluated steady and pulsatile components of afterload and hypothesized that pulsatile components of arterial load actually compensate for the reduction in systemic vascular resistance noted in hyperthyroidism. These data cast doubt on the simplified notion of a single factor such as systemic vascular resistance controlling the observed decrease in ventricular afterload in the hyperthyroid patient (41).

Echocardiographic data have become available to further define the cardiac changes in hyperthyroidism. Specifically, it has been demonstrated that diastolic function improves as evidenced by increased isovolumic relaxation and left ventricular filling in hyperthyroid patients (46). These alterations in hemodynamic parameters may explain many of the cardiovascular signs and symptoms of hyperthyroidism and help to better understand many of the cardiac complications associated with hyperthyroidism, including decreased exercise tolerance and increased risk of CHF.

Cardiac Consequences
Cardiac complications of hyperthyroism include increased risk of atrial fibrillation, CHF, and cardiac ischemia and can lead to even after successful treatment of hyperthyroidism (47). Electrocardiographic changes commonly associated with hyperthyroidism include repolarization abnormalities, atrial and ventricular extrasystolic beats, sinus tachycardia, and atrial fibrillation. Other electrocardiographic findings include ischemia, left ventricular hypertrophy by voltage criteria, and varying degrees of heart block (48–50). A debate continues as to whether hyperthyroidism by itself, even without preexisting structural heart disease, can cause the abnormalities frequently seen in the hyperthyroid patient.

Atrial Fibrillation
An electrophysiologic study demonstrated that the atrial effective refractory period as well as the atrial conduction delay noted in hyperthyroid patients is arrythmogenic and could in

itself account for the predisposition of hyperthyroid patients to develop atrial fibrillation without prior presence of preexisting structural disease (51). A study utilizing 24-hour Holter monitoring of newly diagnosed and untreated patients with hyperthyroidism in whom coexistant cardiac disease was excluded demonstrated the presence of abnormal premature supraventricular depolarizations, episodes of nonsustained supraventricular tachycardia, blunted heart rate oscillations, and decreased heart rate variability consistent with decreased vagal tone. These arrhythmogenic foci were thought to be a causal link between hyperthyroidism and the onset of atrial fibrillation (52). Another mechanism for the development of atrial fibrillation in patients with hyperthyroidism due to Graves' disease is the presence in the blood of activating autoantibodies to β1-adrenergic receptors and to M2 muscarinic receptors, with both autoantibodies present in 82% of patients with atrial fibrillation as compared to only 10% of patients with sinus rhythm (53). These autoantibodies were shown to induce hyperpolarization, decreased action potential duration enhanced early after polarization formation and facilitated triggered firing in pulmonary veins (52).

Previous echocardiographic studies have demonstrated that patients with hyperthyroidism and atrial fibrillation are much more likely to have atrial enlargement than those with hyperthyroidism in sinus rhythm (54). Several studies have demonstrated that most, if not all, of the cardiovascular manifestations associated with hyperthyroidism are reversible with therapy, but long-term follow-up reveals an excess cardiovascular and cerebrovascular mortality (52). This is thought to be most likely due to an increased incidence of supraventricular dysrhythmias (52,55).

Atrial fibrillation occurs in 5–15% of hyperthyroid patients (40). It is notable that a study questioning the usefulness of thyroid function testing in new onset atrial fibrillation found that less than 1% of these patients had hyperthyroidism (56). However, testing is indicated even if the yield is low because multiple studies have shown that treatment of hyperthyroidism may lead to reversion to sinus rhythm; correction of hyperthyroidism is usually recommended before aggressively proceeding with cardioversion for atrial fibrillation (57,58). Although atrial fibrillation secondary to hyperthyroidism is reported to carry a risk of systemic embolism independently of other risk factors for embolization, this risk has not been adequately quantified (14,58).

Congestive Heart Failure

The hemodynamic changes associated with the hyperthyroid state can uncover previously compensated CHF and coronary artery disease. Exertional dyspnea and CHF can result from hyperthyroidism without underlying structural abnormalities in persons of all age groups (6,14). One possibility is that despite the increase in contractility and other increased hemodynamic parameters in hyperthyroidism, there is an inadequate cardiac reserve to allow a further increase in cardiac function during periods of stress (59). A second possible explanation is that the known cardiac hypertrophy that occurs with hyperthyroidism (as evidenced by an increase in left ventricular mass index) leads to systolic dysfunction. This dysfunction is consistent with hyperthyroid cardiomyopathy and is completely reversible with treatment (60,61). Hyperthyroidism can lead to an acute left ventricular dysfunction that mimics ischemic coronary artery disease. This disorder is rapidly reversible with treatment and is termed "myocardial stunning" because of the reversibility of the disease (62).

The clinical entity of resistance to thyroid hormone may lead to multiple cardiovascular changes that are consistent with hyperthyroidism including increased heart rate, cardiac output, and stroke volume. Cardiac symptoms such as palpitations and signs such as tachycardia and atrial fibrillation were observed less frequently in one series of patients with resistance to thyroid hormone. The authors of that study concluded that this syndrome was associated with an incomplete response to thyroid hormone in the heart (63). While this syndrome is thought to be distinct from other syndromes of thyroid dysfunction, clinical findings may be symptomatically treated with β-blockers because of the lower likelihood of developing cardiac complications in this subset of patients.

Mortality

A meta-analysis of 31,138 patients demonstrated a 20% increase in mortality in those who were hyperthyroid as compared to euthyroid patients (64). Specific causes of mortality were not identified (64). Patients over the age of 60 years and those whose hyperthyroidism was due to toxic nodular goiter, usually an older age group, had greater mortality than those under the age of 60 years or whose hyperthyroidism was due to Graves' disease. The increased mortality was due largely to cerebrovascular diseases (65). Another meta-analysis of the relationship between hyperthyroidism and mortality concluded that there were insufficient data to support final conclusions although very old patients might be an exception (66).

Subclinical Hyperthyroidism

Definition and Prevalence

Subclinical hyperthyroidism has been defined by the U.S. Preventive Services Task Force and other authorities as a condition associated with a serum TSH concentration below the lower limit of the reference range, with normal triiodothyronine and thyroxine values (58,67). It should be noted that subclinical hyperthyroidism has been defined variably in different studies with lower limits for serum TSH values ranging from 0.1 to 0.5 making comparison between studies difficult. Etiology ranges from excessive thyroid hormone replacement therapy to thyroid disease, with the most common cause in the elderly person being long-standing multinodular goiter.

The prevalence of subclinical hyperthyroidism appears to vary with geographic area and dietary iodine intake (68). Individuals with low iodine intake are more commonly affected because of compensatory growth of the thyroid gland in response to low iodine and thus the tendency to develop hyperplastic nodules that may become autonomously functioning thyroid tissue. One study in Italy reported that individuals living in iodine deficient areas had an age-related increase in subclinical hyperthyroidism from a prevalence of 0.7% in children to a prevalence of 15.4% in individuals over the age of 75 years (69).

In a study of 1210 persons in England, low TSH was found in 6.3% of women and 5.5% of men (70). However, repeat measurements of serum TSH 1 year later showed a return of TSH to the normal range in the majority of cases. In a study of community-residing persons over the age of 85 years, 3% were found to have suppressed TSH (71). Other studies of large populations confirm a similar prevalence of suppressed TSH ranging from 1.8% to 6%, associated with increasing age and female sex (70,72–75).

Conversion to Overt Hyperthyroidism

In a U.S. population of 2575 persons over the age of 60 years, 101 were found to have low TSH and, of these, 30 had no history of past or present thyroid disease. Over a 4-year follow-up period, most had normal TSH on subsequent testing, but two became overtly hyperthyroid with an increase in serum T4 to above normal values (76). In a prospective study, persons aged 85 years were followed with serum TSH and free T4 until 89 years of age. Of 12 patients with subclinical hyperthyroidism at baseline, 1 became overtly hyperthyroid, 5 had persistent subclinical hyperthyroidism, 5 became euthyroid, and 1 developed subclinical hypothyroidism (71). Several studies suggest that the conversion rate to overt hyperthyroidism ranges from 1.5% to 13% within 1 year (70,76,77). A large study of a population of 272,746 adults identified 2024 cases of subclinical hyperthyroidism (60% over 65 years of age, 77% female), representing a prevalence of 0.63%. On follow-up at 2, 5, and 7 years, 81.8% remained subclinically hyperthyroid at 2 years, 67.5% at 5 years, and 63% at 7 years. Only 0.5–0.7% became overtly hyperthyroid over these time intervals. Return to normal thyroid function occurred in 17.2% in 2 years, 31.5% in 5 years, and 35.6% in 7 years with the greatest likelihood of normalization in those with baseline TSH between 0.1 and 0.4 mU/L (78). Thus, the natural history of subclinical hyperthyroidism is variable, sometimes disappearing over time.

Cardiovascular Consequences

There are many cardiovascular changes that have been described in subclinical hyperthyroidism. These include increased heart rate, increased prevalence of atrial premature beats, shorter isovolumetric contraction time, shorter preejection period, impaired left ventricular diastolic filling, increased left ventricular mass index, increased mean velocity of circumferential fiber shortening, reduced peak overload, reduced peak oxygen uptake and anaerobic threshold during exercise, increased interventricular septum and left ventricular posterior wall thickness, increased left ventricular end-systolic volume, and impaired left ventricular diastolic filling (Table 19.1) (79–84). These alterations can lead to reduced exercise performance.

Decreased large and small artery elasticity was reported in persons with subclinical hyperthyroidism as compared to controls. These findings were associated with echocardiographic data showing significantly increased left ventricular mass index and interventricular septum thickness (85). Corrected QT intervals—a measure of ventricular repolarization and increased risk of arrhythmia and cardiac mortality—were noted to be significantly longer in patients with subclinical hyperthyroidism (86).

Cardiovascular Disease
Atrial Fibrillation

Several large studies have been published which have shown an increased risk of atrial fibrillation in patients with subclinical hyperthyroidism. A retrospective study reported that the risk of atrial fibrillation was five times more likely in patients with subclinical hyperthyroidism, similar to that found in patients with overt hyperthyroidism (60,61,77,87–89). In a prospective study of 3233 community-residing persons over the age of 65 years, 1.5%

Table 19.1 Cardiovascular Findings Associated with Subclinical Hyperthyroidism

Functional alterations	Increased cardiac contractility
	Impaired left ventricular diastolic filling
	Impaired systolic function during exercise
	Increased left ventricular mass index
	Increased intraventricular septal thickness
	Increased left ventricular posterior wall thickness
	Decreased large and small artery elasticity
	Prolonged QTc interval
Clinical consequences	Increased heart rate and frequency of atrial premature beats
	Increased incidence of atrial fibrillation
	Lower serum total and LDL cholesterol concentrations
	Reduced exercise capacity
	Increased all cause mortality and mortality due to cardiovascular disease

Abbreviation: LDL, low-density lipoprotein.

were found to have subclinical hyperthyroidism at baseline. Over the course of 13 years of follow-up, those with subclinical hyperthyroidism had twice the risk of developing atrial fibrillation than those with baseline euthyroidism (90). A recent large meta-analysis of 52,674 persons found that 2188 (4.2%) had subclinical hyperthyroidism and a hazard ration of 1.68 for the development of atrial fibrillation as compared to euthyroid persons, with greatest risk for men and for those with TSH <0.1 mU/L (91). An increase in the number of cardiac L-type Ca^{2+} channels by up to threefold has been reported in patients who are subclinically hyperthyroid, a probable mechanism for the increased rate of atrial fibrillation (92).

Congestive Heart Failure

A recent study of 5316 elderly persons, mean age 75 years, identified 1.3% with subclinical hyperthyroidism. Over a 3.2-year period of follow-up, there was a much greater risk of hospitalization for heart failure, especially in those with TSH <0.1 mU/L, as compared to euthyroid persons (93).

Coronary Heart Disease and Mortality

There are conflicting reports regarding the impact of subclinical hyperthyroidism on mortality. One study reported an increase in all-cause and cardiovascular mortality in individuals over the age of 60 years with subclinical hyperthyroidism with serum TSH concentrations lower than 0.5 mlU/L (94). Another report of elderly persons with untreated subclinical hyperthyroidism who were followed from age 85 through 89 years has demonstrated an increase in both cardiovascular and all-cause mortality (72). A meta-analysis evaluating the risk of coronary heart disease (CHD) events and mortality in persons with subclinical hyperthyroidism found a modestly increased relative risk of 1.21 for CHD and 1.19 for cardiovascular mortality (95). Another large meta-analysis reported hazard ratios of 1.21 for CHD events and 1.29 for cardiovascular heart disease mortality in patients with subclinical hyperthyroidism (91). However, several other studies have shown no association between subclinical hyperthyroidism and risk of CHD events or death (75,90).

Management of Hyperthyroid-Associated Cardiac Disease

Cardiac findings such as palpitations, sinus tachycardia, and even tachyarrhythmias appear to be well tolerated in most hyperthyroid people, rarely produce an immediate crisis, and in most cases are amenable to conservative treatment pending correction of the hyperthyroid state itself. While radioactive iodine is an excellent treatment for the underlying hyperthyroid state, especially in the elderly patient, the time to onset of action can be weeks to months. If an immediate effect is needed, Lugol's solution (potassium iodide) may be administered after an initial dose of antithyroid medication such as propylthiouracil or methimazole. Iodide rapidly reduces circulating levels of thyroid hormone by blocking essential steps in thyroid hormone production. However, propylthiouracil or methimazole must be used in conjunction with the iodide to inhibit thyroid hormone synthesis, and to prevent the possibility of a thyroid nodule or diffuse toxic goiter from converting the iodide to thyroid hormone and effectively worsening the hyperthyroid state (6,14).

In patients who are unstable with signs of cardiac compromise, intravenous β-blockers rapidly decrease heart rate and may reduce the conversion of T4 to T3 by approximately 15%. If the patient presents with CHF, diuretics are still the mainstay of treatment. Digoxin is of use in patients with hyperthyroid mediated CHF, although there may be a Na, K-ATPase-mediated resistance to its action (6).

Treatment of atrial fibrillation should be centered on correcting the hyperthyroidism because of the high rate of spontaneous cardioversion once thyroid hormone concentrations are normalized (57). Most of these conversions take place within 3 weeks of becoming euthyroid and no spontaneous conversions occur if atrial fibrillation is still present after 4 months of euthyroidism or if atrial fibrillation was present for more than 13 months before becoming euthyroid. Patients who remain in atrial fibrillation beyond 16 weeks of return to the euthyroid state are then candidates for cardioversion.

The decision to anticoagulate has not been elucidated in the case of hyperthyroid-associated atrial fibrillation in any randomized controlled trials. However, it has been recommended that older patients with comorbid hypertension, CHF, left atrial enlargement or left ventricular dysfunction or with other conditions increasing the risk of systemic embolization, or those patients with longer duration of atrial fibrillation, should be anticoagulated. On the contrary, it is probably not necessary to anticoagulate young patients without comorbid conditions or with a short duration of atrial fibrillation (14,15,96). Hyperthyroidism increases the sensitivity to the anticoagulant effect of warfarin, resulting in a greater lowering of coagulation factors II and VII and greater increase in prothrombin ratio and partial thromboplastin time (97). When warfarin is used, the dose should be adjusted to keep the international normalization ratio (INR) between 2.0 and 3.0, and continued until euthyroidism has been restored and there is a return to normal sinus rhythm (98). Individual case-by-case review of pertinent risk factors for embolization is appropriate before making the decision to initiate anticoagulaton.

Management of Subclinical Hyperthyroidism

Treatment at this early stage of hyperthyroidism is controversial secondary to the low rates of progression to overt hyperthyroidism. A long-term study of patients with untreated subclinical hyperthyroidism demonstrated an increase in both cardiovascular and all-cause mortality (99). Other studies have demonstrated an increased risk of CHF in patients with subclinical hyperthyroidism (93). These data, coupled with findings of diminished self-reported ratings of quality of life and a higher rate of osteopenia in persons with subclinical hyperthyroidism, make it reasonable to consider earlier, more aggressive treatment, especially in individuals who already manifest these changes or evidence for cardiovascular disease (58,100).

While there have been no randomized prospective trials evaluating the treatment of subclinical hyperthyroidism, there is a consensus that therapy should be initiated in elderly individuals and in younger persons with heart disease or evidence of other problems, such as bone loss, and in particular those persons who have serum TSH levels <0.1 mU/L. A consensus panel of endocrinologists has recommended treatment for those with TSH suppression of <0.1 mU/L, but recommends periodic retesting of thyroid function in patients with partial TSH suppression of 0.1–0.4 mU/L (Table 19.2) (101,102). It has been suggested that all postmenopausal women, individuals over the age of 60 years, and those with a history of heart disease, osteoporosis, or symptoms be treated if the TSH is <0.1 mU/L and that a similar approach be considered if the TSH is between 0.1 and 4 mU/L in this same population. Premenopausal women or those less than 60 years of age without a history of heart disease, osteoporosis, or symptoms but who have a TSH <0.1 mU/L are suggested to have a radioiodine uptake and scan and bone density study, but therapy remains optional as there is little clinical evidence as yet for significant benefit in these patients. Similar individuals with TSH levels between 0.1 and 0.4 mU/L should not be treated though they should have a radioiodine uptake and scan along with periodic TSH testing at 6–12-month intervals (103,104). Treatment leading to the return of serum TSH to normal has been associated with significant improvement in cardiovascular function including a decrease in the heart rate, total number of beats during 24 hours, number of atrial and ventricular premature beats, reduction

Table 19.2   Treatment Recommendations for Subclinical Thyroid Disease

Subclinical hyperthyroidism	Normalization of thyroid function with antithyroid drugs or ^{131}I for patients with: Clinical features of hyperthyroidism Atrial fibrillation Ischemic heart disease Osteopenia/osteoporosis Suppressed TSH <0.1 mU/L Development of increase in T_4, free T_4, or T_3 during follow-up Monitor TSH/free T_4 at 6–12-month intervals in asymptomatic patients with TSH 0.1–0.4 mU/L
Subclinical hypothyroidism	T_4 replacement for patients with: Serum TSH >10 mU/L, Serum TSH 5–10 mU/L, and positive antimicrosomal antibodies or symptoms of mild hypothyroidism Monitor TSH/free T_4 at 6–12-month intervals for patients with serum TSH 5–10 mU/L and negative antimicrosomal antibodies and no evident symptoms of hypothyroidism

Abbreviations: T_4, thyroxine; T_3, triiodothyronine; TSH, thyroid-stimulating hormone.

in left ventricular mass index, interventricular septum thickness, and left ventricular posterior wall thickness at diastole (105).

HYPOTHYROIDISM

Hypothyroidism, defined as an elevated serum TSH along with serum T4 or free T4 below the lower limit of normal, is relatively common in the general population with a well-established relationship to gender and age. The incidence of hypothyroidism in women is three to four times that in men, and there is a clear increase in prevalence with advancing age so that it is found in 15–20% of women over the age of 75 years and in 4–7% of elderly men. The American Thyroid Association now recommends that all persons over the age of 50 years have annual screening for thyroid hormone abnormalities after studies have shown the cost benefit from such practice (106).

Cardiovascular manifestations of hypothyroidism occur as a consequence both of the effects of thyroid hormone deficiency on the myocardium and of hypothyroid-associated dyslipidemia on arterial vasculature. Histologically, swelling of the myofibrillar elements, interstitial fibrosis, basophilic degeneration, and tissue edema have been described (107). There appears to be deposition of mucopolysaccharide, likely reflecting the decline in certain enzymes necessary for the breakdown of these substances. Electron microscopic studies reveal thickening of the capillary basement membrane similar to that observed in diabetes mellitus and in persons of advanced age (108,109). Numerous other ultrastructural changes have been described, including loss of mitochondrial cristae.

At the organ level, the heart in persons with hypothyroidism may be dilated, pale, and flabby as a result of myxedematous infiltration, but there is no evidence of hypertrophy (110). Pericardial effusion may be present.

Thyroid Hormone Deficiency and Cardiovascular Function

Perhaps the most widely accepted change noted in the setting of hypothyroidism is a reduction in myocardial contractility. Using isolated right ventricular papillary muscles from hypothyroid cats and dogs, a decrease was noted in isometric tension and the rate of tension development. The time taken to reach peak tension increased at all muscle lengths and isotonic force–velocity relations shifted downward and to the left, supporting a depressed contractile state (16,111). It has been postulated that decreased myocardial contractility in hypothyroidism may result from a reduction in the thyroid–adrenergic relationship, with either a diminished response to a given amount of catecholamine or a reduced amount of free catecholamine available to interact at the cardiac receptor site. Studies have reported an increase, decrease, and no change in cardiovascular sensitivity to catecholamine stimulation in the setting of hypothyroidism (31,112–114). Levels of norepinephrine in myocardial tissue of hypothyroid cats were not reported to be affected by thyroid status (16), and thus it appears unlikely that a lower level of catecholamine exposure to the cardiac receptor is the cause of significant cardiac effects. Studies have shown a reduction in β-adrenergic receptor activity in atria from hypothyroid rats and an increase in α-receptor activity in the same tissue (115). This reduction in the number and/or affinity of β-receptors in cardiac tissue could result in a depressed myocardial response. Because contractile function is depressed in isolated papillary muscles from hypothyroid rats, thyroid hormone deficiency seems to have a direct effect and is responsible for at least a component of the cardiovascular change induced by the hypothyroid state (16).

The rate of calcium uptake and calcium-dependent ATP hydrolysis by isolated cardiac myocytes is reduced in the setting of hypothyroidism and may be a mechanism for decreased myocardial contractility (116). A reduction in myocyte calcium ATPase activity of the sarcoplasmic reticulum has been described in both rat and mouse models of hypothyroidism, although not in a rabbit model (117–119).

The bradycardia that often occurs in hypothyroidism is thought to result from the lack of thyroid stimulation of sinoatrial (SA) node cells, further impacted by a reduction in sympathoadrenal stimulation (120). A decreased rate of diastolic repolarization and prolonged action potential duration has also been described.

The hemodynamic changes seen in hypothyroidism are opposite to those seen in hyperthyroidism and are less likely to be associated with overt clinical findings. Systemic vascular resistance is increased, heart rate is decreased, isovolumic relaxation time is increased, and there is a decrease in the ejection fraction, blood volume, and cardiac output (14,46,119). An increase in systemic vascular resistance, decrease in heart rate, and decrease in the renin–angiotensin–aldosterone system combined with a slowed diastolic relaxation lead to a decrease in preload and subsequent decrease in stroke volume. Thus, the functional consequence of decreased ventricular contractility, ventricular filling, and stroke volume is reduced cardiac output. The increase in systemic vascular resistance can lead to diastolic hypertension and contribute to an increased risk for adverse cardiovascular events.

Changes in blood lipoprotein composition in hypothyroidism have implications for atherogenesis. Short-term hypothyroidism is associated with an increase in plasma lipoprotein(a) and T3 therapy rapidly lowered lipoprotein(a) together with apolipoprotein B and low-density lipoprotein (LDL) cholesterol. These findings support the hypothesis that thyroid hormone is capable of regulating plasma lipoprotein(a) and apolipoprotein B in a parallel manner. Elevated concentrations of lipoprotein(a) in combination with LDL cholesterol may be involved in the increased risk of cardiovascular disease, which is associated with hypothyroidism (121). Changes in LDL receptor activity are significantly correlated with changes in LDL cholesterol, but not with changes in lipoprotein(a). The LDL receptor pathway appears to be involved in the catabolism of lipoprotein(a) to a limited extent (122). Hypothyroidism has been associated with elevated levels of total and high-density lipoprotein (HDL) cholesterol, total/HDL cholesterol ratio, apolipoprotein AI, and apolipoprotein E. The increase in apolipoprotein AI without a concomitant increase in apolipoprotein AII suggests a selective elevation of HDL2. These effects were found to be reversible with treatment of the hypothyroidism (123).

Pulse wave analysis from recordings at the radial artery in patients with hypothyroidism demonstrates increased augmentation of central aortic pressures and central arterial stiffness. These alterations lead to hypertension and increased cardiac afterload and, along with hypothyroid-associated endothelial dysfunction, contribute to increased cardiovascular risk. These abnormalities are reversed by appropriate thyroid hormone replacement (124).

Other cardiovascular risk factors for patients with hypothyroidism include smoking, elevated levels of homocysteine, elevated C-reactive protein, coagulation abnormalities, and insulin resistance (125).

Clinical Cardiac Manifestations of Hypothyroidism

Clinically evident cardiac manifestations of hypothyroidism occur only in association with a significant reduction in the levels of circulating thyroid hormone. Studies using oxygen consumption as a corollary of thyroid hormone status have reported few cardiac symptoms in otherwise healthy persons until oxygen requirements decline by 75%. This level is highly variable, however. Many persons with hypothyroidism have coexisting medical conditions that compromise the cardiovascular system and may lower the threshold for cardiac problems. The reduced requirement for oxygen by the hypothyroid myocardium may be protective against angina. In fact, angina may develop only after therapy with thyroid hormone has been initiated.

Symptoms due to the effect of hypothyroidism on the heart include dyspnea on exertion and easy fatigability. Less frequent are complaints of orthopnea, paroxysmal nocturnal dyspnea, and angina. Physical findings often present in patients with hypothyroidism include bradycardia, narrowed pulse pressure, mild hypertension, distant heart sounds, and evidence of cardiomegaly. Reduced cardiac output with resultant decrease in glomerular filtration rate can lead to renal sodium retention and peripheral edema in the absence of CHF. In general, there is no change in the jugular venous pressure. In patients with severely diminished thyroid function, however, infiltrative cardiomyopathy, evidence of peripheral edema or nonpitting edema of the lower extremities, pleural effusion, and even ascites may be noted and can produce a clinical picture suggesting CHF. The presence of nonpitting edema raises the possibility that hypothyroidism is present.

The electrocardiogram may be normal in the presence of hypothyroidism but more often there is bradycardia, prolonged QT interval, flattening or inversion of the T wave, particularly in lead II, and low-amplitude P, QRS complex, and T waves (126). These findings may result from a direct effect of thyroid hormone deficiency, but can also be the result of a pericardial effusion that may accompany hypothyroidism. Although not common, incomplete and complete right bundle branch block occur with greater frequency (127). Ventricular arrhythmias may be seen including the ventricular tachycardia of the syndrome of torsades de pointes. With replacement therapy, these changes return to normal and may even precede the return to normal of other clinical features of the disease. The echocardiogram in hypothyroidism demonstrates features of decreased left ventricular contractility with increased systolic time interval and prolongation of isovolumic relaxation time. Small pericardial effusions may be present in as many as 50% of hypothyroid patients but do not affect cardiac function (128,129).

Studies suggest that in the absence of other coexisting diseases, CHF is an extremely uncommon finding in hypothyroidism (130). In the setting of shortness of breath, pleural effusions, cardiomegaly, and other symptoms, it is often difficult to distinguish CHF from what has been termed myxedema heart, a cardiomyopathy resulting from insufficient quantities of thyroid hormone that is reversible with thyroid hormone replacement.

The absence of pulmonary congestion, diminished plasma volume, high protein content of pleural or pericardial effusions, and normal resting venous, atrial, pulmonary artery, and right ventricular end-diastolic pressures are highly suggestive of myxedema. Exercise results in an increase in cardiac output and ejection fraction in persons with myxedema, in contrast to the impaired response in those with congestive failure (131,132). The hemodynamic changes associated with hypothyroidism appear to respond to thyroid hormone, but they are not very responsive to diuretic and digoxin therapy. Since in many persons both conditions occur together, there is a great deal of variability in clinical response.

An increase in the risk for CHD has been associated with hypothyroidism (125). Decreased measures of thyroid function and serum HDL have been observed to be more common in patients with coronary artery disease (133). Treatment of hypothyroidism with hormone replacement has been observed to protect against the angiographic progression of coronary artery disease, perhaps due to metabolic effects of thyroid hormone on plaque progression (134).

Subclinical Hypothyroidism
Definition and Prevalence
Large population surveys have identified a significant proportion of individuals who have serum TSH levels above the accepted upper limit of normal, but in whom serum concentrations of total and free T4 as well as total and free T3 are normal and overt symptoms of hypothyroidism are usually mild or absent. This syndrome, which has been termed subclinical hypothyroidism, is most commonly found in women above the age of 60 years and has been observed in 15–20% of women over the age of 75 years (135–140). Antithyroid antibodies are often present, suggesting an autoimmune etiology (138,139,141). It is thought that the failing thyroid gland responds with an increase in TSH secretion which, in turn, is capable of further driving the thyroid to maintain normal levels of T4 and T3 until true thyroid failure ensues.

In the Framingham study, 5.9% of subjects over the age of 60 years had clearly elevated serum TSH concentrations (>10 mU/L) with normal serum T4 levels and an additional 14.4% had slightly elevated serum TSH (5–10 mU/L) with normal serum T4 (142). A thyroid screening survey of 1149 community-residing women with mean age of 69 ± 7.5 years identified 10.8% as having subclinical hypothyroidism (135). Other studies have established a prevalence rate of between 25 and 104 per 1000 persons with the highest rate occurring in women over the age of 55 years. The incidence in women aged between 40 and 60 years may be as high as 10%.

Data from the Whickham study indicate that 60% of subjects with serum TSH values >6 mU/L and 80% of those with TSH values >10 mU/L had demonstrable antithyroid antibodies in their serum. Of the entire population of women, 5% had both elevated TSH levels and antithyroid antibodies (143).

Progression to Overt Hypothyroidism
One question of clinical importance is what is the likelihood that persons with laboratory criteria for subclinical hypothyroidism will go on to develop clinical hypothyroidism. In a long-term follow-up study, women who initially had antithyroglobulin and antimicrosomal antibodies along with a serum TSH of >6 mU/L developed overt hypothyroidism at the rate of 5% per year. No cases developed in women with borderline elevation of TSH only (6–10 mU/L), and only one case developed in the 67 women who had antithyroid antibodies with normal TSH levels (138).

Other studies support progression to overt hypothyroidism at the rate of 7% per year in women with elevated serum TSH and high titers of antithyroid antibodies with ranges from 1% to 20% per year (141,144). There is a relationship between the degree of elevation of TSH and the long-term risk of progression to overt hypothyroidism with an initial TSH >12 mU/L resulting in 77% incidence of overt hypothyroidism by 10 years of follow-up (145,146). The presence of antithyroid antibodies indicates underlying chronic autoimmune thyroiditis and constitutes a significant risk factor for the development of clinically apparent hypothyroidism in women who are found to have isolated elevated values of serum TSH (145,146).

Cardiovascular Alterations

There is evidence that systolic contractility on effort and left ventricular diastolic contractility at rest are decreased in patients with subclinical hypothyroidism (Table 19.3) (79). These changes may have little functional significance in the resting state, but symptoms can develop during cardiopulmonary exercise. The altered contractility and clinical response to exercise are corrected with thyroid hormone treatment (147–149). Although subclinical hypothyroidism has been associated with a prolongation of the QT interval, little has been reported regarding its clinical consequences.

As in patients with overt hypothyroidism, those with subclinical hypothyroidism have been shown to have alterations in peripheral vasculature. Both diastolic blood pressure and pulse wave velocity were significantly increased in patients with subclinical hypothyroidism compared with euthyroid persons (150). Pulse wave analysis has also demonstrated increased arterial stiffness in patients with subclinical hypothyroidism, which improved after thyroid hormone treatment (151).

There have been many reports indicating that subclinical hypothyroidism is associated with alterations in circulating concentrations of lipids that may enhance the risk for development of vascular disease (149–156). A study of 2108 community-residing persons demonstrated that in the 119-person subgroup (5.6%) with subclinical hypothyroidism, there was a significant increase in total serum cholesterol and in LDL cholesterol with no change in HDL cholesterol (157).

Table 19.3 Cardiovascular Findings Associated with Subclinical Hypothyroidism

Ventricular function	Impaired systolic function on effort
	Impaired left ventricular diastolic function at rest/delayed relaxation time
	Right ventricular systolic and diastolic dysfunction
	Increased risk of CHF
Peripheral vasculature	Increased sytemic vascular resistance
	Impaired vasodilatation
	Increased carotid artery intima-media thickness
	Increased arterial stiffness
	Increased pulse-wave velocity
	Increased diastolic blood pressure
	Increased peripheral vascular disease
Dyslipidemia	Increased total cholesterol
	Increased LDL cholesterol
	Increased apolipoprotein B
	Increased lipoprotein(a)
Atherosclerosis	Increased ischemic/coronary heart disease
	Increased risk of myocardial infarction
	Increased aortic atherosclerosis
Coagulation	Increased factor VII activity
Mortality	Increased cardiac mortality
	Increased all-cause mortality

Abbreviations: CHF, congestive heart failure; LDL, low-density lipoprotein.

Cardiovascular Disease

The relationship between subclinical hypothyroidism and cardiovascular disease has been the subject of many clinical studies that have yielded conflicting results. A study of 1922 patients indicated that subclinical hypothyroidism was not associated with an adverse cardiovascular risk profile (158). This observation was further supported by data from several large longitudinal studies of community-residing persons (90,159). However, a number of other studies suggest that subclinical hypothyroidism is a risk factor for cardiovascular disease.

Coronary Heart Disease and Mortality

The relationship between subclinical hypothyroidism and/or autoimmune thyroid disease and CHD was evaluated in a Japanese population. Ninety-seven patients diagnosed as having CHD by a coronary angiogram (CHD group) and 103 healthy subjects matched for age, sex, and body mass index (control group) were included in the study. Thyroid function, thyroid autoantibodies, and serum lipid concentrations were measured in the CHD and control groups. The CHD group exhibited significantly decreased levels of serum free T3 and free T4 and significantly increased serum TSH levels as compared with the control group, indicating a significant decrease in thyroid function in the CHD patients. Serum HDL cholesterol levels were significantly decreased in the CHD group (133). Another Japanese study of 2550 men and women with mean age of 58.5 years found 10.2% to have subclinical hypothyroidism (mean age 62 years). Men with subclinical hypothyroidism had a prevalence of ischemic heart disease four times greater than euthyroid men but no increase in intracranial hemorrhage or cerebral infarction. Over 12 years of follow-up, there was a significant increase in all-cause mortality in the subclinical hypothyroid men but not in women (160). A longitudinal study of 2108 men and women with a mean age of 50 years found a significant increase in prevalence of CHD in both men and women with subclinical hypothyroidism who had a TSH level >10 mU/L (75). A large meta-analysis had similar results (161). There is evidence to suggest that even mild increase in TSH in women increase the risk for fatal CHD (162).

Age may be a factor in determining the impact of subclinical hypothyroidism on risk for CHD. A meta-analysis of 2531 persons with subclinical hypothyroidism found that there was an increased prevalence of ischemic heart disease and cardiovascular mortality only in patients under the age of 65 years (163). This inverse relationship between age and cardiovascular risk is supported by the findings in a study of persons over the age of 85 years followed over 4 years in whom there was lower all-cause and cardiovascular mortality in those with hypothyroidism as compared to age matched euthyroid persons (71).

Among elderly residents of a nursing home, 6% were found to have subclinical hypothyroidism, and, of these, 83% had dyslipidemia and 56% had evidence of coronary artery disease in contrast to a 16% incidence of coronary artery disease in euthyroid residents (164).

Women with hypercholesterolemia have an increased likelihood of having coexisting subclinical hypothyroidism (165). Patients with subclinical hypothyroidism have been found to have a relative increase in LDL cholesterol and decrease in HDL cholesterol with a corresponding higher prevalence of ischemic heart disease (152). In a large group of elderly women with evidence of aortic atherosclerosis, 13.9% were found to have subclinical hypothyroidism and in those women with a history of myocardial infarction, 21.5% had subclinical hypothyroidism (135). The presence of subclinical hypothyroidism was accompanied by a high prevalence of both aortic athersclerosis and myocardial infarction, with an even higher prevalence in those who also had detectable thyroid antimicrosomal antibodies. A higher rate of adverse events, including reocclusion, has been observed after percutaneous coronary intervention in patients with subclinical hypothyroidism (153). An increase in factor VII activity has been found in a study of patients with subclinical hypo-thyroidism, raising the possibility of a hypercoagulable state that may lead to an increased risk of thromboembolism (166).

Congestive Heart Failure

The alterations in myocardial function seen in patients with subclinical hypothyroidism may predispose these persons to an increased risk for development of CHF. A study of 2730 men and women aged 70–79 years who were followed for a period of 4 years revealed an increased risk for CHF in persons with subclinical hypothyroidism who had TSH levels of 7 mU/L or greater (167). In this population, subclinical hypothyroidism was not associated with an increased risk of CHD, stroke, peripheral arterial disease, or cardiovascular-related or total mortality. A recent study of 5316 elderly persons with a his-tory of cardiovascular disease, mean age 75 years, identified 3.7% with subclinical hypo-thyroidism Over a 3.2-year follow-up period, those persons with TSH levels >10 mU/L had an incidence of heart failure significantly greater than those who were euthyroid (93). Another large study of 3044 persons over the age of 65 years who were followed for 12 years again showed an increased risk of heart failure in those with TSH >10 mU/L. Echo-cardiographic measurements revealed evidence for impaired diastolic function and increased left ventricular mass (168).

Peripheral Vascular Disease

Peripheral vascular disease is also increased in persons with subclinical hypothyroidism. Carotid artery intima-media thickness, a recognized risk factor for cardiovascular disease, was assessed in patients with subclinical hypothyroidism by high-resolution ultrasonogra-phy and found to be increased and positively related to age, TSH, and LDL cholesterol levels. Treatment with thyroid hormone reduced total and LDL cholesterol and carotid intima thickness (169). In a nursing home population of mean age 79 ± 9 years, 78% of persons identified with subclinical hypothyroidism were found to have symptomatic peripheral vascular disease (170).

Effects of Thyroid Hormone Treatment on Cardiovascular Function and Disease

Treatment with L-thyroxine has resulted in improved systolic and diastolic function, improvement in left ventricular ejection fraction with exercise, decrease in systemic vascu-lar resistance, improved endothelial function and measures of quality of life (79,150,171,172). The treatment has also resulted in decrease in total and LDL cholesterol, increase in serum HDL, and decrease in LDL and apolipoprotein B (149,152,153,169,172). A meta-analysis has further demonstrated a modest but effective reduction in total and LDL cholesterol in treated cases of subclinical hypothyroidism (156). A recent study of patients with subclinical hypothyroidism who were treated with thyroxine for 6 months demonstrated an increase in coronary microvascular function as reflected by improved myocardial blood flow and coronary flow reserve (173). A critical question is whether or not early treatment of subclinical hypothyroidism with thyroid hormone replacement will be effective in reducing the risk for subsequent development of atherosclerosis or coronary artery disease. A recent study of a large cohort of patients with subclinical hypothyroidism indicates that treatment is beneficial. Subclinical hypothyroidism was identified in 3093 patients aged 40–70 years and in 1642 patients over the age of 70 years. Over a mean follow-up period of 7.6 years, there was a significant reduction in ischemic heart disease events in the 40–70 year-old patients who were treated with thyroxine but no difference in ischemic events in the treated patients who were over 70 years of age (174).

Thyroid hormone replacement may be of value in the management of patients with CHF. In an experimental study of heart failure patients who also had low T3 levels, T3 given by inravenous infusion over a period of 72 hours resulted in a significant increase in stroke volume and left ventricular end diastolic volume. These changes were also accompanied by an improved neurohumoral profile with a fall in plasma norepinephrine, aldosterone B-type natriuretic peptide levels (175).

Myxedema Coma

Myxedema coma is an extreme, life-threatening form of hypothyroidism that occurs almost exclusively in the elderly, usually in association with infection, severe trauma, cold exposure, or following administration of sedatives, tranquilizers, or narcotics. Cardiac manifestations include bradycardia, hypotension, and shock. The electrocardiogram, in addition to bradycardia, will usually show low voltage and T-wave flattening. Serum creatine kinase (CK) is often markedly elevated and the clinical picture may resemble that of a myocardial infarction.

Management of Overt Hypothyroidism

Younger persons or those with no evidence of cardiovascular compromise may be started on L-thyroxine in an initial dose of 25 µg daily. Because so many elderly persons with hypothyroidism may have underlying cardiovascular abnormalities, initiation of thyroid hormone replacement therapy in this population should be with a smaller dose of L-thyroxine, that is, 12.5 µg daily. The use of diuretic therapy and digoxin should be reserved for persons in whom there is clear evidence of coexisting CHF. The starting dose should be increased by 12.5–25 µg increments at 4–6-week intervals, realizing that both age and hypothyroidism prolong the half-life of L-thyroxine. Because it takes approximately five half-lives to reach a steady state, laboratory monitoring of serum TSH is necessary to avoid too rapid a rise in dosing. Dose adjustments are made until the level of serum TSH has declined to within the normal range or the patient develops signs of toxicity. In general, elderly persons who are hypothyroid require a replacement dose of between 75 and 100 µg daily compared to an approximate dose of 100–125 µg for younger persons. L-thyroxine is the preferred thyroid hormone for replacement because T3 exerts a "burst" effect on the myocardium and is less well tolerated. It also has a shorter half-life, thereby having a less equilibrated metabolic profile. Combination therapies also share the disadvantage of T3, a component in all these medications.

In individuals who have severe ischemic cardiac disease, it may be difficult to return the patient to the euthyroid state without provoking cardiac symptoms. However, in a study of hypothyroid patients who had known symptomatic coronary artery disease, treatment resulted in either no change or an improvement in symptoms in 84% of the patients with only 16% exhibiting an increase in symptoms (176). Attempt should be made to maximize the antianginal regimen, including administration of β-blockers, vasodilators, and calcium channel blockers. If this approach fails, the patient should undergo evaluation for the possibility of angioplasty or coronary artery bypass surgery (125,177).

The patient with myxedema coma should be cared for in an intensive-care unit setting and treatment started promptly with an initial dose of 300–500 µg of L-thyroxine given intravenously. Once there is evidence of a clinical response such as rise in body temperature and heart rate, the daily dose of L-thyroxine should be reduced to 25–50 µg orally and slowly further adjusted by monitoring the serum TSH (178,179).

Management of Subclinical Hypothyroidism

There have been a number of publications dealing with the issue of treatment for subclinical thyroid dysfunction (101,102,104,180,181). Considerable controversy, however, remains. Two reports on subclinical thyroid disease were prepared by a panel of experts appointed by the American Association of Clinical Endocrinologists, the American Thyroid Association, and The Endocrine Society who carried out an exhaustive review of the literature using principles of evidence-based medicine. These reports addressed issues of screening, evaluation, and management of patients with subclinical thyroid disease and culminated in a consensus statement of conclusions and recommendations prepared by the panel members, which was published in 2004 (101,104). Subsequently, a response document from representatives of three organizations was prepared and published in 2005, pointing out areas where there was disagreement with the consensus conference recommendations (102). A rebuttal by the chair of the consensus panel and an editorial have also been published (180,181).

The consensus panel concluded that routine treatment of patients with subclinical hypothyroidism with serum TSH levels of 4.5–10 mU/L was not warranted but indicated that treatment is reasonable for patients with TSH levels >10 mU/L. This recommendation was based on data from patients with TSH above 10 mU/L regarding the projected rate of progression from subclinical to overt hypothyroidism, the observations that patients in this category were at increased risk for cardiovascular events and the effects of thyroxine treatment on symptoms, depression, lipid profiles, and cardiac function (101).

The response of the three sponsoring societies to the consensus panel disagrees with some of the panel's conclusions. Thus, the three societies recommend routine screening for subclinical thyroid disease according to previously published guidelines. Further, they recommend routine treatment of patients with subclinical hypothyroidism who have TSH levels between 4.5 and 10 mU/L (102).

At present, a conservative approach is to monitor patients identified with the syndrome with serum TSH and free T4 at 6–12-month intervals. Replacement therapy with thyroxine should be given to those patients with serum TSH >10 mU/L and to those with TSH between 5 and 10 mU/L, who have either high levels of antimicrosomal antibodies or symptoms consistent with mild hypothyroidism (Table 19.2).

AMIODARONE AND THE THYROID GLAND

Amiodarone, a drug commonly used in the management of patients with supraventricular and ventricular tachyarrhythmias, is also associated with a high prevalence both of thyroid function test abnormalities and of hyperthyroidism and hypothyroidism. It contains approximately 37% iodine by weight and approximately 10% is deiodinated daily liberating 7 mg of iodide for each 200 mg tablet, an amount which is 50–100 times the daily iodine requirement. Because amiodarone is highly lipophilic, it concentrates in adipose tissue, muscle, liver, lung, thyroid gland, and brain from which it is slowly liberated with an elimination half-life of 50–100 days. After discontinuation, amiodarone and its metabolites can persist in the circulation for as long as 9 months (182).

Over 50% of persons treated with amiodarone will develop changes in thyroid function tests within the first month after initial drug administration with the most common charges being slightly elevated total and free T4 levels, low total T3, and transient increase in TSH (183). In most persons, T4 and TSH levels return to normal values within 2–3 months, but T3 levels remain persistently low. Some individuals treated with amiodarone will go on to develop overt hyperthyroidism or hypothyroidism.

Amiodarone-Induced Hyperthyroidism

The overall incidence of amiodarone-induced hyperthyroidism (AIT) varies with the amount of dietary iodine intake. In areas with low environmental iodine, AIT prevalence is as high as 10% while in areas with sufficient iodine intake AIT prevalence is approximately

3% (182,183). Onset of AIT can be sudden or gradual and can occur soon after starting amiodarone or after many years of treatment with an average length of treatment of about 3 years before occurrence of AIT (182). Two forms of AIT have been identified, type 1 and type 2. Type 1 usually occurs in persons who have underlying thyroid abnormalities, often clinically unrecognized, such as thyroid nodules, goiter, or thyroid autoantibodies. In these persons, the hyperthyroidism is caused by iodine-induced excess thyroid hormone synthesis and release (182,183). Type 2 occurs in persons with a previously normal thyroid gland and is typically sudden in onset and may be severe. The hyperthyroidism is due to amiodarone-induced destructive thyroiditis with release of preformed thyroid hormones from the damaged gland (182,183).

Management of type 1 AIT requires administration of high doses of antithyroid drugs such as methimazole 40–60 mg daily or propylthiouracil up to 600–800 mg daily in order to block synthesis of new thyroid hormone. Beta-blockers may also be of value in controlling tachyarrhtmias, especially propranolol which also has the ability to block peripheral conversion of T4 to T3. Antithyroid drugs are not effective in type 2 AIT and management requires the administration of high dose steroids such as prednisone in a starting dose of 30 to 40 mg daily to reduce the inflammatory process in the thyroid and consequently decrease the release of stored thyroid hormone. Once the hyperthyroid state has begun to improve, the steroid dose can be slowly tapered over a period of 2–3 months (182,183). Most type 2 patients will remain euthyroid after resolution of the hyperthyroidism, but a small number may develop hypothyroidism (182).

A critical question is whether or not amiodarone should be discontinued if AIT has developed. Although it is generally recommended that amiodarone be stopped, other study suggests that continuation of amiodarone may not affect long-term outcome. Of 303 patients treated with amiodarone, 8% developed AIT over a follow-up period of 3.3 years. Five out of 12 patients who were continued on amiodarone had spontaneous normalization of thyroid function with a mean time to normalization of 6.2 months and no difference in time from those patients in whom amiodarone was discontinued (184).

Amiodarone-Induced Hypothyroidism

Amiodarone-induced hypothyroidism (AIH) is more likely to occur in areas where environmental iodine is adequate. In the USA, the prevalence of AIH is as high as 22% and is more likely to occur in women and in elderly persons, especially those with underlying thyroid disorders and with circulating thyroid autoantibodies (185). The mechanism is iodine-induced inhibition of thyroid hormone synthesis (182). Persons who develop AIH can be continued on amiodarone while thyroid replacement therapy is initiated with thyroxine. If amiodarone can be discontinued, spontaneous return to a euthyroid state often occurs.

Evaluation of Patients Receiving Amiodarone Therapy

When possible, patients who are to be started on amiodarone should have a careful thyroid gland examination along with thyroid ultrasound in order to detect thyroid abnormalities that may put the patient at increased risk of developing AIT or AIH. In addition, baseline measures of thyroid function should be obtained including TSH, total and free T4, total and free T3, and thyroid peroxidase antibodies (182). Repeat measurement of the thyroid laboratory tests should be done at 6-month intervals or sooner if symptoms of hyperthyroidism or hypothyroidism are suspected.

CONCLUSIONS

Thyroid hormone has multiple effects on the cardiovascular system, acting through a variety of mechanisms. Clinically, these effects are manifest in patients with hyperthyroidism and hypothyroidism, both in the overt forms of the diseases and in the now well-recognized subclinical forms. Treatment aimed at restoration of thyroid function to normal is effective in correcting many of the alterations in cardiovascular function and the clinical expressions which are the consequence of thyroid dysfunction. Evidence continues to accumulate on whether or not there are benefits of treatment of the subclinical stages of thyroid disease, especially subclinical hypothyroidism.

REFERENCES

1. Zhang J, Lazar MA. The mechanism of action of thyroid hormones. Ann Rev Physiol 2000; 62: 439–66.
2. Leng X, Blanco J, Tsai SY, et al. Mechanism for synergistic activation of thyroid hormone receptor and retinoid X receptor on different response elements. J Biol Chem 1994; 269: 31436–42.
3. Brent GA. The molecular basis of thyroid hormone action. N Engl J Med 1994; 331: 847–53.
4. Koshiyama H, Sellitti DF, Akamizu T, et al. Cardiomyopathy associated with Graves' disease. Clin Endocrinol 1996; 45: 111–16.
5. Dillmann WH. Thyroid hormone influences on the cardiovascular system: molecular and clinical studies. Thyroid Today 2001; 24: 1–13.
6. Fadel BM, Ellahham S, Ringel MD, et al. Hyperthyroid heart disease. Clin Cardiol 2000; 23: 402–8.
7. Klein I, Danzi S. Thyroid disease and the heart. Circulation 2007; 116: 1725–35.
8. Ojamaa K, Klemperer JD, MacGilvray SS, et al. Thyroid hormone and hemodynamic regulation of beta-myosin heavy chain promoter in the heart. Endocrinology 1996; 137: 802–8.
9. Morkin E. Regulation of myosin heavy chain genes in the heart. Circulation 1993; 87: 1451–60.
10. Kiss E, Jakab G, Kranias EG, et al. Thyroid hormone-induced alterations in phospholamban protein expression: regulatory effects on sarcoplasmic reticulum Ca2+ transport and myocardial relaxation. Circ Res 1994; 75: 245–51.
11. Ojamaa K, Kenessey A, Klein I. Thyroid hormone regulation of phospholamban phosphorylation in the rat heart. Endocrinology 2000; 141: 2139–44.
12. Zarain-Herzberg A, Marques J, Sukovich D, et al. Thyroid hormone receptor modulates the expression of the rabbit cardiac sarco (endo) plasmic reticulum Ca (2+)-ATPase gene. J Biol Chem 1994; 269: 1460–7.
13. Orlowski J, Lingrel JB. Thyroid and glucocorticoid hormones regulate the expression of multiple Na,K-ATPase genes in cultured neonatal rat cardiac myocytes. J Biol Chem 1990; 265: 3462–70.
14. Klein I, Ojamaa K. Thyroid hormone and the cardiovascular system. N Engl J Med 2001; 344: 501–8.
15. Markowitz C, Yater WM. Response of explanted cardiac muscle to thyroxine. Am J Physiol 1932; 100: 162–6.
16. Buccino RA, Spann JF, Pool PK, et al. Influence of thyroid state on the intrinsic contractile properties and energy stores of the myocardium. J Clin Invest 1967; 46: 1669–182.
17. Klemperer JD, Klein I, Gomez M, et al. Thyroid hormone treatment after coronary-artery bypass surgery. N Engl J Med 1995; 333: 1522–7.
18. Davis PJ, Davis FB. Acute cellular actions of thyroid hormone and myocardial function. Ann Thorac Surg 1993; 56(Suppl): S16–23.
19. Walker JD, Crawford FA, Kato S, et al. The novel effects of 3,5,3'-triiodo-L-thyronine on myocyte contractile function and beta-adrenergic responsiveness in dilated cardiomyopathy. J Thorac Cardiovasc Surg 1994; 108: 672–9.
20. Dudley SC Jr, Baumgarten CM. Bursting of cardiac sodium channels after acute exposure to 3,5,3'-triiodo-L-thyronine. Circ Res 1993; 73: 301–13.
21. Walker JD, Crawford FA Jr, Mukherjee R, et al. The direct effects of 3,5,3'-triiodo-L-thyronine (T3) on myocyte contractile processes. Insights into mechanism of action. J Thorac Cardiovasc Surg 1995; 110: 1369–79.
22. Davis PJ, Davis FB. Nongenomic actions of thyroid hormone. Thyroid 1996; 6: 497–504.
23. Harris DR, Green WL, Craelius W. Acute thyroid hormone promotes slow inactivations of sodium current in neonatal cardiac myocytes. Biochem Biophys Acta 1991; 1095: 175–81.
24. Knight RA. The use of spinal anesthesia to control sympathetic overactivity in hyper-thyroidism. Anesthesiology 1945; 6: 225.
25. Brewster WR, Isaacs JR, Osgood PF, et al. The hemodynamic and metabolic interrelationship in the activity of epinephrine, norepinephrine, and the thyroid hormone. Circulation 1956; 13: 1.
26. Howitt G, Rowlands DJ. Beta-sympathetic blockade in hyperthyroidism. Lancet 1966; 1: 628–31.

27. Shanks RG, Hadden DR, Lowe DC, et al. Controlled trial of propranolol in thyrotoxicosis. Lancet 1969; 1: 993–4.
28. Hellman R, Kelly KL, Mason WD. Propranolol for thyroid storm. N Engl J Med 1977; 297: 671–2.
29. Geffner DL, Hershman JM. Beta-adrenergic blockade for the treatment of hyperthyroidism. Am J Med 1992; 93: 61–8.
30. Hammond HK, White FC, Buxton IL, et al. Increased myocardial beta-receptors and adrenergic responses in hyperthyroid pigs. Am J Physiol 1987; 252: H283–90.
31. Waldstein SS. Thyroid-catecholamine interrelations. Ann Rev Med 1966; 17: 123–32.
32. Levey GS, Klein I. Catecholamine-thyroid hormone interactions and the cardiovascular manifestations of hyperthyroidism. Am J Med 1990; 88: 642–6.
33. Hoit BD, Khoury SF, Shao Y, et al. Effects of thyroid hormone on cardiac beta-adrenergic responsiveness in conscious baboons. Circulation 1997; 96: 592–8.
34. Ojamaa K, Klein I, Sabet A, et al. Changes in adenylyl cyclase isoform as a mechanism for thyroid hormone modulation of cardiac beta-adrenergic receptor responsiveness. Metabolism 2000; 49: 275–9.
35. Polikar R, Burger AG, Scherrer U, et al. The thyroid and the heart. Circulation 1993; 87: 1435–41.
36. Coulombe P, Dussault JH, Walker P. Plasma catecholamine concentrations in hyperthyroidism and hypothyroidism. Metabolism 1976; 25: 973–9.
37. Coulombe P, Dussault JH, Letarte J, et al. Catecholamine metabolism in thyroid diseases. Epinephrine secretion rate in hyperthyroidism and hypothyroidism. J Clin Endocrinol Metab 1976; 42: 125–31.
38. Stoffer SS, Tian NS, Gorman CA, et al. Plasma catecholamines in hypothyroidism and hyperthyroidism. J Clin Endocrinol Metab 1973; 36: 587–9.
39. Trivalle C, Doucet J, Chassagne P, et al. Differences in the signs and symptoms of hyperthyroidism in older and younger patients. J Am Geriatr Soc 1996; 44: 50–3.
40. Boelaert K, Torlinska B, Holder RL, et al. Older subjects with hyperthyroidism present with a paucity of symptoms and signs: a large cross-sectional study. J Clin Endocrinol Metab 2010; 95: 2715–26.
41. Biondi B, Palmieri EA, Lombardi G, et al. Effects of thyroid hormone on cardiac function: the relative importance of heart rate, loading conditions, and myocardial contractility in the regulation of cardiac performance in human hyperthyroidism. J Clin Endocrinol Metab 2002; 87: 968–74.
42. Sun ZQ, Ojamaa K, Nakamura TY, et al. Thyroid hormone increases pacemaker activity in rat neonatal atrial myocytes. J Mol Cell Cardiol 2001; 33: 811–24.
43. Feldman T, Borow KM, Sarne DH, et al. Myocardial mechanics in hyperthyroidism: importance of left ventricular loading conditions, heart rate and contractile state. J Am Coll Cardiol 1986; 7: 967–74.
44. Resnick LM, Laragh JH. Plasma renin activity in syndromes of thyroid hormone excess and deficiency. Life Sci 1982; 30: 585–6.
45. Ojamaa K, Klemperer JD, Klein I. Acute effects of thyroid hormone on vascular smooth muscle. Thyroid 1996; 6: 505–12.
46. Mintz G, Pizzarello R, Klein I. Enhanced left ventricular diastolic function in hyper-thyroidism: noninvasive assessment and response to treatment. J Clin Endocrinol Metab 1991; 73: 146–50.
47. Franklyn JA, Maisonneuve P, Sheppard MC, et al. Mortality after the treatment of hyperthyroidism with radioactive iodine. N Engl J Med 1998; 338: 712–18.
48. Campus S, Rappelli A, Mamavasi A, et al. Heart block and hyperthyroidism. Arch Intern Med 1975; 135: 1091–5.
49. Hoffman I, Lowrey RD. The electrocardiogram in thyrotoxicosis. Am J Cardiol 1960; 6: 893–904.
50. Teoh PC, Cheah JS, Chia BL. Effect of adrenergic blockade and specific antithyroid therapy on electrocardiographic changes in hyperthyroidism. Am J Med Sci 1974; 268: 157–62.
51. Komiya N, Isomoto S, Nakao K, et al. Electrophysiological abnormalities of the atrial muscle in patients with paroxysmal atrial fibrillation associated with hyperthyroidism. Clin Endocrinol 2002; 56: 39–44.
52. Wustmann K, Kucera JP, Zanchi A, et al. Activation of electrical triggers of atrial fibrillation in hyperthyroidism. J Clin Endocrinol Metab 2008; 93: 2104–8.
53. Stavrakis S, Yu X, Patterson E, et al. Activating autoantibodies to the beta-1 adrenergic and M2 muscarinic receptors facilitate atrial fibrillation in patients with Graves' hyperthyrpoidism. J Am Coll Cardiol 2009; 54: 1309–16.
54. Iwasaki T, Naka M, Hiramatsu K, et al. Echocardiographic studies on the relationship between atrial enlargement in patients with hyperthyroidism of Grave's disease. Cardiology 1989; 76: 10–17.
55. Osman F, Gammage MD, Sheppard MC, et al. Cardiac dysrhythmias and thyroid dysfunction: the hidden menace? J Clin Endocrinol Metab 2002; 87: 963–7.

56. Krahn AD, Klein GJ, Kerr CR, et al. How useful is thyroid function testing in patients with recent-onset atrial fibrillation? Arch Intern Med 1996; 156: 2221–4.

57. Nakazawa HK, Sakurai K, Hamada N, et al. Management of atrial fibrillation in the post-thyrotoxic state. Am J Med 1982; 72: 903–6.

58. Toft AD. Subclinical hyperthyroidism. N Engl J Med 2001; 345: 512–16.

59. Forfer JC, Muir AL, Sawers SA, et al. Abnormal left ventricular function in hyperthyroidism: evidence for a possible reversible cardiomyopathy. N Engl J Med 1982; 307: 1165–70.

60. Ching GW, Franklyn JA, Stallard TJ, et al. Cardiac hypertrophy as a result of long-term thyroxine therapy and thyrotoxicosis. Heart 1996; 75: 363–8.

61. Nixon JV, Anderson RJ, Cohen ML. Alteration in left ventricular mass and performance in patients treated effectively for thyrotoxicosis. Am J Med 1979; 67: 268.

62. Pereira N, Parisi A, Dec GW, et al. Myocardial stunning in hyperthyroidism. Clin Cardiol 2000; 23: 298–300.

63. Kahaly GJ, Matthews CH, Mohr-Kahaly S, et al. Cardiac involvement in thyroid hormone resistance. J Clin Endocrinol Metab 2002; 87: 204–12.

64. Brandt F, Green A, Hegedus L, et al. A critical review and meta-analysis of the association between overt hyperthyroidism and mortality. Eur J Endocrinol 2011; 165: 491–7.

65. Metso S, Jaatinen P, Huhtala H, et al. Increased cardiovascular and cancer mortality after radioiodine treatment for hyperthyroidism. J Clin Endocrinol Metab 2007; 92: 2190–6.

66. Volzke H, Schwahn C, Wallaschofski H, et al. The Association of thyroid dysfunction with all-cause and circulatory mortality: is there a causal relationship? J Clin Endocrinol Metab 2007; 92: 2421–9.

67. U.S. Preventive Services Task Force. Screening for thyroid disease: recommendation statement. Ann Intern Med 2004; 140: 125–7.

68. Laurbeg P, Bulow-Pedersen I, Knudsen N, et al. Environmental iodine intake affects the type of non-malignant thyroid disease. Thyroid 2001; 11: 457–69.

69. Belfiore A, Sava L, Runello F, et al. Solitary autonomously functioning thyroid notudles and iodine deficiency. J Clin Endocrinol Metab 1983; 56: 283–7.

70. Parle JV, Franklyn JA, Cross KW, et al. Prevalence and follow-up of abnormal thyrotropin (TSH) concentrations in the elderly in the United Kingdom. Clin Endocrinol (Oxford) 1991; 34: 77–83.

71. Gussekloo J, van Exel E, de Craen AJ, et al. Thyroid status, disability and cognitive function, and survival in old age. JAMA 2004; 292: 2591–9.

72. Canaris GJ, Manowitz NR, Mayor G, et al. The Colorado thyroid disease prevalence study. Arch Intern Med 2000; 160: 525–34.

73. Aghini-Lombardi F, Antonangeli L, Maritino E, et al. The spectrum of thyroid disorders in an iodine-deficient community: the Pescopagano survey. J Clin Endocrinol Metab 1999; 84: 561–6.

74. Vanderpunmp MP, Tunbridge WM, French JM, et al. The incidence of thyroid disorders in the community: a twenty-year follow-up of the Whickham survey. Clin Endocrinol 1995; 43: 55–68.

75. Walsh JP, Bremner AP, Bulsara MK, et al. Subclinical thyroid dysfunction as a risk factor for cardiovascular disease. Arch Intern Med 2005; 165: 2467–72.

76. Sawin CT, Geller A, Kaplan MM, et al. Low serum thyrotropin (thyroid-stimulating hormone) in older persons without hyperthyroidism. Arch Intern Med 1991; 151: 165–8.

77. Sawin CT, Geller A, Wolf PA, et al. Low serum thyrotropin concentrations as a risk factor for atrial fibrillation in older patients. N Engl J Med 1994; 331: 1249–52.

78. Vadiveloo T, Donnan RT, Cochrane L, et al. The epidemiology, audit, and research study (TEARS): the natural history of endogenous subclinical hyperthyroidism. J Clin Endocrinol Metab 2011; 96: E1–8.

79. Biondi B, Palmieri EA, Lombardi G, et al. Effects of subclinical thyroid dysfunction on the heart. Ann Intern Med 2002; 137: 904–14.

80. Donatelli M, Assennato P, Abbadi V, et al. Cardiac changes in subclinical and overt hyperthyroid women: retrospective study. Int J Cardiol 2003; 90: 159–64.

81. Tseng KH, Walfish PG, Persaud JA, et al. Concurrent aortic and mitral valve echocardiography permits measurement of systolic time intervals as an index of peripheral tissue thyroid functional status. J Clin Endocrinol Metab 1989; 69: 633–8.

82. Volzke H, Robinson DM, Schminke U, et al. Thyroid function and carotid wall thickness. J Clin Endocrinol Metab 2004; 89: 2145–9.

83. Gullu S, Altunas F, Dincer I, et al. Effects of TSH suppressive therapy on cardiac morphology and function: beneficial effects of the addition of beta-blockade on diastolic dysfunction. Eur J Endocrinol 2004; 150: 655–61.

84. Biondi B, Palmieri EA, Fazio S, et al. Endogenous subclinical hyperthyroidism affects quality of life and cardiac morphology and function in young and middle-aged patients. J Clin Endocrinol Metab 2000; 85: 4701–5.

85. Shargorodsky M, Serov S, Gavish D, et al. Long-term thyrotropin-suppressive therapy with levothyroxine impairs small and large artery elasticity and increases left ventricular mass in patients with thyroid carcinoma. Thyroid 2006; 16: 381–6.

86. Owecki M, Michalak A, Nikisch E, et al. Prolonged ventricular repolarization measured by corrected QT interval (QTc) in subclinical hyperthyroidism. Horm Metab Res 2006; 38: 44–7.

87. Biondi B, Fazio S, Carella C, et al. Control of adrenergic overactivity by beta-blockade improves the quality of life in patients receiving longterm suppressive therapy with levo-thyroxine. J Clin Endocrinol Metab 1994; 78: 1028–33.

88. Auer J, Schreibner P, Mische T, et al. Subclinical hyperthyroidism as a risk factor for atrial fibrillation. Am Heart J 2001; 142: 838–42.

89. Petretta M, Bonaduce D, Spinelli L, et al. Cardiovascular haemodynamics and cardiac autonomic control in patients with subclinical and overt hyperthyroidism. Eur J Endocrinol 2001; 145: 691–6.

90. Cappola AR, Fried LP, Arnold AM, et al. Thyroid status, cardiovascular risk, and mortality in older adults. JAMA 2006; 295: 1033–41.

91. Collet T-H, Gussekloo J, Bauer DC, et al. Subclinical hyperthyroidism and the risk of coronary heart disease and mortality. Arch Intern Med 2012; 172: 799–809.

92. Kreuzberg U, Theissen P, Schicha H, et al. Single-channel activity and expression of atrial L-type Ca channels in patients with latent hyperthyroidism. Am J Physiol Heart Circ Physiol 2000; 278: H723–30.

93. Gussekloo J, Westendorp RG, Stott DJ, et al. Subclinical thyroid dysfunction and the risk of heart failure in older persons at high cardiovascular risk. J Clin Endocrinol Metab 2012; 97: 852–61.

94. Parle JV, Maisonneuve P, Sheppard MC, et al. Prediction of all-cause mortality and cardiovascular mortality in elderly people from one low serum thyrotropin result: a 10-year cohort study. Lancet 2001; 358: 861–5.

95. Ochs N, Auer R, Bauer DC, et al. Meta-analysis: subclinical thyroid dysfunction and the risk for coronary heart disease and mortality. Ann Intern Med 2008; 148: 832–45.

96. Gilligan DM, Ellenbogen KA, Epstein AE. The management of atrial fibrillation. Am J Med 1996; 101: 413–21.

97. Kellet HA, Sawers JS, Boulton FE, et al. Problems of anticoagulation with warfarin in hyperthyroidism. Quart J Med 1986; 58: 43–51.

98. Aronow WS. The heart and thyroid disease. Clin Ger Med 1995; 11: 219–29.

99. Parle JV, Maisonneuve P, Sheppard MC, et al. Mortality is transiently increased after diagnosis in patients with subclinical hyperthroidism. Lancet 2002; 358: 861–5.

100. Biondi B, Palmieri EA, Fazio S, et al. Endogenous subclinical hyperthyroidism affects quality of life and cardiac morphology and function in young and middle-aged patients. J Clin Endocrinol Metab 2000; 85: 4701–5.

101. Col NF, Surks MI, Daniels GH. Subclinical thyroid disease: clinical applications. JAMA 2004; 291: 239–43.

102. Gharib H, Tuttle RM, Baskin HJ, et al. Consensus Statement: Subclinical thyroid dysfunction: a joint statement on management from the American Association of Clinical Endocrinologists, the American Thyroid Association, and The Endocrine Society. J Clin Endocrinol Metab 2005; 90: 581–5.

103. Cooper DS. Approach to the patient with subclinical hyperthyroidism. J Clin Endocrinol Metab 2007; 92: 3–9.

104. Surks MI, Ortiz E, Daniels GH, et al. Subclinical thyroid disease: scientific review and guidelines for diagnosis and management. JAMA 2004; 291: 228–38.

105. Sgarbi JA, Villaca FG, Garbeline B, et al. The effects of early antithyroid therapy for endogenous subclinical hyperthyroidism in clinical and heart abnormalities. J Clin Endocrinol Metab 2003; 88:1672–7.

106. Ladenson PW, Singer PA, Ain KB, et al. American Thyroid Association guidelines for detection of thyroid dysfunction. Arch Intern Med 2000; 160: 1573–5.

107. Douglas RC, Jacobson SD. Pathologic changes in adult myxedema: survey of 10 necropsies. J Clin Endocrinol Metab 1957; 17: 1354–64.

108. McFadden PM, Berenson GS. Basement membrane changes in myocardial and skeletal muscle capillaries in myxedema. Circ Res 1972; 30: 808–14.

109. Siperstein MD, Unger RH, Madison LL. Studies of muscle capillary basement membranes in normal subjects, diabetic, and prediabetic patients. J Clin Invest 1968; 47: 1973–99.

110. Hamolsky MW, Kurland GS, Freedberg AS. The heart in hypothyroidism. J Chronic Dis 1961; 14: 558–69.

111. Taylor RR, Covell JW, Ross JR. Influence of the thyroid state on left ventricular tension-velocity relations in the intact, sedated dog. J Clin Invest 1969; 48: 775–84.

112. Harrison TS. Adrenal medullary and thyroid relationships. Physiol Rev 1964; 44: 161–85.

113. Leak D, Lew M. Effect of treatment of hypothyroidism on circulatory response to adrenaline. Br Heart J 1963; 25: 30–4.

114. Margolius H, Gaffney TE. Effects of injected norepinephrine and sympathetic nerve stimulation in hypothyroid and hyperthyroid dogs. J Pharmacol Exp Ther 1965; 149: 329–35.

115. Ciaraldi T, Marinetti GV. Thyroxine and propylthiouracil effects in vivo on alpha and beta-adrenergic receptors in rat heart. Biochem Biophys Res Commun 1977; 74: 984–91.

116. Suko J. The calcium pump of cardiac sarcoplasmic reticulum. Functional alterations at different levels of thyroid state in rabbits. J Physiol (Lond) 1973; 228: 563–82.

117. Lifschitz MD, Kayne HL. Cardiac myofibrillar ATPase in hypophysectomized or thyroidectomized rats. Biochem Pharmacol 1966; 15: 405–7.

118. Rovetto MJ, Hjalmarson AC, Morgan HE, et al. Hormonal control of cardiac myosin adenosine triphosphatase in the rat. Circ Res 1972; 31: 397–409.

119. Yazaki Y, Raben MS. Effect of the thyroid state on the enzymatic characteristics of cardiac myosin. A difference in behavior of rat and rabbit cardiac myosin. Circ Res 1975; 36: 208–15.

120. Freedberg AS, Papp JG, Williams EM. The effect of altered thyroid state on atrial intracellular potentials. J Physiol (Lond) 1970; 207: 357–69.

121. Dullaart RP, van Doormaal JJ, Hoogenberg K, et al. Triiodothyronine rapidly lowers plasma lipoprotein (a) in hypothyroid subjects. Neth J Med 1995; 46: 179–84.

122. Hayashi H, Mizushima A, Yoshinaga H, et al. The relationship between lipoprotein (a) and, low density protein receptors during the treatment of hyperthyroidisms. Horm Metab Res 1996; 28: 384–7.

123. O'Brien T, Katz K, Hodge D, et al. The effect of the treatment of hypothyroidism and hyperthyroidism on plasma lipids and apolipoproteins AI, AII, and E. Clin Endocrinol (Oxf) 1997; 46: 17–20.

124. Obuobie K, Smith J, Evans LM, et al. Increased central arterial stiffness in hypothyroidism. J Clin Endocrinol Metab 2002; 87: 4662–6.

125. Cappola AR, Ladenson PW. Hypothyroidism and atherosclerosis. J Clin Endocrinol Metab 2003; 88: 2438–44.

126. Douglas AH, Samuel P. Analysis of electrocardiographic patterns in hypothyroid heart disease. N Y State J Med 1960; 60: 2227–35.

127. Korth C, Schmidt J. Neue beobachtungen zum "myxodemherzen" [Further studies of the heart in myxedema]. Dtsch Arch Klin Med 1955; 202: 437–45.

128. Shenoy MM, Goldman JM. Hypothyroid cardiomyopathy. Echocardiographic documentation of reversibility. Am J Med Sci 1987; 294: 1–9.

129. Kabadi UM, Kumar SP. Pericardial effusion in primary hypothyroidism. Am Heart J 1990; 120: 1393–5.

130. Aber CP, Thompson GS. The heart in hypothyroidism. Am Heart J 1964; 68: 429.

131. Epstein SE, Beiser GD, Stampfer M, et al. Characterization of the circulatory response to maximal upright exercise in normal subjects and patients with heart disease. Circulation 1967; 35: 1049–62.

132. Ertugrul A. A new electrocardiographic observation in infants and children with hypo-thyroidism. Pediatrics 1966; 37: 669–72.

133. Miura S, Iitaka M, et al. Decrease in serum levels of thyroid hormone in patients with coronary heart disease. Endocr J 1996; 43: 657–63.

134. Perk P, ONeill BJ. The effect of thyroid hormone therapy on angiographic coronary artery disease progression. Can J Cardiol 1997; 13: 273–6.

135. Hak AE, Pols HAP, Visser TJ, et al. Subclinical hypothyroidism is an independent risk factor for atherosclerosis and myocardial infarction in elderly women: the Rotterdam Study. Ann Intern Med 2000; 132: 270 8.

136. Cooper DS. Subclinical hypothyroidism. N Engl J Med 2002; 345: 260–5.

137. Evered DC, Ormston BJ, Smith PA, et al. Grades of hypothyroidism. Br Med J 1973; 1: 657–62.

138. Tumbridge WM, Brewis M, French J, et al. Natural History of Autoimmune thyroiditis. Br Med J 1981; 282: 258–62.

139. Jayme JJ, Ladenson PW. Subclinical thyroid dysfunction in the elderly. Trends Endocrinol Metab 1994; 5: 79–86.

140. Biondi B, Cooper DS. The clinical significance of subclinical thyroid dysfunction. Endocr Rev 2008; 29: 76–131.

141. Rosenthal MJ, Hunt WC, Garry PJ, et al. Thyroid failure in the elderly. Microsomal antibodies as discriminant for therapy. JAMA 1987; 258: 209–13.

142. Sawin CT, Castelli WP, Hershman JM, et al. The aging thyroid. Thyroid deficiency in the Framingham study. Arch Intern Med 1985; 145: 1386–8.

143. Tunbridge WM, Evered DC, Hall R, et al. The spectrum of thyroid disease in a community: the Whickham survey. Clin Endocrinol (Oxford) 1977; 7: 481–93.

144. Lazarus JH, Burr ML, McGregor AM, et al. The prevalence and progression of autoimmune thyroid disease in the elderly. Acta Endocrinol 1984; 106: 199–202.

145. Huber G, Staub J-J, Meier C, et al. Prospective study of the spontaneous course of subclinical hypothyroidism: prognostic value of thyrotropin thyroid reserve, and thyroid antibodies. J Clin Endocrinol Metab 2002; 87: 3221–6.

146. Diez JJ, Iglesias P. Spontaneous subclinical hypothyroidism in patients older than 55 years: an analysis of natural course and risk factors for the development of overt thyroid failure. J Clin Endocrinol Metab 2004; 89: 4890–7.

147. Forfar JC, Wathen CG, Todd WT, et al. Left ventricular performance in subclinical hypothyroidism. Q J Med 1985; 57:857–65.

148. Biondi B, Fazio S, Palmieri EA, et al. Left ventricular diastolic dysfunction in patients with subclinical hypothyroidism. J Clin Endocrinol Metab 1999; 84: 2064–7.

149. Cooper D, Halpern R, Wood LC, et al. L-thyroxine therapy in subclinical hypothyroidism: a double-blind, placebo-controlled trial. Ann Intern Med 1984; 101: 18–24.

150. Nagasaki T, Inaba M, Kumeda Y, et al. Increased pulse wave velocity in subclinical hypothyroidism. J Clin Endocrinol Metab 2006; 91: 154–8.

151. Owen PJ, Rajiv C, Vinereanu D, et al. Subclinical hypothyroidism, arterial stiffness, and myocardial reserve. J Clin Endocrinol Metab 2006; 91: 2126–32.

152. Althous BU, Staub JJ, Ryff-de-Leche A, et al. LDL/HDL changes in subclinical hypothyroidism: possible risk factors for coronary heart disease. Clin Endocrinol (Oxford) 1988; 28: 157–63.

153. Kahaly GJ. Cardiovascular and atherogenic aspects of subclinical hypothyroidism. Thyroid 2000; 10: 665–79.

154. Caraccio N, Ferrannini E, Monzani F. Lipoprotein profile in subclinical hypothyroidism: response to levothyroxine replacement, a randomized placebo-controlled study. J Clin Endocrinol Metab 2002; 87: 1533–8.

155. Arem R, Patsch W. Lipoprotein and apolipoprotein levels in subclinical hypothyroidism. Effect of levothyroxine therapy. Arch Intern Med 1990; 150: 2097–100.

156. Danese MD, Ladenson PW, Meinert CL, et al. Effect of thyroxine therapy on serum lipoproteins in patients with mild thyroid failure: a quantitative review of the literature. J Clin Endocrinol Metab 2000; 85: 2993–3001.

157. Walsh JP, Bremner AP, Bulsara MK, et al. Thyroid dysfunction and serum lipids: a community-based study. Clin Endocrinol 2005; 63: 670–5.

158. Pirich C, Mullner M, Sinzinger H. Prevalence and relevance of thyroid dysfunction in 1922 cholesterol screening participants. J Clin Epidemiol 2000; 53: 623–9.

159. Vanderpump MP, Tunbridge WM, French JM, et al. The development of ischemic heart disease in relation to autoimmune thyroid disease in a 20-year follow-up study of an English community. Thyroid 1996; 6: 155–60.

160. Imaizumi M, Akahoshi M, Ichimaru S, et al. Risk for ischemic heart disease and all-cause mortality in subclinical hypothyroidism. J Clin Endocrinol Metab 2004; 89: 3365–70.

161. Rodondi N, den Elzen WPJ, Bauer DC, et al. Subclinical hypothyroidism and the risk of coronary heart disease and mortality. JAMA 2010; 304: 1365–74.

162. Asvold BO, Bjoro T, Ivar T, et al. Thyrotropin levels and risk of fatal coronary heart disease. Arch Intern Med 2008; 168: 855–60.

163. Razvi S, Shakoor A, Vanderpump M, et al. The influence of age on the relationship between subclinical hypothyroidism and ischemic heart disease: a metaanalysis. J Clin Endocrinol Metab 2008; 93: 2998–3007.

164. Mya MM, Aronow WS. Subclinical hypothyroidism is associated with coronary artery disease in older persons. J Gerontol Med Sci 2002; 57A: M658–9.

165. Bindels AJ, Westendorp RG, Frolich M, et al. The prevalence of subclinical hypothyroidism at different total plasma cholesterol levels in middle aged men and women: a need for case finding? Clin Endocrinol (Oxf) 1999; 50: 217–20.

166. Muller B, Tsakiris DA, Roth CB, et al. Haemostatic profile in hypothyroidism as potential risk factor for vascular or thrombotic disease. Eur J Clin Invest 2001; 31: 131–7.

167. Rodondi N, Newman AB, Vittinghoff E, et al. Subclinical hypothyroidism and the risk of heart failure, other cardiovascular events, and death. Arch Intern Med 2005; 165: 2460–6.

168. Rondondi N, Bauer DC, Cappola AR, et al. Subclinical thyroid dysfunction, cardiac function, and the risk of heart failure. J Am Coll Cardiol 2008; 52: 1152–9.

169. Monzani F, Caraccio N, Kozakowa M, et al. Effect of levothyroxine replacement on lipid profile and intima-media thickness in subclinical hypothyroidism: a double-blind, placebo-controlled study. J Clin Endocrinol Metab 2004; 89: 2099–106.

170. Maya MM, Aronow WS. Increased prevalence of peripheral arterial disease in older men and women with subclinical hypothyroidism. J Gerontol Med Sci 2003; 58A: 68–9.

171. Monzani F, Di Bello V, Caraccio N, et al. Effect of levothyroxine on cardiac function and structure in subclinical hypothyroidism: a double blind, placebo-controlled study. J Clin Endocrinol Metab 2001; 86: 1110–15.

172. Razvi S, Ingoe L, Keeka G, et al. The beneficial effect of l-thyroxine on cardiovascular risk factors, endothelial function, and quality of life in subclinical hypothyroidism: randomized, crossover trial. J Clin Endocrinol Metab 2007; 92: 1715–23.

173. Traub-Weidinger T, Graf S, Beheshti M, et al. Coronary vasoreactivity in subjects with thyroid auto-immunity and subcliical hypothyroidism before and after supplementation with thyroxine. Thyroid 2012; 22: 245–51.

174. Ravzi S, Weaver JU, Butler TJ, et al. Levothyroxine treatment of subclinical hypothyroidism, fatal and nonfatal cardiovascular events, and mortality. Arch Intern Med 2012; 172: 811–17.

175. Pingitore A, Galli E, Barison A, et al. Acute effects of triiodothyronine (T3) replacement therapy in patients with chronic heart failure and low-T3 syndrome: a randomized, placebo-controlled study. J Clin Endocrinol Metab 2008; 93: 1351–8.

176. Keating FR Jr, Parkin TW, Selby JB, et al. Treatment of heart disease associated with myxedema. Prog Cardiovasc Dis 1961; 3: 364–81.

177. Becker C. Hypothyroid and atherosclerotic heart disease: pathogenesis, medical management and the role of coronary artery bypass surgery. Endocrinol Rev 1985; 6: 432–40.

178. Jordan RM. Myxedema coma. Pathophysiology, therapy, and factors affecting prognosis. Med Clin North Am 1995; 79: 185–94.

179. Yamamoto T, Fukuyama J, Fujiyoshi A. Factors associated with mortality of myxedema coma: report of eight cases and literature survey. Thyroid 1999; 9: 1167–74.

180. Surks MI. Subclinical thyroid dysfunction: a joint statement on management from the American Association of Clinical Endocrinologists, the American Thyroid Association, and The Endocrine Society. J Clin Endocrinol Metab 2005; 90: 586–7; commentary.

181. Ringel MD, Mazzaferri EL. Subclinical thyroid dysfunction—can there be a consensus about the consensus? J Clin Endocrinol Metab 2005; 90: 588–90; editorial.

182. Martino E, Bartalena L, Bogazzi F, et al. The effects of amiodarone on the thyroid. Endocr Rev 2001; 22: 240–54.

183. Cardenas GA, Cabral JM, Leslie CA. Amiodarone-induced thyrotoxicosis: diagnostic and therapeutic strategies. Clev Clin J Med 2003; 70: 624–31.

184. Ahmed S, Van Gelder IC, Wiesfeld AC, et al. Determinants and outcome of amiodarone-associated thyroid dysfunction. Clin Endocrinol 2011; 75: 388–94.

185. Martino E, Aghini-Lombardi F, Bartalena L, et al. Enhanced susceptibility to amiodarone-induced hypothyroidism in patients with autoimmune thyroid disease. Arch Intern Med 1994; 154: 2722–6.

20

Heart failure in older adults

Ali Ahmed and Jerome L. Fleg

SUMMARY

Heart failure (HF) in older adults is a geriatric syndrome characterized by female predominance, preserved ejection fraction (HFpEF), hypertension, and other comorbidities. The vast majority of HF patients are older adults in whom the etiology and pathophysiology of HF are multifactorial and interactive. HF is the leading cause for hospital admission and readmission for older Americans and is also a leading cause of death. HF symptoms in older adults may be atypical and older adults may attribute their HF symptoms to aging, both of which may result in delayed diagnosis and therapy. Evidence-based therapy with neurohormonal blockade, device, and surgical interventions should be considered for older adults with HF and reduced ejection fraction (HFrEF), keeping in mind there is little data for those 80 years and older, who comprise nearly half of the HF population. Furthermore, there is no evidence-based therapy for HFpEF, which is the more common form of HF in older adults. Thus, prevention of HF in older adults through optimal treatment of HF risk factors such as hypertension, dyslipidemia, hyperglycemia, obesity, and smoking, and promotion of regular physical activity should be encouraged throughout life. Such efforts if successful would likely improve the health and quality of life of older adults to a far greater extent than even the most exciting advances in HF therapy.

EPIDEMIOLOGY AND RISK FACTORS

Heart failure (HF) is predominantly a geriatric syndrome. Geriatric syndromes are a heterogeneous group of disorders, but they share many common features that include multiple etiologies and pathogenetic pathways, a high prevalence in older adults and a substantial adverse impact on quality of life, morbidity, and mortality (Table 20.1) (1). The American Heart Association estimates that based on the findings from the 2005–2008 National Health and Nutrition Examination Surveys (NHANES), approximately 5.7 million or 2.4% of Americans 20 years of age or older have HF and the prevalence increases dramatically with age (2). It has been projected that the prevalence of HF would reach approximately 9 million by 2030. Findings from the Cardiovascular Health Study (CHS) suggest that among community-dwelling Medicare-eligible adults, 65 years of age or older, the prevalence of centrally adjudicated HF was approximately 8.8%, which increases to as high as 14–18% among those 85 years or older (3).

An estimated 670,000 Americans 45 years of age or older develop HF every year (2). Incident HF is uncommon before the age of 50 years and almost exclusively affects African Americans. In the Coronary Artery Risk Development in Young Adults (CARDIA) study, in which 5115 African-American and white young adults 18–30 years of age at baseline were

Table 20.1 Heart Failure in Older Versus Middle-Aged Adults

Characteristic	Older Adults	Middle-Aged Adults
Prevalence	6–18%	<1%
Gender	Predominantly women	Predominantly men
Etiology	Hypertension	Coronary heart disease
Left ventricular systolic function	Normal	Impaired
Left ventricular diastolic function	Impaired	Normal or mildly impaired
Comorbidities	Multiple	Few

Source: Adapted from Ref. 50.

followed for over 20 years, only 27 (0.5%) participants developed HF, and importantly, all but one of these 27 HF patients were African-American (4). Findings from the Framingham Heart Study (FHS) demonstrated that the incidence of HF was about 0.1% and 0.4% for those 45–54 years and 55–64 years, respectively, but increased to about 1%, 1.5% and nearly 3% among those 65–74, 75–84 and ≥85 years, respectively (5). An estimated 1.1 million hospitalizations in the USA are due to HF (2). Most of these hospitalizations occur in older adults, for whom HF is the leading cause for hospital admission and readmission (6,7). In 2008, HF was the underlying cause of death for approximately 56,830 deaths and was associated with another approximately 281,437 deaths (2). Most of the HF deaths occurred in older adults.

Like most other geriatric syndromes, HF has multiple etiologies (1). Findings from the FHS demonstrated that hypertension and coronary artery disease are the two most common pre-existing and prevalent conditions among those who developed new HF, and that hypertension, diabetes, and left ventricular (LV) hypertrophy by electrocardiography were major risk factor in both younger (35–64 years) and older (65–94 years) participants (8). The relative risks of these risk factors are generally higher among younger adults. For example, among men 35–64 years, the presence of hypertension increased the risk of HF by 4.4 times, but only 1.9 times in those ≥65 years. However, because the prevalence of hypertension is much higher among older adults, the overall impact of hypertension as a risk factor is more pronounced in older adults. This concept of population-attributable risk was further clarified from the findings of the CHS, which enrolled community-dwelling older adults. CHS participants with baseline hypertension had 36% increased risk of HF while those with baseline coronary heart disease had 87% increased risk of HF (9). However, the prevalence of hypertension was much higher (41%) than that of coronary artery disease (17%), and as a result, despite its low relative risk, the population-attributable risk of hypertension was similar (about 13%) to that of coronary heart disease (9). This is of enormous public health importance as it suggests that 13% of HF would be prevented if hypertension could be eliminated.

The vast majority of older adults with hypertension have isolated systolic hypertension (ISH), defined as an isolated elevation of systolic blood pressure (SBP) in the absence of elevation of diastolic blood pressure (DBP). In the CHS, 38% of the participants had ISH, defined as SBP ≥140 mmHg and DBP <90 mmHg, and the presence of ISH was associated with a significant 26% increased risk of incident HF (10). Among the CHS participants with hypertension, compared to those with controlled SBP (<140 mmHg), those with SBP ≥140 mmHg had a significant 39% higher risk of incident HF (11), suggesting that control of hypertension in older adults is important. ISH is a manifestation of increased arterial stiffness of large conduit arteries, which explains the wide pulse pressure and low DBP in such older adults (12). Isolated diastolic hypotension (IDH), a mirror image of ISH and defined as an isolated low DBP with a normal or elevated SBP is also common in older adults. In the CHS, about 18% of the participants had IDH, defined as DBP <60 mmHg and SBP ≥100 mmHg, and those with IDH had an independent 33% higher risk of developing new-onset HF (13). The increased risk of incident HF associated with IDH was similar among older adults with and without hypertension. The associations of both ISH and IDH with incident HF were attenuated in older adults with more advanced age, likely due to other competing risk factors.

The CHS also provide insights into many other risk factors and predictors of incident HF in older adults. Among older adults, the presence of diabetes is associated with an independent 45% increased risk of incident HF (14) and among those with diabetes, higher fasting plasma glucose level is associated with higher risk of incident HF (15). Valvular heart disease, peripheral arterial disease, and atrial fibrillation are also potent risk factors for incident HF in older adults (9,16,17). LV hypertrophy and asymptomatic LV systolic dysfunction are also strong predictors of incident HF in older adults (9,18,19). Elevated serum creatinine levels have been shown to be associated with increased risk of HF in older adults (9). However, serum creatinine is an unreliable marker of kidney function in older adults (20). Glomerular filtration rate (GFR) estimated using the Chronic Kidney Disease Epidemiology Collaboration (CKD-EPI) equation is generally more accurate in estimating kidney function, especially in those with higher GFR or normal kidney function (21). When kidney function was estimated using the CKD-EPI formula, older adults with estimated GFR < 45 ml/min/1.73 m^2 appeared to have a significant 44% higher risk of incident HF but not those with estimated GFR 45–59 ml/min/1.73 m^2, who had a non-significant 3% higher risk (22). Elevated serum uric acid levels have unadjusted association with incident HF but lacks independent association (23,24). Several non-traditional risk factors such as low serum albumin and total omega-3 fatty acid levels, elevated levels of transforming growth factor-β-1, N-terminal pro-B-type natriuretic peptide, C-reactive protein, resistin, and various markers of myocardial fibrosis, subclinical hypothyroidism, and impairment of activities of daily living have emerged as potential risk factors for incident HF in older adults (9,25–32).

Among socio-demographic and life-style risk factors, both current smoking and heavy smoking in the past have been associated with a higher risk of incident HF in older adults (33–35). However, moderate alcohol consumption, on the other hand, has been shown to be associated with a lower risk of incident HF (36). Older adults with low income may be at increased risk of developing HF (37). Despite evidence that obesity may be protective in older HF patients (38,39), among older adults without HF, the presence of obesity is associated with a higher risk of incident HF (40,41). In contrast, physical activity has been shown to reduce the risk of HF, regardless of obesity (42,43). Although findings from laboratory animals and human studies suggest that caloric restriction may improve ventricular diastolic function (44,45), currently there is no evidence that caloric restriction is associated with lower risk of incident HF in older adults.

Findings from several population-based studies such as the FHS, the CHS, Olmsted County, and the Strong Heart Study of American-Indians suggest that more than half of older HF patients have preserved left ventricular ejection fraction (HFpEF) (46–49). Findings from these studies indicate that the typical profile of a HF patient in the community is that of an older woman with HFpEF and a history of systolic hypertension (Table 20.1 and Fig. 20.1) (49,50). These patients also tend to have different outcomes compared with older adults with HF and reduced ejection fraction (HFrEF). Older HFpEF patients generally have lower risk of all-cause mortality and HF hospitalizations, although they may have higher risk of non-cardiovascular (CV) hospitalization (51). Some studies have also suggested similar post-discharge mortality in HFpEF and HFrEF patients, in part attributed by

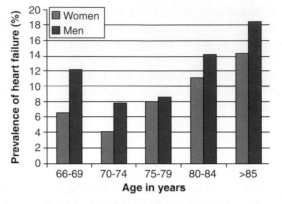

Figure 20.1   Prevalence of heart failure by age and sex in community-dwelling older adults in the Cardiovascular Health Study. *Source*: From Ref. 49.

improved outcomes in HFrEF patients receiving neurohormonal blockade (52). Findings from the Olmsted County, Minnesota suggest that the prevalence of HFpEF might be increasing (53). The health care costs associated with HFpEF are projected to increase dramatically with the aging of the US population.

PATHOPHYSIOLOGY

As a geriatric syndrome, the development of HF in older adults involves multiple etiologies and pathogenetic pathways (Fig. 20.2) (1). Aging is associated with multiple CV and non-CV structural and functional changes (54,55). These age-associated changes, such as diastolic dysfunction, often interact with other HF risk factors such as hypertension, the prevalence of which also increases with age, and play important roles in the pathogenesis of HF (Fig. 20.2). For example, normal aging is associated with increased arterial stiffness, concentric remodeling of the LV myocardium and reduced early diastolic relaxation and filling rates (56–59). Although the progression of hypertension to HF may be similar in young and older adults (60,61), the prevalence of hypertension and LV hypertrophy increase with age and hypertension is generally of longer duration in older adults (62,63). In addition, aging is associated with reduced chronotropic, inotropic, and vasodilator responses to β-adrenergic stimulation (55,64). Reduced maximal stroke volume, reflecting reduced inotropic and lusitropic reserves, may also contribute to HF in some older individuals though not in those screened to exclude occult coronary artery disease (65). These age-related changes, along with various other etiologies and pathogenetic pathways present in older adults interact with each other thus increasing the risk of incident HF.

Despite these pathophysiological age differences in the substrate for HF, relatively few studies have specifically compared younger versus older HF patients in this regard. Neurohormonal activation is felt to play an important fundamental role in the pathophysiology of systolic HF or HFrEF. As in HFrEF, plasma atrial natriuretic peptide and brain natriuretic peptide levels have been shown to be substantially increased in HFpEF at rest and there seems to be an exaggerated response during exercise (66). Compared with age-matched healthy normal subjects, older HFpEF patients had markedly elevated plasma norepinephrine levels, equivalent to those seen in HFrEF, and had levels of atrial and brain natriuretic peptide that were 10-fold higher than those in age-matched controls (67). Findings from older hospitalized HF patients demonstrated lower resting heart rate with a reduced heart rate response to tilt, an age-related increase in plasma norepinephrine levels

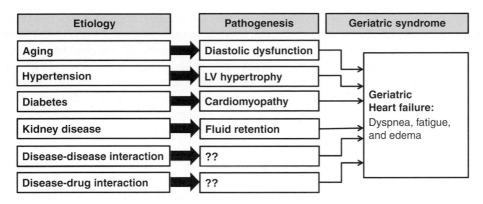

Figure 20.2 Geriatric syndrome model of heart failure in older adults: multiple etiologies and pathogenetic pathways leading to symptoms and signs of heart failure. *Source*: Adapted from Ref. 1.

without similar trends for plasma renin activity or urinary aldosterone, a lower GFR with higher renal vascular resistance (68). In another study that compared ambulatory younger (<65 years) versus older (>75 years) adults with HFrEF, plasma norepinephrine levels were higher in older HF patients (1191, ±80 pg/ml) and older adults without HF (958, ± 84 pg/ml) than younger HF patients (620, ±67 pg/ml) (69). In that study, except for serum aldosterone level, which was higher in older HF patients, serum levels of other neurohormones, such as atrial natriuretic peptide, renin activity, and angiotensin II were higher in younger HF patients (69).

Findings from the CHS suggest that LV hypertrophy may not necessarily be more common in older HFpEF patients than age-matched patients with hypertension but without HFpEF (70). A small study of 36 patients with HFpEF and hypertension suggested two different profiles, one characterized by severe LV hypertrophy and the other by a high rate of regional myocardial ischemia (71). Systolic hypertension precedes the vast majority of incident HFpEF cases and has also been documented in HFpEF patients during acute decompensation with pulmonary edema (49,72). In laboratory animals, diastolic dysfunction develops early in systemic hypertension, and LV diastolic relaxation is very sensitive to increased afterload (73). Increased afterload impairs LV relaxation, leading to increased LV filling pressures, decreased stroke volume, and symptoms of dyspnea and congestion (74). Although it has been hypothesized that HFpEF patients may have transient impairment of left ventricular ejection fraction (LVEF) at the time of acute exacerbation associated with ischemia, a small study of 38 patients found that LVEF was similar both during acute decompensation associated with hypertension and pulmonary edema and 3 days later after resolution of hypertension and pulmonary edema (72). These findings suggest that LVEF measured after acute HF events may accurately reflects LVEF during acute HF. This study and a related study, in which pulmonary edema recurred in about half of such patients despite coronary revascularization, support the concept that acute pulmonary edema in these patients is most likely due to an exacerbation of diastolic dysfunction caused by severe systolic hypertension rather than by ischemia (75).

The etiology and pathogenesis of HFpEF appear to be different from those in HFrEF. As previously discussed, a majority of older HF patients have HFpEF (49), which is relatively uncommon in younger HF patients and little is known about the pathophysiology of HFpEF. Exercise intolerance, manifested as exertional dyspnea and fatigue, is the primary symptom of both forms of HF (Table 20.1) (76). The reduced ability to increase stroke volume through the Frank–Starling mechanism despite severely increased LV filling pressure reflects diastolic dysfunction, which results in reduced cardiac output and exercise capacity in HFpEF (77). Furthermore, peak exercise oxygen consumption (VO_2) in HFpEF and HFrEF show similar impairment (67,77). Compared with age-matched healthy subjects, patients with HFpEF seem to have increased pulse pressure and thoracic aortic wall thickness and markedly decreased aortic distensibility that correlate with their severely decreased peak VO_2 (78). Similar data have been reported for patients with HFrEF (79). With advancing age, there is a modest decline in flow-mediated arterial dilation (FMAD) in large arm and leg arteries. In HFrEF, it had previously been shown that brachial FMAD is severely reduced and may contribute to exercise intolerance in these patients. It has been assumed that HFpEF patients may have similar abnormalities in FMAD as those with HFrEF. However, findings from magnetic resonance measures of flow and cuff occlusion in three well-defined groups of subjects with HFrEF, HFpEF, and age-matched healthy volunteers have demonstrated that compared with normal age-matched controls, FMAD in the femoral artery is substantially reduced in older HFrEF patients but relatively preserved in those with HFpEF (78). Findings from peak exercise tests data from this study confirmed previous reports of similar degree of exercise intolerance in HFpEF and HFrEF, in stark contrast to the FMAD results, thus indicating that abnormalities in FMAD are unlikely to contribute significantly to exercise intolerance in HFpEF.

Another potential contributor to exercise intolerance in HFpEF is chronotropic incompetence (80). In a study of patients with HFpEF and HFrEF, and an age-matched healthy volunteer control group, all participants underwent upright bicycle exercise to exhaustion with detailed physiological measurements, including expired gas analysis (80). The prevalence of chronotropic incompetence, defined by published criteria as the inability of heart rate to increase adequately during physical exertion, was 22% in HFrEF, 20% in HFpEF, and 7% in healthy volunteers (80). Among HF patients, those with chronotropic incompetence had considerable exercise intolerance, assessed as peak oxygen consumption, and in multivariate analyses, chronotropic incompetence was an independent contributor to exercise intolerance (80). Findings from younger HFrEF patients suggest that there are no significant differences in the intensity of exercise performed between patients with and without chronotropic incompetence though there was a trend towards shorter exercise time in those with incompetence (81). Compared with matched subjects with hypertensive cardiac hypertrophy but without HF, those with HFpEF have reduced chronotropic, vasodilator, and cardiac output reserve during exercise that cannot be attributed to diastolic dysfunction (82).

The role of diastolic dysfunction in HFpEF remains unclear (83,84), and that is why the term HFpEF is preferred over the term "diastolic HF". In one study of 63 patients with HFpEF, LV end-diastolic pressure was elevated in 92% of the patients, LV relaxation was abnormal in 79% of the patients, the E/A ratio was abnormal in 48% of the patients, and the E-wave deceleration time was abnormal in 64% of the patients (85). Because one or more indices of diastolic function were abnormal in all patients, the authors of that study concluded that the diagnosis of diastolic HF or HFpEF can be made without the objective measurement of parameters of LV diastolic function. However, noninvasive blood flow Doppler measures of LV diastolic filling has been shown to be rather similar in patients with HFpEF and HFrEF (67). In studies where LV pressures and volume were studied invasively, the LV pressure volume relationship was shifted upward and to the left in most patients, indicative of diastolic dysfunction (77,86,87). Findings from the CHS suggest that overall diastolic LV size tended to be modestly increased in those with HFpEF, rather than decreased, as one would expect with concentric remodeling (70). It seems likely that changes in diastolic function and myocardial mass and composition contribute prominently to HFpEF. However, given the marked heterogeneity in LV function and morphometry seen in the more familiar and well-studied syndrome of HFrEF, the possibility of substantial heterogeneity in HFpEF should not be unexpected, especially given that most HFpEF patients are older adults.

The role of genetic predisposition in the genesis of HFpEF in older adults is not well known. However, data from the Hypertension Genetic Epidemiology Network (Hyper-GEN) study have shown significant heritability of hypertension (88), LV mass and Doppler diastolic filling (89), all risk factors for HFpEF in older adults. In addition, genetic factors have now been identified in patients with hypertrophic cardiomyopathy, a disorder that shares a number of features with HFpEF in older adults. In addition, mutations that result in aldosterone excess or abnormal aldosterone handling result in morphology and symptoms suggestive of early HFpEF. The preponderance of female sex in HFpEF may also help in understanding its pathogenesis. Among healthy normal subjects, older women tend to have smaller chamber size and higher LVEF, compared to men (90). In the Hyper-GEN study, it was found that the deceleration time of early diastolic flow and isovolumic relaxation time were lengthened in hypertensive women than in men, independent of all other factors, indicative of decreased myocardial relaxation (91). Among hypertensive adults in the FHS, the predominant pattern of hypertrophic remodeling in women was concentric, whereas in men it was eccentric; this pattern has also been reported in several other studies, including Hyper-GEN (91) and Losartan Intervention for Endpoint Reduction (LIFE) study (92). However, as mentioned above, in the CHS, LV size was not decreased in HFpEF, as would be expected in concentric remodeling (70).

In rat models of chronic LV pressure overload created by aortic banding, male rats seem to respond with LV dilation and modest wall thickening (eccentric hypertrophy) with resultant increased wall stress and decreased LV contractility (93). In contrast, female rats increased their LV wall thickness and maintained a normal chamber size (concentric hypertrophy), and thereby enjoyed near-normal wall stress, and normal (even a trend toward supra-normal) contractility. As a result, the female rats were able to continue to generate substantially higher systolic pressure, despite the excess afterload. Similar findings have been observed in humans (94,95). Thus, it appears that there is a sex-related variation by which LV responds to pressure load. While male LV, less able to tolerate pressure load, responds to hypertension by dilated cardiomyopathy and low LVEF, the female LV, able to tolerate the pressure load better, develops concentric hypertrophy and maintains normal LV size and LVEF, but at the cost of impaired LV diastolic function. This finding may help to explain why men tend to develop HFrEF, whereas women tend to develop HFpEF. In rodent models, the above interplay between LV remodeling and pressure load has been shown to be influenced substantially by estrogen and androgen, and to be related to gender differences in cardiac angiotensin-converting enzyme (ACE) expression (96).

DIAGNOSIS AND CLINICAL FINDINGS

Because there is no single test or procedure that can definitively diagnose or rule out HF, the diagnosis of HF is based on a constellation of clinical findings (76). The syndrome of HF is characterized by dyspnea, fatigue, and fluid retention, which are manifestations of a reduced cardiac output and compensatory renal and neurohormonal adaptations. A clinical diagnosis of HF should be made before ordering an echocardiogram, given that a diagnosis of HF in older adults should not be ruled out because of normal LVEF. It is also important to remember that the diagnosis of HF may be a process that can span over days to months. Unfortunately, there are many diagnostic criteria for HF for use in clinical and population settings, but none is perfect or universally accepted. Orthopnea and paroxysmal nocturnal dyspnea (PND) are two major criteria for the diagnosis of HF according to modified FHS criteria (48) and the presence of two major criteria is expected to establish a definite diagnosis of HF. However, findings from CHS suggest that many older adults with both orthopnea and PND do not have HF (97). In that study, 7% (388/5771) of the community-dwelling adults ≥65 years of age had both orthopnea and PND, and yet only 20% (76/388) of these individuals had centrally adjudicated HF. Because HF is a clinical syndrome, by definition, all newly diagnosed HF patients are symptomatic and usually have fluid retention and an elevated jugular venous pressure (JVP). However, patients with chronic HF may be euvolemic and may not have classic symptoms and signs. An elevated JVP is the most specific sign of fluid retention in HF and is likely the most important physical examination in the process of diagnosis of HF in older adults (98,99). Both internal jugular vein (IJV) and external jugular vein (EJV) can be used to estimate JVP (76).

Establishing a diagnosis of HF in older adults may be challenging as many of the symptoms and signs of HF can also be found in various non-HF disorders, such as pulmonary conditions, deconditioning, and depression. Further, in early stages of HF, older adults are more likely to present with fatigue than dyspnea. A key distinction between fatigue and dyspnea in older adults is that fatigue is extremely rare at rest, and when present, is more likely to be due to depression than HF. Another subtle distinction is that while both fatigue and dyspnea may occur during exertion, fatigue often sets in at the end of maximal physical activity at patient's own pace, while dyspnea maybe more common during abrupt physical activity, such as rushing across the room to answer a phone. However, low physical activity levels may mask both symptoms. Older adults are also known to attribute their HF symptoms to aging, thus delaying presentation until symptoms are more advanced, which may paradoxically make the diagnosis easier. The diagnosis of HF in older adults may also be delayed due to inadequate history because of cognition or sensory impairments. However, objective determination of an elevated JVP may be particularly helpful in establishing a new diagnosis of HF when historical data are insufficient. B-type natriuretic peptide (BNP) and N-terminal pro-BNP (NT-proBNP) are neurohormones that are secreted by the failing ventricle in HF in response to myocardial wall stress. Several studies have suggested serum levels of these neurohormones may assist in the diagnosis of HF (100,101). However, currently there are no standard cutoffs for these neurohormones to confirm or rule out HF in general, and even less is known about their usefulness in older adults. Further, the accuracy of diagnosis or treatment of HF in real-world HF patients has not been shown to be significantly improved by BNP levels (102–104).

After a clinical diagnosis of HF has been made, the next most important step is to determine an etiology for HF. Just as a clinical diagnosis of fever is incomplete without a search for the underlying cause, a clinical diagnosis of HF is incomplete without a search for an underling etiology. The sequence of steps in evaluation of HF can be conveniently remembered by the mnemonic DEFEAT: Diagnosis, Etiology, Fluid volume, Ejection fraction, And Treatment (105). Although a direct causal association is difficult to establish, the presence of common risk factors such as hypertension, coronary heart disease, or diabetes would suggest that they may have played a role in the multifactorial causal pathways leading to incident HF in older adults. After an appropriate fluid volume assessment, the next most important step in the workup for HF diagnosis is to determine LVEF. This has both prognostic and therapeutic implications (76). Generally speaking, older HFpEF patients tend to have lower mortality than older HFrEF patients, although they have higher mortality compared with older adults without HF (3). However, as clinical presentation of HF is similar regardless of LVEF, morbidity, quality of life, and risk of hospitalizations are rather similar, regardless of LVEF. However, older HFpEF patients tend to have higher non-CV morbidities which account for a larger share of their total hospitalizations. Because life prolonging therapy for HF is only applicable to HFrEF, it is important to make this determination early. Echocardiography is the most convenient, non-invasive and cost-effective way to estimate LVEF, which also provide additional insights about potential HF etiologies such as prior myocardial infarction or valvular heart disease.

PRECIPITANTS

While development of new-onset HF in older adults is often a prolonged process, it may be precipitated by other risk factors. For example, in an older adults with age-related LV diastolic dysfunction and hypertension but without HF, the development of first symptoms and signs of HF may be expedited if hypertension is not well-controlled, or by myocardial ischemia. However, precipitants are often discussed in the context of acute decompensation of chronic HF. Empirical clinical experience and data from clinical studies from mostly younger HF patients suggest that non-adherence to salt and fluid restriction and HF medications may play roles in acute decompensation of chronic HF. In one study of 768 HFrEF patients, mean age 63 years, 180 patients had 323 episodes of decompensation, and 143 patients were hospitalized during 43 weeks of follow-up (106). In that study, 27% of hospitalized patients reported excessive salt intake, 10% reported inappropriate reduction in HF medications, and 7% reported non-adherence to HF medications (106). However, to what extent these associations were causal is unknown. In that study other major causes for hospital admission included arrhythmias (22%), myocardial ischemia (12%), acute myocardial infarction (3%), uncontrolled hypertension (3%), and non-CV causes (24%) (106). In a study of about 100 predominantly African-American HF patients, mean age 59 years, potential reasons for decompensation and hospital admission were: non-adherence with diet (22%), HF drugs (6%), both diet and drugs (37%), and arrhythmias (29%) (107). Similar reasons were observed in another study of 435 hospitalized HF patients: non-adherence to HF medications (15%) and diet (6%), anginal chest pain (33%), respiratory infection (16%), uncontrolled severe hypertension (15%), and arrhythmia (8%) (108). In the latter study, the precipitants were rather similar for both prevalent and incident HF. For example, angina pectoris was present among 30% and 39% of those with prevalent and incident HF, respectively (108).

In a study of 12,640 older hospitalized HF patients, mean age 74 years, 5992 had at least one CV readmission, of which 37% were due to HF (109). In that study, acute myocardial ischemia (11%), acute myocardial infarction (8%), atrial fibrillation (11%), and renal failure or acute respiratory infections (12%) were identified as key precipitants for decompensation. In the Organized Program to Initiate Lifesaving Treatment in Hospitalized Patients with Heart Failure (OPTIMIZE-HF) registry, of the 48,612 hospitalized HF patients, mean age 73 years, 52% women, 29,814 (61%) had one or more precipitating factors leading to decompensation and hospital admission, key of which were acute coronary syndrome (15%), pneumonia and respiratory illnesses (15%), arrhythmias (13%), uncontrolled hypertension (11%), and worsening kidney function (7%) (110). In that study, non-adherence of medications and diet were identified as precipitating factors for 9% and 5% of hospitalizations, respectively.

PROGNOSIS

HF is associated with poor prognosis, especially in older adults (111). In the CHS, of the 5795 Medicare-eligible community-dwelling adults ≥65 years, 274 (4.7%) had centrally adjudicated HF at baseline, who had a mean age 75 (±6) years, 52% were women, and 22% were African American (112). During 13 years of follow-up, 208 (76%) of these HF patients died from all causes, 257 (94%) had all-cause hospitalization, and 111 (41%) had a hospitalization due to HF (112). Of the 111 patients who had a HF hospitalization, 46% had multiple hospitalizations. Cumulative rates for 1-, 5-, and 10-year HF hospitalization were 8%, 27%, and 38%, respectively (112).

Age is a strong predictor of poor outcomes in older HF patients. In a Scottish database of 66,547consecutive first-time admissions for HF, 1-year case-fatality rate increased from 14% in patients <55 years old to 58% in those >84 years (113). Contributing factors to this age-related increased HF mortality include reduced functional reserve, multiple comorbidities, and underutilization of evidence-based medications. Findings from a propensity-matched cohort from the Digitalis Investigation Group (DIG) trial demonstrated that despite a balance in all measured baseline characteristics, during a median follow-up of 40 months, HF patients >65-years old ($n = 4036$) were at a significant higher risk of death due to all causes and CV causes, including progressive HF (114). Although age was not an independent risk factor for hospitalization due to all causes or CV causes, older HF patients had higher risk for hospitalization due to worsening HF (114). In contrast, in more advanced HFrEF patients in the β-Blocker Evaluation of Survival Trial (BEST) trial, age was not an independent predictor of poor outcomes (115).

Among patients with chronic mild to moderate HF in the DIG trial, women appeared to have lower risk of total and CV death, but no difference in death due to progressive HF (116). In contrast, there was no sex difference in total, CV, or HF hospitalization, although there seemed to a lower risk for stroke. Women also had a higher risk for unstable angina hospitalization, which seemed higher among younger patients (116). Race seems to have no independent association with mortality or hospitalization in ambulatory HF patients except that there might be a higher risk for HF hospitalization for African-Americans (117). Functional class and aerobic capacity are strong predictors of mortality in both older and younger HF patients (118–120). Prognosis of HF also appears to vary by LVEF. In the DIG trial, of the 3984 ambulatory chronic HF patients, ≥65 years, 3405 had HFrEF (LVEF ≤ 45%) and 579 had HFpEF (LVEF > 45%) (51). In that study, compared to patients with HFrEF, those with HFpEF had lower risk of all-cause mortality and HF hospitalization, but had no difference in overall hospitalization, and had a higher risk of non-CV hospitalization (51). These findings were confirmed by the Meta-analysis Global Group in Chronic Heart Failure (MAGGIC) investigator who studied 41,347 HF patients from 31 studies, of whom 10,347 had HFpEF and 31,625 had HFrEF (121). In that study, compared with HFrEF, those with HFpEF were older (mean age 71 years, vs. 66 years for HFrEF), but had lower risk of total mortality that was independent of age and other confounders such as sex and comorbidities (121). Of the 48,612 hospitalized older HF patients in OPTIMIZE-HF, 20,118 had HFrEF (LVEF < 40%) and 21,149 had HFpEF (LVEF ≥ 40%), and compared with HFrEF, those with HFpEF had similar length of hospital stay but lower in-hospital mortality (122). In addition, during 60–90 days of follow-up after hospital discharge, HFpEF patients had similar risk for mortality (9.5% vs. 9.8% for HFrEF; $p = 0.459$) and rehospitalization (29.2% vs. 29.9% for HFrEF; $p = 0.591$) (122). In older adults with HFrEF, right ventricular ejection fraction <20% is an independent predictor of poor outcomes (123).

Predictors of higher mortality in older HF patients resemble those in younger HF cohorts and include male sex, higher New York Heart Association (NYHA) class, lower functional capacity (peak VO_2), LV dilation, lower LVEF, diabetes, renal disease, anemia, hyponatremia, and recent HF hospitalization (3,124–126). HF patients with diabetes have higher mortality, which seemed to be more pronounced in women, especially in older women (127). In patients with advanced chronic HFrEF, coronary heart disease has been shown to associated with a higher risk of mortality, which seemed similar in younger and older HF patients (128). Presence of atrial fibrillation seems to have no independent association with mortality but may increase the risk of HF hospitalization (129). Older HF patients with chronic kidney disease are a higher risk for both mortality and hospitalization, although this risk maybe more pronounced when the GFR drops below 45 ml/min/1.73 m^2 (130,131). Hemoglobin levels <13 g/dL have been shown to be associated with poor outcomes (132,133). Hypokalemia is common in HF and is associated with poor outcomes (134–136). Mild hyperkalemia, on the other hand, is less common, and although has unadjusted association with mortality, there appears to have no independent association (137). HF patients with serum magnesium level ≤2 mEq/L may be at higher risk for CV mortality, but not for CV hospitalization (138). Older HF patients with higher levels of NYHA class symptoms were at higher risk for mortality but not for hospitalization (119,120). Elevated serum uric acid is a marker of poor outcomes in HF but lacks independence of association (139).

TREATMENT: GENERAL APPROACH

As for any chronic medical condition, the treatment goals of HF can be classified into three broad categories (1) general approach including life style modifications such as salt and fluid restriction, or system-based interventions such multidisciplinary HF management programs, (2), pharmacotherapy, and (3) device-based therapy. HF pharmacotherapy can be divided into two categories: symptom-relieving therapy and life-prolonging therapy. Because HF symptoms are similar regardless of EF, treatment of HF symptoms is also similar in HFrEF and HFpEF. Life-prolonging therapy using neurohormonal blockade, on the other hand, is currently restricted to HFrEF patients only. This is primarily due to lack of data, as most randomized clinical trials (RCTs) of HF were restricted to mostly younger HFrEF patients. However, findings from two major RCTs that failed to demonstrate clinical benefit of angiotensin-receptor blockers (ARBs) in HFpEF suggest that the role of neurohormonal antagonists may be limited in HFpEF (140,141). Currently, the use of device-based therapies is restricted to HFrEF, although their proper role in older HFrEF is evolving.

Diet

As described earlier, non-adherence to a salt and fluid restricted diet may precipitate acute decompensation of chronic HF. However, there is little prospective data on the role of sodium and fluid on HF exacerbations. It is generally agreed that sodium intake should be restricted to <2 g/day and fluid intake should be restricted to <2 l/day. A more severe sodium restriction may allow a reduction in diuretic dose, but may also lead to non-adherence to salt restriction and acute decompensation, or adherence and malnutrition. Although obesity is associated with a higher risk of incident HF (40,41), obesity has been shown to confer survival benefit to older HF patients (38,39), and weight loss may not be desirable. Hyponatremia is associated with poor outcomes in HF (142). Chronic HF patients with hyponatremia often require a more severe albeit temporary fluid restriction. Most HF patients do not need to monitor their dietary intake of potassium. However, those with hyperkalemia may need to limit their intake of potassium-rich foods, such as tomatoes, bananas, and orange juice.

Physical Activity

Physical activity is associated with reduced risk of HF (42,43) and HF is characterized by exertional fatigue and exercise intolerance. Therefore, physical activity would be expected to improve outcomes and quality of life of older HF patients. Aerobic exercise has been shown to improve peak VO_2, cardiac output, and other physiological parameters in younger patients with HFrEF (143). In one study of 200 HFrEF patients, mean age 72 years (range 60–89 years), combined aerobic and low resistance strength training exercise for 24 weeks improved health-related quality of life, NYHA class, and 6-minute walk distance (144). Limited data suggest that aerobic exercise training can improve exercise capacity and quality of life in patients with HFpEF (145).

Although single center trials have suggested reduced mortality and HF hospitalizations after exercise training, none has been adequately powered for these endpoints. In the multicenter Heart Failure: A Controlled Trial Investigating Outcomes of Exercise Training (HF-ACTION) trial, 2331 chronic HFrEF patients were randomized to usual care plus aerobic exercise training (36 supervised sessions followed by home-based practice) versus usual care alone and followed for a median of 30 months (146). Patients had a median age of 59 years, median LVEF of 25%, 28% were women, 37% had NYHA class III-IV symptoms, and 51% had ischemic heart disease. The composite primary endpoint of all-cause mortality or hospitalization occurred in 759 patients (65%) in the exercise training group and 796 patients (68%) in the usual care group [hazard ratio (HR) = 0.93; 95% confidence interval (CI) = 0.84–1.02; p = 0.13] (146). Findings from this largest and most comprehensive study of exercise training in mild to moderate HFrEF patients suggested that the effect of exercise training on improvement of self-reported health status and depressive symptoms was modest, though statistically significant and of unknown clinical significance (147,148). A post hoc analysis of HF-ACTION suggests that a 6-minute walk test may have similar prognostic efficacy as cardiopulmonary exercise, and neither seem to add much to the prognostic discrimination of traditional models based on important demographic and clinical variables (149). Data based on subgroup analyses in older HF patients are not yet available.

Patient Education

Like other chronic conditions, a great deal of proper HF care depends on patients themselves. Patient participation thus is important for achieving optimal outcomes, and patient education is essential for desired patient participation. Older HF patients should be informed of their diagnosis, including their LVEF, and its prognostic and therapeutic implications. They also should be educated about the role of fluid retention in HF and the importance of salt and fluid restriction in achieving fluid balance. Generally speaking, HF patients should avoid table salt, and limit the use of salt during cooking. They should be encouraged to eat fresh food and avoid canned or processed food. Older HF patients should be encouraged to stay physically active as tolerated. They should also be advised to avoid environments of high temperature or high humidity. A rule of thumb is to stay in environments where the sum of temperature in Fahrenheit and humidity in percentage is less than 160.

Older HF patients should be educated about HF warning symptoms and signs. Because HF decompensation is almost always associated with fluid retention, HF patients should be encouraged to check and document their weight daily, generally in the morning, after emptying bladder and wearing similar clothes. They may be educated to take an extra dose of diuretic for 3–5 days if they gain 3–5 pounds in 3–5 days. If the baseline weight is not achieved in 3–5 days, they should be advised to consult their health care providers. To prevent over-diuresis, patients should be reassured that daily fluctuation in weight by 1 or 2 pounds is not uncommon in HF and does not require extra diuretics. Family members are often involved in the care of older HF patients, and with appropriate permission from the patients, they may assist in proper management of HF at home.

Disease Management Programs

Because a great deal of HF care involves non-drug interventions that require patients and family participation, it would be expected that programs supporting patient and family would improve outcomes, especially hospital admission and readmission. In a prospective, RCT in hospitalized older HF patients, a nurse-directed, multidisciplinary intervention program involving among others comprehensive education of patients and family members and intensive follow-up improved quality of life and reduced hospital readmission during 90 days of follow-up (150). In another RCT of a multidisciplinary, home-based intervention program involving home visits reduced unplanned hospital readmissions and improved quality of life in older HF patients during 6 months of follow-up (151). A meta-analysis of 25 trials and 5942 patients recently hospitalized for HF found that case management interventions, often involving telephone follow-up and home visits, reduced all-cause mortality by 34% after 12 months and reduced HF-related readmissions at both 6 months (HR = 0.64) and 12 months (HR = 0.47) (152). However, telemonitoring has failed to improve outcomes in relatively younger HF patients (153,154). Similarly, dedicated HF clinics have not been shown to reduce hospitalization in HF patients (155).

TREATMENT: PHARMACOTHERAPY FOR HFrEF

Prior to the 1980s, therapy for HFrEF was directed toward symptom control using diuretics and improving the pump function using inotropic drugs. Despite their temporarily beneficial hemodynamic actions, long-term therapy with inotropes was associated with increased morbidity and mortality (156,157). The understanding that HFrEF is characterized by the activation of the renin–angiotensin–aldosterone system and sympathetic nervous system (158,159), led to clinical trials showing that their suppression with drugs such as ACE inhibitors (160,161), ARBs (162,163), β-adrenergic receptor blockers (164–167), and aldosterone antagonists (168–170) reduced mortality and morbidity in these patients. Therefore, pharmacotherapy for HFrEF may be divided into two broader categories: (*i*) symptom-relieving and (*ii*) life-prolonging. It is important to understand the HF care extend well beyond the appropriate use of evidence-based pharmacotherapy. A 79-year-old man with HFrEF receiving evidence-based life-prolonging therapy with enalapril 5 mg twice a day, carvedilol 12.5 mg twice a day, and spironolactone 12.5 mg daily, may still have frequent decompensations, hospital admission, and poor quality of life. Therefore, careful attention to fluid volume status during each follow-up visits and maintenance of euvolemia remains important.

It is also important to avoid over-zealous implementation of evidence-based guidelines in older HFrEF patients, especially among octogenarians. Although octogenarian HF patients comprise nearly half of all older HF patients, most RCTs of neurohormonal blockade in HFrEF excluded such individuals (171). For example, in the Studies Of Left Ventricular Dysfunction (SOLVD)-Treatment trial, only 36% of the HFrEF patients were ≥65 years, but none were ≥81 years of age (161). Similarly, none of the HFrEF patients in MERIT-HF were ≥81 years (167). Mean age of real-world HF patients in HF registries and those enrolled in major RCTs of HFrEF are displayed in Table 20.2. The 10–15 year younger age of patients in these large pivotal HF trials versus real-world HF patients is noteworthy.

Table 20.2 Mean Age of Real-World Heart Failure Patient in Heart Failure Registries and Heart Failure Patients Enrolled in Randomized Clinical Trials

HF Studies	Total, N	Age, Mean (± SD)
Registries of Hospitalized HF Patients		
ADHERE (172)	105,388	72 (± 14)
OPTIMIZE-HF (117)	48,612	73 (± 14)
Alabama HF Project (106)	8049	76 (± 11)
National HF Project (173)	56,924	80 (± 23)
Randomized Clinical Trials of Ambulatory HFrEF Patients		
SOLVD-Treatment (ACE inhibitor) (157)	2569	60 (± 10)
CHARM-Alternative (Angiotensin receptor blocker) (158)	2028	67 (± 11)
US-Carvedilol (Beta-blocker) (160)	1094	58 (± 12)
COPERNICUS (Beta-blocker) (161)	2298	58 (± 11)
MERIT-HF (Beta-blocker) (163)	3991	64 (± 10)
RALES (Aldosterone antagonist) (164)	1663	65 (± 12)
EPHESUS (Aldosterone antagonist) (165)	6632	64 (± 12)
EMPHASIS-HF (Aldosterone antagonist) (166)	2737	69 (± 08)

Diuretics

Nearly all symptomatic HFrEF patients with fluid retention require diuretics to achieve euvolemia and most HF patients with a prior fluid retention may require diuretics to maintain euvolemia (99). This is generally achieved by loop diuretics, most commonly furosemide. Torsemide and bumetanide are less frequently used. It is important for clinicians to become very familiar with one of these three diuretics. Generally speaking, torsemide 20 mg and bumetanide 1 mg are equivalent to furosemide 40 mg. Because older HF patients may suffer from diuretic-related overactive bladder symptoms (174), it is preferable to use diuretics as a single morning dose. Larger doses of diuretics such as furosemide 480 mg daily, however, may be given as 240 mg twice a day, with the afternoon dose around 2 PM to avoid night-time diuresis.

Despite their nearly universal use, there is no RCT data on the long-term effects of chronic therapy with loop diuretics in HF. Findings from propensity-matched studies suggest that prolonged diuretic use may be associated with increased mortality (Fig. 20.3) and hospitalization (175,176). Potential explanation for adverse long-term effects of diuretics include electrolyte imbalance and neurohormonal activation, both associated with poor outcomes (134–136,142,177). Therefore, after euvolemia has been achieved, patients should be encouraged to restrict their salt and fluid intake so that the lower doses of diuretics are needed to maintain euvolemia.

HF patients receiving diuretics often develop hypokalemia, which is associated with poor outcomes (134–136). Therefore, serum potassium levels should be closely monitored and maintained between 4 and 5 mEq/L. Hypokalemia should be corrected with potassium supplements. When patients require chronic therapy with potassium supplements to maintain normokalemia, an aldosterone antagonist should be considered instead. Unlike potassium supplements (178), aldosterone antagonists improve outcomes in HFrEF (168–170). Patients resistant to high dose of loop diuretics (for example, 480 mg of furosemide daily) may respond to a lower dose of furosemide combined with a small dose of metolazone, a thiazide-like diuretic that works primarily at the distal convoluted tubule. However, this combination should be avoided in older HF patient requiring small dose of diuretic to avoid polypharmacy and a higher risk of hypokalemia. Older HF patients resistant to high doses of furosemide may also respond to other loop diuretics such as torsemide or bumetanide. There is some evidence that torsemide is associated with

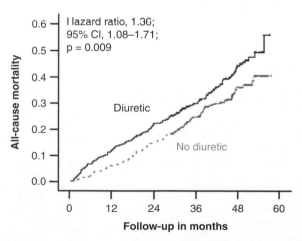

Figure 20.3 Association of chronic diuretic therapy with long-term all-cause mortality in older heart failure patients. *Source*: From Ref. 176.

lower risk of neurohormonal activation and hypokalemia and better outcomes compared to furosemide (179–181).

Angiotensin-Converting Enzyme Inhibitors

Multiple RCTs have conclusively shown the ability of ACE inhibitors to prolong survival and improve symptoms in patients with HFrEF. Therefore, older HFrEF patients without contra-indications should be prescribed an ACE inhibitor as an initial drug of choice for renin–angiotensin inhibition; perhaps, the best data on the efficacy of ACE inhibitors in older adults derives from the Cooperative North Scandinavian ENalapril SUrvival Study (CONSENSUS) trial (160). The mean age in CONSENSUS was 70 years and all patients were NYHA class IV (160). Despite these high-risk characteristics, enalapril 10–20 mg twice daily reduced 6-month mortality from 48% to 29% and markedly improved HF symptoms (160). Further evidence for the benefit of ACE inhibitors is derived from the SOLVD-Treatment trial, in which HFrEF patients randomized to receive enalapril had significant lower risk of death (161). Of note, this mortality benefit was only observed in patients who had a HF hospitalization during the trial, and further, there was no mortality benefit from enalapril beyond the second year of follow-up (161). A subgroup analysis based on the public-use copy of the SOLVD data obtained from the NHLBI by these authors (AA) suggest that ACE inhibitors may be beneficial in older HFrEF patients (Fig. 20.4), although the effect may be more modest in those patients. However, in the SOLVD-Treatment trial, only eight patients were 80 years of age and none were ≥81 years of age (161). Therefore, there is very little data on octogenarian HFrEF patients, who may comprise nearly half of all older HF patients.

In the SOLVD-Treatment trial, enalapril had no effect on sudden cardiac death and most of the mortality benefit was mediated through reductions in death due to progressive HF (161). This is important as the mode of death in HF changes with disease progression (167,182). Because older HFrEF patients may have HF for longer duration or have more advanced HF, they would be more likely to die from progressive pump failure, and thus, are likely to benefit from ACE inhibitors. However, the SOLVD trial was conducted in the pre-β-blocker era of HF therapy, and it remains unclear if the modest mortality reduction benefit of enalapril would still be observed in contemporary HF patients. These nuances need to be considered when prescribing ACE inhibitors to older HFrEF patients as many of these patients are never hospitalized (112,183), and receive β-blockers (122).

There is little data on the benefit and renal effect of ACE inhibitors in HFrEF patients with impaired kidney function (184,185). Finding from propensity-matched studies in

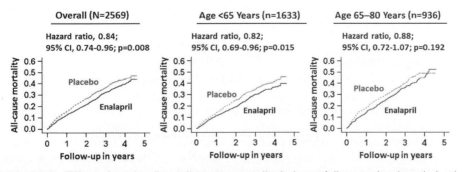

Figure 20.4 Effect of enalapril on all-cause mortality in heart failure and reduced ejection fraction patients in the SOLVD trial, data for all, younger and older patients (Prepared by authors, based on public use copy of the SOLVD data obtained from the NHLBI).

hospitalized older HFrEF patients with and without chronic kidney disease suggest that discharge prescription of ACE inhibitors or ARBs may be associated with a significant modest reduction in all-cause mortality in older patients with HFrEF and chronic kidney disease, including those with more advanced chronic kidney disease (186). Of note, this benefit seemed more modest in those with chronic kidney disease than in those without.

Despite their benefits in improving survival and reducing symptoms, ACE inhibitors have several side effects that are particularly relevant to older adults. These include hypotension, azotemia, and hyperkalemia, all of which are dose-related. Hypotension is a particularly important consideration in older HFrEF patients with low SBP. In addition to causing lethargy and increased risk of falls and fractures, low SBP has been consistently shown to be associated with poor outcomes in HF (187–189). Azotemia often occurs soon after initiation of therapy, especially in patients with compromised baseline renal function. To minimize both hypotension and azotemia, it is often necessary to reduce the diuretic dose soon after ACE inhibitors are begun. Monitoring of electrolytes for hyperkalemia is also useful in this early period.

ACE inhibitors should be considered for older HFrEF patients without prior allergy or intolerance, and needs to be started at low doses, and increased slowly, preferably keeping SBP at or above 120 mmHg. This will allow room for initiation and maintenance of β-blockers without potentially causing hypotension. Cough is the most common side effect of ACE inhibitors. HFrEF patients who cannot tolerate ACE inhibitors may be prescribed an ARB.

Angiotensin-Receptor Blockers

ARBs also antagonize the renin–angiotensin system, but in RCTs of ARBs in HFrEF, most of which were conducted in more contemporary HF patients receiving β-blockers, there was no mortality reduction, and most of the evidence of their benefits is based on significant reduction in combined endpoints (162,163). In Valsartan Heart Failure Trial (Val-HeFT), valsartan significantly reduced the risk for combined endpoint of mortality or morbidity (163). Similarly, in the Candesartan in Heart Failure Assessment of Reduction in Morbidity and Mortality (CHARM)-Alternative Study, candesartan significantly reduced the risk of combined endpoint of CV mortality or HF hospitalization in HFrEF patients who were intolerant of ACE inhibitors (162). In the CHARM-Added trial, addition of candesartan to HFrEF patients receiving ACE inhibitors also reduced this combined endpoint (190). However, patients receiving both drugs had higher risks for hypotension, hyperkalemia, and hypercreatininemia. Therefore, this combination should be avoided in older HFrEF patients. This may also preclude initiation and maintenance of more important drugs such as β-blockers or aldosterone antagonists.

β-Adrenergic Blockers

Evidence for the benefit of β-blockers in older HFrEF is extrapolated from RCTs of much younger HF patients (Table 20.2). Findings from a subgroup analysis of MERIT-HF suggest that metoprolol succinate extended release was equally effective in older and younger HFrEF patients (Fig. 20.5) (191). Among the 490 patients age 75–80 years in MERIT-HF, there was a 29% non-significant reduction in total mortality (191). However, as in most RCTs in HF, MERIT-HF excluded patients ≥81 years of age. Because the inclusion criteria of MERIT-HF would have disqualified 100% of real-world octogenarian HFrEF patients (171), these data should be extrapolated with caution to octogenarian HFrEF patients, who constitute nearly half of all older HF patients.

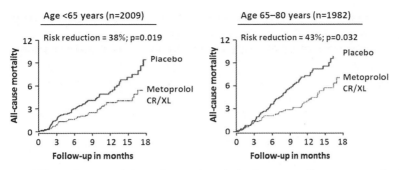

Figure 20.5 Effect of metoprolol succinate extended release on all-cause mortality in heart failure and reduced ejection fraction patients in the MERIT-HF trial, data for younger and older patients. *Source*: From Ref. 191.

Older HFrEF patients without contraindications should be prescribed one of the three β-blockers with RCT evidence of proven benefit (99). These include carvedilol, metoprolol succinate extended release, and bisoprolol (164–167). Based on the findings of the COMET trial, metoprolol tartrate should not be used in HFrEF (192). Nebivolol seems to improve outcomes in older HFrEF patients (193), but it is currently not approved for use in HFrEF in the USA. Carvedilol and metoprolol succinate extended release are the two most commonly used β-blockers in HFrEF and clinicians should be familiar with both of these drugs. Considering the β-1 selective blocker metoprolol succinate extended release does not affect BP, this drug should be considered as the initial β-blocker of choice for older HFrEF patients (194,195). For older HFrEF patients with hypertension, especially if they are receiving another antihypertensive drug, such as amlodipine, their metoprolol succinate extended release may be replaced with carvedilol with the hope that BP may be controlled without amlodipine.

Aldosterone Antagonists

Aldosterone antagonists have emerged as a powerful tool in improving outcomes in HFrEF (168–170). Findings from the Eplerenone in Mild Patients Hospitalization and Survival Study in Heart Failure (EMPHASIS-HF) trial suggest that these drugs are beneficial in contemporary patients with mild to moderate HFrEF (170). A subgroup analysis of EMPHASIS suggest that these drugs were equally effective in younger and older HFrEF patients, although it was not clear how many of these older patient were octogenarians.

Findings from subgroup analysis of the RALES data obtained from RALES investigators (Fig. 20.6) suggest that spironolactone may be equally effective in younger and older HFrEF patients. Unlike many RCTs of HF, RALES participants were real-world-like, with 59% of patients being ≥65 years, although only 143 (9% of 1663) patients were 80–90 years. While this is encouraging, these data need to be extrapolated with caution to real-world octogenarian HFrEF patients as only about 20% of the real-world octogenarians with HF would have been eligible to participate in RALES (171). In a very well-conducted observational study in older (mean age, 78 years) HFrEF (mean EF, 25%), a discharge prescription for an aldosterone antagonist had no independent association with mortality or cardiovascular readmission (196).

Spironolactone may be considered for older HFrEF patients without renal insufficiency and should be started low with 12.5 mg daily and increased to 25 mg daily if tolerated. Serum potassium should be closely monitored and kept between 4 and 5 mEq/L.

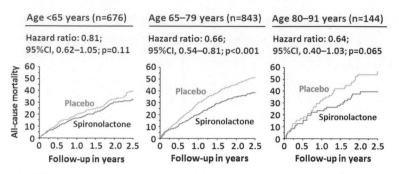

Figure 20.6 Effect of spironolactone on all-cause mortality in heart failure and reduced ejection fraction patients in the RALES trial, data for younger and older patients. *Source*: Courtesy of Faiez Zannad, MD, PhD and Renaud Fay, PhD, INSERIM, Nancy, France.

Male patients with painful gynecomastia should be prescribed eplerenone, a selective aldosterone receptor blocker. When started as initial therapy, eplerenone should be started low at 25 mg daily and increased to 50 mg daily if tolerated.

Hydralazine and Isosorbide Dinitrate
Findings from the African-American Heart Failure Trial (A-HeFT) demonstrated that combined therapy with hydralazine and isosrbide dinitrate may improve outcomes in African-American HFrEF patients receiving ACE inhibitors and β-blockers (197). Although HF occurs at a younger age in African-Americans, the mean age of 57 years in A-HeFT limits the applicability of the results to most real-world older HFrEF patients. Considering that this combination has been shown to be not more beneficial than ACE inhibitors (198), it should not be prescribed to older HFrEF patients receiving ACE inhibitors, before initiating a β-blocker and an aldosterone antagonist, both with superior evidence of benefit.

Digoxin
Findings from the DIG trial demonstrated that digoxin significantly reduced HF hospitalization but had no effect on total mortality (199). Subsequent post hoc analyses of the DIG data have demonstrated that when used in lower doses leading to lower serum digoxin concentration (0.5–0.9 ng/ml), digoxin may also reduce the risk of death (200,201). Digoxin is equally effective in younger and older HFrEF patients (202,203). In the DIG trial, even at the higher dose of 0.25 mg daily, digoxin was very well tolerated in older adults (202). Digoxin dose should generally be 0.125 mg daily in older HF patients. This dose is likely to result in a low serum digoxin concentration, eliminating the need for routine monitoring of serum digoxin concentration (202). Only 5% of the DIG participants were ≥80 years of age, and only 11 patients were ≥90 years. Therefore, digoxin should be used with caution in octogenarian HFrEF patients.

Other Inotropes
The long-term use of oral phosphodiesterase inhibitors, such as amrinone, milrinone, and vesnarinone, are associated with increased mortality (156,204) and are not approved for clinical use. Intravenous milrinone use has also not been shown to be associated with significant mortality benefit (205,206). The calcium-sensitizing phosphodiesterase inhibitor levosimendan has been shown to improve hemodynamic function and symptoms in younger patients with decompensated HF (207), but it does not seem to have a consistent mortality benefit compared with dobutamine (208,209). Synthetic catecholamines such as dobutamine or dopamine may also be used to treat refractory HF symptoms. In one small study of patients in an intensive care setting, dobutamine elicited lesser increases in cardiac output

in patients older than 80 years than in younger patients, consistent with the age-associated decreased sensitivity to catecholamines that occurs in normal (210).

Newer Therapies

Ivabradine reduces heart rate by inhibiting the I_f current but has no effect on contractility. In the Systolic Heart Failure Treatment with I_f Inhibitor Trial (SHIFT), at 30 months of follow-up, compared to placebo, ivabradine reduced the primary composite endpoint of CV death or HF hospitalization by 18% and cumulative hospitalizations by 25% in patients receiving an ACEI or ARB, maximized β-blockade, and a mineralocorticoid antagonist (211). Despite elevated endothelin levels in HF, RCTs have failed to demonstrate clinical benefit of endothelin receptor antagonists in chronic HFrEF (212). Type 5 phosphodiesterase (PDE5) inhibitors increase myocardial contractility, blunt adrenergic stimulation, reduce cardiac afterload, and improve ventilator efficiency and aerobic capacity in short- and intermediate-term studies in HFrEF patients (213–215). However, data from large randomized trials during chronic administration are not yet available for these drugs. Since the beneficial effects of PDE5 inhibitors are thought to be mediated by inhibition of the breakdown of soluble guanylate cyclase (sGC), activators and stimulators of sGC may also have therapeutic potential in HF (216).

Mostly older HF patients have lower hemoglobin levels without evidence of iron deficiency (122). However, there is no evidence that correcting anemia improved outcomes in these patients. In the Ferinject Assessment in Patients with Iron Deficiency and Chronic Heart Failure (FAIR-HF) trial, treatment with intravenous ferric carboxymaltose has been shown to improve symptoms, functional capacity, and quality of life in HF patients (217). In that study, patients had a mean age of 68 years, mean LVEF of 32%, and mean hemoglobin of 12 mg/dL. Iron deficiency was defined as serum ferritin level of <100 μg/L or 100–299 μg/L when the transferrin saturation was <20%, and mean baseline ferritin level and transferrin saturation were about 55 μg/L and 17%, respectively (217). Of note, only 15% of patients in that study were receiving digoxin which has been shown to improve HF symptoms and reduce the risk for HF hospitalization (199,202). Currently, there is no evidence whether these benefits can be achieved by oral iron supplement use. The role of erythropoietin in older HF patients with anemia remains unclear (218). A pilot study of testosterone has shown substantial improvement in exercise tolerance, skeletal muscle performance, and insulin resistance in older adults with HFrEF despite unchanged cardiac function (219).

TREATMENT: DEVICE-BASED THERAPY AND SURGERY FOR HFrEF DEVICES

The high morbidity and mortality associated with HFrEF despite maximal medical therapy has led to the pursuit of additional interventions using devices and surgery in this population. Dyssynchrony in intra-ventricular conduction, manifest as a wide QRS complex on electrocardiogram, is not uncommon in HFrEF and has been shown to be associated with poor outcomes (220). Atrial-synchronized biventricular pacing, also known as cardiac resynchronization therapy (CRT) can synchronize intraventricular conduction and coordinate contraction between the left and right ventricles. Other studies have shown that CRT can improve LV function and enhance functional capacity, quality of life, and survival in HFrEF patients with wide (>120 ms) QRS complex (221–223). Although no randomized trial has specifically addressed the role of CRT in older adults, subgroup analyses of those RCTs suggest that the benefit of CRT may be similar in older versus younger patients. For example, in the Cardiac Resynchronization-Heart Failure (CARE-HF) trial, in HFrEF patients, median age 67 years (34% were >70 years of age), median LVEF 25%, and median QRS 160 ms, CRT reduced the risk of the primary endpoint of all-cause mortality or CV hospitalization by a significant 37% (223). A subgroup analysis of that trials demonstrated that this benefit was significant for both younger (<66 years; $n = 406$) and older

($\geq$66 years; $n = 407$) patients, with 45% and 32% significant reductions in the primary endpoints (223). In that study, of the 407 older patients, about 40 were 80–90 years of age, and none were $\geq$90 years (personal communication from John G. Cleland, Principal Investigator, CARE-HF). These beneficial effects of CRT have also been observed in mild to moderate HFrEF patients. In the Resynchronization–Defibrillation for Ambulatory Heart Failure Trial (RAFT), in HFrEF patients, mean age 66 years, mean LVEF 23%, and mean QRS 158 ms, CRT reduced the risk of the primary endpoint of HF death or HF hospitalization by a significant 25% (224). The beneficial effect of CRT in that trial was similar for younger (<65 years) and older ($\geq$65 years) patients (224). However, what proportion of those age $\geq$65 years were $\geq$80 years is unknown. CRT is a class-I indication in HFrEF patients with LVEF $\leq$35%, a QRS duration $\geq$150 ms with left bundle branch block, and NYHA class II–IV symptoms (225). Thus, CRT should be considered in eligible older HFrEF patients, but should be used with caution in those $\geq$80 years of age.

Given the nearly exponential increase in the risk of sudden cardiac death as LVEF decreases below 30%, it is not surprising that several studies have shown a benefit of an implantable cardioverter defibrillator (ICD) in patients with systolic HF. In the Multicenter Automatic Defibrillator Implantation Trial II (MADIT II), prophylactic implantation of an ICD in patients with a prior myocardial infarction and LVEF < 30% reduced all-cause mortality from 20% to 14% over a 20-month of mean follow-up (226). Of the 1232 MADIT II patients, 370 were <60 years, 426 were 60–69 years and 436 were $\geq$70 years (number of $\geq$80 years unknown), and the benefit of ICD was significant in those <60 and $\geq$70 years. Although HF was not required for study entry and the baseline history of HF was not reported, approximately 75% of patients were receiving diuretics. Of note, the incidence of new or worsened HF was slightly higher in the ICD group (20% vs. 15% in the conventional-therapy group had HF hospitalizations; $p = 0.09$) (226).

The effect of ICDs in a more specific HF population was tested in the Sudden Cardiac Death in Heart Failure Trial (SCD-HeFT). In SCD-HeFT, 2521 HFrEF patients (52% ischemic etiology) with NYHA class II–III symptoms (70% class II), median age 60 years, and median LVEF 25%, were randomized to conventional therapy plus placebo ($n = 847$), conventional therapy plus amiodarone ($n = 845$), or conventional therapy plus a conservatively programmed, shock-only, single-lead ICD ($n = 829$) (227). During a median follow-up of 46 months, the primary endpoint of all-cause mortality occurred in 29% of patients in the placebo group, 28% of those in the amiodarone group, and 22% in the ICD group (227). Although there was no significant interaction between age and ICD benefit in SCD-HeFT, the ICD-associated mortality benefit (vs. placebo) was somewhat more favorable among patients <65 years (HR = 0.68; 95% CI = 0.50–0.93) versus those $\geq$65 years (HR = 0.86; 95% CI = 0.62–1.18). In SCD-HeFT, 31% of the 829 patients in the ICD group received shocks, two thirds of which were considered appropriate (227). Although the use of ICD per se was not associated with any detectable adverse quality of life, those receiving shocks reported significant decline in quality of life (228,229). In SCD-HeFT, quality of life assessment within 1 month after shock revealed significant decrease in perceived general health, physical and emotional functioning, social functioning, and self-rated health, although this perception tended to attenuate with passage of time (228).

The effect of ICDs on outcomes in HFrEF patients due to non-ischemic dilated cardiomyopathy was examined in the Defibrillators in Non-Ischemic Cardiomyopathy Treatment Evaluation (DEFINITE) trial. In that trial, 458 patients with non-ischemic dilated cardiomyopathy and qualifying arrhythmias (premature ventricular complexes or non-sustained ventricular tachycardia, or both), mean age years, and mean LVEF 21% were randomized to receive standard medical therapy ($n = 229$) or standard medical therapy plus a single-chamber ICD ($n = 229$). During a mean follow-up of 29 months, the primary endpoint of all-cause mortality occurred in 17% and 9% of patients in the control and ICD groups, respectively ($p = 0.08$), which was rather similar for those <65 years and ≥65 years (230). Although the overall incidence of sudden cardiac death was low (4% or 17 events), the risk for this pre-specified secondary endpoint was significantly lower in the ICD group (1% or 3 events vs. 6% or 14 events in the standard medical therapy; $p = 0.006$) (230). Of note, the mode of death in HF changes with disease progression (167,182) and HFrEF in older adults are more likely to be more advanced or of longer duration, and thus, more likely to die from progressive pump failure than fatal arrhythmias. In DEFINITE, 41 and 49 patients received appropriate and inappropriate ICD shocks, respectively (230).

The role of CRT and ICDs was examined in the Comparison of Medical Therapy, Pacing, and Defibrillation in Heart Failure (COMPANION) trial, in which 1520 HFrEF patients with wide QRS (≥120 ms), NYHA class III–IV symptoms, mean age 67 years, mean LVEF 22%, and mean QRS duration 160 ms, were randomized to receive optimal medical therapy alone, or additional CRT, or additional CRT plus ICD (222). The 12-month rates of the primary composite endpoint of all-cause death or all-cause hospitalization were 68% (reference group), 56% (HR = 0.81; 95% CI = 0.69–0.96; $p = 0.014$), and 56% (HR = 0.80; 95% CI = 0.68–0.95; $p = 0.010$) in medical therapy, CRT alone and CRT-ICD groups, respectively (222). Analyses of secondary endpoints in COMPANION suggest that CRT use was associated with improvement in symptoms and quality of life and a reduction in hospitalizations, and therapy with ICD provided additional survival benefit. These benefits were similar in younger and older (>65 years) patients, though the proportion of ≥80 years in the study was not reported.

Surgery

Selected older patients with HF may derive major benefits from cardiac surgery. Aortic valve replacement is the treatment of choice for older adults with HF secondary to calcific aortic stenosis (231), although trans-catheter aortic-valve replacement is now available for those considered inoperable severe aortic stenosis (232,233). Coronary revascularization was considered to ameliorate HF symptoms in selected older HF patients with substantial amounts of viable but ischemic myocardium due to coronary artery disease. However, the multicenter Surgical Treatment for Ischemic Heart Failure (STICH) trial failed to show a survival benefit from coronary artery bypass graft (CABG) surgery (234). In STICH, 1212 HFrEF patients with coronary artery disease amenable to CABG and LVEF ≤35%, who had a mean age of 60 years, were randomized to medical therapy alone ($n = 602$) or additional CABG ($n = 610$). During a median follow-up of 56 months, the primary endpoint of all-cause mortality occurred in 41% of patients in the medical-therapy group and 36% of those in the CABG group (HR = 0.86; 95% CI = 0.72–1.04; $p = 0.12$) (234). Although there was significant interaction between age and CABG (p for interaction, 0.41), the effect of CABG was more modest in the 396 STICH participants ≥65 years of age (HR = 0.93; 95% CI = 0.70–1.23) than in the 816 younger (<65 years) patients (HR = 0.80; 95% CI = 0.63–1.01). In STICH, the risk of death within 30 days after randomization was three times higher in patients in the CABG group ($p = 0.006$). Analyses of secondary outcomes suggested that CABG reduced the risk of the combined endpoints of all-cause mortality or all-cause hospitalization and all-cause mortality or CV hospitalization. Patients with viable myocardium, that is those with stunned or hibernating myocardium, were considered to be more amenable to reperfusion and functional recovery. However, in STICH, the effect of CABG did not vary by the presence or absence of viable myocardium (235). Therefore, CABG might be carefully considered in eligible older HFrEF patients with ongoing myocardial ischemia who are refractory to optimal medical and device therapy.

Cardiac transplantation has been successfully employed to treat end-stage HF in carefully selected patients in their seventh decade. In one such series, the 1-year actuarial survival was 84%, only 4% developed a serious infection, and the incidence of rejection was 2.2 episodes per patient (236). These results compared favorably with those in younger individuals. Nevertheless, the shortage of donors and the high likelihood of medical contraindications, such as intrinsic renal or cerebrovascular disease in this age group, markedly limit the applicability of cardiac transplantation in older adults.

A promising therapy in such end-stage older HF patients is the implantation of a permanent LV assist device (LVAD). Although used initially as a temporary bridge for patients undergoing cardiac transplantation (237,238), these devices have been used increasingly for long-term use in patients who are not transplant candidates (238–240). In the Randomized Evaluation of Mechanical Assistance for the Treatment of Congestive Heart Failure (REMATCH) trial, 129 patients with end-stage HF with NYHA class IV symptoms, mean age 67 years, mean LVEF 17%, ineligible for cardiac transplantation, were randomized to optimal medical management ($n = 61$) or receive a LVAD ($n = 68$) (239). Overall, 92 patients died during over 2 years of follow-up, 51 of which was due to pump failure, all but 1 of which occurred in the medial therapy group. During the first year of follow-up, the primary endpoint of all-cause mortality occurred 75% and 48% of patients in the medical therapy and LVAD groups, respectively (HR = 0.52; 95% CI = 0.34–0.78; $p = 0.001$). This benefit appeared to extend through the end of 2 years of follow-up (92% and 77% death among patients in the medical therapy and LVAD groups, respectively; $p = 0.09$) (239). Although patients in the LVAD group reported significant improvement in quality of life at 1 year, they also experience a higher incidence of adverse effects such as infection, bleeding, and device malfunction (239).

The development of continuous flow LVADs has further led to their use as destination therapy in end-stage HF patients with NYHA class IV symptoms despite optimal medical therapy. In the HeartMate II trial, HFrEF patients ineligible for transplantation, mean age 63 years, mean LVEF 17%, 75% with NYHA class IV symptoms an 80% receiving intravenous inotropic drugs, were randomized to receive continuous-flow LVAD ($n = 134$) or pulsatile-flow LVAD ($n = 66$) and followed for an average of 2 years. The primary composite endpoint of survival free from disabling stroke and reoperation to repair or replace the LVAD achieved in 46% of patients in continuous-flow LVAD group and 11% of those in the pulsatile-flow LVAD group (HR = 0.38; 95% CI = 0.27–0.54; $p < 0.001$). At 2 years of follow-up, all-cause mortality occurred in 76% and 42% of patients in the continuous-flow and pulsatile-flow LVAD groups, respectively ($p = 0.008$) (240). Although patients in both groups experienced significant improvements in quality of life and functional capacity, those receiving continuous-flow LVADs experience significantly fewer adverse events and device replacements.

TREATMENT: PHARMACOTHERAPY FOR HFpEF

Despite the widespread recognition during the last two decades of HFpEF as a major clinical entity, the literature base regarding therapy of HFpEF remains sparse, in stark contrast to the numerous studies over the past 30 years that have generated data for evidence-based treatment of HFrEF (99). This situation is incongruous with the high prevalence, substantial morbidity, and significant mortality of HFpEF. Advances in therapy of HFpEF have been hindered by lack of standard case definition, absence of a readily available, reliable test that characterizes and quantitates diastolic function; and relatively poor understanding of the pathophysiology of HFpEF (67,70). Given the importance of the HFpEF syndrome and the paucity of RCT data, this will likely be an area of substantial research activity for many years. On the basis of pathophysiological insights discussed above, future studies might assess physiological pacing in subsets with chronotropic incompetence, weight loss, exercise training, and novel pharmacological agents.

General Approach

The general approaches discussed above for systolic HF are usually applicable to HFpEF (99). There should be a search for a primary etiology. Most such patients will be found to have prominent underlying hypertension (9). A non-invasive stress test or coronary angiography is warranted in selected patients with chest pain and/or "flash pulmonary edema" to exclude severe coronary artery disease since ischemia is not only a therapeutic target in its own right but also strongly impairs diastolic relaxation. Occasional patients will be found to have hypertrophic cardiomyopathy (241) with or without dynamic obstruction, undiagnosed valvular or coronary disease, or, occasionally, amyloid heart disease (242). In addition, each of these underlying etiologies has specific prognostic and therapeutic implications that may supersede concomitant diastolic dysfunction. Given the paucity of data from large definitive trials, recommendations regarding specific agents are considerably less firm than for HFrEF; thus, therapy is largely empiric.

Diuretics

As for systolic HF as discussed above, while powerful loop diuretics are indispensable for rapid resolution of symptoms due to edema and pulmonary congestion, for chronic treatment the lowest possible dose should be employed and many patients with mild or early HF can be managed with as-needed diuretics. The potential adverse effect of long-term diuretic therapy in HF has been reported to be similar in both HFrEF and HFpEF (175).

Digoxin

In the DIG ancillary trial, based on 988 HFpEF (LVEF > 45%) patients, the use of digoxin was associated with a trend toward reduced hospitalizations due to worsening HF, which was countered by a trend toward increased hospitalizations due to unstable angina, but had no effect on total or cause-specific mortalities (243). This largest RCT of digoxin in HFpEF established that there was no net harm from digoxin in patients with HFpEF, contrary to earlier reports based on smaller studies.

ACE Inhibitors

In a group of older HFpEF patients (LVEF > 50%), mean age 80 years, NYHA class III symptoms, enalapril significantly improved functional class, exercise duration, LVEF, diastolic filling, and LV mass (244). In the Perindopril for Elderly People with Chronic Heart Failure (PEP-CHF) trial, 850 older (age >70 years, mean 76 years) HFpEF patients (LVEF ≥ 45%) were randomized to receive perindopril and followed for a median of 2 years. The primary endpoint of all-cause mortality and HF hospitalization occurred in 25% and 24% of patients in the placebo and perindopril groups, respectively (HR = 0.92: 95% CI = 0.70–1.21; $p = 0.545$) (245). Despite this lack of effect, likely due to potential crossover of therapy and lack of statistical power, during the first year of follow-up, there was a trend toward reduction in the primary outcome and a significant reduction in HF hospitalization. In a propensity-matched inception cohort study of hospitalized older (mean age, 81 years) HFpEF (mean LVEF, 55%) patients in OPTIMIZE-HF, a discharge prescription of ACE inhibitors was associated with a modest improvement in the combined endpoint of total mortality or HF hospitalization, but had no significant association with the individual component endpoints (246). Although these data would suggest a modest beneficial effect of ACE inhibitors in HFpEF, their role is yet to be determined in definitive RCTs.

Angiotensin-Receptor Blockers

Two large, multicenter RCTs of ARBs in HFpEF, the CHARM-Preserved and the Irbesartan in Heart Failure with Preserved Ejection Fraction (I-PRESERVE) trials, demonstrated that ARBs have no impact on outcomes in HFpEF (140,141). In the CHARM-Preserved in 3023 HFpEF patients (LVEF > 40%) mean age 67 years, candesartan did not significantly reduce the risk of primary combined endpoint of CV death or HF hospitalization during a median follow-up of 36 months (140). Although there was no effect of CV death, there seemed to a trend toward reduction in the risk of HF hospital admission (140). The I-PRESERVE trial randomized 4128 HFpEF (LVEF $\geq$ 45%) patients, mean age 72 years, to irbesartan or placebo and over a mean follow-up of 50 months, the primary composite endpoint of all-cause death or CV hospitalization was similar in the irbesartan (36%) and placebo (37%) groups (HR = 0.95; 95% CI = 0.86–1.05; p = 0.35) (141). There was no between-group difference in incident CV hospitalization in that trial. Furthermore, there were no significant between-group differences in any pre-specified secondary outcomes, including quality of life and change in NT-proBNP (141). In a propensity-matched inception cohort study of hospitalized older (mean age, 80 years) HFpEF (mean LVEF, 55%) patients in OPTIMIZE-HF, discharge prescription of ABRs had no association with any clinical outcomes (247). In a recent Phase II trial, LCZ396, an angiotensin receptor neprilysin inhibitor structurally resembling valsartan, reduced left atrial volume and improved NYHA class at 36 weeks, but had no significant effect on NT-proBNP in 301 older HFpEF patients (248).

β-Adrenergic Blockers

β-adrenergic receptor blockers substantially improve mortality in HFrEF, attenuate LV hypertrophy, and increase the ischemic threshold, and the time for diastolic filling, all portending potential benefit in HFpEF. However, early diastolic relaxation is impaired by β-adrenergic blockade (249). Regrettably, no adequately powered RCTs of β-blockers have been performed in patients with HFpEF. In the Study of the Effects of Nebivolol Intervention on Outcomes and Rehospitalisation in Seniors with Heart Failure (SENIORS) trial, in older adults with HF, mean age 76 years, mean LVEF 34%, nebivolol, a β-1-selective blocker, reduced the risk of primary endpoint of all-cause mortality or CV hospitalization (HR = 0.86; 95% CI = 0.74–0.99; p = 0.039 (193). However, nebivolol had no effect on the individual endpoints of all-cause mortality and CV hospitalization. Further, about two-thirds of the patients in the SENIORS study had LVEF <35%, which limits generalizability to HFpEF (193). In hospitalized older HF patients in OPTIMIZE-HF, β-blocker use was clinically effective and independently associated with lower risks of death and rehospitalization in HFrEF, but not in those with HFpEF (250).

Aldosterone Antagonists

Aldosterone promotes myocardial hypertrophy and fibrosis (251), both playing important roles in the pathophysiology of HFpEF. The efficacy of aldosterone blockade in improving outcomes in HFrEF is well-established (168–170). Findings from a post hoc analysis of the RALES trial suggest that the effect of spironolactone in HFrEF might be most pronounced in those with the highest baseline concentrations of procollagen biomarkers of fibrosis (252). Aldosterone antagonism also has potential benefits for improvement in vascular fibrosis and stiffness. A placebo-controlled study of 30 patients with hypertension, dyspnea on exertion, and delayed relaxation LV filling pattern by Doppler showed that strain rate and peak strain improved with spironolactone therapy (253). In 44 patients with HFpEF, 6 months of eplerenone treatment improved diastolic function and reduced collagen turnover, but did not increase exercise capacity compared to placebo (254).

The Aldosterone Receptor Blockade in Diastolic Heart Failure (Aldo-DHF) trial randomized 422 HFpEF (LVEF ≥ 50%) patients mean age 67 years to spironolactone or placebo for 1 year (255). In that trial, spironolactone significantly improved diastolic function and ventricular remodeling as well as reduced levels of natriuretic peptides, but these structural benefits did not translate into improvements in exercise capacity, NYHA class, and quality of life (256).

In a propensity-matched inception cohort study of hospitalized older (mean age, 80 years) HFpEF (mean LVEF, 54%) patients in OPTIMIZE-HF, discharge prescription of aldosterone antagonists had no association with any clinical outcomes (257). The effect of spironolactone in HFpEF is currently being studied in the Treatment of Preserved Systolic Cardiac Failure with an Aldosterone Antagonist (TOPCAT) trial (258). The results from this randomized, placebo-controlled, multinational RCT sponsored by the National Institutes of Health are expected in late 2013.

Calcium Antagonists

The role of verapamil was examined in 22 older HFpEF patients (LVEF > 45%) in a randomized, double-blind, placebo-controlled crossover trial (259). There was a 33% improvement in exercise time and significant improvements in HF score and peak filling rate in the absence of a significant difference in BP and LVEF. Verapamil has also been shown to improve diastolic function, symptoms, and exercise capacity in patients with hypertrophic cardiomyopathy (260). In animal models dihydropyridines prevent ischemia-induced increases in LV diastolic stiffness (183) and improve diastolic performance in pacing-induced HF (261). However, negative inotropic calcium antagonists impair early relaxation and have generally shown a tendency toward adverse outcome in patients with HFrEF (262). There have been no adequately powered RCTs of calcium antagonists in HFpEF.

Newer Therapies

Collagen cross-links increase with aging and diabetes, and cause increased vascular and myocardial stiffness. Alagebrium, a novel cross-link breaker, improved vascular and LV stiffness in laboratory animals (263,264). In one small, open label, 4-month study of alagebrium 420 mg/day in 23 patients, mean age 71 years, with stable HFpEF (LVEF > 50%), improved LV mass, quality of life, and tissue Doppler diastolic function indexes, but there were no significant improvements in exercise capacity or aortic distensibility, the primary outcomes of the trial (265). The benefit of reducing chronotropic incompetence by cardiac pacing in HFpEF is being explored in a pilot study.

TREATMENT: ACUTE DECOMPENSATED HEART FAILURE

Acute decompensated heart failure (ADHF) results in 1.1 million hospitalizations, which costs the US economy an estimated $39 billion annually (2). Although HF signs and symptoms generally improve with treatment, rehospitalization and mortality occur in up to 30% and 15%, respectively, within 60–90 days after discharge and are generally higher in older adults (266). Findings from OPTIMIZE-HF registry based on 48,612 hospitalized HF patients, mean age 73 years suggest that 61% had one or more precipitating factors for acute decompensation, and the leading factors were acute coronary syndrome (15%), pneumonia and respiratory illnesses (15%), arrhythmias (13%), uncontrolled hypertension (11%), worsening kidney function (7%), and non-adherence of medications (5%) and diet (5%) (110). Whereas acute treatment varies with the underlying precipitant, common goals are stabilizing hemodynamics and relieving clinical congestion. Intensive diuretic administration is therefore a cornerstone of therapy. The Diuretic Optimization Strategies Evaluation (DOSE) trial found that higher dose furosemide relieved congestion more rapidly than lower doses, with no significant difference between bolus and continuous infusion (267). However, the Evaluation Study of Congestive Heart Failure and Pulmonary Artery Catheterization Effectiveness (ESCAPE) trial demonstrated no benefit of routine pulmonary artery pressure monitoring in reducing hospital morbidity or mortality (268). In a small study of 60 older ADHF patients (mean age 76 years), compared to high dose continuous furosemide infusion, low-dose dopamine infusion added to furosemide bolus provided similar dieuresis (269). In Ultrafiltration Versus Intravenous (IV) Diuretics for Patients Hospitalized for Acute Decompensated Heart Failure (UNLOAD) trial, ultrafiltration was associated with a greater net weight and fluid loss and lower rehospitalization rate compared to diuretics (270). However, the recent Cardiorenal Rescue Study in Acute Decompensated Heart Failure (CARRESS-HF) trial found that diuretic therapy achieved similar weight loss as ultrafiltration, with better preservation of renal function and fewer adverse events (271).

Although elevated levels of blood vasopressin are common in ADHF, the vasopressin antagonist tolvaptan did not reduce hospital stay or mortality in the Efficacy of Vasopressin Antagonism in Heart Failure Outcome Study With Tolvaptan (EVEREST) trial (272). Similarly, the synthetic natriuretic peptide nesiritide had no significant effect on mortality, 30-day rehospitalization, or renal dysfunction in 7141 patients (mean age 67 years) in the Acute Study of Clinical Effectiveness of Nesiritide in Decompensated Heart Failure (ASCEND-HF) trial (273). In the RELAXin in Acute Heart Failure (RELAXAHF) trial, therapy with serelaxin, recombinant human relaxin-2, was associated with improvement in clinical outcomes such as dyspnea, was safe and well-tolerated, and tended to reduce 180-day mortality, but had no effect on hospital readmissions (274). Because most ADHF trials have focused primarily on patients with HFrEF, more data are needed in HFpEF, which is more common in older adults.

END OF LIFE CARE

HF patients who are symptomatic at rest despite optimal medical therapy are considered to have end stage HF (99). Findings from the CHS suggest that despite a very high rate of overall hospitalization and death, less than half of the community-dwelling older HF patients had a hospitalization due to HF (112). Because HF symptoms are often associated with fluid retentions, euvolemia should be achieved with proper dose of diuretics. HF patients at the end of life may also have dyspnea despite euvolemia, and small doses of opioids may be useful in those situations (275). These drugs may also alleviate other symptoms such as cough, pain, and anxiety that may be seen in end of life situations. Therapy with opioids may be initiated with a short-acting opioid on an as-needed-basis, and titrated and given around-the-clock as needed and tolerated. Commonly prescribed short-acting opioids such as morphine and codeine should be used sparingly as these drugs have active metabolites that are renally cleared and may cause delirium and myoclonus (275). To avoid unwanted adverse effects of many long-acting opioids, long-term therapy with long-acting opioids should be given in consultation with palliative care physicians.

Although comfort and relief of symptoms are more important goals than prolongation of life in patients with end-stage HF, therapy with neurohormonal blockade should not be discontinued as many of these drugs also improve symptoms and reduce hospitalizations (276). However, these drugs should be discontinued when necessary to treat specific side effects such as hypotension, bradycardia, worsening kidney function, hyperkalemia, or adverse gastrointestinal effects. Selective patients may benefit from intermittent inotropes or mechanical support. Shocks from ICDs at the end-of-life may be undesirable, and patients should be offered options for elective device deactivation. If primary care physicians are unfamiliar and/or uncomfortable in managing these issues, they should refer patients for hospice and palliative care, who are specially trained and skilled in end-of-life communications with patients and family members and in providing spiritual and bereavement counseling and support (275).

CONCLUSIONS

The HF syndrome constitutes the most common reason for hospitalization among Medicare recipients. Although male predominance, coronary artery disease etiology, reduced LVEF, and little comorbidity characterize most younger HF patients, in older HF population, female sex, hypertension, diabetes and other comorbidies, and preserved LVEF are common. In older HFrEF patients, neurohormonal blockade, device, and surgical interventions may improve prognosis and quality of life as in younger patients. However, no evidence-based therapy currently exists for HFpEF, the more common form of HF in the very old. Notwithstanding all of the advances in the treatment of HF, the dramatic aging of the population dictates that the most practical and cost-effective strategies to combat HF likely reside in better preventive efforts. Public health strategies to reduce the obesity epidemic and smoking rates, increase physical activity, and improve treatment and control of hypertension, dyslipidemia, and hyperglycemia have great potential to reduce the incidence and prevalence of HF.

ACKNOWLEDGEMENT

The authors wish to thank Kanan Patel, MBBS, MPH for her editorial assistance.

REFERENCES

1. Inouye SK, Studenski S, Tinetti ME, Kuchel GA. Geriatric syndromes: clinical, research, and policy implications of a core geriatric concept. J Am Geriatr Soc 2007; 55: 780–91.
2. Roger VL, Go AS, Lloyd-Jones DM, et al. Heart disease and stroke statistics–2012 update: a report from the American Heart Association. Circulation 2012; 125: e2–e220.
3. Gottdiener JS, McClelland RL, Marshall R, et al. Outcome of congestive heart failure in elderly persons: influence of left ventricular systolic function. The Cardiovascular Health Study. Ann Intern Med 2002; 137: 631–9.
4. Bibbins-Domingo K, Pletcher MJ, Lin F, et al. Racial differences in incident heart failure among young adults. N Engl J Med 2009; 360: 1179–90.
5. Kannel WB. Vital epidemiologic clues in heart failure. J Clin Epidemiol 2000; 53: 229–35.
6. Jencks SF, Williams MV, Coleman EA. Rehospitalizations among patients in the Medicare fee-for-service program. N Engl J Med 2009; 360: 1418–28.
7. Stone J, Hoffman GJ. Medicare Hospital Readmissions: Issues, Policy Options and PPACA: Congressional Research Service Report for Congress. Washington, DC: Prepared for Members and Committees of Congress, 2010.
8. Ho KK, Pinsky JL, Kannel WB, Levy D. The epidemiology of heart failure: the Framingham Study. J Am Coll Cardiol 1993; 22: 6A–13A.
9. Gottdiener JS, Arnold AM, Aurigemma GP, et al. Predictors of congestive heart failure in the elderly: the Cardiovascular Health Study. J Am Coll Cardiol 2000; 35: 1628–37.
10. Ekundayo OJ, Allman RM, Sanders PW, et al. Isolated systolic hypertension and incident heart failure in older adults: a propensity-matched study. Hypertension 2009; 53: 458–65.
11. Iyer AS, Ahmed MI, Filippatos GS, et al. Uncontrolled hypertension and increased risk for incident heart failure in older adults with hypertension: findings from a propensity-matched prospective population study. J Am Soc Hypertens 2010; 4: 22–31.
12. Wallace SM, Yasmin McEniery CM, et al. Isolated systolic hypertension is characterized by increased aortic stiffness and endothelial dysfunction. Hypertension 2007; 50: 228–33.
13. Guichard JL, Desai RV, Ahmed MI, et al. Isolated diastolic hypotension and incident heart failure in older adults. Hypertension 2011; 58: 895–901.
14. Roy B, Pawar PP, Desai RV, et al. A propensity-matched study of the association of diabetes mellitus with incident heart failure and mortality among community-dwelling older adults. Am J Cardiol 2011; 108: 1747–53.
15. Barzilay JI, Kronmal RA, Gottdiener JS, et al. The association of fasting glucose levels with congestive heart failure in diabetic adults ≥65 years: the Cardiovascular Health Study. J Am Coll Cardiol 2004; 43: 2236–41.

16. Aronow WS, Ahmed MI, Ekundayo OJ, Allman RM, Ahmed A. A propensity-matched study of the association of peripheral arterial disease with cardiovascular outcomes in community-dwelling older adults. Am J Cardiol 2009; 103: 130–5.

17. Mujib M, Desai RV, Ahmed MI, et al. Rheumatic heart disease and risk of incident heart failure among community-dwelling older adults: a prospective cohort study. Ann Med 2012; 44: 253–61.

18. de Simone G, Gottdiener JS, Chinali M, Maurer MS. Left ventricular mass predicts heart failure not related to previous myocardial infarction: the Cardiovascular Health Study. Eur Heart J 2008; 29: 741–7.

19. Gardin JM, McClelland R, Kitzman D, et al. M-mode echocardiographic predictors of six- to seven-year incidence of coronary heart disease, stroke, congestive heart failure, and mortality in an elderly cohort (the Cardiovascular Health Study). Am J Cardiol 2001; 87: 1051–7.

20. Levey AS, Bosch JP, Lewis JB, et al. A more accurate method to estimate glomerular filtration rate from serum creatinine: a new prediction equation. Modification of Diet in Renal Disease Study Group. Ann Intern Med 1999; 130: 461–70.

21. Levey AS, Stevens LA, Schmid CH, et al. A new equation to estimate glomerular filtration rate. Ann Intern Med 2009; 150: 604–12.

22. Bowling CB, Feller MA, Mujib M, et al. Relationship between stage of kidney disease and incident heart failure in older adults. Am J Nephrol 2011; 34: 135–41.

23. Desai RV, Ahmed MI, Fonarow GC, et al. Effect of serum insulin on the association between hyperuricemia and incident heart failure. Am J Cardiol 2010; 106: 1134–8.

24. Ekundayo OJ, Dell'Italia LJ, Sanders PW, et al. Association between hyperuricemia and incident heart failure among older adults: a propensity-matched study. Int J Cardiol 2010; 142: 279–87.

25. Kalogeropoulos AP, Georgiopoulou VV, deFilippi CR, et al. Echocardiography, natriuretic peptides, and risk for incident heart failure in older adults: the Cardiovascular Health Study. JACC Cardiovasc Imaging 2012; 5: 131–40.

26. Glazer NL, Macy EM, Lumley T, et al. Transforming growth factor beta-1 and incidence of heart failure in older adults: the Cardiovascular Health Study. Cytokine 2012; 60: 341–5.

27. Rodondi N, Bauer DC, Cappola AR, et al. Subclinical thyroid dysfunction, cardiac function, and the risk of heart failure. The Cardiovascular Health study. J Am Coll Cardiol 2008; 52: 1152–9.

28. Bowling CB, Fonarow GC, Patel K, et al. Impairment of activities of daily living and incident heart failure in community-dwelling older adults. Eur J Heart Fail 2012; 14: 581–7.

29. Filippatos GS, Desai RV, Ahmed MI, et al. Hypoalbuminaemia and incident heart failure in older adults. Eur J Heart Fail 2011; 13: 1078–86.

30. Mozaffarian D, Lemaitre RN, King IB, et al. Circulating long-chain omega-3 fatty acids and incidence of congestive heart failure in older adults: the Cardiovascular Health Study: a cohort study. Ann Intern Med 2011; 155: 160–70.

31. Barasch E, Gottdiener JS, Aurigemma G, et al. Association between elevated fibrosis markers and heart failure in the elderly: the Cardiovascular Health Study. Circ Heart Fail 2009; 2: 303–10.

32. Frankel DS, Vasan RS, D'Agostino RB Sr, et al. Resistin, adiponectin, and risk of heart failure the Framingham offspring study. J Am Coll Cardiol 2009; 53: 754–62.

33. Ahmed AA, Ahmed M, Desai RV, et al. Heavy smoking in the past is a risk factor for incident heart failure in older adults despite ≥ 15 years of abstinence: findings from a prospective population study. Circulation 2010; 122: A17788.

34. Ahmed M, Desai RV, Guichard J, et al. Smoking is an independent modifiable risk factor for incident heart failure in community-dwelling older adults: findings from a prospective population study. Circulation 2010; 122: A17098.

35. Gopal DM, Kalogeropoulos AP, Georgiopoulou VV, et al. Cigarette smoking exposure and heart failure risk in older adults: the Health, Aging, and Body Composition Study. Am Heart J 2012; 164: 236–42.

36. Bryson CL, Mukamal KJ, Mittleman MA, et al. The association of alcohol consumption and incident heart failure: the Cardiovascular Health Study. J Am Coll Cardiol 2006; 48: 305–11.

37. Ahmed AA, Zhang Y, Bourge RC, et al. Low income, regardless of education level, is a significant independent predictor of incident heart failure in community-dwelling, Medicare-eligible older adults. Circulation 2011; 124: A12064.

38. Fonarow GC, Srikanthan P, Costanzo MR, et al. An obesity paradox in acute heart failure: analysis of body mass index and inhospital mortality for 108,927 patients in the Acute Decompensated Heart Failure National Registry. Am Heart J 2007; 153: 74–81.

39. Ahmed M, Levitan E, Mujib M, et al. A prospective examination of the obesity paradox in heart failure: Insights from a population study. Circulation 2010; 122: A20596.

40. Kenchaiah S, Evans JC, Levy D, et al. Obesity and the risk of heart failure. N Engl J Med 2002; 347: 305–13.

41. Wannamethee SG, Shaper AG, Whincup PH, Lennon L, Sattar N. Obesity and risk of incident heart failure in older men with and without pre-existing coronary heart disease: does leptin have a role? J Am Coll Cardiol 2011; 58: 1870–7.

42. Hu G, Jousilahti P, Antikainen R, Katzmarzyk PT, Tuomilehto J. Joint effects of physical activity, body mass index, waist circumference, and waist-to-hip ratio on the risk of heart failure. Circulation 2010; 121: 237–44.

43. Wang Y, Tuomilehto J, Jousilahti P, et al. Occupational, commuting, and leisure-time physical activity in relation to heart failure among finnish men and women. J Am Coll Cardiol 2010; 56: 1140–8.

44. Meyer TE, Kovacs SJ, Ehsani AA, et al. Long-term caloric restriction ameliorates the decline in diastolic function in humans. J Am Coll Cardiol 2006; 47: 398–402.

45. Shinmura K, Tamaki K, Sano M, et al. Impact of long-term caloric restriction on cardiac senescence: caloric restriction ameliorates cardiac diastolic dysfunction associated with aging. J Mol Cell Cardiol 2011; 50: 117–27.

46. Devereux RB, Roman MJ, Liu JE, et al. Congestive heart failure despite normal left ventricular systolic function in a population-based sample: the Strong Heart Study. Am J Cardiol 2000; 86: 1090–6.

47. Kannel WB. Epidemiological aspects of heart failure. Cardiol Clin 1989; 7: 1–9.

48. Senni M, Tribouilloy CM, Rodeheffer RJ, et al. Congestive heart failure in the community: a study of all incident cases in Olmsted County, Minnesota, in 1991. Circulation 1998; 98: 2282–9.

49. Kitzman DW, Gardin JM, Gottdiener JS, et al. Importance of heart failure with preserved systolic function in patients ≥65 years of age. CHS Research Group. Cardiovascular Health Study. Am J Cardiol 2001; 87: 413–19.

50. Rich MW, Kitzman DW. Heart failure in octogenarians: a fundamentally different disease. Am J Geriatr Cardiol 2000; 9(Suppl): 97–104.

51. Ahmed A. Association of diastolic dysfunction and outcomes in ambulatory older adults with chronic heart failure. J Gerontol A Biol Sci Med Sci 2005; 60: 1339–44.

52. Ahmed A. 1-year mortality after first hospitalization for heart failure was similar in patients with preserved or reduced ejection fraction. ACP J Club 2006; 145: 78.

53. Owan TE, Hodge DO, Herges RM, et al. Trends in prevalence and outcome of heart failure with preserved ejection fraction. N Engl J Med 2006; 355: 251–9.

54. Fleg JL, Morrell CH, Bos AG, et al. Accelerated longitudinal decline of aerobic capacity in healthy older adults. Circulation 2005; 112: 674–82.

55. Lakatta EG. Deficient neuroendocrine regulation of the cardiovascular system with advancing age in healthy humans. Circulation 1993; 87: 631–6.

56. Desai RV, Ahmed MI, Mujib M, et al. Natural history of concentric left ventricular geometry in community-dwelling older adults without heart failure during seven years of follow-up. Am J Cardiol 2011; 107: 321–4.

57. Fleg JL. Normative Aging changes in cardiovascular structure and function. Am J Geriatr Cardiol 1996; 5: 7–15.

58. Kitzman DW, Sheikh KH, Beere PA, Philips JL, Higginbotham MB. Age-related alterations of Doppler left ventricular filling indexes in normal subjects are independent of left ventricular mass, heart rate, contractility and loading conditions. J Am Coll Cardiol 1991; 18: 1243–50.

59. Schulman SP, Lakatta EG, Fleg JL, et al. Age-related decline in left ventricular filling at rest and exercise. Am J Physiol 1992; 263: H1932–8.

60. Levy D, Larson MG, Vasan RS, Kannel WB, Ho KK. The progression from hypertension to congestive heart failure. JAMA 1996; 275: 1557–62.

61. Wilson PW. From hypertension to heart failure: what have we learned? Clin Cardiol 1999; 22: V1–10.

62. Aronow WS, Fleg JL, Pepine CJ, et al. ACCF/AHA 2011 expert consensus document on hypertension in the elderly: a report of the American College of Cardiology Foundation Task Force on Clinical Expert Consensus Documents. Circulation 2011; 123: 2434–506.

63. Vokonas PS, Kannel WB, Cupples LA. Epidemiology and risk of hypertension in the elderly: the Framingham Study. J Hypertens Suppl 1988; 6: S3–9.

64. Fleg JL, Tzankoff SP, Lakatta EG. Age-related augmentation of plasma catecholamines during dynamic exercise in healthy males. J Appl Physiol 1985; 59: 1033–9.

65. Fleg JL, O'Connor F, Gerstenblith G, et al. Impact of age on the cardiovascular response to dynamic upright exercise in healthy men and women. J Appl Physiol 1995; 78: 890–900.

66. Clarkson PB, Wheeldon NM, MacFadyen RJ, Pringle SD, MacDonald TM. Effects of brain natriuretic peptide on exercise hemodynamics and neurohormones in isolated diastolic heart failure. Circulation 1996; 93: 2037–42.

67. Kitzman DW, Little WC, Brubaker PH, et al. Pathophysiological characterization of isolated diastolic heart failure in comparison to systolic heart failure. JAMA 2002; 288: 2144–50.

68. Cody RJ, Torre S, Clark M, Pondolfino K. Age-related hemodynamic, renal, and hormonal differences among patients with congestive heart failure. Arch Intern Med 1989; 149: 1023–8.

69. Dutka DP, Olivotto I, Ward S, et al. Effects of aging on neuroendocrine activation in subjects and patients in the presence and absence of heart failure with left ventricular systolic dysfunction. Am J Cardiol 1996; 77: 1197–201.

70. Maurer MS, Burkhoff D, Fried LP, et al. Ventricular structure and function in hypertensive participants with heart failure and a normal ejection fraction: the Cardiovascular Health Study. J Am Coll Cardiol 2007; 49: 972–81.

71. Iriarte M, Murga N, Sagastagoitia D, et al. Congestive heart failure from left ventricular diastolic dysfunction in systemic hypertension. Am J Cardiol 1993; 71: 308–12.

72. Gandhi SK, Powers JC, Nomeir AM, et al. The pathogenesis of acute pulmonary edema associated with hypertension. N Engl J Med 2001; 344: 17–22.

73. Gelpi RJ, Pasipoularides A, Lader AS, et al. Changes in diastolic cardiac function in developing and stable perinephritic hypertension in conscious dogs. Circ Res 1991; 68: 555–67.

74. Little WC, Braunwald E. Assessment of cardiac function. In: Braunwald E, ed. Heart Disease. Philadelphia, PA: WB Saunders, 1996: 421–44.

75. Kramer K, Kirkman P, Kitzman D, Little WC. Flash pulmonary edema: association with hypertension and reoccurrence despite coronary revascularization. Am Heart J 2000; 140: 451–5.

76. Ahmed A. Chronic heart failure in older adults. Med Clin North Am 2011; 95: 439–61; ix.

77. Kitzman DW, Higginbotham MB, Cobb FR, Sheikh KH, Sullivan MJ. Exercise intolerance in patients with heart failure and preserved left ventricular systolic function: failure of the Frank-Starling mechanism. J Am Coll Cardiol 1991; 17: 1065–72.

78. Hundley WG, Kitzman DW, Morgan TM, et al. Cardiac cycle-dependent changes in aortic area and distensibility are reduced in older patients with isolated diastolic heart failure and correlate with exercise intolerance. J Am Coll Cardiol 2001; 38: 796–802.

79. Rerkpattanapipat P, Hundley WG, Link KM, et al. Relation of aortic distensibility determined by magnetic resonance imaging in patients ≥60 years of age to systolic heart failure and exercise capacity. Am J Cardiol 2002; 90: 1221–5.

80. Brubaker PH, Joo KC, Stewart KP, et al. Chronotropic incompetence and its contribution to exercise intolerance in older heart failure patients. J Cardiopulm Rehabil 2006; 26: 86–9.

81. Clark AL, Coats AJ. Chronotropic incompetence in chronic heart failure. Int J Cardiol 1995; 49: 225–31.

82. Borlaug BA, Melenovsky V, Russell SD, et al. Impaired chronotropic and vasodilator reserves limit exercise capacity in patients with heart failure and a preserved ejection fraction. Circulation 2006; 114: 2138–47.

83. Burkhoff D, Maurer MS, Packer M. Heart failure with a normal ejection fraction: is it really a disorder of diastolic function? Circulation 2003; 107: 656–8.

84. Zile MR, Lewinter MM. Left ventricular end-diastolic volume is normal in patients with heart failure and a normal ejection fraction: a renewed consensus in diastolic heart failure. J Am Coll Cardiol 2007; 49: 982–5.

85. Zile MR, Gaasch WH, Carroll JD, et al. Heart failure with a normal ejection fraction: is measurement of diastolic function necessary to make the diagnosis of diastolic heart failure? Circulation 2001; 104: 779–82.

86. Maurer MS, Spevack D, Burkhoff D, Kronzon I. Diastolic dysfunction: can it be diagnosed by Doppler echocardiography? J Am Coll Cardiol 2004; 44: 1543–9.

87. Zile MR, Baicu CF, Gaasch WH. Diastolic heart failure abnormalities in active relaxation and passive stiffness of the left ventricle. N Engl J Med 2004; 350: 1953–9.

88. Bella JN, Palmieri V, Liu JE, et al. Relationship between left ventricular diastolic relaxation and systolic function in hypertension: the Hypertension Genetic Epidemiology Network (HyperGEN) Study. Hypertension 2001; 38: 424–8.

89. Tang W, Devereux RB, Rao DC, et al. Associations between angiotensinogen gene variants and left ventricular mass and function in the HyperGEN study. Am Heart J 2002; 143: 854–60.

90. Kane GC, Hauser MF, Behrenbeck TR, et al. Impact of gender on rest Tc-99m sestamibi-gated left ventricular ejection fraction. Am J Cardiol 2002; 89: 1238–41.

91. Bella JN, Palmieri V, Kitzman DW, et al. Gender difference in diastolic function in hypertension (the HyperGEN study). Am J Cardiol 2002; 89: 1052–6.

92. Bella JN, Wachtell K, Palmieri V, et al. Relation of left ventricular geometry and function to systemic hemodynamics in hypertension: the LIFE Study. J Hypertens 2001; 19: 127–34.

93. Douglas PS, Katz SE, Weinberg EO, et al. Hypertrophic remodeling: gender differences in the early response to left ventricular pressure overload. J Am Coll Cardiol 1998; 32: 1118–25.

94. Aurigemma GP, Gaasch WH, McLaughlin M, et al. Reduced left ventricular systolic pump performance and depressed myocardial contractile function in patients > 65 years of age with normal ejection fraction and a high relative wall thickness. Am J Cardiol 1995; 76: 702–5.

95. Aurigemma GP, Silver KH, McLaughlin M, Mauser J, Gaasch WH. Impact of chamber geometry and gender on left ventricular systolic function in patients > 60 years of age with aortic stenosis. Am J Cardiol 1994; 74: 794–8.

96. Freshour JR, Chase SE, Vikstrom KL. Gender differences in cardiac ACE expression are normalized in androgen-deprived male mice. Am J Physiol Heart Circ Physiol 2002; 283: H1997–2003.

97. Ekundayo OJ, Howard VJ, Safford MM, et al. Value of orthopnea, paroxysmal nocturnal dyspnea, and medications in prospective population studies of incident heart failure. Am J Cardiol 2009; 104: 259–64.

98. Butman SM, Ewy GA, Standen JR, Kern KB, Hahn E. Bedside cardiovascular examination in patients with severe chronic heart failure: importance of rest or inducible jugular venous distension. J Am Coll Cardiol 1993; 22: 968–74.

99. Hunt SA, Abraham WT, Chin MH, et al. 2009 focused update incorporated into the ACC/AHA 2005 Guidelines for the Diagnosis and Management of Heart Failure in Adults: a report of the American College of Cardiology Foundation/American Heart Association Task Force on Practice Guidelines: developed in collaboration with the International Society for Heart and Lung Transplantation. Circulation 2009; 119: e391–479.

100. Maisel AS, Krishnaswamy P, Nowak RM, et al. Rapid measurement of B-type natriuretic peptide in the emergency diagnosis of heart failure. N Engl J Med 2002; 347: 161–7.

101. Wright SP, Doughty RN, Pearl A, et al. Plasma amino-terminal pro-brain natriuretic peptide and accuracy of heart-failure diagnosis in primary care: a randomized, controlled trial. J Am Coll Cardiol 2003; 42: 1793–800.

102. Lokuge A, Lam L, Cameron P, et al. B-type natriuretic peptide testing and the accuracy of heart failure diagnosis in the emergency department. Circ Heart Fail 2010; 3: 104–10.

103. Pfisterer M, Buser P, Rickli H, et al. BNP-guided vs symptom-guided heart failure therapy: the Trial of Intensified vs Standard Medical Therapy in Elderly Patients With Congestive Heart Failure (TIME-CHF) randomized trial. JAMA 2009; 301: 383–92.

104. Laramee P, Wonderling D, Swain S, Al-Mohammad A, Mant J. Cost-effectiveness analysis of serial measurement of circulating natriuretic peptide concentration in chronic heart failure. Heart 2013; 99: 267–71.doi:10.1136/heartjnl-2012-302692.

105. Ahmed A. DEFEAT heart failure: clinical manifestations, diagnostic assessment, and etiology of geriatric heart failure. Heart Fail Clin 2007; 3: 389–402.

106. Tsuyuki RT, McKelvie RS, Arnold JM, et al. Acute precipitants of congestive heart failure exacerbations. Arch Intern Med 2001; 161: 2337–42.

107. Ghali JK, Kadakia S, Cooper R, Ferlinz J. Precipitating factors leading to decompensation of heart failure. Traits among urban blacks. Arch Intern Med 1988; 148: 2013–16.

108. Chin MH, Goldman L. Factors contributing to the hospitalization of patients with congestive heart failure. Am J Public Health 1997; 87: 643–8.

109. Khand AU, Gemmell I, Rankin AC, Cleland JG. Clinical events leading to the progression of heart failure: insights from a national database of hospital discharges. Eur Heart J 2001; 22: 153–64.

110. Fonarow GC, Abraham WT, Albert NM, et al. Factors identified as precipitating hospital admissions for heart failure and clinical outcomes: findings from OPTIMIZE-HF. Arch Intern Med 2008; 168: 847–54.

111. Feller MA, Mujib M, Zhang Y, et al. Baseline characteristics, quality of care, and outcomes of younger and older Medicare beneficiaries hospitalized with heart failure: findings from the Alabama Heart Failure Project. Int J Cardiol 2012; 162: 39–44.

112. Bhatia V, Ahmed MI, Desai RV, et al. Incidence and predictors of hospitalization due to heart failure among Medicare-eligible community-dwelling older adults with prevalent heart failure: insights from a prospective population study. Circulation 2010; 122: A20952.

113. MacIntyre K, Capewell S, Stewart S, et al. Evidence of improving prognosis in heart failure: trends in case fatality in 66 547 patients hospitalized between 1986 and 1995. Circulation 2000; 102: 1126–31.

114. Wahle C, Adamopoulos C, Ekundayo OJ, et al. A propensity-matched study of outcomes of chronic heart failure (HF) in younger and older adults. Arch Gerontol Geriatr 2009; 49: 165–71.

115. Ahmed MI, Mujib M, Desai RV, et al. Outcomes in younger and older adults with chronic advanced systolic heart failure: a propensity-matched study. Int J Cardiol 2012; 154: 128–33.

116. Ahmed MI, Lainscak M, Mujib M, et al. Gender-related dissociation in outcomes in chronic heart failure: reduced mortality but similar hospitalization in women. Int J Cardiol 2011; 148: 36–42.

117. Gambassi G, Agha SA, Sui X, et al. Race and the natural history of chronic heart failure: a propensity-matched study. J Card Fail 2008; 14: 373–8.

118. Ahmed A. A propensity matched study of New York Heart Association class and natural history endpoints in heart failure. Am J Cardiol 2007; 99: 549–53.

119. Ahmed A, Aronow WS. A propensity-matched study of the association of physical function and outcomes in geriatric heart failure. Arch Gerontol Geriatr 2008; 46: 161–72.

120. Ahmed A, Aronow WS, Fleg JL. Higher New York Heart Association classes and increased mortality and hospitalization in patients with heart failure and preserved left ventricular function. Am Heart J 2006; 151: 444–50.

121. MAGGIC Investigators. The survival of patients with heart failure with preserved or reduced left ventricular ejection fraction: an individual patient data meta-analysis. Meta-analysis Global Group in Chronic Heart Failure (MAGGIC). Eur Heart J 2012; 33: 1750–7.

122. Fonarow GC, Stough WG, Abraham WT, et al. Characteristics, treatments, and outcomes of patients with preserved systolic function hospitalized for heart failure: a report from the OPTIMIZE-HF Registry. J Am Coll Cardiol 2007; 50: 768–77.

123. Meyer P, Desai RV, Mujib M, et al. Right ventricular ejection fraction <20% is an independent predictor of mortality but not of hospitalization in older systolic heart failure patients. Int J Cardiol 2012; 155: 120–5.

124. Davies LC, Francis DP, Piepoli M, et al. Chronic heart failure in the elderly: value of cardiopulmonary exercise testing in risk stratification. Heart 2000; 83: 147–51.

125. Krumholz HM, Chen YT, Vaccarino V, et al. Correlates and impact on outcomes of worsening renal function in patients ≥65 years of age with heart failure. Am J Cardiol 2000; 85: 1110–13.

126. Croft JB, Giles WH, Pollard RA, et al. Heart failure survival among older adults in the United States: a poor prognosis for an emerging epidemic in the Medicare population. Arch Intern Med 1999; 159: 505–10.

127. Ahmed A, Aban IB, Vaccarino V, et al. A propensity-matched study of the effect of diabetes on the natural history of heart failure: variations by sex and age. Heart 2007; 93: 1584–90.

128. Gheorghiade M, Flaherty JD, Fonarow GC, et al. Coronary artery disease, coronary revascularization, and outcomes in chronic advanced systolic heart failure. Int J Cardiol 2011; 151: 69–75.

129. Ahmed MI, White M, Ekundayo OJ, et al. A history of atrial fibrillation and outcomes in chronic advanced systolic heart failure: a propensity-matched study. Eur Heart J 2009; 30: 2029–37.

130. Campbell RC, Sui X, Filippatos G, et al. Association of chronic kidney disease with outcomes in chronic heart failure: a propensity-matched study. Nephrol Dial Transplant 2009; 24: 186–93.

131. Ahmed A, Rich MW, Sanders PW, et al. Chronic kidney disease associated mortality in diastolic versus systolic heart failure: a propensity matched study. Am J Cardiol 2007; 99: 393–8.

132. Dunlay SM, Redfield MM, Weston SA, et al. Hospitalizations after heart failure diagnosis a community perspective. J Am Coll Cardiol 2009; 54: 1695–702.

133. Go AS, Yang J, Ackerson LM, et al. Hemoglobin level, chronic kidney disease, and the risks of death and hospitalization in adults with chronic heart failure: the Anemia in Chronic Heart Failure: Outcomes and Resource Utilization (ANCHOR) Study. Circulation 2006; 113: 2713–23.

134. Ahmed A, Zannad F, Love TE, et al. A propensity-matched study of the association of low serum potassium levels and mortality in chronic heart failure. Eur Heart J 2007; 28: 1334–43.

135. Alper AB, Campbell RC, Anker SD, et al. A propensity-matched study of low serum potassium and mortality in older adults with chronic heart failure. Int J Cardiol 2009; 137: 1–8.

136. Bowling CB, Pitt B, Ahmed MI, et al. Hypokalemia and outcomes in patients with chronic heart failure and chronic kidney disease: findings from propensity-matched studies. Circ Heart Fail 2010; 3: 253–60.

137. Ahmed MI, Ekundayo OJ, Mujib M, et al. Mild hyperkalemia and outcomes in chronic heart failure: a propensity matched study. Int J Cardiol 2010; 144: 383–8.

138. Adamopoulos C, Pitt B, Sui X, et al. Low serum magnesium and cardiovascular mortality in chronic heart failure: a propensity-matched study. Int J Cardiol 2009; 136: 270–7.

139. Filippatos GS, Ahmed MI, Gladden JD, et al. Hyperuricaemia, chronic kidney disease, and outcomes in heart failure: potential mechanistic insights from epidemiological data. Eur Heart J 2011; 32: 712–20.

140. Yusuf S, Pfeffer MA, Swedberg K, et al. Effects of candesartan in patients with chronic heart failure and preserved left-ventricular ejection fraction: the CHARM-Preserved Trial. Lancet 2003; 362: 777–81.

141. Massie BM, Carson PE, McMurray JJ, et al. Irbesartan in patients with heart failure and preserved ejection fraction. N Engl J Med 2008; 359: 2456–67.

142. Gheorghiade M, Abraham WT, Albert NM, et al. Relationship between admission serum sodium concentration and clinical outcomes in patients hospitalized for heart failure: an analysis from the OPTIMIZE-HF registry. Eur Heart J 2007; 28: 980–8.

143. Fleg JL. Exercise therapy for elderly heart failure patients. Clin Geriatr Med 2007; 23: 221–34.

144. Austin J, Williams R, Ross L, Moseley L, Hutchison S. Randomised controlled trial of cardiac rehabilitation in elderly patients with heart failure. Eur J Heart Fail 2005; 7: 411–17.

145. Smart N, Haluska B, Jeffriess L, Marwick TH. Exercise training in systolic and diastolic dysfunction: effects on cardiac function, functional capacity, and quality of life. Am Heart J 2007; 153: 530–6.

146. O'Connor CM, Whellan DJ, Lee KL, et al. Efficacy and safety of exercise training in patients with chronic heart failure: HF-ACTION randomized controlled trial. JAMA 2009; 301: 1439–50.

147. Flynn KE, Pina IL, Whellan DJ, et al. Effects of exercise training on health status in patients with chronic heart failure: HF-ACTION randomized controlled trial. JAMA 2009; 301: 1451–9.

148. Blumenthal JA, Babyak MA, O'Connor C, et al. Effects of exercise training on depressive symptoms in patients with chronic heart failure: the HF-ACTION randomized trial. JAMA 2012; 308: 465–74.

149. Forman DE, Fleg JL, Kitzman DW, et al. 6-min walk test provides prognostic utility comparable to cardiopulmonary exercise testing in ambulatory outpatients with systolic heart failure. J Am Coll Cardiol 2012; 60: 2653–61.

150. Rich MW, Beckham V, Wittenberg C, et al. A multidisciplinary intervention to prevent the readmission of elderly patients with congestive heart failure. N Engl J Med 1995; 333: 1190–5.

151. Stewart S, Marley JE, Horowitz JD. Effects of a multidisciplinary, home-based intervention on unplanned readmissions and survival among patients with chronic congestive heart failure: a randomised controlled study. Lancet 1999; 354: 1077–83.

152. Takeda A, Taylor SJ, Taylor RS, et al. Clinical service organisation for heart failure. Cochrane Database Syst Rev 2012; 9: CD002752.

153. Chaudhry SI, Mattera JA, Curtis JP, et al. Telemonitoring in patients with heart failure. N Engl J Med 2010; 363: 2301–9.

154. Koehler F, Winkler S, Schieber M, et al. Impact of remote telemedical management on mortality and hospitalizations in ambulatory patients with chronic heart failure: the telemedical interventional monitoring in heart failure study. Circulation 2011; 123: 1873–80.

155. Wilson JR, Smith JS, Dahle KL, Ingersoll GL. Impact of home health care on health care costs and hospitalization frequency in patients with heart failure. Am J Cardiol 1999; 83: 615–7, A10.

156. Packer M, Carver JR, Rodeheffer RJ, et al. Effect of oral milrinone on mortality in severe chronic heart failure. The PROMISE Study Research Group. N Engl J Med 1991; 325: 1468–75.

157. Cohn JN, Goldstein SO, Greenberg BH, et al. A dose-dependent increase in mortality with vesnarinone among patients with severe heart failure. Vesnarinone Trial Investigators. N Engl J Med 1998; 339: 1810–16.

158. Curtiss C, Cohn JN, Vrobel T, Franciosa JA. Role of the renin-angiotensin system in the systemic vasoconstriction of chronic congestive heart failure. Circulation 1978; 58: 763–70.

159. Packer M. Role of the sympathetic nervous system in chronic heart failure. A historical and philosophical perspective. Circulation 1990; 82: I1–6.

160. The CONSENSUS Trial Study Group. Effects of enalapril on mortality in severe congestive heart failure. Results of the Cooperative North Scandinavian Enalapril Survival Study (CONSENSUS). N Engl J Med 1987; 316: 1429–35.

161. The SOLVD Investigators. Effect of enalapril on survival in patients with reduced left ventricular ejection fractions and congestive heart failure. N Engl J Med 1991; 325: 293–302.

162. Granger CB, McMurray JJ, Yusuf S, et al. Effects of candesartan in patients with chronic heart failure and reduced left-ventricular systolic function intolerant to angiotensin-converting-enzyme inhibitors: the CHARM-Alternative trial. Lancet 2003; 362: 772–6.

163. Cohn JN, Tognoni G; Valsartan Heart Failure Trial I. A randomized trial of the angiotensin-receptor blocker valsartan in chronic heart failure. N Engl J Med 2001; 345: 1667–75.

164. Packer M, Bristow MR, Cohn JN, et al. The effect of carvedilol on morbidity and mortality in patients with chronic heart failure. U.S. Carvedilol Heart Failure Study Group. N Engl J Med 1996; 334: 1349–55.

165. Packer M, Coats AJ, Fowler MB, et al. Effect of carvedilol on survival in severe chronic heart failure. N Engl J Med 2001; 344: 1651–8.

166. The CIBIS-II Investigators. The Cardiac Insufficiency Bisoprolol Study II (CIBIS-II): a randomised trial. Lancet 1999; 353: 9–13.

167. The MERIT-HF Investigators. Effect of metoprolol CR/XL in chronic heart failure: Metoprolol CR/XL Randomised Intervention Trial in Congestive Heart Failure (MERIT-HF). Lancet 1999; 353: 2001–7.

168. Pitt B, Zannad F, Remme WJ, et al. The effect of spironolactone on morbidity and mortality in patients with severe heart failure. Randomized Aldactone Evaluation Study Investigators. N Engl J Med 1999; 341: 709–17.

169. Pitt B, Remme W, Zannad F, et al. Eplerenone, a selective aldosterone blocker, in patients with left ventricular dysfunction after myocardial infarction. N Engl J Med 2003; 348: 1309–21.

170. Zannad F, McMurray JJ, Krum H, et al. Eplerenone in patients with systolic heart failure and mild symptoms. N Engl J Med 2011; 364: 11–21.

171. Masoudi FA, Havranek EP, Wolfe P, et al. Most hospitalized older persons do not meet the enrollment criteria for clinical trials in heart failure. Am Heart J 2003; 146: 250–7.

172. Adams KF Jr, Fonarow GC, Emerman CL, et al. Characteristics and outcomes of patients hospitalized for heart failure in the United States: rationale, design, and preliminary observations from the first 100,000 cases in the Acute Decompensated Heart Failure National Registry (ADHERE). Am Heart J 2005; 149: 209–16.

173. Vidán MT, Bueno H, Wang Y, et al. The relationship between systolic blood pressure on admission and mortality in older patients with heart failure. Eur J Heart Fail 2010; 12: 148–55.

174. Ekundayo OJ, Markland A, Lefante C, et al. Association of diuretic use and overactive bladder syndrome in older adults: a propensity score analysis. Arch Gerontol Geriatr 2009; 49: 64–8.

175. Ahmed A, Husain A, Love TE, et al. Heart failure, chronic diuretic use, and increase in mortality and hospitalization: an observational study using propensity score methods. Eur Heart J 2006; 27: 1431–9.

176. Ahmed A, Young JB, Love TE, Levesque R, Pitt B. A propensity-matched study of the effects of chronic diuretic therapy on mortality and hospitalization in older adults with heart failure. Int J Cardiol 2008; 125: 246–53.

177. Francis GS, Benedict C, Johnstone DE, et al. Comparison of neuroendocrine activation in patients with left ventricular dysfunction with and without congestive heart failure. A substudy of the Studies of Left Ventricular Dysfunction (SOLVD). Circulation 1990; 82: 1724–9.

178. Ekundayo OJ, Adamopoulos C, Ahmed MI, et al. Oral potassium supplement use and outcomes in chronic heart failure: a propensity-matched study. Int J Cardiol 2010; 141: 167–74.

179. Lopez B, Querejeta R, Gonzalez A, et al. Effects of loop diuretics on myocardial fibrosis and collagen type I turnover in chronic heart failure. J Am Coll Cardiol 2004; 43: 2028–35.

180. Cosin J, Diez J; TORIC investigators. Torasemide in chronic heart failure: results of the TORIC study. Eur J Heart Fail 2002; 4: 507–13.

181. Murray MD, Deer MM, Ferguson JA, et al. Open-label randomized trial of torsemide compared with furosemide therapy for patients with heart failure. Am J Med 2001; 111: 513–20.

182. Zile MR, Gaasch WH, Anand IS, et al. Mode of death in patients with heart failure and a preserved ejection fraction: results from the Irbesartan in Heart Failure With Preserved Ejection Fraction Study (I-Preserve) trial. Circulation 2010; 121: 1393–405.

183. Ekundayo OJ, Ahmed M, Desai R, et al. A prospective population study of the rate and risk of hospitalization among Medicare-eligible community-dwelling older adults with incident heart failure. Circulation 2010; 122: A21045.

184. Colucci WS. ACE inhibitors in heart failure due to systolic dysfunction: therapeutic use. In: Yeon SB, ed. UpToDate. 3452 Version 9.0 http://www.uptodate.com/contents/ace-inhibitors-in-heart-failure-due-to-systolic-dysfunction-therapeutic-use?source=see_linkTopic Waltham, MA: Wolters Kluwer, 2012.

185. Rose BD, Colucci WS. Renal effects of ACE inhibitors in heart failure. In: Sterns RH, Gottlieb SS, eds. UpToDate. 2365 Version 4.0 http://www.uptodate.com/contents/renal-effects-of-ace-inhibitors-in-heart-failure?source=see_link&anchor=H2#H2. Waltham, MA: Wolters Kluwer, 2012.

186. Ahmed A, Fonarow GC, Zhang Y, et al. Renin-angiotensin inhibition in systolic heart failure and chronic kidney disease. Am J Med 2012; 125: 399–410.

187. Desai RV, Banach M, Ahmed MI, et al. Impact of baseline systolic blood pressure on long-term outcomes in patients with advanced chronic systolic heart failure (insights from the BEST trial). Am J Cardiol 2010; 106: 221–7.

188. Banach M, Bhatia V, Feller MA, et al. Relation of baseline systolic blood pressure and long-term outcomes in ambulatory patients with chronic mild to moderate heart failure. Am J Cardiol 2011; 107: 1208–14.

189. Gheorghiade M, Abraham WT, Albert NM, et al. Systolic blood pressure at admission, clinical characteristics, and outcomes in patients hospitalized with acute heart failure. JAMA 2006; 296: 2217–26.

190. McMurray JJ, Ostergren J, Swedberg K, et al. Effects of candesartan in patients with chronic heart failure and reduced left-ventricular systolic function taking angiotensin-converting-enzyme inhibitors: the CHARM-Added trial. Lancet 2003; 362: 767–71.

191. Deedwania PC, Gottlieb S, Ghali JK, Waagstein F, Wikstrand JC; MERIT-HF Study Group. Efficacy, safety and tolerability of beta-adrenergic blockade with metoprolol CR/XL in elderly patients with heart failure. Eur Heart J 2004; 25: 1300–9.

192. Poole-Wilson PA, Swedberg K, Cleland JG, et al. Comparison of carvedilol and metoprolol on clinical outcomes in patients with chronic heart failure in the Carvedilol Or Metoprolol European Trial (COMET): randomised controlled trial. Lancet 2003; 362: 7–13.

193. Flather MD, Shibata MC, Coats AJ, et al. Randomized trial to determine the effect of nebivolol on mortality and cardiovascular hospital admission in elderly patients with heart failure (SENIORS). Eur Heart J 2005; 26: 215–25.

194. Ahmed A, Dell'Italia LJ. Use of beta-blockers in older adults with chronic heart failure. Am J Med Sci 2004; 328: 100–11.

195. Ahmed A. Myocardial beta-1 adrenoceptor down-regulation in aging and heart failure: implications for beta-blocker use in older adults with heart failure. Eur J Heart Fail 2003; 5: 709–15.

196. Hernandez AF, Mi X, Hammill BG, et al. Associations between aldosterone antagonist therapy and risks of mortality and readmission among patients with heart failure and reduced ejection fraction. JAMA 2012; 308: 2097–107.

197. Taylor AL, Ziesche S, Yancy C, et al. Combination of isosorbide dinitrate and hydralazine in blacks with heart failure. N Engl J Med 2004; 351: 2049–57.

198. Cohn JN, Johnson G, Ziesche S, et al. A comparison of enalapril with hydralazine-isosorbide dinitrate in the treatment of chronic congestive heart failure. N Engl J Med 1991; 325: 303–10.

199. The Digitalis Investigation Group. The effect of digoxin on mortality and morbidity in patients with heart failure. N Engl J Med 1997; 336: 525–33.

200. Ahmed A, Pitt B, Rahimtoola SH, et al. Effects of digoxin at low serum concentrations on mortality and hospitalization in heart failure: a propensity-matched study of the DIG trial. Int J Cardiol 2008; 123: 138–46.

201. Ahmed A, Rich MW, Love TE, et al. Digoxin and reduction in mortality and hospitalization in heart failure: a comprehensive post hoc analysis of the DIG trial. Eur Heart J 2006; 27: 178–86.

202. Ahmed A. Digoxin and reduction in mortality and hospitalization in geriatric heart failure: importance of low doses and low serum concentrations. J Gerontol A Biol Sci Med Sci 2007; 62: 323–9.

203. Rich MW, McSherry F, Williford WO, Yusuf S; Digitalis Investigation Group. Effect of age on mortality, hospitalizations and response to digoxin in patients with heart failure: the DIG study. J Am Coll Cardiol 2001; 38: 806–13.

204. Massie B, Bourassa M, DiBianco R, et al. Long-term oral administration of amrinone for congestive heart failure: lack of efficacy in a multicenter controlled trial. Circulation 1985; 71: 963–71.

205. Cuffe MS, Califf RM, Adams KF Jr, et al. Short-term intravenous milrinone for acute exacerbation of chronic heart failure: a randomized controlled trial. JAMA 2002; 287: 1541–7.

206. Abraham WT, Adams KF, Fonarow GC, et al. In-hospital mortality in patients with acute decompensated heart failure requiring intravenous vasoactive medications: an analysis from the Acute Decompensated Heart Failure National Registry (ADHERE). J Am Coll Cardiol 2005; 46: 57–64.

207. Slawsky MT, Colucci WS, Gottlieb SS, et al. Acute hemodynamic and clinical effects of levosimendan in patients with severe heart failure. Study Investigators. Circulation 2000; 102: 2222–7.

208. Mebazaa A, Nieminen MS, Packer M, et al. Levosimendan vs dobutamine for patients with acute decompensated heart failure: the SURVIVE Randomized Trial. JAMA 2007; 297: 1883–91.

209. Follath F, Cleland JG, Just H, et al. Efficacy and safety of intravenous levosimendan compared with dobutamine in severe low-output heart failure (the LIDO study): a randomised double-blind trial. Lancet 2002; 360: 196–202.

210. Rich MW, Imburgia M. Inotropic response to dobutamine in elderly patients with decompensated congestive heart failure. Am J Cardiol 1990; 65: 519–21.

211. Swedberg K, Komajda M, Bohm M, et al. Ivabradine and outcomes in chronic heart failure (SHIFT): a randomised placebo-controlled study. Lancet 2010; 376: 875–85.

212. Anand I, McMurray J, Cohn JN, et al. Long-term effects of darusentan on left-ventricular remodelling and clinical outcomes in the EndothelinA Receptor Antagonist Trial in Heart Failure (EARTH): randomised, double-blind, placebo-controlled trial. Lancet 2004; 364: 347–54.

213. Guazzi M, Samaja M, Arena R, Vicenzi M, Guazzi MD. Long-term use of sildenafil in the therapeutic management of heart failure. J Am Coll Cardiol 2007; 50: 2136–44.

214. Lewis GD, Lachmann J, Camuso J, et al. Sildenafil improves exercise hemodynamics and oxygen uptake in patients with systolic heart failure. Circulation 2007; 115: 59–66.

215. Guazzi M, Tumminello G, Di Marco F, Fiorentini C, Guazzi MD. The effects of phosphodiesterase-5 inhibition with sildenafil on pulmonary hemodynamics and diffusion capacity, exercise ventilatory efficiency, and oxygen uptake kinetics in chronic heart failure. J Am Coll Cardiol 2004; 44: 2339–48.

216. Lapp H, Mitrovic V, Franz N, et al. Cinaciguat (BAY 58-2667) improves cardiopulmonary hemodynamics in patients with acute decompensated heart failure. Circulation 2009; 119: 2781–8.

217. Anker SD, Comin Colet J, Filippatos G, et al. Ferric carboxymaltose in patients with heart failure and iron deficiency. N Engl J Med 2009; 361: 2436–48.

218. Palazzuoli A, Silverberg D, Iovine F, et al. Erythropoietin improves anemia exercise tolerance and renal function and reduces B-type natriuretic peptide and hospitalization in patients with heart failure and anemia. Am Heart J 2006; 152: 1096 e9–15.

219. Caminiti G, Volterrani M, Iellamo F, et al. Effect of long-acting testosterone treatment on functional exercise capacity, skeletal muscle performance, insulin resistance, and baroreflex sensitivity in elderly patients with chronic heart failure a double-blind, placebo-controlled, randomized study. J Am Coll Cardiol 2009; 54: 919–27.

220. Shamim W, Francis DP, Yousufuddin M, et al. Intraventricular conduction delay: a prognostic marker in chronic heart failure. Int J Cardiol 1999; 70: 171–8.

221. Abraham WT, Fisher WG, Smith AL, et al. Cardiac resynchronization in chronic heart failure. N Engl J Med 2002; 346: 1845–53.

222. Bristow MR, Saxon LA, Boehmer J, et al. Cardiac-resynchronization therapy with or without an implantable defibrillator in advanced chronic heart failure. N Engl J Med 2004; 350: 2140–50.

223. Cleland JG, Daubert JC, Erdmann E, et al. The effect of cardiac resynchronization on morbidity and mortality in heart failure. N Engl J Med 2005; 352: 1539–49.

224. Tang AS, Wells GA, Talajic M, et al. Cardiac-resynchronization therapy for mild-to-moderate heart failure. N Engl J Med 2010; 363: 2385–95.

225. Tracy CM, Epstein AE, Darbar D, et al. 2012; ACCF/AHA/HRS focused update of the 2008 guidelines for device-based therapy of cardiac rhythm abnormalities: a report of the American College of Cardiology Foundation/American Heart Association Task Force on Practice Guidelines. J Am Coll Cardiol 2012; 60: 1297–313.

226. Moss AJ, Zareba W, Hall WJ, et al. Prophylactic implantation of a defibrillator in patients with myocardial infarction and reduced ejection fraction. N Engl J Med 2002; 346: 877–83.

227. Bardy GH, Lee KL, Mark DB, et al. Amiodarone or an implantable cardioverter-defibrillator for congestive heart failure. N Engl J Med 2005; 352: 225–37.

228. Mark DB, Anstrom KJ, Sun JL, et al. Quality of life with defibrillator therapy or amiodarone in heart failure. N Engl J Med 2008; 359: 999–1008.

229. Mishkin JD, Saxonhouse SJ, Woo GW, et al. Appropriate evaluation and treatment of heart failure patients after implantable cardioverter-defibrillator discharge: time to go beyond the initial shock. J Am Coll Cardiol 2009; 54: 1993–2000.

230. Kadish A, Dyer A, Daubert JP, et al. Prophylactic defibrillator implantation in patients with nonischemic dilated cardiomyopathy. N Engl J Med 2004; 350: 2151–8.

231. Levinson JR, Akins CW, Buckley MJ, et al. Octogenarians with aortic stenosis. outcome after aortic valve replacement. Circulation 1989; 80: I49–56.

232. Reynolds MR, Magnuson EA, Lei Y, et al. Health-related quality of life after transcatheter aortic valve replacement in inoperable patients with severe aortic stenosis. Circulation 2011; 124: 1964–72.

233. Makkar RR, Fontana GP, Jilaihawi H, et al. Transcatheter aortic-valve replacement for inoperable severe aortic stenosis. N Engl J Med 2012; 366: 1696–704.

234. Velazquez EJ, Lee KL, Deja MA, et al. Coronary-artery bypass surgery in patients with left ventricular dysfunction. N Engl J Med 2011; 364: 1607–16.

235. Bonow RO, Maurer G, Lee KL, et al. Myocardial viability and survival in ischemic left ventricular dysfunction. N Engl J Med 2011; 364. 1617–25.

236. Aravot DJ, Banner NR, Khaghani A, et al. Cardiac transplantation in the seventh decade of life. Am J Cardiol 1989; 63: 90–3.

237. James KB, McCarthy PM, Thomas JD, et al. Effect of the implantable left ventricular assist device on neuroendocrine activation in heart failure. Circulation 1995; 92: II191–5.

238. McCarthy PM, James KB, Savage RM, et al. Implantable left ventricular assist device. approaching an alternative for end-stage heart failure. Implantable LVAD Study Group. Circulation 1994; 90: II83–6.

239. Rose EA, Gelijns AC, Moskowitz AJ, et al. Long-term use of a left ventricular assist device for end-stage heart failure. N Engl J Med 2001; 345: 1435–43.

240. Slaughter MS, Rogers JG, Milano CA, et al. Advanced heart failure treated with continuous-flow left ventricular assist device. N Engl J Med 2009; 361: 2241–51.

241. Lewis JF, Maron BJ. Elderly patients with hypertrophic cardiomyopathy: a subset with distinctive left ventricular morphology and progressive clinical course late in life. J Am Coll Cardiol 1989; 13: 36–45.

242. Olson LJ, Gertz MA, Edwards WD, et al. Senile cardiac amyloidosis with myocardial dysfunction. Diagnosis by endomyocardial biopsy and immunohistochemistry. N Engl J Med 1987; 317: 738–42.

243. Ahmed A, Rich MW, Fleg JL, et al. Effects of digoxin on morbidity and mortality in diastolic heart failure: the ancillary digitalis investigation group trial. Circulation 2006; 114: 397–403.

244. Aronow WS, Kronzon I. Effect of enalapril on congestive heart failure treated with diuretics in elderly patients with prior myocardial infarction and normal left ventricular ejection fraction. Am J Cardiol 1993; 71: 602–4.

245. Cleland JG, Tendera M, Adamus J, et al. The Perindopril in Elderly People with Chronic Heart Failure (PEP-CHF) study. Eur Heart J 2006; 27: 2338–45.

246. Mujib M, Patel K, Fonarow GC, et al. Angiotensin-converting enzyme inhibitor use and outcomes in older patients with heart failure and preserved ejection fraction. Am J Med 2013; pii: S0002-9343(13)00033-8. doi: 10.1016/j.amjmed.2013.01.004. [Epub ahead of print].

247. Patel K, Fonarow GC, Kitzman DW, et al. Angiotensin receptor blockers and outcomes in real-world older patients with heart failure and preserved ejection fraction: a propensity-matched inception cohort clinical effectiveness study. Eur J Heart Fail 2012; 14: 1179–88.

248. Solomon SD, Zile M, Pieske B, et al. The angiotensin receptor neprilysin inhibitor LCZ696 in heart failure with preserved ejection fraction: a phase 2 double-blind randomised controlled trial. Lancet 2012; 380: 1387–95.

249. Cheng CP, Igarashi Y, Little WC. Mechanism of augmented rate of left ventricular filling during exercise. Circ Res 1992; 70: 9–19.

250. Hernandez AF, Hammill BG, O'Connor CM, et al. Clinical effectiveness of beta-blockers in heart failure: findings from the OPTIMIZE-HF (Organized Program to Initiate Lifesaving Treatment in Hospitalized Patients with Heart Failure) Registry. J Am Coll Cardiol 2009; 53: 184–92.

251. Brilla CG. Aldosterone and myocardial fibrosis in heart failure. Herz 2000; 25: 299–306.

252. Zannad F, Alla F, Dousset B, Perez A, Pitt B. Limitation of excessive extracellular matrix turnover may contribute to survival benefit of spironolactone therapy in patients with congestive heart failure: insights from the randomized aldactone evaluation study (RALES). Rales Investigators. Circulation 2000; 102: 2700–6.

253. Mottram PM, Haluska B, Leano R, et al. Effect of aldosterone antagonism on myocardial dysfunction in hypertensive patients with diastolic heart failure. Circulation 2004; 110: 558–65.

254. Deswal A, Richardson P, Bozkurt B, Mann DL. Results of the Randomized Aldosterone Antagonism in Heart Failure with Preserved Ejection Fraction trial (RAAM-PEF). J Card Fail 2011; 17: 634–42.

255. Edelmann F, Schmidt AG, Gelbrich G, et al. Rationale and design of the 'aldosterone receptor blockade in diastolic heart failure' trial: a double-blind, randomized, placebo-controlled, parallel group study to determine the effects of spironolactone on exercise capacity and diastolic function in patients with symptomatic diastolic heart failure (Aldo-DHF). Eur J Heart Fail 2010; 12: 874–82.

256. Pieske B. Aldo-DHF: aldosterone receptor blockade in diastolic heart failure. European Society of Cardiology 2012 Congress; Hot Line I: Late Breaking Trials on Prevention to Heart Failure. Munich, Germany, 26 August 2012.

257. Patel K, Fonarow GC, Kitzman DW, et al. Aldosterone antagonists and outcomes in real-world older patients with heart failure and preserved ejection fraction. JACC Heart Fail 2013; 1: 40–47.

258. Desai AS, Lewis EF, Li R, et al. Rationale and design of the treatment of preserved cardiac function heart failure with an aldosterone antagonist trial: a randomized, controlled study of spironolactone in patients with symptomatic heart failure and preserved ejection fraction. Am Heart J 2011; 162: 966–72; e10.

259. Setaro JF, Zaret BL, Schulman DS, Black HR, Soufer R. Usefulness of verapamil for congestive heart failure associated with abnormal left ventricular diastolic filling and normal left ventricular systolic performance. Am J Cardiol 1990; 66: 981–6.

260. Bonow RO, Dilsizian V, Rosing DR, et al. Verapamil-induced improvement in left ventricular diastolic filling and increased exercise tolerance in patients with hypertrophic cardiomyopathy: short- and long-term effects. Circulation 1985; 72: 853–64.

261. Cheng CP, Pettersson K, Little WC. Effects of felodipine on left ventricular systolic and diastolic performance in congestive heart failure. J Pharmacol Exp Ther 1994; 271: 1409–17.

262. Brutsaert DL, Sys SU, Gillebert TC. Diastolic failure: pathophysiology and therapeutic implications. J Am Coll Cardiol 1993; 22: 318–25.

263. Vaitkevicius PV, Lane M, Spurgeon H, et al. A cross-link breaker has sustained effects on arterial and ventricular properties in older rhesus monkeys. Proc Natl Acad Sci USA 2001; 98: 1171–5.

264. Asif M, Egan J, Vasan S, et al. An advanced glycation endproduct cross-link breaker can reverse age-related increases in myocardial stiffness. Proc Natl Acad Sci USA 2000; 97: 2809–13.

265. Little WC, Zile MR, Kitzman DW, et al. The effect of alagebrium chloride (ALT-711), a novel glucose cross-link breaker, in the treatment of elderly patients with diastolic heart failure. J Card Fail 2005; 11: 191–5.
266. Gheorghiade M, Peterson ED. Improving postdischarge outcomes in patients hospitalized for acute heart failure syndromes. JAMA 2011; 305: 2456–7.
267. Felker GM, Lee KL, Bull DA, et al. Diuretic strategies in patients with acute decompensated heart failure. N Engl J Med 2011; 364: 797–805.
268. Binanay C, Califf RM, Hasselblad V, et al. Evaluation study of congestive heart failure and pulmonary artery catheterization effectiveness: the ESCAPE trial. JAMA 2005; 294: 1625–33.
269. Giamouzis G, Butler J, Starling RC, et al. Impact of dopamine infusion on renal function in hospitalized heart failure patients: results of the Dopamine in Acute Decompensated Heart Failure (DAD-HF) Trial. J Card Fail 2010; 16: 922–30.
270. Costanzo MR, Guglin ME, Saltzberg MT, et al. Ultrafiltration versus intravenous diuretics for patients hospitalized for acute decompensated heart failure. J Am Coll Cardiol 2007; 49: 675–83.
271. Bart BA, Goldsmith SR, Lee KL, et al. Ultrafiltration in decompensated heart failure with cardiorenal syndrome. N Engl J Med 2012; 367: 2296–304.
272. Konstam MA, Gheorghiade M, Burnett JC Jr, et al. Effects of oral tolvaptan in patients hospitalized for worsening heart failure: the EVEREST Outcome Trial. JAMA 2007; 297: 1319–31.
273. O'Connor CM, Starling RC, Hernandez AF, et al. Effect of nesiritide in patients with acute decompensated heart failure. N Engl J Med 2011; 365: 32–43.
274. Teerlink JR, Cotter G, Davison BA, et al. Serelaxin, recombinant human relaxin-2, for treatment of acute heart failure (RELAX-AHF): a randomised, placebo-controlled trial. Lancet 2013; 381: 29–39. Online first; doi:10.1016/S0140-6736(12)61855-8.
275. Goodlin SJ. Palliative care in congestive heart failure. J Am Coll Cardiol 2009; 54: 386–96.
276. Gheorghiade M, Patel K, Filippatos GS, et al. Effect of oral digoxin in high-risk heart failure patients: a pre-specified subgroup analysis of the DIG trial. Eur J Heart Fail 2013; [Epub ahead of print] doi: 10.1093/eurjhf/hft010.

21

Supraventricular tachyarrhythmias in the elderly

Wilbert S. Aronow, Maciej Banach, and Ali Ahmed

SUMMARY

Atrial fibrillation (AF) is associated with a higher incidence of mortality, stroke, and coronary events than is sinus rhythm. AF with a rapid ventricular rate may cause a tachycardia-related cardiomyopathy. Indications for direct-current cardioversion, drug treatment of AF, and nondrug therapies are discussed. Studies showing the results of ventricular rate control versus drug treatment to maintain sinus rhythm on clinical outcomes are discussed. Patients with chronic or paroxysmal AF at high risk for stroke should be treated with long-term warfarin to achieve an international normalized ratio (INR) of 2.0 to 3.0 or with dabigatran, rivaroxaban, or apixaban. Patients with AF at low risk for stroke or with contraindications to anticoagulants should be treated with aspirin. Management of atrial flutter, paroxysmal supraventricular tachycardia, accelerated atrioventricular junctional rhythm, paroxysmal atrial tachycardia (PAT) with atrioventricular (AV) block, and multifocal atrial tachycardia is also discussed.

ATRIAL FIBRILLATION

Atrial fibrillation (AF) is a cardiac rhythm, which has irregular undulations of the baseline electrocardiogram (ECG) of varying amplitude, contour, and spacing known as fibrillation waves, with the atrial rate between 350 and 600 beats per minute. The fibrillatory waves are seen best in leads V_1, II, III, and aVF. The fibrillation waves may be large and coarse, or they may be fine with an almost flat ECG baseline. The ventricular rate in AF is irregular unless complete atrioventricular (AV) block or dissociation is present. The contour of the QRS complex in AF is normal unless there is prior bundle branch block, an intraventricular conduction defect, or aberrant ventricular conduction.

If AF is associated with a slow regular ventricular response, there is complete AV block with an AV junctional escape rhythm or idioventricular escape rhythm. Myocardial infarction, degenerative changes in the conduction system, and drug toxicity such as digitalis toxicity are major causes of complete AV block. If AF is associated with a regular ventricular response between 60 and 130 beats per minute, there may be complete AV dissociation with an accelerated AV junctional rhythm caused by an acute inferior myocardial infarction, digitalis toxicity, open heart surgery, or myocarditis, usually rheumatic. Regularization of the ventricular response in AF may also occur in patients with complete AV dissociation due to ventricular tachycardia (VT) or a ventricular paced rhythm.

Prevalence

AF is the most common sustained cardiac arrhythmia. The prevalence of AF increases with age (1–5). In the Framingham Study, the prevalence of chronic AF was 2% in persons aged 60–69 years, 5% in persons aged 70–79 years, and 9% in persons aged 80–89 years (1). In a study of 2101 persons, mean age 81 years, the prevalence of chronic AF was 5% in persons aged 60 to 70 years, 13% in persons aged 71–90 years, and 22% in persons aged 91–103 years (2). Chronic AF was present in 16% of 1160 men, mean age 80 years, and in 13% of 2464 women, mean age 81 years (3). In 5201 persons aged 65 years and older in the Cardiovascular Health Study, the prevalence of AF was 6% in men and 5% in women (4). In 1563 persons, mean age 80 years, living in the community, the prevalence of chronic AF was 9% (5). In the Cardiovascular Health Study, the incidence of AF was 19.2 per 1000 person-years (6).

AF may be paroxysmal or chronic. Episodes of paroxysmal AF may last from a few seconds to several weeks. Sixty-eight percent of persons presenting with AF of <72 hours duration spontaneously converted to sinus rhythm (7).

Predisposing Factors

Multiple, small reentrant circuits arising in the atria, exhibiting variable wave lengths, colliding, being extinguished, and arising again usually cause AF (8). Rapidly firing foci are commonly located in or near the pulmonary veins and may also cause AF (9). Factors responsible for onset of AF include triggers that induce the arrhythmia and the substrate that sustains it. Atrial inflammation or fibrosis acts as a substrate for the development of AF. Triggers of AF include acute atrial stretch, accessory AV pathways, premature atrial beats or atrial tachycardia, sympathetic or parasympathetic stimulation, and ectopic foci occurring in sleeves of atrial tissue within the pulmonary veins or vena caval junctions (10). Predisposing factors for AF include age, alcohol, aortic regurgitation and stenosis, atrial septal defect, autonomic dysfunction, cardiac or thoracic surgery, cardiomyopathies, chronic lung disease, cocaine, congenital heart disease, coronary heart disease, congestive heart failure (CHF), diabetes mellitus, drugs (especially sympathomimetics), emotional stress, excess coffee, hypertension, hyperthyroidism, hypoglycemia, hypokalemia, hypovolemia, hypoxia, left atrial enlargement, left ventricular (LV) dysfunction, LV hypertrophy, male gender, mitral annular calcium (MAC), mitral stenosis and regurgitation, myocardial infarction (MI), myocarditis, neoplastic disease, obesity, pericarditis, pneumonia, pulmonary embolism, rheumatic heart disease, sick sinus syndrome, smoking, systemic infection, and the Wolff–Parkinson–White (WPW) syndrome (11). Obesity has been reported to increase the risk of developing AF by 49% in the general population (12,13).

Preoperative AF was a predictor of postoperative complications, including death, and of a significant reduction in 3-year survival in 30000 patients who had coronary artery bypass surgery (CABS) (14). Because of its anti-inflammatory effects, statin therapy might reduce the risk of postoperative AF (15–17). In patients with dilated cardiomyopathy and coexistent AF, atorvastatin had a weaker effect on the reduction of interleukin-6 and N-terminal pro-brain natriuretic peptide concentration in those with AF than in those without AF (18).

In 254 older persons with AF compared to 1445 older persons with sinus rhythm, mean age 81 years, two-dimensional and Doppler echocardiography showed that the prevalence of AF was increased 17.1 times by rheumatic mitral stenosis, 2.9 times by left atrial enlargement, 2.5 times by abnormal LV ejection fraction, 2.3 times by aortic stenosis, 2.2 times by MAC and by ≥1+ mitral regurgitation, 2.1 times by ≥1+ aortic regurgitation, and 2.0 times by LV hypertrophy (19). The Framingham Study demonstrated that low serum thyrotropin levels were independently associated with a 3.1 times increase in the development of new AF in older patients (20).

Numerous drugs can induce AF (21). A meta-analysis of 11 studies including 56,308 patients showed that angiotensin-converting-enzyme inhibitors and angiotensin receptor blockers significantly reduced the risk of AF by 28%, with a 44% significant reduction in AF in patients with CHF (22). This benefit was limited to patients with reduced LV ejection fraction or LV hypertrophy (22).

Associated Risks

In the Framingham Study, the incidence of death from cardiovascular causes was 2.7 times higher in women and 2.0 times higher in men with chronic AF than in women and men with sinus rhythm (23). The Framingham Study also found that after adjustment for pre-existing cardiovascular conditions, the odds ratio for mortality in persons with AF was 1.9 in women and 1.5 in men (24). At 42-month follow-up of 1359 persons with heart disease, mean age 81 years, patients with chronic AF had a 2.2 times increased risk of having new coronary events than patients with sinus rhythm after controlling for other prognostic variables (25). In the Copenhagen City Heart Study, the effect of AF on the risk of cardiovascular death was significantly increased 4.4 times in women and 2.2 times in men (26).

AF was present in 22% of 106,780 persons aged ≥65 years with acute MI in the Cooperative Cardiovascular Project (27). Compared with sinus rhythm, patients with AF had a higher in-hospital mortality (25% vs. 16%), 30-day mortality (29% vs. 19%), and 1-year mortality (48% vs. 33%) (27). AF was an independent predictor of in-hospital mortality (odds ratio = 1.2), 30-day mortality (odds ratio = 1.2), and 1-year mortality (odds ratio = 1.3) (27). Older patients developing AF during hospitalization had a worse prognosis than older patients presenting with AF (27). In the Global Use of Strategies To Open Occluded Coronary Arteries (GUSTO-III) study, 906 of 13,858 patients (7%) developed AF during hospitalization (20). After adjusting for baseline differences, AF increased the 30-day mortality (odds ratio = 1.6) and the 1-year mortality (odds ratio = 1.6) (28).

In the Platelet Glycoprotein IIb/IIIa in Unstable Angina: Receptors Suppression Using Integrilin Therapy (PURSUIT) trial, AF developed in 6.4% of 9432 patients with acute coronary syndromes without ST-segment elevation (29). After adjustment for other variables, patients with AF had a higher 30-day mortality (hazard ratio = 4.0) and 6-month mortality (hazard ratio = 3.0) than patients without AF (29).

AF is also an independent risk factor for stroke, especially in older persons (1,2). In the Framingham Study, the relative risk of stroke in patients with nonvalvular AF compared with patients with sinus rhythm was increased 2.6 times in patients aged 60–69 years, increased 3.3 times in patients aged 70–79 years, and increased 4.5 times in patients aged 80–89 years (1). Chronic AF was an independent risk factor for thromboembolic (TE) stroke with a relative risk of 3.3 in 2101 persons, mean age 81 years (2). The 3-year incidence of TE stroke was 38% in older persons with chronic AF and 11% in older persons with sinus rhythm (2). The 5-year incidence of TE stroke was 72% in older persons with AF and 24% in older persons with sinus rhythm (2). At 37-month follow-up of 1476 patients who had 24-hour ambulatory ECGs (AECGs), the incidence of TE stroke was 43% for 201 patients with AF (relative risk = 3.3), 17% for 493 patients with paroxysmal supra-ventricular tachycardia, and 18% for 782 patients with sinus rhythm (30).

In the Copenhagen City Heart Study, the effect of AF on the risk of stroke was significantly increased 7.6 times in women and 1.7 times in men (26). AF is also a risk factor for impaired cognitive function (31).

In 2384 persons, mean age 81 years, AF was present in 17% of older persons with LV hypertrophy and in 8% of persons without LV hypertrophy (24). Both AF (risk ratio = 3.2) and LV hypertrophy (risk ratio = 2.8) were independent risk factors for new

TE stroke at 44-month follow-up (32). The higher prevalence of LV hypertrophy in older patients with chronic AF contributes to the increased incidence of TE stroke in older patients with AF.

Both AF (risk ratio = 3.3) and 40–100% extracranial carotid arterial disease (ECAD) (risk ratio = 2.5) were independent risk factors for new TE stroke at 45-month follow-up of 1846 persons, mean age 81 years (33). Older persons with both chronic AF and 40–100% ECAD had a 6.9 times higher probability of developing new TE stroke than older persons with sinus rhythm and no significant ECAD (33).

Cerebral infarctions were demonstrated in 22% of 54 autopsied patients aged ≥70 years with paroxysmal AF (34). Symptomatic cerebral infarction was 2.4 times more common in older patients with paroxysmal AF than in older patients with sinus rhythm (34). AF also causes silent cerebral infarction (35).

AF predisposes to CHF in older patients. As much as 30–40% of LV end-diastolic volume may be attributable to left atrial contraction in older persons. Absence of a coordinated left atrial contraction reduces late diastolic filling of the LV because of loss of the atrial kick. In addition, a fast ventricular rate in AF shortens the LV diastolic filling period, further reducing LV filling and stroke volume.

A retrospective analysis of the Studies of Left Ventricular Dysfunction Prevention and Treatment Trials demonstrated that AF was an independent risk factor for all-cause mortality (relative risk = 1.3), progressive pump failure (relative risk = 1.4), and death or hospitalization for CHF (relative risk = 1.3) (36). AF was present in 37% of 355 patients, mean age 80 years, with prior MI, CHF, and abnormal LV ejection fraction and in 33% of 296 patients, mean age 82 years, with prior MI, CHF, and normal LV ejection fraction (37). In this study, AF was an independent risk factor for mortality with a risk ratio of 1.5 (37). In 2708 patients with chronic advanced systolic heart failure, AF was associated with hospitalization for CHF in patients treated with placebo with a hazard ratio of 1.54 (95% CI, 1.17–2.03) (38).

A fast ventricular rate associated with chronic or paroxysmal AF may cause a tachycardia-related cardiomyopathy, which may be an unrecognized curable cause of CHF (39,40). Slowing the rapid ventricular rate by radiofrequency ablation of the AV node with permanent pacing caused an improvement in LV ejection fraction in patients with medically refractory AF (41). In a substudy of the Ablate and Pace Trial, 63 of 161 patients (39%) with AF referred for AV junction ablation and right ventricular pacing had an abnormal LV ejection fraction (42). Forty-eight of the 63 patients had follow-up echocardiograms. Sixteen of the 48 patients (33%) had a marked improvement in LV ejection fraction to a value >45% after ventricular rate control by AV junction ablation (42). In 6 studies of 768 patients with CHF and AF treated with cardiac resynchronization therapy, AV nodal ablation was performed in 339 patients (43). Compared with medical therapy to control ventricular rate, AV nodal ablation was associated with a significant 58% reduction in all-cause mortality, 56% reduction in cardiovascular mortality, and 48% improvement in New York Heart Association functional class (43).

Clinical Symptoms

Patients with AF may be symptomatic or asymptomatic with their arrhythmia diagnosed by physical examination or by an ECG. Examination of a patient after a stroke may lead to the diagnosis of AF. Symptoms caused by AF may include palpitations, skips in heartbeat, exercise intolerance, fatigue on exertion, cough, chest pain, dizziness, and syncope. A rapid ventricular rate and loss of atrial contraction decrease cardiac output and may lead to angina pectoris, CHF, hypotension, acute pulmonary edema, and syncope, especially in patients with aortic stenosis, mitral stenosis, or hypertrophic cardiomyopathy.

Diagnostic Tests

When AF is suspected, a 12-lead ECG with a one-minute rhythm strip should be obtained to confirm the diagnosis. If paroxysmal AF is suspected, a 24-hour AECG should be obtained. All patients with AF should have an M-mode, two-dimensional, and Doppler echocardiogram to determine the presence and severity of the cardiac abnormalities causing AF and to identify risk factors for stroke. Appropriate tests for noncardiac causes of AF should be obtained when clinically indicated. Thyroid function tests should be obtained as AF or CHF may be the only clinical manifestations of apathetic hyperthyroidism in older patients.

Treatment of Underlying Causes

Management of AF should include therapy of the underlying disease (such as hyperthyroidism, pneumonia, or pulmonary embolism) when possible. Surgical candidates for mitral valve replacement should have mitral valve surgery if it is clinically indicated. If mitral valve surgery is not performed in patients with significant mitral valve disease, elective cardioversion should not be attempted in patients with AF since early frequent relapses are common if AF converts to sinus rhythm. Precipitating factors such as CHF, infection, hypoglycemia, hypokalemia, hypovolemia, and hypoxia should be treated immediately. Alcohol, coffee, and drugs (especially sympathomimetics) that precipitate AF should be avoided. Paroxysmal AF associated with the tachycardia–bradycardia (sick sinus syndrome) should be treated with permanent pacing in combination with drugs to decrease a rapid ventricular rate associated with AF (44).

Control of Very Rapid Ventricular Rate

Direct current (DC) cardioversion should be performed immediately in patients who have paroxysmal AF with a very fast ventricular rate associated with an acute MI, chest pain caused by myocardial ischemia, hypotension, severe CHF, syncope, or pre-excitation syndromes. Intravenous β-blockers (45–48), diltiazem (49), or verapamil (50) may be used to reduce immediately a very rapid ventricular rate associated with AF except in patients with pre-excitation syndromes.

Propranolol should be given intravenously in a dose of 1.0 mg over a five-minute period and then administered intravenously at a rate of 0.5 mg/minute to a maximum dose of 0.1 mg/kg. Esmolol administered intravenously in a dose of 0.5 mg/kg over one minute followed by 0.05 to 0.1 mg/kg per minute may also be used to decrease a very rapid ventricular rate in AF. After the very rapid ventricular rate is reduced, oral propranolol should be started with an initial dose of 10 mg given every six hours. This dose may be increased progressively to a maximum dose of 80 mg every six hours if necessary. Other β-blockers can be used with appropriate doses administered.

The initial dose of diltiazem administered intravenously to slow a very rapid ventricular rate in AF is 0.25 mg/kg given over two minutes. If this dose does not slow the very fast ventricular rate or cause adverse effects, a second dose of 0.35 mg/kg administered intravenously over two minutes should be given 15 minutes after the first dose. After slowing the very fast ventricular rate, oral diltiazem should be started with an initial dose of 60 mg given every six hours. If necessary, this dose may be increased to a maximum dose of 90 mg every six hours.

The initial dose of verapamil given intravenously is 0.075 mg/kg (to a maximum dose of 5 mg). If this dose does not decrease the very rapid ventricular rate or cause adverse effects, a second dose of 0.075 mg/kg (to a maximum dose of 5 mg) should be administered intravenously 10 minutes after the first dose. If the second dose of intravenous verapamil does not decrease the very rapid ventricular rate or cause adverse effects, a dose of

0.15 mg/kg (to a maximum dose of 10 mg) should be administered intravenously 30 minutes after the second dose. After slowing the very rapid ventricular rate, oral verapamil should be started with an initial dose of 80 mg every six to eight hours. This dose may be increased to 120 mg every six hours over the next two to three days.

Control of Rapid Ventricular Rate

Digitalis glycosides are ineffective in converting AF to sinus rhythm (51). Digoxin is also ineffective in decreasing a rapid ventricular rate in AF if there is associated fever, hyperthyroidism, acute blood loss, hypoxia or any condition involving increased sympathetic tone (52). However, digoxin should be used to decrease a rapid ventricular rate in AF unassociated with increased sympathetic tone, hypertrophic cardiomyopathy, or the WPW syndrome, especially if there is LV systolic dysfunction.

The usual initial dose of digoxin administered to undigitalized patients with AF is 0.5 mg orally. Depending on the clinical response, a second oral dose of 0.25 mg may be given in six to eight hours, and a third oral dose of 0.25 mg may be given in another six to eight hours to slow a rapid ventricular rate. The usual maintenance oral dose of digoxin given to patients with AF is 0.25–0.5 mg daily, with the dose reduced to 0.125–0.25 mg daily for older patients who are more susceptible to digitalis toxicity (53).

Oral β-blockers (54), diltiazem (55), or verapamil (56) should be added to the therapeutic regimen if a rapid ventricular rate in AF occurs at rest or during exercise despite digoxin. These drugs act synergistically with digoxin to depress conduction through the AV junction. In a study of atenolol 50 mg daily, digoxin 0.25 mg daily, diltiazem-CD 240 mg daily, digoxin 0.25 mg plus atenolol 50 mg daily, and digoxin 0.25 mg plus diltiazem-CD 240 mg daily, digoxin and diltiazem as single drugs were least effective and digoxin plus atenolol was most effective in controlling the ventricular rate in AF during daily activities (57).

Amiodarone is the most effective drug for reducing a rapid ventricular rate in AF (58,59). The noncompetitive β-receptor inhibition and calcium channel blockade are powerful AV nodal conduction depressants. However, the adverse side effect profile of amiodarone limits its use in the treatment of AF. Oral doses of 200 mg to 400 mg of amiodarone daily may be given to selected patients with symptomatic life-threatening AF refractory to other drugs. Vernakalant was more efficacious than amiodarone in converting recent-onset AF to sinus rhythm (60).

Dronedarone was found to be effective in treating patients with intermittent AF (61). However, dronedarone was found in 3236 patients with permanent AF at risk for major vascular events to significantly increase rates of CHF (81%), stroke (232%), and cardiovascular death (211%) and should not be used in patients with permanent AF (62).

Therapeutic concentrations of digoxin do not decrease the frequency of episodes of paroxysmal AF or the duration of episodes of paroxysmal AF diagnosed by 24-hour AECGs (63,64). Digoxin has been shown to increase the duration of episodes of paroxysmal AF, a result consistent with its action in reducing the atrial refractory period (63). Therapeutic concentrations of digoxin also do not prevent a fast ventricular rate from developing in patients with paroxysmal AF (63–65). After a brief episode of AF, digoxin increases the shortening that occurs in atrial refactoriness and predisposes to the reinduction of AF (66). Therefore, digoxin should be avoided in patients with sinus rhythm with a history of paroxysmal AF.

Nondrug Therapies

Radiofrequency catheter modification of AV conduction should be performed in patients with symptomatic AF in whom a rapid ventricular rate cannot be decreased by drugs (67,68). If this procedure does not control the fast ventricular rate associated with AF, complete AV block produced by radiofrequency catheter ablation followed by permanent pacemaker implantation should be performed (69). In a randomized controlled study of 66 persons with CHF and chronic AF, AV junction ablation with implantation of a VVIR pacemaker was superior to drug treatment in controlling symptoms (70). Long-term survival is similar for patients with AF whether they receive radiofrequency ablation of the AV node and implantation of a permanent pacemaker or drug therapy (71). In 44 patients, mean age 78 ± 5 years, radiofrequency catheter ablation followed by pacemaker implantation was successful in ablating the AV junction in 43 of 44 patients (98%) with AF and a rapid ventricular rate not controlled by drug therapy (72).

Surgical techniques have been developed for use in patients with AF in whom the ventricular rate cannot be decreased by drug treatment (73,74). The maze procedure is a surgical dissection of the right and left atrium creating a maze through which the electrical activation is compartamentalized, preventing the formation and perpetuation of the multiple wavelets needed for maintenance of AF. This procedure is typically performed in association with mitral valve surgery or CABS. At 2–3-year follow-up, 74% of 39 patients and 90% of 100 patients undergoing the maze procedure remained in sinus rhythm (75,76). Thirty-five of 43 patients (85%) with drug-refractory, lone paroxysmal AF were arrhythmia free after maze surgery (77). At 29-month follow-up, 18 of 28 patients (64%), mean age 71 years, who had an intraoperative radiofrequency maze procedure for treating AF at the time of valve surgery or CABS were in sinus rhythm (78).

Another intraoperative approach for treating AF in patients undergoing mitral valve surgery is cryoablation limited to the posterior left atrium. Sinus rhythm was restored in 20 of 29 patients (69%) with chronic AF undergoing this procedure (79).

Ablation of pulmonary vein foci that cause AF is a developing area in the treatment of AF. However, recurrent AF develops in 40–60% of patients despite initial efficacy with this procedure (80). Another problem with this approach is a 3% incidence of pulmonary vein stenosis occurring after this procedure (80).

The Randomized studies demonstrated that circumferential pulmonary vein radiofrequency ablation was significantly more effective than antiarrhythmic drug therapy in preventing recurrence of AF (93% vs. 35%) in 198 patients at 1 year (81) and (87% vs. 37%) in 67 patients at 1 year (82). There are no long-term follow-up data showing a reduction in stroke risk in patients apparently cured of AF with radiofrequency catheter ablation. Anticoagulant therapy still needs to be administered to these patients who are at increased risk of developing TE stroke.

In 100 patients, mean age 57 years, with AF (63% with paroxysmal AF), arrhythmia-free survival rates after a single catheter ablation were 40%, 37%, and 29% at 1, 2, and 5 years, respectively (83). Postprocedural cerebral magnetic resonance imaging showed new embolic lesions in 33 of 232 patients (14%), mean age 58 years, with paroxysmal or persistent AF who had radiofrequency left atrial catheter ablation (84).

Modification of the substrate responsible for AF can be accomplished in the right and/or left atrium with linear lesions. This catheter maze-ablation approach is effective in a small percentage of patients (85).

The Atrioverter, an implantable defibrillator connected to right atrial and right coronary sinus defibrillation leads, causes restoration of sinus rhythm by low-energy shock and has an 80% efficacy in terminating AF (86). Further efforts are needed to improve patient tolerability and to prevent earlier recurrence of AF after successful transvenous atrial defibrillation. The implanted atrial defibrillator is currently available only in combination with a ventricular defibrillator. The Atrioverter may also convert atrial tachycardia to sinus rhythm using an atrial pacing overdrive algorhythm before such tachycardias induce AF.

Pacing

Paroxysmal AF associated with the tachycardia–bradycardia (sick sinus) syndrome should be treated with a permanent pacemaker combined with drugs to slow a rapid ventricular rate associated with AF (44). Ventricular pacing is an independent risk factor for the development of chronic AF in patients with paroxysmal AF associated with the tachycardia–bradycardia syndrome (87). Patients with paroxysmal AF associated with the tachycardia–bradycardia syndrome and no signs of AV conduction abnormalities should be treated with atrial pacing or dual-chamber pacing rather than with ventricular pacing because atrial pacing is associated with less AF, fewer TE complications, and a lower risk of AV block than is ventricular pacing (88).

Many older patients are able to tolerate AF without the need for therapy because the ventricular rate is slow due to concomitant AV nodal disease. These patients should not be treated with drugs that depress AV conduction. A permanent pacemaker should be implanted in patients with AF who develop cerebral symptoms such as dizziness or syncope associated with ventricular pauses longer than three seconds which are not drug-induced, as documented by a 24-hour AECG (89). If patients with AF have drug-induced symptomatic bradycardia, and the causative drug cannot be discontinued, a permanent pacemaker must be implanted.

Atrial pacing is effective in treating vagotonic AF (90) and may be considered if treatment with a vagolytic antiarrhythmic drug such as disopyramide is ineffective. Atrial pacing is also effective in treating patients with the sick sinus syndrome (88). However, when bradycardia is not an indication for pacing, atrial-based pacing may not prevent episodes of AF (91). Dual-site atrial pacing is more efficacious than single-site pacing for preventing AF (92). However, the patients in this study had a bradycardia indication for pacing and continued to need antiarrhythmic drugs (92).

Dual-site atrial pacing with continued sinus overdrive for AF in patients with bradycardia prolonged time to AF recurrence and reduced AF burden in patients with paroxysmal AF (93). However, there was no difference in AF checklist symptom scores or overall quality-of-life scores (93). The absence of an effect on symptom control suggests that pacing should be used as adjunctive therapy with other treatment modalities for AF (93).

Biatrial pacing after CABS has also been demonstrated to reduce the incidence of AF (94). All ECGs in patients with paced rhythm should be examined closely for underlying AF to prevent under-recognition of AF and under-treatment with anticoagulants (95). Permanent pacing to prevent AF is not indicated (96).

Percutaneous Left Atrial Appendage Transcatheter Occlusion

In 2 prospective multicenter trials, percutaneous left atrial appendage occlusion using the PLAATO system was attempted in 111 patients, mean age 71 years, with a contraindication to anticoagulant therapy and at least one additional risk factor for stroke (97). Implantation was successful in 108 of 111 patients (97%). At 9.8-month follow-up, two patients (2%) developed stroke (97). At 1065 patient years of follow-up of 707 patients with AF randomized to percutaneous closure of the left atrial appendage with the WATCHMAN left atrial appendage system (463 patients) or to warfarin therapy to maintain an international normalized ratio (INR) between 2.0 and 3.0 (244 patients), the primary endpoint of stroke, cardiovascular death, and systemic embolism was similar in both groups (98). However, primary safety event were 69% significantly higher in the intervention group than in the warfarin control group (98).

Wolff–Parkinson–White Syndrome

DC cardioversion should be performed if a rapid ventricular rate in patients with paroxysmal AF associated with the WPW syndrome is life-threatening or fails to respond to drug therapy. Drug treatment for paroxysmal AF associated with the WPW syndrome includes propranolol plus procainamide, disopyramide, or quinidine (99). Digoxin, diltiazem, and verapamil are contraindicated in patients with AF with the WPW syndrome because these drugs shorten the refractory period of the accessory AV pathway, resulting in more rapid conduction down the accessory pathway. This results in a marked increase in ventricular rate. Radiofrequency catheter ablation or surgical ablation of the accessory conduction pathway should be considered in patients with AF and rapid AV conduction over the accessory pathway (100). In 500 patients with an accessory pathway, radiofrequency catheter ablation of the accessory pathway was successful in 93% of patients (101).

Elective Cardioversion

Elective DC cardioversion has a higher success rate than does medical cardioversion in converting AF to sinus rhythm (102). Table 21.1 shows favorable and unfavorable conditions for elective cardioversion of chronic AF.

The American College of Cardiology (ACC)/American Heart Association (AHA)/European Society for Cardiology (ESC) guidelines state that Class I indications for cardioversion of AF to sinus rhythm include (*i*) immediate DC cardioversion in patients with paroxysmal AF and a rapid ventricular rate who have ECG evidence of acute MI or symptomatic hypotension, angina, or CHF that does not respond promptly to pharmacological measures and (*ii*) DC or drug cardioversion in patients with chronic AF without hemodynamic instability when symptoms of AF are unacceptable (103).

Elective cardioversion of AF either by DC or by antiarrhythmic drugs should not be performed in asymptomatic elderly patients with chronic AF. Rectilinear, biphasic shocks have been found to have greater efficacy and need less energy than the traditional damped sine wave monophasic shocks (104). Therefore, biphasic shocks to cardiovert AF should become the clinical standard.

Antiarrhythmic drugs that have been used to convert AF to sinus rhythm include amiodarone, disopyramide, dofetilide, encainide, flecainide, ibutilide, procainamide,

Table 21.1 Conditions Favorable and Unfavorable for Cardioversion of Atrial Fibrillation

Favorable Conditions	<1 yr duration of AF
	No or minimal cardiomegaly
	Echocardiographic left atrial dimension <45 mm
	After treatment of a precipitating cause such as acute MI, cardiac or thoracic surgery, hyperthyroidism, pneumonia, or pericarditis
	After corrective valvular surgery
	Symptomatic AF with hemodynamic improvement and decrease in symptoms expected from sinus rhythm, especially in patients with valvular aortic stenosis or hypertrophic obstructive cardiomyopathy
Unfavorable Conditions	Duration of atrial fibrillation >1 yr
	Moderate to severe cardiomegaly
	Echocardiographic left atrial dimension >45 mm
	Digitalis toxicity (contraindicated)
	Slow ventricular rate (contraindicated)
	Sick sinus syndrome (contraindicated)
	Chronic obstructive lung disease
	Mitral valve disease
	Heart failure
	Recurrent AF despite antiarrhythmic drugs
	Inability to tolerate antiarrhythmic drugs

Abbreviation: AF, atrial fibrillation.

propafenone, quinidine, and sotalol. None of these drugs is as successful as DC cardioversion, which has a success rate of 80–90% in converting AF to sinus rhythm. All of these drugs are proarrhythmic and may aggravate or cause cardiac arrhythmias.

Encainide and flecainide caused atrial proarrhythmic effects in 6 of 60 patients (10%) (105). The atrial proarrhythmic effects included conversion of AF to atrial flutter with a 1-to-1 AV conduction response and a very fast ventricular rate (105). Flecainide has caused VT and ventricular fibrillation (VF) in patients with chronic AF (106). Antiarrhythmic drugs including amiodarone, disopyramide, flecainide, procainamide, propafenone, quinidine, and sotalol caused cardiac adverse effects in 73 of 417 patients (18%) hospitalized for AF (107). Class IC drugs such as encainide, flecainide, and propafenone should not be used in patients with prior MI or abnormal LV ejection fraction because these drugs may cause life-threatening ventricular tachyarrhythmias in these patients (108).

Dofetilide and ibutilide are Class III antiarrhythmic drugs that have been used for the conversion of AF to sinus rhythm. Eleven of 75 patients (15%) with AF treated with intravenous dofetilide converted to sinus rhythm (109). Torsade de pointes occurred in 3% of patients treated with intravenous dofetilide (109). After 1 - month, 22 of 190 patients (12%) with AF and CHF had sinus rhythm restored with dofetilide compared to 3 of 201 patients (1%) treated with placebo (110). Torsade de pointes developed in 25 of 762 patients (3%) treated with dofetilide and in none of 756 patients (0%) treated with placebo (110). Twenty-three of seventy-nine patients (29%) with AF treated with intravenous ibutilide converted to sinus rhythm (111). Polymorphic VT developed in 4% of patients who received intravenous ibutilide in this study (111). Baseline bradycardia with AF may predispose to ibutilide-induced polymorphic VT.

DC cardioversion of AF has a higher success rate in converting AF to sinus rhythm and a lower incidence of cardiac adverse effects than treatment with any antiarrhythmic drug. However, pretreatment with ibutilide has been found to facilitate transthoracic cardioversion of AF (112).

Unless transesophageal echocardiography has demonstrated no thrombus in the left atrial appendage before cardioversion (113), oral warfarin should be administered for three weeks before elective DC or drug conversion of patients with AF to sinus rhythm (114). Anticoagulant therapy should also be given at the time of cardioversion and continued until sinus rhythm has been maintained for four weeks (114). After DC or drug cardioversion of AF to sinus rhythm, the left atrium becomes stunned and contracts poorly for three to four weeks, predisposing to TE stroke unless the patient is maintained on oral warfarin (115,116). The maintenance dose of oral warfarin should be titrated by serial prothrombin times so that the INR is 2.0–3.0 (116).

In a multicenter, randomized, prospective study, 1222 patients with AF of >2 days duration were randomized to either treatment guided by the findings on transesophageal echocardiography or to management with conventional therapy (117). The primary endpoint was cerebrovascular accident, transient ischemic attack, and peripheral embolism within 8 weeks. The incidence of embolic events at eight weeks was 0.8% in the transesophageal echocardiography treatment group and 0.5% in the conventional treatment group (117). At 8 weeks, there were also no significant differences between the two groups in the rates of death, maintenance of sinus rhythm, or functional status (117). However, there was a trend toward a higher rate of death from any cause in the transesophageal echocardiography treatment group (2.4%) than in the conventional treatment group (1.0%) ($p = 0.06$) (117).

This study showed the importance of maintaining therapeutic anticoagulation in the period after cardioversion even if there is no transesophageal echocardiographic evidence of thrombus (116,118). The best management strategy for patients with evidence of an atrial thrombus on initial transesophageal echocardiography remains controversial (119). In the absence of data from a randomized trial, patients probably should have follow-up transesophageal echocardiography after 1 month of warfarin therapy to document resolution of the atrial thrombus (119,120).

Use of Antiarrhythmic Drugs to Maintain Sinus Rhythm

The efficacy and safety of antiarrhythmic drugs after cardioversion of AF to maintain sinus rhythm has been questioned. A meta-analysis of six double-blind, placebo-controlled studies of quinidine involving 808 patients who had direct-current cardioversion of chronic AF to sinus rhythm demonstrated that 50% of patients treated with quinidine and 25% of patients treated with placebo remained in sinus rhythm at 1-year follow-up (121). However, the mortality was significantly higher in patients treated with quinidine (2.9%) than in patients treated with placebo (0.8%) (121). In a study of 406 patients, mean age 82 years, with heart disease and complex ventricular arrhythmias, the incidence of adverse effects causing drug cessation was 48% for quinidine and 55% for procainamide (122). The incidence of total mortality at 2-year follow-up was insignificantly higher in patients treated with quinidine or procainamide compared with patients not receiving an antiarrhythmic drug (122).

In another study, 85 patients were randomized to quinidine and 98 patients to sotalol after DC cardioversion of AF to sinus rhythm (123). At 6-month follow-up, 48% of quinidine-treated patients and 52% of sotalol-treated patients remained in sinus rhythm (123). At 1-year follow-up of 100 patients with AF cardioverted to sinus rhythm, 37% of 50 patients randomized to sotalol and 30% of 50 patients randomized to propafenone remained in sinus rhythm (124).

In a study of 403 patients with at least one episode of AF in the prior six months, 201 patients were treated with amiodarone and 202 patients were treated with sotalol or propafenone (125). At 16-month follow-up, AF recurred in 35% of patients treated with amiodarone and in 63% of patients treated with sotalol or propafenone (125). Adverse effects causing discontinuation of drug occurred in 18% of patients treated with amiodarone and in 11% of patients treated with sotalol or propafenone (125).

After cardioversion of 394 patients with AF to sinus rhythm, 197 patients were randomized to metoprolol CR/XL and 197 patients to placebo (126). At 6-month follow-up, the percent of patients in sinus rhythm was significantly higher on metoprolol CR/XL (51%) than on placebo (40%) (126). The heart rate in patients who relapsed into AF was also significantly lower in pts treated with metoprolol CR/XL than in patients treated with placebo (126).

In a study of 384 patients with a history of AF or atrial flutter, azimilide lengthened the median time to first symptomatic arrhythmia recurrence from 17 days in the placebo group to 60 days in the azimilide group (127). However, additional data on both efficacy and safety of azimilide are necessary before knowing its role in clinical practice.

Of the 1330 patients in the Stroke Prevention in Atrial Fibrillation (SPAF) Study, 127 persons were taking quinidine, 57 procainamide, 34 flecainide, 20 encainide, 15 disopyramide, and 7 amiodarone (128). Patients who were taking an antiarrhythmic drug had a 2.7 times higher adjusted relative risk of cardiac mortality and a 2.3 times higher adjusted relative risk of arrhythmic death compared with patients not taking an antiarrhythmic drug (128). Patients with a history of CHF who were taking an antiarrhythmic drug had a 4.7 times increased risk of cardiac death and a 3.7 times increased risk of arrhythmic death than patients with a history of CHF not taking an antiarrhythmic drug (128).

A meta-analysis of 59 randomized, controlled trials comprising 23,229 patients that investigated the use of aprindine, disopyramide, encainide, flecainide, imipramine, lidocaine, mexiletine, moricizine, phenytoin, procainamide, quinidine, and tocainide after MI also demonstrated that mortality was significantly higher in patients receiving Class I antiarhythmic drugs (odds ratio = 1.14) than in patients not receiving an antiarrhythmic drug (129). None of the 59 studies showed a decrease in mortality by antiarrhythmic drugs (129).

Amiodarone is the antiarrhythmic drug with the highest success rate in maintenance of sinus rhythm after cardioversion of AF (125). However, in the Cardiac Arrest in Seattle: Conventional Versus Amiodarone Drug Evaluation Study, the incidence of pulmonary toxicity was 10% at 2 years in patients receiving amiodarone in a mean dose of 158 mg daily (130). The incidence of adverse effects from amiodarone also approaches 90% after 5 years of therapy (131).

Ventricular Rate Control

Because maintenance of sinus rhythm with antiarrhythmic drugs may require serial cardioversions, exposes patients to the risks of proarrhythmia, sudden cardiac death, and other adverse effects, and requires the use of anticoagulants in patients in sinus rhythm who have a high risk of recurrence of AF, many cardiologists prefer the management strategy of ventricular rate control plus use of anticoagulants in patients with AF, especially in elderly patients with AF. β-blockers such as propranolol 10–30 mg given three to four times daily can be administered to control ventricular arrhythmias (132) and after conversion of AF to sinus rhythm. Should AF recur, β-blockers have the added advantage of slowing the ventricular rate. β-blockers are also the most effective drugs in preventing and treating AF after CABS (133).

The Pharmacological Intervention in Atrial Fibrillation trial was a randomized trial of 252 patients with AF of between 7 days and 360 days duration which compared ventricular rate control (125 patients) with rhythm control (127 patients) (134). Diltiazem was used as first-line therapy in patients randomized to ventricular rate control. Amiodarone was used as first-line therapy in patients randomized to rhythm control. Amiodarone administration resulted in conversion of 23% of patients to sinus rhythm (134). Symptomatic improvement was reported in a similar percentage of patients in both groups. Assessment of quality of life showed no significant difference between the two treatment groups. The incidence of hospital admission was significantly higher in patients treated with rhythm control (69%) than in patients treated with ventricular rate control (24%) (134). Adverse drug effects caused a change in drug therapy in significantly more patients treated with rhythm control (25%) than in patients treated with ventricular rate control (14%) (134).

The Atrial Fibrillation Follow-Up Investigation of Rhythm Management (AFFIRM) Study randomized 4060 patients, mean age 70 years (39% women), with paroxysmal or chronic AF of less than 6 months duration at high risk for stroke to either maintenance of AF with ventricular rate control or to an attempt to maintain sinus rhythm with antiarrhythmic drugs after cardioversion (135). Patients in both arms of this study were treated with warfarin. All-cause mortality at 5 years was insignificantly increased 15% in the maintenance of sinus rhythm group compared to the ventricular rate control group (24% vs. 21 %, $p = 0.08$) (135). TE stroke was insignificantly reduced in the ventricular rate control group (5.5% vs. 7.1%), and all-cause hospitalization was significantly reduced in the ventricular rate control group (73% vs. 80%, $p < 0.001$) (135). In both groups, the majority of strokes occurred after warfarin was stopped or when the INR was subtherapeutic. There was no significant difference in quality of life or functional status between the two treatment groups (135).

In the AFFIRM Study, the propensity-adjusted hazard ratio for all-cause mortality in patients, mean age 70 years, associated with a recent history of smoking was 1.39,

p = 0.003 (136). In the AFFIRM Study, 2248 patients were aged 70–80 years, 1901 of whom were receiving warfarin (137). All-cause mortality at 3.4-years of follow-up occurred in 18% and 33% of matched patients receiving and not receiving warfarin (hazard ratio = 0.58, p < 0.001) (137).

The Rate Control Versus Electrical Cardioversion for Persistent Atrial Fibrillation Study Group randomized 522 patients with persistent AF after a previous electrical cardioversion to receive treatment aimed at ventricular rate control or rhythm control (138). Both groups were treated with oral anticoagulants. At 2.3-year follow-up, the composite end point of death from cardiovascular causes, heart failure, TE complications, bleeding, implantation of a pacemaker, and severe adverse effects of drugs was 17.2% in the ventricular rate control group versus 22.6% in the rhythm control group (138). In this study, women randomized to rhythm control had a 3.1 times significant increase in cardiovascular morbidity or mortality than women randomized to ventricular rate control (p = 0.002) (139).

The 2-year mortality was similar in 1009 patients with AF and CHF treated with rate control or rhythm control (140).The 37-month mortality was also similar in 1376 patients with AF and CHF treated with rhythm control or rate control (141).

During 19-month follow-up of 110 patients with a history of AF treated with antiarrhythmic drug therapy, recurrent AF was diagnosed by ECG recordings in 46% of the patients and by an implantable monitoring device in 88% of the patients (142). AF lasting longer than 48 hours was detected by the monitoring device in 50 of the 110 patients (46%) (142). Nineteen of these 50 patients (38%) were completely asymptomatic (142).

Risk Factors for Thromboembolic Stroke

Table 21.2 lists risk factors for TE stroke in patients with AF (1,2,32,33,143–154). In the SPAF Study involving patients, mean age 67 years, recent CHF (within three months), a history of hypertension, previous thromboembolism, echocardiographic left atrial enlargement, and echocardiographic LV systolic dysfunction were associated independently with the development of new TE events (148,151). The incidence of new TE events was 18.6% per year if three or more risk factors were present, 6.0% per year if one or two risk factors were present, and 1.0% per year if none of these risk factors was present (148).

In the SPAF Study III involving patients, mean age 72 years, patients were considered at high risk for developing TE stroke if they had either CHF or abnormal LV systolic

Table 21.2   Risk Factors for Stroke in Patients with Atrial Fibrillation

Age (1,32,143–146)
Echocardiographic left ventricular dysfunction (146–149)
History of heart failure (145,149,151)
Hypertension (144,147,149,151)
Prior thromboembolic events (2,32,144–146,148–152)
Women older than 75 yr of age (149)
Rheumatic mitral stenosis (146,147)
Mitral annular calcium (144,153)
Diabetes mellitus (145)
History of myocardial infarction (144,145,147,152)
Echocardiographic left atrial enlargement (147,148)
Echocardiographic left ventricular hypertrophy (32,33,146,147)
Extracranial carotid arterial disease (33)
Hypercholesterolemia (146)
Low serum high-density lipoprotein cholesterol (146)

function, prior thromboembolism, a systolic blood pressure of >160 mm Hg, or the patient was a woman older than age 75 years (149). In a study of 312 patients with chronic AF, mean age 84 years, independent risk factors for the development of new TE stroke were prior stroke (risk ratio = 1.6), rheumatic mitral stenosis (risk ratio = 2.0), LVH (risk ratio = 2.8), abnormal LVEF (risk ratio = 1.8), serum total cholesterol (risk ratio = 1.01 per 1 mg/dL increase), serum high-density lipoprotein cholesterol (risk ratio = 1.04 per 1 mg/dL decrease), and age (risk ratio = 1.03 per 1-year increase) (146).

In the $CHADS_2$ score, 1 point is given for CHF, 1 point for hypertension, 1 point for age older than 75 years, 1 point for diabetes, and 2 points for prior stroke or transient ischemic attack (155). The 1-year adjusted risk for stroke in 1733 Medicare beneficiaries with AF and CHF and no contraindications to warfarin was 1.9% for a $CHADS_2$ score of 0, 2.8% for a score of 1, 4.0% for a score of 2, 5.9% for a score of 3, 8.5% for a score of 4, 12.5% for a score of 5, and 18.2% for a score of 6 (155). At 31-month follow-up of 521 patients with AF, a $CHADS_2$ score of 5 or 6 had a 52 times significantly increased risk for stroke than a score of 0 (156). A CHA_2DS_2-VASc score may also be used for clinical risk stratification for predicting TE events in patients with AF (157). In 441 patients with AF and no contraindications to warfarin, warfarin was used in 8 of 30 patients (27%) with a $CHADS_2$ score of 0, in 82 of 132 patients (62%) with a $CHADS_2$ score of 1, in 121 of 175 patients (70%) with a $CHADS_2$ score of 2, in 72 of 77 patients (94%) with a $CHADS_2$ score of 3, and in 27 of 27 patients (100%) with a $CHADS_2$ of 4 to 6 (158).

Antithrombotic Therapy

Prospective, randomized trials (144,145,149,152,159–165) and prospective, nonrandomized observational data from patients, mean age 83 years (150), and mean age 84 years (166), have documented that warfarin is effective in decreasing the incidence of TE stroke in patients with nonvalvular AF. Analysis of pooled data from five randomized, placebo-controlled studies showed that warfarin significantly decreased the incidence of new TE stroke by 68% and was significantly more effective than aspirin in decreasing the incidence of new TE stroke (145). In the Veterans Affairs Cooperative study, the incidence of new TE events was 4.3% per year in patients on placebo versus 0.9% per year in patients on warfarin in patients with no prior stroke, 9.3% per year in patients on placebo versus 6.1% per year in patients on warfarin in patients with prior stroke, and 4.8% per year in patients on placebo versus 0.9% per year in patients on warfarin in patients older than age 70 year (149). In the European Atrial Fibrillation Trial involving patients with recent transient cerebral ischemic attack or minor ischemic stroke, at 2.3-year follow-up, the incidence of new TE events was 12% per year in patients taking placebo, 10% per year in patients taking aspirin, and 4.0 per year in patients taking warfarin (152).

Nonrandomized observational data from older patients with chronic AF, mean age 83 years, found that 141 patients treated with oral warfarin to achieve an INR between 2.0 and 3.0 (mean INR was 2.4) had a 67% significant decrease in new TE stroke compared with 209 patients treated with oral aspirin (150). Compared with aspirin, warfarin caused a 40% significant decrease in new TE stroke in patients with prior stroke, a 31% significant decrease in new TE stroke in patients with no prior stroke, a 45% significant reduction in new TE stroke in patients with abnormal LVEF, and a 36% significant reduction in new TE stroke in patients with normal LVEF (150).

At 1.1-year follow-up in the SPAF Study III, patients with AF considered to be at high risk for developing new TE stroke who were randomized to treatment with oral warfarin to achieve an INR between 2.0 and 3.0 had a 72% significant decrease in ischemic stroke or systemic embolism compared with patients randomized to treatment with oral aspirin 325 mg daily plus oral warfarin to achieve an INR between 1.2 and 1.5 (149).

Adjusted-dose warfarin caused an absolute decrease in ischemic stroke or systemic embolism of 6.0% per year (149). In the Second Copenhagen Atrial Fibrillation, Aspirin, Anticoagulation (AFASK) Study, low-dose warfarin plus aspirin was also less effective in reducing stroke or systemic TE events in patients with AF (7.2% after 1 year) than was adjusted-dose warfarin to achieve an INR between 2.0 and 3.0 (2.8% after 1 year) (165).

Analysis of pooled data from five randomized controlled studies demonstrated that the annual incidence of major hemorrhage was 1.0% for the control group, 1.0% for the aspirin group, and 1.3% for the warfarin group (145). The incidence of major hemorrhage in patients, mean age 72 years, taking adjusted-dose warfarin to achieve an INR of 2.0 to 3.0 in the SPAF III Study was 2.1% (149). In the Second Copenhagen AFASK Study, the incidence of major hemorrhage in patients, mean age 73 years, was 0.8% per year for patients treated with adjusted-dose warfarin to achieve an INR between 2.0 and 3.0 and 1.0% per year for patients treated with aspirin 300 mg daily (165). The incidence of major hemorrhage in older patients with chronic AF, mean age 83 years, was 4.3% (1.4% per year) in patients treated with warfarin to maintain an INR between 2.0 and 3.0 and 2.9% (1.0% per year) in patients treated with aspirin 325 mg daily (150).

In the SPAF III Study, 892 patients, mean age 67 years, at low risk for developing TE stroke were treated with oral aspirin 325 mg daily (167). The incidence of ischemic stroke or systemic embolism was 2.2% per year (167). The incidence of ischemic stroke or systemic embolism was 3.6% per year in patients with a history of hypertension and 1.1% per year in patients with no history of hypertension (167).

In a study of 13,559 patients with nonvalvular AF hospitalized with an outpatient stroke, compared to an INR of 2.0 or greater, an INR of <2.0 at hospital admission significantly increased the odds of a severe stroke by 1.9 times and the risk of death within 30 days by 3.4 times (168). The 30-day mortality was similar among patients who were taking aspirin or warfarin with an INR of <2.0 (168). Elderly patients taking warfarin should have an INR maintained between 2.0 and 3.0, not one <2.0 or >3.5 (169).

At 2.7-year follow-up of 973 patients, mean age 82 years, with AF randomized to warfarin to maintain an INR between 2.0 and 3.0 or aspirin 75 mg daily, warfarin significantly reduced fatal or disabling stroke, intracranial hemorrhage, or arterial embolism 52% ($p = 0.003$) (170). The yearly risk of extracranial hemorrhage was similar in both treatment groups (170).

Patients with AF and a left atrial thrombus diagnosed by transesophageal echocardiography should be treated with warfarin to maintain an INR level between 2.5 and 3.5 because they are at a high risk for new TE events (171). Of 399 patients with chronic kidney disease and AF (23% on hemodialysis and 33% with an estimated glomerular filtration rate <15 ml/min/1.73 m^2), 232 (58%) were treated with warfarin to maintain an INR between 2.0 and 3.0 (172). At 31-month follow-up of warfarin-treated patients and 23-month follow-up of patients not treated with warfarin, warfarin significantly reduced TE stroke by 72% (9% vs. 26%, $p < 0.001$) without significantly increasing major bleeding (14% vs. 9%) (172).

On the basis of the available data, patients with chronic or paroxysmal AF at high risk for developing TE stroke or with a history of hypertension and who have no contraindications to anticoagulation therapy should be treated with long-term oral warfarin to achieve an INR between 2.0 and 3.0 (114,173). Hypertension must be controlled. Whenever the patient has a prothrombin time taken, the blood pressure should also be checked. The physician prescribing warfarin should be aware of the numerous drugs which potentiate the effect of warfarin causing an increased prothrombin time and risk of bleeding (174). Patients with AF at low risk for developing TE stroke or with contraindications to treatment with long-term oral warfarin should be treated with aspirin 325 mg orally daily (175).

Table 21.3   2011 American College of Cardiology/American Heart Association/Heart Rhythm Society Class I Indications for Treating Patients with Atrial Fibrillation with Antithrombotic Therapy

1. Aspirin 81–325 mg daily or no therapy if aged <60 yr with no heart disease
2. Aspirin 81–325 mg daily if aged <60 yr, heart disease, but no risk factors[a]
3. Aspirin 81–325 mg daily if aged 60–74 yr with no risk factors[a]
4. Warfarin to maintain INR between 2.0–3.0 if aged 65–74 yr with diabetes or coronary artery disease
5. Warfarin to maintain INR between 2.0–3.0 if woman and 75 yr or older
6. Warfarin to maintain INR between 2.0–3.0 or aspirin 81–325 mg daily if man and 75 yr or older with no other risk factors
7. Warfarin to maintain INR between 2.0–3.0 if 65 yr or older with heart failure
8. Warfarin to maintain INR between 2.0–3.0 if left ventricular ejection fraction <35%, or fractional shortening <25%, or hypertension
9. Warfarin to maintain INR between 2.0–3.0 if rheumatic heart disease (mitral stenosis)
10. Warfarin to maintain INR between 2.0–3.0 or higher if prosthetic heart valves
11. Warfarin to maintain INR between 2.0–3.0 or higher if prior thromboembolism
12. Warfarin to maintain INR between 2.0–3.0 or higher if persistent atrial thrombus on transesophageal echocardiography

[a]Risk factors include heart failure, left ventricular ejection fraction <35%, and history of hypertension.
Abbreviation: INR, international normalized ratio.
Source: Adapted from Ref. 173.

Patients younger than age 60 years in Olmstead County, Minnesota with lone AF (no heart disease) had a low risk of TE stroke at 15-year follow-up (176). At 30-year follow-up of this study, increased age and development of hypertension significantly increased the risk of TE events (177). At 30-year follow-up in the Framingham Heart Study, the age-adjusted percentage of patients with lone AF who developed a cerebrovascular event was 28% versus 7% in the control group (178). Table 21.3 shows the ACC/AHA/ Heart Rhythm Society (HRS) Class I indications for antithrombotic therapy in the management of patients with AF (173).

Despite the data showing the efficacy of oral warfarin used in a dose to achieve an INR between 2.0 and 3.0 in reducing the incidence of new TE events in patients with paroxysmal or chronic AF, only about one-third of patients with AF who should be taking warfarin receive it (179). In an academic hospital-based geriatrics practice, only 61 of 124 patients (49%), mean age 80 years, with chronic AF at high risk for developing TE stroke and no contraindications to warfarin were being treated with warfarin therapy (5).

Elderly patients have a higher prevalence and incidence of AF than younger patients (1–6). Elderly patients with AF are at higher risk for developing TE stroke than are younger patients with AF (1,30,32,143–147). However, physicians are more reluctant to treat elderly patients with AF with warfarin therapy. Hopefully, intensive physician education will help solve this important clinical problem.

In the Anticoagulation and Risk Factor in Atrial Fibrillation Study, women off warfarin had significantly higher annual rates of thromboembolism (3.5%) than men (1.8%) (180). Warfarin was associated with significantly lower adjusted TE rates for both women (60% reduction) and men (40% reduction) with similar annual rates of major bleeding (1.0% and 1.1%, respectively) (180).

The Atrial Fibrillation Clopidogrel Trial with Irbersartan for the Prevention of Vascular Events (ACTIVE W) demonstrated in patients with AF that the annual risk of first occurrence of stroke, non-central nervous system systemic embolus, MI, or vascular death was 3.93% in 3371 patients randomized to warfarin to maintain an INR between 2.0 and

3.0 and 5.60% in 3335 patients randomized to clopidogrel 75 mg daily plus aspirin 75–100 mg daily, with a 44% significant reduction in the primary outcome attributed to warfarin (181). The incidence of major bleeding was 10% insignificantly higher in patients treated with clopidogrel plus aspirin than in persons treated with warfarin (181).

Of 2580 patients, mean age 77 years, with hypertension and no history of AF in whom a pacemaker or defibrillator had been implanted, subclinical atrial tachyarrhytmias occurred in 10.1% by three months (182). Of 51 patients who had ischemic stroke or systemic embolism by three months, 11 (22%) had subclinical atrial tachyarrhythmias (182).

New Antithrombotic Drugs

In the Randomized Evaluation of Long-Term Anticoagulation Therapy (RE-LY) study, 18,113 patients, mean age 72 years, with nonvalvular AF and a risk of stroke were randomized in a blinded fashion to the direct thrombin inhibitor dabigatran 150 mg twice daily or 110 mg twice daily or in an unblinded fashion to warfarin to maintain an INR between 2.0 and 3.0 (183). Median follow-up was 2.0 years. The primary outcome was stroke or systemic embolism. Compared with warfarin, dabigatran 150 mg twice daily reduced the primary outcome 34% ($p < 0.001$), reduced all-cause mortality from 4.13% per year to 3.64% per year ($p = 0.051$), and had a similar incidence of major bleeding (Table 21.4)

Table 21.4 Effect of Newer Antithrombotics in Treating Patients with Nonvalvular Atrial Fibrillation

Study	Results
Connolly et al. (183)	At 2-yr follow-up, compared with warfarin, dabigatran 150 mg twice daily reduced stroke or systemic embolism from 1.69% per year to 1.11% per year ($p < 0.001$), reduced mortality from 4.13% per year to 3.64% per year ($p = 0.051$), and had a similar incidence of major bleeding (3.36% per year for warfarin and 3.11% per year for dabigatran)
	Compared with warfarin, dabigatran 110 mg twice daily had a similar incidence of stroke or systemic embolism and of mortality but reduced major bleeding per year from 3.36% to 2.71% ($p = 0.003$)
Patel et al. (185)	At 707-day follow-up, compared with warfarin, rivaroxaban 20 mg daily caused a similar incidence of stroke or systemic embolism and of major bleeding but less intracranial hemorrhage (0.5% vs. 0.7% per year, $p = 0.02$)and less fatal bleeding (0.2% vs. 0.5% per year, $p = 0.003$)
Connolly et al. (186)	Compared with aspirin, apixaban 5 mg twice daily, apixaban reduced stroke or systemic embolism 55% from 3.7% per year to 1.6% per year ($p < 0.001$), reduced mortality 22% from 4.4% per year to 3.5% per year ($p = 0.07$), reduced first hospitalization for cardiovascular causes from 15.9% per year to 12.6% per year ($p < 0.001$), and did not increase major bleeding or intracranial hemorrhage
Granger et al. (187)	Compared with warfarin, apixaban reduced tischemic or hemorrhagic stroke by 21% from 1.60% per year to 1.27% per year ($p = 0.01$), all-cause mortality 11% from 3.94% per year to 3.52% per year ($p = 0.047$), major bleeding 31% from 3.09% per year to 2.13% per year ($p < 0.001$), and hemorrhagic stroke 49% from 0.47% per year to 0.24% per year ($p < 0.001$) (187).

(183). Compared with warfarin, dabigatran 110 mg twice daily had a similar incidence of the primary outcome and of all-cause mortality but reduced major bleeding per year from 3.36% to 2.71% ($p = 0.003$) (Table 21.4) (183). The US Food and Drug Administration (FDA) approved the 150 mg dose of dabigatran but not the 110 mg dose of dabigatran for treating AF because the 150 mg dose reduced TE events better than warfarin (184). The FDA approved a 75 mg dose twice daily of dabgatran in patients with an estimated glomerular filtration rate between 15 and 29 mg/ml/1.73 m^2 although patients with an estimated glomerular filtration rate <30 mg/ml/1.73 m^2 were excluded in the RE-LY trial (184). Dabigatran does not have an antidote.

In the Rivaroxaban Once Daily Oral Direct Factor Xa Inhibition Compared With Vitamin K Antagonism for Prevention of Stroke and Embolism Trial in Atrial Fibrillation (ROCKET AF), 14,264 patients, mean age 73 years, with nonvalvular AF at increased risk for stroke were randomized to the direct factor Xa inhibitor rivaroxaban 20 mg daily or to warfarin to maintain an INR between 2.0 and 3.0 (185). Median follow-up was 707 days. The primary outcome was stroke or systemic embolism. The primary endpoint and major bleeding were similar in both treatment groups. Significant reductions in intracranial hemorrhage (0.5% vs. 0.7% per year, $p = 0.02$) and in fatal bleeding (0.2% vs. 0.5%, $p = 0.003$) occurred in the rivaroxaban group (185). Rivaroxaban does not have an antidote.

In the Apixaban Versus Acetylsalicylic Acid (ASA) to Prevent Stroke in Atrial Fibrillation Patients Who Have Failed or Are unsuitable for Vitamin K Antagonist Treatment (AVERROES) study, 5599 patients, mean age 70 years, with nonvalvular AF at increased risk for stroke for whom vitamin K antagonist therapy was unsuitable were randomized to the direct factor Xa inhibitor apixaban 5 mg twice daily or to aspirin 81–324 mg daily (186). Mean follow-up was 1.1 years. The primary outcome was stroke or systemic embolism. Compared with aspirin, apixaban reduced the primary outcome 55% from 3.7% per year to 1.6% per year ($p < 0.001$), reduced mortality 22% from 4.4% per year to 3.5% per year (p = 0.07), reduced first hospitalization for cardiovascular causes from 15.9% per year to 12.6% per year ($p < 0.001$), and did not increase major bleeding or intracranial hemorrhage (186). Apixaban has no antidote.

In the Apixaban for Reduction in Stroke and Other Thromboembolic Events in Atrial Fibrillation (ARISTOTLE) trial, 18,201 patients, mean age 70 years, with nonvalvular AF and at least one additional risk factor for stroke were randomized to apixaban 5 mg twice daily or to warfarin to maintain an INR between 2.0 and 3.0 (187). Median follow-up was 1.8 years. The primary outcome was ischemic or hemorrhagic stroke or systemic embolism. Compared to warfarin, apixaban reduced tischemic or hemorrhagic stroke by 21% from 1.60% per year to 1.27% per year ($p = 0.01$), all-cause mortality 11% from 3.94% per year to 3.52% per year ($p = 0.047$), major bleeding 31% from 3.09% per year to 2.13% per year ($p < 0.001$), and hemorrhagic stroke 49% from 0.47% per year to 0.24% per year ($p < 0.001$) (187).

ATRIAL FLUTTER

Atrial flutter (AFL) may be paroxysmal or chronic. Episodes of AFL and of AF may occur in the same patient. The AFL waves are usually best seen in leads II, III, aVF, and V_1. The atrial rate usually ranges from 250 to 350 beats per minute and is most commonly 300 beats per minute. There is no isoelectric interval between the AFL waves. In the absence of drug therapy, there is usually a 2:1 AV conduction response.

In the general population, the incidence of AFL increases with age and ranges from 5 per 100,000 persons younger than 50 years of age to 587 per 100,000 persons older than 80 years of age (188). At highest risk of developing AFL are the elderly, men, and patients with CHF or chronic obstructive lung disease (188). Documented structural heart disease or a predisposing condition such as a major surgical procedure or pneumonia was present in 178 of 181 patients (98%) with AFL (188).

The acute onset of AFL with a rapid ventricular rate reduces cardiac output and may lead to angina pectoris, CHF, hypotension, acute pulmonary edema, and syncope. Chronic AFL with a rapid ventricular rate can cause a tachycardia-mediated cardiomyopathy. Patients with AFL are also at increased risk for developing new TE stroke (189,190). Left atrial appendage stunning occurs after cardioversion in patients with AFL, although to a lesser degree than in patients with AF (191).

Management

Management of AFL is similar to management of AF. DC cardioversion is the treatment of choice for converting AFL to sinus rhythm (192). Of 78 patients with AFL, 38% treated with intravenous ibutilide converted to sinus rhythm (111). Fifty-four percent of 16 patients with AFL treated with intravenous dofetilide converted to sinus rhythm (110). Atrial pacing may also be used to try to convert AFL to sinus rhythm (193).

Intravenous verapamil (50), diltiazem (49), or β-blockers (45–48) may be used to immediately slow a very rapid ventricular rate associated with AFL. Oral verapamil (56), diltiazem (55), or β-blockers (57) should be added to the therapeutic regimen if a rapid ventricular rate associated with AFL occurs at rest or during exercise despite digoxin. Amiodarone is the most effective drug for slowing a rapid ventricular rate associated with AFL (59). Digoxin, verapamil, and diltiazem are contraindicated in patients with AFL associated with the WPW syndrome because these drugs shorten the refractory period of the accessory AV pathway, causing more rapid conduction down the accessory pathway. Class I antiarrhythmic drugs such as quinidine should never be used to treat patients with AFL who are not being treated with digoxin, a β-blocker, verapamil, or diltiazem as a 1:1 AV conduction response may develop. Drugs used to treat AFL may also be proarrhythmic (105,106).

Since patients with AFL are at increased risk for developing new TE stroke (189,190), anticoagulant therapy should be administered prior to DC cardioversion or drug cardioversion of patients of AFL to sinus rhythm using the same guidelines as for converting AF (114–118). Patients with chronic AFL should be treated with oral warfarin with the INR maintained between 2.0 and 3.0 (114) or with dabigatran (183), rivaroxaban (185), or apixaban (187). Both $CHADS_2$ and CHA_2DS_2-VASc scores are useful for stroke risk stratification in patients with AFL (194).

Radiofrequency catheter ablation of AFL is a highly successful procedure, especially when the right atrial isthmus is incorporated in the AFL circuit (195,196). Demonstration of bi-directional isthmus block after catheter ablation predicts a high long-term success rate (196). A second radiofrequency catheter ablation may be needed in up to one-third of patients, especially in those with right atrial enlargement (195). Radiofrequency catheter ablation was successful in converting 63 of 70 patients (90%), mean age 78 ± 5 years, with AFL to sinus rhythm (72).

PAROXYSMAL SUPRAVENTRICULAR TACHYCARDIA

Paroxysmal supraventricular tachycardia (PSVT) is a regular narrow complex tachycardia with a rate usually between 140 and 220 beats per minute. A wide QRS complex occurs in the presence of bundle branch block or aberrant ventricular conduction. If aberrant ventricular conduction is present, the QRS complex is usually <140 ms, and a right bundle branch block pattern is present 85% of the time.

PSVT is usually caused by reentry but may be caused by abnormal automaticity or by triggered activity. AV nodal reentrant tachycardia (AVNRT) accounts for 60% of episodes of PSVT (197). Discrete P waves are not seen on the 12-lead ECG in two-thirds of these patients. Retrograde P waves (inverted in leads II, III, and aVF) following the QRS complex occur in approximately 30% of these patients. In approximately 10% of patients, the re-entry circuit is reversed, with anterograde conduction over the fast pathway and retrograde conduction over the slow pathway (197). This type of PSVT is referred to as uncommon AVNRT, and the RP interval is longer than the PR interval.

PSVT secondary to accessory pathway conduction occurs in 30% of patients with sustained PSVT (198). Accessory pathway conduction can be overt as in the WPW syndrome or concealed because accessory pathways are capable of either unidirectional or bidirectional conduction.

PAT includes those forms of PSVT that do not involve the AV node as an obligate part of the tachycardia circuit (199). Atrial tachycardias can be reentrant, automatic, or triggered in origin (199).

The prevalence of short bursts of PSVT diagnosed by 24-hour AECGs in 1476 elderly persons, mean age 81 years, with heart disease was 33% (30). At 42-month follow-up of 1359 persons, mean age 81 years, with heart disease, short bursts of PSVT was not associated with an increased incidence of new coronary events (25). At 43-month follow-up of 1476 persons, mean age 81 years, with heart disease, short bursts of PSVT was not associated with an increased incidence of new TE stroke (30).

Management

Sustained episodes of SVT should first be treated by increasing vagal tone by carotid sinus massage, the Valsalva maneuver, facial immersion in cold water, or administration of phenylephrine (200). If vagal maneuvers are unsuccessful, intravenous adenosine is the drug of choice (201). Intravenous verapamil, diltiazem, or β-blockers may also be used. If these measures do not convert PSVT to sinus rhythm, DC cardioversion should be used.

Most patients with PSVT do not require long-term therapy. If long-term treatment is required because of symptoms due to frequent episodes of PSVT, digoxin, propranolol, verapamil, or diltiazem may be administered (202). These drugs are the initial drug of choice for AVNRT and AV reentrant SVT. For PSVT associated with the WPW syndrome, flecainide or propafenone may be used if there is no associated heart disease (203). If heart disease is present, quinidine, procainamide, or disopyramide plus a β-blocker or verapamil should be used (203). Radiofrequency catheter ablation should be used to treat older persons with symptomatic, drug-resistant SVT and should be considered an early treatment option (204). Radiofrequency catheter ablation can be successfully performed in older patients with low complication rates. Resultant complete heart block for slow pathway ablation in AVNRT occurs in patients exhibiting a significantly prolonged baseline first-degree AV block. Cardiac perforation risk is also increased in elderly women. Radiofrequency catheter ablation was successful in converting 60 of 66 patients, mean age 78 + 5 years, with SVT to sinus rhythm (72).

Accelerated Atrioventricular Junctional Rhythm

Accelerated AV junctional rhythm also called nonparoxysmal AV junctional tachycardia (NPJT) is a form of SVT caused by enhanced impulse formation within the AV junction rather than by reentry (205). This arrhythmia is usually due to recent aortic or mitral valve surgery, acute MI, or digitalis toxicity. The ventricular rate usually ranges between 70 and 130 beats per minute. Treatment of NPJT is directed toward correction of the underlying disorder. Hypokalemia, if present, should be treated with potassium. Digitalis should be stopped if digitalis toxicity is present. β-blockers may be given cautiously if this is warranted by clinical circumstances.

PAT with Atrioventricular Block

Digitalis toxicity causes 70% of cases of PAT with AV block. Digoxin and diuretics causing hypokalemia should be stopped in these persons. If the serum potassium is low or low-normal, potassium chloride is the treatment of choice. Intravenous propranolol will cause conversion to sinus rhythm in about 85% of patients with digitalis-induced PAT with AV block and in about 35% of patients with PAT with AV block not induced by digitalis (200). By increasing AV block, propranolol may also be beneficial in slowing a rapid ventricular rate in PAT with AV block (200).

Multifocal Atrial Tachycardia

Multifocal atrial tachycardia (MAT) is usually associated with acute illness, especially in older persons with pulmonary disease. MAT is best managed by treatment of the underlying disorder. Intravenous verapamil has been reported to be effective in controlling the ventricular rate in MAT, with occasional conversion to sinus rhythm (206). However, Aronow et al. found intravenous verapamil not very effective in treating MAT (207). The tendency of intravenous verapamil to aggravate pre-existing arterial hypoxemia also limits its use in the group of patients most likely to develop MAT (206).

REFERENCES

1. Wolf PA, Abbott RD, Kannel WB. Atrial fibrillation as an independent risk factor for stroke: the Framingham Study. Stroke 1991; 22: 983–8.
2. Aronow WS, Ahn C, Gutstein H. Prevalence of atrial fibrillation and association of atrial fibrillation with prior and new thromboembolic stroke in older patients. J Am Geriatr Soc 1996; 44: 521–3.
3. Aronow WS, Ahn C, Gutstein H. Prevalence and incidence of cardiovascular disease in 1,160 older men and 2,464 older women in a long-term health care facility. J Gerontol Med Sciences 2002; 57A: M45–6.
4. Furberg CD, Psaty BM, Manolio TA, et al. Prevalence of atrial fibrillation in elderly subjects (the Cardiovascular Health Study). Am J Cardiol 1994; 74: 236–41.
5. Mendelson G, Aronow WS. Underutilization of warfarin in older persons with chronic nonvalvular atrial fibrillation at high risk for developing stroke. J Am Geriatr Soc 1998; 46: 1423–4.
6. Psaty BM, Manolio TA, Kuller LH, et al. Incidence of and risk factors for atrial fibrillation in older adults. Circulation 1997; 96: 2455–61.
7. Danias PG, Caulfield TA, Weigner MJ, et al. Likelihood of spontaneous conversion of atrial fibrillation to sinus rhythm. J Am Coll Cardiol 1998; 31: 588–92.
8. Konings KTS, Kirchhof CJ, Smeets JR, et al. High-density mapping of electrically induced atrial fibrillation in humans. Circulation 1994; 89: 1665–80.
9. Jais P, Haissaguerre M, Shah DC, et al. A focal source of atrial fibrillation treated by discrete radio-frequency ablation. Circulation 1997; 95: 572–6.
10. Allessie MA, Boyden PA, Camm AJ, et al. Pathophysiology and prevention of atrial fibrillation. Circulation 2001; 103: 769–77.
11. Aronow WS, Banach M. Atrial fibrillation: the new epidemic of the ageing world. J Atrial Fibrillation 2009; 1: 337–61.
12. Wanahita N, Messerli FH, Bangalore S, et al. Atrial fibrillation and obesity-results of a meta-analysis. Am Heart J 2008; 155: 310–15.
13. Banach M, Goch JH, Ugurlucan M, et al. Obesity and postoperative atrial fibrillation. Is there no connection? Comment on: Wanahita et al. "atrial fibrillation and obesity-results of a meta-analysis". Am Heart J 2008; 156: e5.
14. Banach M, Goch A, Misztal M, et al. Relation between postoperative mortality and atrial fibrillation before surgical revascularization-3-year follow-up. Thorac Cardiovasc Surg 2008; 56: 20–3.
15. Banach M, Ugurlucan M, Mariscalco G, et al. Statins in the prevention of postoperative atrial fibrillation. Is there really no effect? Am Heart J 2008; 155: e53.
16. Banach M, Mikhailidis DP, Ugurlucan M, et al. The significance of statin use in patients subjected to surgical coronary revascularization. Arch Med Sci 2007; 3: S126–32.
17. Rader F, Gajulapalli RD, Pasala T, Einstadter D. Effect of early statin therapy on risk of atrial fibrillation after coronary artery bypass grafting with or without concomitant valve surgery. Am J Cardiol 2011; 108: 220–2.

18. Bielecka-Dabrowa A, Goch JH, Rysz J, et al. Influence of co-existing atrial fibrillation on the efficacy of atorvastatin treatmnt in patients with dilated cardiomyopathy: a pilot study. Lipids Health Dis 2010; 9: 21.

19. Aronow WS, Ahn C, Kronzon I. Echocardiographic findings associated with atrial fibrillation in 1,699 patients aged >60 years. Am J Cardiol 1995; 76: 1191–2.

20. Sawin CT, Geller A, Wolf PA, et al. Low serum thyrotropin concentration as a risk factor for atrial fibrillation in older persons. N Engl J Med 1994; 331: 1249–52.

21. van der Hooft CS, Heeringa J, van Herpen G, et al. Drug-induced atrial fibrillation. J Am Coll Cardiol 2004; 44: 2117–24.

22. Healey JS, Baranchuk A, Crystal E, et al. Prevention of atrial fibrillation with angiotensin-converting enzyme inhibitors and angiotensin receptor blockers. A meta-analysis. J Am Coll Cardiol 2005; 45: 1832–9.

23. Kannel WB, Abbott RD, Savage DD, McNamara PM. Epidemiologic features of chronic atrial fibrillation: the Framingham Study. N Engl J Med 1982; 306: 1018–22.

24. Benjamin EJ, Wolf PA, D'Agostino RB, et al. Impact of atrial fibrillation on the risk of death. The Framingham Heart Study. Circulation 1998; 98: 946–52.

25. Aronow WS, Ahn C, Mercando AD, Epstein S. Correlation of atrial fibrillation, paroxysmal supraventricular tachycardia, and sinus rhythm with incidences of new coronary events in 1,359 patients, mean age 81 years, with heart disease. Am J Cardiol 1995; 75: 182–4.

26. Friberg J, Scharling H, Gadsboll N, et al. Comparison of the impact of atrial fibrillation on the risk of stroke and cardiovascular death in women versus men (The Copenhagen City Heart Study). Am J Cardiol 2004; 94: 889–94.

27. Rathore SS, Berger AK, Weinfurt KP, et al. Acute myocardial infarction complicated by atrial fibrillation in the elderly: prevalence and outcomes. Circulation 2000; 101: 969–74.

28. Wong C-K, White HD, Wilcox RG, et al. New atrial fibrillation after acute myocardial infarction independently predicts death: the GUSTO-III experience. Am Heart J 2000; 140: 878–85.

29. Al-Khatib SM, Pieper KS, Lee KL, et al. Atrial fibrillation and mortality among patients with acute coronary syndromes without ST-segment elevation: results from the PURSUIT trial. Am J Cardiol 2001; 88: 76–9.

30. Aronow WS, Ahn C, Mercando AD, et al. Correlation of paroxysmal supraventricular tachycardia, atrial fibrillation, and sinus rhythm with incidences of new thromboembolic stroke in 1,476 old-old patients. Aging Clin Experimental Res 1996; 8: 32–4.

31. Jozwiak A, Guzik P, Mathew A, et al. Association of atrial fibrillation and focal neurologic deficits with impaired cognitive function in hospitalized patients ≥65 years of age. Am J Cardiol 2006; 98: 1238–41.

32. Aronow WS, Ahn C, Kronzon I, Gutstein H. Association of left ventricular hypertrophy and chronic atrial fibrillation with the incidence of new thromboembolic stroke in 2,384 older persons. Am J Cardiol 1999; 84: 468–9.

33. Aronow WS, Ahn C, Schoenfeld MR, Gutstein H. Association of extracranial carotid arterial disease and chronic atrial fibrillation with the incidence of new thromboembolic stroke in 1,846 older persons. Am J Cardiol 1999; 83: 1403–3.

34. Yamanouchi H, Mizutani T, Matsushita S, Esaki Y. Paroxysmal atrial fibrillation: high frequency of embolic brain infarction in elderly autopsy patients. Neurology 1997; 49: 1691–4.

35. Ezekowitz MD, James KE, Nazarian SM, et al. Silent cerebral infarction in patients with nonrheumatic atrial fibrillation. Circulation 1995; 92: 2178–82.

36. Dries DL, Exner DV, Gersh BJ, et al. Atrial fibrillation is associated with an increased risk for mortality and heart failure progression in patients with asymptomic and symptomatic left ventricular systolic dysfunction: a retrospective analysis of the SOLVD trials. J Am Coll Cardiol 1998; 32: 695–703.

37. Aronow WS, Ahn C, Kronzon I. Prognosis of congestive heart failure after prior myocardial infarction in older persons with atrial fibrillation versus sinus rhythm. Am J Cardiol 2001; 87: 224–5.

38. Ahmed MI, White M, Ekundayo OJ, et al. A history of atrial fibrillation and outcomes in chronic advanced systolic heart failure: a propensity-matched study. Eur Heart J 2009; 30: 2029–37.

39. Shinbane JS, Wood MA, Jensen DN, et al. Tachycardia-induced cardiomyopathy: a review of animal models and clinical studies. J Am Coll Cardiol 1997; 29: 709–15.

40. Schumacher B, Luderitz B. Rate issues in atrial fibrillation: consequences of tachycardia and therapy for rate control. Am J Cardiol 1998; 82: 29N–36N.

41. Wood MA, Brown-Mahoney C, Kay GN, Ellenbogen KA. Clinical outcomes after ablation and pacing therapy for atrial fibrillation: a meta-analysis. Circulation 2000; 101: 1138–44.

42. Redfield MM, Kay GN, Jenkins LS, et al. Tachycardia-related cardiomyopathy: a common cause of ventricular dysfunction in patients with atrial fibrillation referred for atrioventricular ablation. Mayo Clin Proc 2000; 75: 790–5.

43. Ganesan AN, Brooks AG, Roberts-Thomson KC, et al. Role of AV nodal ablation in cardiac resynchronization in patients with coexistent atrial fibrillation and heart failure. A systematic review. J Am Coll Cardiol 2012; 59: 719–26.

44. Pollak A, Falk RH. Pacemaker therapy in patients with atrial fibrillation. Am Heart J 1993; 125: 824–30.

45. Aronow WS, Uyeyama RR. Treatment of arrhythmias with pindolol. Clin Pharmacol Ther 1972; 13: 15–22.

46. Aronow WS, Van Camp S, Turbow M, et al. Acebutolol in supraventricular arrhythmias. Clin Pharmacol Ther 1979; 25: 149–53.

47. Aronow WS. Use of beta-adrenergic blockers in antiarrhythmic therapy. Pract Cardiol 1986; 12: 75–89.

48. Abrams J, Allen J, Allin D, et al. Efficacy and safety of esmolol vs propranolol in the treatment of supraventricular tachyarrhythmias: a multicenter double-blind clinical trial. Am Heart J 1985; 110: 913–22.

49. Salerno DM, Dias VC, Kleiger RE, et al. Efficacy and safety of intravenous diltiazem for treatment of atrial fibrillation and atrial flutter. Am J Cardiol 1989; 63: 1046–51.

50. Aronow WS, Landa D, Plasencia G, et al. Verapamil in atrial fibrillation and atrial flutter. Clin Pharmacol Ther 1979; 26: 578–83.

51. Falk RH, Knowlton AA, Bernard SA, et al. Digoxin for converting recent onset atrial fibrillation to sinus rhythm: a randomized, double-blinded trial. Ann Intern Med 1987; 106: 503–6.

52. Falk RH, Leavitt JI. Digoxin for atrial fibrillation: a drug whose time has gone? Ann Intern Med 1991; 114: 573–5.

53. Aronow WS. Digoxin or angiotensin converting enzyme inhibitors for congestive heart failure in geriatric patients: which is the preferred treatment? Drugs Aging 1991; 1: 98–103.

54. David D, Segni ED, Klein HO, Kaplinsky E. Inefficacy of digitalis in the control of heart rate in patients with chronic atrial fibrillation: beneficial effect of an added beta adrenergic blocking agent. Am J Cardiol 1979; 44: 1378–82.

55. Roth A, Harrison E, Milani G, et al. Efficacy and safety of medium- and high-dose diltiazem alone and in combination with digoxin for control of heart rate at rest and during exercise in patients with chronic atrial fibrillation. Circulation 1986; 73: 316–24.

56. Lang R, Klein HO, Weiss E, et al. Superiority of oral verapamil therapy to digoxin in treatment of chronic atrial fibrillation. Chest 1983; 83: 491–9.

57. Farshi R, Kistner D, Sarma JSM, et al. Ventricular rate control in chronic atrial fibrillation during daily activity and programmed exercise: a crossover open-label study of five drug regimens. J Am Coll Cardiol 1999; 33: 304–10.

58. Gold RL, Haffajee CI, Charos G, et al. Amiodarone for refractory atrial fibrillation. Am J Cardiol 1986; 57: 124–7.

59. Chun SH, Sager PT, Stevenson WG, et al. Long-term efficacy of amiodarone for the maintenance of normal sinus rhythm in patients with refractory atrial fibrillation or flutter. Am J Cardiol 1995; 76: 47–50.

60. Camm AJ, Capucci A, Hohnloser SH, et al. A randomized active-controlled study comparing the efficacy and safety of vernakalant to amiodarone in recent-onset atrial fibrillation. J Am Coll Cardiol 2011; 57: 313–21.

61. Hohnloser SH, Crijns HJGM, van Eickels M, et al. Effect of dronedarone on cardiovascular events in atrial fibrillation. N Engl J Med 2009; 360: 668–78.

62. Connolly SJ, Camm AJ, Halperin JL, et al. Dronedarone in high-risk permanent atrial fibrillation. N Engl J Med 2011; 365: 2268–76.

63. Rawles JM, Metcalfe MJ, Jennings K. Time of occurrence, duration, and ventricular rate of paroxysmal atrial fibrillation: the effect of digoxin. Br Heart J 1990; 63: 225–7.

64. Murgatroyd FD, Gibson SM, Baiyan X, et al. Double-blind placebo controlled trial of digoxin in symptomatic paroxysmal atrial fibrillation. Circulation 1999; 99: 2765–70.

65. Galun E, Flugelman MY, Glickson M, Eliakim M. Failure of long-term digitalization to prevent rapid ventricular response in patients with paroxysmal atrial fibrillation. Chest 1991; 99: 1038–40.

66. Sticherling C, Oral H, Horrocks J, et al. Effects of digoxin on acute, atrial fibrillation-induced changes in atrial refractoriness. Circulation 2000; 102: 2503–8.

67. Morady F, Hasse C, Strickberger SA, et al. Long-term follow-up after radiofrequency modification of the atrioventricular node in patients with atrial fibrillation. J Am Coll Cardiol 1997; 27: 113–21.

68. Feld GK, Fleck P, Fujimura O, et al. Control of rapid ventricular response by radiofrequency catheter modification of the atrioventricular node in patients with medically refractory atrial fibrillation. Circulation 1994; 90: 2299–307.

69. Fitzpatrick AP, Kourouyan HD, Siu A, et al. Quality of life and outcomes after radiofrequency His-bundle catheter ablation and permanent pacemaker implantation: impact of treatment in paroxysmal and established atrial fibrillation. Am Heart J 1996; 131: 499–507.

70. Brignole M, Menozzi C, Gianfranchi L, et al. Assessment of atrioventricular junction ablation and VVIR pacemaker versus pharmacological treatment in patients with heart failure and chronic atrial fibrillation. A randomized, controlled study. Circulation 1998; 98: 953–60.

71. Ozcan C, Jahangir A, Friedman PA, et al. Long-term survival after ablation of the atrioventricular node and implantation of a permanent pacemaker in patients with atrial fibrillation. N Engl J Med 2001; 344: 1043–51.

72. Channamsetty V, Aronow WS, Sorbera C, et al. Efficacy of radiofrequency catheter ablation in treatment of elderly patients with supraventricular tachyarrhythmias and ventricular tachycardia. Am J Ther 2006; 13: 513–15.

73. Cox JL, Boineau JP, Schuessler RB, et al. Successful surgical treatment of atrial fibrillation: review and clinical update. JAMA 1991; 266: 1976–80.

74. Leitch JW, Klein G, Yee R, Guiraudon G. Sinus node-atrioventricular node isolation: long-term results with the "Corridor" operation for atrial fibrillation. J Am Coll Cardiol 1991; 17: 970–5.

75. Handa N, Scaff HV, Morris JJ, et al. Outcome of valve repair and the Cox maze procedure for mitral regurgitation and association atrial fibrillation. J Thorac Cardiovasc Surg 1999; 118: 628–35.

76. McCarthy PM, Gillinov AM, Castle L, et al. The Cox-Maze procedure: the Cleveland Clinic experience. Semin Thorac Cardiovasc Surg 2000; 12: 25–9.

77. Jessurun ER, van Hemel NM, Defauw JAMT, et al. Results of maze surgery for lone paroxysmal atrial fibrillation. Circulation 2000; 101: 1559–67.

78. Naik S, Aronow WS, Fleisher AG. Intraoperative radiofrequency maze procedure for treating atrial fibrillation at the time of valve surgery or coronary artery bypass grafting. Am J Ther 2006; 13: 298–9.

79. Gaita F, Gallotti R, Calo L, et al. Limited posterior left atrial cryoablation in patients with chronic atrial fibrillation undergoing valvular heart surgery. J Am Coll Cardiol 2000; 36: 159–66.

80. Haissaguerre M, Jais P, Shah DC, et al. Electrophysiological end point for catheter ablation of atrial fibrillation initiated from multiple pulmonary venous foci. Circulation 2000; 101: 1409–17.

81. Pappone C, Augello G, Sala S, et al. A randomized trial of circumferential pulmonary vein ablation versus antiarrhythmic drug therapy in paroxysmal atrial fibrillation. The APAF Study. J Am Coll Cardiol 2006; 48: 2340–7.

82. Wazni OM, Marrouche NF, Martin DO, et al. Radiofrequency ablation vs antiarrhythmic drugs as first-line treatment of symptomatic atrial fibrillation. A randomized trial. JAMA 2005; 293: 2634–40.

83. Werasooriya R, Khairy P, Litalien J, et al. Catheter ablation for atrial fibrillation. Are results maintained at 5 years of follow-up. J Am Coll Cardiol 2011; 57: 160–6.

84. Gaita F, Caponi D, Pianelli M, et al. Radiofrequency catheter ablation of atrial fibrillation: a cause of silent thrmboembolism? Magnetic resonance imaging assessment of cerebral thromboembolism in patients undergoing ablation of atrial fibrillation. Circulation 2010; 122: 1667–73.

85. Gaita F, Riccardi R. Catheter maze-ablation for preventing atrial fibrillation: where do we stand? Cardiac Electrophysiol Rev 2001; 5: 231–3.

86. Wellens HJJ, Lau C-P, Luderitz B, et al. Atrioverter: an implantable device for the treatment of atrial fibrillation. Circulation 1998; 98: 1651–6.

87. Sgarbossa EB, Pinski SL, Maloney JD, et al. Chronic atrial fibrillation and stroke in paced patients with sick sinus syndrome. Relevance of clinical characteristics and pacing modalities. Circulation 1993; 88: 1045–53.

88. Andersen HR, Thuesen L, Bagger JP, et al. Prospective randomised trial of atrial versus ventricular pacing in sick-sinus syndrome. Lancet 1994; 344: 1523–8.

89. Aronow WS, Mercando AD, Epstein S. Prevalence of arrhythmias detected by 24-hour ambulatory electrocardiography and value of antiarrhythmic therapy in elderly patients with unexplained syncope. Am J Cardiol 1992; 70: 408–10.

90. Coumel P, Friocourt P, Mugica J, et al. Long-term prevention of vagal atrial arrhythmias by atria pacing at 90/minute: experience with 6 cases. Pacing Clin Electrophysiol 1983; 6: 552–60.

91. Gillis AM, Wyse DG, Connolly SJ, et al. Atrial pacing periablation for prevention of paroxysmal atrial fibrillation. Circulation 1999; 99: 2553–8.

92. Friedman PA, Hill MRS, Hammill SC, et al. Randomized prospective pilot study of long-term dual-site atrial pacing for prevention of atrial fibrillation. Mayo Clin Proc 1998; 73: 848–54.

93. Lau C-P, Tse H-F, Yu C-M, et al. Dual-site atrial pacing for atrial fibrillation in patients without bradycardia. Am J Cardiol 2001; 88: 371–5.

94. Levy T, Fotopoulos G, Walker S, et al. Randomized controlled study investigating the effect of biatrial pacing in prevention of atrial fibrillation after coronary artery bypass grafting. Circulation 2000; 102: 1382–7.

95. Patel AM, Westveer DC, Man KC, et al. Treatment of underlying atrial fibrillation: paced rhythm obscures recognition. J Am Coll Cardiol 2000; 36: 784–7.

96. Knight BP, Gersh BJ, Carlson MD, et al. Role of permanent pacing to prevent atrial fibrillation. science advisory from the American Heart Association Council on Clinical Cardiology (Subcommittee on Electrocardiography and Arrhythmias) and the Quality of Care and Outcomes Research Interdisciplinary Working Group, in collaboration with the Heart Rhythm Society. Circulation 2005; 111: 240–3.

97. Ostermayer SH, Reisman M, Kramer PH, et al. Percutaneous left atrial appendage transcatheter occlusion (PLAATO system) to prevent stroke in high-risk patients with non-rheumatic atrial fibrillation. Results from the international multi-center feasibility trials. J Am Coll Cardiol 2005; 46: 9–14.

98. Holmes DR, Reddy VY, Turi ZG, et al. Percutaneous closure of the left atrial appendage versus warfarin therapy for prevention of stroke in patients with atrial fibrillation: a randomized non-inferiority trial. Lancet 2009; 374: 534–42.

99. Michelson EL. Clinical perspectives in management of Wolff-Parkinson-White syndrome. Part 2: Diagnostic evaluation and treatment strategies. Mod Concepts Cardiovasc Dis 1989; 58: 49–54.

100. Jackman WM, Wang X, Friday KJ, et al. Catheter ablation of accessory atrioventricular pathways (Wolff-Parkinson-White syndrome) by radiofrequency current. N Engl J Med 1991; 324: 1605–11.

101. Calkins H, Yong P, Miller JM, et al. Catheter ablation of accessory pathways, atrioventricular nodal reentrant tachycardia, and the atrioventricular junction. Final results of a prospective, multicenter clinical trial. Circulation 1999; 99: 262–70.

102. Morris JJ Jr, Peter RH, McIntosh HD. Electrical conversion of atrial fibrillation: immediate and long-term results and selection of patients. Ann Intern Med 1966; 65: 216–31.

103. Fuster V, Ryden LE, Asinger RW, et al. ACC/AHA/ESC Guidelines for the Management of Patients With Atrial Fibrillation: Executive Summary. A Report of the American College of Cardiology/American Heart Association Task Force on Practice Guidelines and the European Society of Cardiology Committee for Practice Guidelines and Policy Conferences (Committee to Develop Guidelines for the Management of Patients With Atrial Fibrillation). Developed in collaboration with the North American Society of Pacing and Electrophysiology. J Am Coll Cardiol 2001; 38: 1231–65.

104. Mittal S, Ayati S, Stein KM, et al. Transthoracic cardioversion of atrial fibrillation. Comparison of rectilinear biphasic versus damped sine wave monophasic shocks. Circulation 2000; 101: 1282–7.

105. Feld GK, Chen P-S, Nicod P, et al. Possible atrial proarrhythmic effects of class IC antiarrhythmic drugs. Am J Cardiol 1990; 66: 378–83.

106. Falk RH. Proarrhythmia in patients treated for atrial fibrillation or flutter. Ann Intern Med 1992; 117: 141–50.

107. Maisel WH, Kuntz KM, Reimold SC, et al. Risk of initiating antiarrhythmic drug therapy for atrial fibrillation in patients admitted to a university hospital. Ann Intern Med 1997; 127: 281–4.

108. Cardiac Arrhythmia Suppression Trial. Preliminary report: effect of encainide and flecainide on mortality in a randomized trial of arrhythmia suppression after myocardial infarction. N Engl J Med 1989; 329: 406–12.

109. Falk RH, Pollak A, Singh SN, Friedrich T. Intravenous dofetilide, a Class III antiarrhythmic agent, for the termination of sustained atrial fibrillation or flutter. J Am Coll Cardiol 1997; 29: 385–90.

110. Torp-Pedersen C, Moller M, Bloch-Thomsen PE, et al. Dofetilide in patients with congestive heart failure and left ventricular dysfunction. N Engl J Med 1999; 341: 857–65.

111. Ellenbogen KA, Stambler BS, Wood MA, et al. Efficacy of intravenous ibutilide for rapid termination of atrial fibrillation and atrial flutter: a dose-response study. J Am Coll Cardiol 1996; 28: 130–6.

112. Oral H, Souza JJ, Michaud GF, et al. Facilitating transthoracic cardioversion of atrial fibrillation with ibutilide pretreatment. N Engl J Med 1999; 340: 1849–54.

113. Manning WJ, Silverman DI, Keighley CS, et al. Transesophageal echocardiographically facilitated early cardioversion from atrial fibrillation using short-term anticoagulation: final results of a prospective 4.5-year study. J Am Coll Cardiol 1995; 25: 1354–61.

114. Laupacis A, Albers G, Dalen J, et al. Antithrombotic therapy in atrial fibrillation. Chest 1998; 114: 579S–89S.

115. Fatkin D, Kuchar DL, Thorburn CW, Feneley MP. Transesophageal echocardiography before and during direct current cardioversion of atrial fibrillation: evidence for "atrial stunning" as a mechanism of thromboembolic complications. J Am Coll Cardiol 1994; 23: 307–16.

116. Black IW, Fatkin D, Sagar KB, et al. Exclusion of atrial thrombus by transesophageal echocardiography does not preclude embolism after cardioversion of atrial fibrillation: a multicenter study. Circulation 1994; 89: 2509–13.

117. Klein AL, Grimm RA, Murray RD, et al. Use of transesophageal echocardiography to guide cardioversion in patients with atrial fibrillation. N Engl J Med 2001; 344: 1411–20.

118. Grimm RA, Leung DY, Black IW, et al. Left atrial appendage "stunning" after spontaneous conversion of atrial fibrillation demonstrated by transesophageal Doppler echocardiography. Am Heart J 1995; 130: 174–6.

119. Silverman DI, Manning WJ. Strategies for cardioversion of atrial fibrillation—time for a change? N Engl J Med 2001; 344: 1468–9.

120. Seto TB, Taira DA, Manning WJ. Cardioversion in patients with atrial fibrillation and left atrial thrombi on initial transesophageal echocardiography: should transesophageal echocardiography be repeated before elective cardioversion? A cost-effectiveness analysis. J Am Soc Echocardiogr 1999; 12: 508–16.

121. Coplen SE, Antmann EM, Berlin JA, et al. Efficacy and safety of quinidine therapy for maintenance of sinus rhythm after cardioversion: a meta-analysis of randomized control trials. Circulation 1990; 82: 1106–16.

122. Aronow WS, Mercando AD, Epstein S, Kronzon I. Effect of quinidine or procainimide versus no antiarrhythmic drug on sudden cardiac death, total cardiac death, and total death in elderly patients with heart disease and complex ventricular arrhythmias. Am J Cardiol 1990; 66: 423–8.

123. Juul-Moller S, Edvardsson N, Rehnqvist-Ahlberg N. Sotalol versus quinidine for the maintenance of sinus rhythm after direct current conversion of atrial fibrillation. Circulation 1990; 82: 1932–9.

124. Reimold SC, Cantillon CO, Friedman PL, Antman EM. Propafenone versus sotalol for suppression of recurrent symptomatic atrial fibrillation. Am J Cardiol 1993; 71: 558–63.

125. Roy D, Talajic M, Dorian P, et al. Amiodarone to prevent recurrence of atrial fibrillation. N Engl J Med 2000; 342: 913–20.

126. Kuhlkamp V, Schirdewan A, Stangl K, et al. Use of metoprolol CR/XL to maintain sinus rhythm after conversion from persistent atrial fibrillation. A randomized, double-blind, placebo controlled study. J Am Coll Cardiol 2000; 36: 139–46.

127. Pritchett ELC, Page RL, Connolly SJ, et al. Antiarrhythmic effects of azimilide in atrial fibrillation: efficacy and dose-response. J Am Coll Cardiol 2000; 36: 794–802.

128. Flaker GC, Blackshear JL, McBride R, et al. Antiarrhythmic drug therapy and cardiac mortality in atrial fibrillation. J Am Coll Cardiol 1992; 20: 527–32.

129. Teo KK, Yusuf S, Furberg CD. Effects of prophylactic antiarrhythmic drug therapy in acute myocardial infarction: an overview of results from randomized controlled trials. JAMA 1993; 270: 1589–95.

130. Greene HL; CASCADE Investigators. The CASCADE study: randomized antiarrhythmic drug therapy in survivors of cardiac arrest in Seattle. Am J Cardiol 1993; 72: 70F–4F.

131. Herre J, Sauve M, Malone P, et al. Long-term results of amiodarone therapy in patients with recurrent sustained ventricular tachycardia or ventricular fibrillation. J Am Coll Cardiol 1989; 13: 442–9.

132. Aronow WS, Ahn C, Mercando AD, et al. Effect of propranolol versus no antiarrhythmic drug on sudden death, total cardiac death, and total death in patients ≥ 62 years of age with heart disease, complex ventricular arrhythmias, and left ventricular ejection fraction ≥ 40%. Am J Cardiol 1994; 74: 267–70.

133. Olshansky B. Management of atrial fibrillation after coronary artery bypass graft. Am J Cardiol 1996; 78: 27–34.

134. Hohnloser SH, Cuck K-H, Lilienthal J; PIAF Investigators. Rhythm or rate control in atrial fibrillation—pharmacological intervention in atrial fibrillation (PIAF): a randomised trial. Lancet 2000; 356: 1789–94.

135. The Atrial Fibrillation Follow-Up Investigation of Rhythm Management (AFFIRM) Investigators. A comparison of rate control and rhythm control in patients with atrial fibrillation. N Engl J Med 2002; 347: 1825–33.

136. Pawar PP, Jones LG, Feller M, et al. Association between smoking and outcomes in older adults with atrial fibrillation. Arch Gerontol Geriatr 2012; 54: 85–90.

137. Roy B, Desai RV, Mujib M, et al. Effect of warfarin on outcomes in septuagenarian patients with atrial fibrillation. Am J Cardiol 2012; 109: 370–7.

138. Van Gelder IC, Hagens VE, Bosker HA, et al. A comparison of rate control and rhythm control in patients with recurrent persistent atrial fibrillation. N Engl J Med 2002; 347: 1834–40.

139. Rienstra M, Van Veldhuisen DJ, Hagens VE, et al. Gender-related differences in rhythm control treatment in persistent atrial fibrillation. Data of the rate control versus electrical cardioversion (RACE) study. J Am Coll Cardiol 2005; 46: 1298–306.

140. Al-Khatib SM, Shaw LK, Lee KL, et al. Is rhythm control superior to rate control in patients with atrial fibrillation and congestive heart failure? Am J Cardiol 2004; 94: 797–800.

141. Roy D, Talajic M, Nattel S, et al. Rhythm control versus rate control for atrial fibrillation and heart failure. N engl J Med 2008; 358: 2667–77.
142. Israel CW, Gronefeld G, Ehrlich JR, et al. Long-term risk of recurrent atrial fibrillation as documented by an implantable monitoring device. Implications for optimal patient care. J Am Coll Cardiol 2004; 43: 47–52.
143. Planning and Steering Committees for AFFIRM Study. Atrial fibrillation follow-up investigation of rhythm management—the AFFIRM study design. Am J Cardiol 1997; 79: 1198–202.
144. Boston Area Anticoagulation Trial for Atrial Fibrillation Investigators. The effect of low-dose warfarin on the risk of stroke in patients with nonrheumatic atrial fibrillation. N Engl J Med 1990; 323: 1505–11.
145. Atrial Fibrillation Investigators. Risk factors for stroke and efficacy of antithrombotic therapy in atrial fibrillation. Analysis of pooled data from five randomized controlled trials. Arch Intern Med 1994; 154: 1449–57.
146. Aronow WS, Ahn C, Kronzon I, Gutstein H. Risk factors for new thromboembolic stroke in persons ≥ 62 years old with chronic atrial fibrillation. Am J Cardiol 1998; 82: 119–21.
147. Aronow WS, Gutstein H, Hsieh FY. Risk factors for thromboembolic stroke in elderly patients with chronic atrial fibrillation. Am J Cardiol 1989; 63: 366–7.
148. Stroke Prevention in Atrial Fibrillation Investigators. Predictors of thromboembolism in atrial fibrillation: II. Echocardiocardiographic features of patients at risk. Ann Intern Med 1992; 116: 6–12.
149. Stroke Prevention in Atrial Fibrillation Investigators. Adjusted-dose warfarin versus low-intensity, fixed dose warfarin plus aspirin for high-risk patients with atrial fibrillation: Stroke Prevention in Atrial Fibrillation III randomised clinical trial. Lancet 1996; 348: 633–8.
150. Aronow WS, Ahn C, Kronzon I, Gutstein H. Effect of warfarin versus aspirin on the incidence of new thromboembolic stroke in older persons with chronic atrial fibrillation and abnormal and normal left ventricular ejection fraction. Am J Cardiol 2000; 85: 1033–5.
151. Stroke Prevention in Atrial Fibrillation Investigators. Predictors of thromboembolism in atrial fibrillation: I. Clinical features of patients at risk. Ann Intern Med 1992; 116: 1–5.
152. EAFT (European Atrial Fibrillation Trial) Study Group. Secondary prevention in non-rheumatic atrial fibrillation after transient ischaemic attack or minor stroke. Lancet 1993; 342: 1255–62.
153. Aronow WS, Ahn C, Kronzon I, Gutstein H. Association of mitral annular calcium with new thromboembolic stroke at 44-month follow-up of 2,148 persons, mean age 81 years. Am J Cardiol 1998; 81: 105–6.
154. Peterson P, Kastrup J, Helweg-Larsen S, et al. Risk factors for thromboembolic complications in chronic atrial fibrillation. Arch Intern Med 1990; 150: 819–21.
155. Gage BF, Waterman AD, Shannon W, et al. Validation of clinical classification schemes for predicting stroke. Results from the national registry of atrial fibrillation. JAMA 2001; 285: 2864–70.
156. Khumri TM, Idupulapati M, Rader VJ, et al. Clinical and echocardiographioc markers of mortality risk in patients with atrial fibrillation. Am J Cardiol 2007; 99: 1733–6.
157. Lip GYH, Nieuwlaat R, Pisters R, et al. Refining clinical risk stratification for predicting stroke and thromboembolism in atrial fibrillation using a novel risk factor-based approach. The Euro Heart Survey on Atrial Fibrillation. Chest 2010; 137: 263–72.
158. Desai HV, Aronow WS, Gandhi K, et al. Association of warfarin use with CHADS2 score in 441 patients with nonvalvular atrial fibrillation and no contraindications to warfarin. Prev Cardiol 2010; 13: 172–4.
159. Peterson P, Boysen G, Godtfredsen J, et al. Placebo-controlled, randomised trial of warfarin and aspirin for prevention of thromboembolic complications in chronic atrial fibrillation. Lancet 1989; 1: 175–9.
160. Stroke Prevention in Atrial Fibrillation Investigators. Preliminary report of the Stroke Prevention in Atrial Fibrillation Study. N Engl J Med 1990; 322: 863–8.
161. Stroke Prevention in Atrial Fibrillation Investigators. Stroke prevention in atrial fibrillation study: final results. Circulation 1991; 84: 527–39.
162. Connolly SJ, Laupacis A, Gent M, et al. Canadian Atrial Fibrillation Anticoagulation (CAFA) Study. J Am Coll Cardiol 1991; 18: 345–55.
163. Ezekowitz MD, Bridgers SL, James KE, et al. Warfarin in the prevention of stroke associated with nonrheumatic atrial fibrillation. N Engl J Med 1992; 327: 1406–12.
164. Stroke Prevention in Atrial Fibrillation Investigators. Warfarin versus aspirin for prevention of thromboembolism in atrial fibrillation: Stroke Prevention in Atrial Fibrillation II Study. Lancet 1994; 343: 687–91.
165. Gullov AL, Koefoed BG, Petersen P, et al. Fixed minidose warfarin and aspirin alone and in combination vs adjusted-dose warfarin for stroke prevention in atrial fibrillation. Second Copenhagen Atrial Fibrillation, Aspirin, and Anticoagulation Study. Arch Intern Med 1998; 158: 1513–21.

166. Aronow WS, Ahn C, Kronzon I, Gutstein H. Incidence of new thromboembolic stroke in persons ≥ 62 years old with chronic atrial fibrillation treated with warfarin versus aspirin. J Am Geriatr Soc 1999; 47: 366–8.

167. The SPAF III Writing Committee for the Stroke Prevention in Atrial Fibrillation Investigators. Patients with nonvalvular atrial fibrillation at low risk of stroke during treatment with aspirin. Stroke Prevention in Atrial Fibrillation III Study. JAMA 1998; 279: 1273–7.

168. Hylek EM, Go AS, Chang Y, et al. Effect of intensity of oral anticoagulation on stroke severity and mortality in atrial fibrillation. N Engl J Med 2003; 349: 1019–26.

169. Fang MC, Chang Y, Hylek EM, et al. Advanced age, anticoagulation intensity, and risk for intracranial hemorrhage among patients taking warfarin for atrial fibrillation. Ann Intern Med 2004; 141: 745–52.

170. Mant J, Hobbs R, Fletcher K, et al. Warfarin versus aspirin for stroke prevention in an elderly community population with atrial fibrillation (the Birmingham Atrial Fibrillation Treatment of the Aged Study, BAFTA): a randomised controlled trial. Lancet 2007; 370: 493–503.

171. Nair CK, Holmberg MJ, Aronow WS, et al. Thromboembolism in patients with atrial fibrillation with and without left atrial thrombus documented by transesophageal echocardiography. Am J Ther 2009; 16: 385–92.

172. Lai HM, Aronow WS, Kalen P, et al. Incidence of throboembolic stroke and of major bleeding in patients with atrial fibrillation and chronic kidney disease treated with and without warfarin. Int J Nephrol Renovasc Dis 2009; 2: 33–7.

173. Fuster V, Ryden LE, Cannom DS, et al. ACCF/AHA/HRS focused updates incorporated into the ACC/AHA/ESC 2006 Guidelines for the management of patients with atrial fibrillation. a report of the American College of Cardiology Foundation/American Heart Association Task Force on Practice Guidelines. and the European Society of Cardiology Committee for Practice Guidelines. Developed in partnership with the European Society of Cardiology and in collaboration with the European Heart Rhythm Association and the Heart Rhythm Society. J Am Coll Cardiol 2011; 57: e101–98.

174. Aronow WS, Frishman WH, Cheng-Lai A. Cardiovascular drug therapy in the elderly. Heart Dis 2000; 2: 151–67.

175. Singer DE, Go AS. Antithrombotic therapy in atrial fibrillation. Clin Geriatr Med 2001; 17: 131–47.

176. Kopecky SL, Gersh BJ, McGoon MD, et al. The natural history of lone atrial fibrillation. A population-based study over three decades. N Engl J Med 1987; 317: 669–74.

177. Jahangir A, Lee V, Friedman PA, et al. Long-term progression and outcomes with aging in patients with lone atrial fibrillation. A 30-year follow-up study. Circulation 2007; 115: 3050–6.

178. Brand FN, Abbott RD, Kannel WB, Wolf PA. Characteristics and prognosis of lone atrial fibrillation. 30-year follow-up in the Framingham Study. JAMA 1985; 254: 3449–53.

179. Gage BF, Boechler M, Doggette AL, et al. Adverse outcomes and predictors of underuse of antithrombotic therapy in Medicare beneficiaries with chronic atrial fibrillation. Stroke 2000; 31: 822–7.

180. Fang MC, Singer DE, Chang Y, et al. Gender differences in the risk of ischemic stroke and peripheral embolism in atrial fibrillation. The Anticoagulation and Risk Factors in Atrial Fibrillation (ATRIA) Study. Circulation 2005; 112: 1687–91.

181. The ACTIVE Writing Group on behalf of the ACTIVE Investigators. Clopidogrel plus aspirin versus oral anticoagulation for atrial fibrillation in the atrial fibrillation Clopidogrel Trial with Irbesartan for prevention of Vascular Events (ACTIVE W): a randomised controlled trial. Lancet 2006; 367: 1903–12.

182. Healey JS, Connolly SJ, Gold MR, et al. Subclinical atrial fibrillation and the risk of stroke. N Engl J Med 2012; 366: 120–9.

183. Connolly SJ, Ezekowitz MD, Yusuf S, et al. Dabigatran versus warfarin in patients with atrial fibrillation. N Engl J Med 2009; 361: 1139–51.

184. Beasley BN, Unger EF, Temple R. Anticoagulant options-why the FDA approved a higher but not a lower dose of dabigatran. N Engl J Med 2011; 364: 1788–90.

185. Patel MR, Mahaffey KW, Garg J, et al. Rivaroxaban versus warfarin in nonvalvular atrial fibrillation. N Engl J Med 2011; 365: 883–91.

186. Connolly SJ, Eikelboom J, Joyner C, et al. Apixaban in patients with atrial fibrillation. N Engl J Med 2011; 364: 806–17.

187. Granger CB, Alexander JH, McMurray JJV, et al. Apixaban versus warfarin in patients with atrial fibrillation. N Engl J Med 2011; 365: 981–92.

188. Granada J, Uribe W, Chyou P-H, et al. Incidence and predictors of atrial flutter in the general population. J Am Coll Cardiol 2000; 36: 2242–6.

189. Mehta D, Baruch L. Thromboembolism following cardioversion of common atrial flutter. Chest 1996; 110: 1001–3.

190. Lanzarotti CJ, Olshansky B. Thromboembolism in chronic atrial flutter: is the risk underestimated? J Am Coll Cardiol 1997; 30: 1506–11.

191. Grimm RA, Stewart WJ, Arheart KL, et al. Left atrial appendage "stunning" after electrical cardioversion of atrial flutter: an attenuated response compared with atrial fibrillation as the mechanism for lower susceptibility to thromboembolic events. J Am Coll Cardiol 1997; 29: 582–9.

192. Van Gelder IC, Tuinenburg AE, Schoonderwoerd BS, et al. Pharmacologic versus direct-current electrical cardioversion of atrial flutter and fibrillation. Am J Cardiol 1999; 84: 147R–51R.

193. Orlando J, Del Vicario M, Aronow WS. High reversion of atrial flutter to sinus rhythm after atrial pacing in patients with pulmonary disease. Chest 1977; 71: 580–2.

194. Parikh MG, Aziz Z, Krishnan K, et al. Usefulness of transesophageal echocardiography to confirm clinical utility of CHA2 DS2 -VASc and CHADS2 scores in atrial flutter. Am J Cardiol 2012; 109: 550–5.

195. Saxon LA, Kalman JM, Olgin JE, et al. Results of radiofrequency catheter ablation for atrial flutter. Am J Cardiol 1996; 77: 1014–16.

196. Poty H, Saoudi N, Aziz AA, et al. Radiofrequency of catheter ablation of type 1 atrial flutter: prediction of late success by electrophysiological criteria. Circulation 1995; 92: 1389–92.

197. Akhtar M, Jazayeri MR, Sra J, et al. Atrioventricular nodal reentry: clinical, electrophysiological, and therapeutic considerations. Circulation 1993; 88: 282–95.

198. Josephson ME. Paroxysmal supraventricular tachycardia. An electrophysiologic approach. Am J Cardiol 1978; 41: 1123–6.

199. Stein KM, Mittal S, Slotwiner DJ, et al. Atrial tachycardia: update. Cardiac Electrophysiol Rev 2001; 5: 290–3.

200. Aronow WS. Management of supraventricular tachyarrhythmias. Compr Ther 1989; 15: 11–16.

201. Camm AJ, Garratt CJ. Adenosine and supraventricular tachycardia. N Engl J Med 1991; 325: 1621–9.

202. Winniford MD, Fulton KL, Hillis LD. Long-term therapy of paroxysmal supraventricular tachycardia: a randomized, double-blind comparison of digoxin, propranolol and verapamil. Am J Cardiol 1984; 54: 1138–9.

203. Ganz LI, Friedman PL. Supraventricular tachycardia. N Engl J Med 1995; 332: 162–73.

204. Epstein LM, Chiesa N, Wong MN, et al. Radiofrequency catheter ablation in the treatment of supraventricular tachycardia in the elderly. J Am Coll Cardiol 1994; 23: 1356–62.

205. Rosen KM. Junctional tachycardia: mechanisms, diagnosis, differential diagnosis, and management. Circulation 1973; 47: 654–64.

206. Hazard PB, Burnett CR. Verapamil in multifocal atrial tachycardia. Hemodynamic and respiratory changes. Chest 1987; 91: 68–70.

207. Aronow WS, Plascencia G, Wong R, et al. Effect of verapamil versus placebo on PAT and MAT (paroxysmal atrial tachycardia and multifocal atrial tachycardia). Curr Ther Res 1980; 27: 823–9.

22
Ventricular arrhythmias in the elderly

Wilbert S. Aronow

SUMMARY

Underlying causes of ventricular tachycardia (VT) or complex ventricular arrhythmias (VA) should be treated if possible. Antiarrhythmic drugs should not be used to treat asymptomatic patients with complex VA and no heart disease. Beta blockers are the only antiarrhythmic drugs that have been documented to reduce mortality in patients with VT or complex VA. Radiofrequency catheter ablation of VT has been beneficial in treating selected patients with arrhythmogenic foci of monomorphic VT. The automatic implantable cardioverter-defibrillator (AICD) is the most effective treatment for patients with life-threatening VT or ventricular fibrillation. The American College of Cardiology Foundation/American Heart Association Class I and IIa indications for an AICD are discussed. Patients with AICDs should be treated with biventricular pacing, not with dual-chamber rate-responsive pacing at a rate of 70/minute. Patients with AICDs should be treated with beta blockers, statins, and angiotensin-converting enzyme inhibitors or angiotensin blockers.

The presence of three or more consecutive ventricular premature complexes (VPCs) on an electrocardiogram (ECG) is diagnosed as ventricular tachycardia (VT) (1,2). VT is considered sustained if it lasts ≥30 seconds and nonsustained if its lasts <30 seconds (2). Complex ventricular arrhythmias (VA) include VT or paired, multiform, or frequent VPCs. This author considers frequent VPCs an average of ≥30/hour on a 24-hour ambulatory electrocardiogram (AECG) or ≥6/minute on a 1-minute rhythm strip of an ECG (2,3). Simple VA includes infrequent VPCs and no complex forms.

PREVALENCE OF COMPLEX VENTRICULAR ARRHYTHMIAS

The prevalence of nonsustained VT detected by 24-hour AECGs was 4% in 98 older, disease-free persons in the Baltimore Longitudinal Study of Aging (1), 4% in 106 active older persons (4), 2% in 50 older persons without cardiovascular disease (5), 4% in 729 older women and 13% in 643 older men in the Cardiovascular Health Study (6), 3% in 135 older men and 2% in 297 older women without cardiovascular disease (7), 9% in 385 older men and 8% in 806 older women with hypertension, valvular disease, or cardiomyopathy (7), and 16% in 395 older men and 15% in 771 older women with coronary artery disease (CAD) (7). The prevalence of complex VA in older persons in these studies was 50% (1), 31% (4), 20% (5), 16% in women and 28% in men (6), 31% in older men and 30% in older women without cardiovascular disease (7), 54% in older men and 55% in older women with hypertension, valvular disease, or cardiomyopathy (7), and 69% in older men and 68% in older women with CAD (7).

In 104 older persons, mean age 82 years, without cardiovascular disease who had a 12-lead ECG with a 1-minute rhythm strip obtained within 24 hours of a 24-hour AECG, complex VA were present on the 24-hour AECGs in 33% of persons and on the 1-minute rhythm strips in 2% of persons (3). In this study, in 843 older persons, mean age 82 years, with cardiovascular disease, complex VA were present on the 24-hour AECGs in 55% of persons and on the 1-minute rhythm strips in 4% of persons (3).

In older persons with cardiovascular disease, those with an abnormal left ventricular (LV) ejection fraction (8), with echocardiographic LV hypertrophy (9), or with silent myocardial ischemia (10) have a higher prevalence of VT and of complex VA than those with normal LV ejection fraction, normal LV mass, and no myocardial ischemia.

PROGNOSIS OF VENTRICULAR ARRHYTHMIAS
No Heart Disease

In the Baltimore Longitudinal Study of Aging, nonsustained VT or complex VA were not associated with an increased incidence of new coronary events at 10-year follow-up in 98 older subjects with no clinical evidence of heart disease (11). In addition, in this study, exercise-induced nonsustained VT was not associated with an increased incidence of new coronary events at 2-year follow-up in older persons with no clinical evidence of heart disease (12). And at 5.6-year follow-up in this study, exercise-induced frequent or repetitive VPCs also were not associated with an increased incidence of new coronary events in older persons with no clinical evidence of heart disease (13).

Nonsustained VT or complex VA diagnosed by 24-hour AECGs were not associated with an increased incidence of new coronary events at 2-year follow-up in 76 older persons with no clinical evidence of heart disease (14) and were not associated with an increased incidence of primary ventricular fibrillation (VF) or sudden cardiac death in 86 older persons with no clinical evidence of heart disease (15). Complex VA diagnosed by 24-hour AECGs or by 12-lead ECGs with 1-minute rhythm strips were also not associated with an increased incidence of new coronary events at 39-month follow-up in 104 older persons with no clinical evidence of heart disease (3). Nonsustained VT or complex VA diagnosed by 24-hour AECGs were not associated with an increased incidence of new coronary events at 45-month follow-up of 135 men and at 47-month follow-up of 297 women without cardiovascular disease (7).

Because nonsustained VT or complex VA are not associated with an increased incidence of new coronary events in older persons with no clinical evidence of heart disease, asymptomatic nonsustained VT or complex VA in older persons without heart disease should not be treated with antiarrhythmic drugs. Because simple VA in older persons with heart disease are not associated with an increased incidence of new coronary events (3,7,11,14,15), simple VA in older persons without heart disease should not be treated with antiarrhythmic drugs.

Heart Disease

Numerous studies have documented that patients with VT or with complex VA associated with heart disease are at increased risk for developing new coronary events (16–19). Prospective studies in older persons, mean age 82 years, with heart disease also demonstrated that nonsustained VT and complex VA were significantly associated with an increased incidence of new coronary events and with an increased incidence of primary VF or sudden cardiac death (Table 22.1) (3,7,11,14,15).

Table 22.1 Association of Complex Ventricular Arrhythmias and Ventricular Tachycardia with New Coronary Events in Elderly Patients with Heart Disease

Study	Mean Age [yr]	Cardiac Status	Follow-Up [mo]	Incidence of New Coronary Events
Aronow et al. (n = 843) (3)	82	Heart disease	39	Increased 1.7 times by complex VA
Aronow et al. (n = 391) (14)	82	Heart disease	24	With normal LVEF, increased 2.5 times by complex VA and 3.2 times by VT; increased 7.6 times by complex VA plus abnormal LVEF and increased 6.8 times by VT plus abnormal LVEF
Aronow et al. (n = 468) (15)	82	Heart disease	27	With no LVH, SCD or VF increased 2.4 times by complex VA and 1.8 times by VT; SCD or VF increased 7.3 times by complex VA plus LVH and increased 7.1 times by VT plus LVH
Aronow et al. (n = 404) (10)	82	Heart disease	37	Increased 1.7 times by VT and 2.4 times by complex VA; increased 2.5 times by VT plus SI and 4.0 times by complex VA plus SI
Aronow et al. (n = 395 men) (7)	80	CAD	45	Increased 2.4 times by complex VA and 1.7 times by VT
Aronow et al. (n = 385 men) (7)	80	HT, VD, or CMP	45	Increased 1.9 times by complex VA and 1.9 times by VT
Aronow et al. (n = 771 women) (7)	81	CAD	47	Increased 2.5 times by complex VA and 1.7 times by VT
Aronow et al. (n = 806 women) (7)	81	HT, VD, or CMP	47	Increased 2.2 times by complex VA and 2.0 times by VT

Abbreviations: VA, ventricular arrhythmias; VT, ventricular tachycardia; LVEF, left ventricular ejection fraction; LVH, left ventricular hypertrophy; SCD, sudden coronary death; VF, primary ventricular fibrillation; CAD, coronary artery disease; HT, hypertension; VD, valvular heart disease; CMP, cardiomyopathy; SI, silent ischemia.

MEDICAL THERAPY
General Measures

Underlying causes of complex VA should be treated, if possible. Treatment of congestive heart failure (CHF), digitalis toxicity, hypokalemia, hypomagnesemia, hypertension, LV dysfunction, LV hypertrophy, myocardial ischemia by anti-ischemic drugs such as beta blockers or by coronary revascularization, hypoxia, and other conditions may abolish or reduce complex VA. The older person should not smoke or drink alcohol and should avoid drugs that may cause or increase complex VA.

All older persons with CAD should be treated with aspirin (20–23), with beta blockers (23–28), with angiotensin-converting enzyme (ACE) inhibitors (23,28–33), and with 3-hydroxy-3-methylglutaryl coenzyme A reductase inhibitors (23,34–40) unless there are contraindications to these drugs. The serum low-density lipoprotein (LDL) cholesterol level should be reduced to <70 mg/dl (40). The serum LDL cholesterol level should be reduced at least 30–40% (40).

Age-related physiologic changes may affect absorption, distribution, metabolism, and excretion of cardiovascular drugs (41). There are numerous physiologic changes with aging that affect pharmacodynamics with alterations in end-organ responsiveness to cardiovascular drugs (41). Drug interactions between antiarrhythmic drugs and other cardiovascular drugs are common, especially in older persons (41). There are also important drug-disease interactions that occur in older persons (41). Class I antiarrhythmic drugs have an unacceptable proarrhythmia rate in patients with heart disease and should be avoided. Class III antiarrhythmic drugs should also be used with caution in older patients with heart disease since multiple factors may increase the incidence of proarrhythmia. Except for beta blockers, all antiarrhythmic drugs may cause torsades de pointes (VT with polymorphous appearance associated with prolonged QT interval).

Class I Antiarrhythmic Drugs

Class I antiarrhythmic drugs are sodium channel blockers. Class Ia antiarrhythmic drugs have intermediate channel kinetics and prolong repolarization. These drugs include quinidine, procainamide, and disopyramide. Class Ib antiarrhythmic drugs have rapid channel kinetics and slightly shorten repolarization. These drugs include lidocaine, mexilitine, tocainide, and phenytoin. Class Ic drugs have slow channel kinetics and have little effect on repolarization. These drugs include encainide, flecainide, moricizine, propafenone, and lorcainide. None of the Class I antiarrhythmic drugs have been demonstrated in controlled, clinical trials to reduce sudden cardiac death, total cardiac death, or total mortality.

The International Mexilitine and Placebo Antiarrhythmic Coronary Trial (IMPACT) was a prospective, double-blind, randomized study in survivors of myocardial infarction (MI), mean age 57 years, in whom 317 persons were randomized to mexilitine and 313 persons to placebo (42). Complex VA were present on 24-hour AECGs at study entry in 31% of persons randomized to mexilitine and in 38% of persons randomized to placebo. At 1-year follow-up, mortality was 7.6% for mexilitine-treated patients versus 4.8% for placebo-treated patients (42).

The Cardiac Arrhythmia Suppression Trial (CAST) I was a prospective, double-blind, randomized study in survivors of MI with asymptomatic or mildly symptomatic VA in which 730 patients were randomized to encainide or flecainide and 725 patients to placebo (43). The prevalence of nonsustained VT was 21%. Mean LV ejection fraction was 40%. Thirty-eight percent of patients were 66–79 years of age. Adequate suppression of VA by encainide or flecainide was required before randomization. Despite adequate suppression of VA, at 10-month follow-up, encainide and flecainide significantly increased mortality from arrhythmia or cardiac arrest (relative risk = 3.6; 95% CI 1.7–8.5) and significantly increased total mortality (relative risk = 2.5; 95% CI 1.6–4.5) (41). Older age increased the likelihood of adverse events, including death, in patients receiving encainide and flecainide (44).

CAST II was a prospective, double-blind, randomized study in survivors of MI with asymptomatic or mildly symptomatic VA in which 581 patients were randomized to moricizine and 574 patients to placebo (45). The prevalence of nonsustained VT was 30%. Mean LV ejection fraction was 33%. Thirty-eight percent of patients were 66–79 years of age. Adequate suppression of VA by moricizine was required before randomization.

At 18-month follow-up, the mortality from arrhythmia or cardiac arrest was 8.4% for patients treated with moricizine and 7.3% for patients treated with placebo (45). The 2-year survival rate was 81.7% for patients treated with moricizine and 85.6% for patients treated with placebo (45). The investigators concluded that the use of moricizine in this study was "...not only ineffective but also harmful" (45). Older age increased the likelihood of adverse events, including death, in patients receiving moricizine (44).

An analysis of the CAST I and II studies showed that older age was an independent predictor of adverse events (relative risk 1.30 per decade of age) (44). On the basis of the CAST I and CAST II data, the author would not use encainide, flecainide, or moricizine for the treatment of VT or complex VA in older or younger patients with heart disease.

Aronow et al. (46) performed a prospective study in 406 older persons, mean age 82 years, with heart disease (58% with prior MI) and asymptomatic complex VA diagnosed by 24-hour AECGs. The prevalence of nonsustained VT was 20%. The prevalence of an abnormal ejection fraction was 32%. The incidence of adverse effects causing cessation of drug was 48% for quinidine and 55% for procainamide. Of 406 older persons, 220 were treated with quinidine ($n = 213$) or procainamide ($n = 7$) and 186 with no antiarrhythmic drug. Follow-up 24-hour AECGs in 25 persons with nonsustained VT and in 104 persons with complex VA showed that quinidine or procainamide decreased nonsustained VT more than 90% in 84% of the persons and decreased the average number of VPCs/hour more than 70% in 84% of the persons (46).

At 24-month follow-up, the incidences of sudden cardiac death, total cardiac death, and of total death were not significantly different in persons treated with quinidine or procainamide or with no antiarrhythmic drug (46). The incidence of total mortality was 65% for persons treated with quinidine or procainamide and 63% for persons treated with no antiarrhythmic drug. Quinidine or procainamide did not decrease sudden cardiac death, total cardiac death, or total death in comparison with no antiarrhythmic drug in older patients with ischemic or nonischemic heart disease, abnormal or normal LV ejection fraction, and presence versus absence of VT (46).

Moosvi et al. (47) performed a retrospective analysis of the effect of empiric antiarrhythmic therapy in 209 resuscitated out-of-hospital cardiac arrest patients, mean age 62 years, with CAD. Of the 209 patients, 48 received quinidine, 45 received procainamide, and 116 received no antiarrhythmic drug. The 2-year sudden death survival was 69% for quinidine-treated patients, 69% for procainamide-treated patients, and 89% for patients treated with no antiarrhythmic drug ($p < 0.01$) (47). The 2-year total survival was 61% for quinidine-treated patients, 57% for procainamide-treated patients, and 71% for patients treated with no antiarrhythmic drug ($p < 0.05$) (47).

Hallstrom et al. (48) performed a retrospective analysis of the effect of antiarrhythmic drug use in 941 patients, mean age 62 years, resuscitated from prehospital cardiac arrest attributable to VF between 1970 and 1985. Quinidine was administered to 19% of the patients, procainamide to 18% of the patients, beta blockers to 28% of the patients, and no antiarrhythmic drug to 39% of the patients. There was an increased incidence of death or recurrent cardiac arrest in patients treated with quinidine or procainamide versus no antiarrhythmic drug (adjusted relative risk = 1.17; 95% CI 0.98–1.41). Survival was significantly worse for patients treated with procainamide than for patients treated with quinidine (adjusted relative risk = 1.57; 95% CI 1.21–2.07) (48).

A meta-analysis of six double-blind studies comprising 808 patients with chronic atrial fibrillation who underwent direct-current cardioversion to sinus rhythm showed that the mortality at 1 year was significantly higher in patients treated with quinidine (2.9%) than in patients treated with placebo (0.8%) ($p < 0.05$) (49). Of 1330 patients in the Stroke Prevention in Atrial Fibrillation Study, 127 were receiving quinidine, 57 procainamide, 15 disopyramide,

34 flecainide, 20 encainide, and 7 amiodarone (50). The adjusted relative risk of cardiac mortality was 1.8 times higher (95% CI 0.7–3.7) and the adjusted relative risk of arrhythmic death was 2.1 times higher (95% CI 0.8–5.0) in patients on antiarrhythmic drugs than in patients not on antiarrhythmic drugs (50). In patients with a history of CHF, the adjusted relative risk of cardiac death was 3.3 times higher (95% CI 1.1–8.2) and the adjusted relative risk of arrhythmic death was 5.8 times higher (95% CI 1.2–13.5) in patients receiving antiarrhythmic drugs than in patients not receiving antiarrhythmic drugs (50).

Morganroth and Goin (51) performed a meta-analysis of four randomized, double-blind controlled trials lasting 2–12 weeks in which quinidine ($n = 502$) was compared with flecainide ($n = 141$), mexiletine ($n = 246$), tocainide ($n = 67$), and propafenone ($n = 53$) in the treatment of complex VA. There was an increased risk of mortality in patients treated with quinidine compared with patients treated with the other antiarrhythmic drugs (absolute risk increase = 1.6%; 95% CI 0–3.1%) (51).

Teo et al. (52) analyzed 59 randomized controlled trials comprising 23,229 patients that investigated the use of Class I antiarrhythmic drugs after MI. The Class I drugs investigated included quinidine, procainamide, disopyramide, imipramine, moricizine, lidocaine, tocainide, phenytoin, mexiletine, aprindine, encainide, and flecainide. Mortality was significantly higher in patients receiving Class I antiarrhythmic drugs than in patients receiving no antiarrhythmic drugs (odds ratio = 1.14; 95% CI 1.01–1.28). None of the 59 studies demonstrated that the use of a Class I antiarrhythmic drug decreased mortality in postinfarction patients (52).

On the basis of the data from the studies discussed in this section, none of the Class I antiarrhythmic drugs should be used for the treatment of VT or complex VA in older or younger patients with heart disease.

Calcium Channel Blockers

Calcium channel blockers are not useful in the treatment of complex VA. Although verapamil can terminate a left septal fascicular VT, hemodynamic collapse can occur if intravenous verapamil is administered to patients with the more common forms of re-entry VT. Teo et al. (52) analyzed randomized controlled trials comprising 20,342 patients that investigated the use of calcium channel blockers after MI. Mortality was insignificantly higher in patients receiving calcium channel blockers than in patients receiving no antiarrhythmic drugs (odds ratio = 1.04; 95% CI 0.95–1.14) (52). On the basis of these data, none of the calcium channel blockers should be used in the treatment of VT or complex VA in older or younger patients with heart disease.

Beta Blockers

Teo et al. (52) analyzed 55 randomized controlled trials comprising 53,268 patients that investigated the use of beta blockers after MI. Mortality was significantly reduced in patients receiving beta blockers compared with control patients (odds ratio = 0.81; 95% CI 0.75–0.87) (52).

Beta blockers caused a greater reduction in mortality in older persons after MI than in younger persons after MI (24–27,53). The decrease in mortality after MI in persons treated with beta blockers was due to both a reduction in sudden cardiac death and recurrent MI (24–27,53).

The Beta Blocker Heart Attack Trial was a double-blind, randomized study that included 3290 patients after MI (53–55). Thirty-three percent of the patients were 60–69 years of age. At 25-month follow-up, propranolol decreased sudden cardiac death by 28% in patients with complex VA and by 16% in patients without complex VA. Propranolol significantly reduced total mortality by 34% in patients aged 60–69 years

($p = 0.01$) and insignificantly reduced total mortality by 19% in patients aged 30–59 years (Table 22.2) (53–55).

Beta blockers reduce complex VA including VT (55–57). Beta blockers also increase VF threshold in animal models and have been found to decrease VF in patients with acute MI (58) A randomized, double-blind, placebo-controlled study of propranolol in high-risk survivors of acute MI at 12 Norwegian hospitals showed a 52% significant reduction in sudden cardiac death in patients treated with propranolol for 1 year ($p = 0.038$) (Table 22.2) (58).

Beta blockers reduce myocardial oxygen demand and decrease myocardial ischemia, which may reduce the likelihood of VF. Stone et al. (59) showed by 48-hour AECGs in 50 patients with stable angina pectoris that propranolol, but not diltiazem or nifedipine, caused a significant reduction in the mean number of episodes of myocardial ischemia and in the mean duration of myocardial ischemia compared with placebo. Beta blockers also decrease sympathetic tone, increase vagal tone, and stabilize cardiac membrane potentials, which reduces the likelihood of VF. In addition, beta blockers are antithrombotic (60) and may prevent atherosclerotic plaque rupture (61).

In the retrospective study by Hallstrom et al. (48) in 941 patients, mean age 62 years, resuscitated from prehospital cardiac arrest attributed to VF, beta blockers were administered to 28% of the patients and no antiarrhythmic drug to 39% of the patients. At 108-month follow-up, patients treated with beta blockers had a significant decreased incidence

Table 22.2 Effect of Beta Blockers on Mortality in Patients with Heart Disease and Complex Ventricular Arrhythmias

Study	Results
Hallstrom et al. (48)	At 108-mo follow-up, the adjusted relative risk of death or recurrent cardiac arrest on beta blockers versus no antiarrhythmic drug was 0.62
Beta Blocker Heart Attack Trial (53–55)	At 25-mo follow-up, propranolol decreased sudden cardiac death by 28% in persons with complex VA and by 16% in persons without VA; propranolol significantly reduced total mortality by 34% in persons aged 60–69 yr
Norwegian Propranolol Study (58)	High-risk survivors of acute myocardial infarction treated with propranolol for 1 yr had a 52% significant reduction in sudden cardiac death
Aronow et al. (62)	At 29-mo follow-up, compared with no antiarrhythmic drug, propranolol caused a 47% significant decrease in sudden cardiac death, a 37% significant reduction in total cardiac death, and a 20% borderline significant reduction in total death
Cardiac Arrhythmia Suppression Trial (67)	Persons on beta blockers had a significant reduction in all-cause mortality of 43% at 30 days, of 46% at 1 yr, and of 33% at 2 yr and a significant reduction in arrhythmic death or cardiac arrest of 66% at 30 days, of 53% at 1 yr, and of 36% at 2 yr; beta blockers were an independent factor for reduced arrhythmic death or cardiac arrest by 40% and for reduced all-cause mortality by 33%

Abbreviation: VA, ventricular arrhythmias.

of death or recurrent cardiac arrest compared to patients treated with no antiarrhythmic drug (adjusted relative risk = 0.62; 95% CI 0.50–0.77) (Table 22.2) (48).

Aronow et al. (62) performed a prospective study in 245 older persons, mean age 81 years, with heart disease (64% with prior MI and 36% with hypertensive heart disease), complex VA and no sustained VT diagnosed by 24-hour AECGs, and a LV ejection fraction ≥40%. Nonsustained VT occurred in 32% of patients. Silent myocardial ischemia occurred in 33% of patients. Of the 245 patients, 123 were randomized to propranolol and 122 to no antiarrhythmic drug. Follow-up was 29 months. Propranolol was discontinued because of adverse effects in 14 of 123 patients (11%).

Follow-up 24-hour AECGs were obtained at a median of 6 months in 91% of patients treated with propranolol and in 89% of patients treated with no antiarrhythmic drug (62). Propranolol was significantly more effective than no antiarrhythmic drug in reducing VT >90% (71% vs. 25% of patients) ($p < 0.001$) and in decreasing the average number of VPCs/hour >70% (71% vs. 25% of patients) ($p < 0.001$) (62). The prevalence of silent myocardial ischemia on the follow-up 24-hour AECGs was insignificantly higher on no antiarrhythmic drug. However, silent ischemia was significantly abolished by propranolol, with 37% of patients with silent ischemia on their baseline 24-hour AECGs having no silent ischemia on their follow-up 24-hour AECGs ($p < 0.001$) (62).

Multivariate Cox regression analyses showed that propranolol caused a 47% significant reduction in sudden cardiac death ($p = 0.01$), a 37% significant decrease in total cardiac death ($p = 0.003$), and a 20% insignificant decrease in total death ($p = 0.057$) (Table 22.2) (62). Univariate Cox regression analysis showed that among patients taking propranolol, suppression of complex VA caused a 33% insignificant reduction in sudden cardiac death, a 27% insignificant decrease in total cardiac death, and a 30% insignificant reduction in total death (63). Among patients taking propranolol, abolition of silent myocardial ischemia caused a 70% significant decrease in sudden cardiac death (95% CI 0.12–0.75), a 70% significant reduction in total cardiac death (95% CI 0.14–0.56), and a 69% significant decrease in total death (95% CI 0.18–0.53) (63).

There was also a circadian distribution of sudden cardiac death or fatal MI with the peak incidence occurring from 6 a.m. to 12 p.m. (peak hour was 8 a.m. and a secondary peak occurred around 7 p.m.) in patients treated with no antiarrhythmic drug (64) Propranolol abolished this circadian distribution of sudden cardiac death or fatal MI (64). In this study, propranolol also markedly reduced the circadian variation of complex VA (65) and abolished the circadian variation of myocardial ischemia (66).

In a retrospective analysis of the data from the CAST study, Kennedy et al. (67) found that 30% of patients with a LV ejection fraction ≤40% were receiving beta blockers. Forty percent of the patients were between 66 and 79 years of age. Patients on beta blockers had a significant decrease in all-cause mortality of 43% at 30 days ($p = 0.03$), of 46% at 1 year ($p = 0.001$), and of 33% at 2 years ($p < 0.001$) (Table 22.2) (67). Patients receiving beta blockers had a significant reduction in arrhythmic death or cardiac arrest of 66% at 30 days ($p = 0.002$), of 53% at 1 year ($p = 0.001$), and of 36% at 2 years ($p = 0.001$) (67). Multivariate analysis showed that beta blockers were an independent factor for decreasing arrhythmic death or cardiac arrest by 40% (95% CI 0.36–0.99), for reducing all-cause mortality by 33% ($p = 0.05$), and for decreasing occurrence of new or worsened CHF by 32% (95% CI 0.49–0.94) (Table 22.2) (67).

Angiotensin-Converting Enzyme Inhibitors

ACE inhibitors have been demonstrated to cause a significant reduction in complex VA in patients with CHF in some studies (68,69), but not in other studies (70,71). ACE inhibitors have also been shown to reduce sudden cardiac death in some studies of patients with CHF (32,72).

ACE inhibitors should be administered to reduce total mortality in older and younger patients with CHF (30,32,72,73), an anterior MI (31), an MI with a LV ejection fraction ≤40% (28,29,32), and in all patients with atherosclerotic cardiovascular disease (23,33). ACE inhibitors should be used to treat patients with CHF with abnormal LV ejection fraction (30,32,72,73) or with normal LV ejection fraction (74,75).

On the basis of the available data, ACE inhibitors should be used in treating older or younger patients with VT or complex VA associated with CHF, an anterior MI, an MI with LV systolic dysfunction, or atherosclerotic cardiovascular disease if there are no contraindications to the use of ACE inhibitors. Beta blockers should be used in addition to ACE inhibitors in treating these patients.

Class III Antiarrhythmic Drugs

Class III antiarrhythmic drugs are potassium channel blockers which prolong repolarization manifested by an increase in QT interval on the ECG. These drugs suppress VA by increasing the refractory period. However, prolonging cardiac repolarization and refractory period can trigger after depolarizations and resultant torsade de pointes.

In the Survival With Oral d-Sotalol (SWORD) Trial, 3121 survivors of MI, mean age 60 years, with a LV ejection fraction ≤40% were randomized to d-sotalol, a pure potassium channel blocker with no beta blocking activity, or to double-blind placebo (Table 22.3) (76). At 148-day follow-up, mortality was 5.0% in patients treated with d-sotalol versus 3.1% in patients treated with placebo (relative risk = 1.65; 95% CI 1.15–2.36) (Table 22.3) (76). Presumed arrhythmic deaths accounted for the increased mortality (relative risk = 1.77; 95% CI 1.15–2.74) (76). On the basis of these data, d-sotalol should not be used for the treatment of VT or complex VA in older or younger patients with heart disease.

Table 22.3 Effect of Class III Antiarrhythmic Drugs on Mortality in Patients with Heart Disease and Complex Ventricular Arrhythmias

Study	Results
Waldo et al. (76)	At 148-day follow-up, mortality was 5.0% for d-sotalol versus 3.1% for placebo (relative risk = 1.65;95% CI, 1.15–2.36)
Julian et al. (77)	At 1-yr follow-up, compared with placebo, d,l-sotalol caused an insignificant reduction in mortality
Singh et al. (82)	Compared with placebo, amiodarone significantly suppressed VT and complex VA ($p < 0.001$); 2-yr survival was not significantly different for amiodarone (69.4%) versus placebo (70.8%)
Canadian Amiodarone Myocardial Infarction Arrhythmia Trial (83)	Amiodarone was very effective in suppressing VT and complex VA; at 1.8-yr follow-up, compared with placebo, amiodarone caused an 18% insignificant reduction in mortality
European Myocardial Infarct Amiodarone Trial (85)	At 21-mo follow-up, mortality was similar for amiodarone (13.9%) versus placebo (13.7%)
Sudden Cardiac Death in Heart Failure Trial (86)	At 45.5-mo follow-up, compared with placebo, amiodarone caused a 6% insignificant increase in mortality, and implantable cardioverter-defibrillator therapy reduced mortality by 23% ($p = 0.007$)

Abbrevaition: VA, ventricular arrhythmias.

Studies comparing the effect of d,l-sotalol, a Class III antiarrhythmic drug with beta blocking activity, versus placebo or beta blockers in patients with VT or complex VA have not been performed. In a study of 1486 patients with prior MI, compared with placebo, d,l-sotalol did not significantly reduce mortality in patients followed for 1 year (Table 22.3) (77).

In the Electrophysiologic Study versus Electrocardiographic Monitoring (ESVEM) study, 74% of 486 patients were ≥60 years of age (78). In this study, Holter monitor-guided therapy significantly predicted antiarrhythmic drug efficacy more often than did the electrophysiologic study in patients with sustained VT or survivors of cardiac arrest (77% vs. 45% of patients). However, there was no significant difference in the success of drug therapy selected by the two methods in preventing recurrences of ventricular tachyarrhythmias.

In the ESVEM study, d,l-sotalol was more effective than the other six antiarrhythmic drugs (imipramine, mexiletine, pirmenol, procainamide, propafenone, and quinidine) used in reducing recurrence of arrhythmia, death from arrhythmia, death from cardiac causes, and death from any cause (79). However, 7 of 10 episodes of torsade de pointes during this study occurred in patients receiving d,l-sotalol (79). In 481 patients with VT, d,l-sotalol caused torsade de pointes (12 patients) or an increase in VT episodes (11 patients) in 23 patients (4.9%) (80). Women had a significantly higher risk for drug-induced VF.

On the basis of the available data, the use of beta blockers is recommended over the use of d,l-sotalol in treating older or younger patients with VT or complex VA associated with heart disease.

Amiodarone is very effective in suppressing VT and complex VA associated with heart disease (81–83). Unfortunately, the incidence of adverse effects from amiodarone approaches 90% after 5 years of therapy (84). In the Cardiac Arrest in Seattle: Conventional Versus Amiodarone Drug Evaluation study, the incidence of pulmonary toxicity was 10% at 2 years in patients receiving an amiodarone dose of 158 mg/day (81). Amiodarone can also cause cardiac adverse effects, gastrointestinal adverse effects including hepatitis, hyperthyroidism, hypothyroidism, and neurologic, dermatologic, and ophthalmologic adverse effects.

A double-blind study randomized 674 patients with CHF and complex VA to amiodarone or placebo (Table 22.3) (82). Compared with placebo, amiodarone significantly reduced the number of episodes of VT ($p < 0.001$) and the frequency of complex VA ($p < 0.001$). Twenty-seven percent of patients discontinued amiodarone in this study. At 2-year follow-up, survival was not significantly different in patients treated with amiodarone (69.4%) or placebo (70.8%) (Table 22.3) (82).

The Canadian Amiodarone Myocardial Infarction Arrhythmia Trial (CAMIAT) randomized 1202 survivors of MI with nonsustained VT or complex VA to amiodarone or placebo (Table 22.3) (83). Amiodarone was very effective in suppressing VT and complex VA in this study (Table 22.3) (83). Early permanent discontinuation of amiodarone for reasons other than adverse events occurred in 36% of patients taking this drug (83). At 1.8-year follow-up, amiodarone caused an 18% insignificant reduction in mortality (Table 22.3) (83).

The European Myocardial Infarction Amiodarone Trial (EMIAT) randomized 1486 survivors of MI with a LV ejection fraction ≤40% to amiodarone or placebo (Table 22.3) (85). Early permanent discontinuation of amiodarone occurred in 38.5% of patients taking this drug. At 21-month follow-up, mortality was similar in patients treated with amiodarone (13.9%) or with placebo (13.7%) (Table 22.3) (85).

In the Sudden Cardiac Death in Heart Failure Trial (SCD-HEFT), 2521 patients, mean age 60 years, with New York Heart Association (NYHA) Class II or III CHF due to ischemic or nonischemic heart disease, a LV ejection fraction of 35% or less, and a mean

QRS duration on the resting ECG of 120 ms were randomized to placebo, amiodarone, or an automatic implantable cardioverter-defibrillator (AICD) (Table 22.3) (86). At 45.5-month median follow-up, compared with placebo, amiodarone insignificantly increased mortality by 6% (Table 22.3) (86). At 45.5-month median follow-up, compared with placebo, AICD therapy significantly reduced all-cause mortality by 23% ($p = 0.007$), with an absolute reduction in mortality of 7.2% after 5 years (86).

Since amiodarone has not been found to reduce mortality in older or younger patients with VT or complex VA associated with MI or CHF and has a very high incidence of toxicity, beta blockers should be used rather than amiodarone in treating these patients. A meta-analysis of 10 randomized trials showed that the use of beta blockers significantly reduced 2-year mortality in patients receiving AICD therapy ($p < 0.01$) (87). In a study of 965 patients, mean age 70 years, with AICDs, at 32-month mean follow-up, use of beta blockers significantly reduced all-cause mortality by 46% ($p < 0.001$), whereas use of amiodarone or sotalolol did not significantly affect mortality (88). During 33-month mean follow-up of 1038 patients with AICDs, use of beta blockers significantly reduced appropriate AICD shocks ($p < 0.001$) (89). Use of amiodarone plus a beta blocker was not more effective than beta blocker therapy alone in reducing AICD shocks for any reason (89). In this study, use of sotalol did not decrease appropriate AICD shocks (89).

INVASIVE INTERVENTION

If patients have life-threatening recurrent VT or VF resistant to antiarrhythmic drugs, invasive intervention should be performed. Patients with critical coronary artery stenosis and severe myocardial ischemia should undergo coronary artery bypass graft surgery to reduce mortality (90). In the Coronary Artery Bypass Graft (CABG) Patch Trial, there was no evidence of improved survival among patients with CAD, LV ejection fraction <36%, and an abnormal signal-averaged ECG undergoing complete coronary revascularization in whom an AICD was implanted prophylactically at the time of elective coronary artery bypass graft surgery (91).

Surgical ablation of the arhythmogenic focus in patients with life-threatening ventricular tachyarrhythmias can be curative. This therapy includes aneurysectomy or infarctectomy and endocardial resection with or without adjunctive cryoablation based on activation mapping in the operating room (92–94). However, the perioperative mortality rate is high. Endoaneurysmorrhaphy with a pericardial patch combined with mapping-guided subendocardial resection frequently cures recurrent VT with a low operative mortality and improvement of LV systolic function (95). Radiofrequency catheter ablation of VT has also been beneficial in the therapy of selected patients with arrhythmogenic foci of monomorphic VT (96–98). Catheter ablation has been very effectively used to treat patients with right ventricular outflow tract VT and LV fascicular VT. Prophylactic VT ablation should be considered before implantation of an AICD in patients with stable VT, prior MI, and reduced LV ejection fraction (99).

Automatic Implantable Cardioverter-Defibrillator

However, the AICD has been widely accepted as the most effective treatment for patients with life-threatening VT or VF. Tresch et al. (93,94) showed in retrospective studies that the AICD was very effective in treating life-threatening VT in older as well as in younger patients.

The Multicenter Automatic Defibrillator Implantation Trial (MADIT) randomized 196 patients, mean age 63 years, with a prior MI, a LV ejection fraction ≤35%, a documented episode of asymptomatic nonsustained VT, and inducible nonsuppressible ventricular tachyarrhythmia on electrophysiologic study to receive an AICD or conventional

Table 22.4 Effect of the Automatic Implantable Cardioverter-Defibrillator on Mortality in Patients with Ventricular Tachyarrhythmias

Study	Results
Multicenter Automatic Defibrillator Implantation Trial (100)	At 27-mo follow-up, the AICD caused a 54% significant reduction in mortality (95% CI, 0.26–0.82)
Antiarrhythmics versus Implantable Defibrillators Trial (101)	1-yr survival was 89.3% for AICD versus 82.3% for drug therapy (95% CI, 39 ± 20% decrease in mortality); 2-yr survival was 81.6% for AICD versus 74.7% for drug therapy (95% CI, 27±21% decrease in mortality); 3-yr survival was 75.4% for AICD versus 64.1% for drug therapy (95% CI, 31 ± 21% decrease in mortality)
Canadian Implantable Defibrillator Study (102)	Mortality was 10.2% per year for amiodarone and 8.3% per year for an AICD (risk reduction = 20%; $p = 0.072$)
Cardiac Arrest Study Hamburg (104)	Propafenone was discontinued at 11 mo because mortality from sudden death and cardiac arrest recurrence was 23% for propafenone versus 0% for an AICD ($p < 0.05$)
Cardiac Arrest Study Hamburg (105)	2-year mortality was 12.6% for an AICD versus 19.6% for amiodarone or metoprolol (37% reduction in mortality; $p = 0.047$)
Multicenter Unsustained Tachycardia Trial (106)	Compared with electrophysiologically guided antiarrhythmic drug therapy, the 5-yr total mortality was reduced 20% by an AICD (95% CI, 0.64–1.01), and the 5-yr risk of cardiac arrest or death from an arrhythmia was reduced 76% by an AICD (95% CI 0.13–0.45)
Multicenter Automatic Defibrillator Implantation Trial II (107)	At 20-mo follow-up, the AICD caused a 31% significant reduction in mortality (95% CI, 0.51–0.93)
Multicenter Automatic Defibrillator Implantation Trial II (110)	At 8-yr follow-up, the cumulative probability of all-cause mortality was 49% for patients treated with an AICD versus 62% for patients not treated with an AICD ($p < 0.001$)

Abbreviation: AICD, automatic implantable cardioverter-defibrillator.

medical therapy (Table 22.4) (100). Amiodarone was given to 74% of patients receiving conventional medical therapy versus 2% of patients receiving an AICD. Beta blockers were given to 8% of patients receiving conventional medical therapy versus 26% of patients receiving an AICD. At 27-month follow-up, patients receiving an AICD had a 54% significant reduction in mortality (95% CI 0.26–0.82) (100).

In the Antiarrhythmics versus Implantable Defibrillators (AVID) Trial, 1016 patients, mean age 65 years, were randomized to an AICD or class III antiarrhythmic drug therapy (Table 22.4) (101). Forty-five percent of the patients had been resuscitated from near-fatal VF. The other 55% of the patients had sustained VT with syncope or sustained VT with a LV ejection fraction ≤40% and symptoms suggesting severe hemodynamic compromise due to the arrhythmia (near-syncope, CHF, and angina pectoris).

Amiodarone was administered to 96% of patients randomized to medical therapy and to 2% of patients who had the AICD. Sotalol was administered to 3% of patients randomized to medical therapy and to 0.2% of patients who had the AICD. Beta blockers were administered to 17% of patients randomized to medical therapy and to 42% of patients who had the AICD. The 1-year survival was 89.3% for patients who had the AICD versus 82.3% for patients treated with drug therapy (95% CI, 39 ± 20% decrease in mortality) (Table 22.4) (101). The 2-year survival was 81.6% for patients who had the AICD versus 74.7% for patients treated with drug therapy (95% CI, 27 ± 21% reduction in mortality) (Table 22.4) (101). The 3-year survival was 75.4% for patients who had the AICD versus 64.1% for patients treated with drug therapy (95% CI, 31 ± 21% decrease in mortality) (Table 22.4) (101).

The Canadian Implantable Defibrillator Study (CIDS) randomized 659 patients with VF, cardiac arrest, or hypotensive VT to an AICD or amiodarone therapy (Table 22.4) (102). Cardiac arrhythmic mortality was 4.5% per year in patients treated with amiodarone versus 3% per year in patients treated with an AICD (risk reduction = 33%; p = 0.047). Total mortality was 10.2% per year in patients treated with amiodarone versus 8.3% per year in patients treated with an AICD (risk reduction = 20%; p = 0.072) (Table 22.4) (102). In a subset of CIDS, at 5.6-year follow-up, 47% of patients treated with amiodarone and 27% of patients treated with an AICD had died (103). Amiodarone caused adverse effects in 83% of patients receiving the drug (103).

The Cardiac Arrest Study Hamburg (CASH) randomized 230 patients surviving sudden cardiac death due to documented VT and/or VF to propafenone, metoprolol, amiodarone, or an AICD (Table 22.4) (104). Propafenone was stopped after 11 months because mortality from sudden death and cardiac arrest recurrence was 23% in patients randomized to propafenone versus 0% in patients randomized to an AICD (p < 0.05) (Table 22.4) (104). The 2-year mortality was 12.6% for 99 patients randomized to an AICD versus 19.6% for 189 patients randomized to amiodarone or metoprolol (37% reduction; p = 0.047) (Table 22.4) (105).

The Multicenter Unsustained Tachycardia Trial randomized 704 patients with inducible, sustained ventricular tachyarrhythmias to three treatment groups (Table 22.4) (106). Compared with electrophysiologically guided antiarrhythmic drug therapy, the 5-year total mortality was reduced 20% by an AICD (95% CI 0.64–1.01), and the 5-year risk of cardiac arrest or death from an arrhythmia was reduced 76% by an AICD (95% CI 0.13–0.45) (Table 22.4) (106). Either the total mortality incidence or rate of cardiac arrest or death from arrhythmia was lower in patients randomized to electrophysiologically guided therapy and treated with antiarrhythmic drugs than in patients randomized to no antiarrhythmic treatment (106).

MADIT II randomized 1232 patients, mean age 64 years, with a prior MI and a LV ejection fraction of ≤30% to an AICD or to conventional medical therapy (Table 22.4) (107). Beta blockers were given to 70% of AICD patients versus 70% of conventional medical therapy patients. ACE inhibitors were given to 68% of AICD patients versus 72% of conventional medical therapy patients. Statins were given to 67% of AICD patients versus 64% of conventional medical therapy patients. Amiodarone was given to 13% of AICD patients versus 10% of conventional medical therapy patients. At 20-month follow-up, compared with conventional medical therapy, the AICD reduced all-cause mortality from 19.8% to 14.2%, p = 0.016 (hazard ratio = 0.69; 95% CI 0.51–0.93) (Table 22.4) (107). The effect of AICD therapy in improving survival was similar in patients stratified according to age, sex, LV ejection fraction, New York Heart Association Class, and QRS interval (107).

In MADIT-II, the reduction in sudden cardiac death in patients treated with an AICD was significantly reduced by 68% in 574 patients aged <65 years (p = 0.02), by 65% in 455 patients aged 65–74 years (p = 0.005), and by 68% in 204 patients aged ≥75 years (p = 0.05) (108). The median survival in 348 octogenarians treated with AICD therapy was >4 years (109).

At 8-year follow-up in MADIT II, the cumulative probability of all-cause mortality was 49% for patients treated with an AICD versus 62% for patints not treated with an AICD ($p < 0.001$) (110). AICD treatment caused a 34% reduction in mortality during treatment years 1–4 ($p < 0.001$) and a 26% reduction in mortality during years 5–8 ($p = 0.02$) (110).

After AICD implantation, 35 patients were randomized to treatment with metoprolol and 35 patients to treatment with d,l-sotalol (111). VT recurrence was 17% at 1 year and 20% at 2 years for patients treated with metoprolol versus 43% at 1 year and 49% at 2 years for patients treated with d,l-sotalol ($p = 0.016$). At 26-month follow-up, survival was 91% for patients treated with metoprolol plus an AICD versus 83% for patients treated with d,l-sotalol plus an AICD ($p = 0.287$) (111). In MADIT-II, use of higher doses of beta blockers in patients with ischemic heart disease and an AICD significantly reduced mortality by 56–58% compared with nonuse of beta blockers ($p < 0.01$) (112). These data favor using a beta blocker in patients with an AICD.

At 32-month mean follow-up of 965 patients, death occurred in 73 of 515 patients (13%) treated with beta blockers (group 1), in 84 of 494 patients (17%) treated with ACE inhibitors or angiotensin receptor blockers (ARBs) (group 2), in 56 of 402 patients (14%) treated with statins (group 3), in 40 of 227 patients (18%) treated with amiodarone, in 5 of 26 patients (19%) treated with sotalol (group 5), and in 64 of 265 patients (24%) treated with no beta blocker, ACE inhibitor, ARB, statin, amiodarone, or sotalol (group 6) ($p < 0.001$ for group 1 vs. group 6 and group 3 vs. group 6; $p < 0.02$ for group 2 vs. group 6) (88). These data favor treating patients with AICDs with beta blockers, statins, and ACE inhibitors or ARBs.

The American College of Cardiology Foundation (ACCF)/American Heart Association (AHA) guidelines (Table 22.5) recommend that Class I indications for therapy with an AICD are (*i*) cardiac arrest due to VF or VT not due to a transient or a reversible cause; (*ii*) spontaneous sustained VT; (*iii*) syncope of undetermined origin with clinically relevant, hemodynamically significant sustained VT or VF induced at electrophysiologic study when drug therapy is ineffective, not tolerated, or not preferred; (*iv*) patients with prior MI at least 40 days previously with a LV ejection fraction less than 35% who are in NYHA Class II or III; (*v*) patients with nonischemic dilated cardiomyopathy with a LV ejection

Table 22.5 Class I Indications for Implantation of an Automatic Implantable Cardioverter-Defibrillator

1. Survivors of cardiac arrest due to VF or hemodynamically unstable sustained VT after evaluation to diagnose the cause of the event and to exclude completely reversible causes
2. Structural heart disease and spontaneous sustained VT, whether hemodynamically stable or unstable
3. Syncope of undetermined etiology with clinically relevant, hemodynamically significant sustained VT or VF induced at electrophysiological study
4. LV ejection fraction <35% due to prior myocardial infarction at least 40 days previously and NYHA class II or III
5. Nonischemic dilated cardiomyopathy with LV ejection fraction ≤35% and NYHA class II or III
6. LV ejection fraction <30% due to prior myocardial infarction at least 40 days previously and NYHA class I
7. Nonsustained VT due to myocardial infarction, LV ejection fraction <40%, and inducible VF or sustained VT at electrophysiological study

Abbreviations: VF, ventricular fibrillation; VT, ventricular tachycardia; LV, left ventricular; NYHA, New York Heart Association.
Source: Adapted from Ref. 113.

fraction less than or equal to 35% who are in NYHA class II or III; (*vi*) patients with prior MI at least 40 days previously with a LV ejection fraction less than 30% who are in NYHA Class I; and (*vii*) patients with nonsustained VT due to prior MI with a LV ejection fraction less than 40% and inducible VF or sustained VT at electrophysiological study (113).

The 2009 updated ACCF/AHA guidelines for treatment of CHF (Table 22.6) recommend with a class I indication use of an AICD for (*i*) secondary prevention to increase survival in patients with current or prior symptoms of heart failure and decreased LV ejection fraction who have a history of cardiac arrest, VF, or hemodynamically destabilizing VT; (*ii*) primary prevention of sudden cardiac death to reduce mortality in patients with nonischemic dilated cardiomyopathy or CAD at least 40 days after MI, a LV ejection fraction less than or equal to 35%, and NYHA Class II or III symptoms on optimal medical therapy, with expectation of survival with good functional status for more than 1 year; and (*iii*) may be used in patients receiving cardiac resynchronization therapy (CRT) for NYHA Class III or ambulatory Class IV symptoms despite recommended optimal medical therapy (114,115).

The ACC/AHA guidelines Class IIa indications for treatment with an AICD are listed in Table 22.7 (113). If the patient has no indication for pacing and a normal LV ejection

Table 22.6   Class I Indications for Implantation of an Automatic Implantable Cardioverter-Defibrillator in Patients with Congestive Heart Failure

1. Secondary prevention to increase survival in patients with current or prior symptoms of heart failure and reduced LV ejection fraction who have a history of cardiac arrest, VF, or hemodynamically destabilizing VT
2. Primary prevention of sudden cardiac death to reduce mortality in patients with nonischemic dilated cardiomyopathy or ischemic heart disease at least 40 days after myocardial infarction, a LV ejection fraction less than or equal to 35%, and NYHA Class II or III symptoms on optimal medical therapy, with expectation of survival with good functional status for more than 1 yr
3. May be used in patients receiving cardiac resynchronization therapy for NYHA Class III or ambulatory Class IV symptoms despite recommended optimal medical therapy

Abbreviations: LV, left ventricular; VF, ventricular fibrillation; VT, ventricular tachycardia; NYHA, New York Heart Association.
Source: Adapted from Ref. 114.

Table 22.7   Class IIa Indications for Implantation of an Automatic Implantable Cardioverter-Defibrillator

1. Unexplained syncope, significant LV dysfunction, and nonischemic dilated cardiomyopathy
2. Sustained VT and normal or near normal LV function
3. Hypertrophic cardiomyopathy with one or more major risk factor for SCD
4. Prevention of SCD in patients with arrhythmogenic right ventricular dysplasia/cardiomyopathy who have one or more risk factor for SCD
5. Reduction of SCD in patients with long-QT syndrome who are having syncope and/or VT while using beta blockers
6. Nonhospitalized patients awaiting cardiac transplantation
7. Patients with Brugada syndrome who have had syncope
8. Patients with Brugada syndrome who have had documented VT that has not resulted in cardiac arrest
9. Patients with catecholaminergic polymorphic VT who have syncope and/or documented sustained VT while using beta blockers
10. Patients with cardiac sarcoidosis, giant cell myocarditis, or Chagas disease

Abbreviations: LV, left ventricular; SCD, sudden cardiac death; VT, ventricular tachycardia.
Source: Adapted from Ref. 113.

fraction, CRT should not be performed. If the patient has no indication for pacing and a reduced LV ejection fraction, CRT should not be performed.

An AICD may also be effective in preventing sudden death in patients with hypertrophic cardiomyopathy at high risk for sudden death (116) and in patients at high risk for sudden death because of a long QT interval or the Brugada syndrome (117). An AICD may be useful in preventing sudden death in patients with syncope and ventricular tachyarrhythmias associated with poor LV ejection fraction, regardless of the result of the electrophysiologic study (118). In addition, an AICD may be useful in survivors of VT or VF as a bridge to cardiac transplantation (119).

AICDs were implanted in 378 men and 95 women, mean age 69 ± 12 years (120). At 3.6-year follow-up, survival was 76% in patients who had an AICD because of cardiac arrest due to VF or VT not due to a transient or reversible cause, 85% in patients who had an AICD because of spontaneous sustained VT in association with structural heart disease, 92% in patients who had an AICD because of syncope of undetermined origin with clinically relevant, hemodynamically sustained VT or VF induced at electrophysiological study when drug therapy is ineffective, not tolerated, or not preferred, 84% in patients who had an AICD because of nonsustained VT with CAD, MI, LV dysfunction, and inducible VF or sustained VT at electrophysiological study that is not suppressible by a Class I antiarrhythmic drug, and 85% in all 473 patients (120).

AICDs are not effective in treating patients with LV dysfunction scheduled for elective CABG (91) or in patients who have had an acute MI within 40 days of the procedure (121,122). In patients receiving AICDs early after MI, factors associated with arrhythmias needing AICD therapy are also associated with a high risk of nonsudden death, negating the benefit of AICDs (123). AICDs should also not be used to treat patients with NYHA Class IV CHF despite optimal medical management or in patients with a life expectancy <1 year (114).

Of 209 patients with NYHA Class III or IV heart failure treated with combined CRT-AICD therapy, appropriate cardioverter-defibrillator shocks occurred at 34-month follow-up in 22 of 121 patients (18%) on statins and in 30 of 88 patients (34%) not on statins ($p = 0.009$) (124). Death occurred in 3 of 121 patients (2%) on statins and in 9 of 88 patients (10%) not on statins ($p = 0.017$). Stepwise Cox regression analysis showed that significant independent prognostic factors for appropriate shocks were use of statins (risk ratio = 0.46), smoking (risk ratio = 3.5); and diabetes mellitus (risk ratio = 0.34) (124). Significant independent prognostic factors for the time to mortality were use of statins (risk ratio = 0.05), use of digoxin (risk ratio = 4.2), hypertension (risk ratio = 14.2), diabetes mellitus (risk ratio = 4.3), and LV ejection fraction (risk ratio = 1.1) (124).

Of 529 patients with CHF and a reduced LV ejection fraction, 209 (40%) were treated with CRT plus an AICD and 320 (60%) with an AICD (125). Mean follow-up was 34 months for both groups. Stepwise logistic regression analysis showed that significant independent variables for appropriate AICD shocks were statins (risk ratio = 0.35), smoking (risk ratio = 2.52), and digoxin (risk ratio = 1.92). Significant independent variables for time to deaths were use of CRT (risk ratio = 0.32), statins (risk ratio = 0.18), ACE inhibitors/ARBs (risk ratio = 0.10), hypertension (risk ratio = 24.15), diabetes (risk ratio = 2.54), and age (risk ratio = 1.06) (125).

During 1243 days mean follow-up of 549 patients who had an AICD for CHF, 163 (30%) had appropriate AICD shocks, 71 (13%) had inappropriate AICD shocks, and 63 (12%) died (126). Stepwise logistic regression analysis showed that significant independent prognostic factors for appropriate AICD shocks were smoking (odds ratio = 3.7) and statins (odds ratio = 0.54), for inappropriate AICD shocks were atrial fibrillation (odds ratio = 6.2) and statins (odds ratio = 0.52), and for time to mortality were age (hazard ratio = 1.08 per 1-year increase), ACE inhibitors or ARBs (hazard ratio = 0.25), atrial fibrillation (hazard ratio = 4.1), right ventricular pacing (hazard ratio = 3.6), digoxin (hazard ratio = 2.9), hypertension (hazard ratio = 5.3), and statins (hazard ratio = 0.32) (126).

AICDs were implanted in 485 patients with ischemic cardiomyopathy and in 299 patients with nonischemic cardiomyopathy (127). At 33-month follow-up, appropriate ICD shocks occurred in 179 of 485 patients (37%) with ischemic cardiomyopathy and in 93 of 299 patients (31%) with nonischemic cardiomyopathy (p not significant). All-cause mortality occurred in 162 of 485 patients (33%) with ischemic cardiomyopathy and in 70 of 299 patients (23%) with nonischemic cardiomyopathy ($p = 0.002$) (127).

During implantatation and during 38-month follow-up of 1060 patients who had AICDs, complications occurred in 60 patients (5.7%) (128). These complications consisted of fractured leads requiring lead revision in 36 patients (3.4%), lead infection requiring antibiotics in 5 patients (0.5%), device replacement because of malfunction in 5 patients (0.5%), repositioning of leads in 3 patients (0.3%), a hematoma at the time of implantation in 3 patients (0.3%), pneumothorax at the time of implantation in 2 patients (0.2%), repair of a defective generator in 1 patient (0.1%), replacement of the device because of atrophy of the skin over the device in 1 patient (0.1%), a transient ischemic attack because of atrial fibrillation developing during implantation in 1 patient (0.1%), device replacement because of a recall from Guidant in 1 patient (0.1%), pocket revision because of pain when lying on the side of the pacemaker in 1 patient (0.1%), and pacemaker infection in 1 patient (0.1%) (128). A downloadable algorithm has been developed to reduce inappropriate shocks caused by fractures of implantable AICD leads (129).

Persistent atrial fibrillation is associated with appropriate shocks and with CHF in patients with LV dysfunction treated with an AICD (130). One or more inappropriate AICD shocks occurred in 83 of 719 MADIT II patients (11.5%) and comprised 31.2% of 590 shocks (131). Triggers for inappropriate shocks were atrial fibrillation (44%), supraventricular tachycardia (36%), and abnormal sensing (20%). Patients with inappropriate shocks had a 2.3 times increase in mortality ($p = 0.025$) (131).

In 1193 patients with combined CRT-AICD therapy, atrial tachycardia/atrial fibrillation lasting longer than 10 minutes occurred in 361 patients (30%) (132). Device-detected atrial tachycardia/atrial fibrillation was associated with a 2.16 times increased mortality at 13 months median follow-up ($p = 0.032$) (132).

Of 958 with an AICD, chronic kidney disease was a significant independent predictor of 1-year mortality ($p < 0.001$) (133). The 1-year mortality was 1.8%, 5.3%, 9.0%, 22%, and 38% for stages 1, 2, 3, 4, and 5, respectively, of renal function (133).

Successful radiofrequecy ablation was performed in 22 of 84 patients with an AICD who had inappropriate shocks from atrial tachycardia, atrial flutter, or atrioventricular nodal reentrant tachycardia (134). Ninety-five percent of 22 patients who underwent successful radiofrequency ablation for supraventricular tachycardia had no inappropriate AICD shocks at 21-month follow-up compared to 63% of patients with inappropriate shocks for supraventricular tachycardia who did not have radiofrequency ablation ($p = 0.04$) (134).

In patients with AICDs, compared to patients treated with ventricular backup pacing at a rate of 40/minute, patients treated with dual-chamber rate-responsive pacing at a rate of 70/minute (DDDR-70) had an increase in mortality (135,136), worsening of LV ejection fraction (137), and an increase in new LV wall motion abnormality (137). One reason why DDDR-70 pacing may increase mortality and worsen LV systolic function is that ventricular electrical activation proceeds from the right ventricular apex instead of through the existing conduction system.

In patients with AICDs and no indication for antibradycardia pacing, 22 of 80 patients (28%) treated with right ventricular pacing died at 45-month follow-up, and 8 of 81 patients

(10%) treated with biventricular pacing died at 53-month follow-up ($p < 0.01$) (138). At 23-month follow-up, the LV ejection fraction decreased from 36% to 30% in patients treated with right ventricular pacing and increased at 38-month follow-up from 35% to 40% in patients treated with biventricular pacing ($p < 0.001$) (138). New LV wall motion abnormality developed at 23-month follow-up in 23 of 80 patients (29%) treated with right ventricular pacing and at 38-month follow-up in 7 of 81 patients (9%) treated with biventricular pacing ($p < 0.005$) (138). On the basis of the available data, patients with AICDs should be treated with biventricular pacing, not with DDDR-70 right ventricular pacing (135–138).

REFERENCES

1. Fleg JL, Kennedy HL. Cardiac arrhythmia in a healthy elderly population. Detection by 24-hour ambulatory electrocardiography. Chest 1982; 81: 302–7.
2. Aronow WS, Mercando AD, Epstein S. Prevalence of arrhythmias detected by 24-hour ambulatory electrocardiography and the value of antiarrhythmic therapy in elderly patients with unexplained syncope. Am J Cardiol 1992; 70: 408–10.
3. Aronow WS, Epstein S, Mercando AD. Usefulness of complex ventricular arrhythmias detected by 24-hour ambulatory electrocardiogram and by electrocardiograms with one-minute rhythm strips in predicting new coronary events in elderly patients with and without heart disease. J Cardio vasc Technol 1991; 10: 21–5.
4. Camm AJ, Evans KE, Ward DE, Martin A. The rhythm of the heart in active elderly subjects. Am Heart J 1980; 99: 598–603.
5. Kantelip JP, Sage E, Duchene-Marullaz P. Findings on ambulatory electrocardiographic monitoring in subjects older than 80 years. Am J Cardiol 1986; 57: 398–401.
6. Manolio TA, Furberg CD, Rautaharju PM, et al. Cardiac arrhythmias on 24-h ambulatory electrocardiography in older women and men: the Cardiovascular Health Study. J Am Coll Cardiol 1994; 23: 916–25.
7. Aronow WS, Ahn C, Mercando A, et al. Prevalence and association of ventricular tachycardia and complex ventricular arrhythmias with new coronary events in older men and women with and without cardiovascular disease. J Gerontol A Biol Med Sci 2002; 57A: M178–80.
8. Aronow WS, Epstein S, Schwartz KS, Koenigsberg M. Prevalence of arrhythmias detected by ambulatory electrocardiographic monitoring and of abnormal left ventricular ejection fraction in persons older than 62 years in a long-term health care facility. Am J Cardiol 1987; 59: 368–9.
9. Aronow WS, Epstein S, Schwartz KS, Koenigsberg M. Correlation of complex ventricular arrhythmias detected by ambulatory electrocardiographic monitoring with echocardiographic left ventricular hypertrophy in persons older than 62 years in a long-term health care facility. Am J Cardiol 1987; 60: 730–2.
10. Aronow WS, Epstein S. Usefulness of silent ischemia, ventricular tachycardia, and complex ventricular arrhythmias in predicting new coronary events in elderly patients with coronary artery disease or systemic hypertension. Am J Cardiol 1990; 65: 511–22.
11. Fleg JL, Kennedy HL. Long-term prognostic significance of ambulatory electrocardiographic findings in apparently healthy subjects ≥60 years of age. Am J Cardiol 1992; 70: 748–51.
12. Fleg JL, Lakatta EG. Prevalence and prognosis of exercise-induced nonsustained ventricular tachycardia in apparently healthy volunteers. Am J Cardiol 1984; 54: 762–4.
13. Busby MJ, Shefrin EA, Fleg JL. Prevalence and long-term significance of exercise-induced frequent or repetitive ventricular ectopic beats in apparently healthy volunteers. J Am Coll Cardiol 1989; 14: 1659–65.
14. Aronow WS, Epstein S, Koenigsberg M, Schwartz KS. Usefulness of echocardiographic abnormal left ventricular ejection fraction, paroxysmal ventricular tachycardia, and complex ventricular arrhythmias in predicting new coronary events in patients over 62 years of age. Am J Cardiol 1988; 61: 1349–51.
15. Aronow WS, Epstein S, Koenigsberg M, Schwartz KS. Usefulness of echocardiographic left ventricular hypertrophy, ventricular tachycardia and complex ventricular arrhythmias in predicting ventricular fibrillation or sudden cardiac death in elderly patients. Am J Cardiol 1988; 62: 1124–5.
16. Moss AJ, Davis HT, DeCamilla J, Bayer LW. Ventricular ectopic beats and their relation to sudden and nonsudden death after myocardial infarction. Circulation 1979; 60: 998–1003.
17. Bigger JT, Fleiss JL, Kleiger R, et al. The relationships among ventricular arrhythmias, left ventricular dysfunction, and mortality in the 2 years after myocardial infarction. Circulation 1984; 69: 250–8.

18. Mukharji J, Rude RE, Poole WK, et al. Risk factors for sudden death after acute myocardial infarction: two-year follow-up. Am J Cardiol 1984; 54: 31–6.

19. Kostis JB, Byington R, Friedman LM, et al. Prognostic significance of ventricular ectopic activity in survivors of acute myocardial infarction. J Am Coll Cardiol 1987; 10: 231–42.

20. Antithrombotic Trialists' Collaboration. Collaborative meta-analysis of randomised trials of antiplatelet therapy for prevention of death, myocardial infarction, and stroke in high risk patients. BMJ 2002; 324: 71–86.

21. Goldstein RE, Andrews M, Hall WJ, et al. Marked reduction in long-term cardiac deaths with aspirin after a coronary event. J Am Coll Cardiol 1996; 28: 326–30.

22. Aronow WS, Ahn C. Reduction of coronary events with aspirin in older patients with prior myocardial infarction treated with and without statins. Heart Dis 2002; 4: 159–61.

23. Smith SC Jr, Benjamin EJ, Bonow RO, et al. AHA/ACCF secondary prevention and risk reduction therapy for patients with coronary and other atherosclerotic cardiovascular disease: 2011 update. A guideline from the American Heart Association and American College of Cardiology Foundation. J Am coll Cardiol 2011; 58: 2432–46.

24. Hjalmarson A, Elmfeldt D, Herlitz J, et al. Effect on mortality of metoprolol in acute myocardial infarction. Lancet 1981; 2: 823–7.

25. Gundersen T, Abrahamsen AM, Kjekshus J, et al. Timolol-related reduction in mortality and reinfarction in patients ages 65-75 years surviving acute myocardial infarction. Circulation 1982; 66: 1179–84.

26. Pedersen TR for the Norwegian Multicentre Study Group. Six-year follow-up of the Norwegian Multicentre Study on Timolol after acute myocardial infarction. N Engl J Med 1985; 313: 1055–8.

27. Beta-Blocker Heart Attack Trial Research Group. A randomized trial of propranolol in patients with acute myocardial infarction. JAMA 1982; 247: 1707–14.

28. Aronow WS, Ahn C, Kronzon I. Effect of beta blockers alone, of angiotensin-converting enzyme inhibitors alone, and of beta blockers plus angiotensin-converting enzyme inhibitors on new coronary events and on congestive heart failure in older persons with healed myocardial infarcts and asymptomatic left ventricular systolic dysfunction. Am J Cardiol 2001; 88: 1298–300.

29. Pfeffer MA, Braunwald E, Moye LA, et al. Effect of captopril on mortality and morbidity in patients with left ventricular dysfunction after myocardial infarction. Results of the Survival and Ventricular Enlargement Trial. N Engl J Med 1992; 327: 669–77.

30. The Acute Infarction Ramipril Efficacy (AIRE) Study Investigators. Effect of ramipril on mortality and morbidity of survivors of acute myocardial infarction with clinical evidence of heart failure. Lancet 1993; 342: 821–8.

31. Ambrosioni E, Borghi C, Magnani B; for the Survival of Myocardial Infarction Long-Term Evaluation (SMILE) Study Investigators. The effect of the angiotensin-converting-enzyme inhibitor zofenopril on mortality and morbidity after anterior myocardial infarction. N Engl J Med 1995; 332: 80–5.

32. Kober L, Torp-Pedersen C, Carlsen JE, et al. A clinical trial of the angiotensin-converting-enzyme inhibitor trandolapril in patients with left ventricular dysfunction after myocardial infarction. N Engl J Med 1995; 333: 1670–6.

33. HOPE (Heart Outcomes Prevention Evaluation) Study Investigators. Effects of an angiotensin-converting-enzyme inhibitor, ramipril, on cardiovascular events in high-risk patients. N Engl J Med 2000; 342: 145–53.

34. Miettinen TA, Pyorala K, Olsson AG, et al. Cholesterol-lowering therapy in women and elderly patients with myocardial infarction or angina pectoris. Findings from the Scandinavian Simvastatin Survival Study (4S). Circulation 1997; 96: 4211–18.

35. Lewis SJ, Moye LA, Sacks FM, et al. Effect of pravastatin on cardiovascular events in older patients with myocardial infarction and cholesterol levels in the average range. Results of the Cholesterol and Recurrent Events (CARE) Trial. Ann Intern Med 1998; 129: 681–9.

36. The Long-Term Intervention with Pravastatin in Ischaemic Disease (LIPID) Study Group. Prevention of cardiovascular events and death with pravastatin in patients with coronary heart disease and a broad range of initial cholesterol levels. N Engl J Med 1998; 339: 1349–57.

37. Aronow WS, Ahn C. Incidence of new coronary events in older persons with prior myocardial infarction and serum low-density lipoprotein cholesterol ≥125 mg/dL treated with statins versus no lipid-lowering drug. Am J Cardiol 2002; 89: 67–9.

38. Heart Protection Study Collaborative Group. MRC/BHF Heart Protection Study of cholesterol lowering with simvastatin in 20,536 high-risk individuals: a randomised placebo-controlled trial. Lancet 2002; 360: 7–22.

39. Shepherd J, Blauw GJ, Murphy MB, et al. Pravastatin in elderly individuals at risk of vascular disease (PROSPER): a randomised controlled trial. Lancet 2002; 360: 1623–30.

40. Grundy SM, Cleeman JI, Merz CNB, et al. Implications of recent clinical trials for the National Cholesterol Education Program Adult Treatment Panel III guidelines. Circulation 2004; 110: 227–39.
41. Frishman WH, Aronow WS, Cheng-Lai A. Cardiovascular drug therapy in the elderly. In: Aronow WS, Fleg J, Rich MW, eds. Cardiovascular Disease in the Elderly, 4th edn. New York City: Informa Healthcare, 2008: 99–135.
42. IMPACT Research Group. International Mexiletine and Placebo Antiarrhythmic Coronary Trial: I. Report on arrhythmia and other findings. J Am Coll Cardiol 1984; 4: 1148–63.
43. The Cardiac Arrhythmia Suppression Trial (CAST) Investigators. Preliminary report. Effect of encainide and flecainide on mortality in a randomized trial of arrhythmia suppression after myocardial infarction. N Engl J Med 1989; 321: 406–12.
44. Akiyama T, Pawitan Y, Campbell WB, et al. Effects of advancing age on the efficacy and side effects of antiarrhythmic drugs in post-myocardial infarction patients with ventricular arrhythmias. J Am Geriatr Soc 1992; 40: 666–72.
45. The Cardiac Arrhythmia Suppression Trial II Investigators. Effect of the antiarrhythmic agent moricizine on survival after myocardial infarction. N Engl J Med 1992; 327: 227–33.
46. Aronow WS, Mercando AD, Epstein S, Kronzon I. Effect of quinidine or procainamide versus no antiarrhythmic drug on sudden cardiac death, total cardiac death, and total death in elderly patients with heart disease and complex ventricular arrhythmias. Am J. Cardiol 1990; 66: 423–8.
47. Moosvi AR, Goldstein S, VanderBrug Medendorp S, et al. Effect of empiric antiarrhythmic therapy in resuscitated out-of-hospital cardiac arrest victims with coronary artery disease. Am J Cardiol 1990; 65: 1192–7.
48. Hallstrom AP, Cobb LA, Hui Yu B, et al. An antiarrhythmic drug experience in 941 patients resuscitated from an initial cardiac arrest between 1970 and 1985. Am J Cardiol 1991; 68: 1025–31.
49. Coplen SE, Antmann EM, Berlin JA, et al. Efficacy and safety of quinidine therapy for maintenance of sinus rhythm after cardioversion: a meta-analysis of randomized control trials. Circulation 1990; 82: 1106–16.
50. Flaker GC, Blackshear JL, McBride R, et al. Antiarrhythmic drug therapy and cardiac mortality in atrial fibrillation. J Am Coll Cardiol 1992; 20: 527–32.
51. Morganroth J, Goin JE. Quinidine-related mortalitiy in the short-to-medium term treatment of ventricular arrhythmias. A meta-analysis. Circulation 1991; 84: 1977–83.
52. Teo KK, Yusuf S, Furberg CD. Effects of prophylactic antiarrhythmic drug therapy in acute myocardial infarction. An overview of results from randomized controlled trials. JAMA 1993; 270: 1589–95.
53. Hawkins CM, Richardson DW, Vokonas PS; BHAT Research Group. Effect of propranolol in reducing mortality in older myocardial infarction patients. The Beta-Blocker Heart Attack Trial experience. Circulation 1983; 67: I-94–7.
54. Friedman LM, Byington RP, Capone RJ, et al. Effect of propranolol in patients with myocardial infarction and ventricular arrhythmia. J Am Coll Cardiol 1986; 7: 1–8.
55. Lichstein E, Morganroth J, Harrist R, et al. Effect of propranolol on ventricular arrhythmia. The Beta-Blocker Heart Attack Trial experience. Circulation 1983; 67: I-5–10.
56. Hansteen V. Beta blockade after myocardial infarction: the Norwegian Propranolol Study in high-risk patients. Circulation 1983; 67: I-57–60.
57. de Soyza N, Shapiro W, Chandraratna PAN, et al. Acebutolol for ventricular arrythmia: a randomized, placebo-controlled, double-blind multicenter study. Circulation 1982; 65: 1129–33.
58. Norris RM, Barnaby PF, Brown MA, et al. Prevention of ventricular fibrillation during acute myocardial infarction by intravenous propranolol. Lancet 1984; 2: 883–6.
59. Stone PH, Gibson RS, Glasser SP, et al. Comparison of propranolol, diltiazem, and nifedipine in the treatment of ambulatory ischemia in patients with stable angina. Differential effects on ambulatory ischemia, exercise performance, and anginal symptoms. Circulation 1990; 82: 1962–72.
60. Weksler BB, Gillick M, Pink J. Effects of propranolol on platelet function. Blood 1977; 49: 185–96.
61. Frishman WH, Lazar EJ. Reduction of mortality, sudden death and non-fatal infarction with beta-adrenergic blockers in survivors of acute myocardial infarction: a new hypothesis regarding the cardioprotective action of beta-adrenergic blockade. Am J Cardiol 1990; 66: 66G–70G.
62. Aronow WS, Ahn C, Mercando AD, et al. Effect of propranolol versus no antiarrhythmic drug on sudden cardiac death, total cardiac death, and total death in patients ≥62 years of age with heart disease, complex ventricular arrhythmias, and left ventricular ejection fraction ≥40%. Am J Cardiol 1994; 74: 267–70.
63. Aronow WS, Ahn C, Mercando AD, et al. Decrease of mortality by propranolol in patients with heart disease and complex ventricular arrhythmias is more an anti-ischemic than an antiarrhythmic effect. Am J Cardiol 1994; 74: 613–15.

64. Aronow WS, Ahn C, Mercando AD, Epstein S. Circadian variation of sudden cardiac death or fatal myocardial infarction is abolished by propranolol in patients with heart disease and complex ventricular arrhythmias. Am J Cardiol 1994; 74: 819–21.

65. Aronow WS, Ahn C, Mercando AD, Epstein S. Effect of propranolol on circadian variation of ventricular arrhythmias in elderly patients with heart disease and complex ventricular arrhythmias. Am J Cardiol 1995; 75: 514–16.

66. Aronow WS, Ahn C, Mercando AD, Epstein S. Effect of propranolol on circadian variation of myocardial ischemia in elderly patients with heart disease and complex ventricular arrhythmias. Am J Cardiol 1995; 75: 837–9.

67. Kennedy HL, Brooks MM, Barker AH, et al. Beta-blocker therapy in the Cardiac Arrhythmia Suppression Trial. Am J Cardiol 1994; 74: 674–80.

68. Webster MW, Fitzpatrick MA, Nicholls MG, et al. Effect of enalapril on ventricular arrhythmias in congestive heart failure. Am J Cardiol 1985; 56: 566–9.

69. Fletcher RD, Cintron GB, Johnson G, et al. Enalapril decreases prevalence of ventricular tachycardia in patients with chronic congestive heart failure. Circulation 1993; 87: VI-49–55.

70. Pratt CM, Gardner M, Pepine C, et al. Lack of long-term ventricular arrhythmia reduction by enalapril in heart failure. Am J Cardiol 1995; 75: 1244–9.

71. Aronow WS, Mercando AD, Epstein S. Effect of benazepril on complex ventricular arrhythmias in older patients with congestive heart failure, prior myocardial infarction, and normal left ventricular ejection fraction. Am J Cardiol 1998; 81: 1368–70.

72. Cohn JN, Johnson G, Ziesche S, et al. A comparison of enalapril with hydralazine-isosorbide dinitrate in the treatment of chronic congestive heart failure. N Engl J Med 1991; 325: 303–10.

73. Garg R, Yusuf S; Collaborative Group on ACE Inhibitor Trials. Overview of randomized trials of angiotensin-converting enzyme inhibitors on mortality and morbidity in patients with heart failure. JAMA 1995; 273: 1450–6.

74. Aronow WS, Kronzon I. Effect of enalapril on congestive heart failure treated with diuretics in elderly patients with prior myocardial infarction and normal left ventricular ejection fraction. Am J Cardiol 1993; 71: 602–4.

75. Philbin EF, Rocco TA Jr, Lindenmuth NW, et al. Systolic versus diastolic heart failure in community practice: clinical features, outcomes, and the use of angiotensin-converting enzyme inhibitors. Am J Med 2000; 109: 605–13.

76. Waldo AL, Camm AJ, deRuyter H, et al. Effect of d-sotalol on mortality in patients with left ventricular dysfunction after recent and remote myocardial infarction. Lancet 1996; 348: 7–12.

77. Julian DJ, Prescott RJ, Jackson FS, Szekely P. Controlled trial of sotalol for one year after myocardial infarction. Lancet 1982; 1: 1142–7.

78. Mason JW; Electrophysiologic Study versus Electrocardiographic Monitoring Investigators. A comparison of electrophysiologic testing with Holter monitoring to predict antiarrhythmic-drug efficacy for ventricular tachyarrhythmias. N Engl J Med 1993; 329: 445–51.

79. Mason JW; Electrophysiologic Study versus Electrocardiographic Monitoring Investigators. A comparison of seven antiarrhythmic drugs in patients with ventricular tachyarrhythmias. N Engl J Med 1993; 329: 452–8.

80. Kehoe RF, MacNeil DJ, Zheutlin TA, et al. Safety and efficacy of oral sotalol for sustained ventricular tachyarrhythmias refractory to other antiarrhythmic agents. Am J Cardiol 1993; 72: 56A–66A.

81. Greene HL; CASCADE Investigators. The CASCADE study. Randomized antiarrhythmic drug therapy in survivors of cardiac arrest in Seattle. Am J Cardiol 1993; 72: 70F–4F.

82. Singh SN, Fletcher RD, Fisher SG, et al. Amiodarone in patients with congestive heart failure and asymptomatic ventricular arrhythmia. N Engl J Med 1995; 333: 77–82.

83. Cairns JA, Connolly SJ, Roberts R, et al. Randomised trial of outcome after myocardial infarction in patients with frequent or repetitive ventricular premature depolarisations: CAMIAT. Lancet 1997; 349: 675–82.

84. Herre J, Sauve M, Malone P, et al. Long-term results of amiodarone therapy in patients with recurrent sustained ventricular tachycardia or ventricular fibrillation. J Am Coll Cardiol 1989; 13: 442–9.

85. Julian DG, Camm AJ, Frangin G, et al. Randomised trial of effect of amiodarone on mortality in patients with left-ventricular dysfunction after recent myocardial infarction: EMIAT. Lancet 1997; 349: 667–74.

86. Bardy GH, Lee KL, Mark DB, et al. Amiodarone or an implantable cardioverter-defibrillator for congestive heart failure. N Engl J Med 2005; 352: 225–37.

87. Makikallio TH, Huikuri HV. Association between usage of beta-blocking medication and benefit from implantable cardioverter therapy. Am J Cardiol 2006; 98: 1245–7.

88. Lai HM, Aronow WS, Kruger A, et al. Effect of beta blockers, angiotensin-converting enzyme inhibitors or angiotensin receptor blockers, and statins on mortality in patients with implantable cardioverter-defibrillators. Am J Cardiol 2008; 102: 77–8.

89. Kruger A, Aronow WS, Lai H, et al. Prevalence of appropriate cardioverter-defibrillator shocks in 1038 consecutive patients with implantable cardioverter-defibrillators. Am J Ther 2009; 16: 323–5.

90. O'Rourke RA. Role of myocardial revascularization in sudden cardiac death. Circulation 1992; 85: I-112–17.

91. Bigger JT Jr; Coronary Artery Bypass Graft (CABG) Patch Trial Investigators. Prophylactic use of implanted cardiac defibrillators in patients at high risk for ventricular arrhythmias after coronary artery bypass graft surgery. N Engl J Med 1997; 337: 1569–75.

92. Platia EV, Griffith LSC, Watkins L Jr, et al. Treatment of malignant ventricular arrhythmias with endocardial resection and implantation of the automatic cardioverter-defibrillator. N Engl J Mcd 1986; 314: 213–16.

93. Tresch DD, Platia EV, Guarnieri T, et al. Refractory symptomatic ventricular tachycardia and ventricular fibrillation in elderly patients. Am J Med 1987; 83: 399–404.

94. Tresch DD, Troup PJ, Thakur RK, et al. Comparison of efficacy of automatic implantable cardioverter defibrillator in patients older and younger than 65 years of age. Am J Med 1991; 90: 717–24.

95. Rastegar H, Link MS, Foote CB, et al. Perioperative and long-term results with mapping-guided subendocardial resection and left ventricular endoaneurysmorrhaphy. Circulation 1996; 94: 1041–8.

96. Morady F, Harvey M, Kalbfleisch SJ, et al. Radiofrequency catheter ablation of ventricular tachycardia in patients with coronary artery disease. Circulation 1993; 87: 363–72.

97. Gonska B-D, Cao K, Schaumann A, et al. Catheter ablation of ventricular tachycardia in 136 patients with coronary artery disease: Results and long-term follow-up. J Am Coll Cardiol 1994; 24: 1506–14.

98. Channamsetty V, Aronow WS, Sorbera C, et al. Efficacy of radiofrequency catheter ablation in treatment of elderly patients with supraventricular tachyarrhythmias and ventricular tachycardia. Am J Ther 2006; 13: 513–15.

99. Kuck K-H, Schaumann A, Eckardt L, et al. Catheter ablation of stable ventricular tachycardia before defibrillator implantation in patients with coronary heart disease (VTACH): a multicentre randomised controlled trial. Lancet 2010; 375: 31–40.

100. Moss AJ, Hall WJ, Cannom DS, et al. Improved survival with an implanted defibrillator in patients with coronary disease at high risk for ventricular arrhythmia. N Engl J Med 1996; 335: 1933–40.

101. The Antiarrhythmics versus Implantable Defibrillators (AVID) Investigators. A comparison of antiarrhythmic-drug therapy with implantable defibrillators in patients resuscitated from near-fatal ventricular arrhythmias. N Engl J Med 1997; 337: 1576–83.

102. Roy D, Green M, Talajic M, et al. Mode of death in the Canadian Implantable Defibrillator Study (CIDS) (abstract). Circulation 1998; 98: 1–495.

103. Bokhari F, Newman D, Greene M, et al. Long-term comparison of the implantable cardioverter defibrillator versus amiodarone. Eleven-year follow-up of a subset of patients in the Canadian Implantable Defibrillator Study CIDS. Circulation 2004; 110: 112–16.

104. Siebels J, Cappato R, Ruppel R, et al. Preliminary results of the Cardiac Arrest Study Hamburg (CASH). Am J Cardiol 1993; 72: 109F–13F.

105. Cappato R, Siebels J, Kuck KH. Value of programmed electrical stimulation to predict clinical outcome in the Cardiac Arrest Study Hamburg (CASH) (abstract). Circulation 1998; 98: I-495–6.

106. Buxton AE, Lee KL, Fisher JD, et al. A randomized study of the prevention of sudden death in patients with coronary artery disease. N Engl J Med 1999; 341: 1882–90.

107. Moss AJ, Zareba W, Hall WJ, et al. Prophylactic implantation of a defibrillator in patients with myocardial infarction and reduced ejection fraction. N Engl J Med 2002; 346: 877–83.

108. Goldenberg I, Moss AJ. Treatment of arrhythmias and use of implantable cardioverter-defibrillators to improve survival in elderly patients with cardiac disease. In: Aronow WS, ed. Clinics in Geriatric Medicine on Heart Failure. Vol. 23 Philadelphia: Elsevier, 2007: 205–19.

109. Kaplan BA, Epstein LM, Albert CM, Stevenson WG. Survival in octogenarians receiving implantable defibrillators. Am Heart J 2006; 152: 714–19.

110. Goldenberg I, Gillespie J, Moss AJ, et al. Long-term benefit of primary prevention with an implantable cardioverter-defibrillator. An extended 8-year follow-up study of the MulticenterAutomatic Defibrillator Implantation Trial II. Circulation 2010; 122: 1265–71.

111. Seidl K, Hauer B, Schwick NG, et al. Comparison of metoprolol and sotalol in preventing ventricular tachyarrhythmias after the implantation of a cardioverter/defibrillator. Am J Cardiol 1998; 82: 744–8.

112. Brodine WN, Tung RT, Lee JK, et al. Effects of beta-blockers on implantable cardioverter defibrillator therapy and survival in the patients with ischemic cardiomyopathy (from the Multicenter Automatic Defibrillator Implantation Trial-II. Am J Cardiol 2005; 96: 691–5.

113. Epstein AE, DiMarco JP, Ellenbogen KA, et al. ACC/AHA/HRS guidelines for device-based therapy of cardiac rhythm abnormalities: executive summary. A report of the American College of Cardiology/ American Heart Association Task Force on Practice Guidelines (Writing Committee to Revise the ACC/AHA/NASPE 2002 Guideline Update for Implantation of Cardiac Pacemakers and Antiarrhythmia Devices). Developed in collaboration with the American Association for Thoracic Surgery and Society of Thoracic Surgeons. J Am Coll Cardiol 2008; 51: 2085–105.

114. Jessup M, Abraham WT, Casey DE, et al. 2009 focused update: ACCF/AHA guidelines for the diagnosis and management of heart failure in adults. A Report of the American College of Cardiology Foundation/American Heart Association Task Force on Practice Guidelines. Developed in collaboration with the International Society for Heart and Lung Transplantation. J Am Coll Cardiol 2009; 53: 1343–82.

115. Bristow MR, Saxon LA, Boehmer J, et al. Cardiac-resynchronization therapy with or without an implantable defibrillator in advanced chronic heart failure. N Engl J Med 2004; 350: 2140–50.

116. Maron BJ, Shen W-K, Link MS, et al. Efficacy of implantable cardioverter-defibrillators for the prevention of sudden death in patients with hypertrophic cardiomyopathy. N Engl J Med 2000; 342: 365–73.

117. Brugada P, Brugada R, Brugada J, Geelen P. Use of the prophylactic implantable cardioverter defibrillator for patients with normal hearts. Am J Cardiol 1999; 83: 98D–100D.

118. LeLorier P, Krahn AD, Klein GJ, et al. Comparison of patients with syncope with left ventricular dysfunction and negative electrophysiologic testing to cardiac arrest survivors and patients with syncope and preserved left ventricular function and impact of an implantable defibrillator. Am J Cardiol 2002; 90: 77–9.

119. Lorga-Filho A, Geelen P, Vanderheyden M, et al. Early benefit of implantable cardioverter defibrillator therapy in patients waiting for cardiac transplantation. Pacing Clin Electrophysiol 1998; 21: 1747–51.

120. Aronow WS, Sorbera C, Chagarlamudi A, et al. Indications for and long-term survival in patients with automatic implantable cardioverter-defibrillators. Cardiol Rev 2005; 13: 50–1.

121. Hohnloser SH, Kuck KH, Dorian P, et al. Prophylactic use of an implantable cardioverter-defibrillator after acute myocardial infarction. N Engl J Med 2004; 351: 2481–8.

122. Steinbeck G, Andresen D, Seidl K, et al. Defibrillator implantation early after myocardial infarction. N Engl J Med 2009; 361: 1427–36.

123. Dorian P, Hohnloser SH, Thorpe KE, et al. Mechanisms underlying the lack of effect of implantable cardioverter-defibrillator therapy on mortality in hgh-risk patients with recent myocardial infarction. Insights from the Defibrillation in Acute Myocardial Infarction trial (DINAMIT). Circulation 2010; 122: 2645–52.

124. Desai H, Aronow WS, Tsai FS, et al. Statins reduce appropriate cardioverter-defibrillator shocks and mortality in patients with heart failure and combined cardiac resynchronization and implantable cardioverter-defibrillator therapy. J Cardiovasc Pharmacol Ther 2009; 14: 176–9.

125. Desai H, Aronow WS, Ahn C, et al. Incidence of appropriate cardioverter-defibrillator shocks and mortality in patients with heart failure treated with combined cardiac resynchronization therapy plus implantable cardioverter-defibrillator therapy versus implantable cardioverter-defibrillator therapy. J Cardiovasc Pharmacol Ther 2010; 15: 37–40.

126. Desai H, Aronow WS, Ahn C, et al. Risk factors for appropriate cardioverter-shocks, inappropriate cardioverter shocks, and time to mortality in 549 patients with heart failure. Am J Cardiol 2010; 105: 1336–8.

127. Gandhi K, Aronow WS, Desai H, et al. Incidence of appropriate cardioverter-defibrillator shocks and mortality in patients with implantable cardioverter-defibrillators with ischemic cardiomyopathy versus nonischemic cardiomyopathy at 33-month follow-up. Arch Med Sci 2010; 6: 900–3.

128. Tsai F, Aronow WS, Devabhaktuni S, et al. Prevalence of complications during implantation and during 38-month follow-up of 1060 consecutive patients with implantable cardioverterr-defibrillators. Am J Ther 2010; 17: e8–e10.

129. Swerdlow CD, Gunderson BD, Ousdigian KT, et al. Downloadable algorithm to reduce inappropriate shocks caused by fractures of implantable cardioverter-defibrillator leads. Circulation 2008; 118: 2122–9.

130. Rienstra M, Smit MD, Nieuwland W, et al. Persistent atrial fibrillation is associated with appropriate shocks and heart failure in patients with left ventricular dysfunction treated with an implantable cardioverter defibrillator. Am Heart J 2007; 153: 120–6.

131. Daubert JP, Zareba W, Cannom DS, et al. Inappropriate implantable cardioverter-defibrillator shocks in MADIT II. Frequency, mechanisms, predictors, and survival impact. J Am Coll Cardiol 2008; 51: 1357–65.

132. Santini M, Gasparini M, Landolina M, et al. Device-detected atrial tachyarrhythmias predict adverse outcome in real-world patients with implantable biventricular defibrillators. J Am Coll Cardiol 2011; 57: 167–72.

133. Hager CS, Jain S, Blackwell J, et al. Effect of renal function on survival after implantable cardioverter defibrillator placement. Am J Cardiol 2010; 106: 1297–300.

134. Mainigi SK, Almuti K, Figueredo VM, et al. Usefulness of radiofrequency ablation of supraventricular tachycardia to decrease inappropriate shocks from implantable cardioverter-defibrillators. Am J Cardiol 2012; 109: 231–7.

135. The DAVID Trial Investigators. Dual-chamber pacing or ventricular backup pacing in patients with an implantable defibrillator. The Dual Chamber and VVI Implantable Defibrillator (DAVID) Trial. JAMA 2002; 288: 3115–23.

136. Sukhija R, Aronow WS, Sorbera C, et al. Patients, mean age 70 years, with dual-chamber rate-responsive pacing (DDDR-70) have a higher mortality than patients with backup ventricular pacing (VVI-40) at 3.7-year follow-up. J Gerontol A Biol Sci Med Sci 2005; 60A: M603–4.

137. Sukhija R, Aronow WS, Sorbera C, et al. Left ventricular ejection fraction and prevalence of new left ventricular wall motion abnormality at long-term follow-up in patients treated with dual-chamber rate-responsive pacing at a rate of 70/minute versus backup ventricular pacing at a rate of 40/minute. Am J Cardiol 2005; 96: 412–13.

138. Sukhija R, Aronow WS, Sorbera C, et al. Mortality, left ventricular ejection fraction, and prevalence of new left ventricular wall motion abnormality in patients with implantable cardioverter-defibrillators treated with biventricular pacing versus right ventricular pacing. Am J Ther 2007; 14: 328–30.

23

Bradyarrhythmias and cardiac pacemakers in the elderly

Fernando Tondato and Win-Kuang Shen

SUMMARY

The aging population in USA is growing exponentially, and the number of cardiac implantable electrical devices (CIEDs) is expected to grow proportionally. The most common presentations of bradyarrhythmias are: sinus node dysfunction (SND), atrioventricular block (AVB), and carotid sinus hypersensitivity (CSH). These conditions frequently affect older patients, and pacemaker implantation is the therapy of choice. Few clinical trials have focused exclusively on the elderly; however, the age in most clinical trials of CIEDs ranges between 70 and 75 years. The best pacing mode for each one of the conditions listed above has been a source of debate. Atrial or dual chamber pacing is preferred for SND. Exclusive ventricular pacing is associated with higher risk of atrial fibrillation and possible increased rate of stroke. For patients with AVB, most trials have not shown any significant difference in outcomes between single or dual chamber pacemaker, and the choice should be based on the patient's lifestyle and physical activities. Limited data about pacing in CSH is available; dual chamber pacemaker is the preferred choice for these patients. Current data suggests that very elderly pacemaker recipients have similar outcomes compared to the age-matched general population. Thus, advanced age should not preclude the recommendation of pacing. Health care providers should be aware of end of life issues in pacing therapy. Proactive communication is crucial with very elderly patients or their legal guardians on topics related to withholding or withdrawing such therapy at the end of life.

INTRODUCTION

The aging population in North America has grown exponentially over the past several decades. The 2010 Census revealed that 13% of the US population is above 65 years of age, an increase of 15% when compared to the previous Census in 2000 (1). The need for pacemaker implantation is highly prevalent among elderly, as shown by Kurtz et al. (2), who found that there were 2.4 million pacemakers implanted in the country between 1993 and 2006, and the mean age at implant was 75 ± 12 years. Thus, clinicians will face an increasing aging population presenting with rhythm disorders, many of those requiring the use of cardiac implantable electronic devices (CIEDs).

Several conditions can lead to significant bradycardia, requiring implantation of pacemakers. Sinus node dysfunction (SND) is the leading cause of bradyarrhythmias requiring pacing in the USA, followed by atrioventricular (AV) conduction disorders, and hypersensitivity of the carotid sinus (3). The use of pacing for treatment of neurocardiogenic syncope is still controversial, and its indication is much less frequent. Other conditions that can potentially be managed by cardiac pacing include long QT syndrome and hypertrophic cardiomyopathy; however, these conditions are beyond the scope of this chapter.

SINUS NODE DYSFUNCTION

SND is the most common cause of bradyarrhythmia requiring pacing, and it is predominant among elderly patients (4). The average age of patients at the time of diagnosis of SND is 74 years, with equal distribution between men and women (5). It can be caused by intrinsic abnormalities of the sinus node or extrinsic causes. Mechanisms of SND encompass a wide range of electrophysiologic abnormalities, including failure of impulse generation or failure to transmit impulse from sinus node to the atria (6). The term "sick sinus syndrome" (SSS) can also be used to describe SND.

The most common cause of SND in older patients is idiopathic degeneration of sinus node, with fibrotic infiltration on histology. Other conditions can also be involved, including rheumatic heart disease, Lyme disease, familial sinus node disorders, infiltrative diseases, idiopathic cardiomyopathy, Chagas disease, sarcoidosis, rheumatologic conditions, among others (7). Coronary artery disease is common among patients with SND, but is not necessarily causal (8).

Electrocardiographic Findings of SND

A wide range of electrocardiographic findings can be seen in SND. Sinus bradycardia, defined as heart rate below 60 bpm, is one possible manifestation of SND. Modest sinus bradycardia, defined by heart rates of 40–59 bpm, can be seen in athletes and healthy nonathletic older adults due to a physiologic increase in vagal tone. Sinus rate below 40 bpm, however, is most likely pathological (6).

Sinoatrial (SA) block is another form of SND. It is defined as the inability to propagate impulses generated in the sinus node to adjacent atrial tissue. In these situations, the sinus node impulse formation is appropriate, but the inability to conduct the impulse to atrial tissue results in various degrees of sinus pauses, including sinus arrest. The SA block, similar to AV block, can have different degrees of manifestation. It can present as a simple slowing of conduction to the atria, but with preserved 1:1 conduction. In other words, every impulse generated at the level of sinus node will have a delayed conduction to atrial tissue (first degree SA block). This form of SA block cannot be recognized by the conventional electrocardiogram because the heart rate is preserved. Second-degree SA block type I is characterized by the phenomenon of Wenckebach at the SA junction, leading to progressive prolongation of conduction time from sinus node to atrial tissue, ultimately resulting in conduction block. The SA conduction is then restored, repeating the same cycle of progressive prolongation of conduction time, as described before. The ECG representation of sinoatrial Wenckebach is repetitive group beating, characterized by progressive shortening of PP interval, followed by a sinus pause (blocked SA impulse). With second-degree type II SA block, SA conduction time is stable, but there is intermittent SA block. This phenomenon can be intermittent, and it will manifest as episodic sinus pauses with a specific feature: the PP interval that encompasses the pause will be exactly twice as long as the PP interval during normal sinus rhythm. Complete SA block marks the absence of SA conduction, leading to sinus arrest. This electrocardiographic feature does not allow the differentiation between complete SA block and primary failure of sinus node impulse formation.

Chronotropic incompetence, defined as the inability to reach more than 70% of the maximum predicted rate during exertion, and tachycardia–bradycardia syndrome are other clinical manifestations of SND. The latter condition is characterized by periods of significant bradycardia, and intermittent episodes of atrial tachycardia, atrial fibrillation (AF) or atrial flutter. It is very common to observe marked bradycardia immediately after termination of episodes of tachycardia, which can be associated with presyncope or syncope.

Clinical Manifestations of SND

The clinical manifestation of SND can include a wide range of symptoms, from being asymptomatic to lightheadedness, syncope, exercise intolerance, or heart failure. These symptoms are related to poor cerebral perfusion secondary to low cardiac output in the setting of sinus pauses, intermittent or persistent bradycardia mismatched to the physiologic demand. Palpitation is common among patients with tachycardia–bradycardia syndrome. Up to 50% of patients will present with syncope as the initial symptom of SND. Stroke and thromboembolic events can occur in patients with tachycardia–bradycardia syndrome, commonly associated with paroxysms of AF/atrial flutter. The inability to develop increased sinus rate response in the presence of fever, hypotension, or situations of stress (exercise, anemia) should raise suspicion for the diagnosis of SND. It is important to emphasize that SND can also cause noncardiac symptoms, such as cognitive impairment, memory loss, and lethargy, and subtle symptoms like lack of energy, mild edema and intermittent dyspnea (8,9).

Diagnosis of SND

The diagnosis of SND requires documentation of sinus node pauses or sinus bradycardia. ECG and Holter monitor are useful for documentation when these episodes are frequent or persistent. Transient or reversible causes such as drug effect, especially beta-blockers, and electrolyte or endocrinologic abnormalities need to be excluded. An ambulatory event recorder or implantable loop recorder can be considered when clinical episodes are intermittent or infrequent. A treadmill or cycle exercise test is useful in evaluating the response of sinus rate to exercise. Invasive electrophysiology study is no longer routinely recommended for diagnosis of SND due to its low sensitivity and specificity. The inability to correlate symptoms to sinus node abnormalities induced by programmed stimulation is another limitation of electrophysiologic study for evaluation of SND.

Natural History of SND

The natural history of SND is variable. It is frequently associated with the development of AV block and/or AF (10). Development of AV block occurs at a rate of 1.7%/year among patients with SND, and 8.5% over 5 years, with significant increase to 35% in the same period of time if bundle branch block or bifascicular block was present at initial evaluation (11). The prevalence of AF varies from 40% to 70% at the time of diagnosis of SND. For persons without a history of AF at initial presentation, 4–22% will develop it during long term follow-up (3). SND does not have significant impact on survival when compared to a matched general population, with survival rate of 85%, 79%, and 65% at 1, 2, and 5 years, respectively (12,13). The incidence of sudden death is very low among patients with isolated SND (13,14). Simon et al. did not detect any case of sudden death among untreated patients with SND over 8 years of follow-up (13).

Treatment of SND

In the absence of reversible causes, permanent pacemaker implantation is the only available treatment for SND. Several pacing modes are available for this condition, including single atrial lead (AAI mode), single ventricular lead (VVI mode) or dual-chamber pacemaker (DDD or DDI). Rate-adaptive pacing is currently available in the vast majority of implantable devices, and it can be activated in cases of symptomatic chronotropic insufficiency.

What Is the Ideal Mode of Pacing?

There is a large body of literature from clinical studies assessing the best pacing mode for this condition. The use of exclusive ventricular pacing was a common practice in the past, but several retrospective studies demonstrated increased morbidity and mortality associated with this mode of pacing (15,16). Exclusive ventricular pacing can also cause pacemaker syndrome, which is secondary to loss of AV synchrony. The symptoms related to this pacemaker syndrome can significantly impact the quality of life. Therefore, atrial pacing in SND should be the preferred choice since it promotes a physiologic activation of the ventricles, favoring the propagation of stimulus through the intrinsic conduction system.

The use of dual-chamber pacemaker should be restricted to those patients with combined sinus and AV node disease. Dual-chamber pacemakers allow the use of sinus node as the trigger for ventricular activation. Because this pacing mode preserves the AV synchrony, it is also called "physiologic pacing." The disadvantages of dual-chamber pacing, as compared to single-chamber pacing, include higher costs, longer procedure time during pacemaker implant and increased risk of complications, such as lead dislodgement (17).

Evidence from Clinical Trials of SND

The discussion above clearly shows benefit from exclusive atrial chamber pacing or dual-chamber pacing when compared with ventricular pacing alone. However, some authors question the benefit of physiologic pacing in elderly patients, who are commonly limited in their daily activities, and may not experience full benefit provided by dual-chamber pacing in quality of life and exercise capacity, and are known have higher rates of AF and heart failure, regardless of pacemaker use. Such patients would not experience the benefits of physiologic pacing, but still would be exposed to the increased risks and costs related to implant of dual-chamber pacemakers.

We will review here several seminal trials in pacing for SND, with focus on the elderly population. Few studies focused specifically on elderly patients, but most trials had a large predominance of geriatric patients, with mean age ranging from 70 to 75 years, which is the average age for developing clinical symptoms of SND. Table 23.1 summarizes the results of the major trials in cardiac pacing.

Comparing Atrial and Ventricular Pacing in SND

The DANISH study (18), published in 1994, was the first prospective study to address the concern about increased risk of AF, thromboembolism, and heart failure among patients treated with ventricular pacing when compared with atrial pacing. This study included 225 patients, mean age 76 years, who were randomized to either ventricular pacing only or atrial pacing only and followed for 5 years. This was the first randomized clinical trial to demonstrate significantly higher incidence of AF and thromboembolism among patients receiving ventricular pacing. Mortality and heart failure exacerbation were comparable in both groups. The incidence of AV block in this study was very low, with an annual rate of 0.6%, and the authors concluded that AAI should be the best choice for SND patients.

Andersen et al. (19) re-evaluated the clinical outcomes of the DANISH trial 8 years later; the authors concluded that not only the beneficial aspects of atrial pacing described above (less AF and thromboembolic events) were substantially enhanced over time, but also demonstrated a significant reduction in mortality rate and less heart failure with atrial pacing, which had not been shown in the first study.

Table 23.1 Major Clinical Trials of Pacemakers for SND and/or AV Block

Characteristics	Danish Study (5)	PASE (6)	CTOPP (7,8)	MOST (9)	DANPACE (26)	UKPACE
Patient population	SSS	SSS plus AVB	SSS plus AVB	SSS	SSS	AVB
Patients with SSS/AVB	220/0	175/232	1028/1540	2010/0	1415/0	0/2021
Mean age	76 ± 8 years	76 ± 11.3 years	73 ± 10 years	74 [68–80] years	70 ± 11.3 years	79.9 ± 6 years
Mean follow-up (yr)	5.5	1.5	6.4	2.8	5.4	3.0
Pacing modes	AAI vs. VVI	DDD-R vs. VVIR	DDD/AAI vs. VVI(R)	DDD-R vs. VVIR	AAIR vs. DDD-R	DDD(R) vs. VVI(R)
Primary endpoint	Composite of mortality, thromboembolism and AF	Health-related quality of life as measured by the SF-36	Stroke or CV mortality	All-cause mortality or nonfatal stroke	All-cause mortality	All-cause mortality
Secondary endpoints	CV mortality, HF and AVB	All-cause mortality, nonfatal stroke, AF and pacemaker syndrome	All-cause mortality, AF, HF hospitalization	Composite of all-cause mortality, first stroke, first HF; all-cause mortality; CV mortality; AF; pacemaker syndrome; health-related quality of life; Minnesota Living with HF score	Incidence of paroxysmal and chronic AF, stroke, HF, need for pacemaker re-operation	AF; HF; composite of stroke, transient ischemic attack, or other thromboembolism.

Abbreviations: AAI, single atrial lead; AF, atrial fibrillation; AVB, AV block; DDD, dual-chamber pacing mode; DDD-R, rate-responsive dual-chamber pacing; HF, ; SSS, sick sinus syndrome; VVI, ventricular pacing mode; VVIR, rate-responsive ventricular pacing.

Comparing Dual-Chamber Pacing and Exclusive Ventricular Pacing in SND

The PASE trial (Pacemaker Selection in the Elderly) (20) compared ventricular pacing with dual-chamber pacing with focus on quality-of-life and clinical outcomes in elderly patients (>65 years). The mean age was 76 years, and this study included patients with AV block (49%), SND (43%), and other diagnoses (8%). The authors concluded that dual-chamber pacemaker implantation improves health-related quality of life, but the benefit is limited to patients with SND. The PASE trial showed a nonsignificant trend toward lower rates of AF and embolic events among patients with a dual-chamber pacemaker. These findings were comparable to the results of the DANISH study, previously discussed. However, one of the major criticisms of the PASE trial is that the results were based on the intention-to-treat analysis, and 26% of patients crossed over from ventricular to dual-chamber pacing due to pacemaker syndrome. The large number of crossovers in this study was at least partially explained by the fact that all patients had both atrial and ventricular leads implanted, regardless of the assigned group. This design, in association with loose criteria for pacemaker syndrome, might have accentuated the crossover from VVI to DDD pacing mode, since it involved a simple change in programmable feature, without the need for new surgical intervention.

Similar findings were demonstrated in the CTOPP trial—the Canadian Trial of Physiologic Pacing (17). The authors randomized 1474 patients, with average age of 73 years, with symptomatic bradycardia to ventricular pacing or physiologic pacing (dual-chamber pacemaker). The authors could not demonstrate any significant difference between groups over 3 years with regard to mortality or hospitalization due to heart failure, even though there was a trend in favor of physiologic pacing. There was, however, a reduced rate of AF among patients under physiologic pacing (5.5% among patients under physiologic pacing versus 6.6% in the ventricular pacing group), which was noted only after 2 years of follow-up. The rate of perioperative complications, however, was significantly higher in the physiologic pacing group (9% vs. 4%). In order to assess a possible delayed beneficial response, Kerr et al. (21) extended the follow-up of the CTOPP trial to 6 years. The extended study showed persistent reduction in rate of AF with physiologic pacing, but no delayed benefit on mortality or stroke.

The PASE and CTOPP studies were the first large trials in the field of pacing. However, they included a mixed population of patients with different etiologies for their bradycardia syndromes. Therefore, the specific question about the best pacing mode in SND still remained. In response to that question, the MOST trial—Mode Selection Trial in SND— was developed (22). This study enrolled 2010 patients with SND, with mean age of 74 years, and compared ventricular pacing and dual-chamber pacing with respect to mortality, stroke, hospitalization for heart failure, AF, pacemaker syndrome and quality of life. The study did not show any difference in mortality or stroke. However, patients assigned to dual-chamber pacemaker had lower incidence of AF (27.1% in ventricular pacing versus 21.4% in dual-chamber pacing), better heart failure scores and better quality of life.

The MOST trial investigators were intrigued with the 26% crossover rate in the PASE trial, from VVI to dual-chamber pacing due to pacemaker syndrome. That number of patients with pacemaker syndrome was only 0.9% (2 out of 225 patients) in the DANISH trial, raising questions about the true incidence of this syndrome. One possible explanation is that in PASE, all patients received both atrial and ventricular leads at the time of implant and the pacing mode was easily modified by device programming. In the DANISH trial, patients received either a single atrial or ventricular lead, and the treatment of pacemaker syndrome required an additional surgical intervention in order to implant an atrial lead. To address this question, the MOST investigators created very specific criteria for pacemaker syndrome, and all crossovers had to be adjudicated by a committee. Despite all the efforts to prevent inappropriate diagnosis of pacemaker syndrome, the MOST trial reported a 20% rate of this condition, which was very comparable to other studies without a predetermined definition of pacemaker syndrome, such as PASE. It suggests that patients with SND are more prone to develop pacemaker syndrome when treated with ventricular pacing only.

A meta-analysis (23) of major pacemaker trials (Fig. 23.1) showed that atrial-based pacing did not improve survival or reduce heart failure or cardiovascular death when compared to ventricular-based pacing. However, atrial-based pacing reduced the incidence of AF (HR, 0.80; 95% CI, 0.72 to 0.89; $P = 0.00003$) and stroke (HR, 0.81; 95% CI, 0.67–0.99; $P = 0.035$).

Comparing Dual-Chamber Pacing and Exclusive Atrial Pacing

The clinical trials discussed above compared dual-chamber pacing with exclusive atrial or exclusive ventricular pacing for patients with SND. Even though there was no evident survival benefit from any of those modes of pacing, most studies pointed to worse outcomes among patients receiving exclusive ventricular pacing. However, one question remained: Is exclusive atrial pacing (AAI) better than dual-chamber devices (DDD)? Obviously, this discussion would only apply to patients with preserved AV conduction. The AAI mode would have the advantage of promoting intrinsic conduction at all time, with no risks of exposing the patients to potential deleterious effects of right ventricular pacing. However, if symptomatic AV conduction abnormality developed in the future, a new surgical intervention would be required for implantation of a ventricular lead, increasing the risks of surgical complications and infection.

Nielsen et al. (15) addressed this question by following 1415 patients over 5 years, divided in two groups: (1) AAI-R (exclusive atrial pacing) and (2) DDD-R pacing (dual-chamber pacing) in the DANPACE trial. The mean age was 73 years. Similar to other trials previously discussed, there was no difference in mortality between the two modes of pacing; however, there was a higher incidence of paroxysmal AF (PAF) and twice the number of reoperations in the AAI-R group, suggesting that DDD-R mode is the better choice for patients with SND, even if AV conduction is preserved. The investigators believe that the prolonged PR interval, more commonly observed in the AAI-R group, reduces ventricular preload and results in mitral regurgitation. The DDD-R group, on the other hand, had AV delay programmed at a value high enough to allow intrinsic conduction and significantly reduce the ventricular pacing burden. The AV delay was extended, but not long enough to have negative effects on ventricular filling, as hypothetically happened in the AAI-R group. DANPACE is the largest trial comparing exclusive atrial and dual-chamber pacing over a prolonged follow-up period of 5 years, and provides the strongest evidence to support the use of DDD-R in patients with SND.

Importance of Burden of Ventricular Pacing in SND

Based on the evidence above, it is clear that either atrial or dual-chamber pacing is the preferred method for patients with SND, and exclusive ventricular pacing should be avoided. However, the majority of these studies were somewhat disappointing in not showing a more robust superiority of the so-called "physiologic pacing" over exclusive ventricular pacing, especially with regard to mortality. If dual-chamber pacemaker promotes a more physiologic mode of pacing, why is it so difficult to demonstrate clear superiority of dual-chamber pacing over ventricular pacing only? Sweeney et al. evaluated the effect of ventricular pacing in patients from the MOST trial with SND and a narrow QRS at baseline who received a dual-chamber pacemaker (24). Interestingly, the cumulative percentage of ventricular pacing was higher in the dual-chamber pacing group than in the ventricular pacing (90% vs. 58%), explained by the relatively short AV delay programmed in the

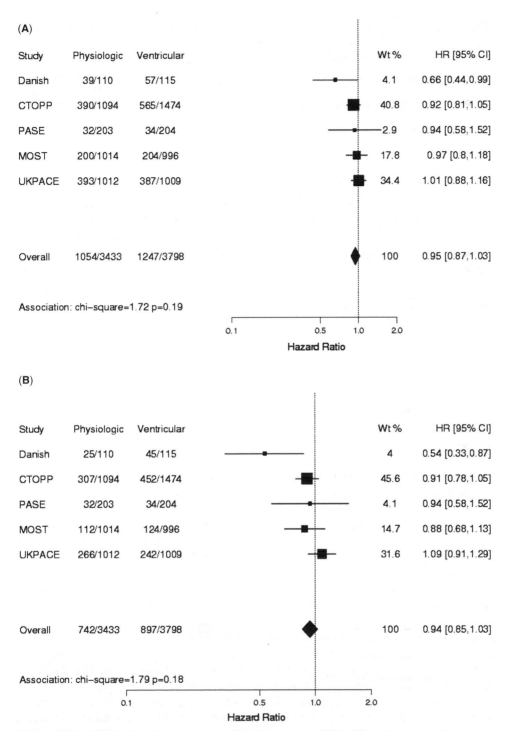

(A)

Study	Physiologic	Ventricular		Wt %	HR [95% CI]
Danish	39/110	57/115		4.1	0.66 [0.44, 0.99]
CTOPP	390/1094	565/1474		40.8	0.92 [0.81, 1.05]
PASE	32/203	34/204		2.9	0.94 [0.58, 1.52]
MOST	200/1014	204/996		17.8	0.97 [0.8, 1.18]
UKPACE	393/1012	387/1009		34.4	1.01 [0.88, 1.16]
Overall	1054/3433	1247/3798		100	0.95 [0.87, 1.03]

Association: chi–square=1.72 p=0.19

Hazard Ratio

(B)

Study	Physiologic	Ventricular		Wt %	HR [95% CI]
Danish	25/110	45/115		4	0.54 [0.33, 0.87]
CTOPP	307/1094	452/1474		45.6	0.91 [0.78, 1.05]
PASE	32/203	34/204		4.1	0.94 [0.58, 1.52]
MOST	112/1014	124/996		14.7	0.88 [0.68, 1.13]
UKPACE	266/1012	242/1009		31.6	1.09 [0.91, 1.29]
Overall	742/3433	897/3798		100	0.94 [0.85, 1.03]

Association: chi–square=1.79 p=0.18

Hazard Ratio

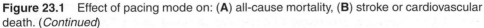

Figure 23.1 Effect of pacing mode on: (**A**) all-cause mortality, (**B**) stroke or cardiovascular death. (*Continued*)

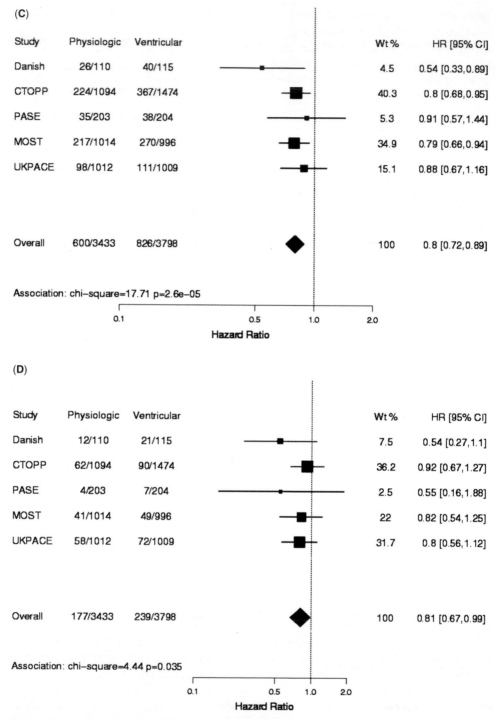

Figure 23.1 (*Continued*) (**C**) atrial fibrillation and (**D**) stroke; expressed as the HR and 95% CI. A HR with upper boundaries <1.0 favors atrial-based pacing. *Source*: From Ref. 23.

dual-chamber pacemakers, which did not allow ventricular activation through the normal conduction system. In this study, there was a direct correlation between cumulative percentage of ventricular pacing and heart failure hospitalization and incidence of AF. The authors concluded that ventricular desynchronization caused by right ventricular pacing increases the risk of hospitalization and AF, mitigating the potential benefit offered by AV synchrony during DDD pacing mode (25).

Similarly, Tang et al. (26) performed a post hoc analysis of the CTOPP trial and evaluated the impact of baseline heart rate preimplantation on clinical outcomes between ventricular and physiologic dual-chamber pacing. This study showed that patients who had baseline HR ≤60 bpm and received exclusive ventricular pacing had worse outcomes for cardiovascular death and stroke than those with higher heart rate, whereas these outcomes were unrelated to baseline bradycardia in the physiological pacing group. This study suggested that patients with bradycardia at baseline will most likely be paced more frequently, and consequently will benefit from physiologic pacing. For the group with HR >60 bpm, the choice of pacing mode does not have a significant impact on outcomes, due to the limited amount of pacing.

These post hoc analyses of two major trials illustrate the important concept that the higher the rate of cumulative ventricular pacing, the higher the chances of complications, including more AF, increased rate of thromboembolic events and worsening heart failure. This concept was well demonstrated later by the DAVID trial (27). Even though this was not primarily a pacemaker trial, it focused on the backup pacing mode selection for implantable cardioverter defibrillator (ICD) candidates. At that time, it was a common practice to implant dual-chamber ICDs. The question was raised whether those patients were receiving unnecessary and potentially harmful ventricular pacing therapy. In DAVID, patients were implanted either with dual-chamber ICD, paced at 70 bpm (DDD mode), or ventricular pacing (VVI at 40 bpm). The study was terminated early when the preliminary results showed significantly worse outcomes in the DDD group with regard to mortality and hospitalization for heart failure. The cumulative percentage of ventricular pacing over time varied from 34% to 36% in DDD group, compared to 1.7–14% in the VVI group.

Current Guidelines for Pacemaker Implantation in SND

Based on the trials discussed above, the American College of Cardiology (ACC), American Heart Association (AHA), and Heart Rhythm Society (HRS) jointly developed the most current guidelines for pacemaker implantation in patients with SND are detailed in Table 23.2 (14).

More recently, the HRS and ACC published a consensus statement on pacemaker device and mode selection (3):

- Class I: Dual-chamber pacing (DDD) or single-chamber atrial pacing (AAI) is recommended over single-chamber ventricular pacing (VVI) in patients with SND and intact AV conduction. Dual-chamber pacing is recommended over single-chamber atrial pacing in patients with SND.
- Class IIa: Rate-adaptive pacing can be useful in patients with significant symptomatic chronotropic incompetence. In patients with SND and intact AV conduction, programming dual-chamber pacemakers to minimize ventricular pacing can be useful for prevention of AF.
- Class IIb: AAI pacing may be considered in selected patients with normal AV and ventricular conduction. Single-chamber VVI pacing may be acceptable if frequent pacing is not expected or the patient has significant comorbidities that are likely to adversely influence survival and clinical outcomes.

Table 23.2 AHA/ACC/HRS Guidelines for Device-Based Therapy of Cardiac Rhythm Abnormalities

	Sinus Node Dysfunction	Atrioventricular Block	Carotid Sinus Hypersensitivity and Autonomic Dysfunction
Class I Pacemaker implant is indicated:	1. Documented symptomatic bradycardia, including frequent sinus pauses that produce symptoms. (*Level of Evidence: C*) 2. Symptomatic chronotropic incompetence. (*Level of Evidence: C*) 3. Symptomatic sinus bradycardia that results from required drug therapy for medical conditions. (*Level of Evidence: C*)	1. Third-degree and advanced second-degree AV block at any anatomic level associated with bradycardia with symptoms (including heart failure) or ventricular arrhythmias presumed to be due to AV block. (*Level of Evidence: C*) 2. Third-degree and advanced second-degree AV block at any anatomic level associated with arrhythmias and other medical conditions that require drug therapy that result in symptomatic bradycardia. (*Level of Evidence: C*) 3. Third-degree and advanced second-degree AV block at any anatomic level in awake, symptom-free patients in sinus rhythm, with documented periods of asystole ≥3.0 sec or any escape rate ≤40 bpm, or with an escape rhythm that is below the AV node. (*Level of Evidence: C*) 4. Third-degree and advanced second-degree AV block at any anatomic level in awake, symptom-free patients with AF and bradycardia with 1 or more pauses of ≥5 sec. (*Level of Evidence: C*) 5. Third-degree and advanced second-degree AV block at any anatomic level after catheter ablation of the AV junction. (*Level of Evidence: C*) 6. Third-degree and advanced second-degree AV block at any anatomic level associated with postoperative AV block that is not expected to resolve after cardiac surgery. (*Level of Evidence: C*)	Recurrent syncope caused by spontaneously occurring carotid sinus stimulation and carotid sinus pressure that induces ventricular asystole of more than 3 sec. (*Level of Evidence: C*)

7. Third-degree and advanced second-degree AV block at any anatomic level associated with neuromuscular diseases with AV block. (*Level of Evidence: B*)

8. Second-degree AV block with symptomatic bradycardia regardless of type or site of block. (*Level of Evidence: B*)

9. Asymptomatic persistent third-degree AV block at any anatomic site with average awake ventricular rates of 40 bpm or faster if cardiomegaly or LV dysfunction is present or if the site of block is below the AV node. (*Level of Evidence: B*)

10. Second- or third-degree AV block during exercise in the absence of myocardial ischemia. (*Level of Evidence: C*)

1. Persistent third-degree AV block with an escape rate >40 bpm in asymptomatic adult patients without cardiomegaly. (*Level of Evidence: C*)

2. Asymptomatic second-degree AV block at intra- or infra-His levels found at electrophysiological study. (*Level of Evidence: B*)

3. First- or second-degree AV block with symptoms similar to those of pacemaker syndrome or hemodynamic compromise. (*Level of Evidence: B*)

4. Asymptomatic type II second-degree AV block with a narrow QRS. When type II second-degree AV block occurs with a wide QRS, including isolated right bundle branch block, pacing becomes a Class I recommendation. (*Level of Evidence: B*)

Class IIa indication— Permanent pacemaker implantation is reasonable if:

1. SND with heart rate less than 40 bpm when a clear association between significant symptoms consistent with bradycardia and the actual presence of bradycardia has not been documented. (*Level of Evidence: C*)

2. Syncope of unexplained origin when clinically significant abnormalities of sinus node function are discovered or provoked in electrophysiological studies. (*Level of Evidence: C*)

Syncope without clear, provocative events and with a hypersensitive cardioinhibitory response of 3 sec or longer. (*Level of Evidence: C*)

(*Continued*)

Table 23.2 AHA/ACC/HRS Guidelines for Device-Based Therapy of Cardiac Rhythm Abnormalities (*Continued*)

	Sinus Node Dysfunction	Atrioventricular Block	Carotid Sinus Hypersensitivity and Autonomic Dysfunction
Class IIb indication: Permanent pacemaker implantation may be considered:	1. Minimally symptomatic patients with chronic heart rate less than 40 bpm while awake.	1. Neuromuscular diseases such as myotonic muscular dystrophy, Erb dystrophy (limb girdle muscular dystrophy), and peroneal muscular atrophy with any degree of AV block (including first degree AV block), with or without symptoms, because there may be unpredictable progression of AV conduction disease. (*Level of Evidence: B*) 2. AV block in the setting of drug use and/or drug toxicity when the block is expected to recur even after the drug is withdrawn. (*Level of Evidence: B*)	Significantly symptomatic neurocardiogenic syncope associated with bradycardia documented spontaneously or at the time of tilt table testing. (*Level of Evidence: B*)
Class III— Pacemaker implantation is not indicated:	1. SND in asymptomatic patients. (*Level of Evidence: C*) 2. SND in patients for whom the symptoms suggestive of bradycardia have been clearly documented to occur in the absence of bradycardia. (*Level of Evidence: C*) 3. SND with symptomatic bradycardia due to nonessential drug therapy. (*Level of Evidence: C*)	1. Asymptomatic first degree AV block. (*Level of Evidence: B*) 2. Asymptomatic type I second-degree AV block at the supra-His (AV node) level or that which is not known to be intra- or infra Hissian. (*Level of Evidence: C*) 3. AV block that is expected to resolve and is unlikely to recur (e.g., drug toxicity, Lyme disease, or transient increases in vagal tone or during hypoxia in sleep apnea syndrome in the absence of symptoms). (*Level of Evidence: B*)	1. Hypersensitive cardioinhibitory response to carotid sinus stimulation without symptoms or with vague symptoms. (*Level of Evidence: C*) 2. Situational vasovagal syncope in which avoidance behavior is effective and preferred. (*Level of Evidence: C*)

Abbreviation: AV, atrioventricular.
Source: Adapted from Ref. 14.

- Class III: There is no indication for dual-chamber pacing or single-chamber atrial pacing in patients with permanent or longstanding persistent AF and no plans to restore or maintain sinus rhythm.

AV BLOCK

AV block is a pathological conduction of an atrial impulse to the ventricles. The block can be partial or complete, and it can happen at any level between atrial and ventricular activation, including intra-atrial, AV nodal, or His-Purkinje abnormalities (28). The causes of block include ischemic heart disease, degenerative and infiltrative diseases, drug toxicities, and excess vagal activity. AV block can be paroxysmal or fixed. A patient can exhibit different degrees of AV block at different times and under different pathophysiological conditions.

Electrocardiographic Evaluation of AV Block

Electrocardiographic criteria are used to define degrees of AV block. First-degree AV block refers to a prolongation in AV conduction, but with consistent conduction of atrial impulse to ventricles, excluding premature atrial beats. On the ECG, normal sinus P waves are followed by QRS complexes, but with a P-R interval that is prolonged at greater than 0.20 seconds. The presence of a narrow QRS usually indicates disease in the AV node, but first-degree AV block with a widened QRS morphology usually suggests conduction delay in the His-Purkinje system with or without a delay in the AV node (28).

Second-degree AV block is manifested by intermittent lack of conduction from atria to ventricles. Mobitz type I second-degree AV block (also called Wenckebach block) is usually, but not always, due to disease in the AV node and produces a gradual prolongation of P-R intervals in successive beats until a P wave is completely blocked for one beat (Fig. 23.2A). Mobitz type II second-degree block, which usually involves disease below the AV node in the His-Purkinje system, produces intermittent block in AV conduction without prior prolongation of the P-R interval (Fig. 23.2B). Type I block is usually considered benign, since AV node disease is the usual site of block and the prognosis is good.

(A)

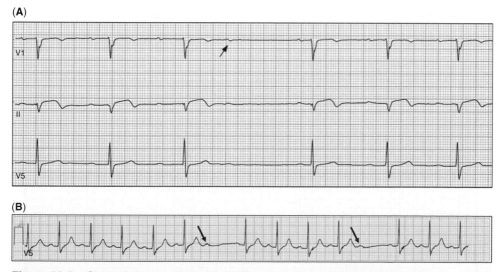

(B)

Figure 23.2 Second-degree AV block. (**A**), Mobitz I. Notice progressive prolongation of PR interval, followed by a blocked P wave (arrow). (**B**) Second degree AV block, type II. The PR interval is constant if AV conduction is present. Intermittent AV block (arrows).

There is lesser tendency for Mobitz I second-degree block to progress to complete heart block (CHB) and syncope. Temporary and permanent pacing is usually indicated for type II block because of its propensity to advance to (CHB).

The term "high-grade AV block" is used by many cardiologists but is not uniformly defined. Usually, the term refers to a situation in which multiple consecutive P waves are blocked. Typically, the P-R interval does not change in conducted beats, so this rhythm resembles type II second-degree AV block. Third-degree or complete AV block is characterized by total failure of all atrial impulses to conduct to the ventricles. The ventricular rhythm is produced by an escape focus in the AV node (junctional escape rhythm) or, more commonly, in the ventricle (idioventricular escape rhythm). The ECG during (CHB) usually exhibits three features: (1) nonconducted P waves, (2) AV dissociation (atrial and ventricular rhythms are independent), and (3) a regular ventricular response produced by the escape rhythm (Fig. 23.3).

Invasive Evaluation of AV Conduction

Electrophysiological testing can be used to identify the site of the AV block. In the non-medicated state, the patient's rhythm is recorded and the P-A, A-H, and H-V intervals are determined. Lack of a His-bundle depolarization following a blocked P wave signifies that the AV node is the site of the block. Presence of the His-bundle signal following a blocked P wave indicates that the impulse has traveled through the AV node, has stimulated the bundle of His, and has blocked below that point. Block below the bundle of His generally requires permanent pacing.

Treatment of AV Block

Cardiac pacing is the only available therapy for symptomatic/advanced AV block. The recommendation for implantation of a permanent pacemaker is based on symptoms. Further details of pacemaker indication and review of current guidelines are addressed below.

For cases of AV block that require pacing therapy, the choices include single ventricular lead or dual-chamber pacing. To determine which is the better pacing mode for the elderly, The UKPACE study (29) enrolled 2021 patients 70 years of age or older with high

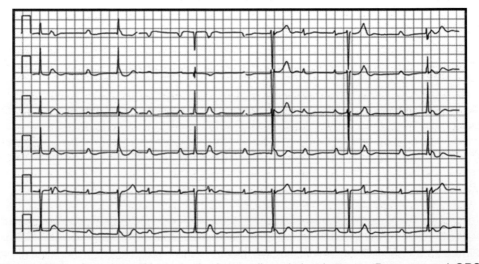

Figure 23.3 Complete AV block. Complete dissociation between P waves and QRS complexes.

grade AV block requiring pacemaker implantation. Patients were randomized to either single-chamber or dual-chamber pacemaker. The single-chamber ventricular pacemaker group was divided in two subgroups: either fixed rate or rate-adaptive pacing. Over a mean follow-up of 4.6 years, there was no difference in mean annual mortality between the single versus dual-chamber pacemaker groups, which was close to 7%. There was also no difference in the rate of AF, heart failure or composite of stroke/transient ischemic attack (TIA) or other thromboembolism. The rate of complications was higher in the dual-chamber group (7.8 percent vs. 3.5 percent, $P < 0.001$), which also required frequent therapeutic interventions and higher rate of operation. The results of UKPACE were disappointing. Despite observational studies demonstrating the benefits of physiologic pacing (30–32), this large randomized clinical trial did not show any prognostic difference between single-chamber and dual-chamber pacemakers. It is possible that the fixed AV interval used in the dual-chamber group promoted more frequent ventricular pacing, counteracting the potential benefits of a more physiologic pacing in patients with intermittent AV block.

The evidence provided by randomized control trials should be the foundation to inform therapeutic decisions. However, it is also important to tailor the therapy to the patient's clinical characteristics. The choice of pacing mode will be strongly influenced by the individual's baseline condition, comorbidities, and other associated rhythm disorders. For instance, for individuals with advanced AV block requiring pacing associated with permanent AF, where there are no plans to restore sinus rhythm, a dual-chamber pacemaker would have no role, and a single ventricular lead would be the appropriate choice (VVI or VVIR). If the treatment is directed to a highly functional older individual with advanced AV block and associated SND with significant chronotropic insufficiency, a dual-chamber pacing would be the best choice, with activation of rate adaptive mode (DDD-R). On the other hand, in cases of sedentary lifestyle, with significant comorbidities and/or very limited functional capacity, the implantation of a single ventricular lead would suffice (VVI or VVIR), without adding the risks of a more complex procedure. The VDD mode is also an alternative for individuals with exclusive AV block and preserved sinus node function. This pacing mode allows both sensing and pacing for the ventricles, but it is limited to exclusive sensing in the atria. A single ventricular lead equipped with a sensing component in its atrial portion can be used, facilitating the implant procedure. This mode is rarely used in the USA, but it is common in Europe and Latin America.

Current Guidelines for Pacing Therapy in AV Block

The ACC, AHA, and HRS jointly developed the current guidelines for pacemaker implantation (14). The current recommendations for pacing in AV block are detailed in Table 23.2.

Once the decision about pacing has been made based on the guidelines listed in Table 23.2, the most recent HRS and ACC Expert Consensus Statement on Pacemaker Device and Mode Selection has the following recommendations (3):

Class I: Dual-chamber pacing is recommended in patients with AV block. Single-chamber ventricular pacing is acceptable in patients with AV block who have specific clinical situations that limit the benefits of dual-chamber pacing (sedentary lifestyle, significant medical comorbidities, vascular access limitations, among others).

Dual-chamber pacing is the choice if there is documented pacemaker syndrome.

Class IIa: Single-lead, dual-chamber VDD pacing can be useful in patients with normal sinus node function and AV block. VVI pacing can be useful in patients following AV junction ablation, or in whom AV junction ablation is planned, for rate control of AF.

Class III: Dual-chamber pacing should not be used in AV block if there are no plans to restore sinus rhythm in a patient with permanent or longstanding persistent AF.

CAROTID SINUS HYPERSENSITIVITY

Carotid sinus hypersensitivity (CSH) is defined as exacerbation of the carotid sinus reflex leading to vagal activation or sympathetic inhibition, with consequent bradycardia and/or hypotension. This condition is commonly seen in the elderly population. When CSH is associated with syncope or presyncope, it defines carotid sinus syndrome (CSS) (33). This syndrome is responsible for 10–25% of syncopal events in elderly (34). Syncope is a classic presentation of CSS. However, only a small proportion will have the classic presentation of symptoms during manipulation of the neck/carotid sinus region, representing less than 1% of all cases of syncope (35). More commonly, patients will present with complaints of unexplained syncope, without a clear trigger, and further tests will reveal the presence of CSH. Up to 37% of patients with CSS will present with dizziness and recurrent falls. These falls can in fact be secondary to true syncope; but some patients, especially at advanced age, will not notice loss of consciousness, either because it was too brief or because they do not recollect the symptoms preceding the event of fall (36).

Diagnosis of CSS

Carotid sinus massage (CSM) can induce a physiologic response, with induction of bradycardia, associated or not with hypotension, especially in individuals above 40 years of age. The diagnostic criteria for CSH has been standardized as a pause >3 seconds (cardioinhibitory component) and/or >50 mmHg drop in systolic blood pressure (vasodepressor component), in response to 3–5 seconds of CSM. It is classified as a mixed response when both criteria are met. The CSM should be performed on both sides and with beat-to-beat monitoring of blood pressure and heart rate. If no abnormal response is detected while the patient is supine, the maneuver should be repeated in the upright position (commonly done during tilt table test, with table inclined at 70 degrees). Up to 30% of patients will have a positive CSM test only in the upright position (33). The CSM is considered positive only if the test reproduces the clinical symptoms (36) because up to 10% of the normal population can have a pronounced physiologic response to CSM, meeting the described criteria for bradycardia and/or hypotension, without relevant clinical significance (36).

CSM is considered safe, even in elderly patients. The rate of neurologic complication is reported between 0.28 and 0.45% (36). This test, however, should not be performed in patients with prior history of TIA or stroke in the past 3 months, carotid bruits or Doppler evidence of significant carotid stenosis (33,36–38).

Atropine can be used to better differentiate true mixed response to CSM from hypotension secondary to intense bradycardia in case of a pure cardioinhibitory response. In a true mixed response, atropine will prevent the induction of bradycardia during CSM, but will not have any effect on the induced hypotension. On the other hand, atropine will prevent hypotension if that was secondary to bradycardia.

The diagnosis of CSS is not always straightforward. As mentioned above, the classic scenario of a syncopal event associated with neck manipulation is quite rare. The investigation of recurrent syncope or fall will include CSM, but in some instances, this test will not be conclusive, either due to lack of response or inability to reproduce the symptoms in the presence of bradycardia and/or hypotension. For those cases, the implantation of ECG recording devices can be helpful for diagnosis of cardioinhibitory form of CSS, which can document asystolic events associated with syncope. Mennozi et al. (39) evaluated a series of 24 patients, mean age of 62 ± 12 years, with recurrent syncope and positive CSM but without reproducibility of symptoms during the test. The implantable ECG recorder detected episodes of asystole in 74% of patients during 2 years of follow-up. From all those events, only 43% of pauses >6 seconds and 0.7% of pauses between 3 and 6 seconds were associated with syncopal or presyncopal symptoms. In a similar study, Maggi et al. (40)

evaluated 18 patients, mean age of 68 ± 12 years, with recurrent syncope, suspected to be neurally mediated, with an implantable event recorder. The results showed a significantly higher number of asystolic syncopal events in patients with a positive CSM test at baseline when compared to patients with a negative test.

CSS Treatment

Despite the high prevalence of CSS in the general population, there are limited data on ideal treatment for this condition. Medical therapy is potentially an option for treatment of CSS, but the data is limited to small series and case reports, and it includes the use of anticholinergic drugs, fludrocortisone, beta-blockers, and serotonin re-uptake inhibitors (SSRI).

Cardiac pacing is widely accepted as the treatment of choice for patients with cardio-inhibitory form or mixed form with predominance of cardioinhibitory component. Peretz et al. (41) followed 89 patients with CSS implanted with VVI pacemaker. The authors did not detect any recurrent syncopal event among patients with cardioinhibitory CSS in 17 years of follow-up.

Maggi et al. (40) proceeded with implantation of a dual-chamber pacemaker in 14 patients (87% of studied population) with positive CSM and recurrent syncope after documentation of symptomatic asystolic events. During follow-up of 35 months, the number of syncopal events decreased dramatically from 1.68/year to 0.04/year after pacing therapy. The study suggested that identification of cardioinhibitory CSH at initial evaluation predicts an asystolic mechanism during syncope and it suggests possible benefit from pacing therapy.

Several other randomized studies have shown that pacing reduces the rate of syncope, falls and the incidence of injury related to fall (42–44). However, it is important to mention that most of these studies were small and unblinded. Up to 15% of patients will continue to present with recurrent syncope and up to 50% will continue to report symptoms of dizziness and orthostatic hypotension after pacemaker implantation (36).

The prognosis of CSS is mostly related to recurrent symptoms, which are quite variable, and can be detected in 25–57% of untreated patients (36). Patients with a vasodepressor response are more prone to recurrence of syncopal events when compared to those with the cardioinhibitory form.

Ideal Pacing Mode in CSS

If a pacemaker is the recommended treatment for patients with symptomatic CSH, what is the best pacing modality? Both sinus bradycardia and/or AV node conduction delay can occur in patients with CSS. Therefore, exclusive atrial pacing (AAI mode) is not recommended, as demonstrated by Morley et al. (43), in 70 patients with syncope and CSS, treated with different pacing modalities. All eight patients treated with AAI mode pacing had recurrence of symptoms due to AV block.

The possible pacing options include VVI, DDI, DDD, or DDD with rate drop response (also called sudden bradycardia response). The latter pacing mode was initially developed to treat patients with vasovagal syndrome. Once a sudden drop in heart rate is detected, the pacemaker is programmed to intervene at a higher rate temporarily, as an attempt to increase cardiac output and compensate for possible hypotension associated with these events. Initial studies in vasovagal patients were promising, but larger randomized double blind studies failed to show benefit from this pacing mode (45,46). The rate-drop response pacing mode was tested in patients with symptomatic CSH and recurrent falls—the SAFEPACE study (44). This single-center trial showed 70% reduction in falls and 75% reduction in injuries after implantation of a pacemaker programmed for rate-drop response. However, a multicenter trial (SAFEPACE 2) (47) failed to show superiority of this pacing mode in comparison to a simple implantable loop recorder. The authors attributed the disappointing result to the population profile, which was older, and patients were physically and cognitively more frail than in the previous trial. Regardless, the results of this study raised doubts about the value of this pacing mode in CSS with recurrent falls.

Observational studies have compared VVI versus DDI or DDD pacing in patients with CSH, with conflicting results, some showing improvement in symptoms regardless of the choice for pacing mode, and other studies showing superiority of dual chamber when compared to VVI in the control of symptoms of syncope (42,43).

In a prospective study, McLeod et al. (34) enrolled 21 patients, mean age of 74 years, with symptomatic CSH without evidence of SND or AV block and compared the impact of three different pacing modes (VVI, DDD-R, and DDD-R with sudden bradycardia response) on recurrence of syncope and quality of life. Patients were exposed to all three modes of pacing in a sequential fashion, spending 6 months in each modality in a double blind study design. The authors found a reduction in episodes of syncope and presyncope in all three pacing modalities after pacemaker therapy, but were unable to demonstrate the superiority of any one pacing mode. There were 29 episodes of syncope before pacemaker implantation, but only two episodes were recorded during all 18 months of follow-up (after patients had gone through all three pacing modes). Similarly, there were 258 episodes of presyncope prior to pacemaker implantation and only 17 episodes during the entire period of observation, and all modes were equally efficacious in reducing these events. The small number of patients is a limitation to this study, but there were a substantial number of events in each group.

Current Pacemaker Guidelines Recommendations in CSS

The current guidelines for device-based therapy of rhythm disorders, published in 2008, include some specific recommendations for patients with CSS (Table 23.2).

The recommendations from HRS/ACC for choice of pacing mode in CSS (3) are quite simple and include the following:

- Class IIa: Dual-chamber or single-chamber ventricular pacing can be useful for patients with hypersensitive CSS.
- Class III: Single-chamber AAI pacing is not recommended for patients with hypersensitive carotid sinus syndrome.

PACEMAKERS IN VERY ELDERLY PATIENTS

The very elderly population is rapidly growing in the USA (48). However, there is a paucity of data on outcomes in octogenarians or nonagenarians after pacemaker implantation. In a series of 149 pacemaker implants in a single center, Stevenson et al. (49) reported that the rate of complications among very elderly patients (>80 years) was comparable with those previously reported in the literature, generally including younger patients (0.7% incidence of major complications in hospital, and 5.4% during 30-day follow-up). However, the 30-day all-cause mortality rate was higher among elderly patients when compared to historical data from other trials including younger patients (cardiovascular mortality of 0.7% and all-cause mortality of 2% in 30 days). This study was limited by a short-term follow-up and modest number of patients. The investigators believe that the higher mortality rate is inherent to the elderly population, and not related to the procedure itself.

In another study, 481 octogenarians (86.2 ± 4.5 years) underwent pacemaker implantation for bradycardia in the Netherlands, and the rates of complications were similar (around 18%) over 5 years of follow-up when compared to patients <80 years old (50). The survival rate was comparable to age- and sex-matched controls, suggesting that pacing for bradycardia can restore life expectancy to normal.

Contradictory to these previous studies, a meta-analysis of 3 major trials in bradycardia pacing (CTOPP, DANISH, and UKPACE) revealed modestly increased rates of acute complications in the elderly (>75 years), most commonly pneumothorax (1.6% versus 0.8%) and lead dislodgement/loss of capture (2.0% vs. 1.1%). The risk of lead fracture, however, was lower among elderly when compared to younger patients (2.7% vs. 3.6%, respectively) (51).

In summary, despite the paucity of data on complications related to pacemaker implantation in the very elderly, the available data does not preclude the recommendation of pacing therapy for these patients.

PACEMAKERS AND END-OF-LIFE

As previously discussed, the number of CIEDs continues to grow in the elderly. Despite proved efficacy of these devices in increasing survival rates, all patients will eventually reach the end of their lives. Once the patient reaches that point, a discussion about device deactivation should be initiated by patients, family members or by health professionals. This discussion encompasses ethical, legal, and many times religious issues, rendering the decision-making process complex and challenging.

A survey performed among internists about cessation of pacing therapy or ICD deactivation in terminally ill patients showed that most internists were less comfortable discussing cessation of pacemaker and ICD therapy compared to other life-sustaining therapies, with only 34% of physicians reporting participation in this decision at some point in their practice (52). Internists commonly reported lack of experience with this practice. Some physicians erroneously classified deactivation of pacemaker in a pacemaker-dependent patient as assisted suicide (19%) or euthanasia (9%) (52).

The HRS has published an Expert Consensus Statement on the Management of Cardiovascular Implantable Electronic Devices in patients nearing end of life or requesting withdrawal of therapy (53). A similar document has also been published by European Heart Rhythm Association (16).

Several key issues are summarized below:

a) Every patient with decision-making capacity has the right to refuse a new therapy or to choose the discontinuation of any medical treatment or intervention, even if its withdrawal will result in death. Patient's autonomy is the fundamental principle in the decision-making process.
b) Patients can refuse any type of therapy and can also request the discontinuation of any type of intervention/therapy. CIEDs are not an exception to this rule.
c) Ethically, CIED deactivation is neither physician-assisted suicide nor euthanasia. The deactivation of these devices will allow the patient to follow the natural course of his/her terminal condition.
d) In some cases, physicians may disagree with the deactivation of device based on the physician's own personal, moral, or religious values. In that case, another physician should become involved in the case and proceed with the patient's wishes.
e) Advance directives are strongly recommended, and ideally should be established as soon as the device is implanted.
f) Patients have the right to refuse any CIED therapy, but do not have the right to demand removal of it, which would impose more risks, and have the same effect as simply turning off the device.

CONCLUSION

The incidence of bradyarrhythmias is high among elderly patients. The geriatric population is growing rapidly, which will result in an increasing number of patients requiring antibradycardia therapy. Pacemakers have been proven to improve the quality of life and reduce symptoms of patients affected by SND, AV conduction abnormalities, or CSH. Large trials comparing different pacing modalities have not shown evident superiority of one pacing mode over another with respect to mortality, regardless of the type of bradyarrhythmias. However, it has been consistently shown that the higher the ventricular pacing burden, the higher is the rate of AF, embolic events and heart failure. Therefore, a physiologic pacing mode should be the first choice if considered a viable option. Deactivation of pacemakers and other CIED at the end of life should be discussed with elderly patients and their families, ideally at an earlier time point.

REFERENCES

1. Howden LM, Meyer JA. United States Census Bureau - Age and Sex Composition: 2010. 2011: 1–16.
2. Kurtz SM, Ochoa JA, Lau E, et al. Implantation trends and patient profiles for pacemakers and implantable cardioverter defibrillators in the United States: 1993–2006. Pacing Clin Electrophysiol 2010; 33: 705–11.
3. Gillis AM, Russo AM, Ellenbogen KA, et al. HRS/ACCF expert consensus statement on pacemaker device and mode selection. J Am Coll Cardiol 2012; 60: 682–703.
4. Menozzi C, Brignole M, Alboni P, et al. The natural course of untreated sick sinus syndrome and identification of the variables predictive of unfavorable outcome. Am J Cardiol 1998; 82: 1205–9.
5. Lamas GA, Lee K, Sweeney M, et al. The mode selection trial (MOST) in sinus node dysfunction: design, rationale, and baseline characteristics of the first 1000 patients. Am Heart J 2000; 140: 541–51.
6. Fuster V, Walsh RA, Harrington RA. Bradyarrhythmias and pacemakers. In: Hurst's the Heart, 13th edn. Fuster V, Walsh RA, Harrington RA, eds. New York: McGraw-Hill Companies, Inc, 2010: 133–44.
7. Wahls SA. Sick sinus syndrome. Am Fam Physician 1985; 31: 117–24.
8. Adan V, Crown LA. Diagnosis and treatment of sick sinus syndrome. Am Fam Physician 2003; 67: 1725–32.
9. Rodriguez RD, Schocken DD. Update on sick sinus syndrome, a cardiac disorder of aging. Geriatrics 1990; 45: 26–30; 3–6.
10. Sutton R, Kenny RA. The natural history of sick sinus syndrome. Pacing Clin Electrophysiol 1986; 9: 1110–14.
11. Brandt J, Anderson H, Fahraeus T, Schuller H. Natural history of sinus node disease treated with atrial pacing in 213 patients: implications for selection of stimulation mode. J Am Coll Cardiol 1992; 20: 633–9.
12. Alt E, Volker R, Wirtzfeld A, Ulm K. Survival and follow-up after pacemaker implantation: a comparison of patients with sick sinus syndrome, complete heart block, and atrial fibrillation. Pacing Clin Electrophysiol 1985; 8: 849–55.
13. Simon AB, Janz N. Symptomatic bradyarrhythmias in the adult: natural history following ventricular pacemaker implantation. Pacing Clin Electrophysiol 1982; 5: 372–83.
14. Epstein AE, DiMarco JP, Ellenbogen KA, et al. ACC/AHA/HRS 2008 guidelines for device-based therapy of cardiac rhythm abnormalities: a report of the American College of Cardiology/American Heart Association Task Force on Practice Guidelines (Writing Committee to Revise the ACC/AHA/ NASPE 2002 Guideline Update for Implantation of Cardiac Pacemakers and Antiarrhythmia Devices): developed in collaboration with the American Association for Thoracic Surgery and Society of Thoracic Surgeons. Circulation 2008; 117: e350–408.
15. Nielsen JC, Thomsen PE, Hojberg S, et al. A comparison of single-lead atrial pacing with dual-chamber pacing in sick sinus syndrome. Eur Heart J 2011; 32: 686–96.
16. Padeletti L, Arnar DO, Boncinelli L, et al. EHRA Expert Consensus Statement on the management of cardiovascular implantable electronic devices in patients nearing end of life or requesting withdrawal of therapy. Europace 2010; 12: 1480–9.
17. Connolly SJ, Kerr CR, Gent M, et al. Effects of physiologic pacing versus ventricular pacing on the risk of stroke and death due to cardiovascular causes. Canadian Trial of Physiologic Pacing Investigators. N Engl J Med 2000; 342: 1385–91.

18. Andersen HR, Thuesen L, Bagger JP, Vesterlund T, Thomsen PE. Prospective randomised trial of atrial versus ventricular pacing in sick-sinus syndrome. Lancet 1994; 344: 1523–8.
19. Andersen HR, Nielsen JC, Thomsen PE, et al. Long-term follow-up of patients from a randomised trial of atrial versus ventricular pacing for sick-sinus syndrome. Lancet 1997; 350: 1210–16.
20. Lamas GA, Orav EJ, Stambler BS, et al. Quality of life and clinical outcomes in elderly patients treated with ventricular pacing as compared with dual-chamber pacing. Pacemaker Selection in the Elderly Investigators. N Engl J Med 1998; 338: 1097–104.
21. Kerr CR, Connolly SJ, Abdollah H, et al. Canadian Trial of Physiological Pacing: effects of physiological pacing during long-term follow-up. Circulation 2004; 109: 357–62.
22. Lamas GA, Lee KL, Sweeney MO, et al. Ventricular pacing or dual-chamber pacing for sinus-node dysfunction. N Engl J Med 2002; 346: 1854–62.
23. Healey JS, Toff WD, Lamas GA, et al. Cardiovascular outcomes with atrial-based pacing compared with ventricular pacing: meta-analysis of randomized trials, using individual patient data. Circulation 2006; 114: 11–17.
24. Sweeney MO, Hellkamp AS, Ellenbogen KA, et al. Adverse effect of ventricular pacing on heart failure and atrial fibrillation among patients with normal baseline QRS duration in a clinical trial of pacemaker therapy for sinus node dysfunction. Circulation 2003; 107: 2932–7.
25. Ellenbogen KA, Wilkoff BL, Kay GN, Lau C-P, eds. Clinical Cardiac Pacing, Defibrillation and Resynchronization Therapy, 4th edn. Philadelphia, PA: Elsevier, 2011: 234–57.
26. Tang AS, Roberts RS, Kerr C, et al. Relationship between pacemaker dependency and the effect of pacing mode on cardiovascular outcomes. Circulation 2001; 103: 3081–5.
27. Wilkoff BL, Cook JR, Epstein AE, et al. Dual-chamber pacing or ventricular backup pacing in patients with an implantable defibrillator: the Dual Chamber and VVI Implantable Defibrillator (DAVID) Trial. JAMA 2002; 288: 3115–23.
28. Schwartzman D. Atrioventricular block and atriovenrticular dissociation. In: Jalife Z, ed. Cardiac Electrophysiology: From Cell to Bedside, 4th edn. Philadelphia: Saunders, 2004: 485–9.
29. Toff WD, Camm AJ, Skehan JD. Single-chamber versus dual-chamber pacing for high-grade atrioventricular block. N Engl J Med 2005; 353: 145–55.
30. Tang CY, Kerr CR, Connolly SJ. Clinical trials of pacing mode selection. Cardiol Clin 2000; 18: 1–23; vii.
31. Lamas GA, Pashos CL, Normand SL, McNeil B. Permanent pacemaker selection and subsequent survival in elderly Medicare pacemaker recipients. Circulation 1995; 91: 1063–9.
32. Petch MC. Who needs dual chamber pacing? Br Med J 1993; 307: 215–16.
33. Moya A, Sutton R, Ammirati F, et al. Guidelines for the diagnosis and management of syncope (version 2009). Eur Heart J 2009; 30: 2631–71.
34. McLeod CJ, Trusty JM, Jenkins SM, et al. Method of pacing does not affect the recurrence of syncope in carotid sinus syndrome. Pacing Clin Electrophysiol 2012; 35: 827–33.
35. Brignole M, Alboni P, Benditt D, et al. Guidelines on management (diagnosis and treatment) of syncope. Eur Heart J 2001; 22: 1256–306.
36. Healey J, Connolly SJ, Morillo CA. The management of patients with carotid sinus syndrome: is pacing the answer? Clin Auton Res 2004; 14: 80–6.
37. Davies AJ, Kenny RA. Frequency of neurologic complications following carotid sinus massage. Am J Cardiol 1998; 81: 1256–7.
38. Munro NC, McIntosh S, Lawson J, et al. Incidence of complications after carotid sinus massage in older patients with syncope. J Am Geriatr Soc 1994; 42: 1248–51.
39. Menozzi C, Brignole M, Lolli G, et al. Follow-up of asystolic episodes in patients with cardioinhibitory, neurally mediated syncope and VVI pacemaker. Am J Cardiol 1993; 72: 1152–5.
40. Maggi R, Menozzi C, Brignole M, et al. Cardioinhibitory carotid sinus hypersensitivity predicts an asystolic mechanism of spontaneous neurally mediated syncope. Europace 2007; 9: 563–7.
41. Peretz DI, Abdulla A. Management of cardioinhibitory hypersensitive carotid sinus syncope with permanent cardiac pacing–a seventeen year prospective study. Can J Cardiol 1985; 1: 86–91.
42. Huang SK, Ezri MD, Hauser RG, Denes P. Carotid sinus hypersensitivity in patients with unexplained syncope: clinical, electrophysiologic, and long-term follow-up observations. Am Heart J 1988; 116: 989–96.
43. Morley CA, Perrins EJ, Grant P, et al. Carotid sinus syncope treated by pacing. Analysis of persistent symptoms and role of atrioventricular sequential pacing. Br Heart J 1982; 47: 411–18.
44. Kenny RA, Richardson DA, Steen N, et al. Carotid sinus syndrome: a modifiable risk factor for nonaccidental falls in older adults (SAFE PACE). J Am Coll Cardiol 2001; 38: 1491–6.
45. Connolly SJ, Sheldon R, Roberts RS, Gent M. The North American Vasovagal Pacemaker Study (VPS). A randomized trial of permanent cardiac pacing for the prevention of vasovagal syncope. J Am Coll Cardiol 1999; 33: 16–20.

46. Connolly SJ, Sheldon R, Thorpe KE, et al. Pacemaker therapy for prevention of syncope in patients with recurrent severe vasovagal syncope: Second Vasovagal Pacemaker Study (VPS II): a randomized trial. JAMA 2003; 289: 2224–9.
47. Ryan DJ, Nick S, Colette SM, Roseanne K. Carotid sinus syndrome, should we pace? A multicentre, randomised control trial (Safepace 2). Heart 2010; 96: 347–51.
48. Perls T. Health and disease in people over 85. Br Med J 2009; 339: b4715.
49. Stevenson RT, Lugg D, Gray R, et al. Pacemaker implantation in the extreme elderly. J Interv Card Electrophysiol 2012; 33: 51–8.
50. Udo EO, van Hemel NM, Zuithoff NP, et al. Long-term outcome of cardiac pacing in octogenarians and nonagenarians. Europace 2012; 14: 502–8.
51. Armaganijan LV, Toff WD, Nielsen JC, et al. Are elderly patients at increased risk of complications following pacemaker implantation? A meta-analysis of randomized trials. Pacing Clin Electrophysiol 2012; 35: 131–4.
52. Kramer DB, Kesselheim AS, Brock DW, Maisel WH. Ethical and legal views of physicians regarding deactivation of cardiac implantable electrical devices: a quantitative assessment. Heart Rhythm 2010; 7: 1537–42.
53. Lampert R, Hayes DL, Annas GJ, et al. HRS Expert Consensus Statement on the Management of Cardiovascular Implantable Electronic Devices (CIEDs) in patients nearing end of life or requesting withdrawal of therapy. Heart Rhythm 2010; 7: 1008–26.

24

Cerebrovascular disease in the elderly patient

Jesse Weinberger

SUMMARY

Stroke is primarily a disease of the elderly. The incidence of stroke under age 65 is less than 2/1000/yr, but rises to 4.6/1000/yr for men and 3.8/1000/yr for women aged 65–74 years, and to 9.4/1000/yr for men and 7.4/1000/yr for women aged 75–84 years (1). Stroke is the third leading cause of death in the USA and is the leading cause of neurological disability. It is often felt to be a fate worse than death by elderly patients.

Stroke is caused by disruption of the circulation of blood to the brain, and can be ischemic due to occlusion of an artery or hemorrhagic due to rupture of an artery. Ischemia accounts for 80–85% of stroke while hemorrhage accounts for 15–20% (2,3). Ischemic stroke is caused primarily by atherosclerotic disease of large extracranial and intracranial vessels, occlusion of intracranial vessels by emboli from a cardiac source, and small vessel intracranial occlusive disease secondary to hypertension and diabetes (Figs. 24.1 and 24.2). Hemorrhage can be intraparenchymal in the brain itself, mainly from hypertension, or subarachnoid from rupture of an aneurysm arising from the vessels of the circle of Willis.

The major risk factor for cerebrovascular disease in studies of patients matched for other cardiovascular risk factors is hypertension (4). Diabetes (5) and cigarette smoking also play a significant role (6), while elevation of serum lipids is less consequential for cerebrovascular disease than for coronary artery disease (7). Control of these risk factors at a young age has contributed to an impressive reduction in the incidence of stroke, but addressing these risk factors in the elderly patient still plays an important role (1). Cardiogenic embolization, particularly from nonvalvular atrial fibrillation, assumes greater importance as an etiology for stroke in the elderly patient, and strategies have currently been developed to reduce the incidence of stroke in these patients (8).

While prevention of stroke is the principal goal in the treatment of patients with cerebrovascular disease, medical therapy for the elderly stroke patient can enhance outcome. New treatment modalities to restore cerebral circulation with thrombolytic therapy have changed the outlook on treatment of stroke, and therapeutic trials are under way to determine if neuroprotective agents can diminish the extent of irreversible brain damage in acute stroke.

ANATOMY AND PHYSIOLOGY OF THE CEREBRAL CIRCULATION

The brain is supplied by an extensive interconnected network of arterial circulation. Each cerebral hemisphere receives blood flow from the ipsilateral internal carotid artery that branches into the middle cerebral artery over the lateral surface of the brain and the anterior cerebral artery over the medial surface of the brain. The brain stem and cerebellum receive blood flow from the vertebral and basilar arteries, which terminate in the posterior cerebral

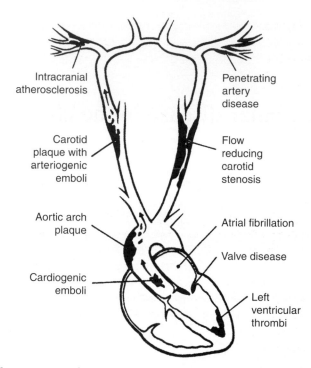

Figure 24.1   The anatomy of the cerebral circulation is diagrammed demonstrating the potential etiologies of ischemic stroke: cardioembolic, carotid atherothrombotic, intracranial atherosclerosis, and small vessel intracranial vascular disease. *Source*: From Ref. 2.

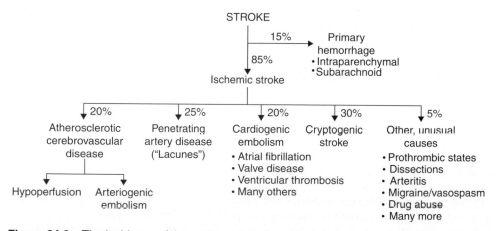
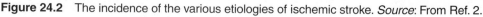

Figure 24.2   The incidence of the various etiologies of ischemic stroke. *Source*: From Ref. 2.

arteries that feed the posterior portions of the cerebral hemisphere including the occipital and posterior parietal lobes and the thalamus.

     Connections exist between the two carotid arteries through the anterior communicating artery and between the basilar artery and the two carotid arteries through the posterior communicating arteries. These collateral channels form a complete circuit of arterial supply known as the circle of Willis. Collateral circulation also can be provided by the external carotid artery that branches from the internal carotid artery at the bifurcation of the cervical common carotid. The external carotid artery can connect to the internal carotid circulation distally through the ophthalmic artery and through anastomoses between the meningeal branches of the external carotid artery and the surface branches of the cerebral arteries. Because of this collateral circulation, the brain can tolerate complete occlusion of a carotid artery without injury or symptoms, and there are case reports of patients with bilateral carotid artery occlusion and unilateral vertebral artery occlusion whose only symptoms are nonspecific dizziness (9).

Another protective mechanism for circulation to the brain is autoregulation. Blood flow is maintained constantly at an average of 50–70 mL/100 g/min in the gray matter containing neuronal cell bodies, and 10–20 mL/100 g/min in the white matter containing the neuronal axons at ranges of mean arterial blood pressure from 60 to 160 mmHg without fluctuations due to changes in pressure (10). Blood flow does fluctuate with the blood partial pressure of carbon dioxide (PCO_2), increasing or decreasing by 4% per 1 torr of PCO_2. This ensures that there will be increased blood supply to metabolically active regions of the brain that are producing large amounts of carbon dioxide so that sufficient oxygen can be delivered.

PATHOPHYSIOLOGY OF ISCHEMIC STROKE

Ischemic stroke is caused by thrombotic or embolic occlusion of arteries supplying the brain. Atherosclerotic disease at the cervical carotid artery bifurcation accounts for about 20% of ischemic stroke (1,2). Because of the extensive collateral circulation of blood to the brain, it is unusual for ischemic stroke to occur on a hemodynamic basis because of occlusive disease in the carotid or vertebrobasilar arteries, unless the channels through the circle of Willis are incomplete. Therefore, the primary mechanism for stroke due to occlusive disease at the carotid artery bifurcation is embolization of thrombus or atherosclerotic debris from plaque at the bifurcation, which occludes an intracerebral artery (11). With complete occlusion of the internal carotid artery (Fig. 24.3), thrombus can propagate distally in the artery and obstruct collateral channels, causing infarction of a large portion of the cerebral hemisphere. Infarction can sometimes occur on a hemodynamic basis because of hypoperfusion in watershed areas, which are supplied by the distal territories of two arterial trees such as the parietal lobe, which receives terminal branches from both the middle and posterior cerebral arteries. Watershed infarcts can also sometimes occur when there is hypoperfusion due to cardiac arrhythmia, syncope, or cardiac arrest (12).

Cardiogenic emboli to occlude the intracranial arteries account for 20–30% of ischemic strokes (Fig. 24.4) (1,2). The largest source of these emboli is thrombus from the left atrium in patients with atrial fibrillation, particularly in patients older than 75 years with a marked preponderance in women older than 80 years (8). Valvular heart disease, thrombus from akinetic ventricular wall with myocardial infarction or cardiomyopathy, right-to-left shunts through a patent foramen ovale or atrial septal defect also contribute to cardioembolic stroke (1,2,13). Artery-to-artery emboli can also arise from atheromatous plaque at the arch of the aorta and may account for up to 4% of strokes (14,15).

Atherosclerotic occlusive disease of the large intracranial arteries is an unusual cause of stroke in white patients, but is more common in African-American and Asian patients (11). Intracranial thrombosis of small penetrating arteries supplying the deep structures of the brain, such as the internal capsule and basal ganglia, account for about 25–50% of ischemic strokes (1,2). These vessels are endarteries that do not have collateral flow to the regions they supply. Thrombosis usually occurs because of proliferative thickening of the walls of these arteries due to fibrinoid necrosis or lipohyalinization caused by diabetes and hypertension (16). When these arteries occlude, they produce small holes in the deep white

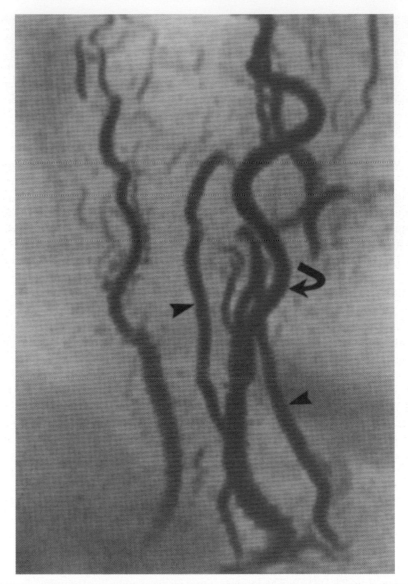

Figure 24.3 Internal carotid artery occlusion. MRA of the extracranial circulation performed using a 2-D time-of-flight sequence. This four-vessel view shows flow in the
left internal carotid artery (*curved arrow*) and in the vertebral arteries (*arrowheads*), but
no flow in the right internal carotid artery.

matter, often referred to as lacunes (Fig. 24.5) (16). While the lesions may be small, if they
are located in significant white matter tracts such as the internal capsule, which carries the
main motor and sensory fibers from the cerebral hemispheres, then a devastating neurological deficit such as complete paralysis of the contralateral arm and leg can result.

Unusual causes of stroke, such as vasculitis, hypercoaguable state from anticardiolipin antibody or protein C and protein S deficiency, arterial dissection, and hematologic
abnormalities such as sickle cell disease occur mainly in younger patients and are less
likely to occur in the elderly (17–21). Even with the advent of noninvasive imaging techniques to identify the nature and causes of ischemic stroke, in 5–10% of strokes the etiology cannot be identified and these are classified as cryptogenic strokes (1,2).

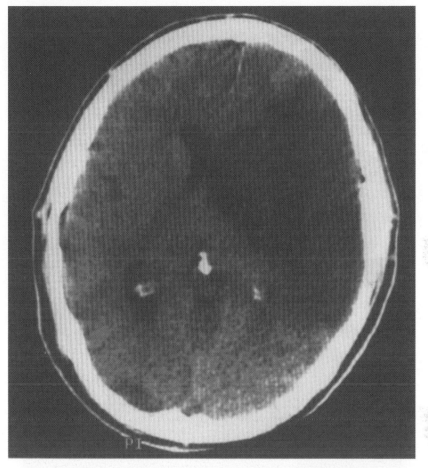

Figure 24.4 Middle cerebral artery occlusion. CAT scan at the level of the frontal horns of the lateral ventricles demonstrates a well-defined wedge-shaped area of low attenuation involving both gray and white matter of the left frontal lobe. There is mass effect demonstrated by shift of the midline to the right. This is consistent with a subacute (3–5-day old) infarct in the middle cerebral artery territory secondary to suggesting middle cerebral artery occlusion.

Intracerebral hemorrhage usually involves the rupture of Charcot Bouchard aneurysm, a microaneurysm formed on the deep penetrating arteries and arterioles caused by hypertension (22). These hypertensive hemorrhages occur mainly in the deep structures of the brain in the region of the basal ganglia and external capsule (Fig. 24.6). In the elderly, more superficial hemorrhages into the lobes of the brain, lobar hemorrhages, become more frequent. Many of these lobar hemorrhages are still due to hypertension or can be hemorrhagic transformation of an embolic infarct (23). Another common cause of lobar hemorrhage in the elderly is amyloid angiopathy (Fig. 24.7), which can occur with or without coincident senile dementia of the Alzheimer's type (24).

Subarachnoid hemorrhage can also occur in the elderly, but a demonstrable berry aneurysm is less frequent than in younger patients (25). There are reports of newly diagnosed arteriovenous malformations (AVM) in elderly patients (26), but these are also a less common source of bleeding in the elderly than in younger patients.

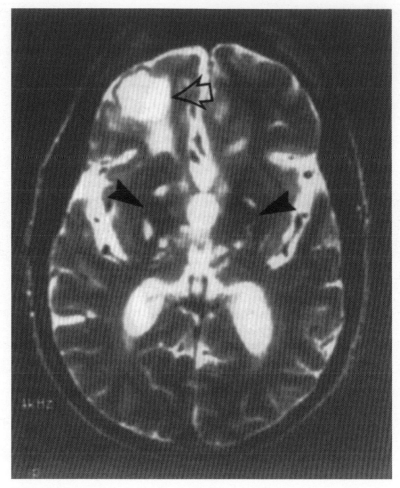

Figure 24.5 Multiple lacular infarcts. Axial T2-weighted MRI sequence demonstrates multiple rounded areas of high signal intensity within the basal ganglia and thalamus (*arrowheads*). There is also an old infarct in the right frontal region (*hollow arrow*).

DIAGNOSIS OF STROKE

The symptoms and signs occurring with a stroke are determined by the anatomical location of the lesion. Most strokes involve the cerebral hemispheres with contralateral hemiparesis or sensory loss, loss of vision in the contralateral visual field, and behavioral and speech disturbances. Strokes involving the brain stem present with ipsilateral deficits of the cranial nerve function such as abnormality of eye movements and a contralateral hemiparesis. Dizziness is a common symptom in the elderly, but dizziness alone is rarely an indication of stroke unless it is accompanied by other signs of dysfunction in the region of the vestibular nuclei in the lateral medulla. Loss of sensation on the ipsilateral face and contralateral body, ipsilateral Horner's syndrome and loss of gag reflex, and difficulty swallowing because of the involvement of the nucleus ambiguous supplying the vagus nerves are signs of lateral medullary infarction, known as Wallenberg's syndrome. Ataxia is found with strokes in the cerebellum as well as the brain stem.

It is important to establish the etiology of the stroke because treatment regimens vary with different subtypes of stroke. The clinical history and physical examination and laboratory analysis are obtained to identify risk factors that could potentially have caused the

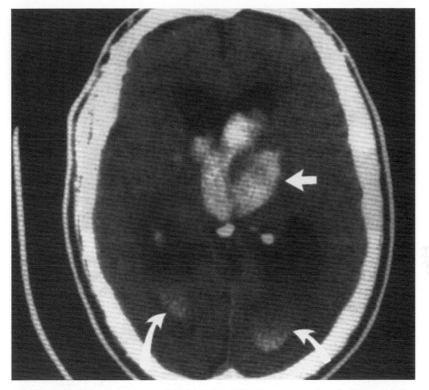

Figure 24.6 Hypertensive hemorrhage. Axial CT scan at the level of the third ventricle shows acute hypertensive hemorrhage in the left side of the thalamus (*arrow*), which has broken through into the third ventricle with blood seen layering in the occipital horns of the lateral ventricles (*curved arrows*).

stroke. The neurological examination is helpful in determining if there is an extensive lesion caused by the occlusion of a large vessel or a major hemorrhage, by determining if there is alteration in level of consciousness along with the focal deficits involved. Lacunar strokes from occlusion of small vessels can also be diagnosed if the typical syndromes of pure motor stroke, pure sensory stroke, dysarthria clumsy hand syndrome, or ataxic hemiparesis are present in an alert patient (16).

The neck is auscultated with the stethoscope to detect a vascular bruit that could signify atherosclerosis at the carotid artery bifurcation as the cause of atheroembolic stroke. The blood pressure is taken to determine if there is hypertension, and the blood glucose is measured to determine if diabetes is present. An electrocardiogram is essential to document if arrhythmias such as atrial fibrillation are present that could predispose to cardioembolic stroke.

Computerized axial tomography (CAT) scan of the brain is usually performed initially to differentiate between hemorrhagic and ischemic stroke. Signs of infarction are often not visualized on CAT scan within the first 4–12 hours after ischemic stroke, and the CAT scan may have to be repeated after 48 hours to determine the location of the stroke. This is important to help differentiate whether the stroke was atherothrombotic or cardioembolic. Thrombotic strokes more frequently occur in the deep structures of the brain. Cardioembolic strokes usually occur by occluding major branches of the internal carotid artery such as the middle cerebral artery (27), producing an infarct in the discrete territory of the artery involved or by occluding distal

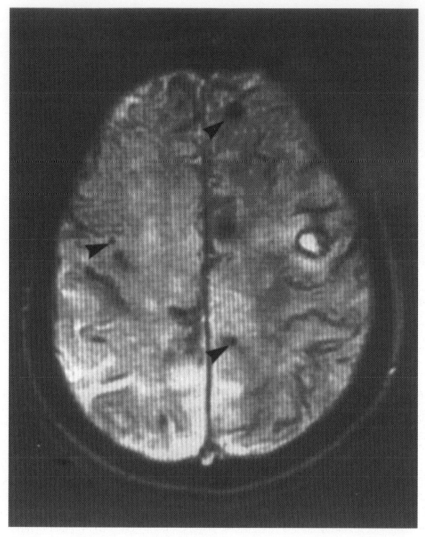

Figure 24.7   Amyloid angiopathy. Axial gradient echo sequence MRI shows an acute lobar hemorrhage in the posterior left frontal region with numerous areas of previous hemorrhage (*arrows*). The appearance of multiple areas of prior hemorrhage is not specific, but in an elderly patient is suggestive of cerebral amyloid angiopathy. *Abbreviation*: MRI, magnetic resonance imaging.

branches resulting in cortical infarctions (Fig. 24.4). Magnetic resonance imaging (MRI) is more sensitive than CAT scan for detecting early signs of infarction in the first 4–12 hours, particularly when the technique of diffusion MRI is employed (Fig. 24.8) (28).

The presence of a small, deep, lacunar infarct in a patient with diabetes and/or hypertension usually indicates that the stroke was caused by small vessel occlusive disease. A cortical infarct in a patient with a known cardiogenic source such as atrial fibrillation is usually sufficient to diagnose a cardioembolic stroke. Carotid duplex ultrasonography is usually performed in all patients with ischemic stroke to determine if atherosclerotic

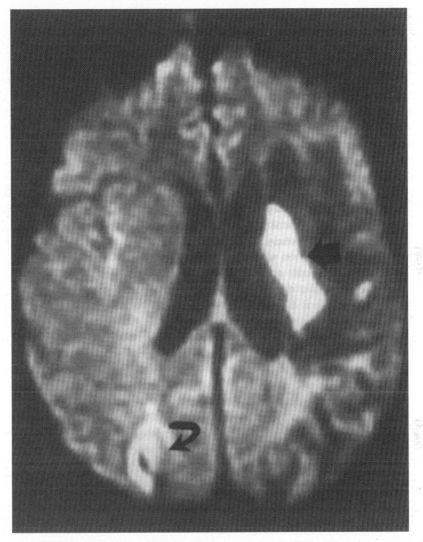

Figure 24.8 Diffusion weighted MRI. A diffusion weighted MRI sequence demonstrates an acute infarct in the region of a previous middle cerebral artery territory infarction (*dark arrow*) as well as an acute watershed type infarct in the right parietal region (*curved arrow*). *Abbreviation*: MRI, magnetic resonance imaging.

disease at the carotid artery bifurcation is the cause, since carotid occlusive disease can produce both superficial and deep cerebral infarction (29). Magnetic resonance angiography (MRA) can also be performed (Fig. 24.3) (30). Transcranial Doppler can identify occlusive disease of large intracranial arteries (31).

Transthoracic echocardiography is employed to rule out a cardiogenic source for stroke. If the suspicion is high that the patient had a cardioembolic stroke and no obvious source is identified, transesophageal echocardiography (TEE) is indicated. TEE is necessary to rule out thrombus in the atrium, right-to-left shunts in the heart such as patent foramen ovale or atrial septal defect, and plaque in the arch of the aorta (32–34).

THERAPY OF ISCHEMIC STROKE

The management of ischemic stroke is summarized in Table 24.1.

Prevention of Ischemic Stroke

At the present time, even with thrombolytic therapy, treatment is limited once an ischemic stroke has already occurred. The major goal for the management of cerebrovascular disease is prevention of stroke. Recent developments indicate that most strokes can be prevented, even when treatment is begun when the patient is already elderly, though early intervention is certainly preferable.

Control of Risk Factors

The modalities for prevention of occlusive cerebrovascular disease are similar to the strategies for prevention of coronary artery disease. Primary prevention is instituted in patients with the primary risk factors for cerebrovascular disease: hypertension, diabetes, atrial fibrillation, smoking, and elevated cholesterol. Secondary prevention is applied to patients who have had warning signs of occlusive cerebrovascular disease: auscultation of a cervical carotid artery bruit, transient ischemic attack (TIA) lasting up to 24 hours, transient monocular blindness (amaurosis fugax), reversible ischemic neurologic deficits (RIND) lasting over 24 hours, or mild stroke from which the patient is not significantly disabled.

Hypertension is the most significant risk factor for stroke. While prevention of stroke is more effective when treatment is started when the patient is young, it is also beneficial to treat hypertension in the elderly (35). Treatment of isolated systolic hypertension to a pressure below 160 mmHg with a thiazide diuretic and additional atenolol 25 mg as necessary (36) or with the calcium channel blocker nitrendipine significantly reduces the risk of stroke in the elderly (37). However, caution must be applied in treating elderly patients, since aggressive lowering of diastolic blood pressure below 65 mmHg may actually increase the risk of stroke. The risk of stroke is also increased with elevated diastolic blood pressure, and the

Table 24.1   Management of Stroke

Stroke Subtype	Etiology	Therapy
Ischemic		
Lacunar	Hypertension	Control of hypertension and diabetes
	Diabetes	aspirin, ticlopidine, tPA
Cardioembolic	Atrial fibrillation	Heparin, warfarin, aspirin, tPA
	Cardiac valve thrombi	
	Cardiac valve replacement	
	Occult (PFO, ASD)	
Large vessel	Atherosclerotic	Extracranial—aspirin, ticlopidine, tPA, carotid endarterectomy Intracranial—aspirin, warfarin, tPA
Hemorrhagic		
Intracranial	Hypertension	Control of hypertension
	Amyloid angiopathy	Steroids?, ventriculostomy?, removal?[a]
Subarachnoid	Aneurysm	Control of hypertension
	Arteriovenous malformation	Nimodipine, malformation epsilonaminocaproic acid?[a], aneurysmclipping, coils.

[a]Question marks indicate controversial therapy.
Abbreviations: PFO, patent foramen ovale; ASD, atrial septal defect.

lowest risk for stroke for elderly patients is in the range of 140/80 mmHg (38). The main factor for prevention of stroke is adequate reduction in blood pressure (39). There is evidence that the angiotensin-converting enzyme inhibitors ramapril and perindopril and the angiotensin-receptor blockers losartan and eprosartan confer an additional protective effect against stroke in addition to regulation of the blood pressure (40–43).

Diabetes causes proliferation of the walls of small arteries in the deep structures of the brain, which can lead to thrombosis (44). Strict control of blood sugar can prevent similar vascular changes observed in the retina (45) and probably does so in the brain as well, although it has never been definitively documented that strict control of blood sugar prevents ischemic stroke. Control of blood sugar may lessen the severity when a stroke occurs, because hyperglycemia at the time of a stroke increases the extent of infarction from an equivalent vascular occlusion (46). Ramipril has been used primarily to reduce the complications of diabetic nephropathy. Treatment with ramipril 10 mg/day reduced the risk of stroke by 33% for diabetic patients older than 55 years with at least one other risk factor for cardiovascular disease (40). Ramipril also reduces the relative risk of stroke by 0.68% in patients with evidence of vascular disease or diabetes plus one other cardiovascular risk factor with no reduction in cardiac ejection fraction or heart failure.

Serum lipids are not as significant a risk factor for stroke as they are for coronary heart disease, but reduction in serum cholesterol with the HMG coreductase inhibitors simvistatin and pravastatin for prevention of myocardial infarction also reduces the incidence of stroke in coronary patients by 33% (47,48). Cholesterol reduction with atorvastatin has been shown to reduce the rate of recurrence of stroke by 33% in patients with an initial stroke (49). High dietary content of the antioxidants β-carotene and vitamin E also have been shown to reduce the incidence of stroke, probably by prevention of propagation of atherosclerosis (50,51).

Maintenance aspirin therapy has been shown to be effective in prevention of myocardial infarction in asymptomatic elderly patients (52), and low-dose aspirin is commonly taken by the elderly on a daily basis. No definite similar reduction in the incidence of stroke in the well elderly patient has been documented with chronic maintenance aspirin therapy (52).

Cigarette smoking is a significant risk factor for stroke. Cessation of smoking reduces the risk of stroke to a level similar to nonsmokers after 3 years of abstinence. Elderly patients should still be encouraged to stop smoking.

MANAGEMENT OF PATIENTS WITH TRANSIENT ISCHEMIC ATTACK
Platelet Antiaggregant Therapy

TIAs are a warning sign of impending stroke. About 25–33% of patients with TIA go on to have a completed stroke (53). The incidence of stroke can be reduced by 50% in male patients with TIA treated with the platelet antiaggregant aspirin 650 mg twice a day, but may not have been effective in women (54). Subsequent studies have demonstrated that lower doses of aspirin ranging from 30 to 325 mg significantly reduce the risk of stroke in both men and women (55–59), but that higher doses may be more effective than lower doses (60).

The platelet antiaggregant ticlopidine (Ticlid) was developed for patients who could not tolerate the gastrointestinal side effects of aspirin. Ticlopidine is actually a stronger platelet antiaggregant than aspirin. It blocks the adenosine diphosphate (ADP) receptor, which is close to the final common pathway for platelet aggregation (61), while aspirin inhibits thromboxane synthesis by cyclooxygenase (62). In a trial comparing aspirin 650 mg twice a day to ticlopidine 250 mg twice a day in TIA patients, ticlopidine conferred a 48% risk reduction of stroke after 1 year and 25% risk reduction after 5 years, compared with therapy with aspirin 650 mg twice a day (63). Subgroup analysis revealed that ticlopidine had an advantage over aspirin in women, African-Americans, and in prevention of lacunar type stroke from small vessel disease (64). However, in the African-American

Stroke Study, ticlopidine did not show any advantage over aspirin therapy alone (65). Ticlopidine is now rarely used because it is associated with significant hematologic complications of leukopenia in 2% of patients (63) and thrombotic thrombocytopenic purpura in one of every 8000 patients (66).

Clopidogrel (Plavix) inhibits platelet aggregation by the same mechanism as ticlopidine, binding to the platelet ADP receptor, but does not have the hematological side effect profile of ticlopidine (67). Clopidogrel 75 mg a day has been shown to decrease the number of ischemic vascular events of all kinds by 8.7% compared with aspirin 325 mg a day in patients with atherosclerotic vascular disease including heart attack, peripheral vascular disease, and stroke (68). However, there was no significant reduction of recurrent stroke with clopidogrel in patients presenting with stroke as the initial event. The addition of aspirin 75–325 mg a day to clopidogrel has been shown to be useful in preventing recurrent myocardial ischemia in patients with acute coronary syndromes (69), but is not more effective than clopidogrel alone (70) or aspirin alone (71) for prevention of recurrent stroke. Clopidogrel has now virtually replaced ticlopidine for treatment of patients with TIA who cannot tolerate aspirin.

Dipyridamole prevents platelet aggregation by inhibiting the enzyme phosphodiesterase (72). Immediate release of dipyridamole has not been shown to be effective alone in preventing stroke in TIA patients (72) and did not appear to have an additive protective effect in combination with aspirin, compared with aspirin alone (72). A timed-release preparation of dipyridamole 200 mg twice a day reduced the risk of stroke in TIA patients by 18% compared with placebo, the same reduction as treatment with 50 mg of aspirin (73). The combination of aspirin 25 mg twice a day with this timed-release preparation of the platelet antiaggregant persantine (Aggrenox) 200 mg reduced the rate of stroke by 37% compared with placebo and 23% compared with aspirin (73). The efficacy of Aggrenox has been confirmed in a second trial where there was a 20% risk reduction in recurrent stroke compared with doses of aspirin ranging from 30 to 325 mg a day (74). Aggrenox has a low side effect profile. Gastrointestinal symptoms are reduced with a low dose of aspirin. The only adverse reaction has been headache, which can be minimized by starting the drug once a day and increasing the dose to twice a day after 1 week. Therefore, Aggrenox appears to be a safe and effective drug for prevention of stroke in elderly TIA patients.

Carotid Artery Disease

Occlusive atherosclerotic disease at the carotid artery bifurcation is found in 50% of patients with TIA. In patients with TIA and less than 40% stenosis, carotid endarterectomy has been shown to be of no benefit compared with aspirin therapy 650 mg twice a day for prevention of stroke. A final resolution has not yet been determined for patients with 40–69% stenosis. For patients with 70% or greater stenosis of the internal carotid artery at the bifurcation ipsilateral to a TIA, surgical therapy has been shown to provide a 20% reduction in the incidence of subsequent stroke compared with medical therapy with aspirin in a center where the risk of the procedure itself is 2% or less (75).

Patients presenting with TIA are initially screened with ultrasonographic examination of the carotid bifurcation employing duplex sonography. The bifurcation is imaged with B-mode sonography to visualize atherosclerotic plaque (76). The degree of stenosis is determined by Doppler sonography, which measures the velocity of the red cells flowing through the artery by the change in frequency shift of the ultrasound, as it reflects back from the red cells as they go by (77). The velocity is increased as the lumen diameter narrows. Identification of stenosis greater than 70% can be obtained with about 90% accuracy compared to angiography (78).

If a stenosis of 70% or greater is established by duplex sonography, or if the results of the testing is not definitive, then MRA is performed to document the degree of stenosis (78). MRA also has an accuracy of 90% compared to angiography (78). When the results of the two studies agree, the accuracy is 99% (79). Performing these two noninvasive studies can avoid the risk of angiography, which can be as high as a 1% incidence of stroke, myocardial infarction, or death in patients with cerebrovascular disease (78). When the two studies do not agree, angiography is usually performed to determine if there is greater than 70% stenosis, or to be certain that there is not an inoperable complete occlusion of the internal carotid. For patients who cannot have an MRA, CT angiography can be performed. This procedure also has a 90% accuracy compared with catheter angiography, but requires injection of a large volume of contrast dye, so that it may not be possible to perform on patients with congestive heart failure or renal disease.

Once the imaging procedures have documented greater than 70% stenosis, the patient is usually treated with carotid endarterectomy unless there are outweighing medical contraindications to performing the surgery. For elderly patients who are not surgical candidates, stenting of carotid stenosis can be performed. The risk of stroke during the procedure is similar to that of carotid endarterectomy, but the systemic complications are reduced (80). The long-term efficacy of carotid stent has not yet been established. Two early studies have determined that there is a greater efficacy and lower complication rate with carotid endarterectomy than with carotid stenting in patients who are not at high risk for carotid endarterectomy (79,81). The larger CREST Trial was completed and indicated that the risk of therapy for carotid endarterectomy and carotid stent for symptomatic stenosis were equivalent. However, the risk for stent was stroke while the risk for endarterectomy was primarily myocardial infarction, usually mild. Complication rates for stent were actually higher for patients over 80-years old than patients under 80. Therefore, the usual practice is to recommend carotid endarterectomy for patients without significant risk of coronary artery disease and stent for patients with too great a risk for myocardial infarction to undergo surgery (82).

The management of asymptomatic carotid artery stenosis remains controversial. The Asymptomatic Carotid Atherosclerosis Study (ACAS) documented a significant benefit of carotid endarterectomy, compared with medical therapy with aspirin 650 mg b.i.d. in patients with greater than 60% stenosis of the internal carotid artery (83). However, the difference was small, with a 10% risk of stroke in the medical group compared with a 5% risk of stroke in the surgical group over a 5-year follow-up period. Furthermore, the results did not diverge until the fifth year of follow-up. This has implications for elderly patients because an immediate risk of complication of carotid surgery may outweigh a risk of stroke 5 years in the future, if the life expectancy of the patient is diminished by other illnesses. A trial demonstrated a higher 16% reduction in stroke with carotid endarterectomy in patients with significant asymptomatic stenosis (84).

Several studies have indicated that acute proliferation of plaque with hemorrhagic changes and plaque growth are implicated in the etiology of thromboembolic events causing stroke from the carotid bifurcation (85–87). Since the overall incidence of stroke is low in asymptomatic patients, endarterectomy after the initial identification of asymptomatic carotid stenosis is usually reserved for patients with a very high-grade lesion or a plaque with large amounts of heterogeneous lucencies, suggestive of recent thrombus (85,86). The remaining patients can be followed with sequential duplex Doppler examinations every 6 months and endarterectomy performed if a progressive stenosis is identified (87,88) or if the patient becomes symptomatic with a TIA.

Prevention of Cardioembolic Stroke

The major risk factor for cardioembolic stroke in the elderly is nonvalvular atrial fibrillation (8). Patients younger than 70 years with atrial fibrillation but no other associated heart disease can be managed with aspirin to effectively prevent stroke (88–91). In elderly patients older than 70 years, all clinical trials for stroke prevention in patients with atrial fibrillation have shown that aspirin is ineffective in preventing embolic stroke due to atrial fibrillation, and anticoagulation with warfarin had a significant protective effect (88,90,92–94). The combination of aspirin and clopidogrel has been shown to be more effective than aspirin for preventing stroke in low-risk patients with atrial fibrillation, but not as effective as warfarin, and further analysis of the data reveals that it is not more effective in high-risk patients than aspirin, which would include patients over 75 (95). In the Stroke Prevention in Atrial Fibrillation (SPAF) trial, the risk of hemorrhagic stroke and other hemorrhagic complications in the elderly over 75 years equaled the risk reduction of cardioembolic stroke induced by warfarin compared with aspirin (88). The degree of anticoagulation in the SPAF trial as measured by the international normalized ratio (INR) was higher than in the other trials of warfarin to prevent stroke in atrial fibrillation, in which a significant reduction in the number of ischemic strokes and poor outcomes was demonstrated (92–94). Therefore, the current recommendation is to treat elderly patients older than 75 years who have atrial fibrillation with warfarin for stroke prophylaxis, keeping the INR between 2.0 and 2.9, with a target of 2.5.

A new category of anticoagulants for primary prevention of stroke in atrial fibrillation have been developed that may have an advantage over anticoagulation with warfarin: The direct thrombin inhibitor dabigatran and the Factor XA inhibitors rivaroxaban and apixaban (96–98). A dose of 110 mg dabigatran twice daily was associated with an equivalent risk of stroke as warfarin with a lower incidence of hemorrhagic complications, while a dose of 150 mg twice daily was associated with a lower incidence of stroke as warfarin with a relative risk of 0.66 (95% CI 0.53–0.82, $p < 0.001$), with an equal incidence of hemorrhagic complications as warfarin (97). However, only the higher dose was approved for use in the USA in order to achieve the increased efficacy. However, in post-marketing experience, the higher dose of dabigatran has been associated with a higher risk of hemorrhagic complications than the original study, particularly in the elderly. Rivaroxaban given 20 mg/day was also more effective than warfarin with a relative risk of 0.88 (95% CI 0.74–1.03, $p < 0.001$) with an equal rate of hemorrhagic complications but a significantly lower rate of intracranial hemorrhage (98). This preparation has currently been approved for use in the USA. Apixaban given 5 mg twice daily reduced the incidence of stroke compared to warfarin by a relative risk reduction of 0.69 (CI 0.60–0.80, $p < 0.001$), with a significantly lower rate of hemorrhagic complications (99). However, apixaban has not as yet been approved for use in the USA. In addition to possible greater efficacy, these medications have the advantage that they are effective immediately without having to establish a therapeutic dosage over a number of days, and they are administered at a fixed dosage instead of having to regulate the dosage based on the INR.

Cardioversion of patients with atrial fibrillation has been employed as a strategy to prevent cerebral emboli. However, these patients may still require anticoagulation. In the Atrial Fibrillation Follow-up Investigation of Rhythm Management (AFFIRM) trial, 3500 patients with atrial fibrillation, mean age 70 years, were randomized to treatment with rate control plus warfarin or maintenance of sinus rhythm plus warfarin. The incidence of stroke was 5.7% in the rate control group, compared with 7.3% in the sinus rhythm group. While this difference was not significant, 78% of the strokes occurred if warfarin was discontinued or the INR was below 2.0, indicating a continuing need for anticoagulation in these patients to prevent stroke (100).

Patients with mechanical cardiac valve replacements are generally treated with warfarin for prevention of embolic stroke with the INR maintained from 3.0 to 3.5. However, in patients with infective endocarditis of a cardiac valve, whether natural or prosthetic, anticoagulation is not used because of the risk of bleeding from mycotic aneurysm (101).

Anticoagulation with warfarin has also been beneficial in preventing stroke during the first 3 months after myocardial infarction (102), although aspirin is usually used for long-term prophylaxis. Patient with heart failure and dilated cardiomyopathy with enlarged left ventricle and are in normal sinus rhythm are at risk for cardioembolic stroke. However, treatment with warfarin was not more effective than aspirin for primary prevention of embolic stroke in these patients (103).

Patent foramen ovale is a major cause of cryptogenic stroke in the young, but does not play a major role as a cause of stroke in the geriatric population. There was no difference in the incidence of recurrent stroke in patients older than 60 years with patent foramen ovale treated with either aspirin or warfarin (104).

Atherosclerotic plaque in the ascending aorta and aortic arch has also been implicated as a potential source of cardioembolic stroke (34). When these plaques are identified as an incidental finding with TEE performed for cardiac disease, then stroke prophylaxis should be instituted, although it has not been documented whether aspirin therapy is sufficient, or anticoagulation with warfarin is necessary. A technique has been developed to image aortic arch plaque with transcutaneous duplex ultrasound, so that patients undergoing carotid duplex sonography can be examined for aortic arch plaque as well (105).

Multi-Infarct Dementia

Elderly patients being evaluated for dementia are often found to have small infarcts or ischemic changes on images of the brain with MRI and CAT scan (Fig. 24.5) (106). Hypertensive patients have small lacunar infarcts in the deep structures, which may not be causing any focal neurological deficits such as hemiparesis, but may cause or contribute to cognitive decline. Patients with atrial fibrillation or other cardioembolic sources of stroke may have silent infarcts that cause cognitive deficits without focal signs. Patients with a history of stroke and mild focal neurological deficits may still have cognitive disturbances. When ischemia is identified as a contributor to the dementia, identification of stroke risk factors and vascular pathology is made and appropriate antithrombotic therapy is instituted.

TREATMENT OF ACUTE ISCHEMIC STROKE

There are four objectives in the treatment of the acute stroke patient: (*i*) diagnosis and prevention of medical complications that could be life threatening, (*ii*) prevention of progression of the current stroke, (*iii*) prevention of recurrent stroke, and (*iv*) reversal of the symptoms of the current stroke.

Medical Complications

The major medical complications associated with stroke are myocardial infarction, pulmonary emboli, aspiration pneumonia, and airway obstruction or reduction in the level of consciousness that compromises respiration. Electrocardiogram is imperative to rule out a concurrent myocardial infarction, and if there is any suggestive history, serial enzymes are obtained. Stroke units with monitored beds are useful in detecting and preventing complications of arrhythmia that could occur with concomitant myocardial infarction, or as the result of the stroke itself. While echocardiographic changes of ST segment depression, U waves, and ventricular fibrillation are more common with hemorrhagic strokes, they can occur with large infarctions severe enough to produce release of catecholamines that can injure the endocarium (107).

Patients who are immobilized from their strokes are treated with low-dose subcutaneous heparin 5000 U b.i.d. or enoxeparin 30 mg q.d. to prevent thrombophlebitis. If there is a substantial risk of bleeding, pressurized air boots can be used instead of low-dose anticoagulation. If there is airway obstruction or obtundation interfering with respiration, prophylactic endotracheal intubation is sometimes initiated. Observation of the oxygen saturation with a pulse oximeter may be sufficient to determine when a patient is becoming hypoxic and intubation is necessary. Patients are generally not fed when there is any obtundation or difficulty in swallowing, usually for a period lasting 48 hours after acute onset of the stroke. However, if there is prolonged inability to swallow, a nasogastric tube or percutaneous gastric tube must be inserted to maintain nutrition for better recovery of the stroke patient.

Prevention of Progression

Prevention of progression of stroke is attained by careful monitoring of the patient. The blood pressure must be maintained at a sufficient level to insure perfusion of the ischemic penumbra, the region of brain around the core area of infarction that is ischemic but not irreversibly damaged. Most stroke patients have an elevation of the blood pressure for the first 48 hours, a response to the ischemic event, which resolves without treatment (108). If the blood pressure rises to a critical level over 200/120, moderate reduction with intravenous labetalol is employed to bring the pressure to the 180/100 range. Drastic reduction in blood pressure with agents such as nitroprusside can cause severe worsening of the stroke.

Progression of stroke can occur in both large vessel occlusive disease and in lacunar or small vessel occlusive disease. Administration of aspirin near onset of ischemic stroke has been shown to improve outcome (109). Acute intravenous anticoagulation with heparin or the low-molecular weight heparinoid Orgaron has not been effective in improving outcome in controlled clinical trials (110,111), although subcutaneous administration of low-molecular weight heparin has shown a small but significant beneficial outcome for stroke patients in one trial (112). Therefore, it is generally not necessary to anticoagulate all stroke patients acutely, while aspirin therapy should be instituted as soon as possible.

Patients with large vessel occlusive disease who show signs of evolving stroke may benefit from anticoagulation with heparin (113,114), particularly when there is brain stem infarction (115). However, the evolution of infarction must be the degree of extent of focal neurological findings, such as a worsening of limb weakness or new cranial nerve deficits. Decline in the level of consciousness of the patient without new focal deficits is common, particularly in patients with middle cerebral artery occlusion from cardioembolic stroke, who develop cerebral edema associated with reperfusion. In this instance, anticoagulation can be associated with adverse outcome because of the hemorrhagic transformation of the infarction and anticoagulation should not be administered. Anticoagulation should be employed judiciously in elderly patients older than 80 years who have a higher risk of hemorrhagic complications.

With mass lesions of the brain, corticosteroid medications such as Decadron and osmotic diuretics such as Mannitol are useful in reducing the amount of vasogenic edema surrounding the lesion. Acute administration of corticosteroids to all stroke patients has been shown to be of no benefit and may actually be deleterious to the patient's outcome (116). In patients with reperfusion, vasogenic edema can develop, but the response to corticosteroids and osmotic agents is poor (117). These agents can have adverse consequences for stroke patients because the hyperglycemia associated with corticosteroids may cause exacerbation of infarction (48), and the dehydration associated with osmotic diuretics may cause reduced perfusion in the ischemic zone. Steroids have not been shown to be beneficial in preventing brain herniation in massive hemispheric strokes with edema. Mannitol 1000 g intravenously over 1 hour can be administered when herniation is imminent, particularly in cases of hyperperfusion with infarction following carotid endarterectomy (118). In extreme cases, hemicraniectomy of the skull on the affected side has been recommended to acutely relieve intracranial pressure and prevent herniation, but has been associated with long-term complications and is not recommended in patients over 60 year of age (119).

In some instances, brain stem stroke that is likely to progress can be diagnosed clinically when a pontine infarct is located rostral to the facial nerve nucleus, with ipsilateral face, arm, and leg weakness (120). This lesion usually involves the ventral anterior pons, where the pyramidal tracts carrying motor fibers from each cerebral hemisphere are located contiguously. Spread of infarction to both sides of the brain stem in this location can result in the locked-in state, where there is quadraparesis and inability to speak, but the patient remains fully conscious. This type of stroke is often associated with basilar artery occlusion and identification, and early heparinization of these types of patients may be beneficial in preventing worsening of the stroke. Carotid and transcranial ultrasound studies can be performed on acute stroke patients to identify large vessel occlusive disease in the carotid or vertebrobasilar circulation because these patients may benefit from early anticoagulation with low molecular heparin, although this has not been definitively established (121).

Prevention of Recurrent Stroke

Prevention of recurrent stroke is particularly important in patients with a cardioembolic source of stroke such as atrial fibrillation or cardiac valve replacement. These patients can have repeat embolization of clot from the heart (122). Cardioembolic stroke almost always causes red infarction, with petechial hemorrhage or hemorrhagic transformation of the infarct when reperfusion occurs with retraction of the embolic clot. Reperfusion usually occurs between 24 and 48 hours after the acute event. Early anticoagulation with heparin can lead to increased size of the hemorrhagic transformation with associated worsening of the neurological condition as well as coma and death from brain herniation. This is particularly applicable to elderly patients, as the risk of major hemorrhagic transformation increases with age (123,124).

In several studies, it has been determined that the risk of re-emoblization in patients with atrial fibrillation is about 2% while the risk of major hemorrhagic transformation resulting in clinical deterioration is about 8% in the first 48 hours after stroke (123,124). Early anticoagulation of stroke patients with atrial fibrillation with heparin or the low-molecular weight heparinoid Orgaron showed no benefit compared with placebo (121,125). Therefore, in patients with atrial fibrillation, anticoagulation is usually held for the first 48 hours, a CAT scan of the brain is repeated, and anticoagulation is initiated if the infarct is not very large and there is no hemorrhagic transformation. In the patients who do have large infarction or hemorrhagic transformation, it is usually safe to anticoagulate from 96 hours to 1 week following the acute stroke (126). A small area of infarction on the initial CAT scan does not indicate that it is safe to anticoagulate acutely because the full extent of the lesion may not be detected until up to 48 hours after the initial event. MRI, particularly with the diffusion weighted imaging technique, is more sensitive in identifying the full extent of early infarction, and when the region of ischemic brain on these studies is small, early anticoagulation can be instituted. When planning to institute maintenance anticoagulation for propyhlaxis of recurrent stroke in atrial fibrillation the new agents dibigatran, rovaroxaban, and apixaban may be considered, since they may have a greater efficacy for prevention of stroke and also take effect immediately without having to adjust the dosage over days with warfarin (97–99).

Early anticoagulation is also necessary in patients with prosthetic cardiac valves who break through with stroke because the risk of early re-emoblization is greater, particularly when noninfectious vegetations are seen on the prosthesis with echocardiography. However, bacterial endocarditis must be ruled out in these instances prior to anticoagulation because mycotic aneurysms can form from infected emboli and can cause hemorrhage when the patient is anticoagulated (127).

Long-term anticoagulation with warfarin can be started at the same time as acute anti-coagulation with heparin to shorten the length of hospital stay. A loading dose of 10 mg/day for 2 days is started and subsequent doses are titrated to the prothrombin time, unless the patient has demonstrated sensitivity to warfarin. As in patients with progressive stroke, anticoagulation should be performed judiciously in elderly patients older than 80 years because of a higher risk of hemorrhagic complications.

The International Stroke Trial demonstrated a beneficial effect of aspirin 300 mg orally given at the time of onset of non-cardioembolic ischemic stroke when outcome was analyzed after 3 months. A 1% reduction in poor outcomes was obtained, primarily from prevention of recurrent stroke. Subcutaneous heparin administration up to 12,500 U b.i.d. had a similar reduction in poor outcome from ischemic strokes, but this reduction was equaled by adverse hemorrhagic events associated with anticoagulation (128).

Reversal of Stroke Symptoms

Administration of the thrombolysin tissue plasminogen activator (tPA) intravenously at a dosage of 0.9 mg/kg over 1 hour with 10% given by bolus within 3 hours after the onset of stroke increases the number of patients with a good outcome from stroke after 3 months. As measured by functional scales, 31% of treated patients had improved outcome compared with 21% of placebo patients (129). There is an immediate improvement in 14% of the stroke patients administered tPA acutely, but there is a 3.6% rate of cerebral hemorrhage causing death, so that the overall difference within the first 24 hours between control and treated patients was not significant. However, after 3 months, the overall mortality rate is equal in treated and untreated patients. tPA can be administered safely to patients older than 80 years without an increase in the incidence of symptomatic cerebral hemorrhage, but the outcome of thrombolytic therapy is not as successful in the elderly as in younger patients (130).

Care must be taken in selecting patients for administration of tPA. To avoid hemorrhagic complications, the prothrombin time and partial thromboplastin time should not be elevated and the platelet count should not be reduced. The patient should not have a history of recent surgery or any other illness that could result in significant systemic bleeding. An unexplained anemia could indicate an occult source of bleeding and is also a contraindication for adminis-tration of tPA. Administration of intravenous tPA to patients more than 3 hours after ischemic stroke or to patients who have changes of infarction on CAT scan of the brain by the time they are ready for treatment leads to an unacceptable degree of hemorrhagic complications and should be avoided (131). Administration of streptokinase had a very high rate of hemorrhagic complications and is not employed in the treatment of acute ischemic stroke (132).

Either tPA or recombinant pro-urokinase (rpro-UK) can also be administered by intra-arterial catheterization directly to the occluded vessel under angiographic control. A randomized trial of 9 mg intra-arterial rpro-UK followed by heparin infusion was per-formed in 180 patients with middle cerebral artery occlusion treated within 6 hours after stroke. A favorable outcome occurred in 40% of 121 patients treated with rpro-UK and 27% of 59 patients treated only with heparin (133). The improvement in outcome was sig-nificant ($p = 0.04$). Recanalization was also significantly improved to 66% in the treated group compared to 19% in the heparin group. However, the risk of symptomatic intracra-nial hemorrhage was 10% in the treated group compared with 2% in the heparin group. Intra-arterial thrombolytic therapy may be more valuable in vertebrobasilar occlusive dis-ease when there are progressive symptoms and the expected outcome is so grave that it outweighs the risk of hemorrhagic complications (134). Clot retraction with mechanical embolus removal devices have been approved for use within 8 hours of onset of cerebral ischemia to restore flow in occluded intracranial arteries (135). However, stent therapy for patients with established intracranial stenosis has not been effective in preventing recurrent stroke compared to medical therapy with aspirin (136).

Another strategy that is under development for the treatment of acute ischemic stroke is the use of neuroprotective agents. Ischemia induces release of excitotoxic neurotransmitters, particularly glutamic acid. In the setting of ischemia, glutamate causes neuronal death by stimulation of the N-methyl-d-aspartate (NMDA) receptor, which induces lethal amounts of calcium to enter the neuron. In experimental animal models, administration of NMDA receptor antagonists protects neurons in the border zone of the infarct from irreversible ischemic necrosis, reducing the infarct volume and improving functional recovery (Fig. 24.9) (137). Several NMDA receptor antagonists have been examined in

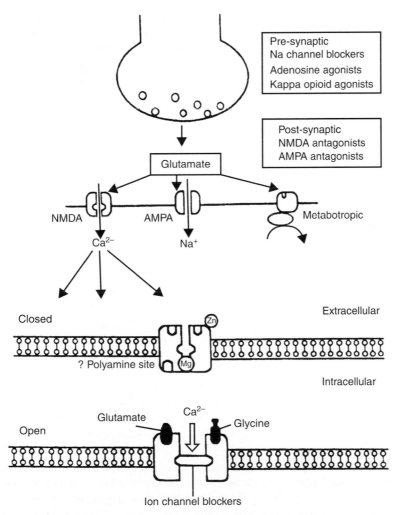

Figure 24.9 The ischemic cascade induced by release of the excitatory amino acids, glutamate and aspartate, which stimulate the NMDA and AMPA receptors is diagrammed. Experimental therapeutic strategies include inhibition of release of the excitatory neurotransmitters (lamotrigine, riluzole), inhibition of sodium influx from stimulation of the AMPA receptor (APV, NBQX), and inhibition of calcium influx from stimulation of the NMDA receptor (aptigenel, dextrorphan, memantine, selfatel, polyamines). *Abbreviations*: NMDA, N-methyl-d-aspartate; AMPA, a-amino-3-hydroxy-5-methylisoxazole-4-propionic acid; APV, ambulatory procedure visit; NBQX, 2,3-dihydroxy-6nitro-sulfamoyl-benzo(f)-quinoxaline. *Source*: From Ref. 138.

controlled treatment trials of ischemic stroke, but so far no significant improvement in outcome of stroke patients with these agents has been documented (138). Future studies may include reperfusion of the ischemic zone by administration of thrombolytic agents followed by administration of neuroprotective agents to prevent ischemic neuronal death.

The relative success of immediate treatment of stroke with tPA within 3 hours after onset has altered the attitude about the management of stroke. Stroke now has to be considered an emergency just like heart attack and is currently referred to as a brain attack. Early recognition of stroke and emergency transport to a hospital facility capable of acute management of stroke patients has become imperative.

MANAGEMENT OF HEMORRHAGIC STROKE

There are two types of hemorrhagic stroke, intracranial and subarachnoid. Intracranial hemorrhage usually commences with severe headache and progressive focal deficit, often leading to obtundation. Most intracranial hemorrhage is due to hypertension and involves the deep structures of the brain around the basal ganglia and internal capsule (Fig. 24.6) (22). Hemorrhage into a superficial lobe in the brain is more common in elderly patients than younger patients, partly due to amyloid angiopathy of the cerebral arteries (Fig. 24.7) (24). Medical therapy of hemorrhage consists primarily of reduction in blood pressure in hypertensive patients and supportive care. Endotracheal intubation may be necessary for airway protection and for impending brain herniation with respiratory failure. Hyper-ventilation may be helpful to reduce increased intracranial pressure. The osmotic diuretic Mannitol can be administered at a dosage of 100 g intravenously to reduce cerebral edema acutely in cases of impending herniation. There is no evidence that steroid medications are of any benefit in improving the outcome of patients with intracranial hemorrhage (139), but they are still occasionally employed for the individual case where reduction of cerebral edema may be helpful. Decadron 10 mg intravenously, acutely followed by 4 mg every 6 hours, is often used. Care must be taken to control blood sugar and prevent gastrointestinal hemorrhage when administering steroid medications.

Surgical management of intracranial hemorrhage is employed in certain instances. Shunting of fluid and removal of blood from the ventricular system can reduce intracranial pressure and prevent hydrocephalus. Deep hemorrhages are usually not benefited by surgical intervention, but occasionally improvement can be obtained with removal of lobar hemorrhage (140,141). The one instance in which surgical management is generally utilized is cerebellar hemorrhage, where drainage of the hematoma can be performed without inordinate risk to prevent compression of the brain stem and death. Cerebellar hemorrhage usually presents initially with dizziness and loss of balance along with headache, progression of focal ataxic symptoms, and, often, somnolence and coma. Early recognition of this condition can improve the outcome considerably with surgery (141).

SUBARACHNOID HEMORRHAGE

The major intracranial vessels are located in the subarachnoid space between the pia mater and dura mater covering the brain. Aneurysms form primarily at branch points from the vessels of the circle of Willis at the base of the brain. Rupture of these aneurysms produces severe headache, photophobia, and stiff neck. The patient may become somnolent or lapse into coma. A third nerve paralysis with ptosis, pupillary dilation, and ophthalmoplegia can result when a hematoma forms on the oculomotor nerve running just below the posterior communicating artery. Focal neurological disturbances such as hemiparesis can also result acutely. Patients with mild-to-moderate deficits have a better prognosis than patients with focal neurological deficit or stupor. CAT scan of the brain can visualize subarachnoid hemorrhage in most cases, but sometimes lumbar puncture is necessary when the CAT scan is negative and there is a high clinical suspicion of subarachnoid hemorrhage. The aneurysm is identified by cerebral angiography.

The optimum care for subarachnoid hemorrhage is prevention of rebleeding by surgical clipping of the aneurysm or by thrombosing the aneurysm with endovascular coils. Surgery should be performed within the first 24 hours in patients with mild-to-moderate deficits. Surgical management after 24 hours is dangerous because of increased ischemic complications due to vasospasm. If surgery cannot be performed within the first 24 hours, it is usually deferred for up to 14 days (142). The ischemic consequences of spasm can be reduced by administration of the calcium channel blocker Nimodipine 60 mg orally for every 6 hours (143,144). In some instances, the antifibrinolysin epsilon amino caproic acid is administered to prevent rebleeding when surgical therapy cannot be performed immediately, but is associated with an increase in ischemic complications (145). Spasm can be detected by measurement of increased flow velocities with transcranial Doppler, which can be employed to monitor patients for the onset of spasm after subarachnoid hemorrhage. When spasm occurs postoperatively, the blood pressure can be elevated to increase cerebral perfusion. Angioplasty can also be performed to dilate vessels when spasm is severe and is causing hemiparesis or stupor (146). When an elderly patient is at high risk for aneurysm surgery, endovascular placement of coils under radiological guidance can be employed to thrombose the aneurysm (147). A study demonstrated that coiling was safer and more effective than surgical management (148), but not all aneurysms are amenable to placement of a coil.

AVM of the brain, in which arteries feed directly into the venous system without going through a capillary bed, can also be a cause of subarachnoid hemorrhage. Surgical extirpation can be performed to eliminate the source of the bleeding, but often the AVM can recur or too much brain parenchyma is at risk for resection to be feasible (149). Embolization of colloidal particles or endovascular insertion of coils can be employed to thrombose the AVM. It is unusual to be able to eliminate the AVM by these methods, but the size can be reduced so that it becomes amenable to surgical removal. Radiosurgery with gamma knife technology can also be performed to eliminate or reduce the volume of the AVM (150).

CONCLUSION

New developments in the understanding of the pathophysiology of stroke and imaging technology for identifying the cause of stroke have dramatically changed the management of cerebrovascular disease. While the main focus remains prevention, new treatments with thrombolysis have changed the concept of stroke from a hopeless condition to a treatable disease. Further developments with neuroprotective agents hold the promise for further advancements in the treatment of stroke. The treatment of stroke as an acute emergency, a brain attack, has introduced a new era in the management of stroke, which can markedly alter the course of the disease in the elderly.

REFERENCES

1. Wolf PA. Cerebrovascular disease in the elderly. In: Tresch DD, Aronow WS, eds. Cardiovascular Disease in the Elderly Patient. New York, NY: Marcel Dekker, 1994: 125–47.
2. Sherman DG, Dyken MJ, Gent M, et al. Antithrombotic therapy for cerebrovascular disorders: an update. Chest 1995; 106: S444–56.
3. Bogousslavsky J, Van Melle G, Regli F. The Lausanne Stroke Registry. Analysis of 1000 consecutive patients with first stroke. Stroke 1988; 19: 1083–92.
4. Kannel WB, Dawber TR, Sorlie P, et al. Components of blood pressure and risk of atherothrombotic brain infarction. The Framingham Study. Stroke 1976; 7: 327–31.
5. Kannel WB, McGee DL. Diabetes and cardiovascular disease. The Framingham Study. JAMA 1979; 241: 2035–8.
6. Wolf PA, Kannel WB, Dawber TR. Prospective investigations: the Framingham Study and the epidemiology of stroke. Adv Neurol 1978; 19: 107–20.

7. Gordon T, Castelli WP, Hjortland MD, et al. High-density lipoprotein as a protective factor against coronary heart disease: the Framingham Study. Am J Med 1987; 62: 707–14.

8. Wolf PA, Dawber TR, Thomas HE, et al. Epidemiologic assessment of chronic atrial fibrillation and risk of stroke: the Framingham Study. Neurology 1978; 28: 973–7.

9. Doniger DE. Bilateral complete carotid and basilar artery occlusion in a patient with minimal deficit: case report and discussion of diagnostic and therapeutic implications. Neurology 1963; 13: 673–6.

10. Obrist WD, Thompson HK, Wang HS, et al. Regional cerebral blood flow estimated by 133 Xenon inhalation. Stroke 1975; 6: 245–56.

11. Fisher CM, Gore I, Okabe N, et al. Atherosclerosis of the carotid and vertebral arteries. Extracranial and intracranial. J Neuropathol Exp Neurol 1965; 24: 455–76.

12. Bosousslavsky J, Regli F. Unilateral watershed cerebral infarcts. Neurology 1986; 36: 373–7.

13. Asinger RW. Incidence of left-ventricular thrombosis after acute transmural myocardial infarction: Serial evaluation by 2-dimensional echocardiography. N Engl J Med 1981; 305: 297–302.

14. Tunick PA, Culliford AT, Lamparello PJ, et al. Atheromatosis of the aortic arch as an occult source of multiple systemic emboli. Ann Intern Med 1991; 114: 391–2.

15. Horowitz DR, Tuhrim S, Budd J, et al. Aortic plaque in patients with brain ischemia: diagnosis by transesophageal echocardiography. Neurology 1992; 42: 1602–4.

16. Fisher CM. Lacunes: Small, deep cerebral infarcts. Neurology 1965; 15: 774–8.

17. Johnson RT, Richardson EP. The neurological manifestations of systemic lupus erythema-tosus. Medicine 1968; 47: 337–69.

18. The Antiphospholipid Antibodies in Stroke Study (APASS) Group. Anticardiolipin antibodies are an independent risk factor for first ischemic stroke. Neurology 1993; 43: 2069–73.

19. Kohier J, Kasper J, Witt L, et al. Ischemic stroke due to protein C deficiency. Stroke 1990; 21: 1077–80.

20. D'Angelo A, Vigano-D'Angelo S, Esmon CT, et al. Acquired deficiencies of proteins. J Clin Invest 1988; 81: 1445–54.

21. Russell MO, Goldberg HI, Hodson A, et al. Effect of transfusion therapy on arteriographic abnormalities and on the recurrence of stroke in sickle cell disease. Blood 1984; 63: 162–9.

22. Cote FM, Yates PO. The occurrence and significance of intracerebral micro-aneurysms. J Pathol Bacteriol 1967; 93: 393–401.

23. Hart RG, Putnam C. Hemorrhagic transformation of cardioembolic stroke. Stroke 1989; 20: 1117–23.

24. Vinters HV. Cerebral amyloid angiopathy: a critical review. Stroke 1987; 18: 311–24.

25. Kassell NF, Torner JC, Haley EC Jr, et al. The International cooperative study on the timing of aneurysm surgery. Part 1: overall management results. J Neurosurg 1990; 73: 18–36.

26. Lusins J, Pinner J, Weinberger J. Disturbance of the visual fields in cerebral vascular malformations. Mt Sinai J Med 1973; 40: 806–11.

27. Llhermitte F, Gautier JC, Derouesne C. Nature of occlusions of the middle cerebral artery. Neurology 1970; 20: 82–8.

28. Warach S, Gaa J, Stewert B, et al. Acute human stroke studied by whole brain echo planar diffusion weighted MRI. Ann Neurol 1995; 37: 231–41.

29. Weinberger J, Tegeler C, McKinney W, et al. Carotid ultrasonography in the management of patients with atherosclerotic disease at the carotid artery bifurcation: a position paper of the American Society of Neuroimaging. J Neuroimaging 1995; 5: 147–57.

30. Polak JF, Bajakian RL, O'Leary DH, et al. Detection of internal carotid artery stenosis: comparison of MR angiography, color Doppler sonography and anteriography. Radiology 1992; 182: 35–40.

31. Aaslid R, Marcwalder TM, Nornes H. Noninvasive transcranial Doppler ultrasound recording of flow velocity in basal cerebral arteries. J Neurosurg 1982; 57: 769–74.

32. Jeanrenaud X, Kappenberger L. Patent foramen ovale and stroke of unknown origin. Cerebrovasc Dis 1991; 1: 184–92.

33. Mas JL. Patent foramen ovale, stroke, and paradoxical embolism. Cerebrovasc Dis 1991; 1: 181–3.

34. Tunick PA, Kronzon I. Protruding atherosclerotic plaque in the aortic arch of patients with systemic embolization: a new finding seen by transesophageal echocardiography. Am Heart J 1990; 120: 658–60.

35. Staessen JA, Fayard R, Thijs L, et al. Systolic Hypertension in Europe (Syst-Eur) Trial Investigators. Randomised double-blind comparison of placebo and active treatment for older patients with isolated systolic hypertension. Lancet 1997; 350: 757–64.

36. Perry HM, Davis BR, Price TR, et al. Randomised double-blind comparison of placebo and active treatment for older patients with isolated systolic hypertension. JAMA 2000; 284: 465–71.

37. Fagard RH, Staessen JA. Treatment of isolated systolic hypertension in the elderly: Systolic Hypertension in Europe (Syst-Eur) Trial Investigators. Clin Exp Hypertens 1999; 21: 491–7.

38. Voko Z, Bots ML, Hofman A, et al. J-shaped relation between blood pressure and stroke in treated hypertensives. Hypertension 1999; 34: 1181–5.

39. Hansson L, Zanchetti A, Carruthers SG, et al. Effects of intensive blood-pressure lowering and low-dose aspirin in patients with hypertension: principal results of the Hypertension Optimal Treatment (HOT) randomized trial. Lancet 1998; 351: 1755–62.

40. The Heart Outcomes Prevention Evaluation Study Investigators. Effects of an angiotensin-converting-enzyme inhibitor, ramipril, on cardiovascular events in high-risk patients. N Engl J Med 2000; 342: 145–53.

41. PROGRESS Collaborative Group. Randomised trial of a perindopril-based blood-pressure-lowering regimen among 6105 individuals with previous stroke or transient ischemic attack. Lancet 2001; 358: 1033–41.

42. Dahlof B, Devereux RB, Kjeldsen SE, et al. Cardiovascular morbidity and mortality in the Losartan Intervention For Endpoint reduction in hypertension study (LIFE): a randomized trial against atenolol. Lancet 2000; 359: 995–1003.

43. Schrader J, Luders S, Kulschewski A, et al. MOSES study group. Morbidity and Mortality after Stroke—Eprosartan compared with nitrendipine for secondary prevention. Principal results of a prospective randomized controlled study. Stroke 2005; 36: 1218–26.

44. Alex M, Baron EK, Goldenberg S, et al. An autopsy study of cerebrovascular accident in diabetes mellitus. Circulation 1962; 25: 663–7.

45. Merimee TJ. Diabetic retinopathy: a synthesis of perspectives. N Engl J Med 1990; 322: 978–83.

46. Woo J, Lam CWK, Kay R, et al. The influence of hyperglycemia and diabetes mellitus on immediate and three month morbidity and mortality after acute stroke. Arch Neurol 1990; 47: 1174–7.

47. The Scandinavian Simvastatin Study Group. Randomised trial of cholesterol lowering in 4444 patients with coronary heart disease: the Scandinavian Simvastatin Survival Study (4S). Lancet 1994; 344: 1383–9.

48. Sheperd J, Cobbe SM, Ford I, et al. Prevention of coronary heart disease with Pravastatin in men with hypercholesterolemia. N Engl J Med 1995; 333: 1301–7.

49. The Stroke Prevention by Aggressive Reduction in Cholesterol Levels (SPARCL) Investigators. High-Dose Atorvastatin after stroke or transient ischemic attack. N Engl J Med 2006; 355: 549–59.

50. Gey KF, Stahelin HB, Eichholzer M. Poor plasma status of carotene and vitamin C is associated with higher mortality from ischemic heart disease and stroke: Basel prospective study. Clin Invest 1993; 71: 3–6.

51. Kushi LH, Folsom AR, Prineas R, et al. Dietary antioxidant vitamins and death from coronary heart disease in postmenopausal women. N Engl J Med 1996; 334: 1156–62.

52. ISIS-2 (Second International Study of Infarct Survival) Collaborative Group. Randomised trial of intravenous streptokinase, oral aspirin, both, or neither among 17,187 cases of suspected myocardial infarction: ISIS-2. Lancet 1988; 2: 349–60.

53. Steering Committee of the Physicians' Health Study Research Group. Final report on the aspirin component of the Ongoing Physicians' Health Study. N Engl J Med 1989; 321: 129–35.

54. Mohr JP. Transient ischemic attacks and the prevention of strokes. N Engl J Med 1978; 299: 93–5.

55. The Canadian Cooperative Study Group. A randomized trial of aspirin and sulfinpyrazone in threatened stroke. N Engl J Med 1978; 299: 53–9.

56. Antiplatelet Trialists' Collaboration. Collaborative overview of randomized trials of antiplatelet therapy: 1. Prevention of death, myocardial infarction, and stroke by prolonged antiplatelet therapy. Br Med J 1994; 308: 81–106.

57. The Dutch TIA Trial Study Group. A comparison of two doses of aspirin (30 mg vs. 283 mg a day) in patients after a transient ischemic attack or minor ischemic stroke. N Engl J Med 1991; 325: 1261–8.

58. The Swedish Aspirin Low-dose Trial (SALT) Collaborative Study Group. Swedish Aspirin Low Dose Trial (SALT) of 75 mg aspirin as secondary prophylaxis after cerebrovascular ischaemic events. Lancet 1991; 338: 1345–9.

59. Farrell B, Godwin J, Richards S, et al. United Kingdom TIA Study Group. The United Kingdom Transient Ischemic Attack (UK-TIA) Aspirin trial: final results. J Neurol Neurosurg Psychiatry 1991; 54: 1044–54.

60. Dyken ML, Barnett HJM, Easton JD, et al. Low-dose aspirin and stroke: "It ain't necessarily so." Stroke. 1992; 23: 1395–9; editorial.

61. Johnson M, Walton PL, Cotton RC, et al. Pharmacological evaluation of ticlopidine, a novel inhibitor of platelet function. Thromb Haemost 1977; 38: 64–9.

62. Roth GJ, Majerus PW. The mechanism of the effect of aspirin on human platelet. I. Acetylation of a particular fraction protein. J Clin Invest 1975; 56: 624–32.
63. Hass WK, Easton JD, Adams HP, et al. A randomized trial comparing ticlopidine hydrochloride with aspirin for the prevention of stroke in high risk patients. N Engl J Med 1988; 321: 501–7.
64. Grotta IC, Norris JW, Karnm B; TASS Baseline and Angiographic Data Subgroup. Prevention of stroke with ticlopidine: Who benefits most? Neurology 1992; 42: 1111–15.
65. Gorclick PB, Richardson DJ, Kelly M, et al. Aspirin and ticlopidine for prevention of recurrent stroke in black patients. A randomized trial. JAMA 2003; 289: 2947–57.
66. Bennet CL, Weinberg PD, Rozenberg-Ben-Dror K, et al. Thrombotic thrombocytopenic purpura associated with ticlopidine: a review of 60 cases. Ann Intern Med 1998; 128: 541–4.
67. Yusuf S, Zhao F, Mehta SR, et al. Effects of Clopidogrel in addition to aspirin in patients with acute coronary syndromes without ST-Segment elevation. N Engl J Med 2001; 345: 494–502.
68. Fitzgerald GA. Dipyridamole. N Engl J Med 1987; 316: 1247–56.
69. Acheson J, Danta G, Hutchinson EC. Controlled trial of dipyridamole in cerebral vascular disease. Br Med J 1969; 1: 614–15.
70. Diener HC, Bogousslavsky J, Brass LM, et al. Aspirin and clopidogrel compared with clopidogrel alone after recent ischaemic stroke or transient ischaemic attack in high-risk patients (MATCH): randomised, double-blind, placebo-controlled trial. Lancet 2004; 364: 331–7.
71. Bhatt DL, Fox KAA, Hackett GI, et al. Clopidogrel and aspirin versus aspirin alone for the prevention of atherothrombotic events. N Engl J Med 2006; 354: 1–12.
72. The America-Canadian Cooperative Study Group. Persantine Aspirin Trial in cerebral ischemia. Part II: endpoint results. Stroke 1985; 16: 406–H5.
73. Diener HC, Cunha L, Forbes C, et al. European Stroke Prevention Study 2. Dipyridamole and acetyl-salicylic acid in the secondary prevention of stroke. J Neurol Sci 1996; 143: 1–13.
74. Halkes PH, van Gijn J, Kappelle LJ, et al. Aspirin plus dipyridamole versus aspirin alone after cerebral ischaemia of arterial origin (ESPRIT): randomized controlled trial. Lancet 2006; 367: 1665–73.
75. North American Symptomatic Carotid Endarterectomy Trial Collaborators. Beneficial effect of carotid endarterectomy in symptomatic patients with high-grade carotid stenosis. N Engl J Med 1991; 325: 445–53.
76. Weinberger J, Robbins A. Neurologic symptoms associated with nonobstructive plaque at carotid bifurcation: analysis by real-time B-mode ultrasonography. Arch Neurol 1983; 40: 489–92.
77. Blackshear WM, Phillips DJ, Chikos PM, et al. Carotid artery velocity patterns in normal and stenotic vessels. Stroke 1979; 11: 67–71.
78. Faught E, Trader SD, Hanna GR. Cerebral complications of angiography for transient ischemia and stroke: predictions of risk. Neurology 1979; 29: 4–15.
79. Ringleb PA, Allenberg J, Bruckmann H, et al. SPACE collaborative group. 30 Day Results from the SPACE Trial of Stent—protected angiogplasty versus carotid endarterectomy in symptomatic patients: a randomized non-inferiority trial. Lancet 2006; 368: 1239–47.
80. Qureshi AI, Luft AR, Janardhan V, et al. Identification of patients at risk for periprocedural neurological deficits associated with carotid angioplasty and stenting. Stroke 2000; 31: 376–82.
81. Mas J-L, Chatellier G, Beyssen B, et al. Endarterectomy versus stenting in patients with symptomatic severe carotid stenosis. N Engl J Med 2006; 355: 1660–71.
82. Brott TG, Hobson RW, Howard G, et al. Stenting vs endarterectomy for treatment of carotid-artery stenosis. N Engl J Med 2010; 363: 11–23.
83. Executive Committee for the Asymptomatic Carotid Atherosclerosis Study. Endarterectomy for asymptomatic carotid artery stenosis. JAMA 1995; 273: 1421–8.
84. Halliday A, Mansfield A, Marro J, et al. MRC Asymptomatic Carotid Surgery Trial (ACST) Collaborative Group. Prevention of disabling and fatal strokes by successful carotid endarterectomy in patients without recent neurological symptoms: randomised controlled trial. Lancet 2004; 363: 1491–502.
85. Imparato AM, Riles TS, Mintzer K, et al. The importance of hemorrhage in the relationship between gross morphologic characteristics and cerebral symptoms in 376 carotid artery plaques. Ann Surg 1983; 197: 195–202.
86. Reillly LM, Lusby RJ, Hughes I, et al. Carotid plaque histology using real-time ultrasonography: Clinical and therapeutic implications. Am J Surg 1983; 46: 188–93.
87. Weinberger J, Ramos L, Ambrose JA, et al. Morphologic and dynamic changes of atherosclerotic plaque at the carotid artery bifurcation: sequential imaging by real time B-mode Ultrasonography. J Am Coll Cardiol 1988; 12: 1515–21.
88. Norris JW, Zhu CZ, Bornstein NM, et al. Vascular risks of asymptomatic carotid stenosis. Stroke 1991; 22: 1485–990.

89. Stroke Prevention in Atrial Fibrillation Investigators. Stroke prevention in atrial fibrillation study. Final results. Circulation 1991; 84: 527–39.

90. Stroke Prevention in Atrial Fibrillation Investigators. Warfarin versus aspirin for prevention of thromboembolism in atrial fibrillation. Stroke Prevention in Atrial Fibrillation II Study. Lancet 1994; 343: 587–91.

91. The Stroke Prevention in Atrial Fibrillation Investigators. Predictors of thromboembolism in atrial fibrillation. I. Clinical features of patients at risk. Ann Intern Med 1992; 116: 1–5.

92. The Stroke Prevention in Atrial Fibrillation Investigators. Predictors of thromboembolism in atrial fibrillation: II. Echocardiographic features of patients at risk. Ann Intern Med 1992; 116: 6–12.

93. Peterson P, Boysen G, Godtfredsen J, et al. Placebo-controlled trial of warfarin and aspirin for prevention of thromboembolic complications in chronic atrial fibrillation. The Copenhaagen AFASAK Study. Lancet 1989; 1: 175–9.

94. Boston Area Anticoagulation Trial for Atrial Fibrillation Investigators. The effect of low-dose warfarin on the risk of stroke in nonrheumatic atrial fibrillation. N Engl J Med 1990; 323: 1505–11.

95. Ezekowitz MD, Bridgers SL, James KE, et al. Warfarin in the prevention of stroke associated with nonrheumatic atrial fibrillation. N Engl J Med 1992; 327: 1406–12.

96. The ACTIVE Investigators. Effect of Clopidogrel added to aspirin in patients with atrial fibrillation. N Engl J Med 2009; 361: 1312–15.

97. Connolly SJ, Ezekowitz MD, Yusuf S, et al. Dabigatran versus warfarin in patients with atrial fibrillation. N Engl J Med 2009; 361: 1139–51.

98. Patel MR, Mahaffey KW, Garg J, et al. Rivaroxaban versus warfarin in nonvalvular atrial fibrillation. N Engl J Med 2011; 365: 883–91.

99. Granger CB, Alexander JH, McMurray JJV, et al. Apixaban versus warfarin in patients with atrial fibrillation. N Engl J Med 2011; 365: 981–9.

100. Wyse DG, Waldo L, DiMarco JP, et al. The Atrial Fibrillation Follow-up Investigation of Rhythm Management (AFFIRM) investigators. A comparison of rate control and rhythm control in patients with atrial fibrillation. N Engl J Med 2002; 1825–33.

101. Szekely P. Systemic embolism and anticoagulant prophylaxis in rheumatic heart disease. Br Med J 1964; 1: 1209–12.

102. Smith P, Arnesen H, Holme I. The effect of warfarin on mortality and reinfarction after myocardial infarction. N Engl J Med 1990; 323: 147–52.

103. Homma SI, Thompson JOP, Pullicino PM. Warfarin and aspirin in patients with heart failure and sinus rhythm. N Engl J Med 2012; 366: 1859–69.

104. Homma S, Sacco RL. Patent foramen ovale and stroke. Circulation 2005; 112: 1063–72.

105. Weinberger J, Azhar S, Danisi F, et al. A new noninvasive technique for imaging atherosclerotic plaque in the aortic arch of stroke patients by transcutaneous real time B-mode ultrasonography. Stroke 1998; 29: 673–6.

106. Gold G, Giannakopoulos P, Montes-Paixao C, et al. Sensitivity and specificity of newly proposed clinical criteria for possible vascular dementia. Neurology 1997; 49: 690–4.

107. Dimant J, Grob D. Electrocardiographic changes and myocardial damage in patients with acute cerebrovascular accidents. Stroke 1977; 8: 448–55.

108. Wallace JD, Levy LL. Blood pressure after stroke. JAMA 1981; 246: 2177–80.

109. International Stroke Trial Collaborative Group. The International Stroke Trial (IST): a randomised trial of aspirin, subcutaneous heparin, both or neither among 19435 patients with acute ischemic stroke. Lancet 1997; 349: 1569–81.

110. Haley EC Jr, Kassell NF, Torner JC. Failure of heparin to prevent progression in progressing ischemic stroke. Stroke 1988; 19: 10–14.

111. The Publication Committee for the Trial of ORG 10172 in Acute Stroke Treatment (TOAST) Investigators. Low molecular weight heparinoid, ORG 10172 (danaproid), and outcome after acute ischemic stroke: a randomized controlled trial. JAMA 1998; 279: 1265–72.

112. Kay R, Wong KS, Yu YL, et al. Low molecular weight heparin for the treatment of acute ischemic stroke. N Engl J Med 1995; 333: 1488–593.

113. Duke RI, Bloch Rf, Alexander GG, et al. Intravenous heparin for the prevention of stroke progression in acute partial stable stroke. A randomized controlled trial. Ann Intern Med 1986; 105: 825–8.

114. Baker RN, Broward JA, Fang HC, et al. Anticoagulant therapy in cerebral infarction. Neurology 1962; 12: 823–30.

115. Fisher CM. The use of anticoagulants in cerebral thrombosis. Neurology 1958; 8: 311–32.

116. Mulley G, Wilcox RG, Mitchell JRA. Dexamethasone in acute stroke. Br Med J 1978; 2: 994–6.

117. Candelise L, Colombo A, Spinner H. Therapy against brain swelling in stroke patients. Stroke 1975; 6: 353–5.
118. Weinberger J. Management of the complications of stroke. In: Adams HP Jr, ed. Handbook of Cerebrovascular Diseases. New York, NY: Marcel Dekker, 1993: 655–72.
119. Schwab S, Steiner S, Aschoff A, et al. Early hemicraniectomy in patients with complete middle cerebral artery infarction. Stroke 1998; 29: 1888–93.
120. Liu J, Tuhrim S, Weinberger J, et al. Premonitory symptoms of stroke in evolution to the locked-in state. J Neurol Neurosurg Psychiatry 1983; 46: 221–6.
121. Adams HP Jr, Bendixen BH, Leira E, et al. Antithrombotic treatment of ischemic stroke among patients with occlusion or severe stenosis of the internal carotid artery: A report of the Trial of ORG 10172 in Acute Stroke Treatment (TOAST). Neurology 1999; 53: 122–5.
122. Koller RL. Recurrent embolic cerebral infarction and anticoagulation. Neurology 1982; 32: 283–5.
123. Cerebral Embolism Study Group. Immediate anticoagulation of embolic stroke: a randomized trial. Stroke 1983; 14: 668–76.
124. Cerebral Embolism Study Group. Immediate anticoagulation of embolic stroke: brain hemorrhage and management options. Stroke 1984; 15: 779–89.
125. Rothrock IF, Dittrich HC, McAllen S, et al. Acute anticoagulation following cardioembolic stroke. Stroke 1989; 20: 730–4.
126. Pessin MS, Estol CJ, LaFranchise F, et al. Safety of anticoagulation after hemorrhagic infarction. Neurology 1993; 43: 1298–303.
127. Pruitt AA, Rubin RH, Karchmer AW, et al. Neurologic complications of bacterial endocarditis. Medicine 1978; 57: 329–51.
128. The International Stroke Trial (IST). International Stroke Trial Collaborative Group. A randomised trial of aspirin, subcutaneous heparin, both or neither among 19,435 patients with acute ischemic stroke. Lancet 1997; 349: 1569–81.
129. The National Institute of Neurological Disorders and Stroke rt-PA Stroke Study Group. Tissue plasminogen activator for acute ischemic stroke. N Engl J Med 1995; 333: 1581–7.
130. Berrouschot J, Rother J, Glahn J, et al. Outcome and severe hemorrhagic complications of intravenous thrombolysis with tissue plasminogen activator in very old (≥80 years) stroke patients. Stroke 2005; 36: 2421–5.
131. Hacke W, Kaste M, Fieschi C, et al. Intravenous thrombolysis with recombinant tissue plasminogen activator for acute hemispheric stroke. The European Cooperative Acute Stroke Study (ECASS). JAMA 1995; 274: 1017–25.
132. Multicenter Acute Stroke Trial: Italy (MAST-I) Group. Randomised controlled trial of streptokinase, aspirin and combination of both in treatment of acute ischaemic stroke. Lancet 1995; 346: 1509–14.
133. Furlan A, Higashida R, Wechsler L, et al. Intra-arterial prourokinase for acute ischemic stroke. The PROACT II Study: a randomized control trial. JAMA 1999; 282: 2003–11.
134. Zeumer H, Hacke S, Ringelstein EF. Local intra-arterial thrombolysis in vertebrobasilar thromboembolic disease. AJNR Am J Neuroradiol 1983; 4: 401–4.
135. Pierot L, van der Bom IM, Wakhloo AK. Advances in stroke: advances in interventional neuroradiology. Stroke 2012; 310–13.
136. Chimowitz MI, Lynn MJ, Derdeyn CP, et al. Stenting versus aggressive medical therapy for intracranial stenosis. N Engl J Med 2011; 365: 993–1003.
137. Rothman S. Synaptic release of excitatory amino acid neurotransmitter mediates anoxic neuronal death. J Neurosci 1984; 4: 1884–91.
138. Muir KW, Lees KR. Clinical experience with excitatory amino acid antagonist drugs. Stroke 1995; 26: 503–13.
139. Poungvarin N, Bhoopat W, Viriyavejakul A, et al. Effects of dexamethasone in primary supratentorial intracerebral hemorrhage. N Engl J Med 1987; 316: 1229–33.
140. Gebel J, Powers WJ. Emergency craniotomy for intracerebral hemorrhage: when doesn't it help and does it ever help? Neurology 2002; 58: 1325–6.
141. Rabinstein AA, Atkinson JL, Wijdicks EFM. Emergency craniotomy in patients worsening due to expanded cerebral hematoma: to what purpose? Neurology 2002; 58: 1367–72.
142. Kassell NF, Tomer IC, Jane IA, et al. The International Cooperative Study on the Timing of Aneurysm Surgery. Part 2: Surgical results. J Neurosurg 1990; 73: 37–47.
143. Teasdale G, Mendelow AD, Graham DI, et al. Efficacy of Nimodipine in cerebral ischemia or hemorrhage. Stroke 1990; 21: 123–5.
144. Allen GS, Han AHS, Preziosi TI, et al. Cerebral arterial spasm—a controlled trial of nimodipine in patients with subarachnoid hemorrhage. N Engl J Med 1983; 308: 619–24.

145. Nibbelink DW. Antihypertensive and antifibrinolytic therapy following subarachnoid hemorrhage from ruptured intracranial aneurysm. In: Sahs AL, Nibbelink DW, Torner IC, eds. Aneurysmal Subarachnoid Hemorrhage. Report of the Cooperative Study. Vol. 13 Baltimore: Urban & Schwarzenberg, 1981: 297–306.
146. Zubkov YN, Nikjforov BM, Shustin VA. Balloon catheter technique for dilatation of constricted cerebral arteries after aneurysmal SAH. Acta Neurochir (Wien) 1984; 70: 65–79.
147. Berenstejn A, Ransohoff J, Kupersmith M, et al. Transvascular treatment of giant aneurysms of the cavernous carotid and vertebral arteries: functional investigation and embolization. Surg Neurol 1984; 21: 3–12.
148. Molyneux AJ, Kerr RSC, Yu L-M, et al. International subarachnoid aneurysm trial (ISAT) of neurosurgical clipping versus endovascular coiling in 2143 patients with ruptured intracranial aneurysms: a randomized comparison of effects on survival, dependency, seizures, rebleeding, subgroups, and aneurysm occlusion. Lancet 2005; 366: 809–17.
149. Spetzler RF, Zabranski JM. Grading and staged resection of cerebral arteriovenous malformations. Clin Neurosurg 1990; 36: 318–37.
150. Dawson RC III, Tarr RW, Hecht ST, et al. Treatment of arteriovenous malformations of the brain with combined embolization and stereotactic radiosurgery: results after one and two years. Am J Neurorad l990; 11: 857–64.

25

Evaluation and management of syncope in the elderly patient

Rose S. Cohen and Mathew S. Maurer

SUMMARY

Syncope, defined as a transient loss of consciousness, is a common syndrome in older adults, with multiple underlying causes. Syncope increases with age, rising sharply in incidence after 70 years. A growing and burdensome public health issue, syncope accounts for 6% of all hospital admissions and 3% of all emergency room visits. The health care cost burden of syncope is estimated at greater than $2.4 billion per year. Among emergency room visits for syncope, 80% are by patients older than 65 years. Given the heterogeneity of conditions that can cause or contribute to cerebral hypoperfusion and the multiple co-morbid conditions that afflict older adults, determination of an underlying cause of syncope is often not accomplished. Pathophysiological classification of syncope falls into 5 major categories: primary cardiac arrhythmias, structural cardiovascular disorder, neurally mediated reflex disorders of blood pressure control, orthostatic/dysautonomic disorders of blood pressure control, and primary neurological or psychiatric disorders. Numerous age-related changes in cardiovascular structure and function (e.g. ventricular and vascular stiffening) as well as changes in other organ systems that regulate salt and water balance, predispose older adults to syncope. Identifying older adults at high risk of an adverse outcome related to syncope as opposed to a majority who are at low risk of adverse outcomes is challenging in clinical practice. Detailed history and physical are the most important tools for evaluating the older adult with syncope, including a careful assessment of hydration status and othostatic changes in vital signs. Initial assessment should also include an ECG. Clinical features that suggest higher risk of adverse outcomes include exertional syncope, aortic stenosis or other structural heart disease, severe anemia or electrolyte abnormality on presentation, absence of prodrome, extremes of systolic blood pressure, abnormal troponin I, and ECG findings suggestive of an arrhythmogenic cause of syncope. Treatment should ideally address the underlying cause of syncope and often includes hydration, elimination of medications such as diuretics or vasodilators and less commonly, implantation of pacemakers or defibrillators, or aortic valve surgery.

INTRODUCTION

Syncope is a sudden transient loss of consciousness (TLOC) and postural tone with rapid and spontaneous recovery. Transient cerebral hypoperfusion results in syncope. The elderly are most vulnerable because of age-associated physiological changes in heart rate and blood pressure regulation, comorbid hypertension and atherosclerosis, reduction in thirst, autonomic dysfunction, and the concurrent use of medications that affect blood pressure regulation.

Syncope is not a disease entity. Rather, it is a symptom resulting from diverse patho-physiological processes, similar to other geriatric syndromes. The assignment of a specific etiology guides the prognosis and treatment of individuals, but is often challenging in real-world practice. The differential diagnosis of syncope spans a spectrum from common benign problems to severe, complex, even life-threatening disorders. When evaluating elderly patients with syncope, the practitioner is faced with multiple possible contributing factors (1). Patients older than 65 years have an average of 3.5 chronic medical comorbidities and use three times as many medications as younger patients on a regular basis. An analysis of elderly institutionalized adults with syncope suggested that 81% had two or more comorbid conditions that could have been implicated (2). Given the often elusive root cause among pathological entities detailed below, it is expected that syncope poses a major challenge for medical professionals and their elderly patients.

EPIDEMIOLOGY

The lifetime prevalence of syncope is 19% among the general population and higher among females than males (3). Large-scale population studies indicate that the incidence of syncope increases with age, rising most sharply after age 70 years. In the Framingham cohort, the overall incidence rate of a first report of syncope was 6.2 per 1000 person-years, incidence rates increased with age, with a sharp rise after 70 years (Fig. 25.1). The incidence of syncope 11.1 events per 1000 person-years in persons aged 70–79 years and 16.9–19.5 events per 1000 person-years in patients older than 80 years (4). Among participants with cardiovascular disease, the age-adjusted incidence rate was nearly twice that among participants without cardiovascular disease (10.6 vs. 6.4 per 1000 person-years). The prevalence of syncope in very elderly (mean age 87 years) institutionalized patients is 23% over 10 years; the yearly incidence is estimated to be at least 6% in this group with a 30% recurrence rate (2). Eighty percent of emergency room patients evaluated for syncope are older than 65 years, and syncope accounts for 1–6% of all hospital admissions and 3% of all emergency room visits (5). Given the increase

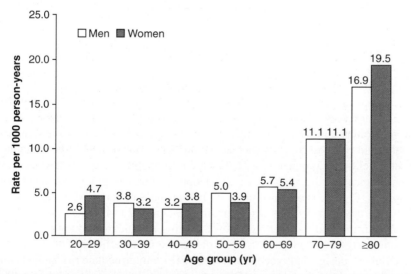

Figure 25.1 Incidence rates of syncope according to age and sex in the Framingham Study. The incidence rates of syncope per 1000 person-years of follow-up increased with age among both men and women. The increase in the incidence rate became steeper starting at the age of 70. Syncope rates were similar in men and women. *Source*: From Ref. 4.

in prevalence of syncope with age, syncope will become a more burdensome public health issue as the segment of over 65-year-olds reaches 12% of the world population and 20% of the US population by 2030 (6).

CONSEQUENCES OF SYNCOPE

The consequences of syncope for the aging population are significant, both on an individual and population basis. Syncope across all age groups accounts for 1–3% of all emergency department (ED) visits and up to 6% hospital admissions (7). Among older individuals presenting with syncope, the 2-year mortality rate was 27% (8). Up to 30% of falls in the elderly may be due to syncope (9). Falls, either with or without loss of consciousness, can result in devastating injuries in the elderly. Five percent to 30% of falls in the community result in injury; approximately 5% of these are fractures and 1% are hip fractures. One in 40 community-dwelling elders who fall will be hospitalized. Only about half of these hospitalized patients will be alive 1 year after the fall (10). Unintentional injury is the fifth leading cause of death, and falls account for 70% of the accidental mortality among people older than 65 years. Even without injury, the fear of falling can be debilitating; elderly patients who fall often restrict their activities and show a higher incidence of depression and dependence in activities of daily living than their peers (11). The overall perception of health is proportional to the number of syncopal events in those with frequent recurrences (12), and such patients have impairment in their quality of life similar to those suffering from arthritis (13).

ETIOLOGIES AND THE IMPORTANCE OF RISK STRATIFICATION

The causes of syncope are traditionally classified into several broad categories. We have found the following pathophysiological classification helpful: (*i*) primary cardiac arrhythmia (bradycardia or tachycardia), (*ii*) structural cardiovascular disorder, (*iii*) neurally mediated reflex disorders of blood pressure control, (*iv*) orthostatic/dysautonomic disorders of blood pressure control, and (*v*) primary neurological or psychiatric diagnoses (Table 25.1). In a majority of the published studies, the term "cardiovascular syncope" is used to refer to the combined diagnoses of structural cardiovascular disease or primary cardiac arrhythmias. The goals of diagnosing and treating patients with syncope are to reduce mortality and morbidity. Risk stratification for causes associated with excess mortality should be performed in all patients, and etiological diagnosis should be made to prevent morbidity associated with syncope recurrence by treating the underlying causes.

Unfortunately, the evaluation of syncope is often nondirected and costly, and frequently leads to great variability in practice and unsatisfying diagnostic conclusions. Examinations diagnostic strategies used in hospitalized elderly patients with syncope identified several relevant issues. Simple, inexpensive, and nonharmful evaluations are vastly underutilized; for example, postural vital signs were recorded in only 27% of one sample. Potentially high-yield provocative tests such as carotid sinus massage (CSM), tilt table testing (TTT) and electrophysiological study (EPS) are infrequently used, while at least one low-yield neurological study, such as carotid Doppler ultrasonography or head computed tomography (CT) scan, is obtained in nearly half of these patients. After an average length of stay of 3–5 days, 42–49% of cases remain undiagnosed (14,15). These results may be contrasted with the findings from trials investigating a standardized approach to syncope diagnosis in emergency room patients that indicate diagnostic efficiency of 76–83% (16,17). Indeed, a trial of a designated syncope unit in the ED for intermediate risk patients improved diagnostic yield in the ED and reduced the rate of hospital admission and the total length of hospital stay without affecting recurrent syncope and all-cause mortality (18).

A logical approach to diagnosis of syncope in the elderly patient begins with an understanding of the differential diagnosis and epidemiology (Table 25.2), although the

Table 25.1 Differential Diagnosis of the Causes of Syncope

Primary Arrhythmic	Neurally Mediated	Dysautonomia/Orthostatic Hypotension	Structural Cardiovascular	Neurological/Psychiatric Mimics of Syncope
Tachyarrhythmias	Simple faint	Hypovolemia	Aortic dissection	Vertebrobasilar TIA
Ventricular including	Vasovagal	Medication-related	Atrial myxoma	Stroke
Ventricular tachycardia	Vasodepressor	Postprandial	Pulmonary embolus	Migraine
Torsades de pointes	Mixed phenotypes	Shy–Drager syndrome	Pulmonary hypertension	Seizure
Supraventricular	Carotid sinus hypersensitivity	Parkinson's disease	Subclavian steal	Narcolepsy
tachycardia	Situational	Spinal cord disease	Hypertrophic cardiomyopathy	Concussion
Atrial fibrillation/flutter	Micturition	Diabetic neuropathy	Aortic stenosis	Panic attacks
Bradyarrhythmias	Cough	Amyloid	Mitral stenosis	Anxiety disorder
Sick sinus syndrome	Swallow	Other peripheral neuropathies	Pump Failure/Cardiogenic Shock	
AV nodal block	Defecation		Myocardial ischemia	
Sinus bradycardia	Laugh		Pericardial disease/tamponade	
Pacemaker malfunctions	Post-exercise			
Pacemaker-mediated				
tachycardia				
Pacemaker syndrome				

Table 25.2 Epidemiology of Syncope in the Elderly Patient

Study Design (Investigators)	Date (Ref.)	N	Mean Age	Clinical Setting	Primary Arrhythmia	Structural Cardiovascular	Neurally Mediated	Orthostatic–Dysautonomic, Drug-Related	Primary Neurological Psychiatric	Unknown, Other Unspecified
Lipsitz et al. (retrospective)	1985 (2)	67	87	Nursing home	3 (4%)	10 (15%)	11 (16%)	15 (22%)	7 (10%)	21 (31%)
Kapoor et al. (prospective)	1986 (19)	210	71	ED, in-patients	54 (26%)	14 (7%)	25 (12%)	25 (12%)	10 (5%)	83 (40%)
McIntosh et al. (prospective)[a]	1993 (20)	65	78	Syncope clinic	14 (21%)	0 (0%)	37 (56%)	21 (32%)	12 (18%)	10 (15%)
Getchell et al. (prospective)	1999 (13)	1516	73	In-patients	217 (14%)	67 (4%)	193 (13%)	254 (17%)	69 (5%)	716 (47%)
Ammirati et al. (prospective)	1999 (15)	195	63	ED	35 (18%)	6 (3%)	69 (35%)	12 (6%)	38 (20%)	35 (18%)
Soteriades et al. (prospective)	2002 (3)	822	66	Community	78 (10%) (reported together in this trial)		174 (21%)	133 (16%)	74 (9%)	363 (44%)
Chen, YL (retrospective)	2003 (21)	987	58	Referral to EP Service	350 (35.5%)	11 (1%)	471 (47.7%)	55 (5.6%)	19 (1.9%)	195 (19.8%)

[a]Percentages add up to more than 100% because some subjects were found to have multiple causes of syncope.
Abbreviation: ED, Emergency department.

true distribution of syncope etiology is difficult to determine because of the differences between populations studied and wide variance in strategies for evaluation. While many studies have examined the etiology of syncope in a variety of clinical settings, few focus on patients older than 65 years or stratify their data by age range.

The percentage of patients with an "unknown" etiology following evaluation was high in early studies. Nonetheless, some conclusions can be drawn from the available data. A large percentage of patients have orthostatic/dysautonomic or neurally mediated disorders of blood pressure control. Primary arrhythmias are fairly common, and structural cardiovascular disorders and primary neurological syncope are comparatively rare. These conclusions are supported by a large multicenter study in which a prospective systematic evaluation of consecutive patients referred to the EDs for syncope established a definite diagnosis in 98%, including neurally mediated syncope in 66% of diagnoses, orthostatic hypotension (OH) in 10%, primary arrhythmias in 11%, structural cardiac or cardiopulmonary disease in 5%, and nonsyncopal attacks in 6%, while only 2% were considered unexplained (22).

Data from cohort and prospective trials have revealed that syncope patients can be stratified into groups with high and low long-term risks of death based on etiology. In a prospective study of 204 primarily hospitalized patients evaluated for syncope and followed for 1 year, the overall mortality rate was 30% and the rate of sudden death was 24% in patients with a cardiovascular cause as compared with 12% and 4%, respectively, in patients with a non-cardiovascular etiology (23). In the Framingham cohort, patients with isolated syncope (i.e., syncope in the absence of prior or concurrent neurological, coronary, or other cardiovascular disease stigmata) did not suffer from excess all-cause or cardiovascular (including sudden death) mortality (24). Similarly, an examination of a community-based sample from the Framingham cohort (average age 66 years) indicates that the excess mortality in patients with syncope is attributable almost entirely to those with a cardiovascular etiology [adjusted hazard ratio for mortality of 2.01; 95% confidence interval (CI) 1.48–2.73], while subjects with neurally mediated, medication-related, or orthostatic/dysautonomic syncope (45% of the sample) did not show increased mortality (adjusted hazard ratio of 1.08; 95% CI 0.88–1.34) (4). A prospective multivariate analysis comparing 940 relatively young (mean age 52.5 years) patients with similar cardiovascular disease severity on a symptom scale, with and without syncope, suggested that mortality was related to underlying cardiac disease severity much more strongly than to the occurrence of a syncopal event itself (25).

ASSESSMENT OF HIGH SHORT-TERM RISK AND NEED FOR HOSPITALIZATION

It is paramount to assess the probability of developing life-threatening events within days and weeks of the initial presentation of syncope. Such an assessment of risk assists in determining which patients among the minority of all syncope patient merit immediate hospitalization and expedited evaluation (26). Overall, the bias in clinical practice is to admit the majority of elderly patients presenting with syncope as suggested by available guidelines, leading to an excess of hospitalizations in the absence of evidence to justify otherwise.

According to the 2009 European Society of Cardiology guidelines, short-term high risk criteria that require prompt hospitalization or early intensive evaluation include severe structural heart disease or coronary artery disease, electrocardiogram (ECG) features to suggest an arrhythmogenic cause of syncope such as nonsustained ventricular tachycardia, bifascicular block, sinus bradycardia, ventricular pre-excitation, ECG suggesting an inherited disease, exertional syncope, syncope in the supine position, palpitations preceding syncope, family history of sudden cardiac death, or severe comorbid anemia or electrolyte disturbance (27). Additionally, the Canadian Cardiovascular Society Position Paper adds the presence of heart failure, hypotension defined as systolic blood pressure less than 90 mmHg, age >60 years (minor risk factor) as compelling features for either prompt hospitalization or early evaluation (28).

In the Short-Term Prognosis of Syncope (STePS) study, among 676 study participants who presented with syncope to the ED, 6.1% experienced severe outcomes at 10 days. Abnormal ECG, concomitant trauma, absence of prodrome, and male gender were associated with short-term unfavorable outcomes (29).

Predictors of 30-day serious events (ranging from death to significant hemorrhage or anemia requiring blood transfusion) have been examined among older adults with syncope. Sun et al. identified a subgroup of patients over age 60 presenting to the ED with a 30-day serious event (7% of the more than 2500 cases reviewed). High risk and low risk predictors were established. Of note, high risk predictors (leading to a 20% 30-day serious event rate) included age greater than 90 years, history of arrhythmia, triage systolic blood pressure greater than 160 mmHg, abnormal ECG, and abnormal troponin I. These factors were used to develop a syncope risk score (one point for each factor). The authors suggest inpatient evaluation for the high risk individual (e.g., those with a syncope risk score of at least 3 points). Interestingly, near syncope rather than true syncope was a low risk predictor (leading to 2.5% 30-day serious event rate) (30). The same group of investigators have subsequently identified patterns and predictors of shorter term 7-day events among 39,943 ED visits for syncope and found positive predictors to include age ≥60, male gender, congestive heart failure (CHF), ischemic heart disease, cardiac arrhythmia, and valvular heart disease. Notably, there was an age-dependent relationship between 7-day outcomes and cardiac arrhythmia and valvular disease, affected patients <60 years old having higher relative risk than older patients (31).

In the San Francisco Syncope Rule study, a prospective study of 684 ED patients with a mean age of 62 years, the following factors predicted 7-day serious outcomes: abnormal ECG, complaint of shortness of breath, hematocrit less than 30%, systolic blood pressure <90 mmHg, and history of CHF (30). A retrospective external validation study was performed of the San Francisco Syncope Rule in a Canadian ED setting, and found that the rule had a sensitivity of 90%, and a specificity of 33%. Physicians failed to predict two deaths, which the rule would have predicted. Most notably however, implementing the rule would have increased the admission rate from 12.3% (the lowest admission rates for syncope in the western world) to 69.5% in a Canadian health system (32), contrary to original estimations that the rule would reduce admission rates.

The prospective observational Risk Stratification of Syncope in the Emergency Department (ROSE) study, found 7.3% of study participants (mean age 63.8 years) to have a serious outcome or all-cause mortality event at 1 month. Independent predictors of such events were brain natriuretic peptide concentration greater than or equal to 300 pg/mL, positive fecal occult blood, hemoglobin less than or equal to 90 g/L, oxygen saturation less than or equal to 94%, and Q-wave on the presenting ECG (33).

The Boston Syncope Criteria include an eight component decision tool to be used by emergency physicians to determine risk for adverse outcome in syncope and thus whether to admit patients with syncope presenting to the ED, including signs and symptoms of acute coronary syndrome, worrisome cardiac history, family history of sudden cardiac death, valvular disease, signs of cardiac conduction disease, volume depletion, persistently abnormal vital signs for greater than 15 minutes, and primary neurological event (34). In a subsequent validation study, the Boston Syncope Criteria was found to safely reduce hospital admissions by 11% (35).

Collectively, these risk assessment tools, summarized in Table 25.3, are difficult to apply to older adults (e.g., >75 years) with syncope because this population was not the

Table 25.3   Risk Stratification Methods for Short-Term Adverse Outcomes in Subjects with Syncope

	Boston Syncope Criteria	Risk Stratification of Syncope in ER	Sun et al. (30)	San Francisco Syncope Rule (36)
High risk	Signs/symptoms of ACS	BNP >300 pg/mL	Age >90 years	History of CHF
	Conduction disease	Positive guaiac	Male gender	Hematocrit <30%
	Worrisome cardiac history	Hemoglobin <90 g/L	History of arrhythmia	Abnormal findings on ECG or
	Valvular heart disease	Oxygen saturation <94%	Triage SBP >160 mm Hg	cardiac monitoring
	Family history of SCD	Q-wave on ECG	Abnormal ECG	Shortness of breath
	Persistent abnormal vital signs in ED		Abnormal troponin	SBP <90 mm Hg
	Volume depletion			
	Primary CNS event			
Low risk		–	Near syncope	–
Outcomes[a]	23%	7.3%	6.7%	11%
Sensitivity	97%	87.2%	NR	96%
Specificity	62%	65.5%	NR	62%
NPV	NR	98.5%	NR	97%
PPV	NR	NR	NR	22%

[a]Prevalence of adverse outcomes or critical intervention.

Abbreviations: ACS, acute coronary syndrome; BNP, b-type natriuretic peptide; CHF, congestive heart failure; CNS, central nervous system; ECG, electrocardiogram; ED, emergency department; NPV, negative predictive value; ROSE, Risk Stratification of Syncope; SBP, systolic blood pressure; SCD, sudden cardiac death.

primary focus of these scores. What they do highlight is that subjects with significant cardio-vascular disease (such as heart failure, abnormal ECGs or previous arrhythmias or abnormal biomarkers) should receive specialized attention often in an inpatient setting. Additionally, markedly abnormal blood pressures and several extra-cardiac conditions, especially anemia, are important indicators of adverse outcomes. These scores have high sensitivity for identifying individuals with high risk of short-term outcomes but limited specificity. Thus, the application of these scores is likely most useful to identify a cohort of older adults who do not require inpatient evaluation, avoiding unnecessary hospitalizations in this cohort.

CURRENT CLINICAL GUIDELINES: COMMENT ON THE ELDERLY

The AHA/ACCF issued a Scientific Statement on the Evaluation of Syncope in 2006. The most recent clinical guidelines were issued by the European Society of Cardiology in 2009. These guidelines outline the definition of syncope, risk stratification, diagnostic testing, and recommended treatments (27). Both documents address special considerations in the elderly population and are highlighted below in Table 25.4. Additionally, a point is made that the evaluation of mobile independent, cognitively normal elderly patients should be comparable to the workup of younger patients (37).

INITIAL WORKUP

The initial diagnostic workup should consist of history, physical examination, and 12-lead ECG. Studies across a wide range of subjects indicate that the history and physical examination alone can directly make a diagnosis in up to 50% of patients with syncope, and can suggest possible etiologies in many more. The ECG makes a definitive diagnosis in only a few patients (usually <5%), but is helpful in identifying patients likely to have underlying structural heart disease and/or cardiac conduction disturbances (39) and thus is a standard of care for older adults presenting with syncope. Laboratory tests are rarely definitive and probably can be limited to those patients in whom a particular disorder (anemia, hypoglycemia, severe dehydration) is suspected as a contributing factor. While we do not recommend routine measurement of biomarkers (e.g., troponin or b-type natriuretic peptides) in older adult patients with syncope, clinicians should be aware of their prognostic significance when abnormal.

Table 25.4   European Society of Cardiology Guidelines for the Diagnosis and Management of Syncope (27) and the AHA/ACCF Scientific Statement on the Evaluation of Syncope (38): Comments Particular to the Elderly Population

	ESC	AHA/ACCF
Recommended workup	Orthostatic blood pressure measurements, carotid sinus massage, TTT Mini–mental state examination if suspect cognitive deficit, consider implantable loop recorder if arrhythmia strongly suspected	Orthostatic blood pressure and heart rate measurement
Comment on falls	Modification of risk for fall/syncope may reduce future events in community dwelling frail elderly	Up to 30% falls in the elderly may be related to syncope
Most common causes	OH, CSH, reflex syncope cardiac arrhythmias	OH, postprandial hypotension, CSH, neurally mediated (consider Parkinson's disease), cardiovascular medications

Abbreviations: CSH, carotid sinus hypersensitivity; OH, orthostatic hypotension; TTT, tilt table testing.

Patient History

In evaluating patients, it is essential to differentiate syncope from other pathological entities. Conditions such as vertigo, substance intoxication, and hypoglycemia that do not result in a transient loss of consciousness (LOC) with spontaneous recovery are not syncope. Sustained arrhythmic events requiring electrical or chemical cardioversion present with a spectrum ranging from syncope to sudden cardiac death; in these cases the diagnosis is usually not in question, and the evaluation strategy to follow is clear.

Seizures are another common cause of unexplained loss of consciousness, but also do not constitute true syncope. Distinguishing between syncope and seizure is a common diagnostic challenge, but can usually be accomplished from the history. However, many patients with syncope have myoclonic jerks that can be mistaken for seizure activity by witnesses. In one series of patients with neurally mediated syncope during TTT, 8% of patients with positive tests had apparent neurological events (40). In a study of 94 consecutive patients who had transient loss of consciousness, the best discriminatory finding was orientation immediately after the event according to the eyewitness. Nausea and sweating before the event were useful to exclude a seizure but, contrary to common clinical teaching, incontinence and trauma were not discriminatory findings (41). Another study found that lateral tongue biting had a sensitivity of 24% and a specificity of 99% for the diagnosis of generalized tonic–clonic seizures (42). A standardized evaluation of 671 patients with LOC revealed head turning and unresponsiveness during unconsciousness to be predictive of seizures, while dizziness or diaphoresis prior to the event or LOC after prolonged sitting or standing were suggestive of syncope (43). In addition, patients with seizures often have a history of prior seizures or other neurological symptoms or findings on neurological examination that suggest the diagnosis.

Distinguishing between syncope and falls can be difficult. There is considerable clinical overlap among these entities in the elderly. Discriminating between syncope and falls relies upon accurate accounts from patients and/or witnesses of the event. Classically, patients postsyncope recall the circumstances and events immediately preceding LOC, possibly up to the initial loss of postural tone, and then recall finding themselves on the ground after the gap in consciousness but, unlike patients with simple falls, they cannot recall actually striking the ground. In contrast, patients with simple falls complicated by transient LOC due to head trauma (i.e., concussion) should distinctly recall striking their head before blacking out.

Unfortunately, many elderly patients have retrograde amnesia regarding the event; one study demonstrated that 32% of cognitively normal older adults could not remember falling 3 months afterward (44). Other trials have shown that 21–32% of subjects with witnessed syncope during CSM have amnesia for the LOC (45,46). A witnessed account is unavailable in many cases of falls brought to medical attention. Falls that are not clearly mechanical often have an attributable cardiovascular cause, particularly bradycardia or neurally mediated blood pressure control disorders (40). Thus, in the elderly, syncope and unexplained falls may be indistinguishable clinical manifestations of the same pathophysiological process, and for this reason we treat any unexplained fall in an elderly adult as potential syncope. Additionally, cognitive impairment may lessen an elderly patient's ability to recall a syncopal or fall event. The European Society of Cardiology guidelines recommend performing a mini–mental state examination be performed if cognitive impairment is suspected (30).

Once it has been established that the patient has had syncope, the primary history taking should focus on precipitating factors, prodromal symptoms, and symptoms following the event. Chronology of recurrence, if applicable, can aid in evaluation. Parallel history is often invaluable. Historical factors associated with particular etiologies of syncope are detailed in Table 25.5. A thorough evaluation of cardiovascular symptoms (i.e., angina, dyspnea, edema, and exercise intolerance) should be obtained in all patients. In a multicenter

Table 25.5   Historical Factors Associated with Various Etiologies of Syncope

Historical Feature	Associated Diagnosis
Nausea, diaphoresis, warmth, long prodrome, total duration of episodes greater than 4 yr	Neurally mediated syndrome
Absence of cardiovascular disease	
Nausea or vomiting associated with syncope	
Syncope occurs after sudden, unexpected, or unpleasant sight, sound, smell, or paint	
During or after micturition, defecation, coughing, laughing, and swallowing	Neurally mediated situational syncope
Syncope occurs during a meal or in the absorptive state after a meal	Postprandial hypotension
With neck pressure (tight collar, shaving, and head turning)	Carotid sinus hypersensitivity
Postepisode confusion, lateral tongue biting, and head turning during episode	Seizure
Diplopia, ataxia, vertigo, and dysarthria	Neurological (transient ischemic attack, migraine, and stroke) or subclavian steal
With arm exercise	Subclavian steal
Upon assuming upright posture or after prolonged standing, especially in crowded or hot places	Orthostatic hypotension
During or after exertion	Aortic stenosis, myocardial ischemia, and vasodepressor response to exercise
While supine	Arrhythmia
History of myocardial infarction or congestive heart failure	Arrhythmia

cross-sectional observational study, The Italian Group for the Study of Syncope in the Elderly, greater than 70% of patients had symptoms prior to syncope. Multivariate regression analysis showed that prodromal symptoms nausea (RR = 3.7, 95% CI 1.26–11.2), blurred vision (RR = 3.5, 95% CI 1.34–9.59) were predictive of noncardiac syncope, while symptoms of dyspnea (RR = 5.5, 95% CI 1.0–30.2) was predictive of cardiac syncope in the elderly (47). Residual symptoms are uncommon in patients with arrhythmia-induced syncope, while those with neurally mediated disorders of blood pressure control may describe moderate-to-severe fatigue afterward (48). In patients with suspected or known structural heart disease, the most specific historical elements for cardiovascular syncope are syncope while supine or during exertion, blurred vision, and duration of symptoms less than 4 years. In patients without suspected heart disease, palpitations are the only predictor of a cardiovascular etiology (49). The use of vasodilating, antiarrhythmic, diuretic, or bradycardic medications should be noted and considered.

Despite the wealth of data demonstrating the value of historical information in guiding the diagnostic and management strategy for patients with syncope, the medical history has a reduced diagnostic specificity in older individuals. In one study, the diagnosis of the cause of syncope was possible on the basis of the history alone in 26% of younger patients and 5% of older patients, with older individuals having fewer prodromal symptoms and signs (50).

Physical Examination

A detailed physical examination should be performed in all patients with syncope. Hydration status and orthostatic changes in vital signs should be assessed. A careful cardiovascular examination should be performed with attention to significant cardiac murmurs and their alteration with body position and various maneuvers, evidence of left ventricular enlargement, and delayed or diminished carotid upstrokes. The extremities should be examined for diminished or absent peripheral arterial pulsations and for bruits. A meticulous neurological examination with attention to the presence of nystagmus, aniscoria, facial asymmetry, plegia, ataxia, and dysmetria should be performed in all patients with syncope. Neurological findings that are focal, especially if recent in onset, suggest central nervous system (CNS) pathology.

Electrocardiogram

The ECG is most commonly normal following a syncopal episode. Definitive diagnoses on initial ECG include marked sinus bradycardia, Mobitz II second- or third-degree atrioventricular (AV) block, alternating left and right bundle branch block, ventricular tachycardia (VT), pacemaker malfunction, paroxysmal supraventricular tachycardia (PSVT), sinus bradycardia, sinoatrial block, or pauses, if associated with symptoms. Such findings are rare (<5%) because arrhythmias resulting in syncope are often self-limited. Other electrocardiographic rhythm and conduction abnormalities can guide further evaluation. For example, first-degree or Mobitz type I second-degree AV block, sinus node dysfunction (SND), and bundle branch and fascicular blocks may suggest a bradycardic event, while evidence of prior myocardial infarction (MI) or left ventricular hypertrophy raises the possibility of VT.

RESULTS OF THE INITIAL EVALUATION

The simple initial evaluation described above is very effective in identifying patients at risk for a cardiovascular etiology for syncope (and therefore increased mortality). A large, prospectively followed cohort of ED patients presenting with syncope demonstrated that the four factors independently predicting increased risk of death in the following year are age greater than 45 years, history of CHF, history of ventricular arrhythmias, and abnormal ECG (not including sinus bradycardia, sinus tachycardia and nonspecific ST segment or T-wave abnormalities) at presentation (51). In patients with none of these four risk factors, mortality at 1 year was 1%, while it was 9%, 16%, and 27% for subjects with one, two, three, or more risk factors, respectively. Unfortunately, because age greater than 45 years is a risk factor, this method is unable to identify any low risk older individuals. Another method for predicting risk in patients with syncope, the San Francisco Syncope Rule (52–55) relies on five risk factors: systolic blood pressure less than 90 mmHg, shortness of breath, non-sinus rhythm or new changes on ECG, history of CHF, or hematocrit less than 30%. Only one of 371 patients (0.3%) with no risk factors had a serious event within 30 days, whereas 52 of 342 patients (15.2%) with one or more of these risk factors had a serious event within 30 days.

In another investigation, only four of 146 patients not suspected to have structural heart disease following history, physical examination, and ECG were found to have had cardiovascular syncope after extensive evaluation (49). Patients with evidence of structural heart disease by history, physical examination, or ECG or those identified as high risk by the aforementioned risk scores should be admitted to the hospital for further evaluation. Diagnostic testing in this group should be aimed at defining the type of underlying heart disease as well as identifying whether a spontaneous arrhythmia is the cause of syncope. Among subjects with syncope and without structural heart disease, long-term follow-up is associated with an excellent outcome and relatively low (~15%) recurrence rate (56), obviating the need for inpatient evaluation.

THE ROLE OF ECHOCARDIOGRAPHY IN INITIAL EVALUATION

An echocardiogram may be beneficial in confirming or excluding structural heart disease, but may not be required in all patients. Echocardiography can directly diagnose a variety of uncommon cardiovascular conditions including severe valvular abnormalities, ventricular hypertrophy with outflow obstruction, severe pulmonary hypertension, and atrial myxoma or thrombus, but such findings are rare in the absence of a suggestive initial evaluation. In one study of 650 consecutive syncope patients (average age 60 years, with 44% >75 years), echocardiography was useful mainly in confirming suspected severe aortic stenosis (AS) and in risk-stratifying patients with known cardiac disease by ejection fraction (EF). Echocardiography was normal or non-relevant in all patients without cardiac disease by history, physical, or ECG in this study group (57).

The role of routine echocardiography in the evaluation of all patients with possible syncope remains to be fully defined, but data suggest that echocardiography is most useful for assessing the severity of the underlying cardiac disease and for risk stratification in patients with unexplained syncope who also have a positive cardiac history or an abnormal ECG (57). Accordingly, it seems reasonable to defer echocardiography in patients without suggestion of structural heart disease from history, physical examination, or ECG, when an alternate diagnosis is identified. However, current guidelines support the use of echocardiography when the etiology of syncope is not identified from the initial workup.

ETIOLOGICAL CATEGORIES AND DIAGNOSTIC TESTING

The remainder of this chapter will focus on the separate etiological categories of syncope as described above. A general description and salient pathophysiological information will be presented for each, followed by an examination of specific testing strategies and their efficacy. The frequency of use of typical diagnostic tests at our medical center and the estimated diagnostic efficacy of each from the literature are detailed in Table 25.6. These data highlight the discrepancy between the tests that are likely to yield definitive diagnoses, based on the published literature (58), and the current practice patterns that largely focus on low-yield non-provocative testing.

STRUCTURAL CARDIOVASCULAR DISORDERS

Most of the etiologies in this category (such as subclavian steal syndrome, pulmonary embolism, and aortic dissection) can be directly diagnosed or at least strongly suggested by the initial clinical evaluation. A careful history and physical examination can guide specific confirmatory testing such as echocardiography, ventilation-perfusion or CT imaging, and angiography. Many of these conditions are relatively uncommon causes of syncope; the

Table 25.6   Diagnostic Utility of Commonly Used Tests in Elderly Patients with Syncope

Test	Frequency of Ordering	Diagnostic Yield From Literature
History and physical exam	100%	20–50%
Electrocardiogram	100%	2–11%
Telemetry monitoring	81%	2–15%
Echocardiogram	55%	5–10%
CT scan of head	40%	1%
Holter monitoring	30%	2–15%
Carotid Doppler	19%	1%
Electroencephalogram	13%	1%
Electrophysiological study	10%	15–25%
Tilt table test	6%	30–60%
Carotid sinus massage	5%	14–68%

Data from a series of consecutive patients (mean age 68 years, with 65% >65 years) admitted to Columbia Presbyterian Medical Center over a 2-year period (1995–1996). Representative data on diagnostic yield as evaluated from published literature (see text for details).

full diagnostic workup of these disorders is beyond the scope of this chapter and will not be discussed further here. The most common etiology in this category among the elderly is AS, myocardial ischemia resulting in cardiac pump failure, or arrhythmia, which is a rare primary cause of isolated syncope.

AORTIC STENOSIS

Calcific or degenerative AS is the most common valvular lesion in the elderly. Risk factors include advancing age, congenital bicuspid valve, smoking, and hypertension; the estimated prevalence of critical AS approaches 6% by 86 years of age (59). Syncope occurs in up to 42% of patients with severe valvular AS, commonly with exercise (60). When patients with AS experience syncope not linked to exertion, the symptom may be unrelated to the valve disease (61). Dehydration or the use of vasodilating drugs may predispose individuals with AS to a decreased cardiac output and syncope. In patients with AS, syncope has prognostic significance with an average survival of 2–3 years in affected patients after its onset, in the absence of valve replacement. Physical findings in severe AS may include decreased amplitude and rate of the carotid pulse, paradoxical splitting of S2, and a very late-peaking systolic murmur heard best at the right upper sternal border (occasionally at the apex in the elderly), as well as manifestations of pulmonary hypertension and CHF, if present (62). The diagnosis of critical AS is usually suggested by history and physical examination and may be confirmed with transthoracic echocardiography or left-sided cardiac catheterization.

MYOCARDIAL ISCHEMIA

The bulk of data suggest that cardiac enzymes may be of little value when obtained routinely on elderly patients with syncope in the absence of signs or symptoms suggestive of myocardial ischemia. Although one report suggests that syncope as a presenting manifestation of MI may increase in incidence with age, particularly in the oldest old (>80 years) (63), in a large observational series of hospitalized syncope patients (average age 73 years, with prevalence of known coronary artery disease 34%), syncope was caused by myocardial ischemia in only 1% (12). In another group of elderly patients, 77% had serial measurement of cardiac enzymes following admission for syncope; only one of 80 patients "ruled in" for MI, and this patient presented with unstable angina and syncope in the setting of chest pain (64). Although most patients admitted for syncope via the ED do not have an MI, serial cardiac enzymes are often obtained; in one series in 62% of subjects (65). However, only 2.1% (95% CI, 0.04–6.09%) had positive cardiac enzymes were obtained during their hospitalization in this study. Of the three patients with positive enzymes, two had chest discomfort and ST segment and T-wave abnormalities on ECG, and the third patient had dementia and could not recall the details surrounding her syncopal event, but had a left bundle branch block on baseline ECG. We would suggest that the diagnostic utility of "ruling out" active ischemia with serial cardiac enzyme testing in all elderly patients admitted with syncope is low in the absence of new ECG changes, symptoms of myocardial ischemia, or a history of ischemic events.

Cardiac stress testing in syncope has not been prospectively studied, but is unlikely to add to the diagnostic evaluation unless patients present with anginal features or exertional syncope. Even among patients who have syncope during exertion, severe AS, hypertrophic obstructive cardiomyopathy, pulmonary hypertension, or a vasodepressor response to exercise are probably more common (causes) than myocardial ischemia.

PRIMARY ARRHYTHMIC SYNCOPE
Tachyarrhythmias

Ventricular tachyarrhythmias are a relatively infrequent, but life-threatening etiology of syncope in the elderly. The increased prevalence of hypertension, diabetes mellitus, hypercholesterolemia, and coronary artery disease in the elderly increases the likelihood of associated left ventricular dysfunction from MI or cardiomyopathy in this cohort. Elderly patients also more commonly have left ventricular hypertrophy and AS, two conditions that predispose to ventricular dysrhythmias. The presence of a cardiomyopathy, ischemic or non-ischemic in etiology, in the setting of syncope is a critical finding associated with a significant rate of malignant events and outcomes, which may justify consideration of automatic implantable cardioverter defibrillator (AICD) implantation even if a malignant arrhythmia is never documented (66). The use of QT-interval-prolonging medication or drugs that predisposes to hypokalemia or hypomagnesemia places elderly patients at risk for torsades de pointes.

Supraventricular tachyarrhythmias (SVT) are a rare cause of syncope, but may be more likely to result in cerebral hypoperfusion in elderly patients with dehydration, on venodilating agents, or with diastolic dysfunction, where reliance on cardiac preload is high. These arrhythmias should always be correlated with symptoms prior to assuming that they are the cause of syncope.

Bradyarrhythmias

Bradycardia is a much more common etiology of syncope in the elderly population compared with the young. While bradycardia has traditionally been grouped with ventricular tachyarrhythmias and structural cardiovascular disorders under the heading of "cardiovascular syncope" in epidemiological studies, the excess mortality in patients with bradycardia is likely small in comparison. Bradycardia may result from intrinsic disease of the cardiac conduction system and/or extrinsic factors such as medications or autonomic influences.

Intrinsic conduction system disease may lead to SND and AV nodal block. SND has several presentations including sinus bradycardia, sinus pauses, and tachy–brady syndromes. Common tachy–brady syndromes include (1) paroxysmal SVTs alternating with sinus bradycardia, (2) paroxysmal SVTs followed immediately by pauses due to delayed sinus node recovery, and (3) persistent atrial fibrillation with slow or highly variable rates (indicating AV nodal block rather than SND). Interestingly, in patients with posttachycardia pauses, syncope is likely related to the transient pause rather than the more obvious tachycardia.

Risk factors for the development of SND include age, structural heart disease (including infiltrative cardiomyopathies such as amyloid), and cardiac surgery. Symptomatic SND is an indication for permanent cardiac pacing (67), but survival in the elderly is related to the underlying structural cardiac disease and not to the presence of SND itself (68). High-grade AV block is another common cause of syncope in the elderly and indication for pacemaker placement (52) in the absence of contributing medications. Mortality in the oldest old (>80 years of age) is increased regardless of the presence of structural heart disease; in those aged between 65 and 79 years the picture is less clear, but syncope has been identified as an independent contributor to mortality (36).

Extrinsic causes of bradycardia include various medications (including donepezil, an anticholinesterase inhibitor used commonly to treat cognitive dysfunction) and metabolic disorders, including hyperkalemia, acidosis, hypothyroidism, and hypothermia. Generally, these factors must be corrected before determining whether permanent pacing is indicated, unless bradycardic medication is required for concurrent tachyarrhythmias (tachy–brady syndrome). In elderly patients, bradycardic medications, including β-blockers and rate-lowering calcium blockers, must be dosed cautiously and these two classes generally should not be used in combination. To avoid digoxin toxicity, current practice involves relatively low maintenance doses, which must be further adjusted according to the estimated glomerular filtration rate and drug interactions, notably with amiodarone. Reflex bradycardia is mediated by alterations in autonomic tone and is seen in neurally mediated syncope such as carotid sinus hypersensitivity (CSH) and the common "vasovagal faint."

In patients with reflex bradycardia, it is important to identify those with a significant vasodepressor component of a neurally mediated syndrome (see below), who may not derive much clinical benefit from standard pacemaker placement.

General indications for permanent pacing include (*i*) symptomatic bradycardia, (*ii*) advanced conduction disease with a high risk of progression to symptomatic bradycardia, and (*iii*) need for medical therapy that risks provoking symptomatic bradycardia (67). Elderly patients often resist pacer implantation because they did not think they wanted such aggressive care. These concerns can be addressed by explaining the relative ease of the procedure, recovery, and aftercare. Also, device replicas are available so patients can see how small and unobtrusive they are. Ambulatory patients who still request conservative treatment of serious bradycardias may finally consent after considering the facial trauma and other injuries that can result from unexpected nonfatal syncope. The do-not-resuscitate (DNR) status is not an absolute contraindication to pacing, but the surgeon and anesthesiologist may request temporary suspension of DNR, so that they may treat unlikely procedural complications like ventricular arrhythmias or cardiac perforation.

SHORT-TERM ECG MONITORING
Short-term continuous ECG monitoring, whether as inpatient telemetry or outpatient Holter monitoring, is often utilized in an attempt to diagnose syncope etiology. However, patients with arrhythmia-related syncope may go weeks, months, or even years between recurrent events reducing the yield of short-term ECG monitoring. Another central problem in attributing syncope to arrhythmias is that the vast majority of detected arrhythmias in patients with syncope are brief and result in no symptoms (69). Particularly in the case of bradycardia, abnormal rhythms on monitoring should be correlated with episodes of presyncope or syncope prior to initiating pacemaker therapy.

In one series of 649 syncope inpatients, telemetry monitoring was used in 100% of admissions. Abnormalities were found in only 7% of patients, with only 1% being diagnostic of syncope etiology (15). The duration of telemetry monitoring in hospital for an older individual with syncope has not been well studied, but data suggests that 24-hour monitoring may be insufficient (70) whereas durations longer than 48 hours are rarely necessary (71).

Outpatient Holter monitoring is similarly low-yield, with an incidence of symptom-correlated arrhythmias of approximately 4% in selected patients and less in unselected subjects (72). However, a study among individuals aged 80 and older yielded a higher diagnostic yield of 11.2% in a tertiary care center in Switzerland over a 10-year period where 475 Holter studies were performed. The diagnostic yield further increased in the presence of heart disease, low left ventricular EF, male gender, and in individuals aged 90 years or older (73). Nevertheless, the efficacy of short-term ECG monitoring in diagnosing or ruling out arrhythmic causes of syncope remains limited, although the presence of frequent ventricular ectopy or nonsustained VT can be used to identify patients at higher risk for malignant arrhythmias and guide further testing (74).

LONG-TERM ECG MONITORING
In patients with multiple episodes of syncope separated by relatively long time intervals, extended ECG monitoring is useful. Patient-activated intermittent loop recorders may capture the rhythm during syncope after the patient has regained consciousness, since several minutes of retrograde ECG recording can be obtained. External event monitors are superior to Holter monitoring in distinguishing between arrhythmias during syncope versus alternate diagnoses when symptoms occur in the absence of any documented arrhythmia (75,76). Compliance with external event monitors for longer than 1 month is problematic, however, as patients must wear fixed electrodes during the entire monitoring interval.

Moreover, as event monitors record only a five-minute interval of data, elderly patients or their caregivers must be able to activate recording shortly after an event.

The implantable loop recorder (ILR), which is placed in a subcutaneous pouch using local anesthesia (similar to a pacemaker) and has a battery life of 18 to 24 months, has increased the diagnostic yield of patients with unexplained syncope. In one series of 64 patients, syncope was correlated with ECG evidence of arrhythmia in 27% of them (77). An excellent diagnostic yield has been suggested even in patients with recurrent syncope of unknown etiology after extensive testing. A small study of patients with negative workup including ambulatory ECG, TTT, and EPS demonstrated that 46% had symptom-correlated arrhythmias captured by ILR during a 2-year follow-up period; most of these events were bradycardic in origin. Only 14% of patients had recurrence of symptoms during the first month, illustrating the limitation of external monitoring (78).

Among patients referred for investigation of unexplained syncope, older adults (e.g., >65 years old) were more likely to have an indication for ILR implantation than those younger than 65 years; ILR also had a higher diagnostic value, with an arrhythmia being more likely to be detected and successfully treated (79). Up-front costs of implantation are high, and the procedure carries a small risk of local complications. However, cost–benefit analyses suggest that the increased diagnostic yield from ILR in the long run may lead to decreased overall expenditure in syncope diagnosis (80). A randomized assessment of ILR versus a "conventional" diagnostic strategy, including EPS and TTT, in elderly patients with syncope showed significantly improved (52% vs. 20%) diagnostic accuracy in the ILR group. However, patients with left ventricular EF less than 35% and patients with clinical symptoms suggesting neurally mediated syncope were excluded from the study group, biasing the results in favor of ILR (81). While the optimal duration of monitoring with ILR is unknown, a 12-month monitoring period identified 90% of episodes, suggesting that this is a reasonable duration (82).

Advances in monitoring technology have led to the development of simple, sophisticated, hygienic, single use devices that employ easy-to-wear adhesive patches which can provide high fidelity recordings for up to 2 weeks. These devices are waterproof and can thus be used by frail older adults, eliminating the need for daily application of multiple leads that make traditional long term monitoring problematic for a large percentage of older adults. Studies using these novel technologies are ongoing.

ELECTROPHYSIOLOGICAL STUDY

The diagnostic yield of EPS in patients with unexplained syncope is much greater in those with preexisting heart disease (83) [i.e., those with a previous MI, EF <0.40, and/or an abnormal rest ECG (especially, bundle branch block)] (84). EPS is unlikely to demonstrate a potential cause of syncope in patients who have no structural heart disease, a left ventricular EF greater than 0.40, no ventricular ectopic activity during cardiac monitoring, and a normal ECG. Such a clinical profile in a patient with multiple syncopal episodes predicts with a high degree of certainty (>99%) that the EPS will be negative and the risk of sudden death low (70).

While EPS may be a high-yield diagnostic test in the elderly patient with structural heart disease and syncope, the decision to undergo EPS should be made on a case-by-case basis. Patients with poor functional capacity, severe cognitive impairment, or comorbidities likely to result in death within a relatively short period of time are probably not appropriate candidates. Likewise, patients who do not want definitive therapy such as permanent pacemaker or AICD implantation may have an unacceptable risk-benefit ratio with EPS as well. Furthermore, in patients who already have received an AICD for primary or secondary prevention, the device does not prevent progression of the underlying heart disease. As the end of life approaches, palliative options, including device inactivation, should be discussed to avoid repeated, ineffective shocks for terminal arrhythmias.

ORTHOSTATIC HYPOTENSION AND DYSAUTONOMIC DISORDERS OF BLOOD PRESSURE CONTROL

Orthostatic hypotension (OH) is an extremely common cause of syncope in the elderly. Following the assumption of a standing position, gravity induces pooling of blood in the lower extremities. Blood pressure is normally maintained in this setting of decreased circulatory volume by vasoconstriction and increased heart rate. Numerous age-related changes in cardiovascular structure and function, including impaired baroreflex function, diastolic dysfunction, a higher prevalence of disorders that directly or indirectly impair autonomic function, the common use of vasoactive medications, and impairment in salt and water balance, all contribute to an increase in the incidence and prevalence of OH in the elderly.

All elderly patients with syncope should have measurement of orthostatic vital signs. The most commonly accepted definition is a decline of ≥20 mmHg in systolic blood pressure or ≥10 mmHg in diastolic blood pressure on standing (85). In the vast majority of patients with OH, the drop in blood pressure is detected within 2 minutes of assuming upright posture (86). However, in certain patients, there is a delayed orthostatic intolerance and blood pressure progressively falls over 15 to 45 minutes. This response, which can be detected during TTT, is termed a dysautonomic response to upright posture.

OH is frequently not associated with symptoms (87). In one prospective study of 223 patients with syncope, OH was detected in 69 patients (31%), but was common in patients for whom other probable causes of syncope were assigned following evaluation (79). Syncope should not be attributed to orthostatic changes alone unless orthostatic symptoms are present or systolic blood pressure declines to less than 90 mmHg on postural change (88).

Decreased intravascular volume and adverse effects of drugs are the most common causes of symptomatic OH in the elderly (80). The status of the patient's hydration preceding the syncopal event should be assessed along with the daily intake of salt and alcohol. The medications most commonly contributing to orthostasis in the elderly are nitrates, diuretics, antihypertensives, anti-Parkinsonian drugs, antidepressants, and antipsychotics. Potent vasodilators must be titrated very cautiously in this population. Certain situational factors may predispose elderly patients to orthostasis, notably the redistribution of circulatory volume to the splanchnic circulation following a meal. An evaluation of 47 community-dwelling elders and three patients admitted for syncope evaluation indicated that symptomatic hypotension during TTT occurred earlier and increased in incidence from 12% to 22% in the postprandial state (89).

OH may also be an important manifestation of autonomic dysfunction resulting from a wide variety of diseases and drugs. The Shy–Drager syndrome is associated with autonomic failure and involvement of the corticospinal, extrapyramidal, and cerebellar tracts, including a Parkinson-like syndrome. Parkinson's disease itself can be associated with autonomic dysfunction. Lesions of the spinal cord caused by cervical trauma and other disorders, such as transverse myelitis, syringomyelia, and various tumors, may result in severe OH. OH may also be a manifestation of peripheral neuropathy that involves sympathetic fibers. This may be associated with such diseases as diabetes mellitus, amyloidosis, porphyria, chronic alcoholism, and pernicious anemia.

TREATMENT OF ORTHOSTATIC HYPOTENSION AND DYSAUTONOMIAS

Treatment for OH and dysautonomias includes mechanical interventions (e.g., compressive devices such as stockings or abdominal bands, counterpressure maneuvers like squatting or leg crossing); pharmacological interventions including both the withdrawal of potentially exacerbating medications (e.g., diuretics, vasodilators); and institution of pharmacological therapy [salt (NaCl) pills, mineralocorticoids, midodrine, and possibly pyridostigmine]. The management initially consists of education, advice, and training on various factors that influence blood pressure. Increased water and salt ingestion effectively improves orthostatic blood pressure. Subsequent treatment options discussed below include physiological interventions such as leg crossing, squatting, elastic abdominal binders, and stockings. Among the available pharmacological therapies, salt pills and the mineralocorticoid fludrocortisone are often employed initially; second-line therapy may include sympathomimetics such as midodrine. In older individuals, supine hypertension may coexist with OH and may be exacerbated by treatment of the latter condition. Some degree of supine hypertension may have to be tolerated to minimize the short-term risk of orthostasis and associated falls. Additionally, pyridostigmine may be a useful agent in such patients (90). Mineralocorticoids also may cause hypokalemia.

In elderly individuals with syncope, review of medications with special attention to agents that can cause or contribute to dehydration and vasodilation are essential first steps in the treatment algorithm for OH and dysautonomias. Indeed, following the adage that "less is more,"clinicians should first consider which pharmacological agents could be discontinued or reduced in dosage prior to adding pharmacological therapy. While salt and fludrocortisones have been initial therapy for patients with disordered blood pressure regulation, they have not been subjected to rigorous controlled clinical trials and carry the risk of exacerbating hypertension and other states common in older individuals associated with abnormal volume regulation, including renal insufficiency, cirrhosis, and heart failure.

Compressive devices for the lower limbs (e.g., compression stockings, bandage wrap, and others) are an effective nonpharmacological therapy especially for older individuals with OH (91). Randomized data have demonstrated that elastic compression stockings of the legs and abdomen are associated with the amelioration of declines in tilt induced blood pressure, with improvement in symptoms (90% asymptomatic in the active therapy versus 53% in the control arm), and with improvements in symptoms over the first month (92). Another study demonstrated similar efficacy using abdominal compression alone, which increases standing blood pressure to a varying degree by increasing stroke volume (93). Compression of all compartments is the most efficacious, followed by abdominal compression, whereas leg compression alone has been shown in a small study to be less effective (94), presumably reflecting the large venous capacity of the abdomen relative to the legs. We have found that older individuals have difficulty applying commonly available over-the-counter compressive stockings secondary to arthritic limitations and concomitant peripheral vascular disease and often express concern about the inability to regulate the degree of compression applied by such devices. Accordingly, the use of elastic bandages, which are available in a roll (e.g., ACE bandages) may facilitate application and provide the ability to self-regulate how tightly such devices are applied.

Squatting, bending forward, and leg crossing can improve orthostatic blood pressure in patients with OH, primarily by augmenting venous return, thereby increasing cardiac output. Studies suggest that targeting the splanchnic circulation has the greatest effect on orthostatic blood pressure changes (95), again presumably because of the larger capacitance of the splanchnic versus limb beds. Suitability and effectiveness of a specific counter maneuver depend on the orthopedic or neurological limitations of each older individual with syncope and probably should be individually evaluated for efficacy before recommending long-term adherence.

The α-adrenergic agonist, midodrine, was approved by the Food and Drug Administration for the treatment of OH but has recently been under intense scrutiny (96). In a multicenter, randomized, placebo-controlled study, 10-mg dose of midodrine or placebo three times per day for 6 weeks improved standing systolic blood pressure and symptoms, independent of the severity of OH, use of fludrocortisone, or compression garments. The main adverse effects were those of pilomotor reactions, urinary retention, and supine hypertension.

A prospective registry study of 135 consecutive elderly adults (mean age 84) examined the utility of midodrine for treatment of neurocardiogenic syncope at an initial dose of 2.5 mg orally three times daily and monitored over a median period of 2.7 years. Findings supported that midodrine was safe and well tolerated in patients with symptomatic OH, vasovagal syncope, and vasodepressor or mixed carotid sinus syndrome when standard therapies were attempted first (97). Cautious administration of midodrine to older individuals who are at risk of supine hypertension with dosing early in the morning and early afternoon, when orthostatic symptoms are at their worst, is advised. This schedule permits 2–3 hours of upright activity after each dose. Patients must be instructed to avoid lying down after drug treatment with midodrine and to rest in a seated, rather than supine, position if they grow tired during the day. Symptoms of OH tend to lessen during the evening, and it is recommended to avoid pressor agents at that time of day. Rarely, midodrine induced supine hypertension has been suggested to cause or contribute to severe cerebrovascular complications.

Acetylcholinesterase inhibition with pyridostigmine has emerged as a potentially novel treatment for patients with both OH and supine hypertension (98). There have been several small trials involving approximately 100 individuals. Trials in patients with neurogenic OH found statistically significant improvement in standing diastolic blood pressures (99–101). In one study, a single 60-mg dose of pyridostigmine bromide compared with placebo, with or without midodrine, did not affect supine blood pressure but did prevent the decline in diastolic blood pressure (101). However, long-term data has shown significant rates of discontinuation (90). At this time, further data are needed prior to supporting a definitive role for pyridostigmine in patients with OH and supine hypertension.

NEURALLY MEDIATED DISORDERS OF BLOOD PRESSURE CONTROL

This collection of disorders involves a neural reflex mediated by the nucleus tractus solitarius, an area in the brain stem that regulates blood pressure. The receptors for the afferent limb of the reflex are contained in several possible locations; examples include the left ventricle (vasovagal syncope), carotid sinus body (carotid sinus hypersensitivity [CSH]), pharynx, or trachea (cough syncope), and the bladder (postmicturition syncope). In susceptible individuals, stimulation of the reflex results in withdrawal of sympathetic vasomotor tone and vasodilatation with resultant syncope. When accompanied by bradycardia, the term "vasovagal" is used, while the term "vasodepressor" is employed for reflex reactions that are not accompanied by significant bradycardia.

Vasovagal Syncope

The "simple faint" has traditionally been considered a disease of the young patient. Early studies of elderly institutionalized and community-dwelling patients indicated that syncope was neurally mediated in only 1–5% of cases (2,19). Neurally mediated syncope in early studies was diagnosed with the classical features of a precipitating event followed by nausea, pallor, and sweating. The elderly more commonly have syncope without a prodrome, or with retrograde amnesia for the event, making diagnosis by history alone problematic. More recently, use of TTT has suggested that neurally mediated syncope is much more common in the elderly than previously believed, and likely constitutes a significant fraction of those previously carrying an "unknown" diagnosis.

Carotid Sinus Hypersensitivity

Carotid sinus hypersensitivity is an underappreciated cause of unexplained falls and syncope in the elderly, with a prevalence in elderly adults presenting to the ED with unexplained falls of 34% in one trial (102). However, a significant percentage (39%) of older adults without syncope meet criteria for CSH (103), indicating that the finding of a hypersensitive response should not necessarily preclude further investigation for other causes of syncope (104). Attacks may be precipitated by factors that exert pressure on the carotid sinus (tight collars, shaving, sudden head turning), a history of which is obtained in one-quarter of patients with this syndrome. Syncope from CSH occurs predominantly in men, 70% of whom are older than 50 years; the majority of patients have coronary artery disease or hypertension. Other predisposing factors include cervical pathology such as enlarged lymph nodes, scars resulting from neck surgery; carotid body tumors, and parotid, thyroid, or head and neck tumors.

CSH can produce bradycardia and/or vasodilatation, and is classified according to its predominant hemodynamic manifestation. Cardioinhibitory CSH is defined as sinus pauses greater than 3 seconds, while vasodepressor CSH is denoted as a fall in systolic blood pressure greater than 50 mmHg; if both mechanisms are noted, then the disorder is termed mixed-type CSH. The diagnosis is made with CSM, which some investigators consider positive only if symptoms are also reproduced during the examination (105).

CAROTID SINUS MASSAGE

Carotid sinus hypersensitivity is diagnosed by CSM if there is an asystole of 3 seconds or longer and/or a fall in systolic blood pressure of 50 mmHg or more (85). Many physicians have been hesitant to perform CSM because of the theoretical risk of stroke. However, after excluding patients with clinical history of stroke, or transient ischemic attack, and/or audible carotid artery bruits, the risk of neurological complications was 0.17–0.45% in two studies on the safety of the maneuver (106,107). Patients with history of VF or VT should be excluded, as ventricular dysrhythmias during CSM have been reported, albeit rarely, in this setting.

CSM should be performed on one side at a time by applying gentle digital pressure for five to 10 seconds at the bifurcation of the carotid artery, below the angle of the jaw at the level of the cricothyroid cartilage. The procedure was initially performed only in the supine position, but CSM in the upright position (usually performed during a TTT session) increases sensitivity (108). The distinction between cardioinhibitory and vasodepressor types is important, so the test should be performed with continuous beat-to-beat blood pressure monitoring in addition to continuous ECG if possible. Dual-chamber pacing has been shown to prevent falls in patients with cardioinhibitory CSH (109), but the benefits in mixed-type and vasodepressor forms of CSH are less clear.

TILT TABLE TESTING

During TTT, patients are secured to a motorized table with a footboard, and brought quickly to an upright position at an angle of 60° to 80° while undergoing ECG and beat-to-beat blood pressure monitoring. Various protocols have been evaluated for the provocation of neurally mediated syncope through TTT, either in the drug-free state or with various pharmacological agents (nitroglycerin, isoproterenol, and adenosine). In general, sensitivity of TTT increases with the use of pharmacological agents, longer duration of TTT, and a greater angle of head up tilt. However, with the addition of pharmacological agents, the specificity declines (110,111).

In patients with negative EPS, rates of hypotension on upright TTT (without pharmacological provocation) of 27–67% are reported as compared to approximately 10% in controls without syncope (112–115). A retrospective evaluation of TTT in 352 subjects with unexplained syncope (including 133 patients >65 years and 43 patients >80 years) showed an age-related decline in positive responses. However, a surprisingly high proportion of elderly patients with unexplained syncope had a positive TTT (37% of patients aged >65 years, and 23% of patients aged >80 years). Notably in this study and another (116), the hemodynamic response in those subjects with neurally medicated syncope differed by the age of the subjects. In younger patients, a cardioinhibitory response is more often demonstrated (e.g., vasovagal response), while in the elderly, a vasodepressor response is more common. These data demonstrate that a large proportion of elderly patients may have neurally mediated syncope that may be difficult to diagnose based on clinical grounds alone (117). Upright TTT can confirm the diagnosis in these patients and can help reassure patients that they have an excellent long-term survival.

TREATMENT OF NEURALLY MEDIATED SYNCOPE

Treatment of neurally mediated reflex syncope consists of the following: (*i*) reassurance regarding the benign nature of the problem, (*ii*) education about avoidance of predisposing factors and triggering events, (*iii*) recognition of preceding symptoms and maneuvers to abort the episode, and (*iv*) avoidance of volume depletion and prolonged upright posture. Salt supplements and water intake are often part of this initial approach. When these initial efforts are ineffective and a more aggressive treatment strategy is needed, pharmacological and pacing therapies can be employed (Table 25.7).

In older individuals, because of concerns for treatment related side effects, especially in frail older adults, and because of the lack of definitive controlled data in this population, physiological interventions (e.g., compressive devices such as stockings or abdominal bands, counterpressure maneuvers including squatting, leg crossing, and isometric hand grip) are preferred initial strategies, while pharmacological interventions (β-blockers, salt pills, fludrocortisone, midodrine) and electrical therapies should be reserved for more severe cases. Among the multitude of drugs that have been used for the treatment of neurally mediated syncope, uncontrolled or short-term controlled trials have shown satisfactory or favorable results that unfortunately have not been confirmed in the majority of long-term, placebo-controlled, prospective trials. These trials also have generally failed to randomize a representative population of older individuals (118).

Table 25.7 Syncope Treatment Options

Bradycardia
   Correct reversible causes
   Pacing
Tachycardia
   Correct reversible causes
   Anti-arrhythmic drugs
   ICD
Structural cardiac disease
   Medical therapy
   Coronary revascularization
   Aortic valve surgery and valvuloplasty
Orthostatic hypotension
   Compressive devices
   Salt and fluids
   Mineralocorticoids
   Midodrine
Neurogenic syncope
   Avoid precipitants
   Options for OH as above
   Consider pacing for reflex bradycardia

Abbreviations: ICD, implantable cardioverter defibrillator; OH, orthostatic hypotension.

β-blockers were traditionally used to treat neurally mediated syncope, in part because tilt table-induced faints generally are preceded by increased blood levels of cate-cholamines (119). Due to their negative inotropic effect, β-blockers, have been proposed to lessen the degree of ventricular mechanoreceptor activation associated with an abrupt decrease in venous return and to block the effects of elevated circulating adrenaline, but several studies raise questions about their routine use. A case control study of patients with neurally mediated syncope demonstrated that recurrent syncope was actually more frequent in those receiving β-blockers (120). Atenolol 50 mg/day has been shown to be ineffective in preventing syncopal recurrences in a double-blind, randomized clinical trial (121); there was a trend toward a better outcome in patients treated with placebo, and adverse events occurred more frequently in the active arm of this study. Additionally, the multicenter Prevention of Syncope Trial (POST), a randomized, placebo-controlled, double-blind trial designed to assess the effects of metoprolol in preventing vasovagal syncope over a 1-year period, demonstrated that metoprolol was not effective (122). Accordingly, we have stopped employing β-blockers as initial therapy for neurally mediated syncope.

While α-agonists have a clear and well-defined role in treating patients with OH and dysautonomias (see Treatment of OH above), their role in patients with neurally mediated syncope is less clear. Etilefrine, an α-agonist, was not effective in preventing syncopal recurrences in a large, multicenter, double-blind study [Vasovagal Syncope International Study (VASIS)] (123). Midodrine, another α-agonist, has been shown to be effective in reducing symptoms and improving quality of life in the short-term in patients with very frequent "hypotensive" symptoms (e.g., >1 syncope/mo) (124,125). However, the data supporting the use of midodrine in neurally mediated syncope are far less compelling than those presently available for OH.

The role of pacemakers in managing patients with neurally mediated syncope characterized by prolonged (e.g., >3 sec) sinus pauses is not clear. Four randomized clinical trials of pacing therapy have been conducted to date; three of these were positive (126–128), while the only one that was blinded was negative (129). When the 289 patients from all four studies are analyzed collectively, syncope recurred in 18% (25/140) of the paced patients and in 45% (67/149) of non-paced patients. The International Study on Syncope of Uncertain Etiology (ISSUE-3) (130) was a double-blind, randomized placebo-controlled study among patients ≥40 years of age who had experienced ≥3 syncopal episodes in the previous 2 years and were found to have on ILR a ≥3-second period of asystole or ≥6 sec asystole without syncope. Of the 511 subjects who had ILRs, 89 met these criteria, of which 77 of 89, mean age 63 years, had dual chamber pacemaker implantation with rate drop response or to sensing only. Syncope recurred in 27 patients, 19 of whom had been assigned to pacemaker OFF and eight to pacemaker ON. The 2-year estimated syncope recurrence rate was 57% (95% CI, 40–74) with pacemaker OFF and 25% (95% CI, 13–45) with pacemaker ON (log rank: $p = 0.039$). The risk of recurrence was reduced by 57% (95% CI, 4–81). However, five patients had procedural complication including lead dislodgment in 4 requiring correction and subclavian vein thrombosis in one patient. Thus, in this relatively young cohort dual-chamber permanent pacing was effective in reducing recurrence of syncope with severe asystolic neurally mediated syncope. However, despite the observed 32% absolute and 57% relative reduction in syncope recurrence, whether this invasive treatment is required for the relatively benign neurally mediated syncope is not clear (130). At present, pacing therapy appears effective in some, but certainly not in all patients with neurally mediated syncope. Pacing is only effective for neurally mediated syncope associated with asystole and has no role in treating the vasodilation that is frequently the dominant hemodynamic event in neurally mediated syncope. At present, cardiac pacing probably should be reserved after other therapies have failed and only as a last resort in a highly selected subgroup of patients affected by severe and recurrent neurally mediated syncope.

For patients with carotid sinus syndrome (CSH and symptoms), cardiac pacing may be beneficial, with its efficacy demonstrated by two randomized, controlled trials (102,131). However, neither of these trials was blinded, and thus the true treatment effect of pacing for patients with CSH remains unknown. Interestingly, in patients with abnormal asystolic responses induced by CSM, spontaneous asystolic episodes during long-term follow-up occurred in 74% of subjects, with asystolic episodes of greater than 3 seconds and greater than 6 seconds after 2 years of follow-up occurring in 82% and 53%, respectively (132). Accordingly, an asystolic response to carotid sinus stimulation may predict the occurrence of spontaneous asystolic episodes during follow-up and thus could be useful in identifying elderly subjects in whom pacing therapy would be ultimately beneficial.

SEIZURES AND ELECTROENCEPHALOGRAPHY

In patients with a clinical history compatible with a seizure or suggestive findings such as tongue biting, electroencephalography (EEG) may be beneficial in confirming the diagnosis. However, EEG should not be performed routinely in the evaluation of patients with syncope. In one study of the 99 patients referred for EEG because of syncope, near-syncope, or related complaints, 15 had abnormal findings, but in only one patient was the final diagnosis or treatment of the syncope affected by the EEG. In addition, almost all patients with abnormal EEG had clinical histories compatible with seizures or focal neurological findings on examination (133).

STROKES, TRANSIENT ISCHEMIC ATTACKS, AND SPECIFIC TESTING

Cerebrovascular atherosclerosis and impaired cerebrovascular autoregulation secondary to hypertension can contribute to cerebral hypoperfusion among the elderly. However, syncope is generally not a primary manifestation of cerebrovascular disease unless disease of the posterior circulation is present. When secondary to vertebrobasilar disease, syncope is almost always accompanied by other neurological symptoms traced to ischemia in the same territory, such as vertigo and ataxia (134,135). The common practice of cerebrovascular imaging via ultrasonography or other methods has not been extensively studied in this setting, but in the absence of suggestive history, probably contributes little to diagnosis (136).

Brain imaging in the evaluation of syncope yields helpful information only in the setting of a suggestive history or abnormal findings on neurological examination. A review of 195 patients estimated the diagnostic yield of head CT at 4%; in all of these patients, a witnessed seizure or focal neurological examination was present (18). In the setting of syncope and suspected head trauma, CT scanning may be indicated to exclude a subdural hematoma.

DRIVING AND SYNCOPE IN THE ELDERLY

The risk of a syncopal episode while driving has obvious consequences with respect to personal and public safety. The European Society of Cardiology (ESC), the American Heart Association, and the Heart Rhythm Society made recommendations related to patients with primary cardiac arrhythmias and neurocardiogenic conditions associated with syncope, in the setting of limited data. They placed the ultimate responsibility of determination of risk of recurrent syncopal events while driving on the judgment of the physician. Restrictions to driving differ between private drivers and commercial vehicle drivers. Driving was generally recommended to be resumed in private driver syncope patients post pacemaker implantation after 1 week, post AICD on a case-by-case basis, and after single mild reflex syncope there were no restrictions recommended (38). Complete driving restrictions were recommended for patients with severe untreated arrhythmias and severe untreated neurocardiogenic syncope (137).

In a case-control study of consecutive patients at the Mayo Clinic (including outpatient clinics and the ED) evaluated for syncope, cases were reviewed for causes, characteristics and recurrent cases of syncope (138). Among 3877 patients identified, 9.8% had syncope while driving. Although the mean age at presentation was 56 years, both in the general syncope group as well as the syncope with driving group, age had a bimodal distribution, with a peak at age of 65 to 75 years. This corresponds to an age range in which a high frequency of automobile accidents is observed. Other characteristics more common in the subset with syncope while driving included male sex and), a history of cardiovascular disease and stroke. The most common causes of syncope while driving included neurally mediated syncope (37.3%) and cardiac arrhythmias (11.8%). Notably, 13.8% of syncope recurrences recurred while driving. Prodromal symptoms of nausea, palpitations, chest pain, dyspnea, and ear ringing were also more common in the syncope while driving subset ($p \leq 0.05$). While survival was comparable to age and sex matched controls, syncope recurred in 18.8% of patients with syncope while driving and among those who had recurrences, 48% of recurrences occurred greater than 6 months after the initial evaluation, challenging the current recommendation that driving can be resumed if syncope does not recur in 3–6 months (139). For older adults with syncope, the decision whether to drive must take into account the aforementioned factors that suggest a high risk for recurrence, presence or lack of prodromal symptoms, and other extra-cardiac factors such as cognitive dysfunction, especially executive function, which has a high correlation with the ability to perform multiple complex tasks that are required to safely operative a motor vehicle.

COST-EFFECTIVENESS OF SYNCOPE ASSESSMENT AND MANAGEMENT

It is estimated that the health care cost burden of syncope is estimated at greater than $2.4 billion per year (32). Part of this cost is driven by the inappropriate use of healthcare resources. The proposal of a syncope unit in the 2004 ESC guidelines was borne from the lack of a standardized assessment of syncope as well as to reduce the overall healthcare costs associated with the high rate of hospitalization among syncope patients (139). The issue of health care cost becomes particularly relevant among the elderly, who are highly likely to be admitted to the hospital and undergo unnecessary testing when presenting with syncope. While rate of recurrent syncope and all-cause mortality were not affected, Shen et al. (18) demonstrated in a randomized clinical trial that a syncope unit in the ED improved diagnostic yield, reduced hospital admissions, and reduced total length of stay compared to standard care for syncope. In a prospective study by Mitro et al. of 501 patients (mean age 65 years) evaluated in a syncope unit, standardized diagnostic workup based on the European Society of Cardiology guidelines yielded a diagnosis in 89% of all patients (140), much higher than is traditionally reported (71).

An evaluation of cost per test yield among 2106 consecutive patients found the cost per test affecting diagnosis were highest for electroencephalography ($32, 973), CT scans ($24, 881) and cardiac enzymes ($22, 397) and the lowest for postural blood pressure recordings ($17–20), highlighting that many unnecessary tests are obtained to evaluate syncope and less expensive, higher yield tests should be more heavily utilized by clinicians. Additionally, these data demonstrated the diagnostic yields and costs for cardiac tests were improved when patients met the San Francisco Syncope Rule (7).

Data suggest that the use of decision making software based on ESC guidelines may significantly reduce unnecessary admissions while not increasing the prevalence of serious cardiovascular events among discharged patients (141). Reductions in cost were also observed related to less frequent use of unnecessary head CT scanning and magnetic resonance brain imaging with increased use of provocative measures including orthostatic blood pressure measurements, TTT and CSM (26).

SUGGESTED DIAGNOSTIC ALGORITHM

Determining the underlying cause and risk stratification for subjects with syncope relies on the performance of a complete history, physical examination (especially orthostatic blood pressure measurements), and ECG. Approximately one-third of patients have a clear diagnosis evident at presentation. Another third of patients have a most likely etiology after initial evaluation, and directed testing can be performed in this group to confirm the suspected diagnoses. Since primary neurological causes of syncope are unlikely, specific neurological tests are rarely useful in the absence of a suggestive history and physical examination. A suggested strategy for the diagnosis of syncope in the elderly patient is detailed below and in Figure 25.2 (139). However, strict adherence to a guideline is contrary to the basic principles of geriatric medicine and geriatric cardiology, in which heterogeneity and complexity prevail. Accordingly, every practitioner must place this strategy in the context of the individual patient and modify it according to individual nuances and personal preferences.

In the remaining patients with unexplained syncope, cardiac testing, specifically to evaluate for malignant tachyarrhythmias, should be performed in patients with structural heart disease. For patients with recurrent unexplained syncope without structural heart or cardiac conduction system disease (or patients with structural heart disease and negative cardiac testing), TTT to evaluate for OH and neurally mediated causes is appropriate. This test should be performed prior to long-term ECG monitoring to identify the significant percentage of subjects with neurally mediated syncope and resultant bradycardia who do not require pacing. If the etiology of syncope is still undetermined following directed cardiac and autonomic testing, long-term ECG monitoring should be employed. The ILR has

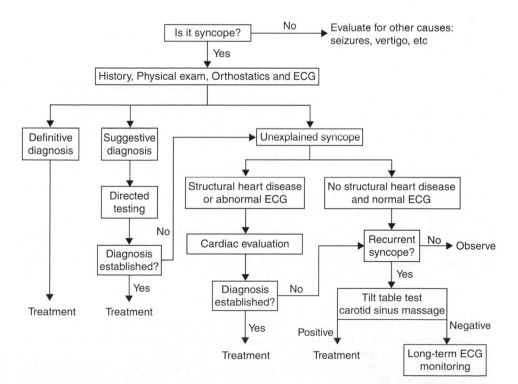

Figure 25.2   Suggested diagnostic algorithm for elderly patients with syncope. *Source*: From Ref. 139.

the potential to obtain a diagnosis in these patients even if external monitoring is negative, particularly if episodes are separated by long time intervals.

CONCLUSIONS

Syncope is common in the elderly and is associated with significant morbidity and mortality. It is a symptom or syndrome, not a disease, and has a complex differential diagnosis ranging from benign to malignant causes; elderly patients commonly have multiple possible contributing factors. The assignment of the underlying etiology can be greatly facilitated through an understanding of syncope epidemiology and the utility of relevant diagnostic tests. Identifying patients with underlying structural heart disease is important for risk stratification. In the elderly, multiple origins of syncope frequently coexist and need to be addressed. Particular emphasis should be given to the impact of polypharmacy, OH, postprandial hypotension, and CSH (38). For patients with unexplained syncope, provocative tests (EPS, TTT, and CSM) are more likely to yield a definitive diagnosis than observational testing strategies. Table 25.7 summarizes the treatment options for different causes of syncope.

ACKNOWLEDGMENTS

Dr. Maurer was supported by the National Institute on Aging, Bethesda, Maryland (K24 AG036778-03). Carol Raymond, MLIS Contra Costa Health Services Degnan Medical Library was instrumental in performing literature searches and obtaining articles for this chapter. Dr. Denis J. Mahar, Medical Director, Cardiology Department Contra Costa Health Services provided valuable support for the drafting of the manuscript. Dr. Oliver Z. Graham, Department of Internal Medicine Contra Costa Health Services provided valuable support and insight into refining the content of this chapter.

REFERENCES

1. Ungar A, Morrione A, Rafanelli M, et al. The management of syncope in older adults. Minerva Med 2009; 100: 247–58.
2. Lipsitz LA, Wei JY, Rowe JW. Syncope in an elderly, institutionalised population: prevalence, incidence, and associated risk. Q J Med 1985; 55: 45–54.
3. Chen LY, Shen WK, Mahoney DW, et al. Prevalence of syncope in a population aged more than 45 years. Am J Med 2006; 119: 1088; e1–7.
4. Soteriades ES, Evans JC, Larson MG, et al. Incidence and prognosis of syncope. N Engl J Med 2002; 347: 878–85.
5. Day SC, Cook EF, Funkenstein H, et al. Evaluation and outcome of emergency room patients with transient loss of consciousness. Am J Med 1982; 73: 15–23.
6. Forman DE, Rich MW, Alexander KP, et al. Cardiac care for older adults. Time for a new paradigm. J Am Coll Cardiol 2011; 57: 1801–10.
7. Mendu ML, McAvay G, Lampert R, et al. Yield of diagnostic tests in evaluating syncopal episodes in older patients. Arch Intern Med 2009; 169: 1299–305.
8. Kapoor W, Snustad D, Peterson J, et al. Syncope in the elderly. Am J Med 1986; 80: 419–28.
9. Tinetti ME, Williams CS, Gill TM. Dizziness among older adults: a possible geriatric syndrome. Ann Intern Med 2000; 132: 337–44.
10. Kane RL, Ouslander JG, Abrass IB. Essentials of Clinical Geriatrics, 4th edn. Vol. xxvi New York: McGraw-Hill, Health Professions Division, 1999: 621.
11. Murphy SL, Williams CS, Gill TM. Characteristics associated with fear of falling and activity restriction in community-living older persons. J Am Geriatr Soc 2002; 50: 516–20.
12. Rose MS, Koshman ML, Spreng S, et al. The relationship between health-related quality of life and frequency of spells in patients with syncope. J Clin Epidemiol 2000; 53: 1209–16.
13. Linzer M, Pontinen M, Gold DT, et al. Impairment of physical and psychosocial function in recurrent syncope. J Clin Epidemiol 1991; 44: 1037–43.
14. Getchell WS, Larsen GC, Morris CD, et al. Epidemiology of syncope in hospitalized patients. J Gen Intern Med 1999; 14: 677–87.
15. Pires LA, Ganji JR, Jarandila R, et al. Diagnostic patterns and temporal trends in the evaluation of adult patients hospitalized with syncope. Arch Intern Med 2001; 161: 1889–95.

16. Sarasin FP, Louis-Simonet M, Carballo D, et al. Prospective evaluation of patients with syncope: a population-based study. Am J Med 2001; 111: 177–84.

17. Ammirati F, Colivicchi F, Santini M. Diagnosing syncope in clinical practice. Implementation of a simplified diagnostic algorithm in a multicentre prospective trial - the OESIL 2 study (Osservatorio Epidemiologico della Sincope nel Lazio). Eur Heart J 2000; 21: 935–40.

18. Shen WK, Decker WW, Smars PA, et al. Syncope Evaluation in the Emergency Department Study (SEEDS): a multidisciplinary approach to syncope management. Circulation 2004; 110: 3636–45.

19. Purser JL, Kuchibhatla MN, Fillenbaum GG, et al. Identifying frailty in hospitalized older adults with significant coronary artery disease. J Am Geriatr Soc 2006; 54: 1674–81.

20. McIntosh S, Da Costa D, Kenny RA. Outcome of an integrated approach to the investigation of dizziness, falls and syncope in elderly patients referred to a 'syncope' clinic. Age Ageing 1993; 22: 53–8.

21. Chen LY, Gersh BJ, Hodge DO, et al. Prevalence and clinical outcomes of patients with multiple potential causes of syncope. Mayo Clin Proc 2003; 78: 414–20.

22. Brignole M, Menozzi C, Bartoletti A, et al. A new management of syncope: prospective systematic guideline-based evaluation of patients referred urgently to general hospitals. Eur Heart J 2006; 27: 76–82.

23. Kapoor WN, Karpf M, Wieand S, et al. A prospective evaluation and follow-up of patients with syncope. N Engl J Med 1983; 309: 197–204.

24. Savage DD, Corwin L, McGee DL, et al. Epidemiologic features of isolated syncope: the Framingham Study. Stroke 1985; 626–9.

25. Kapoor WN, Hanusa BH. Is syncope a risk factor for poor outcomes? Comparison of patients with and without syncope. Am J Med 1996; 100: 646–55.

26. Brignole M, Hamdan MH. New concepts in the assessment of syncope. J Am Coll Cardiol 2012; 59: 1583–91.

27. Task Force for the Diagnosis and Management of Syncope; European Society of Cardiology (ESC); European Heart Rhythm Association (EHRA); Heart Failure Association (HFA); Heart Rhythm Society (HRS). Moya A, Sutton R, Ammirati F, et al. Guidelines for the diagnosis and management of syncope (version 2009). Eur Heart J 2009; 30: 2631–71.

28. McCarthy F, McMahon CG, Geary U, et al. Management of syncope in the Emergency Department: a single hospital observational case series based on the application of European Society of Cardiology Guidelines. Europace 2009; 11: 216–24.

29. Costantino G, Perego F, Dipaola F, et al. Short- and long-term prognosis of syncope, risk factors, and role of hospital admission: results from the STePS (Short-Term Prognosis of Syncope) study. J Am Coll Cardiol 2008; 51: 276–83.

30. Sun BC, Derose SF, Liang LJ, et al. Predictors of 30-day serious events in older patients with syncope. Ann Emerg Med 2009; 54: 769–78; e1–5.

31. Gabayan GZ, Derose SF, Asch SM, et al. Predictors of short-term (seven-day) cardiac outcomes after emergency department visit for syncope. Am J Cardiol 2010; 105: 82–6.

32. Thiruganasambandamoorthy V, Hess EP, Alreesi A, et al. External validation of the San Francisco Syncope Rule in the Canadian setting. Ann Emerg Med 2010; 55: 464–72.

33. Reed MJ, Newby DE, Coull AJ, et al. The ROSE (risk stratification of syncope in the emergency department) study. J Am Coll Cardiol 2010; 55: 713–21.

34. Grossman SA, Fischer C, Lipsitz LA, et al. Predicting adverse outcomes in syncope. J Emerg Med 2007; 33: 233–9.

35. Grossman SA, Bar J, Fischer C, et al. Reducing admissions utilizing the Boston Syncope Criteria. J Emerg Med 2012; 42: 345–52.

36. Saccilotto RT, Nickel CH, Bucher HC, et al. San Francisco Syncope Rule to predict short-term serious outcomes: a systematic review. CMAJ 2011; 183: E1116–26.

37. Sutton R, Brignole M, Benditt D, et al. The diagnosis and management of syncope. Curr Hypertens Rep 2010; 12: 316–22.

38. Strickberger SA, Benson DW, Biaggioni I, et al. AHA/ACCF Scientific Statement on the evaluation of syncope: from the American Heart Association Councils on Clinical Cardiology, Cardiovascular Nursing, Cardiovascular Disease in the Young, and Stroke, and the Quality of Care and Outcomes Research Interdisciplinary Working Group; and the American College of Cardiology Foundation: in collaboration with the Heart Rhythm Society: endorsed by the American Autonomic Society. Circulation 2006; 113: 316–27.

39. Linzer M, Yang EH, Estes NA III, et al. Diagnosing syncope. Part 1: value of history, physical examination, and electrocardiography. Clinical Efficacy Assessment Project of the American College of Physicians. Ann Intern Med 1997; 126: 989–96.

40. Passman R, Horvath G, Thomas J, et al. Clinical spectrum and prevalence of neurologic events provoked by tilt table testing. Arch Intern Med 2003; 163: 1945–8.

41. Hoefnagels WA, Padberg GW, Overweg J, et al. Transient loss of consciousness: the value of the history for distinguishing seizure from syncope. J Neurol 1991; 238: 39–43.

42. Benbadis SR, Wolgamuth BR, Goren H, et al. Value of tongue biting in the diagnosis of seizures. Arch Intern Med 1995; 155: 2346–9.

43. Sheldon R, Rose S, Ritchie D, et al. Historical criteria that distinguish syncope from seizures. J Am Coll Cardiol 2002; 40: 142–8.

44. Cummings SR, Nevitt MC, Kidd S. Forgetting falls. The limited accuracy of recall of falls in the elderly. J Am Geriatr Soc 1988; 36: 613–16.

45. McIntosh SJ, Lawson J, Kenny RA. Clinical characteristics of vasodepressor, cardioinhibitory, and mixed carotid sinus syndrome in the elderly. Am J Med 1993; 95: 203–8.

46. Shaw FE, Kenny RA. The overlap between syncope and falls in the elderly. Postgrad Med J 1997; 73: 635–9.

47. Galizia G, Abete P, Mussi C, et al. Role of early symptoms in assessment of syncope in elderly people: results from the Italian group for the study of syncope in the elderly. J Am Geriatr Soc 2009; 57: 18–23.

48. Calkins H, Shyr Y, Frumin H, et al. The value of the clinical history in the differentiation of syncope due to ventricular tachycardia, atrioventricular block, and neurocardiogenic syncope. Am J Med 1995; 98: 365–73.

49. Alboni P, Brignole M, Menozzi C, et al. Diagnostic value of history in patients with syncope with or without heart disease. J Am Coll Cardiol 2001; 37: 1921–8.

50. Del Rosso A, Alboni P, Brignole M, et al. Relation of clinical presentation of syncope to the age of patients. Am J Cardiol 2005; 96: 1431–5.

51. Martin TP, Hanusa BH, Kapoor WN. Risk stratification of patients with syncope. Ann Emerg Med 1997; 29: 459–66.

52. Quinn JV, Stiell IG, McDermott DA, et al. Derivation of the San Francisco Syncope Rule to predict patients with short-term serious outcomes. Ann Emerg Med 2004; 43: 224–32.

53. Quinn JV, McDermott D. Medical decisionmaking and the San Francisco Syncope Rule. Ann Emerg Med 2006; 48: 762–3; author reply 763.

54. Quinn J, McDermott D, Stiell I, et al. Prospective validation of the San Francisco Syncope Rule to predict patients with serious outcomes. Ann Emerg Med 2006; 47: 448–54.

55. Quinn JV, Stiell IG, McDermott DA, et al. The San Francisco Syncope Rule vs physician judgment and decision making. Am J Emerg Med 2005; 23: 782–6.

56. Gatzoulis K, Sideris S, Theopistou A, et al. Long-term outcome of patients with recurrent syncope of unknown cause in the absence of organic heart disease and relation to results of baseline tilt table testing. Am J Cardiol 2003; 92: 876–9.

57. Sarasin FP, Junod AF, Carballo D, et al. Role of echocardiography in the evaluation of syncope: a prospective study. Heart 2002; 88: 363–7.

58. Garcia-Civera R, Ruiz-Granell R, Morell-Cabedo S, et al. Selective use of diagnostic tests inpatients with syncope of unknown cause. J Am Coll Cardiol 2003; 41: 787–90.

59. Lindroos M, Kupari M, Heikkilä J, et al. Prevalence of aortic valve abnormalities in the elderly: an echocardiographic study of a random population sample. J Am Coll Cardiol 1993; 21: 1220–5.

60. Grech ED, Ramsdale DR. Exertional syncope in aortic stenosis: evidence to support inappropriate left ventricular baroreceptor response. Am Heart J 1991; 121: 603–6.

61. Wilmshurst PT, Willicombe PR, Webb-Peploe MM. Effect of aortic valve replacement on syncope in patients with aortic stenosis. Br Heart J 1993; 70: 542–3.

62. Braunwald E, Zipes D, Libby P. Heart Disease: A Textbook of Cardiovascular Medicine, 6th edn. Vol. xx Philadelphia: Saunders, 2001: 2297.

63. Bayer AJ, Chadha JS, Farag RR, et al. Changing presentation of myocardial infarction with increasing old age. J Am Geriatr Soc 1986; 34: 263–6.

64. Link MS, Lauer EP, Homoud MK, et al. Low yield of rule-out myocardial infarction protocol in patients presenting with syncope. Am J Cardiol 2001; 88: 706–7.

65. Grossman SA, Van Epp S, Arnold R, et al. The value of cardiac enzymes in elderly patients presenting to the emergency department with syncope. J Gerontol A Biol Sci Med Sci 2003; 58: 1055–8.

66. Phang RS, Kang D, Tighiouart H, et al. High risk of ventricular arrhythmias in patients with nonischemic dilated cardiomyopathy presenting with syncope. Am J Cardiol 2006; 97: 416–20.

67. Gregoratos G, Abrams J, Epstein AE, et al. ACC/AHA/NASPE 2002 guideline update for implantation of cardiac pacemakers and antiarrhythmia devices: summary article. A report of the American College of Cardiology/American Heart Association Task Force on Practice Guidelines (ACC/AHA/NASPE Committee to Update the 1998 Pacemaker Guidelines). J Cardiovasc Electrophysiol 2002; 13: 1183–99.

68. Tung RT, Shen WK, Hayes DL, et al. Long-term survival after permanent pacemaker implantation for sick sinus syndrome. Am J Cardiol 1994; 74: 1016–20.
69. DiMarco J, Philbrick JT. Use of ambulatory electrocardiographic (Holter) monitoring. Ann Intern Med 1990; 113: 53–68.
70. Bass EB, Curtiss EI, Arena VC, et al. The duration of Holter monitoring in patients with syncope. Is 24 hours enough? Arch Intern Med 1990; 150: 1073–8.
71. Kapoor WN. Evaluation and management of the patient with syncope. JAMA 1992; 268: 2553–60.
72. Gibson TC, Heitzman MR. Diagnostic efficacy of 24-hour electrocardiographic monitoring for syncope. Am J Cardiol 1984; 53: 1013–17.
73. Kühne M, Schaer B, Sticherling C, et al. Holter monitoring in syncope: diagnostic yield in octogenarians. J Am Geriatr Soc 2011; 59: 1293–8.
74. Kapoor WN, Cha R, Peterson JR, et al. Prolonged electrocardiographic monitoring in patients with syncope. Importance of frequent or repetitive ventricular ectopy. Am J Med 1987; 82: 20–8.
75. Kus T, Nadeau R, Costi P, et al. Comparison of the diagnostic yield of Holter versus transtelephonic monitoring. Can J Cardiol 1995; 11: 891–4.
76. Cumbee SR, Pryor RE, Linzer M. Cardiac loop ECG recording: a new noninvasive diagnostic test in recurrent syncope. South Med J 1990; 83: 39–43.
77. Krahn AD, Klein GJ, Yee R, et al. Use of an extended monitoring strategy in patients with problematic syncope. Reveal Investigators. Circulation 1999; 99: 406–10.
78. Krahn AD, Klein GJ, Yee R, et al. Final results from a pilot study with an implantable loop recorder to determine the etiology of syncope in patients with negative noninvasive and invasive testing. Am J Cardiol 1998; 82: 117–19.
79. Brignole M, Menozzi C, Maggi R, et al. The usage and diagnostic yield of the implantable loop-recorder in detection of the mechanism of syncope and in guiding effective antiarrhythmic therapy in older people. Europace 2005; 7: 273–9.
80. Krahn AD, Klein GJ, Yee R, et al. The high cost of syncope: cost implications of a new insertable loop recorder in the investigation of recurrent syncope. Am Heart J 1999; 137: 870–7.
81. Krahn AD, Klein GJ, Yee R, et al. Randomized assessment of syncope trial: conventional diagnostic testing versus a prolonged monitoring strategy. Circulation 2001; 104: 46–51.
82. Assar MD, Krahn AD, Klein GJ, et al. Optimal duration of monitoring in patients with unexplained syncope. Am J Cardiol 2003; 92: 1231–3.
83. Doherty JU, Pembrook-Rogers D, Grogan EW, et al. Electrophysiologic evaluation and follow-up characteristics of patients with recurrent unexplained syncope and presyncope. Am J Cardiol 1985; 55: 703–8.
84. Krol RB, Morady F, Flaker GC, et al. Electrophysiologic testing in patients with unexplained syncope: clinical and noninvasive predictors of outcome. J Am Coll Cardiol 1987; 10: 358–63.
85. Cooke J, Carew S, Costelloe A, et al. The changing face of orthostatic and neurocardiogenic syncope with age. QJM 2011; 104: 689–95.
86. Atkins D, Hanusa B, Sefcik T, et al. Syncope and orthostatic hypotension. Am J Med 1991; 91: 179–85.
87. Lipsitz LA. Orthostatic hypotension in the elderly. N Engl J Med 1989; 321: 952–7.
88. Thomas JE, Schirger A, Fealey RD, et al. Orthostatic hypotension. Mayo Clin Proc 1981; 56: 117–25.
89. Maurer MS, Karmally W, Rivadeneira H, et al. Upright posture and postprandial hypotension in elderly persons. Ann Intern Med 2000; 133: 533–6.
90. Sandroni P, Opfer-Gehrking TL, Singer W, Low PA. Pyridostigmine for treatment of neurogenic orthostatic hypotension [correction of hypertension]–a follow-up survey study. Clin Auton Res 2005; 15: 51–3.
91. Henry R, Rowe J, O'Mahony D. Haemodynamic analysis of efficacy of compression hosiery in elderly fallers with orthostatic hypotension. Lancet 1999; 354: 45–6.
92. Podoleanu C, Maggi R, Brignole M, et al. Lower limb and abdominal compression bandages prevent progressive orthostatic hypotension in elderly persons: a randomized single-blind controlled study. J Am Coll Cardiol 2006; 48: 1425–32.
93. Smit AA, Wieling W, Fujimura J, et al. Use of lower abdominal compression to combat orthostatic hypotension in patients with autonomic dysfunction. Clin Auton Res 2004; 14: 167–75.
94. Denq JC, Opfer-Gehrking TL, Giuliani M, et al. Efficacy of compression of different capacitance beds in the amelioration of orthostatic hypotension. Clin Auton Res 1997; 7: 321–6.
95. Tutaj M, Marthol H, Berlin D, et al. Effect of physical countermaneuvers on orthostatic hypotension in familial dysautonomia. J Neurol 2006; 253: 65–72.
96. Dhruva SS, Redberg RF. Accelerated approval and possible withdrawal of midodrine. JAMA 2010; 304: 2172–3.

97. Paling D, Vilches-Moraga A, Akram Q, et al. Midodrine hydrochloride is safe and effective in older people with neurocardiogenic syncope. J Am Geriatr Soc 2010; 58: 2026–7.

98. Gales BJ, Gales MA. Pyridostigmine in the treatment of orthostatic intolerance. Ann Pharmacother 2007; 41: 314–18.

99. Singer W, Opfer-Gehrking T, McPhee B, et al. Acetylcholinesterase inhibition: a novel approach in the treatment of neurogenic orthostatic hypotension. J Neurol Neurosurg Psychiatry 2003; 74: 1294–8.

100. Singer W, Opfer-Gehrking TL, Nickander KK, et al. Acetylcholinesterase inhibition in patients with orthostatic intolerance. J Clin Neurophysiol 2006; 23: 476–81.

101. Singer W, Sandroni P, Opfer-Gehrking TL, et al. Pyridostigmine treatment trial in neurogenic orthostatic hypotension. Arch Neurol 2006; 63: 513–18.

102. Kenny RA, Richardson DA, Steen N, et al. Carotid sinus syndrome: a modifiable risk factor for non-accidental falls in older adults (SAFE PACE). J Am Coll Cardiol 2001; 38: 1491–6.

103. Kerr SR, Pearce MS, Brayne C, et al. Carotid sinus hypersensitivity in asymptomatic older persons: implications for diagnosis of syncope and falls. Arch Intern Med 2006; 166: 515–20.

104. Coplan NL. Carotid sinus hypersensitivity and syncope: cause/effect or true/true/unrelated. Arch Intern Med 2006; 166: 491–2.

105. Puggioni E, Guiducci V, Brignole M, et al. Results and complications of the carotid sinus massage performed according to the "method of symptoms". Am J Cardiol 2002; 89: 599–601.

106. The Antiarrhythmics versus Implantable Defibrillators (AVID) Investigators. A comparison of antiarrhythmic-drug therapy with implantable defibrillators in patients resuscitated from near-fatal ventricular arrhythmias. N Engl J Med 1997; 337: 1576–83.

107. Munro NC, McIntosh S, Lawson J, et al. Incidence of complications after carotid sinus massage in older patients with syncope. J Am Geriatr Soc 1994; 42: 1248–51.

108. Morillo CA, Camacho ME, Wood MA, et al. Diagnostic utility of mechanical, pharmacological and orthostatic stimulation of the carotid sinus in patients with unexplained syncope. J Am Coll Cardiol 1999; 34: 1587–94.

109. Sheldon R, Connolly S, Krahn A, et al. Identification of patients most likely to benefit from implantable cardioverter-defibrillator therapy: the Canadian Implantable Defibrillator Study. Circulation 2000; 101: 1660–4.

110. Mussi C, Tolve I, Foroni M, et al. Specificity and total positive rate of head-up tilt testing potentiated with sublingual nitroglycerin in older patients with unexplained syncope. Aging (Milano) 2001; 13: 105–11.

111. Kumar NP, Youde JH, Ruse C, et al. Responses to the prolonged head-up tilt followed by sublingual nitrate provocation in asymptomatic older adults. Age Ageing 2000; 29: 419–24.

112. Calkins H, Kadish A, Sousa J, et al. Comparison of responses to isoproterenol and epinephrine during head-up tilt in suspected vasodepressor syncope. Am J Cardiol 1991; 67: 207–9.

113. Grubb BP, Temesy-Armos P, Hahn H, et al. Utility of upright tilt-table testing in the evaluation and management of syncope of unknown origin. Am J Med 1991; 90: 6–10.

114. Strasberg B, Rechavia E, Sagie A, et al. The head-up tilt table test in patients with syncope of unknown origin. Am Heart J 1989; 118: 923–7.

115. Raviele A, Gasparini G, Di Pede F, et al. Usefulness of head-up tilt test in evaluating patients with syncope of unknown origin and negative electrophysiologic study. Am J Cardiol 1990; 65: 1322–7.

116. Kurbaan AS, Bowker TJ, Wijesekera N, et al. Age and hemodynamic responses to tilt testing in those with syncope of unknown origin. J Am Coll Cardiol 2003; 41: 1004–7.

117. Bloomfield D, Maurer M, Bigger JT Jr. Effects of age on outcome of tilt-table testing. Am J Cardiol 1999; 83: 1055–8.

118. Brignole M. Randomized clinical trials of neurally mediated syncope. J Cardiovasc Electrophysiol 2003; 14: S64–9.

119. Almquist A, Goldenberg IF, Milstein S, et al. Provocation of bradycardia and hypotension by isoproterenol and upright posture in patients with unexplained syncope. N Engl J Med 1989; 320: 346–51.

120. Alegria JR, Gersh BJ, Scott CG, et al. Comparison of frequency of recurrent syncope after beta-blocker therapy versus conservative management for patients with vasovagal syncope. Am J Cardiol 2003; 92: 82–4.

121. Madrid AH, Ortega J, Rebollo JG, et al. Lack of efficacy of atenolol for the prevention of neurally mediated syncope in a highly symptomatic population: a prospective, double-blind, randomized and placebo-controlled study. J Am Coll Cardiol 2001; 37: 554–9.

122. Sheldon R, Connolly S, Rose S, et al. Prevention of Syncope Trial (POST): a randomized, placebo-controlled study of metoprolol in the prevention of vasovagal syncope. Circulation 2006; 113: 1164–70.

123. Raviele A, Brignole M, Sutton R, et al. Effect of etilefrine in preventing syncopal recurrence in patients with vasovagal syncope: a double-blind, randomized, placebo-controlled trial. The Vasovagal Syncope International Study. Circulation 1999; 99: 1452–7.

124. Ward CR, Gray JC, Gilroy JJ, et al. Midodrine: a role in the management of neurocardiogenic syncope. Heart 1998; 79: 45–9.

125. Perez-Lugones A, Schweikert R, Pavia S, et al. Usefulness of midodrine in patients with severely symptomatic neurocardiogenic syncope: a randomized control study. J Cardiovasc Electrophysiol 2001; 12: 935–8.

126. Connolly SJ, Sheldon R, Roberts RS, Gent M. The North American Vasovagal Pacemaker Study (VPS). A randomized trial of permanent cardiac pacing for the prevention of vasovagal syncope. J Am Coll Cardiol 1999; 33: 16–20.

127. Sutton R, Brignole M, Menozzi C, et al. Dual-chamber pacing in the treatment of neurally mediated tilt-positive cardioinhibitory syncope : pacemaker versus no therapy: a multicenter randomized study. The Vasovagal Syncope International Study (VASIS) Investigators. Circulation 2000; 102: 294–9.

128. Ammirati F, Colivicchi F, Santini M; Syncope Diagnosis and Treatment Study Investigators. Permanent cardiac pacing versus medical treatment for the prevention of recurrent vasovagal syncope: a multicenter, randomized, controlled trial. Circulation 2001; 104: 52–7.

129. Connolly SJ, Sheldon R, Thorpe KE, et al. Pacemaker therapy for prevention of syncope in patients with recurrent severe vasovagal syncope: Second Vasovagal Pacemaker Study (VPS II): a randomized trial. JAMA 2003; 289: 2224–9.

130. Brignole M, Menozzi C, Moya A, et al. Pacemaker therapy in patients with neurally mediated syncope and documented asystole: Third International Study on Syncope of Uncertain Etiology (ISSUE-3): a randomized trial. Circulation 2012; 125: 2566–71.

131. Brignole M, Menozzi C, Lolli G, et al. Long-term outcome of paced and nonpaced patients with severe carotid sinus syndrome. Am J Cardiol 1992; 69: 1039–43.

132. Menozzi C, Brignole M, Lolli G, et al. Follow-up of asystolic episodes in patients with cardioinhibitory, neurally mediated syncope and VVI pacemaker. Am J Cardiol 1993; 72: 1152–5.

133. Davis TL, Freemon FR. Electroencephalography should not be routine in the evaluation of syncope in adults. Arch Intern Med 1990; 150: 2027–9.

134. Ausman JI, Shrontz CE, Pearce JE, et al. Vertebrobasilar insufficiency. A review. Arch Neurol 1985; 42: 803–8.

135. Davidson E, Rotenberg Z, Fuchs J, et al. Transient ischemic attack-related syncope. Clin Cardiol 1991; 14: 141–4.

136. Maurer M, Rivadeneira H, Bloomfield D, et al. Underutilization of cardiovascular testing in elderly patients with syncope. Am J Cardiol 1998; 7: 58.

137. Epstein AE, Miles WM, Benditt DG, et al. Personal and public safety issues related to arrhythmias that may affect consciousness: implications for regulation and physician recommendations. A medical/scientific statement from the American Heart Association and the North American Society of Pacing and Electrophysiology. Circulation 1996; 94: 1147–66.

138. Sorajja D, Nesbitt GC, Hodge DO, et al. Syncope while driving: clinical characteristics, causes, and prognosis. Circulation 2009; 120: 928–34.

139. Brignole M, Alboni P, Benditt DG, et al. Guidelines on management (diagnosis and treatment) of syncope. Update 2004. Executive summary. Rev Esp Cardiol 2005; 58: 175–93.

140. Mitro P, Kirsch P, Valožik G, et al. A prospective study of the standardized diagnostic evaluation of syncope. Europace 2011; 13: 566–71.

141. Daccarett M, Jetter TL, Wasmund SL, et al. Syncope in the emergency department: comparison of standardized admission criteria with clinical practice. Europace 2011; 13: 1632–8.

26
Pericardial disease in the elderly

Lovely Chhabra and David H. Spodick

SUMMARY
The various forms of pericardial diseases include congenital pericardial defects, pericarditis (acute, chronic and recurrent forms), constrictive pericarditis, pericardial effusion, cardiac tamponade, neoplasms and cysts. The spectrum of pericardial diseases thus varies from a commonly occurring benign entity, acute pericarditis, to ominous and imminently life-threatening cardiac tamponade. The current chapter provides a comprehensive evidence-based review of pericardial diseases to help guide clinicians in answering difficult diagnostic and management questions. There is little data regarding the effects of aging on the etiologic spectrum and management of pericardial diseases. Future prospective studies are warranted to provide better insight about the etiopathogenesis and targeted approach to pericardial disease management in the elderly.

INTRODUCTION

The pericardium is a thin covering around the heart that separates it from other mediastinal structures and provides structural support to the heart. The pericardium has substantial hemodynamic and metabolic impacts on the heart; however it is not essential for one's survival. The normal pericardium consists of two sacs: an outer (fibrous) pericardium and an inner double-layered serous pericardium. The serous pericardium comprises visceral pericardium (or epicardium) and parietal pericardium. The visceral pericardium surrounds the heart and proximal great vessels and is reflected to form a parietal layer which lines the fibrous pericardium. The visceral pericardium has an external layer of flat mesothelial cells, which lies on a stroma of fibrocollagenous support tissue. The parietal pericardium contains elastic fibers, as well as the large arteries supplying blood to the heart wall, and the larger venous tributaries carrying blood from the heart wall. The visceral and parietal pericardial layers are separated by a pericardial cavity, which in the healthy population contains about 20–50 ml of pericardial fluid produced by the visceral layer. The pericardium provides lubrication to prevent friction between the heart and surrounding structures, and also serves as a mechanical and immunological barrier. The spectrum of the pericardial diseases includes congenital pericardial defects, pericarditis (acute, chronic and recurrent forms), neoplasms and cysts (1,2). Acute pericarditis is the most common form of pericardial disease, constituting approximately 5% of nonischemic chest pain presentations to the emergency room (3).

AGE-RELATED CHANGES IN PERICARDIAL ANATOMY
AND SPECTRUM OF PERICARDIAL DISORDERS

Like any other structure, the pericardium undergoes changes with aging. There is little prospective data to suggest the effects of aging on pericardial anatomy and variations of etiologic spectrum of the pericardial diseases. The published data on this subject is meager and mostly based on retrospective studies or consensus opinion of experts. With aging, there is a decrease in pericardial elastic tissue (1). Since the amount of the elastic tissue facilitates stretching of the pericardium, one may conceptually project that the elderly are more hemodynamically sensitive to the ill effects of pericardial effusion (4). Thus, the likelihood of having pericardial tamponade with the same amount of pericardial effusion should be higher in the elderly as compared to younger populations. However, a retrospective analysis aimed to assess the possible differences in etiologic spectrum and clinical course of pericardial effusion in elderly patients found no significant differences in the etiology, clinical course and prognosis of moderate and large pericardial effusions in elderly and younger patients and advocated use of similar management strategy in different age groups (5). Certain diseases, such as Dressler's syndrome and neoplasms, may be more frequently seen in elderly patients. The etiologic agent causing idiopathic/viral pericarditis also varies among age groups. Though the most common viral infections causing pericarditis have been reported to be coxsackievirus (types A and B) and echovirus, however most of this data comes from children diagnosed by serologic testing in the 1960s. Other data suggest that adult patients are more commonly infected with cytomegalovirus and herpes viruses as well as HIV (6,7). Geriatric patients may also be subjected to the risk of experiencing purulent, mycobacterial or fungal pericarditis relatively more common than young adults because of age related immunosuppression. Acute pericarditis is largely a benign condition, however it is not uncommon for pericarditis chest pain to have an overlapping spectrum with myocardial ischemia. It can sometimes be clinically difficult to differentiate pericarditis from AMI especially in elderly patients with angina-like pain, who fall in high coronary risk factor profile (due to increased incidence of CAD with age (8), thus these patients may be subjected to an urgent diagnostic coronary angiography more often than younger populations to exclude transmural infarction. Age is also an independent risk predictor for increased mortality, cardiovascular events and heart failure exacerbations in constrictive pericarditis patients after pericardiectomy and thus elderly patients are at a higher risk of having these events post-pericardiectomy (9). A Mayo-Clinic study reported a higher incidence of post-cardiac surgery pericardial effusions requiring pericardiocentesis in older adults. The prevalence of posterior extra echocardiographic spaces is higher in the elderly population (15% for those in their 80s vs. <1% in subjects in the 20- to 30-year age decade) which may represent subepicardial fat masquerading as pericardial fluid and producing a posterior extra echocardiographic space, especially in obese elderly subjects (10). Optimal management of any pericardial disease in the elderly must take into account frequent and occasionally severe comorbidities, for example, adjustment of dosing of NSAIDs and colchicine in elderly as they often have impaired renal function. One should also account occasional complex social situations in the elderly requiring careful hospital discharge planning.

CONGENITAL PERICARDIAL DEFECTS

The most common congenital defect of the pericardium is partial absence, mostly on the left (about 70%), followed by the right side (about 17%) (1). Complete pericardial absence is quite rare and mostly asymptomatic; however, homolateral cardiac displacement and increased cardiac mobility predispose to an increased risk for traumatic type A aortic dissection (11). About 30% of patients may have additional congenital abnormalities like atrial septal defect, bicuspid aortic valve, and bronchogenic cysts. Partial left sided pericardial absence may be complicated by cardiac strangulation caused by herniation of the left atrium (LA), left atrial appendage or left ventricle (LV) through the defect causing chest pain, dyspnea, syncope or even sudden death. Echocardiography may suggest the diagnosis by showing prominence of right-sided cardiac chambers associated with abnormal septal motion; however, cardiac computed tomography (CT), or cardiac magnetic resonance imaging (CMR) are often required for confirmation (12,13).

PERICARDIAL CYSTS

A pericardial cyst is usually a benign structural abnormality which is usually detected as an incidental finding on chest radiography, most commonly at the right cardiophrenic angle (1,14). Pericardial cysts can be congenital or acquired (often due to inflammation). Inflammatory cysts comprise pseudocysts as well as encapsulated and loculated pericardial effusions, caused by bacterial infection (usually tuberculosis in endemic areas), rheumatic heart disease, trauma and cardiac surgery (14,15). Echinococcal cysts usually occur from ruptured hydatid cysts in the liver and lungs. Most cysts are small and asymptomatic, and need no specific treatment. However, some patients may experience symptoms like chest pain/discomfort and dyspnea. Echocardiography is the initial investigation of choice but cardiac CT or CMR are often required.

In symptomatic patients, the treatment of choice is percutaneous aspiration and ethanol sclerosis (16). If this is not feasible, videoassisted thoracoscopy or surgical resection is needed with exception of echinococcal cysts where surgical excision is not recommended. Echinococcal cysts are treated with percutaneous aspiration and instillation of ethanol or silver nitrate after pre-treatment with albendazole.

ACUTE PERICARDITIS

Acute pericarditis refers to inflammation of the pericardial sac and is the commonest form of pericardial disease. It can occur in isolation or may be a manifestation of an underlying systemic disease (17–19).

Etiology

The etiologic spectrum of acute pericarditis is very wide, but in most patients (about 85–90%) it is thought to be idiopathic because the yield of diagnostic tests to confirm etiology has been relatively low. With the conventional diagnostic approach, based on noninvasive techniques, such cases are presumed to be viral in the developed world (17–19). The etiologies are summarized in Table 26.1.

Clinical Presentation and Diagnosis

The diagnosis of pericarditis is suggested by the presence of at least two of four simple clinical criteria: typical pericardial chest pain, pericardial friction rub, characteristic electrocardiographic (ECG) changes, and new or worsening pericardial effusion (17–23).

Typical chest pain of pericarditis is usually sharp, of sudden onset, pleuritic, located substernally with radiation to one or both the trapezial ridges, improves on sitting up and leaning forward, worse on recumbency and not relieved by nitroglycerine but responds to nonsteroidal anti-inflammatory drugs (NSAIDs). In practice it is, however, not uncommon for pericarditic chest pain to have an overlapping spectrum with myocardial ischemia (1,17,22,23). Other common associated symptoms are nonproductive cough and dyspnea.

A pericardial friction rub is usually a high-pitched, scratchy or squeaky sound heard best at the left lower sternal border; it is thought to be generated by friction of the two inflamed layers of the pericardium, corresponding to the movement of the heart within the

Table 26.1 Etiology of Pericarditis

Idiopathic Pericarditis (most cases; about 85–90%)–though presumably believed to be viral in origin

Infectious Pericarditis (about 2/3 of cases in established diagnosis)

a. Viral: [most common though diagnostic yield low, about 1–2%: Coxsackie, CMV, EBV, Echovirus, Influenza, Varicella, Rubella, Hepatitis B and C, HIV, Mumps, HHV6, Parvovirus B19]

b. Bacterial: [Tuberculosis (most common in endemic regions), Coxiella, Pneumo-, Meningo-, Gonococci, Staphylococcus, Chalmydia, Mycoplasma, Legionella, Leptospira, Listeria, Lyme]

c. Fungal: [Histoplasmosis, Aspergillosis, Blastomycosis, Candida]

d. Parasitic: [Very rare: Echinococcus, Toxoplasmosis]

Non-Infectious Pericarditis (about 1/3 of cases)

a. Systemic autoimmune diseases (about 3–5%): [rheumatoid arthritis, systemic lupus erythematosus, sjogren syndrome, systemic sclerosis, systemic vasculitis, mixed connective tissue diseases, sarcoidosis, Behchet syndrome, familial Mediterranean fever]

b. Pericardial injury syndromes: [early post-myocardial infarction pericarditis, Late post-myocardial infarction (Dressler's syndrome), post-pericardiotomy syndrome, post-traumatic pericarditis]

c. Neoplastic Pericarditis (about 5–7%): [primary tumors (pericardial mesothelioma, sarcoma), secondary (metastatic or by direct extension; lung and breast cancer, lymphoma are most common)].

d. Metabolic/Endocrine: [uremia, dialysis pericarditis, hypothyroidism, gout, scurvy]

e. Drug/Toxin-induced: [procainamide, hydralazine, methyldopa, isoniazid, phenytoin, penicillins, tetracyclines, yellow fever vaccine, scorpion fish sting, talc etc.].

f. Radiation-induced pericarditis.

g. Post-thoracic surgery.

h. Myocarditis with pericardial involvement (myopericarditis).

Abbreviations: CMV, Cytomegalovirus; EBV, Epstein-Barr Virus; HIV, Human Immunodeficiency Virus; HHV-6, Human Herpes Virus-6.

pericardial sac (24). The rub can be transient, mono-, bi- or triphasic and variable in intensity. An audible friction rub is highly specific for pericarditis.

ECG changes associated with pericarditis have been classified in four stages, though not all the stages are observed in all pericarditis patients due to that treatment can accelerate or alter ECG progression and also the duration of the ECG changes in pericarditis depends upon its cause and the extent of any associated myocardial damage (25,26). In stage 1, diffuse concave ST-segment elevation (secondary to epicardial inflammation) and PR-segment depression is seen within the first hours to days with corresponding ST-segment depression in aVR and usually V1. There can also be PR-segment elevation in aVR suggestive of an atrial current of injury. The TP-segment should be considered as the isoelectric segment in defining the ST-segment deviation (27). ST-segment normalization is noted in stage 2 followed by T-wave flattening and inversion in stage 3. Stage 4 is characterized by the return of the ECG to either prepericarditis state or indefinitely persistent T-wave inversions (common in cases destined to constrict). The two most common clinical conditions where ECG findings may mimic pericarditis are acute myocardial ischemia (AMI) and generalized early repolarization (28). As opposed to pericarditis, AMI usually causes localized convex ST-elevation usually associated with reciprocal ST-depression which may also be frequently accompanied by Q-waves, T-wave inversions (while ST is still elevated unlike pericarditis), arrhythmias and conduction abnormalities. In AMI, PR-depressions are almost never present. Early repolarization usually occurs in young males (age <40 years) and ECG changes are often characterized by terminal R–S slurring, temporal stability of ST-deviations and J-height/T-amplitude ratio in V5 and V6 of <25% as opposed to pericarditis where terminal R–S slurring is very uncommon and J-height/T-amplitude ratio is ≥25% (28). Very rarely, ECG changes in hypothermia may mimic pericarditis; however, differentiation can be helpful by a detailed history and presence of an Osborne wave in hypothermia (29).

The finding of a new or worsening pericardial effusion on transthoracic echocardiography supports the diagnosis and guides further management in a patient with known or suspected pericarditis, though the absence of an effusion or other echocardiographic abnormalities does not exclude the diagnosis (21–23).

Initial Diagnostic Evaluation and Work-up

The diagnosis of acute pericarditis is usually suspected based on a history of characteristic chest pain, and confirmed if a pericardial friction rub is present. ECG serves as one of the most important parts of the diagnostic toolkit for pericarditis. The detailed diagnostic algorithm is in Figure 26.1. An initial history and physical examination should be performed with particular attention to physical signs of cardiac tamponade, such as pulsus paradoxus and elevated jugular venous pressure (JVP). Kussmaul's sign occurs in constrictive pericarditis, though rarely can be found in cardiac tamponade (9,30), necessitating consideration of effusive-constrictive pericarditis.

Initial diagnostic work-up should include an ECG, chest radiograph, complete blood cell count, cardiac biomarkers (creatinine kinase and troponin), inflammatory markers (sedimentation rate and/or C-reactive protein) and echocardiography for most patients.

Chest radiography findings are normal in most patients with acute pericarditis and is done to exclude other diagnoses. The chest radiograph however may apparent cardiomegaly if patients have a pericardial effusion.

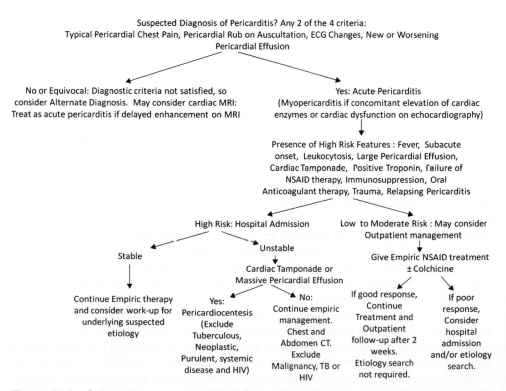

Figure 26.1   Schematic representation of diagnostic and management approach to Acute Pericarditis.

Serum cardiac enzyme levels may often be elevated in pericarditis, presumably as a result of the involvement of the epicardium in the inflammatory process (myopericarditis) (31,32). It can sometimes be clinically difficult to differentiate pericarditis from AMI especially in patients with angina like pain, high coronary artery risk factor profile, ST-segment elevation, and elevated troponin T values, thus urgent diagnostic coronary angiography may be needed to exclude the more ominous diagnosis of infarction. Most younger and some older patients with an elevated troponin level and acute pericarditis have normal findings on coronary angiography (32). Although patients with ST-segment elevation myocardial infarction must receive prompt reperfusion, clinicians must also consider the diagnosis of pericarditis to avoid unnecessary coronary angiography. Urgent echocardiography can be helpful in this regard by demonstrating normal LV regional contractility (22).

Leukocytosis and raised concentration of *inflammatory markers* can be supportive to the diagnosis; however, they are neither sensitive nor specific for acute pericarditis. Blood cultures should be ordered for patients presenting with high-grade fever (>38°C).

Echocardiography is reasonable in all cases of pericarditis, with urgent echocardiography if there is hemodynamic compromise or suspicion of cardiac tamponade (33).

Cardiac CT and CMR are highly sensitive in the detection of generalized or loculated effusions and can also measure pericardial thickness. The most sensitive method for the diagnosis of acute pericarditis is delayed enhancement of the pericardium on CMR. CMR is also helpful in determining any myocardial involvement in case of significant myopericarditis (34,35).

Since most patients with acute pericarditis have a benign self-limiting clinical course and the yield of routine viral studies is low, routine viral antibody titers and cultures are not recommended as the management is not usually altered (36,37). For patients in whom an autoimmune etiology is suspected, an antinuclear antibody titer, rheumatoid factor or anti-neutrophil cytoplasmic antibody (ANCA) should be ordered. Tuberculin skin test or QuantiFERON-TB assay and human immunodeficiency virus serology should be ordered in patients with suspected tuberculous pericarditis, in areas with endemic prevalence of TB and/or suspected immunosuppression. If the history and physical examination suggest a specific cause such as malignancy (relatively common in elderly pericardial disease patients), then appropriate additional tests should be performed. In cases in which the diagnosis of acute pericarditis remains uncertain, CMR may be useful (22).

Pericardiocentesis is indicated in suspected purulent, tuberculous, or neoplastic pericarditis. Pericardiocentesis can also be performed for patients with persistent symptomatic pericardial effusions (38–40). Diagnostic studies of the pericardial fluid should include measurement of adenosine deaminase for tuberculosis, tumor markers (carcinoembryonic antigen, cytokeratin 19 etc) and cytology for suspected neoplasms, and polymerase chain reactions (PCR) and cultures for suspected infectious etiology. Other markers like cell count, glucose, proteins and LDH are rarely useful in determining a specific etiology though useful in distinguishing exudative from transudative effusion (1).

Abdominal and Thoracic CT-scan is warranted in suspected lymphomas, other neoplasms or metastatic disease. A normal CT-scan would help in excluding neoplastic or tuberculous disease.

In cases of pleuropericardial effusions, a diagnostic thoracocentesis may be useful and pleural fluid analysis should be performed similarly as pericardial fluid.

Pericardial Biopsy used to be generally performed as a part of surgical drainage in patients with cardiac tamponade who relapsed after pericardiocentesis (therapeutic biopsy) and as a diagnostic procedure in patients with unclear diagnosis and pericardial effusion lasting for >3 weeks (41,42). With the advent of modern pericardioscopy, diagnostic pericardial biopsy can be performed for patients with persistent disease but unclear diagnosis. Targeted biopsy has particularly proven helpful for the diagnosis of neoplastic pericarditis (43).

Who needs Hospitalization?

Initial diagnostic evaluation should also focus on risk-stratification in order to determine which patients need hospitalization. High-risk features include fever (temperature >38°C), leukocytosis, a large pericardial effusion (echo-free space >20 mm), subacute onset, cardiac tamponade, acute trauma, immunosuppressed state, concurrent oral anticoagulation, failure of NSAID therapy, elevated troponin levels, and recurrent or incessant pericarditis. Patients with such high-risk features should be considered for in-hospital management (17,44).

Treatment

Therapy for pericarditis or myopericarditis should be aimed at the specific etiology, when known. For the majority of cases which are either idiopathic or presumed viral, an empiric medical management approach is used which centers around three major agents—NSAIDs, colchicine, and corticosteroids (17–19,45).

NSAID's are recommended as the first line of therapy for idiopathic or viral pericarditis, in the absence of any contraindication for their use. The goal of therapy is relief of pain and resolution of the inflammation (1,17,22,23). Inflammatory markers may be used as a guide for therapy, though not always essential. Commonly recommended NSAIDs are ibuprofen, aspirin, indomethacin or ketorolac. Ibuprofen is most commonly used (400–600 mg three times a day for 2–4 weeks in uncomplicated cases). Aspirin (800 mg orally every 6–8 hours for 7–10 days followed by gradual tapering of the dose by 800 mg per week for 3 additional weeks) should be used preferentially in patients with acute pericarditis in the setting of myocardial infarction because of the requirement for antiplatelet therapy; other NSAIDs have a potential of interference with myocardial healing and scar formation (46).

Colchicine, which has been essential to treat recurrent pericarditis, has been supported for routine use in acute pericarditis by prospective studies (COPE trial) (47). Colchicine can be given 0.6 mg twice a day (0.6 mg daily for patients <70 kg) for 3 months following an acute attack. It should be considered in all patients with acute pericarditis, especially in patients who have not benefitted from NSAID therapy after 1 week (48,49). However, it should be avoided or used with caution in patients with severe renal insufficiency, hepatobiliary dysfunction, blood dyscrasias, and gastrointestinal motility disorders.

Corticosteroids should not be used as first line therapy in acute pericarditis due to increased risk of disease recurrence (47,50,51). Steroids should be considered if the patient has clearly received no benefit from NSAID and colchicine therapy and a specific cause for pericarditis has been excluded. Other conditions when systemic corticosteroids should be considered as an initial treatment of acute pericarditis are: an immune-mediated disease, a connective tissue disorder, or uremic pericarditis. Recommended initial dose of prednisone is 0.2–0.5 mg/kg/day followed by weekly dose tapering after the normalization of CRP levels and to be continued for total of 2–4 weeks.

RECURRENT PERICARDITIS

Relapsing pericarditis is a challenging complication of acute pericarditis, which can be frustrating for both the patient and the clinician. No optimal treatment regimen has been definitely established for this entity. This term encompasses the two broad spectrums of this disease: (*i*) *Intermittent relapsing type* (where patients may have widely varying symptom-free intervals, usually of more than 6 weeks without therapy) and (*ii*) *Incessant type* (where discontinuation of anti-inflammatory therapy always results in a relapse within 6 weeks) (52). The onset of first symptoms of recurrent pericarditis is usually within 18–20 months after the initial attack (47,53). The use of corticosteroids as a first line treatment in acute pericarditis is a strong risk factor for future episodes of relapsing pericarditis and reduces the efficacy of colchicine. Possible mechanisms proposed for the causation of relapsing pericarditis include: (*i*) early use of steroids may augment viral replication causing increased viral antigen exposure in viral/idiopathic pericarditis thus increasing the risk for relapsing pericarditis, (*ii*) reinfection, (*iii*) insufficient dosing or duration of anti-inflammatory (NSAID) therapy in acute idiopathic pericarditis or insufficient steroid therapy in case of autoimmune disease, (*iv*) exacerbation of connective tissue disease and (*v*) autoimmune phenomena (like the presence of anti-heart antibodies, etc.) (23). Most cases of recurrent pericarditis are considered to be autoimmune. Other predisposing factors which may play a role include genetic or familial factors (usually autosomal dominant pattern of inheritance) (54) and sex-linked inheritance (e.g., chronic recurrent pericarditis associated with ocular hypertension) (55). The reported frequency of recurrent pericarditis averages around 24%; however, the number of recurrences and the intervals between them vary considerably among individual patients (22,52,56–58).

Diagnosis of recurrent pericarditis requires a prior documented episode of acute pericarditis followed by symptoms of recurrent pleuritic chest pain and often association with one of the following signs or symptoms: fever, pericardial friction rub, ECG changes, echocardiographic evidence of pericardial effusion, and elevation in the white blood cell count, erythrocyte sedimentation rate, or C-reactive protein. Many cases merely repeat the symptoms of the index attack with some or without any of these acute phase reactants (1,2,22,23).

The *initial treatment* of recurrent pericarditis is similar to that of the initial acute episode. Outpatient management is feasible in almost all cases. Hospitalization may be required for patients with high-risk features as in acute pericarditis. Aspirin (or another NSAID) and colchicine are recommended as the initial therapy for recurrent pericarditis due to idiopathic or viral causes. In patients with an identified etiology, specific therapy targeting the underlying disorder should be utilized. The NSAIDs should be preferably given thrice daily at the same dosing as in acute pericarditis. Colchicine should be used preferably in combination with NSAIDs, at up to 2 mg on the first day, followed by 0.6 mg once or twice daily for 6 months after the last episode of pericarditis (49,59). Caution is necessary with the use of colchicine in patients with severe renal insufficiency, hepatobiliary dysfunction, blood dyscrasias, and gastrointestinal motility disorders. Along with the initial medical therapy, exercise restriction is found to immensely help reduce the exacerbations or recurrent attacks (52). Glucocorticoids are a double-edged sword in patients with pericarditis; they may have specific but rare indications, but they should be the last resort. The use of glucocorticoid therapy should be limited to the patients who fail NSAID and colchicine therapy; those with definite rheumatologic disease; presumed autoimmune etiology; and intolerance or contraindications to aspirin or NSAIDs (e.g., severe peptic ulcer disease, etc.). Lower doses of prednisone (0.2–0.5 mg/kg/day; i.e., 25 mg for the average patient) is recommended for 4 weeks until symptom resolution and C-reactive protein normalization (60). Dose tapering should be done slowly and colchicine should be added. Some experts suggest that if the patients are already receiving corticosteroid therapy for relapsing pericarditis, then combination of high-dose NSAIDs or aspirin for several months with a very slow taper of prednisone by 1-mg decrements weekly or even monthly may be effective in preventing recurrences (61). The use of intrapericardial glucocorticoid therapy (triamcinolone) has been employed by Maisch and colleagues; this achieves high local glucocorticoid concentrations which maintains efficacy while minimizing systemic toxicity (62–64). Practical application of intrapericardial steroid therapy, however, is largely limited due to technical considerations especially in patients with a small, or no pericardial effusion, where pericardioscopy or the PerDUCER technique must be available to utilize this form of treatment; the availability of such techniques is very limited in the USA (65). Other immunosuppressive agents like azathioprine, cyclophosphamide or mycophenolate may be tried in patients who have shown poor tolerance or inadequate response to other therapies including steroids (66). Pericardiectomy has been employed for end-stage or refractory recurrent pericarditis; however, its reported efficacy is very variable (67–69). Thus, we recommend pericardiectomy to be reserved for only very few selected patients: (*i*) if more than one recurrence is accompanied by cardiac tamponade (which is usually uncommon) or (*ii*) if a recurrence is principally manifested by persistent pain despite an intensive trial with medical treatment and evidence of serious glucocorticoid or immunosuppressive toxicity.

CONSTRICTIVE PERICARDITIS
Constrictive pericarditis can be acute, subacute, or chronic and is a severely disabling complication of pericardial inflammation, where the heart is imprisoned in a thick and sometimes calcified pericardium, leading to impaired ventricular filling and reduced ventricular function (1). It is a potentially curable entity in patients with heart failure with normal ejection fraction; however, it is often underdiagnosed because of the difficulty in differentiating it from restrictive cardiomyopathy or other etiologies responsible for predominantly right-sided heart failure. The diagnosis may sometimes remain equivocal even after extensive testing including 2-dimensional and Doppler echocardiography, cardiac CT and CMR, and conventional cardiac catheterization (70,71).

Etiology
Constrictive pericarditis can occur after virtually any pericardial disease process (rarely follows acute recurrent pericarditis) (72). The most common causes are idiopathic or viral (42–49%) and post-cardiac surgery (11–37%) in the developed world. In the developing world and in immunocompromized patients, tuberculosis is a major cause (9,73,74). Other causes include radiation therapy, connective tissue disorders, infectious (tuberculous or purulent) and miscellaneous (malignancy, trauma, drug-induced, asbestosis, sarcoidosis, and uremic pericarditis). If we account the risk of developing constrictive pericarditis following a first episode of acute pericarditis (as cases per 1,000 person–years), then the strongest predisposition is associated with acute purulent and tuberculous pericarditis (72).

Pathophysiology
Constrictive pericarditis as similar to restrictive cardiomyopathy limits the diastolic filling and results in diastolic heart failure, with relatively preserved global systolic function. In constrictive pericarditis, diastolic filling is restricted by an inelastic pericardium (initial myocardial expansion unaffected) whereas in restrictive cardiomyopathy, there is usually a non-dilated ventricle with a rigid myocardium that causes a major decrease in the effective operative compliance of the heart muscle itself. Table 26.2 enlists the generalities and distinguishing features among these two entities, including the ventricular interaction and summary of catheterization findings.

Clinical Presentation
Symptoms in constrictive pericarditis are either related to a fluid overload state (ranging from peripheral edema to anasarca) or diminished cardiac output on exertion causing

Table 26.2 Constrictive Pericarditis Versus Restrictive Cardiomyopathy

Generalities:

1. Positive diagnosis essential; negative test for one does not imply probability of the other.
2. Eventual endomyocardial and/or pericardial biopsy occasionally inescapable.
3. Both may co-exist, esp. postirradiation.
4. Physical examination unhelpful (unless residual pericardial rub).
5. Hemodynamics generally unhelpful.
6. Echo-Doppler and computed tomography nearly always make the diagnosis.

	Constrictive Pericarditis	Restrictive Cardiomyopathy
Markedly different diastolic pressures	Absent	Occasional
Septal myocardium	Normal	Stiff
Systolic function	Normal	Reduced or normal
Ventricular filling	Very rapid in early diastole	Variable
Endomyocardial biopsy	Usually normal (except fibrosis, postirradiation or vasculitides)	Abnormal: infiltration, fibrosis, inflammation, amyloidosis
Physical findings	Kussmaul's sign +, apical impulse −, pericardial knock +, regurgitant murmurs −	Kussmaul's sign ±, apical impulse +++, S3 (advanced), S4 (early disease), regurgitant murmurs ++
ECG	Usually only ST-T and P abnormalities	May have QRS changes: abnormal Q waves and conduction defects
Chest X-ray	Pericardial calcification, pleural effusion	Pericardial calcification-absent
2D-Echocardiogram	Pericardial thickening and calcifications with indirect signs of constriction: RA and LA enlargement with normal appearing ventricles, normal systolic function, early rapid pathological outward and inward movement of IV septum (dip-plateau phenomenon), flattening wave at posterior LV wall, LV diameter not increasing after the early rapid filling phase, Dilated IVC and hepatic veins with restricted respiratory fluctuations.	Pericardial thickening-absent. Small LV cavity with large atria. Increased ventricular wall thickness sometimes + (esp. thickened interatrial septum in amyloidosis). Thickened valves and granular sparkling seen in amyloidosis.

(Continued)

Table 26.2 Constrictive Pericarditis Versus Restrictive Cardiomyopathy (*Continued*)

Doppler Echo	Constrictive Pericarditis	Restrictive Cardiomyopathy
Ventricular filling	Restricted bi-ventricular filling with respiratory variation >25% over the AV-valves.	Rare or minimal respiratory variation across AV- valves.
Mitral inflow velocity (E)	Increased with significant respiratory variation (Insp E < Exp E).	Mitral inflow velocity (E) usually increased with no respirophasic variation.
Mitral Annular motion in early filling	Velocity > 8 cm/s.	Velocity (<8 cm/s)..
Tricuspid Flow velocity	Inspiratory (E) > Expiratory E flow velocity.	Tricuspid flow velocity has minimal respirophasic variation.
Hepatic vein forward flow	Greatly decreased in diastole in expiration and increased diastolic reversal in expiration.	Systolic > diastolic forward flow. Increased diastolic and systolic reversals in inspiration.
Tissue Doppler Echo	Negative findings (see opposite column)	Peak early velocity of longitudinal expansion (peak Ea) of ≥ 8 cm/s (Sens-89%, Spec-100%)
TEE	Pericardial wall thickening	Absent
CT/MRI	Thickened/Calcified pericardium, tube-like configuration of one or both ventricles, AV-groove narrowing, caval veins congestion, uni-/bi-atrial enlargement	Pericardium is usually normal.
Cardiac catheterization	"Dip and plateau" or square root sign in the pressure curve of the right and/or left ventricle, Equalization of LV/RV end-diastolic pressures (EDP) in the range of 5 mmHg or less. In Inspiration: Increase in RV systolic pressure and decrease in LV diastolic pressure. With expiration: opposite.	Dip and plateau seen. LVEDP often > 5 mmHg greater than RVEDP (may be identical). RV systolic pressure > 50 mmHg and RVEDP <1/3 RVSP

fatigability and dyspnea or both. The majority of patients (nearly 95%) with constrictive pericarditis have elevated JVP with a deep, steep y descent. Kussmaul's sign (paradoxical rise of JVP during inspiration) and pericardial "knock" (an accentuated heart sound occurring slightly earlier than other S3) are present less frequently (in about 20% and 45% of cases respectively), but usually favor the diagnosis of constrictive pericarditis (1,23). Pulsus paradoxus (a drop in systemic blood pressure greater than 10 mmHg during normal inspiration) is also an occasional finding in constrictive pericarditis and usually present if accompanied with a large pericardial effusion or tamponade (i.e., *effusive-constrictive pericarditis*). Profound cachexia, ascites, peripheral edema/anasarca, pulsatile hepatomegaly and pleural effusion may occur more commonly with chronic constrictive pericarditis (23).

Diagnostic Evaluation

Initial evaluation in patients with suspected constrictive pericarditis should include an ECG, chest radiograph and echocardiogram. The diagnosis of constrictive pericarditis is often made by echocardiography; however patients may have to undergo cardiac catheterization. Cardiac catheterization can support the diagnosis with the aid of invasive hemodynamic evaluation and concurrent angiography helps define the coronary anatomy prior to a possible surgical intervention. Cardiac CT and CMR are often required as a part of the workup especially if the patients are being evaluated for a pericardiectomy (e.g., with prior radiation exposure), as these modalities offer detailed anatomic information about the adjacent mediastinal/vascular structures and the extent of pericardial thickening, calcification, and scarring.

The ECG in constrictive pericarditis does not have any specific diagnostic findings. It may often reveal non-specific ST-T abnormalities, low QRS voltage and interatrial block. Patients with restrictive cardiomyopathy often have depolarization abnormalities, such as bundle branch block, ventricular hypertrophy, pathological Q-waves and impaired AV-conduction. Some elderly patients with constrictive pericarditis may have these findings from other diseases.

Chest radiograph showing pericardial calcification is highly supportive of constrictive pericarditis, especially in conjunction with a relevant clinical presentation. However, the absence of calcification does not exclude the diagnosis, and in fact, the majority of these patients will not have evident pericardial calcification on a chest radiograph (75).

Echo-Dopplercardiography is usually the initial diagnostic imaging and indirect hemodynamic study in patients with suspected constrictive pericarditis. Two-dimensional and M-mode echocardiography allow structural visualization while Doppler echocardiography provides indirect hemodynamic information. *Doppler echocardiography is critical for the diagnosis of constrictive pericarditis*. Two-dimensional and M-mode echocardiographic findings seen in constrictive pericarditis are: increased pericardial thickness, abnormal ventricular septal motion, dilatation and absent or diminished collapse of the IVC and hepatic veins, ventricular and atrial septal bounce, frequent moderate biatrial enlargement (severe enlargement being more compatible with restrictive cardiomyopathy) and a sharp halt in ventricular diastolic filling (76–78). Doppler echo findings suggestive of constrictive pericarditis are: (*i*) restrictive mitral and tricuspid inflow velocities, typically (but not always) with respiratory variation; (*ii*) preserved or increased medial mitral annulus early diastolic (e′) velocity, which is an important distinction from restrictive cardiomyopathy in which the e′ is diminished with a cutoff value of 7 cm/s; and (*iii*) increased hepatic vein flow reversal with expiration, reflecting the ventricular interaction and the dissociation of the intracardiac and intrathoracic pressures (Fig. 26.2) (1,22,23). In restrictive cardiomyopathy, the mitral inflow velocity rarely shows respiratory variation, and therefore the

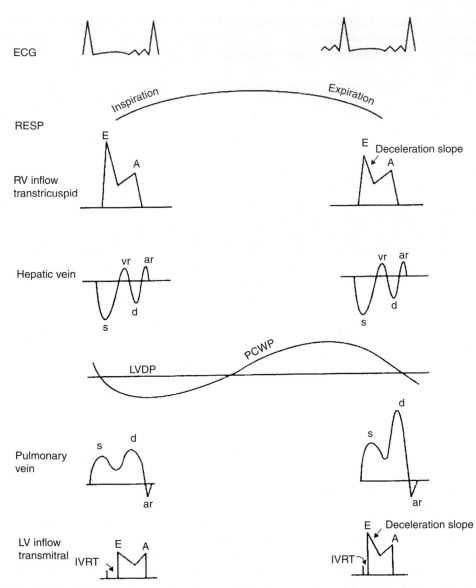

Figure 26.2   Schemata of doppler flows in constrictive pericarditis. Constrictive Pericarditis: schemata of Doppler flows across tricuspid valve, in hepatic veins, in pulmonary veins and across mitral valve. Top: ECG and Respiratory traces. Middle: LVDP = constant elevated level of left ventricular diastolic pressure; PCWP = respiratory variation of Pulmonary capillary wedge pressure; s and d = systolic and diastolic waves of hepatic and pulmonary veins; ar = atrial reversal; vr = ventricular reversal; E= peak early filling velocity in right (RV) and left (LV) ventricles; A = peak presystolic filling velocities due to atrial contraction; IVRT = isovolumic relaxation time of left ventricle (sharply decreased in expiration indicating more rapid relaxation). *Source*: Adapted from Ref. 1.

differentiation of restrictive cardiomyopathy from constrictive pericarditis should be based on the respiratory patterns of ventricular filling. Also, mitral annular velocity is markedly decreased in restrictive cardiomyopathy (due to impaired myocardial relaxation); however, it is well preserved or even increased in constrictive pericarditis because the longitudinal motion of the heart is the main mechanism of diastolic filling in this condition (79).

Cardiac CT findings which are commonly seen in constrictive pericarditis are increased pericardial thickness and pericardial calcification. It is the most sensitive modality in detecting pericardial calcifications (80). CT may assist in the preoperative planning of pericardiectomy in patients with a history of previous cardiothoracic surgery given its ability to identify critical mediastinal/vascular structures. Other advantages which cardiac CT may offer are: (*i*) assessment of the extent of lung injury in patients with previous radiation exposure; (*ii*) evaluation of the location and extent of pericardial calcification and (*iii*) to avoid the need for invasive coronary angiography in those with normal CT coronary angiography (81).

Characteristic CMR findings in patients with constrictive pericarditis are: increased pericardial thickening and dilatation of the inferior vena cava. CMR better differentiates small effusions from pericardial thickening and is better to identify pericardial inflammation and pericardial-myocardial adhesion (82,83).

Invasive hemodynamic monitoring may sometimes be required to establish the diagnosis especially in cases where doppler echocardiographic findings have remained equivocal or nondiagnostic. It can be used to support the diagnosis in patients who are scheduled to undergo diagnostic coronary angiography before a planned surgical intervention (pericardiectomy). The major hemodynamic findings suggestive of constrictive pericarditis include: increased atrial pressure, equalization of end-diastolic pressure, dip-and-plateau or square-root-sign of ventricular diastolic pressure (an early diastolic dip followed by a plateau of diastasis, the last stage of diastole just before contraction), enhanced ventricular interdependence, respiratory variation in LV and RV filling and discordant change in LV and RV systolic pressure with respiration (1,2). In most patients with the restrictive pattern, there is no ventricular interdependence and there is concordant change in LV and RV systolic pressure with respiration.

Treatment

The symptoms of untreated constrictive pericarditis are often permanent and progressive. In a very small group of patients affected by this disease, constriction may be transient or reversible and this most commonly occurs in the setting of pericardial inflammation related to post-pericardiotomy or post-viral pericarditis (84,85). In patients with newly diagnosed constrictive pericarditis and who are hemodynamically stable, a trial of conservative medical management with NSAIDs is recommended for about 2–3 months. In patients where the condition is clearly chronic (e.g., presence of severe cachexia, hepatic dysfunction, dense pericardial calcification, etc.) and patients who have failed initial conservative medical management, pericardiectomy is the treatment of choice (86). Operative mortality associated with pericardiectomy is more than 6% at the most experienced medical centers around the globe. Due to the complex nature of this surgical procedure and a higher rate of associated operative mortality, surgery should be considered cautiously after weighing the risk/benefit ratio. In patients with either mild or very advanced disease and in those with radiation-induced constriction, myocardial dysfunction, significant renal dysfunction, or mixed constrictive-restrictive disease, pericardiectomy may not be beneficial. Cardiac transplantation may be considered in patients with very advanced disease or with associated severe myocardial dysfunction.

EFFUSIVE-CONSTRICTIVE PERICARDITIS

Effusive-constrictive pericarditis is a relatively uncommon pericardial condition where both pericardial effusion and constrictive pericarditis coexist. In this condition, the scarred pericardium not only constricts the cardiac volume, but can also put pericardial fluid under increased pressure, leading to signs of cardiac tamponade. In effusive-constrictive pericarditis, it is mainly the visceral layer of pericardium, (rarely the parietal layer), which causes constrictive physiology (87,88). Like other forms of pericarditis, the most common etiology is idiopathic. Tuberculosis is a frequent cause in the developing world. Other causes include malignancy, radiation, chemotherapy, bacterial infections, and post-surgical pericardial disease.

It differs from classical constrictive pericarditis in clinical examination in a few ways: (*i*) pulsus paradoxus is often present; this is in contrast to classical constrictive pericarditis where pulsus paradoxus is a relatively uncommon finding because the inspiratory decline in the intrathoracic pressure is not transmitted to the right heart chambers; and (*ii*) pericardial knock and Kussmaul's sign are usually absent in effusive-constrictive pericarditis.

The diagnosis of effusive-constrictive pericarditis is often revealed during pericardiocentesis in patients who were initially considered to have uncomplicated cardiac tamponade (87,88). The diagnosis is usually supported by the presence of persistently elevated right atrial pressures despite lowering of the pericardial pressure after pericardiocentesis, subsequent development of a rapidly descent and the lack of an inspiratory decline in right atrial pressures. Two other common clinical conditions where a persistently elevated right atrial pressure after pericardiocentesis may be present are right heart failure and tricuspid regurgitation (not rare in constriction); thus these must be excluded before diagnosing effusive-constrictive pericarditis.

Pericardiocentesis may alone be therapeutic in patients with effusive-constrictive pericarditis, although it usually does not fully reverse the underlying condition in all the patients. In patients where no significant benefit is achieved after pericardiocentesis, pericardiectomy must be performed (1,2,87,88). Usually, these patients require a visceral pericardiectomy which is often more difficult as it requires a sharp dissection of many small fragments until an improvement in ventricular motion is observed. Thus, this procedure should be performed only at centers with sufficient expertise for surgical treatment of constrictive pericarditis. In very few patients, constrictive pericarditis may be due to a reversible inflammation of the pericardium (like post-viral pericarditis), the pericardial effusion may often resolve after treatment with anti-inflammatory medications; this condition is known as *transient constrictive pericarditis*. In these patients, a trial of NSAIDs or corticosteroids for 2–3 weeks is reasonable before considering an invasive approach.

PERICARDIAL EFFUSION

Pericardial effusion refers to an excess fluid collection over the normal physiologic amounts in the pericardial cavity. A pericardial effusion can occur as a result of almost any pericardial disorder, including acute pericarditis and a variety of other systemic disorders including malignancy. The symptoms and prognosis of a pericardial effusion depend on the onset, underlying etiology and its associated hemodynamic impact. Pericardial effusions may develop rapidly (acute) or more gradually (subacute or chronic). With increasing pericardial fluid accumulation, intrapericardial pressure continues to rise and when the pressure becomes high enough to impede cardiac filling, cardiac function becomes impaired and cardiac tamponade ensues.

Etiology

A pericardial effusion can result from almost any pericardial disorder, however the majority of pericardial effusions are not found to have an identifiable cause (idiopathic) and thus frequently such cases are presumed to be viral, mostly secondary to acute viral pericarditis. In cases where an etiology is established, one of these conditions is most common: acute infectious pericarditis, malignancy (particularly metastatic spread of noncardiac tumors), autoimmune disease, post-myocardial infarction or cardiac surgery, sharp or blunt chest trauma (including a cardiac diagnostic or interventional procedure), mediastinal radiation, renal failure with uremia, hypothyroidism (especially myxedema), aortic dissection extending into the pericardium and certain drugs. Hydropericardium resulting from the transudation of fluid in the setting of congestive heart failure is also probably one of the commonest causes for mild grade non-inflammatory transudative pericardial effusions (1).

The underlying cause of a pericardial effusion may be suspected by its clinical setting. One of the previous studies suggested that accounting for presence or absence of three major factors can strongly suggest the etiology, though not confirm the diagnosis, which are: (*i*) size of the effusion; (*ii*) presence or absence of tamponade and (*iii*) inflammatory signs (defined as two or more of the following features: characteristic chest pain; pericardial friction rub; fever >37°C; and diffuse ST segment elevation) (89):

1. The presence of inflammatory signs was found to be associated with acute idiopathic (presumably viral) pericarditis (with a likelihood ratio of 5.4: i.e., the probability of finding an idiopathic/viral cause in a patient with the presence of inflammatory signs will be 5.4 times more than in a patient without inflammatory signs).
2. A large effusion without inflammatory signs or tamponade was found to be associated with a chronic idiopathic pericardial effusion (with a likelihood ratio of 20).
3. A large tamponade without inflammatory signs was associated with a malignant effusion (likelihood ratio 2.9).

Clinical Findings

Most patients with small pericardial effusions and without associated hemodynamic instability are usually asymptomatic from the effusion itself, but may have mild symptoms related to the underlying cause (e.g., fever, pleuritic chest pain etc. in the setting of acute pericarditis). Some patients with smaller effusions may experience a pressure or achy sensation in the chest possibly due to the stretching of the pericardium. Large effusions associated with some hemodynamic impairment can usually present with signs and symptoms related to impaired cardiac function (i.e., fatigue, dyspnea, elevated JVP, edema, etc). Other physical symptoms may result from the encroachments on neighboring structures: dyspnea on exertion produced by displacement and compression of lung tissue causing a restrictive pulmonary defect, dysphagia, or choking throat sensation from esophageal compression, cough from bronchial encroachment, hiccups from esophageal compression and involvement of vagi and phrenic nerves; and hoarseness from compression of the recurrent laryngeal nerve (1).

Almost all the patients with very large pericardial effusions or with impending tamponade physiology will have tachycardia, an elevated JVP, and pulsus paradoxus. Other physical signs are usually of little use and are more of historic interest because they are insensitive and nonspecific. Heart sounds may not be muffled sometimes even in large pericardial effusions. The ability to percuss cardiac dullness beyond the apical point of maximal impulse is consistent with pericardial effusion, but depends upon the absence of disease of the lower lobe of the left lung or left pleura and the expertise of the examiner. The Bamberger–Pins–Ewart's sign (an area of dullness at the left infrascapular area due to bronchial compression by a large effusion) also suffers from similar limitations (1,90).

Asymptomatic pericardial effusions are often incidentally diagnosed during diagnostic work-up for another suspected ailment. In general, pericardial effusions should always be suspected in some specific clinical settings, particularly when that disease condition is known to involve the pericardium; for example, cases of acute pericarditis, history of recurrent pericarditis, unexplained new radiographic cardiomegaly without pulmonary congestion, unexplained persistent high-grade fever with signs/symptoms of recent peri-carditis (purulent pericarditis), presence of isolated left (or left larger than right) pleural effusion and fever or hemodynamic deterioration in a patient with another disease process that can involve the pericardium (1,91).

Diagnostic Evaluation

Whenever clinical suspicion of a pericardial effusion is raised, the subsequent diagnostic approach should be followed in three major steps: confirming the presence of a pericardial effusion; assessing its hemodynamic impact and, whenever possible, establishing the underlying etiology of the effusion. Besides a good history and physical examination, an initial diagnostic work-up should include basic labs (hemogram and chemistry panel), TSH, an electrocardiogram, cardiac biomarkers, chest radiograph and echocardiogram. Other diagnostic modalities include cardiac CT, CMR, and pericardial fluid analysis/biopsy, which may be required in certain special situations.

ECG findings suggestive of a pericardial effusion are low QRS voltage and electrical alternans. Electrical alternans is usually present in very large pericardial effusions and especially cardiac tamponade and is often accompanied by sinus tachycardia. Cardiac bio-markers form an integral part of the intial work-up and can often be elevated if the pericar-dial effusion occurs as a result of acute pericarditis.

The chest radiograph may appear largely normal in case of small pericardial effu-sions. The cardiac silhouette usually does not enlarge until at least 200–250 mL of pericar-dial fluid has accumulated. In case of large pericardial effusions, the chest X-ray shows cardiomegaly and in case of very large effusions, a classic bottle-shaped heart.

Echocardiography, by far, is the most important and readily available investigation for pericardial effusion. It is highly specific and sensitive in detecting a pericardial effu-sion and can also provide information regarding its hemodynamic significance. Pericar-dial fluid appears on an echocardiogram as an echolucent space between the pericardium and the epicardium. The echocardiogram is highly useful in roughly estimating the size of an effusion but unlike a cardiac CT or CMR, it cannot precisely quantify the fluid amount as it is usually difficult to visualize and measure the entire pericardial sac in any one sector scan plane by an echocardiogram. Small effusions (<100 mL) may be localized (only seen posteriorly), typically <5 mm in thickness, and only cause minimal separation between the visceral pericardium and the thicker parietal pericardial sac. Moderate effusions (100–500 mL) usually tend to be seen along the length of the posterior wall but not anteriorly and the echo-free space is ≤1 cm at its greatest width. Large effusions (>500 mL) tend to be seen circumferentially and the echo-free space is >1 cm at its great-est width (1).

Cardiac CT or CMR are both superior to echocardiography in detecting loculated effusions and pericardial fluid quantification. One of them may also be required before a planned surgical intervention (like a thoracotomy-approach pericardial window or pericardiectomy) as both of these modalities offer an additional information about the thoracic anatomy and neighboring vascular structures, which is not provided by echocardiography.

Pericardial fluid analysis is often performed when the patient is undergoing a thera-peutic pericardiocentesis, say in case of cardiac tamponade. Pericardiocentesis for pri-mary diagnostic purposes should be performed only in very rare clinical situations and must be critically weighed for a risk–benefit ratio of the procedure. The diagnostic yield of the procedure is relatively low, and many low-risk patients can be managed empiri-cally without making a specific diagnosis. In about 60% of the patients, diagnosis can be made using a suspected etiology-based approach accounting the three factors described previously (89). Pericardiocentesis should be reserved for the following conditions in pericardial effusion: (*i*) cardiac tamponade or impending hemodynamic instability; (*ii*) suspected malignancy or metastatic disease; (*iii*) clinically suspected purulent or tuberculous pericarditis; (*iv*) large pericardial effusions (>20 mm) if the effusion persists for more than a month or if there is associated right-sided chamber collapse; and (*v*) moderate-to-large pericardial effusions of unknown etiology that do not respond rapidly to anti-inflammatory therapy.

Pericardial fluid should be analyzed by cultures, for cytology, adenosine deaminase (for tuberculous pericarditis), and PCR (92,93). Parameters such as white cell count, proteins, glucose and LDH which are often used to determine the nature of the effusion (transudative vs. exudative) are mostly not helpful in distinguishing the etiology in case of pericardial effusions and thus are not recommended for routine testing (1,94).

For small to moderate-sized asymptomatic pericardial effusions without associated hemodynamic instability, regular follow-up with clinical examination and/or echocardiography is preferred. Most of the small pericardial effusions are idiopathic (presumably postviral) and resolve spontaneously or with NSAIDs in a few weeks.

CARDIAC TAMPONADE

Cardiac tamponade refers to significant compression of the heart caused by the accumulated pericardial contents. Tamponade occurs when all cardiac chambers are compressed as a result of increased intrapericardial pressure to the point of compromising systemic venous return to the right atrium (RA). The increased intrapericardial pressure reduces the myocardial transmural pressure, and the cardiac chambers become smaller, with reduced chamber diastolic compliance and a decrease in cardiac output and blood pressure. In contrast to constrictive pericarditis, during tamponade, most of the inspiratory decline in the intrathoracic pressure is able to get transmitted through the pericardium to the right side of the heart which results in an increase in systemic venous return with inspiration and distention of the right ventricle (RV). Due to very high intrapericardial pressure, the pericardium prevents the free wall of the RV from expanding and thus the expansion is limited to the interventricular and interatrial septa, resulting in bulging of the RV and RA into the LV and LA. This bulging results in reduced LV and LA compliance and decreased filling of the LV and LA during inspiration and this mechanism contributes to pulsus paradoxus (decrease in systolic blood pressure by >10 mmHg during inspiration), which is one of the important clinical signs of cardiac tamponade.

Types of Cardiac Tamponade

Cardiac tamponade may be *acute, subacute, low-pressure type or regional. Acute cardiac tamponade* is often sudden in onset and life threatening if not treated promptly (3). *Subacute cardiac tamponade* is less dramatic process than acute tamponade. Patients may be asymptomatic in early course, but, once intrapericardial pressure reaches a critical value, they experience classical symptoms related to decreased heart function or encroachment on neighboring structures. *Low pressure tamponade* occurs in severely hypovolemic patients (like traumatic hemorrhage, overdiuresis, etc.) at presentation and these patients have both intracardiac and pericardial diastolic pressures in range of 6–12 mmHg (95). Initial fluid resuscitation with intravenous fluid boluses will usually elicit typical tamponade hemodynamics. *Regional tamponade* refers to a loculated, eccentric effusion or localized hematoma causing compression of only selected chambers. As a result, the typical physical, hemodynamic, and echocardiographic signs of cardiac tamponade are often absent. Regional cardiac tamponade is mostly seen after a pericardiotomy or, rarely, myocardial infarction.

Clinical Findings

Classical physical findings seen in cardiac tamponade are sinus tachycardia, elevated JVP, muffled heart sounds, systemic hypotension and pulsus paradoxus. The first three clinical signs together are popularly referred to as Beck's triad. Some previous studies have suggested that it is not uncommon for patients to have a normal blood pressure or even hypertension during tamponade and this is often due to significantly increased sympathetic activity outweighing the co-existent compressive physiology. Hypertension may be more commonly present in patients who present with subacute rather than acute tamponade (96,97). Kussmaul's sign is usually not seen in cardiac tamponade, unless patients have severe co-existent constrictive pericarditis (98).

Diagnostic Evaluation

The diagnostic approach in a patient with suspected cardiac tamponade should be on the same lines as for a patient with suspected pericardial effusion, as described previously.

The typical electrocardiogram (ECG) findings seen in cardiac tamponade include sinus tachycardia, low voltage and frequently electrical alternans. Electrical alternans in tamponade is due to an alternation in the position of the heart with relation to the recording electrodes. Presence of total electrical alternans (P-wave, PR-segment, QRS-complex, and ST-segment alternans) is highly specific for cardiac tamponade, however the sensitivity is very low, as it is seen in only 5–10% of patients with cardiac tamponade (99). Presence of lone QRS alternans is more common; however, it is not very specific for tamponade. The presence of QRS vector alternans (i.e., a beat-to-beat QRS axis-shift), as opposed to QRS amplitude alternans (i.e., beat-to-beat amplitude variation) favors the diagnosis of tamponade (1,99).

Urgent echocardiography is often needed in a case of suspected cardiac tamponade. Typical echocardiographic findings in tamponade include late diastolic collapse of the RA and early diastolic collapse of the RV, especially when the intrapericardial pressure exceeds the intracavitary pressure (100–102). The maximal pericardial pressure in tamponade occurs during end-diastole, when the RA volume is minimal, causing right atrial buckling. Persistence of RA collapse for more than one-third of the cardiac cycle is highly sensitive and relatively specific for tamponade. Left ventricular collapse, which can also occur in tamponade, is highly specific (though not as sensitive) for tamponade. Reciprocal changes occur in the RV and LV during respiration which indicate ventricular interdependence. The interventricular septum bulges into the LV during inspiration due to an increased systemic venous return to the RV and limited expansion of the RV free wall due to the increased intrapericardial pressure. The transmitral pressure gradient increases during expiration and subsequently, the systemic venous return decreases with reversal of diastolic flow in the hepatic veins. These findings contribute to pulsus paradoxus. Other echocardiographic findings in tamponade include inferior vena cava (IVC) dilatation, (with less than a 50% reduction in its diameter during inspiration) and the "swinging motion of the heart" within the pericardial sac.

Cardiac CT or magnetic resonance imaging (MRI) are often not required for evaluation of cardiac tamponade and usually echocardiography is sufficient to guide the management approach (103). Cardiac CT or CMR are needed only in special conditions for the evaluation of a pericardial effusion, as described previously. Cardiac CT or CMR may sometimes serve as a superior modality for the evaluation of a loculated pericardial effusion or localized tamponade physiology.

Treatment

The definitive treatment of cardiac tamponade is decompression of the pericardial sac, thereby relieving the elevated intrapericardial pressure and improving hemodynamic status. Cardiac tamponade with overt hemodynamic compromise always requires urgent fluid removal, which produces a rapid and dramatic improvement in cardiac and systemic hemodynamics. In occasional cases with cardiac tamponade but no overt hemodynamic instability, close serial clinical follow-up by physical examination and echocardiogram can be done; most patients however would eventually need the pericardial drainage. In hypotensive patients, volume expansion with saline, blood, plasma, and dextran can be used as a temporary measure (104), but often fails. Positive-pressure mechanical ventilation should be avoided in acute tamponade because it further reduces cardiac filling. The use of inotropic therapy (like dobutamine) is controversial because endogenous sympathetic stimulation is usually maximal in tamponade.

Pericardial fluid removal can be performed by either catheter pericardiocentesis or open surgical drainage with or without a pericardial "window", or video-assisted thoracoscopic pericardiectomy (105). Catheter pericardiocentesis should always be attempted first as it is more rapid and a less invasive approach. Surgical drainage has the advantages of permitting diagnostic pericardial biopsies and pericardiectomy, if needed. Surgical drainage is also required for loculated effusions which are often not amenable to pericardiocentesis. Pericardial fluid obtained after drainage should be examined for gram staining, bacterial cultures, acid-fast bacilli stain and culture, PCR, cytology, and carcinoembryonic antigen.

SPECIAL FORMS OF PERICARDITIS

A few etiology-specific forms of pericarditis are discussed here separately as they are probably of more common occurrence in geriatric patients than in the general adult patient population.

Neoplastic Pericarditis

The most common cause of neoplastic pericarditis is secondary metastasis (106). Primary pericardial tumors, like pericardial mesothelioma, are rare (about 40 times less common than metastases). The most common metastatic tumor involving the pericardium is lung cancer; others include breast and esophageal cancer, melanoma, lymphoma, and leukemia (107). Kaposi's sarcoma in HIV patients used to be a common cause, however its incidence has decreased in the current era due to available potent antiretroviral therapy. Malignant involvement of the pericardium can present as pericarditis, pericardial effusion, cardiac tamponade, or pericardial constriction (constrictive pericarditis). Presentation in case of a neoplastic pericardial effusions may range from an asymptomatic large effusion to cardiac tamponade. Patients often have a history of previous cancer or advanced metastatic disease. Initial diagnostic evaluation should include an ECG, chest radiograph, and echocardiogram. CT and MRI are useful adjuncts in the diagnostic workup and are often required eventually. Pericardiocentesis with cytologic and/or flow cytometric analysis of the pericardial fluid should always be performed in patients whenever a malignant/neoplastic pericardial effusion is suspected (23).

The goal of therapy in neoplastic pericardial disease is to treat the manifestations of the pericardial disease (like pericardial effusion) and treat the underlying malignancy (107). Patients with large pericardial effusions and cardiac tamponade should receive pericardiocentesis. Neoplastic pericardial effusions are often recurrent, requiring a pleuro-pericardial or peritoneo-pericardial window for palliative drainage (108,109). Intrapericardial instillation of sclerosing agents (like tetracycline, doxycycline, bleomycin, or talc, etc.), in conjunction with prolonged catheter drainage, has been tried in the past, to produce inflammation and scarring of the pericardial surfaces, thereby eliminating the potential space for fluid reaccumulation (110). However, due to potential toxicity with sclerosing therapy and its short-lasting effects, it is not usually recommended in current practice. Intrapericardial instillation of chemotherapeutic agents in cases of confirmed malignant pericardial effusions has been attempted with some success (cisplatin in cases of secondary lung cancer and thiotepa in breast cancer pericardial metastases) (111,112). This approach allows for relatively high doses of chemotherapy to be administered locally with minimal systemic side effects and palliation of symptoms from a hemodynamically significant effusion.

Uremic Pericarditis

Patients with end-stage renal disease may develop pericarditis, pericardial effusions, and rarely, constrictive pericarditis. Two types of pericarditis have been described with renal failure (113,114):

(i) Uremic pericarditis: incidence is about 6–10% of patients with renal failure before dialysis had been instituted. It correlates with the degree of azotemia (BUN usually >60 mg/dL).
(ii) Dialysis-associated pericarditis: in about 13% of patients on maintenance hemodialysis and occasionally with peritoneal hemodialysis. This is usually due to inadequate dialysis or fluid overload.

Another type of pericarditis has also been reported in the patients post-renal transplantation and is usually related to uremia and less commonly to cytomegalovirus or other infections like nocardia.

The treatment of uremic or dialysis-associated pericarditis is the initiation or intensification of the dialysis regimen, as long as there is no circulatory compromise or evidence of impending tamponade. Most patients respond to the dialysis (either hemodialysis or peritoneal) with resolution of chest pain and a decrease in the pericardial effusion. Heparin-free hemodialysis is preferred in order to prevent hemopericardium. The size of the pericardial effusion should be monitored by serial echocardiography. Excess fluid removal with hemodialysis can lead to cardiovascular collapse in patients with tamponade or impending tamponade. Patients presenting with large effusions, evidence of diastolic collapse or who have failed intensive hemodialysis need pericardiocentesis. Pericardiocentesis may also be recommended for rapidly developing moderate-sized pericardial effusions. Patients with large, non-resolving, and recurrent pericardial effusions would benefit from surgical drainage: subxiphoid pericardiotomy (with or without the instillation of intrapericardial corticosteroids) or pericardiectomy. An intrapericardial catheter can also be placed for drainage and steroid instillation.

FUTURE DIRECTIONS

The effect of age on the pericardial disease spectrum remains underinvestigated and clearly deserves more attention. Future prospective studies are warranted to provide a better insight about the etiopathogenesis and targeted approach to the pericardial diseases in the elderly.

REFERENCES

1. Spodick DH. The Pericardium: A Comprehensive Textbook. New York: Marcel Dekker, 1997.
2. Spodick DH. Pericardial disease. In: Braunwald E, Zipes D, Libby P, eds. Heart Disease: A Textbook of Cardiovascular Medicine. New York: Saunders, 2001.
3. Spodick DH. Acute cardiac tamponade. N Engl J Med 2003; 349: 684–90.
4. Kindelan J, de Hoyos A. Surgical treatment of pericardial disease in the elderly. In: Katlic MR. Cardiothoracic Surgery in the Elderly. New York: Springer, 2011: 437–42.

5. Mercé J, Sagristà Sauleda J, Permanyer Miralda G, et al. Pericardial effusion in the elderly: A different disease? Rev Esp Cardiol 2000; 53: 1432–6.

6. Corey GR, Campbell PT, Van Trigt P, et al. Etiology of large pericardial effusions. Am J Med 1993; 95: 209.

7. Campbell PT, Li JS, Wall TC, et al. Cytomegalovirus pericarditis: a case series and review of the literature. Am J Med Sci 1995; 309: 229.

8. Tzivoni D, Licht A, Eliakim M. Acute idiopathic pericarditis in the aged. Eur J Cardiol 1975; 2: 327–35.

9. Ling LH, Oh JK, Schaff HV, et al. Constrictive pericarditis in the modern era: evolving clinical spectrum and impact on outcome after pericardiectomy. Circulation 1999; 100: 1380–6.

10. Savage DD, Garrison RJ, Brand F, et al. Prevalence and correlates of posterior extra echocardiographic spaces in a free-living population based sample (the Framingham study). Am J Cardiol 1983; 51: 1207–12.

11. Meunier JP, Lopez S, Teboul J, Jourdan J. Total pericardial defect: risk factor for traumatic aortic type A dissection. Ann Thorac Surg 2002; 74: 266.

12. Nasser WK, Helmen C, Tavel ME, Feigenbaum H, Fisch C. Congenital absence of the left pericardium: clinical, electrocardiographic, radiographic, hemodynamic, and angiographic findings in six cases. Circulation 1970; 41: 469–78.

13. Connolly HM, Click RL, Schattenberg TT, Seward JB, Tajik AJ. Congenital absence of the pericardium: echocardiography as a diagnostic tool. J Am Soc Echocardiogr 1995; 8: 87–92.

14. Satur CM, Hsin MK, Dussek JE. Giant pericardial cysts. Ann Thorac Surg 1996; 61: 208 10.

15. Borges AC, Gellert K, Dietel M, et al. Acute right-heart failure due to hemorrhage into a pericardial cyst. Ann Thorac Surg 1997; 63: 845–7.

16. Kinoshita Y, Shimada T, Murakami Y, et al. Ethanol sclerosis can be a safe and useful treatment for pericardial cyst. Clin Cardiol 1996; 19: 833–5.

17. Spodick DH. Acute pericarditis: current concepts and practice. JAMA 2003; 289: 1150.

18. Lange RA, Hillis LD. Clinical practice. Acute pericarditis. N Engl J Med 2004; 351: 2195.

19. Troughton RW, Asher CR, Klein AL. Pericarditis. Lancet 2004; 363: 717.

20. Spodick DH. The normal and diseased pericardium: current concepts of pericardial physiology, diagnosis and treatment. J Am Coll Cardiol 1983; 1: 240.

21. Imazio M, Spodick DH, Brucato A, et al. Diagnostic issues in the clinical management of pericarditis. Int J Clin Pract 2010; 64: 1384–92.

22. Khandaker MH, Espinosa RE, Nishimura RA, et al. Pericardial disease: diagnosis and management. Mayo Clin Proc 2010; 85: 572–93.

23. Maisch B, Seferovic PM, Ristic AD, et al. Guidelines on the diagnosis and management of pericardial diseases executive summary: The task force on the diagnosis and management of pericardial diseases of the European Society of Cardiology. Eur Heart J 2004; 25: 587–610.

24. Spodick DH. Pericardial rub. Prospective, Multiple observer investigation of pericardial friction in 100 patients. Am J Cardiol 1975; 35: 357.

25. Spodick DH. Diagnostic electrocardiographic sequences in acute pericarditis: significance of PR segment and PR vector changes. Circulation 1973; 48: 575–80.

26. Baljepally R, Spodick DH. PR-segment deviation as the initial electrocardiographic response in acute pericarditis. Am J Cardiol 1998; 81: 1505–6.

27. Chhabra L, Spodick DH. Ideal isoelectric reference segment in pericarditis: a suggested approach to a commonly prevailing clinical misconception. Cardiology 2012; 122: 210–12.

28. Spodick DH. Differential characteristics of the electrocardiogram in early repolarization and acute pericarditis. N Engl J Med 1976; 295: 523–6.

29. Chhabra L, Spodick DH. Hypothermia masquerading as pericarditis: an unusual electrocardiographic analogy. J Electrocardiol 2012; 45: 350–2.

30. Myers RB, Spodick DH. Constrictive pericarditis: clinical and pathophysiologic characteristics. Am Heart J 1999; 138: 219–32.

31. Bonnefoy E, Godon P, Kirkorian G, et al. Serum cardiac troponin I and ST-segment elevation in patients with acute pericarditis. Eur Heart J 2000; 21: 832–6.

32. Imazio M, Demichelis B, Cecchi E, et al. Cardiac troponin I in acute pericarditis. J Am Coll Cardiol 2003; 42: 2144–8.

33. Cheitlin MD, Armstrong WF, Aurigemma GP, et al. ACC/AHA/ASE 2003 guideline update for the clinical application of echocardiography—summary article: a report of the American College of Cardiology/American Heart Association Task Force on Practice Guidelines (ACC/AHA/ASE Committee to Update the 1997 Guidelines for the Clinical Application of Echocardiography). J Am Coll Cardiol 2003; 42: 954–70.

34. Rienmuller R, Gurgan M, Erdmann E, et al. CT and MR evaluation of pericardial constriction: a new diagnostic and therapeutic concept. J Thorac Imaging 1993; 8: 108–21.

35. Zurick AO, Bolen MA, Kwon DH, et al. Pericardial delayed hyperenhancement with CMR imaging in patients with constrictive pericarditis undergoing surgical pericardiectomy: a case series with histopathological correlation. JACC Cardiovasc Imaging 2011; 4: 1180–91.

36. Permanyer-Miralda G, Sagrista-Sauleda J, Soler-Soler J. Primary acute pericardial disease: a prospective series of 231 consecutive patients. Am J Cardiol 1985; 56: 623–30.

37. Zayas R, Anguita M, Torres F, et al. Incidence of specific etiology and role of methods for specific etiologic diagnosis of primary acute pericarditis. Am J Cardiol 1995; 75: 378–82.

38. Imazio M, Spodick DH, Brucato A, Trinchero R, Adler Y. Controversial issues in the management of pericardial diseases. Circulation 2010; 121: 916–28.

39. Imazio M, Trinchero R. Clinical management of acute pericardial disease: a review of results and outcomes. Ital Heart J 2004; 5: 803.

40. Imazio M, Brucato A, Derosa FG, et al. Aetiological diagnosis in acute and recurrent pericarditis: when and how. J Cardiovasc Med (Hagerstown) 2009; 10: 217.

41. Tsang TS, Enriquez-Sarano M, Freeman WK, et al. Consecutive 1127 therapeutic echocardiographically guided pericardiocenteses: clinical profile, practice patterns, and outcomes spanning 21 years. Mayo Clin Proc 2002; 77: 429–36.

42. Nugue O, Millaire A, Porte H, et al. Pericardioscopy in the etiologic diagnosis of pericardial effusion in 141 consecutive patients. Circulation 1996; 94: 1635–41.

43. Seferovic PM, Ristic AD, Maksimovic R, et al. Diagnostic value of pericardial biopsy: improvement with extensive sampling enabled by pericardioscopy. Circulation 2003; 107: 978–83.

44. Spodick DH. Risk prediction in pericarditis: who to keep in hospital? Heart 2008; 94: 398–9.

45. Lorbar M, Spodick DH. 'Idiopathic' pericarditis–the clinician's challenge [nothing is idiopathic]. Int J Clin Pract 2007; 61: 138–42.

46. Spodick DH. Safety of ibuprofen for acute myocardial infarction pericarditis. Am J Cardiol 1986; 57: 896.

47. Imazio M, Bobbio M, Cecchi E, et al. Colchicine in addition to conventional therapy for acute pericarditis: results of the COlchicine for acute PEricarditis (COPE) trial. Circulation 2005; 112: 2012–16.

48. Imazio M, Brucato A, Trinchero R, Spodick D, Adler Y. Colchicine for pericarditis: hype or hope? Eur Heart J 2009; 30: 532–9.

49. Spodick DH. Colchicine effectively and safely treats acute pericarditis and prevents and treats recurrent pericarditides. Heart 2012; 98: 1035–6.

50. Lange RA, Hillis LD. Clinical practice: acute pericarditis [published correction appears in N Engl J Med 2005;352(11):1163]. N Engl J Med 2004; 351: 2195–202.

51. Imazio M, Demichelis B, Parrini I, et al. Recurrent pain without objective evidence of disease in patients with previous idiopathic or viral acute pericarditis. Am J Cardiol 2004; 94: 973–5.

52. Soler-Soler J, Sagrista-Sauleda J, Permanyer-Miralda G. Relapsing pericarditis. Heart 2004; 90: 1364–8.

53. Imazio M, Demichelis B, Parrini I, et al. Management, risk factors, and outcomes in recurrent pericarditis. Am J Cardiol 2005; 96: 736.

54. DeLine JM, Cable DG. Clustering of recurrent pericarditis with effusion and constriction in a family. Mayo Clin Proc 2002; 77: 39–43.

55. Erdol C, Erdol H, Celik S, et al. Idiopathic chronic pericarditis associated with ocular hypertension: probably an unknown combination. Int J Cardiol 2003; 87: 293–5.

56. Brucato A, Brambilla G, Moreo A, et al. Long term outcomes in difficult-to-treat patients with recurrent pericarditis. Am J Cardiol 2006; 98: 267–71.

57. Maisch B. Recurrent pericarditis: mysterious or not so mysterious? Eur Heart J 2005; 26: 631–3.

58. Fowler NO, Harbin AD III. Recurrent acute pericarditis: follow-up study of 31 patients. J Am Coll Cardiol 1986; 7: 300–5.

59. Imazio M, Brucato A, Cemin R, CORP (COlchicine for Recurrent Pericarditis) Investigators. Colchicine for recurrent pericarditis (CORP): a randomized trial. Ann Intern Med 2011; 155: 409–14.

60. Markel G, Imazio M, Brucato A, Adler Y. Colchicine for the prevention of recurrent pericarditis. Isr Med Assoc J 2008; 10: 69.

61. Marcolongo R, Russo R, Laveder F, et al. Immunosuppressive therapy prevents recurrent pericarditis. J Am Coll Cardiol 1995; 26: 1276.

62. Maisch B, Ristić AD, Pankuweit S. Intrapericardial treatment of autoreactive pericardial effusion with triamcinolone; the way to avoid side effects of systemic corticosteroid therapy. Eur Heart J 2002; 23: 1503–8.

63. Spodick DH. Intrapericardial treatment of persistent autoreactive pericarditis/myopericarditis and pericardial effusion. Eur Heart J 2002; 23: 1481–2.

64. Maisch B, Ristić AD, Seferovic PM, Spodick DH. Intrapericardial treatment of autoreactive myocarditis with triamcinolon. Successful administration in patients with minimal pericardial effusion. Herz 2000; 25: 781–6.

65. Maisch B, Ristić AD, Rupp H, Spodick DH. Pericardial access using the PerDUCER and flexible percutaneous pericardioscopy. Am J Cardiol 2001; 88: 1323–6.

66. Asplen CH, Levine HD. Azathioprine therapy of steroid-responsive pericarditis. Am Heart J 1970; 80: 109–11.

67. Hatcher CR Jr, Logue RB, Logan WD Jr, et al. Pericardiectomy for recurrent pericarditis. J Thorac Cardiovasc Surg 1971; 62: 371–8.

68. Miller JI, Mansour KA, Hatcher CR. Pericardiectomy: current indication, concept, and results in a university center. Ann Thorac Surg 1982; 84: 40–5.

69. Greason K, Danielson GK, Oh JK, Nishimura RA. Pericardiectomy for chronic relapsing pericarditis [abstract 1005-1204]. J Am Coll Cardiol 2001; 37: 478A–479A.

70. Hatle LK, Appleton CP, Popp RL. Differentiation of constrictive pericarditis and restrictive cardiomyopathy by Doppler echocardiography. Circulation 1989; 79: 357–70.

71. Oh JK, Hatle LK, Seward JB, et al. Diagnostic role of Doppler echocardiography in constrictive pericarditis. J Am Coll Cardiol 1994; 23: 154–62.

72. Imazio M, Brucato A, Maestroni S, et al. Risk of constrictive pericarditis after acute pericarditis. Circulation 2011; 124: 1270–5.

73. Schwefer M, Aschenbach R, Heidemann J, Mey C, Lapp H. Constrictive pericarditis, still a diagnostic challenge: comprehensive review of clinical management. Eur J Cardiothorac Surg 2009; 36: 502–10.

74. Mayosi BM. Contemporary trends in the epidemiology and management of cardiomyopathy and pericarditis in sub-Saharan Africa. Heart 2007; 93: 1176–83.

75. Ling LH, Oh JK, Breen JF, et al. Calcific constrictive pericarditis: is it still with us? Ann Intern Med 2000; 132: 444.

76. Engel PJ, Fowler NO, Tei CW, et al. M-mode echocardiography in constrictive pericarditis. J Am Coll Cardiol 1985; 6: 471.

77. Hoit BD. Imaging the pericardium. Cardiol Clin 1990; 8: 587.

78. D'Cruz IA, Dick A, Gross CM, et al. Abnormal left ventricular-left atrial posterior wall contour: a new two-dimensional echocardiographic sign in constrictive pericarditis. Am Heart J 1989; 118: 128.

79. Veress G, Ling LH, Kim KH, et al. Mitral and tricuspid annular velocities before and after pericardiectomy in patients with constrictive pericarditis. Circ Cardiovasc Imaging 2011; 4: 399.

80. Rienmüller R, Doppman JL, Lissner J, et al. Constrictive pericardial disease: prognostic significance of a nonvisualized left ventricular wall. Radiology 1985; 156: 753.

81. Verhaert D, Gabriel RS, Johnston D, et al. The role of multimodality imaging in the management of pericardial disease. Circ Cardiovasc Imaging 2010; 3: 333.

82. Masui T, Finck S, Higgins CB. Constrictive pericarditis and restrictive cardiomyopathy: evaluation with MR imaging. Radiology 1992; 182: 369.

83. Zurick AO, Bolen MA, Kwon DH, et al. Pericardial delayed hyperenhancement with CMR imaging in patients with constrictive pericarditis undergoing surgical pericardiectomy: a case series with histopathological correlation. JACC Cardiovasc Imaging 2011; 4: 1180.

84. Haley JH, Tajik AJ, Danielson GK, et al. Transient constrictive pericarditis: causes and natural history. J Am Coll Cardiol 2004; 43: 271.

85. Sagristà-Sauleda J, Permanyer-Miralda G, Candell-Riera J, et al. Transient cardiac constriction: an unrecognized pattern of evolution in effusive acute idiopathic pericarditis. Am J Cardiol 1987; 59: 961.

86. DeValeria PA, Baumgartner WA, Casale AS, et al. Current indications, risks, and outcome after pericardiectomy. Ann Thorac Surg 1991; 52: 219.

87. Hancock EW. A clearer view of effusive-constrictive pericarditis. N Engl J Med 2004; 350: 435.

88. Sagristà-Sauleda J, Angel J, Sánchez A, et al. Effusive-constrictive pericarditis. N Engl J Med 2004; 350: 469.

89. Sagristà-Sauleda J, Mercé J, Permanyer-Miralda G, Soler-Soler J. Clinical clues to the causes of large pericardial effusions. Am J Med 2000; 109: 95.

90. Ewart W. Practical aids in the diagnosis of pericardial effusion, in connection with the question as to surgical treatment. Br Med J 1896; 1: 717.

91. Weiss JM, Spodick DH. Association of left pleural effusion with pericardial disease. N Engl J Med 1983; 308: 696.

92. Tuon FF, Litvoc MN, Lopes MI. Adenosine deaminase and tuberculous pericarditis–a systematic review with meta-analysis. Acta Trop 2006; 99: 67.

93. Levy PY, Fournier PE, Charrel R, et al. Molecular analysis of pericardial fluid: a 7-year experience. Eur Heart J 2006; 27: 1942.

94. Ben-Horin S, Bank I, Shinfeld A, et al. Diagnostic value of the biochemical composition of pericardial effusions in patients undergoing pericardiocentesis. Am J Cardiol 2007; 99: 1294.

95. Sagristà-Sauleda J, Angel J, Sambola A, et al. Low-pressure cardiac tamponade: clinical and hemodynamic profile. Circulation 2006; 114: 945.

96. Shabetai R. Pericardial effusion: haemodynamic spectrum. Heart 2004; 90: 255.

97. Brown J, MacKinnon D, King A, Vanderbush E. Elevated arterial blood pressure in cardiac tamponade. N Engl J Med 1992; 327: 463.

98. Meyer TE, Sareli P, Marcus RH, et al. Mechanism underlying Kussmaul's sign in chronic constrictive pericarditis. Am J Cardiol 1989; 64: 1069.

99. Spodick DH. Images in cardiology. Truly total electric alternation of the heart. Clin Cardiol 1998; 21: 427–8.

100. Himelman RB, Kircher B, Rockey DC, Schiller NB. Inferior vena cava plethora with blunted respiratory response: a sensitive echocardiographic sign of cardiac tamponade. J Am Coll Cardiol 1988; 12: 1470.

101. Mercé J, Sagristà-Sauleda J, Permanyer-Miralda G, et al. Correlation between clinical and Doppler echocardiographic findings in patients with moderate and large pericardial effusion: implications for the diagnosis of cardiac tamponade. Am Heart J 1999; 138: 759.

102. Restrepo CS, Lemos DF, Lemos JA, et al. Imaging findings in cardiac tamponade with emphasis on CT. Radiographics 2007; 27: 1595.

103. Kolski BC, Kakimoto W, Levin DL, Blanchard DG. Echocardiographic assessment of the accuracy of computed tomography in the diagnosis of hemodynamically significant pericardial effusions. J Am Soc Echocardiogr 2008; 21: 377.

104. Sagristà-Sauleda J, Angel J, Sambola A, Permanyer-Miralda G. Hemodynamic effects of volume expansion in patients with cardiac tamponade. Circulation 2008; 117: 1545.

105. Uramoto H, Hanagiri T. Video-assisted thoracoscopic pericardiectomy for malignant pericardial effusion. Anticancer Res 2010; 30: 4691.

106. Klatt EC, Heitz DR. Cardiac metastases. Cancer 1990; 65: 1456.

107. Maisch B, Ristic A, Pankuweit S. Evaluation and management of pericardial effusion in patients with neoplastic disease. Prog Cardiovasc Dis 2010; 53: 157.

108. Olson JE, Ryan MB, Blumenstock DA. Eleven years' experience with pericardial-peritoneal window in the management of malignant and benign pericardial effusions. Ann Surg Oncol 1995; 2: 165.

109. Hankins JR, Satterfield JR, Aisner J, et al. Pericardial window for malignant pericardial effusion. Ann Thorac Surg 1980; 30: 465.

110. Liu G, Crump M, Goss PE, et al. Prospective comparison of the sclerosing agents doxycycline and bleomycin for the primary management of malignant pericardial effusion and cardiac tamponade. J Clin Oncol 1996; 14: 3141.

111. Tomkowski WZ, Wiśniewska J, Szturmowicz M, et al. Evaluation of intrapericardial cisplatin administration in cases with recurrent malignant pericardial effusion and cardiac tamponade. Support Care Cancer 2004; 12: 53.

112. Martinoni A, Cipolla CM, Cardinale D, et al. Long-term results of intrapericardial chemotherapeutic treatment of malignant pericardial effusions with thiotepa. Chest 2004; 126: 1412.

113. Gunukula SR, Spodick DH. Pericardial disease in renal patients. Semin Nephrol 2001; 21: 52.

114. Banerjee A, Davenport A. Changing patterns of pericardial disease in patients with end-stage renal disease. Hemodial Int 2006; 10: 249.

27

Venous thromboembolic disease in older adults

Marina Shcherba, Henny H. Billett, and Laurie G. Jacobs

SUMMARY

Venous thromboembolic (VTE) disease, comprising deep venous thrombosis and pulmonary embolism (PE), is a common and potentially morbid or fatal condition in older adults. The increase in risk observed in the elderly is usually associated with concurrent conditions rather than intrinsic hypercoagulability. Clinical data support thromboprophylaxis for the majority of patients in the hospital setting. Recommendations for continuing preventative therapy after hospital discharge are less well defined. Treatment and secondary prevention of VTE are discussed during three periods of time—acute treatment beginning with suspicion of the diagnosis through stabilization on an anticoagulant, long-term therapy following diagnosis (usually 3–6 months), and extended therapy which may continue indefinitely for some patients.

EPIDEMIOLOGY

Venous thromboembolic (VTE) disease, comprising deep vein thrombosis (DVT) and pulmonary embolism (PE), is a common medical condition, particularly among the elderly. It is considered to be the third most common cardiovascular disorder after acute coronary syndromes and stroke. There were about 247,000 admissions for PE in the USA in 2006 (1), with an estimated 3 month mortality of 10–18%. The majority of deaths occur during the first week following the diagnosis (2). Due to more rapid recognition and better treatment, in-hospital case-fatality rates have declined from 5.9% in 2001–2002 to 2.4% in 2007–2008 for the first PE, and from 11.4% (2001–2002) to 7.1% for any PE (2007–2008), but this level is still clearly too high.

VTE disease is much more common in the elderly. The Worcester Venous Thromboembolism study suggested that adults over the age of 75 years have a 16-fold increase in the incidence of VTE as compared with adults under the age of 55 years (3). A study of male inpatients at 16 short-stay hospitals identified a 10-fold increase in the annual incidence of DVT for hospitalized medical patients from age 55 to 75 years old (4). A large community-based study from France supports this; they identified the annual incidence of symptomatic VTE to be 1.83 per 1000 (1.24 for DVT and 0.60 for PE) in patients <55 years, which rose with age, regardless of gender, to 10 per 1000 in those older than 75 years (5).

PATHOPHYSIOLOGY

Virchow's triad is a widely accepted theory delineating the pathophysiology of venous thromboembolic disease. It postulates that venous stasis, vascular injury, and hypercoagulability lead to the development of thrombosis.

Venous stasis can occur during periods of immobility, or due to internal or external obstruction to blood flow. Most venous thrombi occur in the venous sinuses of lower extremities and at the bifurcations of the venous system in areas with the slowest blood flow. Venous stasis due to decreased mobility, such as that associated with limb paralysis after a stroke or an orthopedic procedure, is more frequently associated with thrombosis in elderly patients. Chronic medical conditions, including congestive heart failure, recent myocardial infarction, chronic pulmonary disease, osteoarthritis, varicose veins, and other debilitating diseases, decrease mobility and increase venous stasis, increasing the VTE risk. Diseases that more often affect the elderly such as polycythemia, hypergammaglobulinemia, dysproteinemia, or cryoglobulinemia can also promote venous stasis and thrombosis.

Vascular injury plays an important role in the elderly patient, and can occur directly with endothelial disruption from trauma, or indirectly from burns, endotoxin exposure, and/or the increased release of inflammatory cytokines accompanying many medical and surgical conditions (6). Endothelial damage leads to the expression of tissue factor, either directly from endothelial cells or from monocytes attracted to the site of damage, which promotes factor VII activation and coagulation. Endothelial damage also results in subendothelial exposure of collagen and von Willebrand factor, which in turn lead to platelet adhesion and aggregation, resulting in local hypercoagulability at the site of injury (7).

Genetic abnormalities producing *hypercoagulability* are rarely first identified in the elderly patient, as most present at an earlier age. The most frequent causes of an inherited (primary) hypercoagulable state are the factor V Leiden mutation and the prothrombin gene mutation, which together account for 50% to 60% of cases. Defects in protein S, protein C, and antithrombin III account for the majority of the remaining cases. Testing for genetic causes of hypercoagulability is generally not recommended in elderly patients with VTE as it rarely changes the overall management. Testing for antiphospholipid syndrome in an elderly patient with history of multiple VTEs, miscarriage, and a positive family history of thrombosis, however, is a justifiable exception.

Acquired rather than congenital hypercoagulability predominates in the geriatric population due to the increased incidence of malignancy, trauma, surgery, and systemic infection. Malignancy induces a hypercoagulable state by several mechanisms. Malignant cells can produce a procoagulant protein that directly stimulates factor X, bypassing the intrinsic and extrinsic coagulation systems, and resulting in accelerated conversion of prothrombin to thrombin. Tissue trauma associated with cancer surgery increases tissue thromboplastin, leading to increased levels of procoagulants and thrombosis (8). Cancer cells also have the ability to activate platelets directly, further promoting thrombosis.

Thus, conditions that predispose to venous stasis, vascular injury, and hypercoagulability, are common in the elderly and appear to play an important pathophysiological role, explaining much of the epidemiologic increase in incidence of VTE in this population. Despite the identifiable underlying conditions which predispose elderly to VTE, it should be noted that 26–45% of VTE cases have no identifiable cause (9).

THROMBOPROPHYLAXIS

Identification of appropriate patients and selection of effective and safe agents for VTE prophylaxis are areas of much investigation. The role of thromboprophylaxis in patients at the highest risk for VTE, particularly hospitalized medical patients, including those with cancer, surgical patients, and orthopedic patients, has been extensively evaluated over the past decade (10–12) and the efficacy of VTE thromboprophylaxis in selected groups of patients has been confirmed by randomized controlled studies.

Age alone is often considered sufficient criteria for thromboprophylaxis in hospitalized patients. A recent prospective multicenter study showed that elderly patients with VTE were more likely to have been hospitalized (75% vs. 52%, $p < 0.001$) or to have been immobilized for more than 3 days. They were also more likely to have infections, respiratory, renal or heart dysfunction, diabetes, stroke history, and cancer-associated VTE (30% vs. 20%) (13).

Hospitalized Medical Patients

As acutely ill medical patients may have as much as an eightfold increase in the incidence of VTE, it would seem appropriate to administer thromboprophylaxis to all patients, but the attendant increased bleeding risk, cost, and adverse effects of therapy may offset the apparent gains. The risk versus benefit ratio for anticoagulation must be constantly assessed. One approach to deciding whether to prescribe VTE prophylaxis for hospitalized patients is to "objectively" assess VTE risk with an established risk assessment instrument such as the Padua Prediction Score (Fig. 27.1) (14). The Padua Prediction Score stratifies hospitalized patients into high and low risk groups by assigning points to the 11 most common risk factors. Patients with fewer than four points have been found to have a very low incidence of VTE (0.3%) and do not require prophylaxis. Patients with >4 points have a higher risk for VTE (11%), suggesting the need for prophylaxis.

Table 27.1 summarizes many of the American College of Chest Physicians (ACCP) Clinical Practice Guidelines' major recommendations for thromboprophylaxis in hospitalized medical patients. Either low molecular weight heparin (LMWH) or unfractionated heparin (UFH) is recommended for thromboprophylaxis for medical patients, as both have been found to reduce the incidence of DVT in patients admitted to a medical service, including the elderly (15–18).

Patients with cancer have been found to have a four to sixfold increase in the incidence of DVT (19). The incidence of VTE in elderly cancer patients is higher than that in younger cancer patients, mirroring the increased risk due to age-associated comorbid conditions, frequent hospitalizations, and prolonged immobilization. The risk of VTE depends on the type of cancer, stage, administration of chemotherapy and/or hormonal therapy, surgical interventions, presence of an indwelling central venous catheter, age, immobilization,

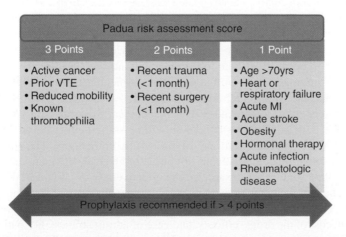

Figure 27.1 Padua risk assessment score for thromboprophylaxis (14). *Abbreviations*: MI, myocardial infarction; VTE, venous thromboembolism.

Table 27.1 Summary of the American College of Chest Physicians (ACCP) Clinical Practice Guidelines for Thromboprophylaxis for Elderly Hospitalized Medical Patients (10)

Thromboprophylaxis for the Elderly Hospitalized Medical Patient	
Acutely ill at low risk of thrombosis and age <70 years	No pharmacologic prophylaxis or mechanical prophylaxis (1B)
Acutely ill at increased risk of thrombosis	LMWH, LDUH, or fondaparinux (1B) during acute hospital stay (2B)
Increased risk of thrombosis with risk for major bleeding	Mechanical thromboprophylaxis with GCS/IPC (2C)
Critically ill	LMWH or LDUH thromboprophylaxis (2C)
Critically ill at risk for major bleeding	GCS and/or IPC at least until the bleeding risk decreases (2C)

Abbreviations: IPC, intermittent pneumatic compression; GCS, graduated compression stockings; LDUH, low dose unfractionated heparin; LMWH, low molecular weight heparin.

and prior history of VTE. Clinical decision-making regarding VTE prophylaxis must be done in the context of an assessment of prognosis and definition of the goals of care. LMWH, UFH, and fondaparinux are anticoagulants recommended for thromboprophylaxis in hospitalized cancer patients with acute illness and expected immobility (20).

Elderly patients admitted with an acute ischemic or hemorrhagic stroke for whom a prolonged immobilization may be anticipated are also at increased risk of VTE. Options for VTE prophylaxis in patients with acute ischemic stroke include anticoagulants or mechanical methods of thromboprophylaxis. The selection is dependent on an evaluation of the risk of hemorrhage as compared to the risk of recurrent stroke (21).

Surgical Patients

As increasing numbers of the elderly are undergoing major surgery, either electively or urgently, perioperative VTE prevention in this group of patients becomes even more important. Postoperative VTE risk depends upon a number of factors, some of which are related to the surgical procedure itself, such as the degree of invasiveness, type and duration of anesthesia, and requirement for immobilization. Patient-related adverse risk factors include, but are not limited to, increasing age, history of prior DVT, presence of malignancy, obesity, thrombophilia, or one or more significant medical conditions such as heart disease, infection, or recent stroke.

The presence or absence of procedural and individual risk factors described enables surgical patients to be stratified into low, moderate, and high risk for the development of VTE. Table 27.2 summarizes the current ACCP recommendations for surgical thromboprophylaxis as applicable to an older adult population. For surgical patients, anticoagulant prophylaxis is generally recommended over mechanical methods unless the patient is at high risk for bleeding. Ideally prophylaxis should be started either before or shortly after surgery, and continued at least until the patient is fully ambulatory. The administration of prophylaxis for longer than a month has not been studied. Several meta-analyses and randomized controlled studies have examined the effectiveness of UFH, LMWH, mechanical prophylaxis, and antiplatelet therapy in reducing the incidence of VTE in hospitalized surgical patients. The actual choice of agent is usually driven by consideration of the patient's renal function, cost of the drugs, efficacy, and ease of administration. For patients undergoing neuraxial anesthesia or analgesia, special precautions are required to mitigate the risk of bleeding and cord compression from a spinal hematoma (22).

Table 27.2 Summary of Current ACCP Recommendations for Surgical Thromboprophylaxis for the Elderly (11)

Thromboprophylaxis for the Elderly Surgical Patient	
Low risk of thrombosis and age <70 years	Mechanical thromboprophylaxis with IPC over GCS (2C) If early ambulation, no pharmacologic prophylaxis or mechanical prophylaxis needed (1B)
Moderate risk of thrombosis	LMWH (2B), LDUH (2B), or IPC (2C)
High risk of thrombosis	LMWH (1B) or LDUH (1B) and IPC/GCS (2C)
High risk and undergoing abdominal/pelvic surgery for cancer	Extended-duration, postoperative LMWH for 4 weeks (Grade 1B)
Moderate to high risk of thrombosis and high risk for major bleeding	GCS and/or IPC at least until the bleeding risk decreases (2C)

Abbreviations: IPC, intermittent pneumatic compression; GCS, graduated compression stockings; LDUH, low dose unfractionated heparin; LMWH, low molecular weight heparin.

For vascular surgery patients, the ACCP has recommended that anticoagulant prophylaxis not be used unless additional risk factors are present (11). If present, then low dose UFH or LMWH is preferred. In contrast, elderly patients undergoing general, thoracic, abdominal, or pelvic surgery, including major open urologic and gynecologic surgery, usually require VTE prophylaxis due to age and other comorbid risk factors.

Orthopedic Surgery Patients

Orthopedic surgery is commonly performed in older adults, particularly hip fracture surgery and elective total knee and hip replacement. These patients have an especially high risk for VTE due to a combination of procedure-associated and individual risk factors. Due to increased attention to VTE prophylaxis, the incidence of in-hospital VTE in orthopedic patients admitted for total hip and total knee replacement decreased from 15–50% in the 1980s to 1–2% in 2001 (23). It has become clear that greater than 50–70% of all VTEs in orthopedic patients, however, occur following discharge, with hip replacement-associated VTEs often occurring more than 1 month after discharge, while most post-knee replacement VTEs occur in the first 2 weeks (24). This evidence supports a growing interest in extending postoperative thromboprophylaxis for patients undergoing orthopedic or major abdominal surgery (24,25).

In contrast to medical patients, there appears to be a significant difference in the benefit of thromboprophylaxis with one type of heparin over another. Several randomized trials have studied the use of UFH or LMWH for VTE prophylaxis in orthopedic surgery patients and have found that LMWH is consistently associated with a superior efficacy and reduction in asymptomatic DVT by 50% (12).

The new oral anticoagulant (NOAC) agents—rivaroxaban, dabigatran, and apixaban—have demonstrated efficacy for thromboprophylaxis. Pooled analyses of four major phase III studies comparing oral rivaroxaban (a factor Xa inhibitor) with subcutaneous enoxaparin (LMWH) for the prevention of VTE after total hip or knee arthroplasty have shown significant reductions in symptomatic VTE and all-cause mortality (odds ratio 0.48; 95% CI 0.30–0.76) and a nonsignificant increase in bleeding (2.8% vs. 2.5% with LMWH) (26). Dabigatran has been studied in patients undergoing total hip or knee replacement surgery in three large randomized trials, RE-MODEL (27), RE-NOVATE (28), and RE-MOBILIZE (29), and was found to be noninferior to enoxaparin in the first two trials, with comparable bleeding risks. However, in RE-MOBILIZE, which used a higher dose of LMWH heparin comparable to that used in the USA, dabigatran failed to reach the noninferiority end point. Clinical trials evaluating apixaban for VTE prophylaxis are currently underway in the USA (30).

Elderly Patients in NonHospital Institutional Settings

A few large observational studies have found the incidence of VTE in long-term nursing home residents to be about 1% (31). As a result, routine use of thromboprophylaxis in chronically immobilized persons residing at home or in a nursing home is not recommended. For those in postacute (subacute) care, the risk is only slightly higher, 1.0–2.4% (32). For patients recovering from orthopedic surgery in the subacute setting of a nursing home, however, specifically total hip replacement or hip fracture surgery, thromboprophlaxis is recommended to be continued for 35 days postoperatively (12). Data are limited regarding the benefits, risks, and costs of the use of prophylaxis for orthopedic patients or those with a new hemiparesis who have not regained ambulatory status by 35 days.

Community-Dwelling Patients with Cancer

Patients with cancer often have several risk factors for VTE including conditions causing stasis and hypercoagulability, and may also suffer endovascular injury as the result of the use of transvenous catheters and procedures. In addition, a prior history of VTE, hormonal therapy, use of angiogenesis inhibitors such as thalidomide or lenalidomide, may impose additional risk. The 2012 ACCP guidelines (10) and the 2011 Clinical Practice Guidelines in Oncology from the National Comprehensive Cancer Network (NCCN) do not recommend routine VTE prophylaxis in ambulatory patients with cancer, except for those with multiple myeloma receiving thalidomide or lenalidomide plus chemotherapy or dexamethasone, due to the lack of definitive evidence for efficacy in cancer patients (33). Moreover, routine prophylaxis with anticoagulants, such as LMWH, low dose UFH (LDUH) or warfarin, with the use of indwelling central venous catheters in cancer patients, is not recommended (34).

VTE DIAGNOSIS
Clinical Presentation
Deep Venous Thrombosis

DVTs may be asymptomatic or present with leg pain, tenderness, swelling, erythema, and/or skin discoloration. Other clinical features can include venous distension, a palpable cord representing a thrombosed vessel, and/or the prominence of superficial veins or cyanosis. Due to the variety of clinical findings, the clinical diagnosis of DVT is nonspecific and requires further testing for confirmation. Moreover, the degree of clinical symptomatology does not correlate with the extent of thrombosis. The differential diagnosis for patients suspected of having a DVT includes a muscle strain or tear, twisting injury, lymphangitis or lymphatic obstruction, venous reflux, popliteal cyst, cellulitis, chronic venous stasis, or abnormality of the knee joint. In an elderly population, chronic medical conditions, including heart failure, kidney disease, peripheral vascular disease with venous stasis, leg swelling in a paralyzed limb, and severe osteoarthritis, may also raise the suspicion of DVT.

Pulmonary Embolism

PE is underrecognized and underdiagnosed in the elderly. PEs may be asymptomatic or present with dyspnea (73–78%), tachypnea (60–70%), pleuritic chest pain (44–65%), cough (30–37%), tachycardia (24–30%), or hemoptysis (9–13%) (35). Cardiovascular collapse, hypotension, syncope, and coma are usually associated with a massive PE. Other more subtle findings include an unexplained arrhythmia, fever, wheezing, anxiety, and confusion. Electrocardiographic (ECG) findings such as the new onset of atrial fibrillation, right bundle branch block, or signs of right heart strain with an $S_1Q_3T_3$ pattern may also be observed (36). The differential diagnosis of PE includes the whole spectrum of cardiopulmonary diseases from pneumonia and myocardial infarction to congestive heart failure and cardiac tamponade. Absent the classic features of PE, such symptoms are commonly attributed to exacerbations of chronic underlying cardiopulmonary conditions by both physicians and elderly patients (37,38). Elderly patients present less often with chest or pleuritic pain, and more often with tachycardia and syncope when compared with younger patients (39).

Chest pain and abnormalities in vital signs are often present in younger patients with VTE, but are less common in the elderly (40). One study indicated that elderly patients tend to develop acute pulmonary hypertension more often than younger patients, which may account for the increased incidence of syncope (40). It is estimated that about 10% of all hospital deaths are attributed to PE; about 80% of those aged 60 years or greater occur in patients without any prior surgery or immobility. Heightened clinical suspicion and an understanding of the different presentations of PE in the elderly will result in appropriate testing and treatment of this disease.

Elderly patients diagnosed with a DVT during an outpatient visit have a similar incidence of an associated acute PE to that observed in younger patients, but the elderly require hospitalization at the time of diagnosis more often than their younger counterparts (74% vs. 65%) (41). Elderly in-patients with acute PE more frequently have an elevation in cardiac biomarkers (troponin and brain naturetic protein [BNP]) when compared with younger patients (41). Massive PE in the elderly is estimated to comprise 5–6% of PEs but more than two-thirds of elderly patients with a massive PE do not undergo thrombectomy or thrombolytic therapy, presumably due to their risk of bleeding and comorbidities (14,41,42).

Clinical Decision Rules

Due to the variable and nonspecific nature of the clinical symptoms of both DVT and PE in general, and in elderly patients in particular, all patients require further evaluation upon clinical suspicion of VTE. Frequently, the first step is to assess the pretest probability of DVT or PE based upon the clinical presentation through the use of a clinical prediction rule. These rules weigh signs, symptoms, and other risk factors to either increase or decrease the likelihood of the diagnosis of DVT or PE. Two widely accepted and validated instruments are the Wells' score for DVT (43,44) and PE (45) and the Geneva score (46,47).

The modified Wells' score is a point system based on nine clinical characteristics with one point assigned for each as shown in Figure 27.2. DVT is likely if the score is >2 and unlikely if the score is ≤1. Since it is critical to determine whether another diagnosis is more or less likely, the subjective assessment is dependent on the clinical acumen of the physician. The Wells' score for suspected PE is based upon seven similar clinical parameters: three points each for clinical signs and symptoms of DVT (leg swelling, pain with palpation) or if "PE as likely as or more likely than an alternative diagnosis"; one and a half points each for heart rate higher than 100 beats/min, immobilization (bedrest for three consecutive days), surgery in the previous 4 weeks, or previous objectively diagnosed VTE; and one point each for the presence of hemoptysis or malignancy. A score of <2 signifies a low pretest probability; 2–6, an intermediate probability; and a score of >6, a high pretest probability of PE, correlating with a confirmed diagnosis of PE in 1.3%, 16.2%, and 37.5% of patients through further testing (46).

The Geneva score (47) and modified Geneva score (48) are alternative validated clinical decision rules for the diagnosis of PE, which take into consideration the patient's age and the presence or absence of unilateral leg edema. They are based on eight clinical characteristics only, but are complex. The modified Geneva score is used more frequently and has a scoring system as follows: 1 point each for age >65 years, prior history of DVT, active malignancy, surgery or fracture within 1 month, unilateral limb pain, hemoptysis, pain on deep vein palpation of lower limb and unilateral edema, or a heart rate 75–94 beats per minute. If the heart rate is greater than 94 beats per minute, an additional point is added. A score of <2 suggests that PE is unlikely, whereas a score ≥2 suggests that PE is a likely diagnosis. The Wells' and Geneva modified scoring systems are compared in Figure 27.3.

A number of prognostic indicators have been studied to identify unstable PE patients who may be at high risk of mortality. Patients with a coexisting DVT, elevated cardiac markers (troponin and BNP), right ventricular thrombus, or right ventricular dysfunction on echocardiogram, are at an increased risk of early mortality from PE (48,49). The most well-known of these assessment indicators is called the PE Severity Index (PESI), which estimates the risk of 30-day mortality in patients with an acute PE. A simplified PESI score (41) assigns one point for each of the following variables: age >80 years, a history of cancer,

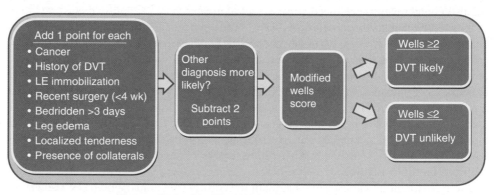

Figure 27.2   Modified Wells' Score for DVT (43).

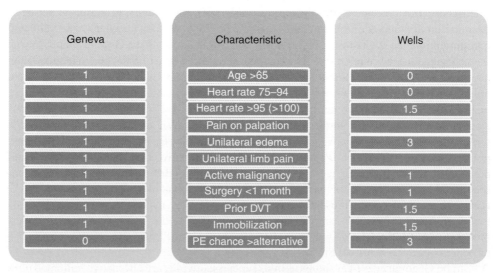

Geneva	Characteristic	Wells
1	Age >65	0
1	Heart rate 75–94	0
1	Heart rate >95 (>100)	1.5
1	Pain on palpation	
1	Unilateral edema	3
1	Unilateral limb pain	
1	Active malignancy	1
1	Surgery <1 month	1
1	Prior DVT	1.5
1	Immobilization	1.5
0	PE chance >alternative	3

<2 for each = unlikely diagnosis

Figure 27.3   Comparison of the Geneva Score and the Wells' clinical probability score for PE (45,47).

chronic cardiopulmonary disease, a heart rate greater than or equal to 110 beats per minute, a systolic blood pressure less than 100 mmHg, and an arterial oxygen saturation less than 90%. A total point score of zero indicates a low 30-day mortality risk (1.1%) from VTE, while a score of one or more indicates high 30-day mortality (8.9%) (41).

D-Dimer Testing

As noted, a clinical prediction rule in itself is not sufficient to exclude or accept the diagnosis of VTE and depends, particularly for the Wells' scoring system, on the subjective ability to assess alternative diagnoses correctly. Additional testing for confirmation is required. For patients who fall into a low pretest probability grouping for DVT and/or PE, D-dimer testing is recommended to exclude DVT or PE. The high negative predictive value of the D-dimer makes further testing unnecessary.

The D-dimer is a degradation product of cross-linked fibrin. It is formed when cross-linked fibrin undergoes proteolysis by plasmin. The D-dimer can be detected in the blood by variety of different assays. The quantitative enzyme-linked immunosorbent assay (ELISA) is most commonly used, with a level of greater than 500 ng/mL considered to be abnormal (50). D-dimer assays have been studied extensively, and in general, they are characterized by having a good sensitivity and negative predictive value but poor specificity and positive predictive value. The sensitivity of the D-dimer is about 95%; abnormal levels are found in 95% of patients with PE when measured by ELISA, rapid quantitative ELISA and semiquantitative ELISA techniques. D-dimer levels are normal in only 40–68% of patients who do not have a PE, regardless of the assay used, attesting to the low specificity for PE. Abnormal D-dimer levels are common in hospitalized patients due to a number of chronic and acute medical conditions. Specificity decreases further with increasing age. In one study, the specificity of D-dimer decreased from 67% in patients ≤40 years of age to 10% in those ≥80 years (51).

A normal D-dimer level in combination with low pretest probability, as assessed by clinical prediction rules, effectively rules out a DVT or PE. The 2012 ACCP guidelines recommend testing for the D-dimer level rather than proceeding to the use of a compression ultrasound of the proximal veins as the initial diagnostic modality for all patients with low pretest probability of a first lower extremity DVT. In patients with moderate pretest probability of DVT, the D-dimer test or a compression ultrasound of proximal veins is recommended, but the D-dimer is preferred as the initial test. If the D-dimer is positive in either case, then compression ultrasound is recommended to diagnose thrombosis and assess its site and extent. In patients with high pretest probability, D-dimer testing is not recommended as a "stand alone" test (52).

Although prediction rules have been validated in clinical studies, they are generally more applicable for use in younger patients. Two studies analyzing the applicability of the pretest probability combined with D-dimer testing to rule out PE have noted that elderly patients are more likely to be assigned to the high pretest probability category. About 71–78% in those aged >60 years were assigned to high pretest probability for PE as compared to 40–64% in those younger than age sixty due to similarity in presentation of PE to many other acute and chronic conditions in elderly (53,54).

Imaging Modalities
Imaging Modalities for DVT

A number of noninvasive and invasive imaging modalities can be used to diagnose DVT. In patients with high pretest probability of DVT, the ACCP recommends *proximal compression ultrasonography (CUS)* or *whole-leg ultrasound* as the initial diagnostic test (52). CUS remains the most commonly used diagnostic test for the diagnosis of lower and upper extremity DVT. The diagnosis of DVT by CUS is established by a number of findings such as abnormal compressibility of the vein, abnormal color Doppler flow, or the presence of an echogenic band. The inability to compress a vein using B-mode ultrasonography has high sensitivity (97%) and specificity (98%) for proximal thromboses but a reduced sensitivity (73%) for distal clots (55,56), which can be enhanced by using color Doppler or triplex scanning. In symptomatic patients, color-flow scanning was 100% sensitive and 98% specific for clots in veins above the knee, and 94% sensitive and 75% specific for those below the knee (57). The presence of an echogenic band, however, has a specificity of only 50% even though it is considered sensitive for the diagnosis of DVT. CUS has some limitations: it does not detect thrombi in the iliac vein and has limited value in patients with leg deformities, excessive fluid, or a plaster cast. Moreover, patients with pelvic neoplasms or abscesses may demonstrate isolated noncompressibility of the vein even when a thrombosis is absent (58).

In patients with a high pretest probability and a positive proximal CUS or whole-leg ultrasound, treatment is recommended. In patients with a high pretest probability but a negative proximal CUS, additional testing is warranted with either whole-leg ultrasound, highly-sensitive D-dimer or repeat CUS in 1 week. In patients with an initial negative CUS but a positive D-dimer, whole-leg ultrasound or repeat CUS in 1 week is recommended by the ACCP. For patients with a high pretest probability but negative serial proximal CUSs, a negative single proximal CUS and a negative highly sensitive D-dimer, or a negative whole-leg ultrasound, no further testing is recommended. If the whole-leg ultrasound detects isolated distal DVT, then serial testing should be done to rule out proximal extension (52).

Contrast venography, long considered the gold standard for the diagnosis of DVT, is no longer recommended as an initial screening test due to patient discomfort, difficulty in obtaining an adequate study, dye load, and the potential for causing a thrombosis due to the procedure. *Magnetic resonance venography (MRV)*, on the other hand, is as accurate as contrast venography and is a noninvasive but more expensive approach to the diagnosis of DVT. One study evaluated eighty-five patients with suspected DVT who underwent contrast venography and MRV from the inferior vena cava to the popliteal veins. MRV had a sensitivity of 100%, a specificity of 96%, and negative predictive value of 100% (59). Changes in the signal from the clot over time may also allow estimation of the age of the thrombus (60). This noninvasive diagnostic modality has not gained widespread popularity due to its high cost but is useful in difficult diagnostic situations.

Imaging Modalities for PE

The accurate diagnosis of PE is important in elderly patients due to the increased prevalence of disease and often atypical presentation. Although a number of preliminary findings might raise the suspicion for PE, including ECG abnormalities, abnormal oxygen saturation, tachycardia, and elevated cardiac markers, confirmatory tests are necessary to establish a diagnosis. As with the diagnosis of DVT, clinical prediction rules and pretest assessment of the probability of PE are important. In the case of a low or moderate pretest probability of PE, D-dimer testing is recommended. If negative, the diagnosis of PE is unlikely (61). If a D-dimer test is positive, the physician should proceed to an imaging modality, preferably helical CT pulmonary angiography (CT-PA), also known as CT angiography (CTA) (62).

Helical CT pulmonary angiography (CT-PA) has increasingly become the preferred diagnostic modality for the diagnosis of PE as it is relatively safe, provides a rapid diagnosis, and detects alternative diagnoses for patient's symptoms such as pneumonia, atelectasis, or other pulmonary disease (63,64). In the PIOPED II study, the sensitivity of CT-PA was 83% (65). Importantly, 96% of patients without a PE had a negative CT-PA, demonstrating good specificity for the test. Venous-phase imaging improves the sensitivity to 90%, while maintaining a similar specificity of 95%. PEs that are not identified by this diagnostic test tend to be more peripheral in the lung and smaller. Studies suggest that specificity, sensitivity, negative, and positive predictive values for CT-PA do not change with age (66,67). This modality is preferred for elderly patients but may be limited in those with morbid obesity, renal insufficiency, or contrast allergy.

The *ventilation/perfusion (V/Q) lung scan* was extensively studied for use in the diagnosis of PE in the PIOPED study, in which it was compared with the gold standard pulmonary angiography (68). The accuracy of the V/Q scan was greatest when the test was combined with a prior clinical probability assessment. In the PIOPED study, patients with a high clinical probability of PE and a high probability V/Q scan had a 95% likelihood of having a PE. Those who had low probability of PE and a low probability V/Q scan had only a 4% likelihood of having a PE. Most patients fell into the intermediate probability range, however, where the diagnostic accuracy of the V/Q scan ranged from 15% to 86%, and additional testing was required to make a diagnosis. In a study of unselected elderly patients, the rate of nondiagnostic V/Q scans was found to be higher than in a younger population (69). Another study noted that in patients over the age of 80 years, the diagnostic yield of V/Q lung scans was only 42%, as compared to 68% under the age of 40 years (51). In contrast to CT-PA, PEs missed by V/Q scan tended to be the clinically more important central PEs. In addition, the V/Q scan is often of limited value in elderly patients due to the high prevalence of coexistent cardiopulmonary disease. In elderly patients without cardiopulmonary disease and with contraindications to CT-PA, the V/Q lung scan remains a diagnostic option.

Like venography, *pulmonary angiography*, once considered the "gold standard" for diagnosis of PE, is no longer widely used due to the invasiveness and morbidity associated with catheter insertion and contrast load and reactions, including, cardiac arrhythmias and respiratory insufficiency. It is strictly reserved for patients with high clinical probability of PE, nondiagnostic imaging modalities, normal renal function, and very few comorbidities who are being considered for thrombolysis.

Echocardiography is not recommended as a routine imaging test to diagnose PE. However, its use has increased because it can identify patients with PE who are at risk for severe morbidity or mortality and who may therefore benefit from more aggressive initial treatment, such as thrombolysis or thrombectomy. It is estimated that 30–40% of patients with an acute PE have echocardiographic abnormalities, which include decreased right ventricular function (especially free wall hypokinesis with preserved contractility at the apex, McConnell's sign), increased right ventricular size and tricuspid regurgitation (70). Patients with a massive PE are more likely to demonstrate these abnormalities. Thus, the echocardiogram can assist in diagnosing a hemodynamically significant PE and help justify the use of thrombolytic therapy (71).

VTE THERAPY

Treatment usually requires a clinical decision regarding the use of anticoagulants. Anticoagulant therapy is recommended for the treatment of DVT or PE, but the decision to anticoagulate should always involve consideration of the potential risks and benefits. To emphasize this analysis, the ACCP has recently changed their guidelines regarding therapy for isolated distal VTE. The current guideline no longer recommends routine anticoagulation for all distal VTE. If the thrombosis is isolated to the distal veins of the lower extremity, symptoms are mild or lacking, the risk of progression is low, and there are no associated risk factors, serial diagnostic imaging over 2 weeks can be considered and a decision regarding anticoagulation can be made on the basis of progression. In patients with symptomatic distal DVT, anticoagulation is recommended for 3 months (72).

Acute medical therapies for VTE, except for thrombolytics, do not dissolve the clot. Rather, acute treatment is intended to prevent clot extension and embolization and to manage symptoms and prevent or mitigate the postthrombotic syndrome (PTS). Anticoagulant therapy should be initiated when there is a strong clinical suspicion of a DVT or PE while diagnostic testing is pursued, as the risk of extension or embolization of the thrombosis generally outweighs the potential short-term harm unless there is evidence or strong potential for acute bleeding. For patients with low probability of VTE, diagnostic testing can be pursued without initiating anticoagulation as long as results are obtained in a timely manner (73).

Treatment decisions are usually considered with regard to three sequential time periods—*initial therapy*, *long-term therapy*, and *extended therapy*. *Initial therapy* bridges the time from an initial clinical suspicion of a DVT or PE, through clinical diagnostic evaluation and confirmation, and concluding with the achievement of stable anticoagulation (if chosen). Initial therapy usually spans the first 5–7 days of treatment. *Long-term therapy* follows initial therapy for the majority of patients, and continues for at least 3 months, at which time, *extended therapy* with an anticoagulant is considered. Extended therapy may continue indefinitely. At each point, an individualized assessment of the risks of anticoagulation, principally bleeding, should be weighed against the potential benefits, including prevention of progression, cardiovascular and pulmonary compromise, recurrence, PTS, pulmonary hypertension and death.

Acute Symptom Management

Pain from venous distension and pressure due to obstruction from the thrombus can be aggravated by upright posture as well as by local inflammation causing erythema and induration. The application of heat to the site of pain and inflammation may palliate these initial symptoms. Although nonsteroidal anti-inflammatory drugs (NSAIDs) are commonly prescribed for pain and inflammation, they are relatively contraindicated in the treatment of DVT as their use increases the risk of bleeding. Pain medications such as acetaminophen may be prescribed but their efficacy is limited.

Early ambulation in patients with a DVT had been controversial but is now recommended. Clinical study indicates that ambulation is not associated with an increased risk for embolization, may reduce the risk for early extension of a proximal thrombosis, either improves or has no impact upon pain and edema, and may reduce the incidence of PTS (72).

Compression of the leg (venous system and soft tissues) is also recommended in the management of lower extremity DVT (73). It should be initiated early, certainly within 1 month of diagnosis, as compression has been demonstrated to reduce the incidence of the PTS in patients with symptomatic proximal DVT and may also reduce pain and edema. Compression is accomplished by knee high graduated elastic compression stockings exerting a pressure of 30 to 40 mmHg at the ankle, thigh high stockings (which may be superior to knee high in efficacy but are often difficult to apply), or careful application of an ACE bandage with graduated compression but allowing arterial flow. Compression therapy should be continued for 1–2 years, and indefinitely for patients who develop chronic venous insufficiency and the PTS.

Patients with an acute PE may present with hemodynamic instability and dyspnea, which can progress to cardiovascular collapse, respiratory failure, and death. Management of patients presenting with hypotension parallels that of other critically ill patients requiring hemodynamic support with fluids and vasopressors. Supplemental oxygen should be provided for treatment of hypoxemia; intubation with mechanical ventilation is indicated for severe hypoxemia and impending respiratory failure.

Anticoagulant Therapy
Heparins
Initial therapy for the majority of patients with either a DVT or PE currently includes an immediate acting anticoagulant, such as UFH, LMWH, or a synthetic heparin like fondaparinux, along with initiation of vitamin K antagonist therapy (most commonly warfarin in the USA). The parenteral agent provides immediate anticoagulation, "bridging", the period between clinical suspicion and achievement of full therapeutic anticoagulation, which if provided by a vitamin K antagonist, may take 5–7 days. Rapid and consistent achievement of a therapeutic intensity of anticoagulation is essential, as inadequate therapy with UFH, as indicated by a subtherapeutic partial thromboplastin time (PTT), in the first 24 hours, has been associated with a higher recurrence rate (5% vs. 23%) (74).

UFH administered as an intravenous infusion or by subcutaneous injection several times daily has been successfully used for initial therapy of VTE. It is less costly and less effective than LMWH or fondaparinux and is preferred for patients with significant renal insufficiency, high bleeding risk, or impending procedures which might require anticoagulation discontinuation as it has a shorter half-life (about 4 hours) than LMWHs. The major limitation of UFH is the need to achieve rapid and consistent therapeutic anticoagulation, indicated by a PTT 1.5–2.5 times greater than the control value. Due to the unpredictable binding of UFH to plasma proteins and cells, dosing is challenging, and although weight-based nomograms (75) can assist, the PTT must be monitored often with frequent adjustments in dose.

Achievement of a stable therapeutic level of anticoagulation is most problematic with the use of UFH. LMWHs, including enoxaparin, tinzaparin, and dalteparin, have more predictable pharmacokinetics than UFH, and have been associated with lower risks of bleeding, thrombocytopenia, VTE recurrence and death. They are therefore preferred for the initial treatment of both DVT (73) and PE (76). Once daily dosing, as compared with twice daily, is recommended, due to cost concerns and the ease of administration, with comparable outcomes of recurrence, bleeding, and mortality (77). LMWHs are excreted via the kidney, which can be problematic for older adults with decreased renal function. LMWHs are relatively contraindicated for those with a calculated creatinine clearance less than 30 mL/min. Enoxaparin is approved for DVT treatment whether a PE is present, or not; tinzaparin for DVT treatment; and dalteparin for extended therapy but not initial therapy for DVT. However, in practice, all three LMWHs are often prescribed interchangeably but they should not be considered equivalent in therapeutic efficacy as head-to-head trials have not been performed.

Fondaparinux, a synthetic very LMW pentasaccharide heparin is administered subcutaneously once daily. It is comparable or superior to LMWH in efficacy for initial therapy for DVT (78), and to UFH for PE (79). It has a longer half-life than UFH and LMWHs, requires dosage adjustment based upon weight, and is excreted by the kidney; as a result, significant caution is warranted in older adults.

For patients in whom VTE occurs in the setting of a malignancy, the current recommendation is to extend the initial therapy with LMWH through the period of long-term therapy, rather than bridging to warfarin therapy, as this regimen was found to achieve superior results in cancer patients (74).

New Oral Anticoagulants
The NOACs discussed earlier have been studied not only for VTE prophylaxis but also for VTE treatment. These drugs achieve a rapid state of therapeutic anticoagulation and can, in

theory, be used as initial therapy or follow bridging therapy from UFH or LMWH. All these drugs have been approved for anticoagulation in patients with nonvalvular atrial fibrillation but, as of this writing, only one drug, rivaroxaban, has been approved for VTE therapy, such approval may soon be forthcoming. Dabigatran, an oral thrombin (factor IIa) inhibitor, has been studied in patients with VTE and found to be noninferior to warfarin in a 6 month clinical trial of long-term therapy following initial parenteral anticoagulation in both groups. Compared to warfarin, dabigatran had comparable incidences of VTE recurrence (2%), major bleeding (2%), and any bleeding (17–22%) (80). Rivaroxaban, an oral factor Xa inhibitor, has been studied for use as therapy for acute symptomatic DVT (81) and PE (82). In an-open label randomized trial, it was found to be noninferior to standard enoxaparin bridged to warfarin therapy during 3–6 months of treatment. The recurrence rate in patients treated with rivaroxaban (2.1%) versus enoxaparin (3%) and the safety (8.1% major and clinically relevant bleeding in both groups), were comparable. A study of extended therapy compared rivaroxaban to placebo following long-term therapy and found it to be superior (1.3% events vs. 7.1% with placebo; hazard ratio, 0.18; 95% CI, 0.09–0.39; $p < 0.001$); bleeding was not statistically different. A parallel clinical study of PE demonstrated similar results (83). Apixaban, also an oral Xa inhibitor has undergone clinical trials for long-term anticoagulant treatment for DVT. Although there is limited clinical experience using these agents for VTE in the USA, several have been approved and are in current use for VTE in Europe.

Vitamin K Antagonists

Warfarin, a vitamin K antagonist, is still the most widely prescribed oral anticoagulant for VTE therapy, but this may change with development and increasing use of the NOACs. Warfarin should be prescribed coincidently with an immediate acting agent, such as heparin or LMWH, since it requires several days to achieve the desired anticoagulant intensity as indicated by the international normalized ratio (INR). LMWH is administered coincidently with warfarin (bridging) until 2 days of the desired therapeutic INR level (target 2.5; range 2–3) has been achieved, at which time LMWH is discontinued. This commonly requires 5–14 days. Warfarin has a narrow therapeutic index—a low INR is associated with VTE recurrence, and a high INR with bleeding. Although the risk of bleeding increases with an INR above 4.5, in clinical practice the incidence of spontaneous bleeding is low. Four randomized clinical trials compared observation to vitamin K treatment (which reverses the anticoagulant effect of warfarin) for patients with an INR of 4.5–10. No significant difference in bleeding (2% vitamin K vs. 0.8% placebo) was found (74). Warfarin has multiple drug and dietary interactions, and the maintenance dosage is unpredictable in a given individual as it is influenced by genetic factors, diet, drug use, and clinical status. These factors have made warfarin a difficult drug to manage, particularly in elderly patients who often have multiple acute and chronic conditions and medications.

Initial and chronic warfarin dosing has undergone significant study. Larger loading doses have not been proven to be advantageous in achieving a more timely sustainable therapeutic level. Although an initial dosage of 10 mg for 2 days is now recommended, (74), the 5 mg dose may be preferred for elderly patients as warfarin's pharmacokinetics are altered with age causing a greater response in INR for a given dosage. Older adults require a lower acute and chronic dosage to achieve and maintain therapeutic INR. On a population basis, a study of patients treated in an anticoagulation clinic found that the chronic dosage required to maintain a therapeutic level declines with age, with 4.9 mg as the average for adults aged 75 or less, 4 mg for those aged 75–84 years, and 3.5 mg for those aged 85 years or more (83). The timing of monitoring of the INR should be driven by the results and dosing. For patients who achieve and consistently maintain a therapeutic INR, the interval for testing can be extended to a 12-week period (74).

Community Versus Hospital Setting for Initial Therapy

The use of LMWHs, which are administered daily by subcutaneous injection (as contrasted with intravenous or multiple daily injections of UFH) and the use of the oral NOACs, has enabled the treatment of VTE to occur in the community or long-term care setting as long as appropriate clinical assessment and stability is achievable. Treatment at home has achieved comparable outcomes compared to that administered in the hospital in selected patient subgroups (84). Clinical assessment includes obtaining a medical history incorporating thrombosis and bleeding risk factors, performing a physical examination, and accessing diagnostic test results quickly. For LMWH, there must be established methods of administration of the subcutaneous injections, and, for warfarin, a means of obtaining therapeutic monitoring of the INR during bridging to vitamin K antagonist therapy. Elderly patients with PE may have more instability in vital signs, ECG, and pulse oxygenation, and may therefore be less suitable for home therapy (85). Contraindications for outpatient treatment include active bleeding, bleeding history, significant alterations in blood pressure or respiration, significant anemia, thrombocytopenia, a history of heparin-induced thrombocytopenia (HIT) or heparin (or LMWH) allergy, severe renal insufficiency (creatinine clearance <30 mL/min) or the inability to obtain or administer the drug reliably. The daily LMWH injections can be administered in the office, by self-injection, or by a home care nurse or other caregiver for the duration of bridging therapy. Although the cost of LMWH therapy may be substantial if borne by the patient, it may be covered by insurance or alternative coverage arrangements that seek to avoid the costly hospital admissions required for the standard therapies for VTE.

The use of the NOACs, which produce stable drug levels and have far fewer food and drug interactions, would further enable treatment in the community setting as no injections or INR monitoring would be necessary; however, the same initial clinical assessment is required. These drugs have not entered clinical practice for the treatment of DVT in the USA at this time, so their role remains to be established.

Inferior Vena Cava Filters

Placement of an inferior vena cava filter is recommended only for the patient in whom anticoagulation is contraindicated due to active hemorrhage or a very high risk of serious bleeding. If the bleeding risk is mitigated, anticoagulation should subsequently be initiated. A single randomized trial (86) examined the use of inferior vena cava filters placed in patients with DVT who were also treated with anticoagulation. At 8 years of follow-up, the use of inferior vena cava filters decreased the rate of subsequent PE but increased the incidence of subsequent DVT. A case series evaluating the use of filters in patients with and without anticoagulation failed to show any difference in outcomes (87).

The use of inferior vena cava filters without anticoagulation in patients with DVT who have a high risk of bleeding is a common practice, particularly in the elderly, but has not been well studied. The literature suggests that the incidence of PTS is increased. This has led to increased use of removable inferior vena cava filters, which must be extracted early in the course of treatment before the filters endothelialize. As filter retrieval in elderly patients is infrequent in clinical practice, the advantage that these filters may provide is offset by their greater migration rate before they endothelialize and fully embed, and by their increased incidence of the PTS.

Thrombolysis and Operative Thrombectomy

Treatments aimed at dissolving or removing a proximal DVT, systemic thrombolytic therapy or catheter-directed thrombolysis (CDT), for example, with or without mechanical thrombus fragmentation, may be considered for patients who are at high risk for the PTS, such as those with proximal iliac and common femoral vein thrombi. Catheter-directed therapy appears to result in a lower incidence of bleeding than systemic thrombolysis, although the evidence is limited, particularly in the elderly. Case series and a few clinical trials suggest that these therapies may more effectively reduce VTE recurrence, mortality and PTS (74). Conversely, thrombolytic therapy for VTE may be associated with increased risk for bleeding (as compared with systemic anticoagulation) in older adults due to age-related factors in conjunction with associated comorbidities. Operative thrombectomy for DVT has been even less well studied, but has yielded similar results to thrombolysis. The ACCP consensus clinical practice guidelines (72) recommend CDT over thrombectomy or operative therapy, but only for patients with an iliofemoral DVT who have had symptoms for less than 7 days, good functional status, life expectancy of greater than 1 year, and at centers with both the resources and expertise to perform the procedure.

Thrombolysis (as compared to standard systemic anticoagulation) for patients with a PE leads to more rapid resolution of the clot, but is associated with a comparable increase in the risk of bleeding. Patients with unstable or massive PE and signs of cardiopulmonary compromise (hypotension, tachycardia, tachypnea, fever, hypoxemia, elevated cardiac troponin, and abnormal ECG or echocardiographic findings) have an unfavorable prognosis and may be candidates for systemic thrombolysis or CDT, but the potential benefits must be balanced against the increased bleeding risk in older adults. Patients undergoing thrombolysis for DVT or PE must be transitioned to immediate acting anticoagulation and then bridged to long term anticoagulation.

COMPLICATIONS OF THERAPY
Bleeding Risk Assessment

An individualized assessment of the risk for bleeding is required for all patients with VTE as anticoagulation is the mainstay of therapy. This risk must be weighed against the potential benefits of anticoagulant therapy—the prevention of short and long term cardiopulmonary compromise, death, recurrent VTE, venous insufficiency, and the PTS. Clinical decision-making regarding anticoagulation in older adults is complex and nuanced by both their clinical status and their goals of care and must be explicitly discussed with the patient and, often, with their caregivers. It should also be considered carefully for patients who have a very poor prognosis or a high risk of bleeding, and for those in whom the burden (drug administration, monitoring and cost) may outweigh the potential benefits.

The discussion and clinical decision-making regarding anticoagulation therapy should reoccur at several points in the clinical course. The initial assessment of bleeding risk is undertaken and the risks and benefits weighed upon clinical suspicion or diagnosis of a DVT or PE prior to obtaining the results of the laboratory evaluation. These issues should be reassessed with any bleeding episode, prior to initiating long-term therapy, after the initial 3 months of long-term therapy (usually with warfarin), and again at the conclusion of long-term therapy, when extended therapy may be contemplated, and at least yearly thereafter if anticoagulant therapy is continued.

Although major bleeding on warfarin therapy is reported to occur in only 1–3% of patients per year, this statistic is derived from clinical trials undertaken for a variety of conditions. Often these studies have excluded patients with moderate or high risk of bleeding. The most common sites for bleeding are the gastrointestinal tract, genitourinary tract, and soft tissues, but intracranial bleeding is associated with the greatest morbidity. Age is associated with an increased risk for bleeding in general, and for intracranial hemorrhage in particular. Risk factors for bleeding include age, the intensity of anticoagulation, use of medications that may be independently associated with bleeding or interact with the prescribed anticoagulant, selected medical conditions, history of bleeding, personal risk for trauma (e.g., falls), medication adherence, and duration of anticoagulant therapy.

Concurrent use of other medications and herbals which influence platelet function such as aspirin, clopidogrel, NSAIDs, selective serotonin reuptake inhibitors (SSRIs), vitamin E and ginkgo biloba, among others, also increase the risk for bleeding, sometimes substantially. One study of patients with atrial fibrillation who were treated with both warfarin and clopidogrel reported a bleeding rate three times greater than that of patients treated with warfarin alone (88). Recent hemorrhage and concomitant medical conditions, including renal and liver disease, uncontrolled hypertension, stroke, and cancer, which may impact platelet function or coagulation factor synthesis, also increase bleeding risk.

Falls are often cited by physicians as a relative contraindication for anticoagulation. However, the risk of falling (generally about 30% per year in older adults) and sustaining further injury due to bleeding, is often outweighed by the potential benefits of anticoagulant therapy for VTE, at least during the initial and first 3 months of therapy, but this must be individualized. In a study of patients with atrial fibrillation treated with anticoagulants, the risk of an intracranial hemorrhage in a faller was twice that of a nonfaller, but the actual risk was low (2.8% vs. 1.1%) and not related to treatment with warfarin, aspirin, or no antithrombotic agent (89). In addition, some factors contributing to the risk for falls may be modifiable, such as the prescription of sedative-hypnotics and psychotropics, alcohol use, low vision, poor shoes, muscle weakness and gait problems, and orthostatic hypotension. Conversely, other fall risk factors may not be amenable to modification, for example, deficits related to stroke, parkinsonism, or dementia.

The evaluation of bleeding risk includes elements of the history, physical, and laboratory examination as described in Table 27.3. The HAS-BLED score is a commonly used instrument to evaluate bleeding risk (90). Additional items such as gait and cognitive assessment are recommended for older adults as their risk for bleeding while on anticoagulation therapy is increased.

Heparin-Induced Thrombocytopenia

Thrombocytopenia caused by heparin can occur through nonimmune (Type 1) mediated and immune (Type 2) mediated mechanisms. Type I heparin-associated thrombocytopenia occurs in 10–20% of patients (91). The decline in the platelet count is commonly seen within the first few days after initiation of heparin use, with a nadir of about $100 \times 10^9/L$. It is not a progressive thrombocytopenia and is not usually associated with bleeding. This type of heparin-associated thrombocytopenia is managed conservatively by discontinuation of heparin and monitoring of the platelet count, which usually rises to pretreatment levels within several days.

Type 2 heparin-induced thrombocytopenia, or HIT, is less common and occurs in about 1–3% of patients treated with UFH and in 0–0.8% of patients treated with LMWH (92). Clinical criteria for HIT include a fall in the platelet count by greater than 50% or to less than $100 \times 10^9/L$ within 5–14 days of initiating UFH. HIT with thrombosis or "HITT" is accompanied by a new thrombotic or thromboembolic event. Both arterial and venous events occur, but most events are venous, and include DVT, PE, and dural sinus thrombosis. Arterial thromboses, which occur in 25% of patients, include aortic occlusion, myocardial infarction, stroke, and peripheral artery thrombosis (93). Skin necrosis at the site of injection of UFH or LMWH is considered a manifestation of the HIT syndrome, even in the absence of thrombocytopenia as defined above (93). Early onset HIT may occur in up to 30% of patients with persistent antibodies due to heparin therapy within the prior 3 months (94).

Although the pathogenesis of HIT has not been fully elucidated, heparin initiates an antibody response directed against the complex of heparin and platelet factor 4 (PF4) which activates the platelets, causing thrombosis (95). An assessment of the presence and

Table 27.3 Evaluation of Bleeding Risk: The HAS-BLED Score (90)

Letter	Clinical Characteristic	Points
H	Hypertension	1
A	Abnormal liver or renal function	
	Renal: dialysis, transplant, serum creatinine>2.6 mg/dL	1
	Liver: cirrhosis, bilirubin >2×ULN, AST/ALT >3×ULN	1
S	Stroke	1
B	Bleeding (prior history or predisposition)	1
L	Labile or unstable INRs	1
E	Elderly (>65 years)	1
D	Drugs (NSAIDs/Antiplatelet agents)	1
	alcohol	1

Bleeding risk score of 0: 0.9% bleeding risk, 1: 3.4%, 2: 4.1%, 3: 5.8%, 4: 8.9% 5: 9.1%.
Scores >5 are too rare and have not been calculated.
Abbreviations: ALT, alanine transaminase; AST, aspartate transaminase; INR, international normalized ratio; NSAIDs, nonsteroidal anti-inflammatory drugs; ULN, upper limits of normal.

titer of this heparin-PF4 antibody response is important in the diagnosis of HIT and is usually performed by ELISA techniques. As the false positive rate is high, patients with a positive ELISA test should have serotonin release assay (SRA) performed for confirmation.

The diagnosis of HIT requires both clinical and serological findings; the finding of anti-heparin-PF4 antibodies alone is not sufficient. Clinical prediction rules to assess the probability of HIT, such as the "4Ts score," are useful (96). The 4Ts score is based on assessment of the degree of thrombocytopenia, timing of platelet fall, presence of thrombosis, and evidence for other causes of thrombocytopenia. Several studies examined the validity of the 4Ts score in predicting which patients are at high or low risk of clinically significant HIT. Patients with a low 4Ts score have very low probability of HIT (0–3%). Many patients (24–61%) with a high 4Ts score, however, do not have HIT (97). As the 4Ts score has low positive predictive value, clinical assessment plays a major role in the diagnosis of HIT, because diagnostic laboratory test results are usually not immediately available and management decisions must be made promptly due to the high risk of thrombosis.

The ACCP recommends discontinuing heparin in patients with a moderate or high 4Ts score and sending an ELISA test for HIT antibody (98). Alternative medications for anticoagulation, including direct thrombin inhibitors or indirect factor Xa inhibitors, such as fondaparinux, should be administered while waiting for laboratory results. Patients with a positive SRA should continue to receive treatment with nonheparin anticoagulants, but those with a negative SRA can be restarted on heparin, since the SRA assay has high sensitivity and specificity. Patients with a low 4Ts score should be assumed not to have HIT and heparin can usually be continued.

Surgical patients are at highest risk for HIT, perhaps due to the prevalence of heparin use for thromboprophylaxis. Patients undergoing cardiac surgery often have 40–50% decrease in the platelet count within the first 72 hours after surgery due to prolonged exposure of platelets to the artificial membrane oxygenator, but only thrombocytopenia that begins 5–10 days after surgery is likely to be due to HIT. In contrast, early onset and persistent thrombocytopenia is usually caused by non-HIT factors but may be associated with coincident heparin-dependent antibody seroconversion (99).

HIT is a common problem in the hospital setting. It is estimated that 25,000–50,000 people in the USA develop HIT annually (97). Of note, in up to 25% of patients with HIT, the development of thrombosis precedes the development of thrombocytopenia (100). Venous thrombosis occurs in approximately one out of eight patients (101), and some studies suggest that over 50% of patients with HITT develop thrombosis within 1 month (102). Thus, anticoagulant therapy is required during the management of HIT and HITT for at least 3 months. Direct thrombin inhibitors such as argatroban or bivalirudin are usually prescribed. In patients with HITT and normal renal function, the ACCP recommends argatroban or lepirudin in preference to other nonheparin anticoagulants (98). Fondaparinux can also be safely used in this setting as shown in several studies (103). In patients with HITT and renal insufficiency, argatroban is recommended due to its hepatic clearance.

Due to the prevalence of type I thrombocytopenia and the morbidity of type II thrombocytopenia, the ACCP recommends that the platelet count be monitored every 2–3 days from day 4 to 14, or until heparin is stopped, for patients who are considered to have a HIT risk of more than 1% (orthopedic or surgical patients). If the risk of HIT is considered to be less than 1%, platelet monitoring is not recommended. For patients exposed to heparin within the past 100 days, obtaining a baseline platelet count prior to starting heparin or LMWH therapy is recommended, with a repeat platelet count 24 hours later.

DURATION OF THERAPY

The duration of long term anticoagulation therapy for VTE is based upon an estimated risk of recurrence, as well as patient preference and bleeding risk. This risk of recurrence is influenced by many factors, most importantly whether the clot was "provoked" (i.e., associated with an identifiable and reversible risk factor), whether it occurred in the setting of an active malignancy, and whether it is a recurrent VTE. Location appears to be important for lower extremity DVT, with the risk of recurrence associated with a proximal vein DVT twice that associated with a distal clot (104). Recurrence rates for DVT and PE are similar, but patients who initially present with PE are more likely to have PE on recurrence. If the thrombosis is a recurrence, the rate of yet another recurrence is significantly (50%) greater.

In a landmark study, the odds of developing a recurrence for patients with DVT who discontinued therapy after 6 weeks was twice that of those treated for 6 months (105). This led to evaluations of longer durations of therapy, which have supported longer periods of anticoagulation to reduce recurrent VTE, as well as the need to identify higher risk patients (104). Current recommendations are to reassess all patients with VTE after 3 months of anticoagulant therapy when additional information from diagnostic testing, bleeding experience on anticoagulation, and patient preferences may be available. Longer term therapy is generally considered at the 3–6-month point following diagnosis. Therapy prescribed beyond 3–6 months is considered "extended therapy."

VTE related to surgery is associated with a relatively lower risk for recurrence (1% after 1 year, 3% after 5 years) than other "reversible" risk factors such as trauma, air travel for more than 8 hours, estrogen use (5% after 1 year, 15% after 5 years) (106), "unprovoked VTE" (10% after 1 year and 30% after 5 years) or active cancer (estimated to be 15% per year but highly variable due to type and treatment) (72). Risk factors for recurrence identified during the initial diagnostic evaluation (Fig. 27.4) can be categorized as epidemiologic, situational, genetic, or clinical. Recommendations for duration of therapy depend in part upon whether risk factors occur in isolation or in combination. Male gender, non-Asian ethnicity, hereditary thrombophilia, and presence of an antiphospholipid antibody are examples of epidemiologic and clinical factors associated with increased risk for VTE recurrence (72). Consensus guidelines have attempted to utilize these risk factors to provide general recommendations for the duration of therapy.

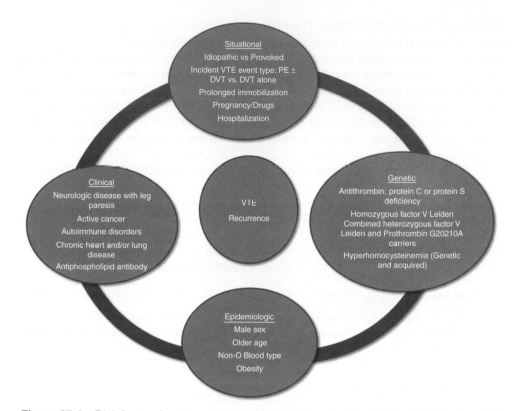

Figure 27.4   Risk factors for recurrence—epidemiologic, situational and clinical factors (78).

The presence of residual thrombosis on duplex imaging at the conclusion of 3 months of therapy for patients with an initial unprovoked DVT may indicate a higher risk of recurrence (107). The D-dimer test, described initially for use in the diagnosis of VTE, may also be useful in identifying patients at higher or lower risk for recurrence. These two tests performed during or at the conclusion of long-term therapy (3–6 months) may be helpful in deciding whether or not to continue anticoagulant treatment. In general, patients with an unprovoked VTE have a higher rate of recurrence than those with a provoked VTE and may require therapy for a longer duration.

In a patient-level meta-analysis, the risk of recurrent VTE was 2.59 times greater among patients with an elevated D-dimer 1 month after anticoagulation discontinuation (108). Another study examined the usefulness of monthly D-dimer testing after discontinuation of anticoagulation for patients with a first unprovoked VTE (109). A normal result was found in 68% of patients 1 month after discontinuation and was associated with a low risk of recurrence (4.4 per 100 patient years). Patients who subsequently developed an elevated D-dimer level that was sustained for 1 year had a higher rate of recurrence (7/31; 27 per 100 patient years) than patients in whom the level remained normal (4/149; 2.9 per 100 patient years).

Continuation of anticoagulant therapy beyond 3 months should be considered for patients in whom the estimated risk of recurrence is high, if cardiopulmonary compromise occurred with the prior episode, or if the risk of PTS is significant. Bleeding risk, overall prognosis, and patient preferences also influence the decision on duration of treatment. Patients on extended therapy should be reassessed at least annually with review of their clinical status, prognosis and preferences, bleeding history, and alternatives to continued therapy.

POSTTHROMBOTIC SYNDROME

PTS reportedly occurs within 2 years in almost half of patients who suffer a DVT. The definition of PTS is somewhat nonspecific, but includes chronic edema, skin discoloration, associated pain on standing, pruritis, and occasionally, varicosities of the veins, as well as other signs and symptoms often associated with lower extremity DVT. Similar signs and symptoms can occur with other conditions. The skin discoloration is often described as "brawny" due to iron staining from red cell stasis. The tenderness of the medial lower leg is called "lipodermatosclerosis." Venous stasis ulcers may develop which heal slowly and are prone to recurrence. Due to the similarity of symptoms and signs, it may be difficult to distinguish recurrent DVT from chronic PTS. Because PTS may be associated with significant morbidity, prevention is critical. Preventive measures include early compression, ambulation, and optimal anticoagulation in terms of intensity and duration. PTS is managed primarily with compression therapy and local care, but the condition often becomes chronic.

REFERENCES

1. Tsai J, Grosse SD, Grant AM, et al. Trends in in-hospital deaths among hospitalizations with pulmonary embolism. Arch Intern Med 2012; 172: 960–1.
2. Conget F, Otero R, Jimenez R, et al. Short-term clinical outcome after acute symptomatic pulmonary embolism. Thromb Haemost 2008; 100: 937–42.
3. Spencer FA, Emery C, Lessard D, et al. The Worcester Venous Thromboembolism study. A population-based study of the clinical epidemiology of venous thromboembolism. J Gen Intern Med 2006; 21: 722–7.
4. Anderson FA Jr, Wheeler HB, Goldberg RJ, et al. A population-based perspective of the hospital incidence and case-fatality rates of deep vein thrombosis and pulmonary embolism. The Worcester DVT Study. Arch Intern Med 1991; 151: 933–8.
5. Oger E. Incidence of venous thromboembolism: a community-based study in Western France. EPI-GETBP Study Group. Groupe d'Etude de la Thrombose de Bretagne Occidentale. Thromb Haemost 2000; 83: 657–60.
6. Morris CD, Creevy WS, Einhorn TA. Pulmonary distress and thromboembolic conditions affecting orthopaedic practice. In: Buckwalter JA, Einhorn TA, Simon SR, eds. Orthopaedic Basic Science: Biology and the Biomechanics of the Musculoskeletal System, 2nd edn. Vol. 12 Rosemont, IL: American Academy of Orthopaedic Surgeons, 2000: 347–60.
7. Mammen EF. Pathogenesis of venous thrombosis. Chest 1992; 102: 640S–4S.
8. Behranwala KA, Williamson RC. Cancer-associated venous thrombosis in the surgical setting. Ann Surg 2009; 249: 366–75.
9. Kroegel C, Reissig A. Principle mechanisms underlying venous thromboembolism: epidemiology, risk factors, pathophysiology and pathogenesis. Respiration 2003; 70: 7–30.
10. Kahn SR, Lim W, Dunn AS, et al. Prevention of VTE in nonsurgical patients: Antithrombotic Therapy and Prevention of Thrombosis, 9th ed: American College of Chest Physicians Evidence-Based Clinical Practice Guidelines. Chest 2012; 141: e195S–226S.
11. Gould MK, Garcia DA, Wren SM, et al. Prevention of VTE in nonorthopedic surgical patients. Antithrombotic Therapy and Prevention of Thrombosis, 9th ed: American College of Chest Physicians Evidence-Based Clinical Practice Guidelines. Chest 2012; 141: e227–77.
12. Falck-Ytter Y, Francis CW, Johanson NA, et al. Prevention of VTE in orthopedic surgery patients. Antithrombotic Therapy and Prevention of Thrombosis, 9th ed: American College of Chest Physicians Evidence-Based Clinical Practice Guidelines. Chest 2012; 141: e278S–325S.
13. Spirk D, Hussman M, Hayoz D, et al. Predictors of in-hospital mortality in elderly patients with acute venous thrombo-embolism: the SWIss Venous ThromboEmbolism Registry (SWIVTER). Eur Heart J 2012; 33: 921–6.
14. Barbar S, Noventa F, Rossetto V, et al. A risk assessment model for the identification of hospitalized medical patients at risk for venous thromboembolism: the Padua Prediction Score. J Thromb Haemost 2010; 8: 2450–7.
15. Belch JJ, Lowe GD, Ward AG, et al. Prevention of deep vein thrombosis in medical patients by low dose heparin. Scott Med J 1981; 26: 115–17.
16. Spyropoulos AC, Anderson FA Jr, Fitzgerald G, et al. IMPROVE Investigators. Predictive and associative models to identify hospitalized medical patients at risk for VTE. Chest 2011; 140: 706–14.

17. Samama MM, Cohen AT, Darmon JY, et al. Prophylaxis in Medical Patients with Enoxaparin Study Group. A comparison of enoxaparin with placebo for the prevention of venous thromboembolism in acutely ill medical patients. N Engl J Med 1999; 341: 793–800.

18. Dahan R, Houlbert D, Caulin C, et al. Prevention of deep vein thrombosis in elderly medical in-patients by a low molecular weight heparin: a randomized double-blind trial. Haemostasis 1986; 16: 159–64.

19. Johnson MJ, Sproule MW, Paul J. The prevalence and associated variables of deep venous thrombosis in patients with advanced cancer. Clin Oncol (R Coll Radiol) 1999; 11: 105–10.

20. Mandala M, Falanga A, Roila F. Venous thromboembolism in cancer patients: ESMO Clinical Practice Guidelines for the management. Ann Oncol 2010; 21: v274–6.

21. Raslan AM, Fields JD, Bhardwaj A. Prophylaxis for venous thrombo-embolism in neurocritical care: a critical appraisal. Neurocrit Care 2010; 12: 297–309.

22. Green L, Machin SJ. Managing anticoagulated patients during neuraxial anaesthesia. Br J Haematol 2010; 149: 195–208.

23. Bjørnarå BT, Gudmundsen TE, Dahl OE. Frequency and timing of clinical venous thromboembolism after major joint surgery. J Bone Joint Surg Br 2006; 88: 386–91.

24. Huo MH, Muntz J. Extended thromboprophylaxis with low-molecular-weight heparins after hospital discharge in high-risk surgical and medical patients: a review. Clin Ther 2009; 31: 1129–41.

25. Rasmussen MS, Jørgensen LN, Wille-Jørgensen P. Prolonged thromboprophylaxis with low molecular weight heparin for abdominal or pelvic surgery. Cochrane Database Syst Rev 2009: C004318.

26. Turpie AG, Lassen MR, Eriksson BI, et al. Rivaroxaban for the prevention of venous thromboembolism after hip or knee arthroplasty. Pooled analysis of four studies. Thromb Haemost 2011; 105: 444–53.

27. Eriksson BI, Dahl OE, Rosencher N, et al. RE-MODEL Study Group. Oral dabigatran etexilate vs. subcutaneous enoxaparin for the prevention of venous thromboembolism after total knee replacement: the RE-MODEL randomized trial. J Thromb Haemost 2007; 5: 2178–85.

28. Eriksson BI, Dahl OE, Rosencher N, et al. RE-NOVATE Study Group. Dabigatran etexilate versus enoxaparin for prevention of venous thromboembolism after total hip replacement: a randomised, double-blind, non-inferiority trial. Lancet 2007; 370: 949–56.

29. Ginsberg JS, Davidson BL, Comp PC, et al. RE-MOBILIZE Writing Committee. Oral thrombin inhibitor dabigatran etexilate vs North American enoxaparin regimen for prevention of venous thromboembolism after knee arthroplasty surgery. J Arthroplasty 2009; 24: 1–9.

30. Goldhaber SZ, Leizorovicz A, Kakkar AK, et al. ADOPT Trail Investigators. Apixaban versus enoxaparin for thromboprophylaxis in medically ill patients. N Engl J Med 2011; 365: 2167–77.

31. Gomes JP, Shaheen WH, Truong SV, et al. Incidence of venous thromboembolic events among nursing home residents. J Gen Intern Med 2003; 18: 934–6.

32. Scannapieco G, Ageno W, Airoldi A, et al. TERSICORE Study Group. Incidence and predictors of venous thromboembolism in post-acute care patients. A prospective cohort study. Thromb Haemost 2010; 104: 734–40.

33. Palumbo A, Rajkumar SV, Dimopoulos MA, et al. International Myeloma Working Group. Prevention of thalidomide- and lenalidomide-associated thrombosis in myeloma. Leukemia 2008; 22: 414–23.

34. Akl E, Vasireddi S, Gunukula S, et al. Anticoagulation for cancer patients with central venous catheters. Cochrane Database Syst Rev 2011: CD006468.

35. Miniati M, Prediletto R, Fromichi B. Accuracy of clinical assessment in the diagnosis of pulmonary embolism. Am J Respir Crit Care Med 1999; 159: 864–71.

36. Wells PS, Anderson DR, Rodger M. Excluding pulmonary embolism at the bedside without diagnostic imaging: management of patients with suspected pulmonary embolism presenting to the emergency department by using a simple clinical model and D-dimer. Ann Intern Med 2001; 135: 98–107.

37. Rogers RL. Venous thromboembolic disease in the elderly patients: atypical, subtle, and enigmatic. Clin Geriatr Med 2007; 23: 413–23.

38. Busby W, Bayer A, Pathy J. Pulmonary embolism in the elderly. Age Ageing 1998; 17: 205–9.

39. Timmons S, Kingston M, Hussain M, et al. Pulmonary embolism: differences in presentation between older and younger patients. Age Aging 2003; 32: 601–5.

40. Goldhaber S, Visani L, De Rosa M. Acute pulmonary embolism: clinical outcomes in the International Cooperative Pulmonary Embolism Registry. Lancet 1999; 352: 1386–9.

41. Jimenez D, Aujesky D, Moores L, et al. Simplification of the pulmonary embolism severity index for prognostication in patients with acute symptomatic pulmonary embolism. Arch Intern Med 2010; 170: 1383–9.

42. Kucher N, Rossi E, De Rosa M, et al. Massive pulmonary embolism. Circulation 2006; 113: 577–82.

43. Wells PS, Anderson DR, Bormanis J, et al. Value of assessment of pretest probability of deep-vein thrombosis in clinical management. Lancet 1997; 350: 1795–8.

44. Wells PS, Anderson DR, Rodger M, et al. Evaluation of D-dimer in the diagnosis of suspected deep-vein thrombosis. N Engl J Med 2003; 349: 1227–35.

45. Wells PS, Anderson DR, Rodger M. Excluding pulmonary embolism at the bedside without diagnostic imaging: management of patients with suspected pulmonary embolism presenting to the emergency department by using a simple clinical model and D-dimer. Ann Intern Med 2001; 135: 98–107.

46. van Belle A, Büller HR, Huisman MV, et al. Christopher Study Investigators. Effectiveness of managing suspected pulmonary embolism using an algorithm combining clinical probability, D-dimer testing, and computer tomography. JAMA 2006; 295: 172–9.

47. Le Gal G, Righini M, Roy PM, et al. Prediction of pulmonary embolism in the emergency department: the revised Geneva score. Ann Intern Med 2008; 144: 165–71.

48. Sanchez O, Trinquart L, Colombet I, et al. Prognostic value of right ventricular dysfunction in patients with haemodynamically stable pulmonary embolism: a systematic review. Eur Heart J 2008; 29: 1569–77.

49. Jiménez D, Aujesky D, Díaz G, et al. RIETE Investigators. Prognostic significance of deep vein thrombosis in patients presenting with acute symptomatic pulmonary embolism. Am J Respir Crit Care Med 2010; 181: 983–91.

50. Stein PD, Hull RD, Patel KC, et al. D-dimer for the exclusion of acute venous thrombosis and pulmonary embolism: a systematic review. Ann Intern Med 2004; 140: 589–602.

51. Righini M, Goehring C, Bounameaux H, et al. Effects of age on the performance of common diagnostic tests for pulmonary embolism. Am J Med 2000; 109: 357–61.

52. Bates SM, Jaeschke R, Stevens SM, et al. Diagnosis of DVT: Antithrombotic Therapy and Prevention of Thrombosis, 9th ed: American College of Chest Physicians Evidence-Based Clinical Practice Guidelines. Chest 2012; 141: e351S–418S.

53. Söhne M, Kamphuisen PW, van Mierlo PJ, et al. Diagnostic strategy using a modified clinical decision rule and D-dimer test to rule out pulmonary embolism in elderly in- and outpatients. Thromb Haemost 2005; 94: 206–10.

54. Righini M, LeGal G, Perrrier A, et al. Effect of age on the assessment of clinical probability of pulmonary embolism by prediction rules. J Thromb Haemost 2004; 5: 1206–8.

55. Monreal M, Montserrat E, Salvador R, et al. Real-time ultrasound for diagnosis of symptomatic venous thrombosis and for screening of patients at risk: correlation with ascending conventional venography. Angiology 1989; 40: 527–33.

56. Lensing AW, Prandoni P, Brandjes D, et al. Detection of deep-vein thrombosis by real-time B-mode ultrasonography. N Engl J Med 1989; 320: 342–5.

57. Mattos MA, Londrey GL, Leutz DW, et al. Color-flow duplex scanning for the surveillance and diagnosis of acute deep venous thrombosis. J Vasc Surg 1992; 15: 366–75.

58. Birdwell BG, Raskob GE, Whitsett TL, et al. Predictive value of compression ultrasonography for deep vein thrombosis in symptomatic outpatients: clinical implications of the site of vein noncompressibility. Arch Intern Med 2000; 160: 309–13.

59. Carpenter JP, Holland GA, Baum RA, et al. Magnetic resonance venography for the detection of deep venous thrombosis: comparison with contrast venography and duplex Doppler ultrasonography. J Vasc Surg 1993; 18: 734–41.

60. Moody AR, Pollock JG, O'Connor AR, et al. Lower-limb deep venous thrombosis: direct MR imaging of the thrombus. Radiology 1998; 209: 349–55.

61. Stein PD, Woodard PK, Weg JG, et al. Diagnostic pathways in acute pulmonary embolism: recommendations of the PIOPED II Investigators. Am J Med 2006; 119: 1048–55.

62. Goldhaber SZ, Elliott CG. Acute pulmonary embolism: part I. epidemiology, pathophysiology and diagnosis. Circulation 2003; 108: 2726–9.

63. Garg K, Sieler H, Welsh CH, et al. Clinical validity of helical CT being interpreted as negative for pulmonary embolism: implications for patient treatment. Am J Roentgenol 1999; 172: 1627–31.

64. Hall WB, Truitt SG, Scheunemann LP, et al. The prevalence of clinically relevant incidental findings on chest computed tomographic angiograms ordered to diagnose pulmonary embolism. Arch Intern Med 2009; 169: 1961–5.

65. Stein PD, Fowler SE, Goodman LR, et al. PIOPED II Investigators. Multidetector computed tomography for acute pulmonary embolism. N Engl J Med 2006; 354: 2317–27.

66. Righini M, Nendaz M, Le Gal G, et al. Influence of age on the cost-effectiveness of diagnostic strategies for suspected pulmonary embolism. J Thromb Haemost 2007; 5: 1869–77.

67. Stein PD, Beemath A, Quinn DA, et al. Usefulness of multidetector spiral computer tomography according to age and gender for diagnosis of acute pulmonary embolism. Am J Cardiol 2007; 99: 1303–5.

68. The PIOPED Investigators. Value of the ventilation/perfusion scan in acute pulmonary embolism. Results of the prospective investigation of pulmonary embolism diagnosis (PIOPED). JAMA 1990; 263: 2753–9.

69. Calvo-Romero JM, Lima-Rodriguez BM, Bureo-Dacla P, et al. Predictors of the intermediate ventilation/perfusion lung scan in patients with suspected pulmonary embolism. Eur J Emerg Med 2005; 12: 129–31.

70. Gibson NS, Sohne M, Buller HR. Prognostic value of echocardiography and spiral computed tomography in patients with pulmonary embolism. Curr Opin Pulm Med 2005; 11: 380–4.

71. Goldhaber SZ. Echocardiography in the management of pulmonary embolism. Ann Intern Med 2002; 136: 691–700.

72. Kcaron C, Akl EA, Comcrota AJ, ct al. Antithrombotic therapy for VTE disease: Antithrombotic Therapy and Prevention of Thrombosis, 9th ed: American College of Chest Physicians Evidence-Based Clinical Practice Guidelines. Chest 2012; 141: e419S–94S.

73. Erkens PM, Prins MH. Fixed dose subcutaneous low molecular weight heparins versus adjusted dose unfractionated heparin for venous thromboembolism. Cochrane Database Syst Rev 2010; 9: CD001100.

74. Hull RD, Raskob GE, Brant RF, et al. Relation between the time to achieve the lower limit of the APTT therapeutic range and recurrent venous thromboembolism during heparin treatment for deep vein thrombosis. Arch Intern Med 1997; 157: 2562–8.

75. Raschke R, Reilly BM, Srinivas S, et al. The weight based heparin dosing nomogram versus a standard care nomogram: a randomized controlled trial. Ann Intern Med 1993; 119: 874–81.

76. Quinlan DJ, McQuillan A, Eikelboom JW. Low-molecular weight heparin compared with intravenous unfractionated heparin for treatment of pulmonary embolism: a metaanalysis of randomized, controlled trials. Ann Intern Med 2004; 140: 175–83.

77. van Dongen CJ, MacGillavry MR, Prins MH. Once versus twice daily LMWH for the initial treatment of venous thromboembolism. Cochrane Database Syst Rev 2005: CD003074.

78. Büller HR, Davidson BL, Decousus H, et al. Matisse Investigators. Fondaparinux or enoxaparin for the initial treatment of symptomatic deep venous thrombosis: a randomized trial. Ann Intern Med 2004; 140: 867–73.

79. Büller HR, Davidson BL, Decousus H, et al. Matisse Investigators. Subcutaneous fondaparinux versus intravenous unfractionated heparin in the initial treatment of pulmonary embolism. N Engl J Med 2003; 349: 1695–702.

80. Schulman S, Kearon C, Kakkar AK, et al. RE-COVER Study Group. Dabigatran versus warfarin in the treatment of acute venous thromboembolism. N Engl J Med 2009; 361: 2342–52.

81. The EINSTEIN Investigators. Oral rivaroxaban for symptomatic venous thromboembolism. N Engl J Med 2010; 363: 2499–510.

82. The EINSTEIN-PE Investigators. Oral rivaroxaban for the treatment of symptomatic pulmonary embolism. N Engl J Med 2012; 366: 1287–97.

83. Singla DA. Warfarin doses in the very elderly. Am J Health Syst Pharm 2005; 62: 1062–6.

84. Koopman MMW, Prandoni P, Piovella F, et al. The TasmanStudy Group. Treatment of venous thrombosis with intravenous unfractionated heparin administered in the hospital as compared with subcutaneous low-molecular-weight heparin administered at home. N Engl J Med 1996; 334: 682–7.

85. Otero R, Uresandi F, Jiménez D, et al. Home treatment in pulmonary embolism. Thromb Res 2010; 126: e1–5.

86. Decousus H, Leizorovicz A, Parent F, et al. A clinical trial of vena caval filters in the prevention of pulmonary embolism in patients with proximal deep-vein thrombosis. Prévention du Risque d'Embolie Pulmonaire par Interruption Cave Study Group. N Engl J Med 1998; 338: 409–15.

87. Billett HH, Jacobs LG, Madsen EM, et al. Efficacy of inferior vena cava filters in anticoagulated patients. J Thromb Haemost 2007; 5: 1–6.

88. Hansen ML, Sørensen R, Clausen MT, et al. Risk of bleeding with single, dual, or triple therapy with warfarin, aspirin, and clopidogrel in patients with atrial fibrillation. Arch Intern Med 2010; 170: 1433–41.

89. Gage BF, Birman-Deych E, Kerzner R, et al. Incidence of intracranial hemorrhage in patients with atrial fibrillation who are prone to fall. Am J Med 2005; 118: 612–17.

90. Pisters R, Lane DA, Nieuwlaat R, et al. A novel user-friendly score (HAS-BLED) to assess 1-year risk of major bleeding in patients with atrial fibrillation: the Euro Heart Survey. Chest 2010; 138: 1093–100.

91. Menajovsky LB. Heparin-induced thrombocytopenia: clinical manifestations and management strategies. Am J Med 2005; 118: S21–30.

92. Martel N, Lee J, Wells PS. Risk for heparin-induced thrombocytopenia with unfractionated and low-molecular-weight heparin thromboprophylaxis: a meta-analysis. Blood 2005; 106: 2710–15.

93. Warkentin TE, Roberts RS, Hirsh J, et al. Heparin-induced skin lesions and other unusual sequelae of the heparin-induced thrombocytopenia syndrome: a nested cohort study. Chest 2005; 127: 1857–61.

94. Lubenow N, Kempf R, Eichner A, et al. Heparin-induced thrombocytopenia: temporal pattern of thrombocytopenia in relation to initial use or the exposure to heparin. Chest 2002; 122: 37–42.

95. Newman PM, Chong BH. Heparin-induced thrombocytopenia. New evidence for the dynamic binding of purified anti-PF4 antibodies to platelets and the resultant platelet activation. Blood 2000; l96: 182–7.

96. Lo GK, Juhl D, Warkentin TE, et al. Evaluation of pretest clinical score (4T's) for the diagnosis of heparin-induced thrombocytopenia in two clinical settings. J Thromb Haemost 2006; 4: 759–65.

97. Ohman EM, Granger CB, Rice L, et al. Identification, diagnosis and treatment of HITT: a registry of prolonged heparin use and thrombocytopenia among hospitalized patients with and without cardiovascular disease. J Thromb Thrombolysis 2005; 19: 11–19.

98. Linkins LA, Dans AL, Moores LK, et al. Treatment and prevention of heparin-induced thrombocytopenia: Antithrombotic Therapy and Prevention of Thrombosis, 9th ed: American College of Chest Physicians Evidence-Based Clinical Practice Guidelines. Chest 2012; 141: e495S–530S.

99. Selleng S, Malowsky B, Strobel U, et al. Early-onset and persisting thrombocytopenia in post-cardiac surgery patients is rarely due to heparin-induced thrombocytopenia, even when antibody tests are positive. J Thromb Haemost 2010; 8: 30–6.

100. Greinacher A, Farner B, Kroll H, et al. Clinical features of heparin-induced thrombocytopenia including risk factors for thrombosis. A retrospective analysis of 408 patients. Thromb Haemost 2005; 94: 132–5.

101. Levine RL, McCollum D, Hursting MJ. How frequently is venous thromboembolism in heparin treated patients associated with heparin-induced thrombocytopenia? Chest 2006; 130: 631–2.

102. Warkentin TE, Pai M, Sheppard JI, et al. Fondaparinux treatment of acute heparin-induced thrombocytopenia confirmed by the serotonin-release assay: a 30-month, 16-patient case series. J Thromb Haemost 2011; 9: 2389–96.

103. Prandoni P, Prins MH, Lensing AW, et al. AESOPUS Investigators. Residual thrombosis on ultrasonography to guide the duration of anticoagulation in patients with deep venous thrombosis: a randomized trial. Ann Intern Med 2009; 150: 577–85.

104. Boutitie F, Pinede L, Schulman S, et al. Influence of preceding duration of anticoagulant treatment and initial presentation of venous thromboembolism on risk of recurrence after stopping therapy: analysis of individual participants' data from seven trials. BMJ 2011; 342: d3036–41.

105. Schulman S, Rhedin A-S, Lindmarker P, et al. A comparison of six weeks with six months of oral anticoagulant therapy after a first episode of venous thromboembolism. N Engl J Med 1995; 332: 1661–5.

106. Baglin T, Luddington R, Brown K, et al. Incidence of recurrent venous thromboembolism in relation to clinical and thrombophilic risk factors: prospective cohort study. Lancet 2003; 362: 523–6.

107. Carrier M, Rodger MA, Wells PS, et al. Residual vein obstruction to predict the risk of recurrent venous thromboembolism in patients with deep vein thrombosis: a systematic review and meta-analysis. J Thromb Haemost 2001; 9: 1119–25.

108. Douketis J, Tosetto A, Marcucci M, et al. Patient-level meta-analysis: effect of measurement timing, threshold, and patient age on ability of D-dimer testing to assess recurrence risk after unprovoked venous thromboembolism. Ann Intern Med 2010; 153: 523–31.

109. Cosmi B, Legnani C, Tosetto A, et al. PROLONG Investigators. Usefulness of repeated D-dimer testing after stopping anticoagulation for a first episode of unprovoked venous thromboembolism: the PROLONG II prospective study. Blood 2010; 115: 481–8.

28

Management of peripheral arterial disease in the elderly

Wilbert S. Aronow

SUMMARY

Patients with peripheral arterial disease (PAD) are at increased risk for all-cause mortality, cardiovascular mortality, and mortality from coronary artery disease (CAD). Smoking should be stopped and hypertension, dyslipidemia, diabetes mellitus, and hypothyroidism treated. Statins reduce the incidence of intermittent claudication and improve exercise duration until the onset of intermittent claudication in patients with PAD and hypercholesterolemia. The serum low-density lipoprotein (LDL) cholesterol should be reduced to <70 mg/dl. Antiplatelet drugs such as aspirin or clopidogrel, angiotensin-converting enzyme (ACE) inhibitors, and statins should be given to patients with PAD. Beta blockers should be given if CAD is present. Cilostazol improves exercise time until intermittent claudication. Exercise rehabilitation programs should be used. Revascularization should be performed if indicated. Patients with an infrarenal or juxtarenal abdominal aortic aneurysm (AAA) measuring 5.5 cm or larger should undergo repair to eliminate the risk of rupture. Patients with an infrarenal or juxtarenal AAA measuring 4.0–5.4 cm in diameter should be monitored by ultrasound or computed tomographic scans every 6–12 months to detect expansion Patients with an AAA should undergo intensive risk factor modification, be treated with ACE inhibitors, statins, and beta blockers, and undergo surgery if indicated.

INTRODUCTION

Peripheral arterial disease (PAD) is chronic arterial occlusive disease of the lower extremities caused by atherosclerosis. PAD may cause intermittent claudication which is pain or weakness with walking that is relieved with rest. The muscle pain or weakness after exercise occurs distal to the arterial obstruction. Since the superficial femoral and popliteal arteries are most commonly affected by atherosclerosis, the pain of intermittent claudication is most commonly localized to the calf. Atherosclerotic obstruction of the distal aorta and its bifurcation into the two iliac arteries may cause pain in the buttocks, hips, thighs, or the inferior back muscles as well as the calves.

The Rutherford classification of PAD includes seven stages (1). PAD is classified as stage 0 if the person is asymptomatic, stage 1 if mild intermittent claudication is present, stage 2 if moderate intermittent claudication is present, stage 3 if severe intermittent claudication is present, stage 4 if ischemic rest pain is present, stage 5 if the person has minor tissue loss, and stage 6 if the person has ulceration or gangrene (1).

Only one-half of elderly persons with documented PAD are symptomatic. Persons with PAD may not walk far or fast enough to induce muscle ischemic symptoms because of comorbidities such as pulmonary disease or arthritis, may have atypical symptoms unrecognized as intermittent claudication (2), may fail to mention their symptoms to their physician, or may have sufficient collateral arterial channels to tolerate their arterial obstruction. Women with PAD have a higher prevalence of leg pain on exertion and at rest, poorer functioning, and greater walking impairment from leg symptoms than men with PAD (3). Poorer leg strength in women contributes to poorer lower extremity functioning in women with PAD than in men with PAD (3). Women with PAD develop a faster functional decline than men with PAD (4). More sedentary hours and slower outdoor walking speed are associated with faster decreases in functioning and adverse calf muscle changes in PAD (5). Increased physical activity levels during daily life are associated with less functional decline in patients with PAD (6).

Upper extremity PAD will cause unequal blood pressure measurements in each arm. PAD patients also have a higher prevalence of cognitive impairment and erectile dysfunction.

If the arterial flow to the lower extremities cannot meet the needs of resting tissue metabolism, critical lower extremity ischemia occurs with pain at rest or tissue loss. Critical ischemia causes rest pain in the toes or foot with progression to ulceration or gangrene. Chronic arterial insufficiency ulcers commonly develop at the ankle, heel, or leg. Mummified, dry, black toes or devitalized soft tissue covered by a crust is gangrene caused by ischemic infarction. Suppuration often develops with time, and dry gangrene changes to wet gangrene.

PHYSICAL EXAMINATION

The vascular physical examination includes: (*i*) measurement of the blood pressure in both arms, (*ii*) palpation of the carotid pulses and listening for carotid bruits, (*iii*) auscultation of the abdomen and flank for bruits, (*iv*) palpation of the abdomen and notation of the presence of the aortic pulsation and its maximal diameter, (*v*) palpation of pulses at the brachial, radial, ulnar, femoral, popliteal, dorsalis pedis, and posterior tibial sites, and (*vi*) auscultation of both femoral arteries for femoral bruits (4).

The shoes and socks should be removed and the feet were inspected. The color, temperature, and integrity of the skin should be evaluated and the presence of distal hair loss, trophic skin changes, hypertrophic nails, and ulcerations noted (7).

NON-INVASIVE DIAGNOSIS

Persons with PAD of the lower extremities have reduced or absent arterial pulses. Non-invasive tests used to assess lower extremity arterial blood flow include measurement of ankle and brachial artery systolic blood pressures, characterization of velocity wave form, and duplex ultrasonography. Measurement of ankle and brachial artery systolic blood pressures using a Doppler stethoscope and blood pressure cuffs allows calculation of the ankle-brachial index (ABI) which is normally 0.9–1.2. An ABI of less than 0.90 is 95% sensitive and 99% specific for the diagnosis of PAD (8). The lower the ABI, the more severe the restriction of arterial blood flow, and the more serious the ischemia. ABIs of 0.6–0.9 usually correlate with mild to moderate intermittent claudication. ABIs of 0.4–0.6 usually correlate with severe intermittent claudication. With ABIs between 0.25 and 0.4, rest pain and tissue loss are often found. Patients with calcified arteries from diabetes mellitus or renal failure occasionally have relatively non-compressible arteries leading to falsely elevated ABI values in the normal range. Patients with an ABI of 1.4 or higher also have an increased incidence of cardiovascular events (9) and less quality of life (10).

In addition to measuring arterial pressure in non-palpable arteries, Doppler ultrasound methods allow characterization of the flow versus time velocity waveform. Finding biphasic flow at the groin or monophasic flow more distally is evidence of arterial obstruction even when ABI measurements are falsely increased to normal levels because of calcification.

Duplex ultrasonography combines Doppler frequency measurements with two-dimensional images of blood vessels. The severity of flow restriction caused by an arterial stenosis can be accurately assessed by this most comprehensive non-invasive method (11).

Dupex ultrasonography, computed tomographic angiography, and magnetic resonance angiography are useful in assessing the anatomic location and severity of PAD and in selecting suitable candidates for endovascular or surgical revascularization (7).

Treadmill exercise testing with and without pre-exercise and post-exercise ABIs helps differentiate claudication from pseudoclaudication in patients with exertional leg symptoms (7). Treadmill exercise testing may be useful to diagnose PAD with a normal resting ABI but a reduced post-exercise ABI (7). Treadmill exercise testing may objectively document the magnitude of symptom limitation in patients with claudication (7). The post-exercise ABI is a powerful independent predictor of all-cause mortality and provides additional risk stratification than the resting ABI (12).

PREVALENCE

The prevalence of PAD increases with age. Schroll and Munck reported that the prevalence of PAD was 16% in men and 13% in women aged 60 years (Table 28.1) (13). Criqui et al. showed that the prevalence of PAD was 5.6% in persons aged 38–59-years old, 15.9% in persons aged 60–69-years old, and 33.8% in persons aged 70–82-years old (Table 28.1) (14). In the Cardiovascular Health Study, PAD was present in 13.9% of 2214 men aged ≥65 years and in 11.4% of 2870 women aged ≥65 years without cardiovascular disease

Table 28.1   Prevalence of Peripheral Arterial Disease

Study	Prevalence
360 men aged 60 years (13)	16%
306 women aged 60 years (13)	13%
158 persons aged 38–59 years (14)	5.6%
161 persons aged 60–69 years (14)	15.9%
294 persons aged 70–82 years (14)	33.8%
2214 women aged ≥65 years (15)	13.9%
2870 women aged ≥65 years (15)	11.4%
467 men, mean age 80 years (16)	20%[a]
1444 women, mean age 81 years (16)	13%[a]
2589 men aged ≥55 years (17)	16.9%
3861 women aged ≥55 years (17)	20.5%
1160 men, mean age 80 years (18)	32%[a]
2464 women, mean age 81 years (18)	26%[a]
268 blacks, mean age 81 years (19)	29%[a]
71 Hispanics, mean age 81 years (19)	24%[a]
1310 whites, mean age 82 years (19)	23%[a]
386 men, mean age 72 years (20)	26.7%[a]
620 women, mean age 72 years (20)	17.1%[a]
6979 men and women, mean age 69 years (21)	29%

[a]Symptomatic peripheral arterial disease.

(Table 28.1) (15). Symptomatic PAD was present in 20% of 467 men, mean age 80 years, and in 13% of 1444 women, mean age 81 years, living in the community and being seen in a geriatrics clinic (Table 28.1) (16). In the Rotterdam Study, PAD was present in 16.9% of 2589 men aged ≥55 years and in 20.5% of 3861 women aged ≥55 years (Table 28.1) (17). The prevalence of symptomatic PAD was 32% in 1160 men, mean age 80 years, and 26% in 2464 women, mean age 81 year, living in a nursing home (Table 28.1) (18). The prevalence of symptomatic PAD in persons living in a nursing home was also 29% in 268 blacks, mean age 81 years, 24% in 71 Hispanics, mean age 81 years, and 23% in 1310 whites, mean age 82 years (Table 28.1) (19). The prevalence of symptomatic PAD was 26.7% in 386 men, mean age 72 years, and 17.1% in 620 women, mean age 72 years, living in the community and being seen in a university general medicine clinic (Table 28.1) (20). The prevalence of PAD in 6979 men and women, mean age 69 years, screened for PAD by an ABI because they were aged 70 years or older or because they were aged 50–69 years with a history of cigarette smoking or diabetes mellitus was 29% (Table 28.1) (21). Among these patients with PAD, classic claudication was present in only 11% (21).

RISK FACTORS

Modifiable risk factors that predispose to PAD include cigarette smoking (13,16,20,22–30), diabetes mellitus (13,16,20,22–29,31), hypertension (13,14,16,20,26–29,32), dyslipidemia (13,16,20,22,24–29,31,33–35), increased plasma homocysteine levels (36–39), and hypothyroidism (40). Obesity is associated with a high ABI (41). A reduced glomerular filtration rate (42–44), microalbuminuria (44), the metabolic syndrome in women (45), inflammation (45,46), and a family history of PAD (47) are also associated with PAD.

Table 28.2 indicates that significant independent risk factors for PAD in 467 men, mean age 80 years, and in 1444 women, mean age 81 years, living in the community and seen in an academic geriatrics practice were age (odds ratio = 1.05 for each 1-year increase in age in men and 1.03 for each 1-year increase in age in women); current cigarette smoking (odds ratio = 2.6 for men and 4.6 for women); systolic or diastolic hypertension (odds ratio = 2.2 for men and 2.8 for women); diabetes mellitus (odds ratio = 6.1 for men and 3.6 for women); serum high-density lipoprotein cholesterol (odds ratio = 0.95 for each 1 mg/dl increase in men and 0.97 for each 1 mg/dl increase in women); and serum low-density lipoprotein (LDL) cholesterol (odds ratio = 1.02 for each 1 mg/dl increase in men and in women) (16).

In 147 men and women with PAD and 373 men and women without PAD, mean age 81 years, plasma homocysteine was a significant independent risk factor for PAD with an odds ratio of 1.13 for each 1 μmol/l increase (39). In 249 men and women, mean age

Table 28.2 Significant Independent Risk Factors for Symptomatic Peripheral Arterial Disease in 467 Men, Mean Age 80 Years, and in 14,444 Women, Mean Age 81 Years

	Odds Ratio	
Risk Factor	Men	Women
Age (each 1-year increase)	1.05	1.03
Current cigarette smoking	2.6	4.6
Systolic or diastolic hypertension	2.2	2.8
Diabetes mellitus	6.1	3.6
High-density lipoprotein cholesterol	0.95 for 1 mg/dl increase	0.97 for 1 mg/dl increase
Low-density lipoprotein cholesterol	1.02 for 1 mg/dl increase	1.02 for 1 mg/dl increase

Source: Adapted from Ref. 16.

79 years, the prevalence of PAD was significantly higher in persons with subclinical hypothyroidism (14 of 18 persons or 78%) than in persons with euthyroidism (40 of 231 persons
or 17%) (40).

COEXISTENCE OF OTHER ATHEROSCLEROTIC DISORDERS

PAD coexists with other atherosclerotic disorders (Table 28.3) (20,29,48–53). In a study
of 1886 men and women, mean age 81 years, 270 of 468 persons (58%) with PAD had
coexistent CAD and 159 of 468 persons (34%) with PAD had prior ischemic stroke
(Table 28.3) (48). In a study of 1802 men and women, mean age 80 years, living in the
community and seen in an academic geriatrics practice, 161 of 236 persons (68%) with
PAD had coexistent CAD and 100 of 236 persons (42%) with PAD had coexistent prior
ischemic stroke (Table 28.3) (49).

In 924 men, mean age 80 years, the prevalence of PAD was 1.5 times significantly higher in 336 men with mitral annular calcium than in 588 men without mitral
annular calcium (43% vs. 28%) (Table 28.3) (50). In 1881 women, mean age 81 years,
the prevalence of PAD was 1.6 times significantly higher in 985 women with mitral
annular calcium than in 896 women without mitral annular calcium (31% vs. 19%)
(Table 28.3) (50).

Table 28.3 Coexistence of Peripheral Arterial Disease with Other Atherosclerotic Disorders
in Older Persons

Study	Result
1886 persons, mean age 81 years (48)	If PAD was present, 58% had coexistent CAD and 34% had prior ischemic stroke
1802 persons, mean 80 years (49)	If PAD was present, 68% had coexistent CAD and 42% had prior ischemic stroke
924 men, mean age 80 years (50)	PAD was 1.5 times higher in men with mitral annular calcium than in men without mitral annular calcium
1881 women, mean age 81 years (50)	PAD was 1.6 times higher in women with mitral annular calcium than in women without mitral annular calcium
989 men, mean age 80 years (51)	PAD was 1.6 times higher in men with aortic stenosis than in men without aortic stenosis
1998 women, mean age 81 years (51)	PAD was 1.7 times higher in women with aortic stenosis than in women without aortic stenosis
279 persons with PAD, mean age 71 years, undergoing coronary angiography for suspected CAD (29)	Obstructive CAD was present in 98% of persons, left main CAD in 18% of persons, and 3- or 4-vessel CAD in 63% of persons
218 persons without PAD, mean age 70 years, undergoing coronary angiography for suspected CAD (29)	Obstructive CAD was present in 82% of persons, left main CAD in <1% of persons, and 3- or 4-vessel CAD in 11% of persons
1006 persons, mean age 72 years (20)	If PAD was present, 63% had coexistent CAD, and 43% had prior ischemic stroke
336 patients, mean age 73 years (52)	CAD was present in 75% of patients with a decreased ABI and in 29% of age- and gender-matched patients with a normal ABI
273 patients, mean age 71 years, with CAD (53)	The lower the ABI, the higher the prevalence of 3- or 4-vessel CAD

Abbreviations: PAD, peripheral arterial disease; CAD, coronary artery disease.

In 989 men, mean age 80 years, the prevalence of PAD was 1.6 times significantly higher in 141 men with valvular aortic stenosis than in 848 men without valvular aortic stenosis (48% vs. 30%) (Table 28.3) (51). In 1998 women, mean age 81 years, the prevalence of PAD was 1.7 times significantly higher in 321 women with valvular aortic stenosis than in 1677 women without valvular aortic stenosis (39% vs. 23%) (Table 28.3) (51).

In 279 men and women, mean age 71 years, with documented PAD and in 218 men and women, mean age 70 years, without PAD with normal ABIs undergoing coronary angiography for suspected CAD, the prevalence of obstructive CAD was significantly higher in persons with PAD (98%) than in persons without PAD (81%) (Table 28.3) (29). The prevalence of left main CAD was significantly higher in persons with CAD (18%) than in persons without CAD (<1%) (Table 28.3) (29). The incidence of 3- or 4-vessel CAD was significantly higher in persons with PAD (63%) than in persons without PAD (11%) (Table 28.3) (29).

In 1006 men and women, mean age 72 years, if PAD was present, 63% had coexistent CAD, and 43% had prior ischemic stroke (Table 28.3) (20). In 118 patients, mean age 73 years, with a decreased ABI, the prevalence of CAD was 75%, whereas in 118 age-matched and gender-matched patients with a normal ABI, the prevalence of CAD was 29% (Table 28.3) (52). The prevalence of aortic valve calcium or mitral annular calcium was also higher in the patients with a decreased ABI (69%) than in the patients with a normal ABI (36%) (Table 28.3) (52).

In 273 patients, mean age 71 years, with CAD, the lower the ABI, the higher the prevalence of 3- or 4-vessel CAD (Table 28.3) (53). Patients with PAD and CAD have more extensive and calcified coronary atherosclerosis, constrictive arterial remodeling, and greater disease progression (54). Patients with PAD also have a higher prevalence of left ventricular systolic dysfunction than patients without PAD (55).

CARDIOVASCULAR MORTALITY AND MORBIDITY

Persons with PAD are at increased risk for all-cause mortality, cardiovascular mortality, and cardiovascular events (9,24,56–72). At 10-year follow-up of 565 men and women, mean age 66 years, PAD significantly increased the risk of all-cause mortality (relative risk = 3.1), of mortality from cardiovascular disease (relative risk = 5.9), and of mortality from CAD (relative risk = 6.6) (56). At 4-year follow-up of 1492 women, mean age 71 years, an ABI of 0.9 or less was associated with a relative risk of 3.1 for all-cause mortality after adjustment for age, smoking, and other risk factors (59).

In a prospective study of 291 men and women, mean age 82 years, with PAD, CAD was present in 160 persons (55%) (58). Silent myocardial ischemia detected by 24-hour ambulatory electrocardiography was present in 60 of 160 persons (38%) with PAD and CAD and in 26 of 131 persons (20%) with PAD and no clinically evident CAD (58). At 43-month follow-up, new coronary events developed in 54 of 60 persons (90%) with PAD, CAD, and silent myocardial ischemia and in 59 of 100 persons (59%) with PAD, CAD, and no silent myocardial ischemia (58). New coronary events also developed in 18 of 26 persons (69%) with PAD, no CAD, and silent myocardial ischemia and in 34 of 105 persons (32%) with PAD, no CAD, and no silent myocardial ischemia (58).

A pooled analysis of mortality in eight large randomized percutaneous coronary intervention (PCI) trials of 19,867 patients showed that the presence of PAD was associated with higher rates of post-PCI death and myocardial infarction (50). PAD was an independent predictor of short- and long-term mortality (64).

At 7.5-year follow-up of persons in the Cardiovascular Health study in a propensity-matched study of community dwelling older adults, matched hazard ratios for PAD for all-cause mortality, incident heart failure, and symptomatic PAD were 1.57, 1.32, and 3.92, respectively (67). In a well-balanced propensity-matched population of 2689 patients with advanced chronic systolic heart failure, during 4.1 years of follow-up, PAD was significantly associated with increased mortality and hospitalization (70).

At 33-month follow-up of 414 patients with PAD and at 48-month follow-up of 89 patients without PAD followed in a vascular surgery clinic, the incidence of death, new stroke/transient ischemic attack, new myocardial infarction, new coronary revascularization, new carotid endarterectomy, or new PAD revascularization was significantly higher in patients with PAD (63%) than in patients without PAD (24%) (72). PAD was a significant independent risk factor for all-cause mortality with a hazard ratio of 2.2.

Dipyridamole thallium scintigraphy also has prognostic value in the pre-operative assessment of patients with PAD undergoing vascular surgery (73).

RISK FACTOR MODIFICATION

Continuing smoking increases the risk of amputation in patients with intermittent claudication (74). Patency in lower extremity bypass grafts is also worse in smokers than in non-smokers (75). Smoking cessation reduces the progression of PAD to critical leg ischemia and reduces the risk of myocardial infarction and death from vascular causes (76). Smoking cessation programs should be strongly encouraged in persons with PAD (Table 28.4). Patients should be assisted with counseling and developing a plan for quitting that may include pharmacotherapy and/or referral to a smoking cessation program (77,78).

Approaches to smoking cessation include use of nicotine patches or nicotine polacrilex gum, which are available over the counter (79). If this therapy is unsuccessful, nicotine nasal spray or treatment with the antidepressant buproprion should be considered (79,80). A nicotine inhaler may also be used (81). The dosage and duration of treatment of each of these pharmacotherapies are discussed in detail elsewhere (81). Concomitant behavioral therapy may also be needed (82). Repeated physician advice is very important in the treatment of smoking addiction.

Hypertension should be adequately controlled to decrease cardiovascular mortality and morbidity in persons with PAD (Table 28.4) (32,83–85). The blood pressure should be reduced to <140/90 mmHg (32). In the Heart Outcomes Prevention Evaluation (HOPE) Study, 1715 persons had symptomatic PAD, and 2118 persons had asymptomatic PAD with an ABI less than 0.9 (84). In the HOPE Study, compared with placebo, ramipril 10 mg daily significantly reduced cardiovascular events by 25% in persons with symptomatic PAD (84). In this study, ramipril reduced the absolute incidence of cardiovascular events by

Table 28.4 Medical Management of Peripheral Arterial Disease

1. Smoking cessation program
2. Treatment of hypertension with blood pressure reduced to <140/90 mmHg and to <130/80 mmHg in patients with diabetes mellitus or chronic renal insufficiency
3. Control diabetes mellitus with the hemoglobin A_{1c} level reduced to <7%
4. Treat dyslipidemia and reduce serum low-density lipoprotein cholesterol to <70 mg/dl
5. Antiplatelet drug therapy with aspirin or preferably clopidogrel
6. Treatment with an angiotensin-converting enzyme inhibitor
7. Treatment with beta blockers in patients with coronary artery disease in the absence of contraindications to these drugs
8. Use of statins
9. Treatment with cilostazol in patients with intermittent claudication
10. Exercise rehabilitation program
11. Foot care

5.9% in persons with asymptomatic PAD and by 2.3% in persons with a normal ABI (62). In the HOPE Study, the antihypertensive properties of ramipril did not completely account for the observed risk reduction (84).

Among persons with PAD in the Appropriate Blood Pressure Control in Diabetes trial, the incidence of cardiovascular events in persons treated with antihypertensive drug therapy with enalapril or nisoldipine was 13.6% if the mean blood pressure was reduced to 128/75 mmHg versus 38.7% if the mean blood pressure was reduced to 137/81 mmHg (85).

Elderly persons with diabetes mellitus and PAD and no CAD have a 1.5 times higher incidence of new coronary events than elderly non-diabetics with PAD and prior MI (86). The higher the hemoglobin A_{1c} levels in patients with diabetes mellitus and PAD, the higher the prevalence of severe PAD (87). Diabetes mellitus should be treated with the hemoglobin A_{1c} level decreased to less than 7% to decrease the incidence of myocardial infarction (88). The blood pressure should be reduced to less than 140/90 mmHg in elderly persons with PAD and diabetes mellitus (32) although earlier guidelines recommended less than 130/80 mmHg (89). Elderly diabetics with PAD should also be treated with statins (90) and the serum LDL cholesterol reduced to <70 mg/dl (91).

Treatment of dyslipidemia with statins has been documented to reduce the incidence of mortality, cardiovascular events, and stroke in persons with PAD with and without CAD (34,35,91–100). At 5-year follow-up of 4444 men and women with CAD and hypercholesterolemia in the Scandinavian Simvastatin Survival Study, compared with placebo, simvastatin significantly decreased the incidence of intermittent claudication by 38% (92).

In a study of 264 men and 396 women, mean age 80 years, with symptomatic PAD and a serum LDL cholesterol of 125 mg/dl or higher, 318 of 660 persons (48%) were treated with a statin and 342 of 660 persons (52%) with no lipid-lowering drug (97). At 39-month follow-up, treatment with statins caused a significant independent reduction in the incidence of new coronary events of 58%, of 52% in persons with prior myocardial infarction, and of 59% in persons with no prior myocardial infarction (97).

In the Heart Protection Study, 6748 of the 20,536 persons (33%) had PAD (93). At 5-year follow-up, treatment with simvastatin 40 mg daily caused a significant 19% relative reduction and a 6.3% absolute reduction in major cardiovascular events independent of age, gender, or serum lipids levels (93). These data favor administration of statins to elderly persons with PAD regardless of serum lipids levels.

On the basis of the available data, elderly persons with PAD and hypercholesterolemia should be treated with statins to reduce cardiovascular mortality and morbidity and progression of PAD (34,35,90–97) and to improve exercise time until intermittent claudication (Table 28.4) (98–100). Statins also reduce perioperative myocardial infarction and mortality (101,102) and 2-year mortality (102) in patients undergoing non-cardiac vascular surgery.

Since lipid-lowering therapy is underutilized in persons with PAD (103,104), intensive educational programs are needed to educate physicians to use lipid-lowering therapy in elderly persons with cardiovascular disease and dyslipidemia (104–106). On the basis of data from the Heart Protection Study, persons with PAD should be treated with statins regardless of age, gender, or initial serum lipids levels (93).

Increased plasma homocysteine level is a risk factor for PAD (36–39). Reduction of increased plasma homocysteine levels can be achieved by administering a combination of folic acid, vitamin B6, and vitamin B12. However, we do not have double-blind, randomized, placebo-controlled data showing that reduction of increased plasma homocysteine levels will reduce coronary events and slow progression of PAD in elderly persons with PAD.

Hypothyroidism is a risk factor for PAD (40). Elderly persons with clinical or sub-clinical hypothyroidism should be treated with l-thyroxine to decrease the development of CAD (107) and possibly of PAD (40). There is no evidence showing that treatment with l-thyroxine will reduce the development of PAD or improve symptoms.

ANTIPLATELET DRUGS

Antiplatelet drugs that have been shown to decrease the incidence of vascular death, non-fatal myocardial infarction, and non-fatal stroke in persons with PAD are aspirin, ticlodip-ine, and clopidogrel (108). Aspirin plus dipyridamole has not been shown to be more efficacious than aspirin alone in the treatment of persons with PAD (108). Oral platelet glycoprotein IIb/IIIa inhibitors have been shown to increase mortality in the treatment of persons with CAD and have not been investigated in the treatment of persons with PAD (109). Adverse hematologic effects associated with ticlodipine limit the use of this drug in the treatment of elderly persons with PAD (110).

Thromboxane A_2 induces platelet aggregation and vasoconstriction. Aspirin decreases the aggregation of platelets exposed to thrombogenic stimuli by inhibiting the cyclo-oxygenase enzyme reaction within the platelet and thereby blocking the conversion of arachidonic acid to thromboxane A_2 (111,112). Clopidogrel is a thienopyridine derivative that inhibits platelet aggregation by inhibiting the binding of adenosine 5'-diphosphate to its platelet receptor (112).

The Antithrombotic Trialists' Collaboration Group (ATCG) reported a meta-analysis of 26 randomized studies of 6263 persons with intermittent claudication due to PAD (108). At follow-up, the incidence of vascular death, non-fatal myocardial infarction, and non-fatal stroke was 6.4% in patients randomized to antiplatelet drugs versus 7.9% in the con-trol group, a significant reduction of 23% caused by antiplatelet therapy. The reductions are significant for all subgroups.

The ATCG reported a meta-analysis of 12 randomized studies of 2497 persons with PAD undergoing peripheral arterial grafting (108). At follow-up, the incidence of vascular death, non-fatal myocardial infarction, and non-fatal stroke was 5.4% in persons random-ized to antiplatelet drugs versus 6.5% in the control group, a significant reduction of 22% caused by antiplatelet therapy.

The ATCG also reported a meta-analysis of four randomized studies of 946 persons with PAD undergoing peripheral angioplasty (108). At follow-up, the incidence of vascular death, non-fatal myocardial infarction, and non-fatal stroke was 2.5% in patients random-ized to antiplatelet drugs versus 3.6% in the control group, a significant reduction of 29% caused by antiplatelet therapy.

If one combines the 42 randomized studies of 9706 patients with intermittent claudi-cation, peripheral arterial grafting, or peripheral angioplasty, the incidence of vascular death, non-fatal myocardial infarction, and non-fatal stroke at follow-up was significantly decreased 23% by antiplatelet drugs, with similar benefits among patients with intermittent claudica-tion, those having peripheral arterial grafting, and those having peripheral angioplasty (108). These data favor the use of aspirin in men and women with PAD (Table 28.4) (108).

Aspirin

Table 28.5 shows the efficacy of different doses of aspirin in reducing in high-risk persons the incidence of vascular death, non-fatal myocardial infarction, and non-fatal stroke (108). Since aspirin doses greater than 150 mg daily do not reduce vascular death, non-fatal myo-cardial infarction, and non-fatal stroke more than does a dose of 75–150 mg daily and cause more gastrointestinal bleeding than the lower doses, this author prefers an aspirin dose of 81 mg daily in treating elderly persons with atherosclerotic vascular disease.

Table 28.5 Efficacy of Aspirin Doses in Decreasing Vascular Death, Nonfatal Myocardial Infarction, and Nonfatal Stroke in High-Risk Patients

Aspirin Dose	Decrease in Vascular Death, Myocardial Infarction, or Stroke
500–1500 mg (34 trials)	19%
160–325 mg (19 trials)	26%
75–150 mg (12 trials)	32%
<75 mg (3 trials)	13%

Source: Adapted from Ref. 108.

Clopidogrel

In the Clopidogrel versus Aspirin in Patients at Risk for Ischaemic Events (CAPRIE) trial, 5795 persons with PAD were randomized to clopidogrel 75 mg daily and 5797 persons with PAD were randomized to aspirin 325 mg daily (113). At 1.9-year follow-up, the annual incidence of vascular death, non-fatal myocardial infarction, and non-fatal stroke was 3.7% in persons randomized to clopidogrel versus 4.9% in persons randomized to aspirin, a 24% significant decrease with the use of clopidogrel (113).

On the basis of these data, it is reasonable to conclude that clopidogrel is superior to aspirin in the management of patients with PAD. On the basis of these data, the author also recommends the use of clopidogrel 75 mg daily in the treatment of patients with PAD (Table 28.4). However, clopidogrel is much more expensive than is aspirin. In a vascular surgery clinic, 501 of 506 persons (83%) with PAD were treated with aspirin or clopidogrel (114). Aspirin 75–325 mg daily or clopidogrel 76 mg daily are recommended by the 2011 American College of Cardiology Foundation (ACCF)/American Heart Association (AHA) guidelines to reduce the risk of myocardial infarction, stroke, or vascular death in patients with PAD (77).

ORAL ANTICOAGULANTS

In the Dutch Bypass Oral Anticoagulants or Aspirin Study, 2690 persons were randomized after infrainguinal bypass surgery to aspirin 80 mg daily or to oral anticoagulation with phenprocoumon or acenocoumarol to maintain an INR of 3.0–4.5 (115). At 21-month follow-up, there was no significant difference between the two treatments in the primary outcome of infrainguinal graft occlusion (115). There was no significant difference between the two treatments in the secondary outcomes of myocardial infarction, stroke, amputation, or vascular death (115). However, persons treated with oral anticoagulant therapy had 1.96 times more major bleeding episodes than persons treated with oral aspirin (115). The American College of Cardiology (ACC)/AHA guidelines state that oral anticoagulant therapy with warfarin should not be given to reduce the risk of adverse cardiovascular ischemic events in persons with atherosclerotic lower extremity PAD (7,77).

ANGIOTENSIN-CONVERTING ENZYME INHIBITORS

Data from the HOPE Study showed that ramipril 10 mg daily significantly decreased cardiovascular events in persons with symptomatic PAD and in persons with asymptomatic PAD (84). Angiotensin-converting enzyme (ACE) inhibitors as well as statins also have many pleotropic effects to account for their vascular protective properties beyond their primary mode of action including inhibition of cellular proliferation, restoration of endothelial activity, inhibition of platelet reactivity, and an antioxidant potential (116). The

ACC/AHA guidelines recommend treating persons with PAD with ACE inhibitors unless there are contraindications to the use of these drugs to reduce cardiovascular mortality and morbidity (Table 28.4) (117).

BETA BLOCKERS

Persons with PAD are at increased risk for developing new coronary events (24,56–72). Many physicians have been reluctant to use beta blockers in persons with PAD because of concerns that beta blockers will aggravate intermittent claudication. However, a meta-analysis of 11 randomized controlled studies found that beta blockers do not adversely affect walking capacity or the symptoms of intermittent claudication in persons with mild-to-moderate PAD (118).

An observational study was performed in 575 men and women, mean age 80 years, with symptomatic PAD and prior myocardial infarction (119). Of the 575 persons, 85 persons (15%) had contraindications to the use of beta blockers. Of the 490 persons without contraindications to the use of beta blockers, 257 persons (52%) were treated with beta blockers. Adverse effects causing cessation of beta blockers occurred in 31 of the 257 persons (12%). At 32-month follow-up, use of beta blockers caused a 53% significant independent decrease in the incidence of new coronary events in elderly persons with PAD and prior myocardial infarction (119). In a vascular surgery clinic, 301 of 364 persons (83%) with PAD and CAD were treated with beta blockers (114). Beta blockers should be used to treat CAD in patients with PAD in the absence of contraindications to these drugs (Table 28.4).

STATINS

On the basis of data from the Heart Protection Study, persons with PAD should be treated with statins regardless of age, gender, or initial serum lipids levels (Table 28.4) (93). Three double-blind, randomized, placebo-controlled studies have also demonstrated that statins improve walking performance in persons with PAD (Table 28.6) (98–100).

In a study of 69 persons, mean age 75 years, with intermittent claudication, a mean ABI of 0.63, and a serum LDL cholesterol of 125 mg/dl or higher, 3 of 34 persons (9%)

Table 28.6 Effects of Statins on Walking Performance in Patients with Intermittent Claudication

Study	Results
69 persons, mean age 75 years, with intermittent claudication and hypercholesterolemia (98)	Compared with placebo, simvastatin 40 mg daily significantly increased treadmill exercise time until the onset of intermittent claudication by 24% at 6 months and by 42% at 1 year
354 persons, mean age 68 years, with intermittent claudication and hypercholesterolemia (99)	At 1-year follow-up, compared with placebo, atorvastatin 80 mg daily significantly increased pain-free treadmill walking distance by 40% and community-based physical activity
86 persons, mean age 67 years, with intermittent claudication and hypercholesterolemia (100)	At 6-month follow-up, compared with placebo, simvastatin 40 mg daily significantly increased pain-free walking distance and total walking distance on a treadmill, the mean ankle-brachial index at rest and after exercise, and symptoms of claudication

treated with simvastatin and 6 of 35 persons (17%) treated with placebo died before the 1-year study was completed (98). Compared with placebo, simvastatin significantly increased the treadmill exercise time until the onset of intermittent claudication by 24% at 6 months and by 42% at 1-year after therapy (Table 28.6) (98).

In a study of 354 persons, mean age 68 years, with intermittent claudication and hypercholesterolemia, at 1-year follow-up, compared with placebo, atorvastatin 80 mg daily significantly improved pain-free treadmill walking distance by 40% and significantly improved community-based physical activity (Table 28.6) (99). In a study of 86 persons, mean age 67 years, with intermittent claudication and hypercholesterolemia, at 6-month follow-up, compared with placebo, simvastatin 40 mg daily significantly improved pain-free walking distance and total walking distance on a treadmill, significantly improved the mean ABI at rest and after exercise, and significantly improved symptoms of claudication (Table 28.6) (100).

Statin use is also associated with superior leg functioning independent of cholesterol levels and other potential confounders (120). The data suggest that non-cholesterol-lowering properties of statins may favorably influence functioning in persons with and without PAD (120).

Despite the data recommending use of statins, aspirin, and ACE inhibitors or angiotensin receptor blockers for secondary prevention in patients with PAD, millions of adults in the USA with PAD are not receiving these drugs (121). Use of these drugs in patients with PAD and no other cardiovascular disease was associated with a 65% significant reduction in all-cause mortality (121).

DRUGS TO INCREASE WALKING DISTANCE

Chelation therapy has been demonstrated to be ineffective in the therapy of PAD (122). Numerous drugs have been shown to be ineffective in improving walking distance in persons with intermittent claudication (123,124). Beraprost sodium, an orally active prostaglandin I_2 analog, was demonstrated to be no more effective than placebo in persons with intermittent claudication (125). Naftidrofuryl (126) and propionyl levocarnitine (127) have been reported to improve exercise walking distance in persons with intermittent claudication but have not been approved for use in the USA (123).

Two drugs, pentoxifylline and cilostazol, have been approved by the US Food and Drug Administration for symptomatic treatment of intermittent claudication. However, many studies have found no consistent improvement with pentoxifylline in patients with intermittent claudication in comparison with placebo (128–130). In a vascular surgery clinic, all the 301 persons (100%) with intermittent claudication were treated with cilostazol or pentoxifylline (114).

Cilostazol inhibits phosphodiesterase type 3, increasing intracellular concentration of cyclic adenosine monophosphate. Cilostazol suppresses platelet aggregation and also acts as a direct arterial vasodilator. Cilostazol has been documented in numerous trials to improve exercise capacity in patients with intermittent claudication (124,131–134), and in a dose of 100 mg twice daily, was shown to be superior to both placebo and pentoxifylline (133).

Cilostazol should be administered to patients with PAD to increase walking distance (Table 28.4), but should not be given to persons with PAD who also have heart failure. Other contraindications to the use of cilostazol include a creatinine clearance <25 ml/min, a known predisposition for bleeding, or coadministration of CYP3A4 or CYP2C19 inhibitors such as cimetidine, diltiazem, erythromycin, ketoconazole, lansoprazole, omeprazole, and HIV-1 protease inhibitors.

EXERCISE REHABILITATION

Exercise rehabilitation programs have been demonstrated to increase walking distance in persons with intermittent claudication through improvements in peripheral circulation, walking economy, and cardiopulmonary function (135,136). The optimal exercise program for improving claudication pain distance in persons with PAD uses intermittent walking to near-maximal pain during a program of at least 6 months (137). Strength training is less effective than treadmill walking (138). The ACC/AHA guidelines recommend a supervised exercise program for patients with intermittent claudication (Table 28.4) (7).

Supervised exercise training is recommended for a minimum of 30–45 minutes in sessions performed at least three times per week for a minimum of 12 weeks (4) and preferably for 6 months or longer (137). Among persons with PAD, self-directed walking exercise performed at least three times weekly is associated with significantly less functional decline during the subsequent year (139).

FOOT CARE

Persons with PVD must have proper foot care (Table 28.4) (7,140). They must wear properly fitted shoes. Careless nail clipping or injury from walking barefoot must be avoided. Feet should be washed daily and the skin kept moist with topical emollients to prevent cracks and fissures, which may have portals for bacterial infection. Fungal infection of the feet must be treated. Socks should be wool or other thick fabrics, and padding or shoe inserts may be used to prevent pressure sores. When a wound of the foot develops, specialized foot gear, including casts, boots, and ankle foot arthoses may be helpful in unweighting the affected area (140).

LOWER EXTREMITY ANGIOPLASTY AND BYPASS SURGERY

Table 28.7 states that the indications for lower extremity percutaneous transluminal angioplasty or bypass surgery are (*i*) incapacitating claudication in persons interfering with work or lifestyle; (*ii*) limb salvage in persons with limb-threatening ischemia as manifested by rest pain, nonhealing ulcers, and/or infection or gangrene; and (*iii*) vasculogenic impotence (141). Percutaneous transluminal angioplasty can be performed if there is a skilled vascular interventionalist and the arterial disease is localized to a vessel segment less than 10 cm in length (141). Compared to percutaneous transluminal angioplasty alone, stenting improves 3-year patency by 26% (142) After infrainguinal bypass surgery, oral anticoagulant therapy is preferable in persons with venous grafts, whereas aspirin is preferable in persons with non-venous grafts (115).

Percutaneous balloon angioplasty and/or stenting is indicated for short-segment stenoses, whereas multisegment disease and occlusions are most effectively treated with surgical revascularization (143). Revascularization of PAD is discussed extensively elsewhere (7,140). In patients presenting with severe limb ischemia caused by infra-inguinal disease and who are suitable for either surgery or angioplasty, by-pass surgery and balloon-angioplasty are associated with similar outcomes in terms of amputation-free

Table 28.7 Indications for Angioplasty or Bypass Surgery in Lower Extremities

---

1. Incapacitating intermittent claudication in persons interfering with work or lifestyle
2. Limb salvage in persons with limb-threatening ischemia as manifested by rest pain, non-healing ulcers, and/or infection or gangrene
3. Vasculogenic impotence

Source: Adapted from Ref. 141.

survival (144). Patients with intermittent claudication should be considered for revascularization to improve symptoms only in the absence of other disease that would limit exercise improvement such as angina pectoris, heart failure, chronic pulmonary disease, or orthopedic limitations (7).

However, 6-month outcomes from 111 patients with claudication due to aortoiliac PAD randomized to optimal medical therapy, optimal medical therapy plus supervised exercise, or optimal medical therapy plus stent revascularization showed that the greatest increase in treadmill walking performance occurred in the patients randomized to optimal medical therapy plus supervised exercise (145).

AMPUTATION

Non-randomized studies have demonstrated that both immediate and long-term survival are higher in patients having revascularization rather than amputation for limb-threatening ischemia (146,147). However, amputation of lower extremities should be performed if tissue loss has progressed beyond the point of salvage, if surgery is too risky, if life expectancy is very low, or if functional limitations diminish the benefit of limb salvage (140).

ABDOMINAL AORTIC ANEURYSM

The prevalence of abdominal aortic aneurysm (AAA) increases with advancing age, smoking, hypercholesterolemia, hypertension, male gender, and family history (7,148–150). The prevalence of an AAA varies from 1.3% for men aged 45–54 years to 12.5% for men aged 75–84 years (7). The prevalence of an AAA varies from 0% for women aged 45–54 years to 5.2% for women aged 75–84 years (7). Most patients with an AAA are asymptomatic, with their AAA noted on studies performed for other reasons rather than on physical examination. Of 110 men with an AAA, 71% had CAD, 46% had lower extremity PAD, and 27% had cerebrovascular disease (151). The prognosis of an AAA in women is worse than in men (152).

In patients that have evidence of back, abdominal, or groin pain in the presence of a pulsatile abdominal mass, the aorta needs to be evaluated immediately, preferably with computed tomographic scanning. In one study, the mortality rates were 35% for ruptured AAAs, 26% for symptomatic AAAs, and 5% for asymptomatic AAAs undergoing repair (153). In another study, treatment of 96 high-risk patients, mean age 72 years, with an AAA with an endovascular stent-graft prosthesis was associated with a 100% survival at 90-day follow-up (154).

The ACCF/AHA guidelines recommend that patients with infrarenal or juxtarenal AAAs measuring 5.5 cm or larger should undergo repair to eliminate the risk of rupture (7). Patients with infrarenal or juxtarenal AAAs measuring 4.0–5.4 cm in diameter should be monitored by ultrasound or computed tomographic scans every 6–12 months to detect expansion (7).

Patients with AAA should undergo intensive risk factor modification. In one study, use of ACE inhibitors was associated with a reduced risk of ruptured AAA (155). Of 130 patients with AAAs not treated surgically, patients treated with statins (58% of the group) had a significantly lower mortality at 45-month follow-up (5% for statin-treated patients vs. 16% for patients not treated with statins) (156). The size of the AAA was 4.6 cm at baseline versus 4.5 cm at 23-month follow-up in patients treated with statins versus 4.5 cm at baseline and 5.3 cm at 24-month follow-up in patients not treated with statins (156). Use of statins also reduced perioperative and 2-year mortality in patients undergoing surgical AAA repair (101,102). In addition, long-term statin use was associated with decreased all-cause mortality and cardiovascular mortality after successful AAA surgery irrespective of clinical risk factors and use of beta blockers (157).

In 400 patients ineligible for open repair of an AAA randomized to no repair or endovascular repair, at 8-year follow-up, endovascular repair was associated with a significant 47% reduction in aneurysm-related mortality but was not associated with a reduction in all-cause mortality (158).

REFERENCES

1. Dormandy JA, Rutherford RB; TASC Working Group. TransAtlantic Inter-Society Consensus (TASC). Management of Peripheral Arterial Disease (PAD). J Vasc Surg 2000; 31: S1–S296.
2. McDermott MM, Greenland P, Liu K, et al. Leg symptoms in peripheral arterial disease. Associated clinical characteristics and functional impairment. JAMA 2001; 286: 1599–606.
3. McDermott MM, Greenland P, Liu K, et al. Sex differences in peripheral arterial disease: leg symptoms and physical functioning. J Am Geriatr Soc 2003; 51: 222–8.
4. McDermott MM, Ferrucci L, Liu K, et al. Women with peripheral arterial disease experience faster functional decline than men with peripheral arterial disease. J Am Coll Cardiol 2011; 57: 707–14.
5. McDermott MM, Liu K, Ferrucci L, et al. Greater sedentary hours and slower walking speed outside the home predict faster declines in functioning and adverse calf muscle changes in peripheral arterial disease. J Am Coll Cardiol 2011; 57: 2356–64.
6. Garg PK, Liu K, Tian L, et al. Physical activity during daily life and functional decline in peripheral arterial disease. Circulation 2009; 119: 251–60.
7. Hirsch AT, Haskal ZJ, Hertzer NR, et al. ACC/AHA 2005 Practice Guidelines for the management of patients with peripheral arterial disease (lower extremity, renal, mesenteric, and abdominal aortic): Executive Summary. Circulation 2006; 113: 1474–547.
8. McDermott MM, Greenland P, Liu K, et al. The ankle brachial index is associated with leg function and physical activity: the Walking and Leg Circulation Study. Ann Intern Med 2002; 136: 873–83.
9. Criqui MH, McClelland RL, McDermott MM, et al. The ankle-brachial index and incident cardiovascular events in the MESA (Multi-Ethnic Study of Atherosclerosis). J Am Coll Cardiol 2010; 56: 1506–12.
10. Allison MA, Hiatt WR, Hirsch AT, Coll JR, Criqui MH. A high ankle-brachial index is associated with increased cardiovascular morbidity and lower quality of life. J Am Coll Cardiol 2008; 51: 1292–8.
11. Kohler TR, Nance DR, Cramer MM, et al. Duplex scanning for diagnosis of aortoiliac and femoropopliteal disease: a prospective study. Circulation 1987; 76: 1074–80.
12. Sheikh MA, Bhatt DL, Li J, Lin S, Bartholomew JR. Usefulness of postexercise ankle-brachial index to predict all-cause mortality. Am J Cardiol 2011; 107: 778–82.
13. Schroll M, Munck O. Estimation of peripheral arteriosclerotic disease by ankle blood pressure measurements in a population of 60 year old men and women. J Chron Dis 1981; 34: 261–9.
14. Criqui MH, Fronek A, Barrett-Connor E, et al. The prevalence of peripheral arterial disease in a defined population. Circulation 1985; 71: 510–15.
15. Newman A, Siscovick DS, Manolio TA, et al. Ankle-arm index as a marker of atherosclerosis in the Cardiovascular Health Study. Circulation 1993; 88: 837–45.
16. Ness J, Aronow WS, Ahn C. Risk factors for peripheral arterial disease in an academic hospital-based geriatrics practice. J Am Geriatr Soc 2000; 48: 312–14.
17. Meijer WT, Hoes AW, Rutgers D, et al. Peripheral arterial disease in the elderly. The Rotterdam Study. Arterioscler Thromb Vasc Biol 1998; 18: 185–92.
18. Aronow WS, Ahn C, Gutstein H. Prevalence and incidence of cardiovascular disease in 1160 older men and 2464 older women in a long-term health care facility. J Gerontol Med Sci 2002; 57A: M45–6.
19. Aronow WS. Prevalence of atherothrombotic brain infarction, coronary artery disease and peripheral arterial disease in elderly blacks, Hispanics and whites. Am J Cardiol 1992; 70: 1212–13.
20. Ness J, Aronow WS, Newkirk E, McDanel D. Prevalence of symptomatic peripheral arterial disease, modifiable risk factors, and appropriate use of drugs in the treatment of peripheral arterial disease in older persons seen in a university general medicine clinic. J Gerontol Med Sci 2005; 60A: M255–7.
21. Hirsch AT, Criqui MH, Treat-Jacobson D, et al. Peripheral arterial disease detection, awareness, and treatment in primary care. JAMA 2001; 286: 1317–24.
22. Hughson WG, Mann JI, Garrod A. Intermittent claudication: prevalence and risk factors. Br Med J 1978; 1: 1379–81.
23. Beach KW, Brunzell JD, Strandness DE Jr. Prevalence of severe arteriosclerosis obliterans in patients with diabetes mellitus: relation to smoking and form of therapy. Arteriosclerosis 1982; 2: 275–80.
24. Reunanen A, Takkunen H, Aromaa A. Prevalence of intermittent claudication and its effect on mortality. Acta Med Scand 1982; 211: 249–56.

25. Pomrehn P, Duncan B, Weissfeld L, et al. The association of dyslipoproteinemia with symptoms and signs of peripheral arterial disease: the Lipid Research Clinics Program Prevalence Study. Circulation 1986; 73: I-100–7.

26. Stokes J III, Kannel WB, Wolf PA, et al. The relative importance of selected risk factors for various manifestations of cardiovascular disease among men and women from 35 to 64 years old: 30 years of follow-up in the Framingham Study. Circulation 1987; 75: V-65–73.

27. Aronow WS, Sales FF, Etienne F, Lee NH. Prevalence of peripheral arterial disease and its correlation with risk factors for peripheral arterial disease in elderly patients in a long-term health care facility. Am J Cardiol 1988; 62: 644–6.

28. Murabito JM, Evans JC, Nieto K, et al. Prevalence and clinical correlates of peripheral arterial disease in the Framingham Offspring Study. Am Heart J 2002; 143: 961–5.

29. Sukhija R, Yalamanchili K, Aronow WS. Prevalence of left main coronary artery disease, of 3-vessel or 4-vessel coronary artery disease, and of obstructive coronary artery disease in patients with and without peripheral arterial disease undergoing coronary angiography for suspected coronary artery disease. Am J Cardiol 2003; 92: 304–5.

30. Conen D, Everet BM, Kurth T, et al. Smoking, smoking status, and risk for symptomatic peripheral arterial disease in women. A cohort study. Ann Intern Med 2011; 154: 719–26.

31. Beach KW, Brunzell JD, Conquest LL, Strandness DE. The correlation of arteriosclerosis obliterans with lipoproteins in insulin-dependent and non-insulin-dependent diabetes. Diabetes 1979; 28: 836–40.

32. Aronow WS, Fleg JL, Pepine CJ, et al. ACCF/AHA 2011 expert consensus document on hypertension in the elderly. a report of the American College of Cardiology Foundation Task Force on Clinical Expert Consensus Documents. Developed in collaboration with the American Academy of Neurology, American Geriatrics Society, American Society for Preventive Cardiology, American Society for Hypertension, American Society of Nephrology, Association of Black Cardiologists, and European Society of Hypertension. J Am Coll Cardiol 2011; 57: 2037–114.

33. Aronow WS, Ahn C. Correlation of serum lipids with the presence or absence of atherothrombotic brain infarction and peripheral arterial disease in 1,834 men and women aged ≥62 years. Am J Cardiol 1994; 73: 995–7.

34. Aronow WS. Treatment of older persons with hypercholesterolemia with and without cardiovascular disease. J Gerontol Med Sci 2001; 56A: M138–45.

35. Aronow WS. Should hypercholesterolemia in older persons be treated to reduce cardiovascular events? J Gerontol Med Sci 2002; 57A: M411–13.

36. Boushey CJ, Beresford SAA, Omenn GS, Motulsky AG. A quantitative assessment of plasma homocysteine as a risk factor for vascular disease. Probable benefits of increasing folic acid intakes. JAMA 1995; 274: 1049–57.

37. Malinow MR, Kang SS, Taylor IM, et al. Prevalence of hyperhomocyst(e)inemia in patients with peripheral arterial occlusive disease. Circulation 1989; 79: 1180–8.

38. Clarke R, Daly L, Robinson K, et al. Hyperhomocysteinemia: an independent risk factor for vascular disease. N Engl J Med 1991; 324: 1149–55.

39. Aronow WS, Ahn C. Association between plasma homocysteine and peripheral arterial disease in older persons. Coronary Artery Dis 1998; 9: 49–50.

40. Mya MM, Aronow WS. Increased prevalence of peripheral arterial disease in older men and women with subclinical hypothyroidism. J Gerontol Med Sci 2003; 58A: M68–9.

41. Tison GH, Ndumele CE, Gerstenblith G, et al. Usefulness of baseline obesity to predict development of a high ankle brachial index from the Multi-Ethnic Study of Atherosclerosis. Am J Cardiol 2011; 107: 1386–91.

42. Joseph J, Koka M, Aronow WS. Prevalence of moderate and severe renal insufficiency in older persons with hypertension, diabetes mellitus, coronary artery disease, peripheral arterial disease, ischemic stroke, or congestive heart failure in an academic nursing home. J Am Med Dir Assoc 2008; 9: 257–9.

43. Duncan K, Aronow WS, Babu S. Prevalence of moderate or severe chronic kidney disease in patients with severe peripheral arterial disease versus mild or moderate peripheral arterial disease. Med Sci Monit 2010; 16: CR584–7.

44. Baber U, Mann D, Shimbo D, et al. Combined role of reduced estimated glomerular filtration rate and microalbuminuria on the prevalence of peripheral arterial disease. Am J Cardiol 2009; 104: 1446–51.

45. Conen D, Rexrode KM, Creager MA, et al. Metabolic syndrome, inflammation, and risk of symptomatic peripheral arterial disease in women. A prospective study. Circulation 2009; 120: 1041–7.

46. Brevetti G, Giugliano G, Brevetti L, et al. Inflammation in peripheral arterial disease. Circulation 2010; 122: 1862–75.

47. Wassel CL, Loomba R, Ix JH, et al. Family history is associated with prevalence and severity of peripheral arterial disease. The San Diego Population study. J Am Coll Cardiol 2011; 58: 1386–92.

48. Aronow WS, Ahn C. Prevalence of coexistence of coronary artery disease, peripheral arterial disease, and atherothrombotic brain infarction in men and women ≥62 years of age. Am J Cardiol 1994; 74: 64–5.

49. Ness J, Aronow WS. Prevalence of coexistence of coronary artery disease, ischemic stroke, and peripheral arterial disease in older persons, mean age 80 years, in an academic hospital-based geriatrics practice. J Am Geriatr Soc 1999; 47: 1255–6.

50. Aronow WS, Ahn C, Kronzon I. Association of mitral annular calcium with symptomatic peripheral arterial disease in older persons. Am J Cardiol 2001; 88: 333–4.

51. Aronow WS, Ahn C, Kronzon I. Association of valvular aortic stenosis with symptomatic peripheral arterial disease in older persons. Am J Cardiol 2001; 88: 1046–7.

52. Park H, Das M, Aronow WS, et al. Relation of decreased ankle-brachial index to prevalence of atherosclerotic risk factors, coronary artery disease, aortic valve calcium, and mitral annular calcium. Am J Cardiol 2005; 95: 1005–6.

53. Sukhija R, Aronow WS, Yalamanchili K, et al. Association of ankle-brachial index with severity of angiographic coronary artery disease in patients with peripheral arterial disease and coronary artery disease. Cardiology 2005; 103: 158–60.

54. Hussein AA, Uno K, Wolski K, et al. Peripheral arterial disease and progression of coronary atherosclerosis. J Am Coll Cardiol 2011; 57: 1220–5.

55. Ward RP, Goonewardena SN, Lammertin G, Lang RM. Comparison of the frequency of abnormal cardiac findings by echocardiography in patients with and without peripheral arterial disease. Am J Cardiol 2007; 99: 499–503.

56. Criqui MH, Langer RD, Fronek A, et al. Mortality over a period of 10 years in patients with peripheral arterial disease. N Engl J Med 1992; 326: 381–6.

57. Smith GD, Shipley MJ, Rose G. Intermittent claudication, heart disease risk factors, and mortality: the Whitehall study. Circulation 1990; 82: 1925–31.

58. Aronow WS, Ahn C, Mercando AD, Epstein S. Prognostic significance of silent ischemia in elderly patients with peripheral arterial disease with and without previous myocardial infarction. Am J Cardiol 1992; 69: 137–9.

59. Vogt MT, Cauley JA, Newman AB, et al. Decreased ankle/arm blood pressure index and mortality in elderly women. JAMA 1993; 270: 465–9.

60. Eagle KA, Rihal CS, Foster ED, et al. Long-term survival in patients with coronary artery disease: importance of peripheral vascular disease. J Am Coll Cardiol 1994; 23: 1091–5.

61. Farkouh ME, Rihal CS, Gersh BJ, et al. Influence of coronary heart disease on morbidity and mortality after lower extremity revascularization surgery: a population-based study in Olmsted County, Minnesota (1970-1987). J Am Coll Cardiol 1994; 24: 1290–6.

62. Simonsick EM, Guralnik JM, Hennekens CH, et al. Intermittent claudication and subsequent cardiovascular disease in the elderly. J Gerontol Med Sci 1995; 50A: M17–22.

63. Newman AB, Tyrrell KS, Kuller LH. Mortality over four years in SHEP participants with a low ankle-arm index. J Am Geriatr Soc 1997; 45: 1472–8.

64. Saw J, Bhatt DL, Moliterno DJ, et al. The influence of peripheral arterial disease on outcomes. A pooled analysis of mortality in eight large randomized percutaneous coronary intervention trials. J Am Coll Cardiol 2006; 48: 1567–72.

65. Criqui MH, Ninomiya JK, Wingard DL, Ji M, Fronck A. Progression of peripheral arterial disease predicts cardiovascular disease morbidity and mortality. J Am Coll Cardiol 2008; 52: 1736–42.

66. Schouten O, van Kujik J-P, Flu W J, et al. Long-term outcome of prophylactic coronary revascularization in cardiac high-risk patients undergoing major vascular surgery (from the Randomized DECREASE-V Pilot Study). Am J Cardiol 2009; 103: 897–901.

67. Aronow WS, Ahmed MI, Ekundayo OJ, Allman RM, Ahmed A. A propensity-matched study of the association of peripheral arterial disease with cardiovascular outcomes in community-dwelling older adults. Am J Cardiol 2009; 103: 130–5.

68. Diehm C, Allenberg JR, Pittrow D, et al. Mortality and vascular morbidity in older adults with asymptomatic versus symptomatic peripheral arterial disease. Circulation 2009; 120: 2053–61.

69. Popovic B, Arnould MA, Selton-Suty C, et al. Comparison of two-year outcomes in patients undergoing isolated coronary artery bypass grafting with and without peripheral arterial disease. Am J Cardiol 2009; 104: 1377–82.

70. Ahmed MI, Aronow WS, Criqui MH, et al. Effect of peripheral arterial disease on outcomes in advanced chronic systolic heart failure. A propensity-matched study. Circ Heart Fail 2010; 3: 118–24.

71. Parikh SV, Saya S, Divanji P, et al. Risk of death and myocardial infarction in patients with peripheral arterial disease undergoing percutaneous coronary intervention (from the National Heart, Lung and Blood Institute Dynamic Registry). Am J Cardiol 2011; 107: 959–64.

72. Chhabra A, Aronow WS, Ahn C, et al. Incidence of new cardiovascular events in patients with and without peripheral arterial disease seen in a vascular surgery clinic. Med Sci Monit 2012; 18: CR131–4.

73. Hendel RC, Whitfield SS, Villegas BJ, et al. Prediction of late cardiac events by dipyridamole thallium imaging in patients undergoing elective vascular surgery. Am J Cardiol 1992; 70: 1243–9.

74. Juergens IL, Barker NW, Hines EA. Arteriosclerosis of veterans: a review of 520ses with special reference to pathogenic and prognostic factors. Circulation 1960; 21: 188–99.

75. Myers KA, King RB, Scott DF, et al. The effect of smoking on the late patency of arterial reconstructions in the legs. Br J Surg 1978; 65: 267–71.

76. Quick CRG, Cotton LT. The measured effect of stopping smoking on intermittent claudication. Br J Surg 1982; 69: S24–6.

77. Rooke TW, Hirsch AT, Misra S, et al. 2011ACCF/AHA focused update of the guideline for the management of patients with peripheral artery disease (updating the 2005 guideline). A report of the American College of Cardiology Foundation/American Heart Association Task Force on Practice Guidelines. Developed in collaboration with the Society for Cardiovascular Angiography and Interventions, Society of Interventional Radiology, Society for Vascular Medicine, and Society for Vascular Surgery. J Am Coll Cardiol 2011; 58: 2020–45.

78. Creager MA, Belkin M, Bluth EI, et al. 2012 ACCF/AHA/ACRSCAI/SIR/STS/SVM/SVN/SVS key data elements and definitions for peripheral atherosclerotic vascular disease. A report of the American College of Cardiology Foundation/American Heart Association Task Force on Clinical Data Standards (Writing Committee to develop clinical data standards for peripheral atherosclerotic vascular disease). Developed in collaboration with the American Association of Cardiovascular and Pulmonary Rehabilitation, American Academy of Neurology, American Association of Neurological surgeons, American Diabetes Association, Society of Atherosclerosis Imaging and Prevention, Socioety of Cardiovascular Computed Tomography, Society for Cardiovascular Magnetic Resonance, and Vascular Disease Foundation. J Am Coll Cardiol 2012; 59: 294–357.

79. Benowitz NL. Treating tobacco addiction: nicotine or no nicotine. N Engl J Med 1997; 337: 1230–1.

80. Hurt RD, Sachs DPL, Glover ED, et al. A comparison of sustained-release buproprion and placebo for smoking cessation. N Engl J Med 1997; 337: 1195–202.

81. Frishman WH, Ky T, Ismail A. Tobacco smoking, nicotine, and non-nicotine replacement therapies. Heart Dis 2001; 3: 365–77.

82. Tonnesen P, Fryd V, Hansen M, et al. Effect of nicotine chewing gum in combination with group counseling on the cessation of smoking. N Engl J Med 1988; 318: 15–18.

83. Adler AI, Stratton IM, Neil HAW, et al. Association of systolic blood pressure with macrovascular and microvascular complications of type 2 diabetes (UKPDS 36): prospective observational study. Br Med J 2000; 321: 412–19.

84. Ostergren J, Sleight P, Dagenais G, et al. Impact of ramipril in patients with evidence of clinical or subclinical peripheral arterial disease. Eur Heart J 2004; 25: 17–24.

85. Mehler PS, Coll JR, Estacio R, et al. Intensive blood pressure control reduces the risk of cardiovascular events in patients with peripheral arterial disease and type 2 diabetes. Circulation 2003; 107: 753–6.

86. Aronow WS, Ahn C. Elderly diabetics with peripheral arterial disease and no coronary artery disease have a higher incidence of new coronary events than elderly nondiabetics with peripheral arterial disease and prior myocardial infarction treated with statins and with no lipid-lowering drug. J Gerontol A Biol Sci Med Sci 2003; 58: M573–5.

87. Aronow WS, Ahn C, Weiss MB, Babu S. Relation of increased hemoglobin A1c levels to severity of peripheral arterial disease in patients with diabetes mellitus. Am J Cardiol 2007; 99: 1468–9.

88. Stratton IM, Adler AI, Neil HAW, et al. Association of glycaemia with macrovascular and microvascular complications of type 2 diabetes (UKPDS 35): prospective observational study. Br Med J 2000; 321: 405–12.

89. Chobanian AV, Bakris GL, Black HR, et al. The seventh report of the joint national committee on prevention, detection, evaluation, and treatment of high blood pressure: the JNC 7 report. JAMA 2003; 289: 2560–72.

90. Aronow WS, Ahn C, Gutstein H. Reduction of new coronary events and of new atherothrombotic brain infarction in older persons with diabetes mellitus, prior myocardial infarction, and serum low-density lipoprotein cholesterol ≥125 mg/dL treated with statins. J Gerontol Med Sci 2002; 57A: M747–50.

91. Grundy SM, Cleeman JI, Merz CN, et al. Implications of recent clinical trials for the National Cholesterol Education Program Adult Treatment Panel III guidelines. Circulation 2004; 110: 227–39.

92. Pedersen TR, Kjekshus J, Pyorala K, et al. Effect of simvastatin on ischemic signs and symptoms in the Scandinavian Simvastatin Survival Study (4S). Am J Cardiol 1998; 81: 333–6.

93. Heart Protection Study Collaborative Group. MRC/BHF Heart Protection Study of cholesterol lowering with simvastatin in 20,536 high-risk individuals: a randomised placebo-controlled trial. Lancet 2002; 360: 7–22.

94. Aronow WS, Ahn C. Incidence of new coronary events in older persons with prior myocardial infarction and serum low-density lipoprotein cholesterol ≥125 mg/dL treated with statins versus no lipid-lowering drug. Am J Cardiol 2002; 89: 67–9.

95. Aronow WS, Ahn C, Gutstein H. Incidence of new atherothrombotic brain infarction in older persons with prior myocardial infarction and serum low-density lipoprotein cholesterol ≥125 mg/dL treated with statins versus no lipid-lowering drug. J Gerontol Med Sci 2002; 57A: M333–5.

96. Aronow WS, Ahn C. Frequency of congestive heart failure in older persons with prior myocardial infarction and serum low-density lipoprotein cholesterol ≥125 mg/dl treated with statins versus no lipid-lowering drug. Am J Cardiol 2002; 90: 147–9.

97. Aronow WS, Ahn C. Frequency of new coronary events in older persons with peripheral arterial disease and serum low-density lipoprotein cholesterol ≥125 mg/dl treated with statins versus no lipid-lowering drug. Am J Cardiol 2002; 90: 789–91.

98. Aronow WS, Nayak D, Woodworth S, Ahn C. Effect of simvastatin versus placebo on treadmill exercise time until the onset of intermittent claudication in older patients with peripheral arterial disease at 6 months and at 1 year after treatment. Am J Cardiol 2003; 92: 711–12.

99. Mohler ER III, Hiatt WR, Creager MA; Study Investigators. Cholesterol reduction with atorvastatin improves walking distance in patients with peripheral arterial disease. Circulation 2003; 108: 1481–6.

100. Mondillo S, Ballo P, Barbati R, et al. Effects of simvastatin on walking performance and symptoms of intermittent claudication in hypercholesterolemic patients with peripheral vascular disease. Am J Med 2003; 114: 359–64.

101. Poldermans D, Bax JJ, Kertai MD, et al. Statins are associated with a reduced incidence of perioperative mortality in patients undergoing major noncardiac vascular surgery. Circulation 2003; 107: 1848–51.

102. Desai H, Aronow WS, Ahn C, et al. Incidence of perioperative myocardial infarction and of 2-year mortality in 577 elderly patients undergoing noncardiac vascular surgery treated with and without statins. Arch Gerontol Geriatr 2010; 51: 149–51.

103. Ghosh S, Ziesmer V, Aronow WS. Underutilization of aspirin, beta blockers, angiotensin-converting enzyme inhibitors, and lipid-lowering drugs and overutilization of calcium channel blockers in older persons with coronary artery disease in an academic nursing home. J Gerontol Med Sci 2002; 57A: M398–400.

104. Ghosh S, Aronow WS. Utilization of lipid-lowering drugs in elderly persons with increased serum low-density lipoprotein cholesterol associated with coronary artery disease, symptomatic peripheral arterial disease, prior stroke, or diabetes mellitus before and after an educational program to treat dyslipidemia. J Gerontol Med Sci 2003; 58A: M432–5.

105. Sanal S, Aronow WS. Effect of an educational program on the prevalence of use of antiplatelet drugs, beta blockers, angiotensin-converting enzyme inhibitors, lipid-lowering drugs, and calcium channel blockers prescribed during hospitalization and at hospital discharge in patients with coronary artery disease. J Gerontol Med Sci 2003; 58A: M1046–8.

106. Nayak D, Aronow WS. Effect of an ongoing educational program on the use of antiplatelet drugs, beta blockers, angiotensin-converting enzyme inhibitors, and lipid-lowering drugs in patients with coronary artery disease seen in an academic cardiology clinic. Cardiol Rev 2005; 13: 95–7.

107. Mya MM, Aronow WS. Subclinical hypothyroidism is associated with coronary artery disease in older persons. J Gerontol Med Sci 2002; 57A: M658–9.

108. Antithrombotic Trialists' Collaboration. Collaborative meta-analyis of randomised trials of antiplatelet therapy for prevention of death, myocardial infarction, and stroke in high risk patients. BMJ 2002; 324: 71–86.

109. Chew DP, Bhatt DL, Sapp S, Topol EJ. Increased mortality with oral platelet glycoprotein IIb/IIIa antagonists. A meta-analysis of phase III multicenter randomized trials. Circulation 2001; 103: 201–6.

110. Bennett CL, Weinberg PD, Rozenberg-Ben-Dror K, et al. Thrombotic thrombocytopenic purpura associated with ticlopidine; a review of 60 cases. Ann Intern Med 1998; 128: 541–4.

111. Roth GJ, Majerus PW. The mechanism of the effect of aspirin on human platelets: I. Acetylation of a particulate fraction protein. J Clin Invest 1975; 56: 624–32.

112. Mills DC, Puri R, Hu CJ, et al. Clopidogrel inhibits the binding of ADP analogues to the receptor mediating inhibition of platelet adenylate cyclase. Arterioscl Thromb 1992; 12: 430–6.

113. CAPRIE Steering Committee. A randomised, blinded, trial of clopidogrel versus aspirin in patients at risk of ischaemic events (CAPRIE). Lancet 1996; 348: 1329–39.

114. Sukhija R, Yalamanchili K, Aronow WS, et al. Clinical characteristics, risk factors, and medical treatment of 561 patients with peripheral arterial disease followed in an academic vascular surgery clinic. Cardiol Rev 2005; 13: 108–10.

115. Dutch Bypass Oral Anticoagulants or Aspirin (BOA) Study Group. Efficacy of oral anticoagulants compared with aspirin after infrainguinal bypass surgery (The Dutch Bypass Oral Anticoagulants or Aspirin Study): a randomized trial. Lancet 2000; 355: 346–51.

116. Faggiotto A, Paoletti R. Statins and blockers of the renin-angiotensin system. Vascular protection beyond their primary mode of action. Hypertension 1999; 34: 987–96.

117. Smith SC Jr, Blair SN, Bonow RO, et al. A statement for healthcare professionals from the American Heart Association and the American College of Cardiology. J Am Coll Cardiol 2001; 38: 1581–3.

118. Radack K, Deck C. Beta-aderenergic blocker therapy does not worsen intermittent claudication in subjects with peripheral arterial disease: meta-analysis of randomized controlled trials. Arch Intern Med 1991; 151: 1769–76.

119. Aronow WS, Ahn C. Effect of beta blockers on incidence of new coronary events in older persons with prior myocardial infarction and symptomatic peripheral arterial disease. Am J Cardiol 2001; 87: 1284–6.

120. McDermott MM, Guralnik JM, Greenland P, et al. Statin use and leg functioning in patients with and without lower-extremity peripheral arterial disease. Circulation 2003; 107: 757–61.

121. Pande RL, Perlstein TS, Beckman JA, Creager MA. Secondary prevention and mortality in peripheral artery disease. National Health and Nutrition Examination Study, 1999 to 2004. Circulation 2011; 96: 1031–3.

122. Ernst E. Chelation therapy for peripheral arterial occlusive disease: a systematic review. Circulation 1997; 96: 1031–3.

123. Hiatt WR. Medical treatment of peripheral arterial disease and claudication. N Engl J Med 2001; 344: 1608–21.

124. Eberhardt RT, Coffman JD. Drug treatment of peripheral vascular disease. Heart Dis 2000; 2: 62–74.

125. Mohler ER III, Hiatt WR, Olin JW, et al. Treatment of intermittent claudication with beraprost sodium, an orally active prostaglandin I2 analogue. A double-blinded, randomized, controlled trial. J Am Coll Cardiol 2003; 41: 1679–86.

126. Lehert P, Comte S, Gamand S, Brown TM. Naftidrofuryl in intermittent claudication: a retrospective analysis. J Cardiovasc Pharmacol 1994; 23: S48–52.

127. Brevetti G, Perna S, Sabba C, et al. Propionyl-L-carnitine in intermittent claudication: a double-blind, placebo-controlled, dose titration, multicenter study. J Am Coll Cardiol 1999; 26: 1411–16.

128. Radack K, Wyderski RJ. Conservative management of intermittent claudication. Ann Intern Med 1990; 113: 135–46.

129. Porter JM, Cutler BS, Lee BY, et al. Pentoxifylline efficacy in the treatment of intermittent claudication: multicenter controlled double-blind trial with objective assessment of chronic occlusive arterial disease patients. Am Heart J 1982; 104: 66–72.

130. Eberhardt RT, Coffman JD. Drug treatment of peripheral vascular disease. In: Frishman WH, Sonnenblick EH, Sica DA, eds. Cardiovascular Pharmacotherapeutics, 2nd edn. New York: McGraw Hill, 2003: 919–34.

131. Dawson DL, Cutler BS, Meissner MH, Strandness DE Jr. Cilostazol has beneficial effects in treatment of intermittent claudication. Results from a multicenter, randomized, prospective, double-blind trial. Circulation 1998; 98: 678–86.

132. Thompson PD, Zimet R, Forbes WP, Zhang P. Meta-analysis of results from eight randomized, placebo-controlled trials on the effect of cilostazol on patients with intermittent claudication. Am J Cardiol 2002; 90: 1314–19.

133. Dawson DL, Cutler BS, Hiatt WR, et al. A comparison of cilostazol and pentoxifylline for treating intermittent claudication. Am J Med 2000; 109: 523–30.

134. Money SR, Herd JA, Isaacsohn JL, et al. Effect of cilostazol on walking distances in patients with intermittent claudication caused by peripheral vascular disease. J Vasc Surg 1998; 27: 267–74.

135. Gardner AW, Katzel LI, Sorkin JD, et al. Improved functional outcomes following exercise rehabilitation in patients with intermittent claudication. J Gerontol Med Sci 2000; 55A: M570–7.

136. Hamburg NM, Balady GJ. Exercise rehabilitation in peripheral artery disease. Functional impact and mechanisms of benefit. Circulation 2011; 123: 87–97.

137. Gardner AW, Poehlman ET. Exercise rehabilitation programs for the treatment of claudication pain. A meta-analysis. JAMA 1995; 274: 975–80.

138. Hiatt WR, Wolfel EE, Meier RH, Regensteiner JG. Superiority of treadmill walking exercise versus strength training for patients with peripheral arterial disease. Implications for the mechanism of the training response. Circulation 1994; 90: 1866–74.

139. McDermott MM, Liu K, Ferrucci L, et al. Physical performance in peripheral arterial disease: a slower rate of decline in patients who walk more. Ann Intern Med 2006; 144: 10–20.

140. Fujitani RM, Gordon IL, Perera GB, Wilson SE. Peripheral vascular disease in the elderly. In: Aronow WS, Fleg JL, eds. Cardiovascular Disease in the Elderly Patient, 3rd edn. New York City: Marcel Dekker, Inc, 2003: 707–63.

141. Weitz JI, Byrne J, Clagett GP, et al. Diagnosis and treatment of chronic arterial insufficiency of the lower extremities: a critical review. Circulation 1996; 94: 3026–49.

142. Palmaz JC, Garcia OJ, Schatz RA, et al. Placement of balloon-expandable intraluminal stents in iliac arteries. First 171 procedures. Radiology 1990; 174: 969.

143. Comerota AJ. Endovascular and surgical revascularization for patients with intermittent claudication. Am J Cardiol 2001; 87: 34D–43D.

144. BASIL trial participants. Bypass versus angioplasty in severe ischaemia of the leg (BASIL): multi-centre, randomised controlled trial. Lancet 2005; 366: 1925–34.

145. Murphy TP, Cutlip DE, Regensteiner JG, et al. Supervised exercise versus primary stenting for claudication resulting from aortoiliac peripheral artery disease. Six-month outcomes from the Claudication: Exercise Versus Endoluminal Revascularization (CLEVER) Study. Circulation 2012; 125: 130–9.

146. Ouriel K, Fiore WM, Geary JE. Limb-threatening ischemia in the medically compromised patient: amputation or revascularization? Surgery 1988; 104: 667–72.

147. DeFrang RD, Taylor LM Jr, Porter JM. Basic data related to amputations. Ann Vasc Surg 1991; 5: 202–7.

148. Rodin MB, Daviglus ML, Wong GC, et al. Middle age cardiovascular risk factors and abdominal aortic aneurysm in older age. Hypertension 2003; 42: 61–8.

149. Sule S, Aronow WS, Babu S. Prevalence of risk factors and of coronary artery disease, ischemic stroke, carotid arterial disease and lower extremity peripheral arterial disease in 96 patients undergoing elective surgery for an abdominal aneurysm. Int J Angiol 2008; 17: 141–2.

150. Forsdahl SH, Singh K, Solberg S, Jacobsen BK. Risk factors for abdominal aortic aneurysms. A 7-year prospective study: The Tromso Study, 1994–2001. Circulation 2009; 119: 2202–8.

151. Sukhija R, Aronow WS, Yalamanchili K, et al. Prevalence of coronary artery disease, lower extremity peripheral arterial disease, and cerebrovascular disease in 110 men with an abdominal aortic aneurysm. Am J Cardiol 2004; 94: 1358–9.

152. Norman PE, Powell JT. Abdominal aortic aneurysm. The prognosis in women is worse. Circulation 2007; 115: 2865–9.

153. Sullivan CA, Rohrer MJ, Cutler BS. Clinical management of the symptomatic but unruptured abdominal aortic aneurysm. J Vasc Surg 1990; 11: 799–803.

154. Sukhija R, Aronow WS, Mathew J, et al. Treatment of abdominal aortic aneurysms with an endovascular stent-graft prosthesis in 96 high-risk patients. Cardiol Rev 2005; 13: 165–6.

155. Hackam DG, Thiruchelvam D, Redelmeier DA. Angiotensin-converting enzyme inhibitors and aortic rupture: a population-based case-control study. Lancet 2006; 368: 659–65.

156. Sukhija R, Aronow WS, Sandhu R, et al. Mortality and size of abdominal aortic aneurysm at long-term follow-up of patients not treated surgically and treated with and without statins. Am J Cardiol 2006; 97: 279–80.

157. Kertai MD, Boersma E, Westerhout CM, et al. Association between long-term statin use and mortality after successful abdominal aortic aneurysm surgery. Am J Med 2004; 116: 96–103.

158. The United Kingdom EVAR Trial Investigators. Endovascular repair of aortic aneurysm in patients physically ineligible for open repair. N Engl J Med 2010; 362: 1872–80.

29

Perioperative cardiovascular evaluation and treatment of elderly patients undergoing noncardiac surgery

Vikram Prasanna, Andrew J. Litwack, and Lee A. Fleisher

SUMMARY

Perioperative cardiovascular morbidity and mortality continues to be a significant source of complications after surgery in the elderly. The evaluation of the patient integrates clinical risk assessment, the risk of surgery and the exercise capacity in the decision to undergo further diagnostic testing. In patients with previous coronary stent, optimal management of anti-platelet agents incorporates the risks of surgical bleeding versus the benefits of continuation of the medication. The type of intraoperative anesthesia: general versus regional and inhaled versus intravenous, does not appear to affect perioperative mortality or major cardiac morbidity. The optimal perioperative management of the high risk patient includes continuation of the patient's chronic cardiovascular medications, particularly β-blockers and statins, and monitoring for cardiac myonecrosis during the perioperative period (8).

Over 30 million patients undergo noncardiac surgery annually in the USA, 4 million of whom are at risk of having coronary artery disease (CAD) on the basis of clinical risk factors. More than 1 million patients have cardiovascular complications postoperatively (1). The health care costs associated with these adverse cardiac outcomes have been estimated to be in excess of $10 billion annually in the USA. With the shifting demographics of the US population, increasingly the elderly represent the majority on whom surgical procedures are performed. Up to 80% of patients over 80 years have identifiable cardiovascular diseases and that is the leading cause of mortality (2).

With aging, there are several important physiologic cardiovascular changes that occur that can play a key role in management of these patients. The left ventricular (LV) wall thickness increases largely due to an increase in the size of cardiac myoctes. Also, there is an increase in left atrial (LA) size and decreased atrial compliance such that with small changes in volume, there is a drastic rise in LA pressure. Outside the heart, there are significant changes to the vasculature with increases intimal thickening and increased vascular stiffness. Together these changes impart a decreased ability of the cardiovascular system to cope with stress (2).

Cardiovascular complications continue to be a significant etiology of adverse outcome in elderly patients undergoing noncardiac procedures in spite of improvements in surgical and anesthetic techniques and perioperative medical management. These complications are related to a high prevalence of CAD in older patients and to the changes in the cardiovascular system that occurs with aging. The mortality of acute myocardial infarction (MI) increases dramatically in the aged.

The preoperative evaluation and preparation of the elderly patient undergoing noncardiac surgery represents a unique challenge for the primary care physician, cardiologist, anesthesiologist, and surgeon. The elderly not only have a higher prevalence of cardiovascular disease but also are more likely to need urgent or emergent noncardiac surgical procedures. They also represent a population that is not well represented in current clinical trial data. Therefore, the preoperative evaluation is frequently more complicated and may need to be performed on a more urgent basis than in younger patients. In approaching the elderly surgical patient, the fundamental assumption is that the preoperative evaluation will result in changes in perioperative management. In determining the extent of the preoperative evaluation, it is important not to perform testing unless the results will affect perioperative management.

It is important to realize that the preoperative evaluation may also represent the patient's initial cardiovascular, and sometimes medical, evaluation. Therefore, strategies to assess and modify perioperative cardiac risk may also have important long-term consequences for the patient. To provide the practitioner with an understanding of some of the issues and concerns for the anesthesiologist and medical caregivers, this chapter will review those factors that identify the high-risk elderly patient and the preoperative and perioperative interventions that may modify that risk.

ASSESSMENT OF THE PATIENT BEFORE NONCARDIAC SURGERY
History
Since the highest risk to any elderly patient undergoing noncardiac surgery is related to cardiovascular complications, a thorough history should focus on cardiovascular risk factors and symptoms of active cardiac conditions (Table 29.1). Determining the risk of adverse perioperative cardiac events may be useful in determining whether the proposed surgery is the ideal approach to achieving the individual patient's longer-term goals. Several approaches can be used to estimate perioperative cardiac risk in patients before noncardiac surgery. The most widely used model is the revised cardiac risk index (RCRI), which is based on six independent predictors of complications: high-risk type of surgery, history of ischemic heart disease, history of heart failure (HF), history of cerebrovascular disease, preoperative treatment with insulin, and preoperative serum creatinine >2 mg/dL (3). It assigns one point each for the presence of six independent risk factors for major cardiac complications in patients having nonemergency surgery. The incidence of major cardiac events in patients with 0, 1, 2, or 3 risk factors was 0.4%, 0.9%, 7%, and 11%, respectively, in the validation cohort. This risk stratification system predicts outcome, but also identifies patients who need additional testing or medical interventions. Patients with active cardiac conditions (unstable coronary syndromes, decompensated HF, significant arrhythmias, severe valvular disease) should generally have these conditions corrected before proceeding with elective noncardiac surgery.

Exercise tolerance is one of the most important determinants of perioperative risk. A high exercise tolerance, even in patients with stable angina, is associated with a low perioperative cardiac risk. Estimated energy requirements for various activities can be defined by metabolic equivalent (MET) levels, where 1 MET equals resting energy expenditure of approximately 3.5 mL oxygen/kg/min. Perioperative cardiac risk is increased in patients unable to achieve 4 METs during normal daily activities (4). Estimation of MET capacity can be done accurately and simply by asking specific questions during the preoperative interview that assess functional capacity (Table 29.2) or by using simple questionnaires

Table 29.1   Clinical Predictors of Increased Perioperative Cardiovascular Risk (MI, CHF, Death)

Active cardiac conditions
Unstable coronary syndromes
- Unstable or severe angina[b] (CCS class III or IV) (7)
- Recent MI[a]

Decompensated HF (NYHA functional class IV; worsening or new onset HF)
Significant arrhythmias
- High-grade atrioventricular block
- Mobitz II atrioventricular block
- Third-degree atrioventricular heart block
- Symptomatic ventricular arrhythmias
- Supraventricular arrhythmias (including atrial fibrillation) with uncontrolled ventricular rate
- Sinus tachycardia at rest
- Symptomatic bradycardia
- Newly recognized VT

Severe valvular disease
- Severe aortic stenosis (mean pressure gradient >40 mmHg, aortic valve area <1.0 cm^2, or symptomatic)
- Symptomatic mitral stenosis (progressive dyspnea on exertion, exertional presyncope, or HF)

Clinical predictors of risk
History of ischemic heart disease
History of compensated or prior HF
History of cerebrovascular disease
Diabetes mellitus
Renal insufficiency

[a]The American College of Cardiology National Database Library defines recent MI as >7 days but <30 days.
[b]May include "stable" angina in patients who are unusually sedentary.
Abbreviations: CCS, Canadian Cardiovascular Society; CHF, congestive heart failure; ECG, electrocardiogram; HF, heart failure; LOE, level of evidence; MI, myocardial infarction; NYHA, New York Heart Association; VT, ventricular tachycardia.
Source: From Ref. 8.

Table 29.2   Estimated Energy Requirement for Various Activities

1 MET	Can you take care of yourself?
	Eat, dress, or use the toilet?
	Walk indoors around the house?
	Walk a block or two on level ground at 2–3 mph or 3.2–4.8 km/h?
	Do light work around the house like dusting or washing dishes?
4 METs	Climb a flight of stairs or walk up a hill?
	Walk on level ground at 4 mph or 6.4 km/h?
	Run a short distance?
	Do heavy work around the house like scrubbing floors or lifting, or moving heavy furniture?
	Participate in moderate recreational activities like golf, bowling, dancing, doubles tennis, or throwing a baseball or football?
>10 METs	Participate in strenuous sports like swimming, singles tennis, football, basketball, or skiing?

Abbreviation: MET, metabolic equivalent.
Source: From Ref. 8.

that have been developed for this purpose (5). Patients who could not walk four blocks and could not climb two flights of stairs were considered to have poor exercise tolerance, and had twice as many perioperative cardiovascular complications as those with better functional status (4). An alternative approach is to perform a 6-minute walk test, which has been shown to be predictive in cardiac surgery (6).

Disease-Specific Approach
Coronary Artery Disease
Symptoms of cardiovascular disease should be carefully determined, especially characteristics of chest pain, if present. In patients with symptomatic CAD, the preoperative evaluation may lead to the recognition of an increase in the frequency or pattern of anginal symptoms. It is important to realize that certain populations of patients, such as the elderly, women, or those with diabetes mellitus (DM), may present with more atypical symptoms of angina pectoris. Advanced age is a special risk, not only because of the increased likelihood of coronary disease, but also because of the effects of aging on the myocardium. The mortality of acute MI increases dramatically in the aged. Often comorbidities may cloud the detection of angina in older individuals. For example, the patient with lung disease may have dyspnea on exertion that could be multifactorial, and the debilitated individual may be unable to exercise sufficiently to detect angina. If unstable angina is present, there is associated high perioperative risk of MI (9). Even when angina symptoms are "stable," there may be a sizeable risk of perioperative myocardial ischemia that correlates with the functional limitation, so that additional preoperative cardiovascular testing or perioperative monitoring may be useful.

In addition to identifying the severity and stability of CAD, if present, it is also necessary to know any prior medical or surgical cardiac interventions that have been performed. In patients with known CAD, as well as those with previously occult coronary disease, the questions become (1) What is the amount of myocardium in jeopardy? (2) What is the ischemic threshold, i.e., the amount of stress required to produce ischemia? (3) What is the patient's ventricular function? (4) Is the patient on his or her optimal medical regimen? Given evidence regarding the limited value of coronary revascularization before noncardiac surgery, the indication for preoperative testing is limited to the group in whom coronary revascularization may be beneficial independent of noncardiac surgery (8).

Traditionally, perioperative risk assessment for noncardiac surgery was based upon the time interval between an MI and the surgery. Although many earlier studies demonstrated an increased incidence of reinfarction if surgery is performed within 6 months of an MI, this time interval is no longer valid in the current era of thrombolytics, endovascular stenting, and aggressive medical management options after an acute MI (10–12). The American College of Cardiology/American Heart Association (ACC/AHA) Task Force on Perioperative Evaluation of the Cardiac Patient Undergoing Noncardiac Surgery considers those with an acute MI within 7 days of the surgical procedure to be at highest risk, while those with a prior MI within 7–30 days are considered to have an increased, but somewhat lower, risk (8). Current management of MI provides for risk stratification during convalescence. If a recent stress test does not indicate residual myocardium at risk, the likelihood of reinfarction after noncardiac surgery is low. Claims data suggests that the risk of reinfarction remains elevated for at least 2 months after an MI, and that coronary artery bypass grafting (CABG) may reduce that risk while coronary stent placement soon after an MI does not (13,14).

Hypertension
Hypertension (HTN) is common and its prevalence increases with age. Although mild to moderate HTN is not an independent predictor of postoperative cardiac complications,

a hypertensive crisis in the postoperative period, defined as a diastolic blood pressure greater than 120 mmHg, and clinical evidence of impending or actual end-organ damage increases the risk of MI and cerebrovascular accident. Several precipitants of hypertensive crises have been identified, including pheochromocytoma, abrupt clonidine withdrawal prior to surgery, and the use of chronic monoamine oxidase inhibitors with or without sympathomimetic drugs in combination. If the initial evaluation establishes HTN as mild or moderate, antihypertensive medications should be continued perioperatively, and blood pressure (BP) should be maintained near preoperative levels to reduce the risk of myocardial ischemia. In patients unable to take oral medications, parenteral β-blockers and transdermal clonidine may be used. In patients with more severe HTN, such as diastolic BP higher than 110 mm Hg, the potential benefits of delaying surgery to optimize antihypertensive medications should be weighed against the risk of delaying the surgical procedure. A randomized trial of treated hypertensive patients without known CAD who presented the morning of surgery with an elevated diastolic blood pressure was unable to demonstrate any difference in outcome between those who were actively treated with intranasal nifedipine versus those in whom surgery was delayed (15).

Valvular Heart Disease

Valvular heart disease is frequently encountered in elderly patients undergoing surgical procedures. The ACC/AHA guidelines indicate that severe valvular disease is a major clinical predictor of increased perioperative cardiovascular risk (16). Aortic stenosis places a patient at increased risk, with those with critical stenosis associated with the highest risk of cardiac decompensation in patients undergoing elective noncardiac surgery. Two of the main issues in the perioperative management of patients with valvular heart disease are antibiotic prophylaxis against infective endocarditis and the management of anticoagulation in the perioperative period in patients with prosthetic heart valves. The new guidelines only recommend antibiotic prophylaxis before dental procedures "that involve manipulation of gingival tissue or the periapical region of teeth or perforation of the oral mucosa" for certain patients considered to be at highest risk of acquiring endocarditis. These patients include those who have a prosthetic heart valve, those who have had a previous episode of infective endocarditis, individuals with certain types of congenital heart disease, or those who have received a heart transplant and have developed cardiac valvulopathy.

Aortic Stenosis

Aortic stenosis is more common in men, is particularly a condition of the elderly, and usually results from degenerative calcific aortic valve disease in this population. The patient with suspected aortic stenosis merits further evaluation prior to noncardiac surgery, since those with severe aortic stenosis are considered to be at high risk (17). Kertai has reported a substantially higher rate of perioperative complications in patients with severe aortic stenosis, compared with patients with moderate aortic stenosis—31% (5/16) versus 11% (10/92) (18). If the aortic stenosis is symptomatic, elective noncardiac surgery should generally be postponed or canceled. Such patients require aortic valve replacement (AVR) before elective but necessary noncardiac surgery. A transcatheter AVR might be an option for patients that are at high risk or prohibitive risk for open aortic valve surgery. If a patient is not a candidate for AVR, percutaneous balloon aortic valvuloplasty may be reasonable as a bridge to surgery in hemodynamically unstable adult patients with aortic stenosis who require urgent noncardiac surgery.

Calleja and colleagues showed that elderly patients (mean age >75 years) with asymptomatic, severe AS can undergo moderate-risk, noncardiac surgery without major cardiac events (19). They do caution that the occurrence of intraoperative hypotension should be recognized promptly and treated aggressively with vasopressors, such as phenylephrine. The use of pulmonary artery catheters has shown benefit in such high-risk cardiac populations perioperatively in situations where hypotension and fluid-shifts can pose significant morbidity. Adequate preload should be maintained throughout the perioperative period. Maintenance of sinus rhythm is important since the atrial contraction contributes significantly to ventricular filling in patients with severe aortic stenosis.

General anesthesia may be preferable to spinal anesthesia in patients with aortic stenosis since the hemodynamic effects of spinal anesthesia may be undesirable. Patients with severe aortic stenosis may also benefit from close postoperative hemodynamic monitoring in an intensive care unit (19).

Mitral Stenosis

The major concerns in the patient with mitral stenosis undergoing noncardiac surgery are (1) maintaining hemodynamic stability; (2) decreasing the incidence of perioperative arrhythmia such as atrial fibrillation; and (3) prevention of infective endocarditis Increases in heart rate reduce LV filling across the stenotic mitral valve and increase the transmitral pressure gradient. Patients with mitral stenosis can become symptomatic with tachycardia, which frequently manifest during the perioperative period. Beta-blockers may be used to reduce heart rate in an attempt to optimize hemodynamic conditions. Antiarrhythmic agents may be considered to prevent the development of atrial fibrillation since this arrhythmia is particularly likely in these patients.

Prosthetic Heart Valves

More than 60,000 cardiac valve replacements are performed each year in the USA. Issues important in the perioperative period for those with prosthetic valves include the management of chronic anticoagulation therapy, reducing the risk of infective endocarditis, preventing valve thrombosis, and identifying valve-related hemolysis (20).

There are two major types of mechanical prosthetic heart valves, the caged-ball and the tilting-disk valves. While mechanical prosthetic valves have greater durability than bioprosthetic valves, they are more thrombogenic. The risk of valve thrombosis is greatest in patients with caged-ball prosthetic valves (Starr-Edwards). Single-tilting-disk prosthetic valves (Bjork-Shiley, Medtronic-Hall, and Omnicarbon) have an intermediate risk of valve thrombosis, and bileaflet tilting-disk prostheses (St. Jude, Carbomedics, Edwards Duromedics) pose the lowest risk of the mechanical prosthetic valves. The possibility of prosthetic valve dysfunction may be suggested by new cardiac symptoms and abnormal auscultatory findings on physical examination. Mechanical prosthetic valves may be evaluated with cine-fluoroscopy, echocardiography, or cardiac catheterization. The management of chronic warfarin anticoagulation in the perioperative period is of major importance in patients with mechanical prosthetic heart valves. The risk of temporarily discontinuing anticoagulation must be weighed against the benefit of a reduced risk of perioperative bleeding for all patients on chronic anticoagulation, especially those with prosthetic heart valves. In general, the incidence of thromboembolism in patients with valvular heart disease depends on the position of the valve involved, the type of prosthetic heart valve, the existence of concomitant heart disease, the presence of LA enlargement, and whether atrial fibrillation is present (16).

In patients at low risk of thrombosis, defined as those with a bileaflet mechanical AVR with no risk factors (atrial fibrillation, previous thromboembolism, LV dysfunction, hypercoagulable conditions, older-generation thrombogenic valves, mechanical tricuspid valves, or more than 1 mechanical valve) it is recommended that warfarin be stopped 48–72 h before the procedure (so the INR falls to less than 1.5) and restarted within 24 h after the procedure. Heparin is usually unnecessary. In patients at high risk of thrombosis, defined as those with any mechanical mitral valve replacement or a mechanical AVR with any risk factor, therapeutic doses of intravenous unfractionated heparin should be started when the INR falls below 2.0 (typically 48 h before surgery), stopped 4–6 h before the procedure, restarted as early after surgery as bleeding stability allows, and continued until the INR is again therapeutic with warfarin therapy (16).

The use of low-molecular-weight heparins (LMWHs) in preoperative warfarin anti-coagulation bridging was investigated in a multicenter, single-arm cohort study (21) of 224 high-risk patients (prosthetic valves, atrial fibrillation, and a major risk factor). Warfarin was held for 5 days; LMWHs were given 3 days preoperatively and at least 4 days postoperatively. The overall rate of thromboembolism was 3.6%, and the overall rate of cardio-embolism was 0.9%. Major bleeding was seen in 6.7% of subjects, although only 8–15 episodes occurred during LMWH administration. Whatever form of heparin is used as bridging therapy, it is recommended that warfarin should be restarted as soon as possible following surgery, and that heparin should be resumed and continued until oral anticoagulation is in the therapeutic range.

Congestive Heart Failure

In virtually all studies to date, the presence of symptomatic congestive HF preoperatively has been associated with an increased incidence of perioperative cardiac morbidity (3,17). Stabilization of symptoms of pulmonary congestion is prudent prior to elective surgery. It is important to determine the etiology of the left-sided HF since the type of perioperative monitoring and treatments would be different for such conditions as ischemic or nonisch-emic cardiomyopathy, systolic or nonsystolic HF, or mitral or aortic valvular insufficiency and/or stenosis. Diastolic filling abnormalities are particularly common in older patients and may increase the risk of developing symptomatic HF or atrial fibrillation in the periop-erative period.

Hypertrophic Cardiomyopathy

It is estimated that the prevalence of hypertrophic cardiomyopathy in the adult population is 0.2%. Patients with this condition typically have marked degrees of LV hypertrophy, reduced ventricular compliance, hyperdynamic LV systolic function and systolic anterior motion of the mitral valve leaflet, with or without a dynamic pressure gradient in the sub-aortic area. It is important to identify this condition preoperatively since there may be increased risk of hemodynamic compromise in the perioperative period. Atrial fibrillation is also more common in patients with hypertrophic cardiomyopathy. The overall preva-lence of this arrhythmia among patients with hypertrophic cardiomyopathy is greater than 20%, and the occurrence of atrial fibrillation increases with age.

Hreybe et al. searched the National Hospital Discharge Survey database from 1996 to 2002 for patients with a diagnosis of hypertrophic cardiomyopathy who had undergone noncardiac surgery (22). They matched 227 patients with hypertrophic cardiomyopathy with 554 controls by age, gender, and year of surgery. The in-hospital incidence of death or MI was higher in patients with hypertrophic cardiomyopathy than in controls. Even after controlling for age, gender, race, presence of HTN, DM, history of CAD, history of HF, atrial fibrillation, and ventricular arrhythmias in a multivariate binary logistic regression model, the presence of hypertrophic cardiomyopathy significantly increased the odds of death by 61% and almost tripled the odds of the combined end point of death or MI. It had been recommended that spinal anesthesia be avoided in these patients because it can decrease systemic vascular resistance and increase venous capacitance; although the evi-dence is very weak, regional anesthesia has been used successfully in these patients (23,24).

As a result of the pathophysiology of hypertrophic cardiomyopathy, patients with this condition are particularly susceptible to factors that alter LV filling, such as diminished intravascular volume, alterations in systemic vascular resistance, and increases in heart rate. Special care should be taken to maintain adequate intravascular volume, minimize pain and anxiety, and avoid treatment with catecholamines. If hypotension does occur in a patient with hypertrophic cardiomyopathy, hydration is indicated, as is consideration of treatment with an $\alpha 1$-adrenergic agonist like phenylephrine. Positive inotropic drugs such as dopamine and dobutamine and drugs that reduce the preload, such as nitroglycerin, should be avoided. Intensive care unit monitoring, which may include pulmonary artery catheter monitoring, may be useful postoperatively to limit periods of hypotension and avoid volume depletion, although its usefulness has not been established.

Diastolic Dysfunction
The hypertensive heart is typically characterized by concentric LV hypertrophy, normal or above-normal systolic function, and diastolic dysfunction. In the elderly patient with marked concentric LV hypertrophy and small end-systolic chamber sizes, diastolic dysfunction can lead to pulmonary congestion. The pathophysiology of this condition lies in impaired relaxation and increased LV diastolic stiffness. Increases in LV diastolic stiffness will mandate higher LA pressures to maintain filling and thus promote elevated pulmonary venous pressures and pulmonary congestion when LA pressures are elevated or reduced cardiac output when LA pressures are not elevated. This population may be particularly sensitive to factors that affect diastolic filling of the left ventricle, such as increased heart rate, atrial fibrillation, or volume depletion. Identifying chronically hypertensive patients with diastolic dysfunction with reliable echocardiography parameters could guide optimal perioperative fluid and blood pressure management.

Increased sympathetic nervous system activity producing increases in blood pressure and heart rate may occur as the patient emerges from anesthesia. This response may compromise diastolic filling, so it is critical to assess volume status at this time. In certain patients, this may be extremely difficult without continuous invasive hemodynamic monitoring. While a pulmonary artery catheter cannot be routinely recommended, it may provide important information in special circumstances in which patients are hemodynamically unstable.

Obstructive Sleep Apnea
It is believed by some authorities that approximately 1 in 5 American adults have at least mild obstructive sleep apnea (OSA). This figure is likely to increase as the population becomes older and more obese. In the perioperative period, adult patients with OSA, even if asymptomatic, present special challenges that must be addressed to minimize risk of morbidity and mortality. Most experts agree that in the absence of a sleep study, a presumptive diagnosis of OSA may be made based on consideration of the following criteria: increased body mass index, increased neck circumference, snoring, daytime hypersomnolence, and tonsillar hypertrophy. Preoperative initiation of continuous positive airway pressure should be considered particularly if OSA is severe. Patients with increased perioperative risk from OSA should be extubated when fully awake and in the semiupright position after full reversal of neuromuscular blockade.

Arrhythmias
Cardiac arrhythmias and conduction disturbances are not uncommon findings in the perioperative period particularly in the elderly. High-grade atrioventricular block, symptomatic ventricular arrhythmias in the presence of underlying heart disease, and supraventricular arrhythmias with an uncontrolled ventricular response are considered major clinical

predictors of increased perioperative risk (8). The management of perioperative ventricular arrhythmias is not well studied and is generally considered to be the same as that for the nonsurgical patient. Reversible causes such as electrolyte disturbances, acid–base abnormalities, or decompensated HF should be corrected. A search for underlying cardiac or pulmonary disease or for potential drug toxicity is essential. More recent detailed studies using continuous electrocardiogram (ECG) monitoring found that asymptomatic ventricular arrhythmias, including couplets and nonsustained ventricular tachycardia (VT), were not associated with an increase in cardiac complications after noncardiac surgery (25). Nonsustained ventricular arrhythmias, whether single premature ventricular contractions, complex ventricular ectopy, or nonsustained VT, usually do not require therapy unless they result in hemodynamic compromise. No studies support the suppression of preoperative arrhythmias with antiarrhythmics to reduce surgical morbidity and mortality.

Atrial Fibrillation

The incidence of atrial fibrillation doubles with each decade beginning at 60 years, so that by the age of 80–89 years, the prevalence of atrial fibrillation is currently estimated to be 8–10%. Median age of patients with atrial fibrillation in the USA is about 75 years, with approximately 70% of patients with atrial fibrillation between the ages of 65 and 85 years. Atrial fibrillation is projected to increase 2.5-fold in prevalence during the next 50 years. Winkel and colleagues evaluated 317 patients without atrial fibrillation undergoing major vascular surgery to determine the incidence of new-onset atrial fibrillation and its association with adverse cardiovascular outcomes (26). They reported a 4.7% incidence of postoperative atrial fibrillation and a more than sixfold increase in cardiovascular death, MI, unstable angina, and stroke in the first 30 days, and a fourfold increase over the next 12 months. Early treatment to restore sinus rhythm or to control the ventricular response is therefore indicated. Prophylactic intravenous diltiazem in randomized, placebo-controlled trials in high-risk thoracic surgery has reduced the incidence of clinically significant atrial arrhythmias. Other useful agents in the elderly include digoxin, β-blockers, and amiodarone or dronedarone with dose adjustments for age, weight, and diseases. Anticoagulation with warfarin should be initiated per published guidelines when the risk of bleeding is reasonably safe. Aspirin should be considered in older patients who are unable to tolerate or who are not candidates for oral anticoagulation. Aspirin combined with clopidogrel (75 mg/day) may further reduce the risk of major vascular events, but as with warfarin, the risk of major hemorrhage is increased.

Physical Examination

A complete preoperative physical examination is necessary for every patient undergoing noncardiac surgery. Blood pressure and heart rate should be determined in both the supine and standing positions to assess intravascular volume status and autonomic dysfunction. Careful cardiac auscultation should be performed to detect clinically important cardiac findings, including the presence of an S_3 gallop suggestive of HF and murmurs suggestive of significant valvular disease, particularly aortic stenosis. The pulmonary exam and evaluation of the jugular venous pulsations and lower extremity edema can also help determine intravascular volume status and the presence of HF. Reduced or absent peripheral arterial pulses suggest the presence of occult atherosclerotic disease. Carotid bruits suggest carotid stenosis and may require changes in perioperative blood pressure management.

Identifying Surgery-Specific Risk

The surgical procedure influences the extent of the preoperative evaluation required by determining the potential range of changes in perioperative management (Table 29.3).

Table 29.3   Cardiac Risk[a] Stratification for Noncardiac Surgical Procedures

High risk	Aortic and other major vascular
	Peripheral vascular
Intermediate risk	Reported cardiac risk generally <5%
	Carotid endarterectomy
	Endovascular Procedures
	Head and neck
	Intraperitoneal and intrathoracic
	Orthopedic
	Prostate
Low risk[b]	Reported cardiac risk generally <1%
	Endoscopic procedures
	Superficial procedure
	Cataract
	Breast

[a]Combined incidence of cardiac death and nonfatal myocardial infarction.
[b]Do not generally require further preoperative cardiac testing.
Source: From Ref. 8.

Knowledge of the urgency, type, and anticipated duration of the surgical procedure and the expected blood loss and intravascular volume shifts is necessary to make perioperative management plans.

Surgical procedures that are neither emergent nor associated with significant blood loss are not associated with a high risk of cardiac ischemia. For example, cataract surgery is associated with minimal cardiac stress and exceedingly low cardiac morbidity and mortality rates, even after a recent MI (27). Similarly, outpatient procedures have also been shown to be associated with a low incidence of cardiac morbidity and mortality (28). In such patients, changes in perioperative management are rarely needed unless the patient demonstrates unstable angina or signs or symptoms of CHF.

Vascular surgery represents a unique group of patients in whom there is extensive evidence regarding preoperative testing and perioperative interventions. Since further determination of cardiac status may alter perioperative care, the benefit of further evaluation and treatment in this population would be expected to be greater than the associated costs or risks of such testing, and has been studied most extensively.

APPROACH TO THE PATIENT

In 1996, an ACC/AHA Task Force developed Guidelines for Perioperative Cardiovascular Evaluation for Noncardiac Surgery. These guidelines were developed to provide a framework for cardiac risk stratification for those undergoing noncardiac surgery, acknowledging the lack of prospective, randomized trials in this area. The guidelines were updated in 2002 and most recently in 2009 (8). These guidelines assess clinical risk predictors (Table 29.1), type of surgery (Table 29.3), and exercise tolerance (Table 29.2) to be performed in an algorithm model to assist in decision-making for further preoperative cardiac testing. The decision to undertake further testing depends upon the interaction of the clinical risk factors, surgery-specific risk, and functional capacity.

The identification of perioperative cardiac risk has been studied for three decades, and much of the work has focused on the development of clinical risk indices. The RCRI, described previously, has become the standard tool for assessing the probability of perioperative cardiac risk in a given individual, and directs the decision to perform cardiovascular testing and implement perioperative management protocols.

More recently, Gupta and colleagues have proposed a new perioperative MI and cardiac arrest risk calculator (MICA) (29). On multivariate logistic regression analysis, five predictors of perioperative MI or cardiac arrest were identified: type of surgery, dependent functional status, abnormal creatinine, American Society of Anesthesiologists' class, and increasing age. The risk model was subsequently validated on multiple data sets and was found to outperform the RCRI (29).

DIAGNOSTIC TESTING

Some studies raise questions about the usefulness of preoperative noninvasive stress testing before noncardiac surgery, while other studies consider it useful in specific populations. In general, the negative predictive values of the specific stress testing modalities studied in these patient populations are high. Therefore, in a patient with a negative stress test for myocardial ischemia, the risk of a perioperative cardiac event is relatively low. On the other hand, the positive predictive values of available stress tests are consistently low, so that a patient with evidence of stress-induced myocardial ischemia often still has a good perioperative outcome. This may be explained by the fact that an acute MI is sometimes caused by the rupture of a non-flow-limiting, unstable coronary artery plaque. Stress testing detects flow-limiting coronary artery stenoses (>50–70% arterial lumen narrowing), but cannot detect stenoses that are non-flow limiting.

The low risk of a major cardiac event in patients undergoing low-risk surgery generally does not require an assessment of CAD to further stratify risk. Likewise, patients that have reasonably good functional status, that is, those who can perform ≥4 METs of activity, can generally proceed with surgery without the need for preoperative noninvasive stress testing. Conversely, stress testing should be considered in patients with poor or unknown functional status, with clinical risk predictors, undergoing intermediate or high-risk operations if the results of the stress test, will change the decision whether to proceed with surgery or the approach to the patient.

Figure 29.1 presents in algorithmic form a framework for determining which patients are candidates for preoperative cardiac testing (8). The AHA/ACC Writing Committee chose to include the level of the recommendations and strength of evidence for many of the pathways. Importantly, the value of adopting the algorithm depends upon local factors such as current perioperative risk and rate of utilization of testing.

1. Step 1: The individual should determine the urgency of noncardiac surgery. In many instances, patient- or surgery-specific factors dictate an obvious strategy (e.g., emergent surgery) that may not allow for further cardiac assessment or treatment.
2. Step 2: Does the patient have one of the active cardiac conditions? In patients being considered for elective noncardiac surgery, the presence of unstable coronary disease, decompensated HF, or severe arrhythmia or valvular heart disease usually leads to cancellation or delay of surgery until the cardiac problem has been clarified and treated appropriately. Examples of unstable coronary syndromes include previous MI with evidence of important ischemic risk by clinical symptoms or noninvasive study, unstable or severe angina, and new or poorly controlled ischemia-mediated HF. Depending on the results of the test or interventions and the risk of delaying surgery, it may be appropriate to proceed to the planned surgery with maximal medical therapy.
3. Step 3: Is the patient undergoing low-risk surgery? In these patients, interventions based on cardiovascular testing in stable patients would rarely result in a change in management, and it would be appropriate to proceed with the planned surgical procedure.

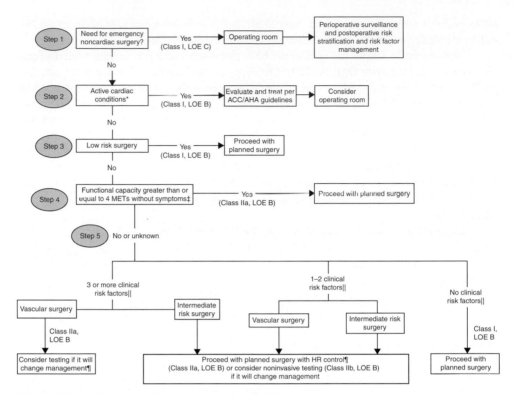

Figure 29.1   Cardiac evaluation and care algorithm for noncardiac surgery based on active clinical conditions, known cardiovascular disease, or cardiac risk factors for patients 50 years of age or greater. ‡: See Table 29.2 for estimated MET level. ||: Clinical risk factors include ischemic heart disease, compensated or prior heart failure, DM, renal insufficiency, and cerebrovascular disease. ¶: Consider perioperative beta blockade for populations in which this has been shown to reduce cardiac morbidity/mortality (see section on β-blockers).

4. Step 4: Does the patient have moderate functional capacity without symptoms? In highly functional asymptomatic patients, management will rarely be changed on the basis of results of any further cardiovascular testing and it is therefore appropriate to proceed with the planned surgery. If the patient has poor functional capacity, is symptomatic, or has unknown functional capacity, then the presence of clinical risk factors will determine the need for further evaluation. If the patient has no clinical risk factors, then it is appropriate to proceed with the planned surgery, and no further change in management is indicated.

If the patient has one or two clinical risk factors, then it is reasonable either to proceed with the planned surgery, with heart rate control, or to consider testing if it will change management. In patients with three or more clinical risk factors, if the patient is undergoing vascular surgery, recent studies suggest that testing should only be considered if it will change management. In nonvascular surgery in which the perioperative morbidity related to the procedures ranges from 1% to 5% (intermediate-risk surgery), there are insufficient data to determine the best strategy (proceeding with the planned surgery with tight heart rate control with β-blockade or further cardiovascular testing if it will change management).

Resting Electrocardiography

A routine ECG before noncardiac surgery solely on the basis of age is no longer recommended based on the literature (30). Therefore, the clinical history of the patient and surgical risk should be utilized to determine the need for an immediate preoperative ECG. A preoperative resting ECG should also be performed in any patient undergoing vascular surgical procedures who has at least one clinical risk factor; it is reasonable for an ECG to be performed in patients without clinical indicators undergoing vascular surgery. A preoperative resting ECG is recommended for patients with known CAD, peripheral arterial disease, or cerebrovascular disease who are undergoing intermediate-risk surgical procedures.

It has been estimated that up to 30% of MIs are silent and only detected on routine ECG, especially in patients with diabetes or HTN. The baseline ECG has limited applicability in the assessment of myocardial ischemia but may be useful to detect significant conduction disturbances and arrhythmias. ECG abnormalities may not always lead to delay of a noncardiac surgical procedure but may lead to increased vigilance by the anesthesiologist intraoperatively.

High-grade atrioventricular block, symptomatic ventricular arrhythmias in the presence of underlying heart disease, and supraventricular arrhythmias with uncontrolled ventricular rate are considered high-risk clinical predictors by the ACC/AHA guidelines (8). Pathological Q waves are also associated with an increased risk. The presence of LV hypertrophy, left bundle branch block, ST-segment abnormalities, and rhythm other than sinus are considered minor risk predictors. Despite the absence of evidence to suggest that a 12-lead ECG is required in all patients immediately prior to noncardiac surgery, the availability of an old ECG may be useful for comparison.

Assessment of LV Function

In general, an assessment of baseline LV function should be reserved for those with unexplained cardiopulmonary symptoms. This can be accomplished using echocardiography, radionuclide angiography, and/or contrast ventriculography. Most commonly, however, echocardiography is used when assessment of LV function is felt to be warranted. LV ejection fraction has been correlated with short- and long-term prognosis in multiple studies in patients undergoing noncardiac surgery; in general, the lower the ejection fraction, the greater the perioperative risk. Importantly, Halm and colleagues were unable to demonstrate that preoperative echocardiographic information added to clinical risk factors for risk stratification (31). However, Flu and colleagues performed echocardiography preoperatively in 1005 consecutive vascular surgery patients (32). LV dysfunction was diagnosed in 506 (50%) patients of which 80% were asymptomatic. In open vascular surgery ($n = 649$), both asymptomatic systolic and isolated diastolic LV dysfunction were associated with 30-day cardiovascular events and long-term cardiovascular mortality. In endovascular surgery ($n = 356$), only symptomatic HF was associated with 30-day cardiovascular events and long-term cardiovascular mortality. The key question is whether information from an echocardiogram would actually add incremental value above clinical assessment.

The ACC/AHA Task Force guidelines recommend that preoperative assessment of LV systolic function prior to noncardiac surgery should be limited to patients with current or poorly controlled HF, but not as a routine test in patients without prior HF. Among patients with a history of HF and with dyspnea of unknown etiology, the indications are less clear.

Noninvasive Cardiac Stress Testing

The ultimate goal of a preoperative cardiac stress test is to identify patients with myocardial ischemia in whom further cardiac interventions would significantly lower perioperative cardiac risks. As noted above, testing should only be performed in a subset of patients with poor exercise capacity, moderate to high clinical risk and undergoing major vascular or intermediate surgery.

An important aspect of cardiac stress testing relies on Bayes' theorem, which states that the correct interpretation of the results of noninvasive stress testing requires estimating the pretest probability of CAD in the patient being studied. False-positive stress test results are more common in those in whom CAD is unlikely to be present and false-negative results are more common in those with a high likelihood of CAD. Therefore, estimating the probability of CAD in a specific patient will often guide decision-making even before a stress test is considered.

A limited number of prospective studies have investigated the predictive value of noninvasive cardiac stress tests in determining the risk of postoperative cardiac events. The positive predictive values of all stress testing modalities are poor (10–20%). On the other hand, negative predictive values of most cardiac stress testing modalities are high (95%–100%), so that patients without evidence of ischemia are at the lowest risk for an adverse perioperative outcome. If noninvasive cardiac stress testing is recommended before non-cardiac surgery in ambulatory patients, the optimal test is the exercise treadmill ECG, to determine functional capacity and to detect myocardial ischemia. In patients with baseline ECG abnormalities that render the exercise ECG uninterpretable (e.g., left bundle branch block, LV hypertrophy with repolarization abnormality, digitalis effect) or in those who are unable to ambulate, an imaging study needs to be added. The choice between nuclear myo-cardial perfusion imaging or echocardiographic imaging should be based on availability and local expertise.

Exercise ECG Cardiac Stress Testing

The sensitivity of exercise ECG testing for detecting obstructive coronary disease is dependent on severity of stenosis and extent of disease, as well as the criteria used for a positive test. As many as 50% of patients with single-vessel coronary disease and adequate levels of exercise can have a normal exercise ECG. The mean sensitivity and specificity of exercise testing for obstructive CAD are 68% and 77%, respectively. The sensitivity and specificity are 81% and 66% for multivessel disease and 86% and 53% for three-vessel or left main CAD, respectively. The older age of patients undergoing noncardiac and vascu-lar surgery may reduce the prognostic utility of exercise stress testing in this group (33). Often these patients will have a submaximal treadmill exercise study, not being able to achieve their maximum predicted heart rate due to medical therapy, such as β-blocker use, or to comorbid states. Indeed, when considering the utility of preoperative noninvasive cardiac stress testing in an elderly individual undergoing noncardiac surgery, clinicians must ask whether the study sample on which recommendations are based is relevant to the individual patient. A patient's performance on a treadmill or bicycle ergometer may also be predictive of postoperative cardiac outcomes. The level at which ischemia is evident on the exercise ECG can be used to estimate an "ischemic threshold" for a patient to guide perioperative medical management. The onset of a myocardial ischemic response at low exercise workloads is associated with a significantly increased risk of perioperative and long-term cardiac events. This may support further intensification of perioperative medi-cal therapy in high-risk patients, which may impact on perioperative cardiovascular events.

Pharmacological Cardiac Stress Testing

Pharmacological stress testing has been advocated for preoperative cardiac risk assessment for patients in whom exercise tolerance is limited. Often, these patients may not exercise sufficiently during daily life to provoke symptoms of myocardial ischemia or HF. Pharma-cological stress tests with echocardiographic or nuclear scintigraphic imaging have been studied extensively in preoperative cardiac risk assessment for noncardiac, and especially vascular, surgery and will be briefly reviewed here.

A preoperative dipyridamole-thallium scintigraphy scan has been shown to be a sensitive predictor of postoperative cardiac events (34–37). Pooled data, though, show that the positive predictive value for adverse cardiac outcomes is low, ranging from 36% to 45%. The negative predictive value, on the other hand, is high (up to 97%). In several studies, the presence of a fixed defect was shown to have no predictive value for adverse postoperative cardiac outcomes, although, in two studies, there was a higher risk compared to patients with no ischemic defect. Importantly, the risk of perioperative cardiac events as a function of stress nuclear myocardial perfusion imaging is continuous rather than categorical. Some studies have shown that the risk of cardiac events increases as the extent of reversible defects increases (35,38). Abnormal imaging studies with a small degree of reversible defect carry a small risk of cardiac events, whereas the cardiac risk increases significantly as the size of the reversible defect increases to a moderate degree (20–25% of LV mass).

Several studies support the use of preoperative dipyridamole-thallium scintigraphy, in combination with clinical parameters, to identify patients at high risk for adverse cardiac outcomes after noncardiac surgery. Dipyridamole-thallium scintigraphy was found to be most useful in further stratifying patients considered at intermediate clinical risk (one or two clinical variables). In this group, the presence of a redistribution defect was associated with a 30% event rate compared to a 3% event rate in those without a thallium redistribution defect. In more than 50% of cases, the dipyridamole-thallium stress test did not add incremental information to the preoperative assessment after clinical variables were evaluated. Many studies have found that dipyridamole-thallium scintigraphy scans with a large number and size of redistribution defects, presence of LV dilatation after stress, or pulmonary radiotracer uptake are predictive of a higher postoperative cardiac risk (35).

There are few studies that evaluate the long-term postoperative outcomes of patients with abnormal dipyridamole-thallium scans. In one study, an abnormal dipyridamole-thallium scan was associated with a significantly increased risk of cardiac death in the perioperative period and in late follow-up in comparison to those with a normal scan (37). A reversible defect was the only predictor of death or MI during late follow-up and was associated with a twofold greater risk of a cardiac event than if the defect was fixed. The number of perfusion defects, a history of angina, and the presence of chest pain during the study were independent predictors of perioperative cardiac events. Fleisher et al. utilized criteria from the Thrombolysis in Myocardial Infarction IIIB (TIMI-IIIB) trials for quantification of dipyridamole-thallium results (35). They reported a significantly increased long-term risk only in the subset of patients with high-risk thallium markers, including increased lung uptake and multiple segments with reversible defects.

Dobutamine stress echocardiography (DSE) involves the identification of new or worsening myocardial wall motion abnormalities (WMAs) using two-dimensional echocardiography during infusion of intravenous dobutamine. This technique has been shown to have similar accuracy as dipyridamole-thallium scintigraphy for the detection of CAD. DSE has been found to be useful for the assessment of preoperative cardiac risk among patients undergoing noncardiac surgery particularly in patients with intermediate clinical risk (39). The estimated low positive predictive values (17–43%) and high negative predictive values (93–100%) are similar to those for dipyridamole-thallium. There are several advantages to DSE compared with dipyridamole-thallium scintigraphy. DSE can assess valvular abnormalities, the cost of DSE is significantly lower, there is no radiation exposure, and the duration of the study is significantly shorter.

There are a few studies that report long-term cardiac outcomes after noncardiac surgery among patients with abnormal preoperative DSE. In one study, patients were followed for up to 2 years after major vascular surgery (40). There were two cardiac events (3%)

among patients with negative DSE. Among 23 patients with positive DSE, 68% subsequently underwent coronary revascularization before the noncardiac surgery was performed. There were no perioperative events in the group of patients with positive DSE who underwent coronary revascularization before noncardiac surgery. By contrast, 40% of those with positive DSE who did not undergo coronary revascularization had perioperative adverse cardiac outcomes. In this study, DSE predicted perioperative and long-term outcome among patients undergoing major vascular surgery, with a high negative predictive value. In a second study, patients undergoing major vascular surgery were evaluated by clinical parameters and results of DSE and followed for an average of 19 months postoperatively. The presence of extensive dobutamine-induced WMAs and a previous history of MI independently predicted late cardiac events, increasing risk up to sixfold (41).

CORONARY ANGIOGRAPHY AND REVASCULARIZATION BEFORE NONCARDIAC SURGERY

Coronary Angiography

An abnormal noninvasive study in the preoperative period may lead to coronary angiography and revascularization, changes in anesthetic technique, utilization of expensive resources such as intensive care units, and aggressive treatment of hemodynamic fluctuations. Historically, the use of coronary angiography as a screening procedure before elective peripheral vascular surgical procedures was advocated due to the high perioperative mortality associated with the high prevalence of CAD in this patient group (12). Many argue that using coronary angiography as a preoperative screening tool is too costly and places patients at further risk due to the cumulative risks of these procedures, especially in the elderly with significant comorbid diseases. This has led to increased interest in preoperative noninvasive cardiac stress testing to assist in risk-stratifying patients before elective noncardiac surgery and to the increased use of perioperative β-blocker therapy, particularly in high-risk patients based on clinical parameters.

The present indications for coronary angiography in the preoperative evaluation before noncardiac surgery are adapted from the ACC/AHA guidelines for coronary angiography in the general population and will likely be updated with the publication of the new guidelines (42). Coronary angiography should be considered in patients with unstable angina pectoris, recent MI, or large areas of myocardium at risk on noninvasive stress tests if coronary revascularization would be considered.

Coronary Revascularization

The Coronary Artery Revascularization Prophylaxis (CARP) trial showed that coronary artery revascularization before elective vascular surgery did not significantly alter long-term outcome (43). In this trial, 510 patients at increased risk for perioperative cardiac complications were randomized to undergo either coronary artery revascularization or no revascularization before elective major vascular surgery. Among the patients assigned to undergo revascularization, percutaneous coronary intervention (PCI) was performed in 59% and CABG in 41%. There was no difference between groups in either postoperative MI or in mortality at 2.7 years after randomization. Of note, however, only a minority of patients in this trial had three-vessel CAD. In a follow-up analysis, Ward and colleagues reported improved outcome in the subset who underwent CABG compared to PCI (44). When patients who underwent coronary angiography in both the randomized and nonrandomized portion of the CARP trial, only the subset of patients with unprotected left main disease showed a benefit with preoperative coronary artery revascularization (45).

In the DECREASE II study, Poldermans et al. enrolled 770 patients undergoing major vascular surgery and at intermediate cardiac risk, defined as the presence of one or two cardiac risk factors (age >70 years, angina, history of MI, a history of or compensated CHF, diabetes, creatinine >2.0 mg/dL, or previous transient ischemic attack or cerebrovascular accident) (46). Patients were randomized to either undergo further risk stratification with DSE or proceed to surgery. Patients with three or more risk factors were excluded from the study and considered for further risk stratification. All patients received preoperative bisoprolol that was continued after surgery, with a targeted heart rate of 60–65 beats per minute. Physicians were not blinded to the results of DSE, and heart rate was kept below the ischemic threshold with tight perioperative β-blocker control. Of the 34 patients who were considered for revascularization because of extensive ischemia on DSE, 12 underwent revascularization (10 PCI and 2 CABG), with complete revascularization in only 6. The 30-day incidence of cardiac death and nonfatal MI was similar in both groups (1.8% in the no testing group vs. 2.3% in the tested group). Poldermans et al. published results from the Dutch Echocardiographic Cardiac Risk Evaluation Applying Stress Echo (DECREASE)-V pilot study, which randomized 101 patients, the majority of whom had three-vessel or left main CAD, to undergo coronary revascularization or no revascularization before major vascular surgery (47). In this population of patients with severe coronary disease, extensive stress-induced ischemia on noninvasive testing, and an average age of approximately 70 years, coronary revascularization did not affect the composite end point of death or MI at either 30 days or 1 year. In those patients in whom there was successful revascularization, there was significant improvement in long-term outcome (48). The quality of the data in the DECREASE trials has recent been questioned by an internal investigation at Erasmus University which has led to questions regarding the robustness of the conclusions of these trials.

Percutaneous Coronary Intervention

The benefit of PCI before noncardiac surgery has also been examined in several cohort studies. Posner and colleagues utilized an administrative data set of patients who underwent PCI before noncardiac surgery (49). They matched patients with coronary disease undergoing noncardiac surgery with and without prior PCI and looked at cardiac complications. In this nonrandomized design, they noted a significantly lower rate of 30-day cardiac complications in patients who underwent PCI at least 90 days before the noncardiac surgery. Importantly, PCI within 90 days of noncardiac surgery did not improve outcome. Although the explanation for these results is unknown, they may support the notion that PCI performed "to get the patient through surgery" may not improve perioperative outcome. Cardiac complications usually do not occur in patients with stable and/or asymptomatic coronary stenosis, and PCI may actually destabilize coronary plaques, resulting in acute coronary events in the days or weeks after noncardiac surgery.

PCI using coronary stenting poses several special issues. Kaluza and colleagues reported on the outcome in 40 patients who underwent prophylactic coronary stent placement less than 6 weeks before major noncardiac surgery requiring general anesthesia (50). There were 7 MIs, 11 major bleeding episodes, and 8 deaths. All deaths and MIs, as well as 8 of 11 bleeding episodes, occurred in patients subjected to surgery fewer than 14 days after stenting. Four patients expired after undergoing surgery 1 day after stenting. Wilson and colleagues reported on 207 patients who underwent noncardiac surgery within 2 months of stent placement (51). Eight patients died or suffered an MI, all of whom were among the 168 patients undergoing surgery 6 weeks after stent placement. Vincenzi et al. studied 103 patients and reported that the risk of suffering a perioperative cardiac event was 2.11-fold greater in patients with recent stents (<35 days before surgery) as compared with PCI more than 90 days before surgery (52). Leibowitz et al. studied 216 consecutive patients who had a PCI within 3 months of noncardiac surgery (122 balloon

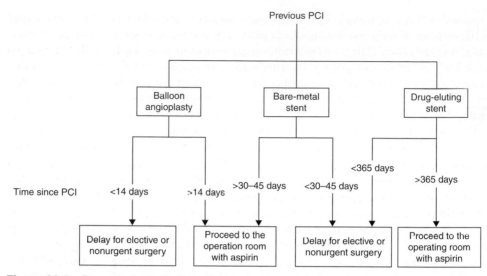

Figure 29.2 Proposed approach to the management of patients with previous PCI requiring noncardiac surgery (based upon expert opinion). PCI indicates percutaneous coronary intervention. *Source*: Adapted from Ref. 8.

angioplasty and 94 stent) (53). A total of 26 patients (12%) died, 13 in the stent group (14%) and 13 in the balloon angioplasty group (11%), a nonsignificant difference. The incidence of acute MI and death within 6 months were not significantly different (7% and 14% in the stent group and 6% and 11% in the PTCA group, respectively). Significantly, more events occurred in the two groups when noncardiac surgery was performed within 2 weeks of PCI. On the basis of the accumulating data, elective noncardiac surgery after PCI, with or without stent placement, should be delayed for 4–6 weeks.

Drug-eluting stents (DES) may represent an even greater problem during the perioperative period due to a delay in endothelialization. Late stent thrombosis in the perioperative period in patients who have had coronary interventions with DES has been described. Drug-eluting stents may create an additional risk of adverse cardiac events over a prolonged period (up to 12 months), particularly if antiplatelet agents are discontinued (54). However, a recent case series suggests that an elevated risk continues beyond 1 year (55). The new guidelines suggest continuing aspirin therapy in all patients with a coronary stent and discontinuing clopidogrel for as short a time interval as possible for patients with bare-metal stents inserted after 30 days or DES after 1 year. Based upon the nonperioperative literature, there is a suggestion that holding clopidogrel for the traditional 8 days before surgery may actually increase cardiac risk associated with a hypercoagulable rebound, suggesting that a shorter discontinuation period may be optimal. A recent cohort study suggests that withdrawal of antiplatelet agents >5 days is associated with increased major adverse cardiac events (56).

For patients who have undergone successful coronary intervention with or without stent placement before planned or unplanned noncardiac surgery, there is uncertainty regarding how much time should pass before the noncardiac procedure is performed. One approach is outlined in Figure 29.2, which is based on expert opinion.

PERIOPERATIVE INTERVENTIONS TO REDUCE RISK
Intra-Aortic Balloon Counterpulsation
Among patients with unstable angina or severe CAD, placement of an intra-aortic balloon counterpulsation device has been used before induction of anesthesia in patients

considered high-risk for noncardiac surgical procedures. In several small case series, peri-operative morbidity and mortality were low (57). In clinical practice, however, intra-aortic balloon counterpulsation is seldom used before noncardiac surgery except in the most unstable patients with ongoing myocardial ischemia and a need for an emergency surgical procedure.

β-Blockers

Several studies in the late 1970s indicated that β-blocker therapy could be safely continued preoperatively, often resulting in a reduction in the incidence of perioperative myocardial ischemia. These studies, and the concern for β-blocker withdrawal-induced tachycardia, HTN, and myocardial ischemia, led to recommendations to continue β-blocker therapy preoperatively. By decreasing adrenergic stimulation of the heart, β-blockers may reduce the incidence of perioperative arrhythmias and myocardial ischemia.

The first randomized, placebo-controlled study of β-blockers in high-risk non-cardiac surgical patients involved the perioperative use of atenolol, which was adminis-tered beginning 2 days preoperatively and continued for 7 days postoperatively (58,59). A significantly lower incidence of perioperative ischemia and improved event-free 6-month survival was observed in the atenolol group. No difference in perioperative MI or cardiac death was noted between groups. Of note, several risk factors and medications were not equally distributed in the two groups, with the placebo group having a higher risk profile. In a study of the perioperative use of bisoprolol in elective major vascular surgery in patients with at least one risk factor for CAD and a positive stress test, bisoprolol was administered at least 7 days preoperatively, titrated to achieve a resting heart rate of 60 bpm or less, and continued postoperatively for 30 days (60). Patients with large zones of myo-cardial ischemia were excluded from the trial. Bisoprolol led to an approximate 80% reduc-tion in perioperative MI or cardiac death. Importantly, the quality of the data from the Erasmus group has been questioned.

The same data were then reevaluated with respect to clinical factors, DSE results, and β-blocker usage (61). A clinical risk score was calculated by assigning one point for each of the following characteristics: age 70 years or older, current angina, MI, CHF, prior cere-brovascular events, DM, and renal failure. Importantly, DSE was performed only in patients with a significant number of risk factors. Those patients who demonstrated new WMAs had higher event rates than those without new WMAs, for the same clinical risk score. When the risk of death or MI was stratified by perioperative β-blocker usage, there was no significant improvement in those without any of the prior risk factors. In those with fewer than three clinical risk factors, the use of β-blockers was associated with a lower rate of cardiac events (0.8% vs. 2.3%), and β-blocker therapy was very effective in reducing car-diac events in those with limited stress-induced ischemia on DSE (33% vs. 2.8%). By contrast, β-blocker therapy had no effect in patients with more extensive stress-induced ischemia on DSE.

Lindenauer et al. published a retrospective cohort study conducted by searching a database used by 329 participating hospitals for quality assessment (62). A total of 119,454 patients were given β-blockers within the first or second day of hospitalization for major noncardiac surgery. There was no effect on in-hospital mortality for the entire cohort (2.3% vs. 2.4%). For patients with an RCRI score of 3 or higher, β-blockers were protective; patients with an RCRI score of 1 had no mortality benefit. For those with an RCRI of 0, in-hospital mortality increased with the use of perioperative β-blockade.

In the POISE trial, Devereaux and colleagues randomized 8351 high-risk patients undergoing noncardiac surgery to metoprolol succinate 200 mg daily, or matching placebo (63). The long-acting metoprolol was first administered at 100 mg 2–4 hours before surgery, within 6 hours after surgery, and then at 200 mg daily thereafter. Active treatment with a β-blocker reduced the composite of cardiovascular death, nonfatal MI, and nonfatal cardiac arrest at 30 days after randomization by 1.1%, but increased mortality by 0.8% and stroke by 0.5%. Two possible explanations for the increased mortality and stroke rate are (1) timing of medication administration and (2) lack of titration of the medication. Patients at intermediate risk were randomized to statin therapy, β-blocker therapy, both (started on average 30 days in advance) or double placebo. β-blocker therapy was associated with significantly decreased cardiovascular events, while statin therapy was not (64). Wallace et al. reported that perioperative β-blockade administered according to the Perioperative Cardiac Risk Reduction protocol is associated with a reduction in 30-day and 1-year mortality (65). Perioperative withdrawal of β-blockers is associated with increased mortality. Atenolol is associated with improved outcome compared to metoprolol in several large administrative datasets (66).

In 2009, an update to the ACC/AHA guidelines on perioperative β-blockade modified previous recommendations based on recent evidence (8). The continuation of β-blockers in patients undergoing surgery who are receiving β-blockers remains a Class I recommendation. No other Class I recommendations are stated. The use of β-blockers titrated to heart rate and blood pressure are all Class IIa recommendations for the following: (1) patients undergoing vascular surgery who are at high cardiac risk because of CAD; (2) the finding of cardiac ischemia on preoperative testing in patients for whom preoperative assessment for vascular surgery identified high cardiac risk, as defined by the presence of more than one RCRI clinical risk factor; and (3) for patients in whom preoperative assessment identified CAD or high cardiac risk, as defined by the presence of more than one clinical risk factor, who are undergoing intermediate-risk surgery. A new Class III recommendation is that the routine administration of high-dose β-blockers in the absence of dose titration is not useful, and may be harmful to patients not currently taking β-blockers who are undergoing noncardiac surgery. Ideally, β-blocker therapy should be initiated more than 7 days in advance, titrated to a heart rate of less than 70 beats per minute, and longer-acting agents such as atenolol or bisoprolol should be used. The ESC Guidelines continue to advocate that both recommendations are Class I. Flu et al. demonstrated that β-blocker treatment initiated >1 week before surgery is associated with lower preoperative heart rate and improved outcomes compared with treatment initiated <1 week preoperatively (67).

Statins

In addition to their cholesterol-lowering properties, statins have anti-inflammatory and plaque-stabilizing properties. In a case-controlled study, Poldermans and colleagues were able to show that statin therapy was associated with reduced mortality after vascular surgery, even in the subset of patients on β-blocker therapy (68). Durazzo and colleagues published a randomized trial of 200 vascular surgery patients in which statins were started an average of 30 days prior to vascular surgery (69). A significant reduction in cardiovascular complications was demonstrated using this protocol. Hindler and colleagues conducted a meta-analysis to evaluate the overall effect of preoperative statin therapy on postoperative outcomes (70). Preoperative statin therapy was associated with 59% reduction in mortality (1.7% vs. 6.1%; $p = 0.0001$) after vascular surgery. When including noncardiac surgery, a 44% reduction in mortality (2.2% vs. 3.2%; $p = 0.0001$) was observed. Le Manach and colleagues studied patients undergoing infrarenal aortic surgery and compared those on chronic statin therapy who had their statin continued immediately postoperatively versus those who had a period in which it was discontinued (71). They demonstrated that postoperative statin withdrawal (>4 days) was an independent predictor of postoperative myonecrosis (odds ratio 2.9, 95% CI, 1.6–5.5) (71). It is therefore critical that statins be continued perioperatively. Most recently, a total of 250 patients were assigned to fluvastatin, and 247 to placebo, a median of 37 days before vascular surgery (72). Perioperative fluvastatin therapy was associated with an improvement in postoperative cardiac outcome. However, a recent small randomized trial questions the value of statin therapy in reducing perioperative inflammation (73).

Nitroglycerin

Continuous intravenous infusions of nitroglycerin, a venodilator, are most useful for the management of perioperative HTN. The postoperative patient with HF and/or ischemic heart disease may also benefit from its use. Nitroglycerin may also reduce preload and improve myocardial oxygen supply.

Nitroglycerin has been a mainstay of anti-ischemic therapy, but its value during the perioperative period is controversial. Two randomized clinical trials have focused on high-risk noncardiac surgery patients. Coriat et al. studied a cohort of patients undergoing carotid endarterectomy using a high-dose narcotic anesthetic technique (74). They demonstrated a significantly reduced incidence of myocardial ischemia with 1.0 μg/kg/min of nitroglycerin compared to 0.5 μg/kg/min; no patients sustained a perioperative MI. Another study compared nitroglycerin at 1.0 μg/kg/min to placebo in high-risk patients undergoing noncardiac surgery and demonstrated no difference in perioperative myocardial ischemia or infarction (75). Many of the effects of nitroglycerin are mimicked by the anesthetic agents, minimizing some of the potential beneficial effects of nitroglycerin and potentially leading to more profound hypotension. Therefore, the evidence does not support the routine prophylactic use of this agent.

α-2-Adrenergic Agonists

Alpha-2-adrenergic agonists have received a great deal of attention as adjuvants to anesthetic management. Clonidine stimulates central α-2-adrenergic receptors and thereby decreases sympathetic nervous outflow to the vasculature, producing vasodilation and lowering blood pressure. Clonidine may be useful for the management of postoperative HTN. It is available for oral and transdermal use and should be continued in the patient taking clonidine preoperatively in order to avoid a withdrawal syndrome. Clonidine should not be used in patients with high-grade atrioventricular conduction disturbances.

Clonidine has been shown to significantly decrease the incidence of intra-operative ischemia compared with placebo in patients undergoing noncardiac surgery. In patients undergoing elective vascular surgery, clonidine reduced the incidence of perioperative myocardial ischemia, and there were fewer nonfatal MIs among patients treated with clonidine compared to those who received placebo (76). In one prospective, randomized, double-blinded, clinical trial, 190 patients with, or at risk for, CAD received clonidine or placebo in the perioperative period. Clonidine significantly decreased the incidence of perioperative myocardial ischemia and significantly reduced mortality for up to 2 years postoperative. A meta-analysis of 23 randomized trials comparing preoperative, intraoperative, or postoperative (within the first 48 hours) administration of α-2-adrenergic agonists with controls found that α-2-adrenergic agonists significantly reduced ischemia and mortality after noncardiac surgery (77). Alpha-2-adrenergic agonists also significantly reduced mortality and MI incidence during vascular surgery (78). Although these results suggest that α-2-adrenergic agonists may have a role in reducing cardiac complications of noncardiac surgery, their use has not been widely adopted in perioperative care.

Calcium Channel Antagonists

Calcium channel blockers may be useful in the management of postoperative HTN, but some may produce reflex tachycardia; this is particularly true of the dihydropyridine compounds like nifedipine. In one systematic review of 11 studies of calcium channel blockers before noncardiac surgery, these drugs were found to significantly reduce the development of myocardial ischemia and supraventricular tachycardia (79). Use of calcium channel blockers was associated with a trend toward reduced death and MI, and in post hoc analyses, they significantly reduced the combined end points of death and MI. The majority of these benefits were attributable to diltiazem. Further studies of calcium channel blockers, and perhaps of diltiazem in particular, appear warranted in the perioperative setting.

Cardiac Devices

Temporary or Permanent Pacemaker Placement Prior to Surgery

In general, perioperative temporary pacemaker placement is indicated for high-grade conduction abnormalities and marked bradycardia with associated symptoms. In cases where symptoms are not present, easy access to temporary transvenous pacemaker equipment in the operating room is advised. Recommendations for temporary or permanent pacemaker implantation in patients undergoing noncardiac surgery are the same as those for elective pacemaker implantations for patients not undergoing surgical procedures. As with all invasive procedures, the risk of temporary pacemaker placement must be considered.

Management of Permanent Pacemakers

Over 460,000 individuals in the USA have permanent pacemakers, 85% of whom are over the age of 65. It is important that the type of pacemaker implanted is known in order to guide perioperative management if issues arise. Major pacemaker manufacturers provide technical support for particular devices, as should the cardiologist who implanted the device, if available. A conservative recommendation is that a pacemaker be interrogated at least 2 months prior to an elective procedure. Indications for use of perioperative pacemakers and management of preexisting devices are generally based on expert opinion. No established evidence-based guidelines are available. In general, noncardiac surgery should be delayed for 48 hours after permanent pacemaker implantation, if possible, to minimize the risk of acute dislodgment of the pacemaker leads.

The American Society of Anesthesiologists has issued recommendations for the perioperative care of patients with cardiac rhythm management devices. Based on these recommendations and those reviewed elsewhere, once it has been determined that a patient has a cardiac rhythm management device (i.e., a permanent pacemaker or an implantable cardioverter defibrillator) based on the history, physical examination, and review of chest radiographs and ECGs, the type of device must be determined (80). This can generally be done by contacting the patient's cardiologist or the clinic responsible for regular device checks. Patients also typically have a card or other form that indicates the manufacturer of the device. It is important to determine the extent to which the patient is pacemaker dependent. If the patient is known to have complete heart block with an inadequate ventricular rate or severe symptomatic bradycardia, he or she should be considered dependent on the device to sustain an adequate heart rhythm. If the pacemaker was implanted after atrioventricular node ablation (e.g., to control a rapid ventricular response to atrial fibrillation), the patient should also be considered device dependent. This information can also be obtained from the patient's cardiologist or the clinic responsible for regular device checks. Preoperative evaluation involves several steps, which are reviewed in the American Society of Anesthesiologists Task Force practice advisory cited earlier (79). These include determining whether electromagnetic interference is likely to occur during the planned surgical procedure; determining whether reprogramming pacing function to asynchronous mode or disabling rate responsive function is advantageous given the likelihood of such interference; and suspending anti-tachyarrhythmia functions that may be present.

Electrocautery may interfere with pacemakers by causing oversensing in patients with unipolar and, rarely, bipolar systems. In this case, it is recommended that the electrocautery electrode be kept at least four to six inches away from the pacemaker to minimize electrical interference. A pacemaker could be programmed to a fixed-rate mode to avoid reprogramming problems. In cases of emergent surgery or situations in which the pacemaker cannot be interrogated and reprogrammed, a magnet should be placed over the pacemaker and maintained in place intraoperatively if the use of electrocautery is anticipated and an ECG recorded to evaluate the backup mode and function of the pacemaker. A programming device specific for the interrogation of the pacemaker being used should be available in the operating room when the potential for electrocautery interference is high, the use of defibrillation or cardioversion is expected, or when there has been a noted change in the function and pacing mode of the pacemaker. Pacing thresholds may be decreased because of hypoxia and myocardial ischemia and may be raised because of hyperkalemia and acid/base disturbances.

Management of Automatic Implantable Cardiac Defibrillators

Management of the automatic implantable cardiac defibrillator (AICD) in the perioperative setting is based on the recommendations outlined above (80). However, although application of a magnet over the AICD prevents unecessary shocks caused by electrocautery, it does not convert the pacemaker function to a fixed rate mode and may lead to inappropriate inhibition of pacing during electrocautery. It is therefore important to reprogram the pacemaker to a fixed rate mode prior to surgery in pacemaker dependent patients. If the device is inactivated by reprogramming then the patient needs to be monitored and appropriate resuscitation equipment should be available. The cardiologist who cares for the patient should provide expert assistance in perioperative mangagement of the AICD. Also, the technical support provided by the major AICD manufacturers may provide specific recommendations. If the AICD is reprogrammed, it should be put back in the activated mode prior to the patient being transferred to an unmonitored bed or when resuscitation equipment is no longer readily available. Endocarditis prophylaxis for patients with an AICD is not indicated.

INTRAOPERATIVE MANAGEMENT
Anesthetic Agents

There are many different approaches to the anesthetic care and intraoperative monitoring of the patient with CAD, depending on the integration of patient- and surgery-specific factors. The type of anesthesia used was not found to be an independent predictor of 30-day mortality in a multivariate analysis (81).

There are three classes of anesthesia: general, regional, and local/sedation or monitored anesthetic care (MAC), defined as local anesthesia administration by the surgeon, both with and without sedation. Outcome studies specifically addressing anesthetic technique in high-risk patients will be discussed after a review of the pharmacology of specific agents.

General Anesthesia

General anesthesia can best be defined as a state including unconsciousness, amnesia, analgesia, immobility, and attenuation of autonomic responses to noxious stimulation, which can be achieved with inhalational agents, intravenous agents, or their combination. General anesthesia can be achieved with or without an endotracheal tube. Traditionally, laryngoscopy and intubation were thought to be the time of greatest stress and risk for myocardial ischemia, but there is evidence to suggest that extubation is the time of greatest risk.

There are four approved and commonly used inhalational anesthetic agents in the USA, all of which have reversible myocardial depressant effects and decrease myocardial oxygen demand, depending on their concentration and effects on systemic vascular resistance and baroreceptor responsiveness (Table 29.4). Overall, there appears to be no one best inhalation anesthetic for patients with CAD. The available agents are briefly reviewed below.

Isoflurane has become the most widely used anesthetic, even for patients with CAD. Isoflurane is a potent vasodilator and has minimal effects on baroreceptor function. Large-scale studies of these inhalational agents in patients undergoing CABG have not demonstrated any increased incidence of myocardial ischemia or infarction (82).

Two newer inhalation agents, desflurane and sevoflurane, are available. Desflurane has the fastest onset and is commonly used in the outpatient setting, although it is associated with airway irritability leading to tachycardia. In a large-scale study comparing a narcotic-based anesthetic with desflurane, the desflurane group had a significantly higher incidence of myocardial ischemia (83). By including narcotics with desflurane, this tachycardia can be avoided. Sevoflurane is the newest approved agent for use in the USA.

There are theoretical advantages to the use of inhalational anesthetics in patients with CAD. Several investigative groups have demonstrated in vitro and in animal models that theses agents possess protective effects on the myocardium similar to ischemic preconditioning. This favorable effect on myocardial oxygen demand would serve to offset the theoretical effects of coronary steal in patients with chronic coronary occlusion.

High-dose narcotics are an alternative form of anesthesia and offer an advantage of hemodynamic stability and lack of myocardial depression. The disadvantage is the

Table 29.4 Clinical Qualities of Inhaled Anesthetics

Agent	Advantages	Disadvantages
Nitrous oxide	Rapid uptake and elimination Minimal respiratory depression Minimal circulatory depression Odorless, nonpungent	Supports combustion Expansion of closed air spaces Inactivates vitamin B_{12} Lack of anesthetic potency Suggestion of increased cardiac morbidity
Isoflurane Desflurane	Decreases cerebral metabolic rate Cardiac output maintained Rapid uptake and elimination	Tachycardia at greater concentration Airway irritation Tachycardia with rapid increase in inspired concentration Requires specialized vaporizer for administration Expensive unless low flows are used
Sevoflurane	Rapid uptake and elimination Nonpungent Less depression of myocardial contractility Stable heart rate	Reacts with CO_2 absorbents Inorganic fluoride release Expensive unless low flows are used

requirement for postoperative ventilation. Alternatively, remifentanil, which is an ultra short-acting narcotic, can be used, thus negating the need for prolonged ventilation. There has been no difference in survival or major morbidity between a high-dose narcotic technique and inhalation-based technique. Therefore, most anesthesiologists use a "balanced" technique of lower doses of narcotics with an inhalational agent.

An alternative anesthetic agent is intravenous propofol, which is an alkyl phenol that can be used for both induction and maintenance of general anesthesia. It can result in profound hypotension secondary to reduced arterial blood pressure with no change in heart rate. It has a rapid clearance with few residual effects on awakening; however, it is expensive.

Regional Anesthesia

Regional anesthesia includes the techniques of spinal and epidural anesthesia, as well as peripheral nerve blocks. Peripheral techniques offer the advantage of minimal or no hemodynamic effects. In contrast, spinal or epidural techniques are associated with sympathetic blockade, which can lead to reduction in blood pressure, reflex sympathetic activation above the level of the blockade, and slowing of heart rate.

The associated autonomic effects of spinal anesthesia occur sooner than the same anesthetic agent administered epidurally. Since a catheter is usually left in place for epidural anesthesia, it can be more easily titrated. Improved outcomes have been demonstrated with a combined regional and general anesthetic approach for patients with CAD, particularly in those undergoing vascular surgery (84,85). One study noted a decreased incidence of all-cause cardiac morbidity with no difference in acute MI or cardiac death in patients receiving combined general plus regional anesthesia compared to general anesthesia alone for infrainguinal surgery. Another study using epidural anesthesia for infrainguinal surgery, followed by epidural analgesia versus general anesthesia plus postoperative intravenous patient-controlled analgesia, showed no difference in cardiac morbidity between the two groups (84). A third study randomized patients to epidural, spinal, and general anesthesia and found no difference in cardiac outcome (86). Importantly, those patients who had a failed regional technique had the highest incidence of cardiac morbidity. The same findings are true for patients undergoing aortic surgery (87,88).

Monitored Anesthetic Care

In a large-scale epidemiological study, MAC was associated with increased 30-day mortality in a univariate analysis, although it did not remain significant in multivariate analysis (81). The major concern with MAC is the inability to adequately block the stress response, including tachycardia. Although MAC can supplement analgesia, the ability to provide good local anesthesia is important.

Pulmonary Artery Catheterization

Historically, pulmonary artery (PA) catheters were widely used in high-risk patients undergoing major noncardiac surgery, with the assumption that better understanding of cardiac filling pressures and cardiac output would lead to improved outcomes. However, in randomized studies placement of a PA catheter perioperatively did not alter cardiac morbidity (89). The American Society of Anesthesiologists advocates reserving use of the PA catheter for those circumstances in which there is a high-risk patient undergoing a high-risk surgery, when the PA catheter will make a difference in medical management.

Anemia

Anemia has also been associated with an increased incidence of perioperative myocardial ischemia. In a small retrospective study of patients undergoing infrainguinal bypass surgery, a hematocrit lower than 27% was associated with a significantly increased risk of postoperative MI (90). A higher rate of myocardial ischemia was noted in patients undergoing radical prostatectomy who had a hematocrit 28% or less compared with those with a higher hematocrit, although there was no difference in the rate of major morbidity (91). Carson et al. enrolled 2016 patients who were 50 years of age or older, who had either a history of or risk factors for cardiovascular disease, and whose hemoglobin level was below 10 g per deciliter after hip-fracture surgery (92). A liberal transfusion strategy, as compared with a restrictive strategy, did not reduce rates of death or inability to walk independently on 60-day follow-up or reduce in-hospital morbidity in elderly patients at high cardiovascular risk.

Maintenance of Body Temperature

Hypothermia has also been associated with an increased incidence of myocardial ischemia in vascular surgery patients. In a randomized trial involving patients either undergoing vascular surgery or with known risk factors for CAD, use of forced air warming to maintain normothermia was associated with a significant reduction in cardiac morbidity and myocardial ischemia for the first 24 postoperative hours (93). Therefore, maintenance of normothermia should be a goal of perioperative management.

Surveillance for Perioperative MI

The optimal and most cost-effective strategy for monitoring high-risk patients for major cardiac morbidity after noncardiac surgery is unknown. Postoperative myocardial ischemia or infarction is often clinically silent, most likely due to the confounding effects of analgesics. Creatine kinase (CK)-MB has been shown to be less specific than cardiac troponins for the detection of MI postoperatively. Non-ST-elevation MI occurs more often than ST-elevation MI perioperatively.

Myocardium-specific enzymes such as cardiac troponins (I or T) are quite sensitive in the detection of perioperative MI. In one study of 96 patients undergoing vascular surgery, eight patients sustained a perioperative MI, as confirmed by the presence of new segmental WMAs, and all had elevations of cardiac troponin I (cTn-I), while six patients had elevated CK-MB (94). Troponin I had a specificity of 99%, while CK-MB had a specificity of 81%. Other studies have confirmed the clinical utility of cardiac troponins in the perioperative setting (95–98).

Historically, perioperative MI was associated with a 30–50% short-term mortality. With greater perioperative surveillance and more sensitive troponin assays, more asymptomatic MIs are being detected. More recent series have reported that perioperative MI is associated with a short-term mortality of up to 20% (77). In a study of patients undergoing vascular surgery, where cTn-I levels were measured immediately after surgery and on three consecutive postoperative days, 12% had elevated troponin I levels, which was associated with a sixfold increased risk of 6-month mortality and a 27-fold increased risk of MI (99). Le Manach and colleagues studied 1152 consecutive patients who underwent abdominal infrarenal aortic surgery, and identified four patterns of cTn-I release after surgery (100). One group had no abnormal levels, while a second group had only mild elevations of cTn-I. Two groups demonstrated elevations of cTn-I consistent with a perioperative MI. One demonstrated acute (<24 hours) and early elevations of cTn-I above threshold, and the other demonstrated prolonged low levels of cTn-I release, followed by a delayed (>24 hours) elevation of cTn-I. The authors suggest that these two different patterns represent two distinct pathophysiologies: acute coronary occlusion for early morbidity and prolonged myocardial ischemia for late events. The VISION trial determined the relationship between the peak fourth-generation troponin T (TnT) measurement in the first 3 days after noncardiac surgery and 30-day mortality in a total of 15,133 patients (101). Multivariable analysis demonstrated that peak TnT values of at least 0.02 ng/mL, occurring in 11.6% of patients, were associated with higher 30-day mortality compared with the reference group. Peak TnT measurement added incremental prognostic value to discriminate those likely to die within 30 days. The ACC/AHA guidelines recommend the use of cardiac biomarkers for patients at high risk and those with clinical, ECG, or hemodynamic evidence of cardiovascular dysfunction.

Postoperative Analgesia

If postoperative tachycardia and catecholamine surges lead to cardiac events, the more intense analgesia regimens may be beneficial in improving perioperative outcomes. Additionally, there is growing interest in the role of postoperative analgesia in reducing the hypercoagulable state, as well as providing other benefits to the geriatric patient, such as reduced delirium. Studies comparing general with regional anesthesia have demonstrated reduced platelet aggregability in the epidural group (102).

REFERENCES

1. Mangano DT. Perioperative cardiac morbidity. Anesthesiology 1990; 72: 153–84.
2. Colloca G, Santoro M, Gambassi G. Age-related physiologic changes and perioperative management of elderly patients. Surg Oncol 2010; 19: 124–30.
3. Lee TH, Marcantonio ER, Mangione CM, et al. Derivation and prospective validation of a simple index for prediction of cardiac risk of major noncardiac surgery. Circulation 1999; 100: 1043–9.
4. Reilly DF, McNeely MJ, Doerner D, et al. Self-reported exercise tolerance and the risk of serious perioperative complications. Arch Intern Med 1999; 159: 2185–92.
5. Hlatky MA, Boineau RE, Higginbotham MB, et al. A brief self-administered questionnaire to determine functional capacity (the Duke Activity Status Index). Am J Cardiol 1989; 64: 651–4.
6. de Arenaza DP, Pepper J, Lees B, et al. Preoperative 6-minute walk test adds prognostic information to Euroscore in patients undergoing aortic valve replacement. Heart 2010; 96: 113–17.
7. Campeau L. Grading of angina pectoris. Circulation 1976; 54: 522–3.
8. Fleisher LA, Beckman JA, Brown KA, et al. 2009 ACCF/AHA focused update on perioperative beta blockade incorporated into the ACC/AHA 2007 guidelines on perioperative cardiovascular evaluation and care for noncardiac surgery: a report of the American college of cardiology foundation/American heart association task force on practice guidelines. Circulation 2009; 120: e169–276.
9. Shah KB, Kleinman BS, Rao T, et al. Angina and other risk factors in patients with cardiac diseases undergoing noncardiac operations. Anesth Analg 1990; 70: 240–7.
10. Rao TLK, Jacobs KH, El-Etr AA. Reinfarction following anesthesia in patients with myocardial infarction. Anesthesiology 1983; 59: 499–505.
11. Shah KB, Kleinman BS, Sami H, Patel I, Rao T. Reevaluation of perioperative myocardial infarction in patients with prior myocardial infarction undergoing noncardiac operations. Anesth Analg 1990; 71: 231–5.
12. Hertzer NR, Bevan EG, Young JR, et al. Coronary artery disease in peripheral vascular patients: a classification of 1000 coronary angiograms and results of surgical management. Ann Surg 1984; 199: 223–33.
13. Livhits M, Gibbons MM, de Virgilio C, et al. Coronary revascularization after myocardial infarction can reduce risks of noncardiac surgery. J Am Coll Surg 2011; 212: 1018–26.
14. Livhits M, Ko CY, Leonardi MJ, et al. Risk of surgery following recent myocardial infarction. Ann Surg 2011; 253: 857–64.
15. Weksler N, Klein M, Szendro G, et al. The dilemma of immediate preoperative hypertension: to treat and operate, or to postpone surgery? J Clin Anesth 2003; 15: 179–83.
16. Nishimura RA, Carabello BA, Faxon DP, et al. American College of Cardiology/American Heart Association Task F. ACC/AHA 2008 guideline update on valvular heart disease: focused update on infective endocarditis: a report of the American College of Cardiology/American Heart Association Task Force on Practice Guidelines: endorsed by the Society of Cardiovascular Anesthesiologists, Society for Cardiovascular Angiography and Interventions, and Society of Thoracic Surgeons. Circulation 2008; 118: 887–96.
17. Goldman L, Caldera DL, Nussbaum SR, et al. Multifactorial index of cardiac risk in noncardiac surgical procedures. N Engl J Med 1977; 297: 845–50.

18. Kertai MD, Bountioukos M, Boersma E, et al. Aortic stenosis: an underestimated risk factor for perioperative complications in patients undergoing noncardiac surgery. Am J Med 2004; 116: 8–13.

19. Calleja AM, Dommaraju S, Gaddam R, et al. Cardiac risk in patients aged >75 years with asymptomatic, severe aortic stenosis undergoing noncardiac surgery. Am J Cardiol 2010; 105: 1159–63.

20. Wilson W, Taubert KA, Gewitz M, et al. Prevention of infective endocarditis. Guidelines from the American Heart Association. A guideline from the American Heart Association Rheumatic Fever, Endocarditis, and Kawasaki Disease Committee, Council on Cardiovascular Disease in the Young, and the Council on Clinical Cardiology, Council on Cardiovascular Surgery and Anesthesia, and the Quality of Care and Outcomes Research Interdisciplinary Working Group. Circulation 2007; 116: 1736–54.

21. Kovacs MJ, Kearon C, Rodger M, et al. Single-arm study of bridging therapy with low-molecular weight heparin for patients at risk of arterial embolism who require temporary interruption of warfarin. Circulation 2004; 110: 1658.

22. Hreybe H, Zahid M, Sonel A, et al. Noncardiac surgery and the risk of death and other cardiovascular events in patients with hypertrophic cardiomyopathy. Clin Cardiol 2006; 29: 65–8.

23. Haering JM, Comunale ME, Parker RA, et al. Cardiac risk of noncardiac surgery in patients with asymmetric septal hypertrophy. Anesthesiology 1996; 85: 254–9.

24. Thompson R, Liberthson R, Lowenstein E. Perioperative anesthetic risk of noncardiac surgery in hypertrophic obstructive cardiomyopathy. J Am Med Assoc 1985; 254: 2419–21.

25. OKelly B, Browner WS, Massie B, et al. Ventricular arrhythmias in patients undergoing noncardiac surgery. The Study of Perioperative Ischemia Research Group [see comments]. JAMA 1992; 268: 217–21.

26. Winkel TA, Schouten O, Hoeks SE, et al. Prognosis of transient new-onset atrial fibrillation during vascular surgery. Eur J Vasc Endovasc Surg 2009.

27. Schein OD, Katz J, Bass EB, et al. The value of routine preoperative medical testing before cataract surgery. Study of Medical Testing for Cataract Surgery. N Engl J Med 2000; 342: 168–75.

28. Warner MA, Shields SE, Chute CG. Major morbidity and mortality within 1 month of ambulatory surgery and anesthesia. JAMA 1993; 270: 1437–41.

29. Gupta PK, Gupta H, Sundaram A, et al. Development and validation of a risk calculator for prediction of cardiac risk after surgery. Circulation 2011; 124: 381–7.

30. Committee on Standards and Practice Parameters, Apfelbaum JL, Connis RT, Nickinovich DG; American Society of Anesthesiologists Task Force on Preanesthesia Evaluation, Pasternak LR, Arens JF, Caplan RA, et al. Practice advisory for preanesthesia evaluation: an updated report by the American Society of Anesthesiologists Task Force on Preanesthesia Evaluation. Anesthesiology 2012; 116: 522–38.

31. Halm EA, Browner WS, Tubau JF, Tateo IM, Mangano DT. Echocardiography for assessing cardiac risk in patients having noncardiac surgery. Study of Perioperative Ischemia Research Group. Ann Intern Med 1996; 125: 433–41.

32. Flu WJ, van Kuijk JP, Hoeks SE, et al. Prognostic implications of asymptomatic left ventricular dysfunction in patients undergoing vascular surgery. Anesthesiology 2010; 112: 1316–24.

33. Gianrossi R, Detrano R, Mulvihill D, et al. Exercise-induced ST depression in the diagnosis of coronary artery disease: a meta-analysis. Circulation 1989; 80: 87–98.

34. Cutler BS, Leppo JA. Dipyridamole thallium 201 scintigraphy to detect coronary artery disease before abdominal aortic surgery. J Vasc Surg 1987; 5: 91–100.

35. Fleisher LA, Rosenbaum SH, Nelson AH, et al. Preoperative dipyridamole thallium imaging and Holter monitoring as a predictor of perioperative cardiac events and long tem outcome. Anesthesiology 1995; 83: 906–17.

36. Mangano DT, London MJ, Tubau JF, et al. Dipyridamole thallium-201 scintigraphy as a preoperative screening test. A reexamination of its predictive potential. Study of Perioperative Ischemia Research Group. Circulation 1991; 84: 493–502.

37. Younis LT, Aguirre F, Byers S, et al. Perioperative and long-term prognostic value of intravenous dipyridamole thallium scintigraphy in patients with peripheral vascular disease. Am Heart J 1990; 119: 1287–92.

38. Landesberg G, Wolf Y, Schechter D, et al. Preoperative thallium scanning, selective coronary revascularization, and long-term survival after carotid endarterectomy. Stroke 1998; 29: 2541–8.

39. Beattie WS, Abdelnaem E, Wijeysundera DN, Buckley DN. A meta-analytic comparison of preoperative stress echocardiography and nuclear scintigraphy imaging. Anesth Analg 2006; 102: 8–16.

40. Davila-Roman V, Waggoner A, Sicard G, et al. Dobutamine stress echocardiography predicts surgical outcome in patients with an aortic aneurysm and peripheral vascular disease. J Am Coll Cardiol 1993; 21: 957–63.

41. Poldermans D, Arnese M, Fioretti PM, et al. Sustained prognostic value of dobutamine stress echo-cardiography for late cardiac events after major noncardiac vascular surgery. Circulation 1997; 95: 53–8.

42. Hillis LD, Smith PK, Anderson JL, et al. 2011 ACCF/AHA guideline for coronary artery bypass graft surgery: executive summary: a report of the American College of Cardiology Foundation/American Heart Association Task Force on Practice Guidelines. Circulation 2011; 124: 2610–42.

43. McFalls EO, Ward HB, Moritz TE, et al. Coronary-artery revascularization before elective major vascular surgery. N Engl J Med 2004; 351: 2795–804.

44. Ward HB, Kelly RF, Thottapurathu L, et al. Coronary artery bypass grafting is superior to percutaneous coronary intervention in prevention of perioperative myocardial infarctions during subsequent vascular surgery. Ann Thorac Surg 2006; 82: 795–800; discussion 800-1.

45. Garcia S, Moritz TE, Ward HB, et al. Usefulness of revascularization of patients with multivessel coronary artery disease before elective vascular surgery for abdominal aortic and peripheral occlusive disease. Am J Cardiol 2008; 102: 809–13.

46. Poldermans D, Bax JJ, Schouten O, et al. Should major vascular surgery be delayed because of pre-operative cardiac testing in intermediate-risk patients receiving beta-blocker therapy with tight heart rate control? J Am Coll Cardiol 2006; 48: 964–9.

47. Poldermans D, Schouten O, Vidakovic R, et al. A clinical randomized trial to evaluate the safety of a noninvasive approach in high-risk patients undergoing major vascular surgery: the DECREASE-V Pilot Study. J Am Coll Cardiol 2007; 49: 1763–9.

48. Schouten O, van Kuijk JP, Flu WJ, et al. Long-term outcome of prophylactic coronary revascularization in cardiac high-risk patients undergoing major vascular surgery (from the randomized DECREASE-V Pilot Study). Am J Cardiol 2009; 103: 897–901.

49. Posner KL, Van Norman GA, Chan V. Adverse cardiac outcomes after noncardiac surgery in patients with prior percutaneous transluminal coronary angioplasty. Anesth Analg 1999; 89: 553–60.

50. Kaluza GL, Joseph J, Lee JR, Raizner ME, Raizner AE. Catastrophic outcomes of noncardiac surgery soon after coronary stenting. J Am Coll Cardiol 2000; 35: 1288–94.

51. Wilson SH, Fasseas P, Orford JL, et al. Clinical outcome of patients undergoing non-cardiac surgery in the two months following coronary stenting. J Am Coll Cardiol 2003; 42: 234–40.

52. Vicenzi MN, Meislitzer T, Heitzinger B, et al. Coronary artery stenting and non-cardiac surgery–a prospective outcome study. Br J Anaesth 2006; 96: 686–93.

53. Leibowitz D, Cohen M, Planer D, et al. Comparison of cardiovascular risk of noncardiac surgery following coronary angioplasty with versus without stenting. Am J Cardiol 2006; 97: 1188–91.

54. Schouten O, van Domburg RT, Bax JJ, et al. Noncardiac surgery after coronary stenting: early surgery and interruption of antiplatelet therapy are associated with an increase in major adverse cardiac events. J Am Coll Cardiol 2007; 49: 122–4.

55. Rabbitts JA, Nuttall GA, Brown MJ, et al. Cardiac risk of noncardiac surgery after percutaneous coronary intervention with drug-eluting stents. Anesthesiology 2008; 109: 596–604.

56. Albaladejo P, Marret E, Samama CM, et al. Non-cardiac surgery in patients with coronary stents: the RECO study. Heart 2011; 97: 1566–72.

57. Masaki E, Takinami M, Kurata Y, Kagaya S, Ahmed A. Anesthetic management of high-risk cardiac patients undergoing noncardiac surgery under the support of intraaortic balloon pump. J Clin Anesth 1999; 11: 342–5.

58. Mangano DT, Layug EL, Wallace A, Tateo I. Effect of atenolol on mortality and cardiovascular morbidity after noncardiac surgery. Multicenter Study of Perioperative Ischemia Research Group. N Engl J Med 1996; 335: 1713–20.

59. Wallace A, Layug B, Tateo I, et al. Prophylactic atenolol reduces postoperative myocardial ischemia. McSPI Research Group [see comments]. Anesthesiology 1998; 88: 7–17.

60. Poldermans D, Boersma E, Bax JJ, et al. The effect of bisoprolol on perioperative mortality and myocardial infarction in high-risk patients undergoing vascular surgery. Dutch Echocardiographic Cardiac Risk Evaluation Applying Stress Echocardiography Study Group [see comments]. N Engl J Med 1999; 341: 1789–94.

61. Boersma E, Poldermans D, Bax JJ, et al. Predictors of cardiac events after major vascular surgery: Role of clinical characteristics, dobutamine echocardiography, and beta-blocker therapy. JAMA 2001; 285: 1865–73.

62. Lindenauer PK, Pekow P, Wang K, et al. Perioperative beta-blocker therapy and mortality after major noncardiac surgery. N Engl J Med 2005; 353: 349–61.

63. Devereaux PJ, Yang H, Yusuf S, et al. Effects of extended-release metoprolol succinate in patients undergoing non-cardiac surgery (POISE trial): a randomised controlled trial. Lancet 2008; 371: 1839–47.

64. Dunkelgrun M, Boersma E, Schouten O, et al. Bisoprolol and fluvastatin for the reduction of perioperative cardiac mortality and myocardial infarction in intermediate-risk patients undergoing noncardiovascular surgery: a randomized controlled trial (DECREASE-IV). Ann Surg 2009; 249: 921–6.

65. Wallace AW, Au S, Cason BA. Association of the pattern of use of perioperative beta-blockade and postoperative mortality. Anesthesiology 2010; 113: 794–805.

66. Wallace AW, Au S, Cason BA. Perioperative beta-blockade: atenolol is associated with reduced mortality when compared to metoprolol. Anesthesiology 2011; 114: 824–36.

67. Flu WJ, van Kuijk JP, Chonchol M, et al. Timing of pre-operative Beta-blocker treatment in vascular surgery patients: influence on post-operative outcome. J Am Coll Cardiol 2010; 56: 1922–9.

68. Poldermans D, Bax JJ, Kertai MD, et al. Statins are associated with a reduced incidence of perioperative mortality in patients undergoing major noncardiac vascular surgery. Circulation 2003; 107: 1848–51.

69. Durazzo AE, Machado FS, Ikeoka DT, et al. Reduction in cardiovascular events after vascular surgery with atorvastatin: a randomized trial. J Vasc Surg 2004; 39: 967–75.

70. Hindler K, Shaw AD, Samuels J, et al. Improved postoperative outcomes associated with preoperative statin therapy. Anesthesiology 2006; 105: 1260–72.

71. Le Manach Y, Godet G, Coriat P, et al. The impact of postoperative discontinuation or continuation of chronic statin therapy on cardiac outcome after major vascular surgery. Anesth Analg 2007; 104: 1326–33.

72. Schouten O, Boersma E, Hoeks SE, et al. Fluvastatin and perioperative events in patients undergoing vascular surgery. N Engl J Med 2009; 361: 980–9.

73. Neilipovitz DT, Bryson GL, Taljaard M. STAR VaS–Short Term Atorvastatin Regime for Vasculopathic Subjects: a randomized placebo-controlled trial evaluating perioperative atorvastatin therapy in noncardiac surgery. Can J Anaesth 2012; 59: 527–37.

74. Coriat P, Daloz M, Bousseau D, et al. Prevention of intraoperative myocardial ischemia during noncardiac surgery with intravenous nitroglycerin. Anesthesiology 1984; 61: 193–6.

75. Dodds TM, Stone JG, Coromilas J, Weinberger M, Levy DG. Prophylactic nitroglycerin infusion during noncardiac surgery does not reduce perioperative ischemia. Anesth Analg 1993; 76: 705–13.

76. Wallace AW, Galindez D, Salahieh A, et al. Effect of clonidine on cardiovascular morbidity and mortality after noncardiac surgery. Anesthesiology 2004; 101: 284–93.

77. Fleisher LA, Nelson AH, Rosenbaum SH. Postoperative myocardial ischemia: etiology of cardiac morbidity or manifestation of underlying disease. J Clin Anesth 1995; 7: 97–102.

78. Wijeysundera DN, Naik JS, Beattie WS. Alpha-2 adrenergic agonists to prevent perioperative cardiovascular complications: a meta-analysis. Am J Med 2003; 114: 742–52.

79. Wijeysundera DN, Beattie WS. Calcium channel blockers for reducing cardiac morbidity after noncardiac surgery: a meta-analysis. Anesth Analg 2003; 97: 634–41.

80. American Society of A: Practice advisory for the perioperative management of patients with cardiac implantable electronic devices: pacemakers and implantable cardioverter-defibrillators. An updated report by the american society of anesthesiologists task force on perioperative management of patients with cardiac implantable electronic devices. Anesthesiology 2011; 114: 247–61.

81. Cohen M, Duncan PG, Tate RB. Does anesthesia contribute to operative mortality? JAMA 1988; 260: 2859–63.

82. Leung JM, Goehner P, O'Kelly BF, et al. Isoflurane anesthesia and myocardial ischemia: comparative risk versus sufentanil anesthesia in patients undergoing coronary artery bypass graft surgery. The SPI (Study of Perioperative Ischemia) Research Group. Anesthesiology 1991; 74: 838–47.

83. Helman JD, Leung JM, Bellows WH, et al. The risk of myocardial ischemia in patients receiving desflurane versus sufentanil anesthesia for coronary artery bypass graft surgery. The S.P.I. Research Group. Anesthesiology 1992; 77: 47–62.

84. Christopherson R, Beattie C, Frank SM, et al. Perioperative morbidity in patients randomized to epidural or general anesthesia for lower extremity vascular surgery. Perioperative Ischemia Randomized Anesthesia Trial Study Group [see comments]. Anesthesiology 1993; 79: 422–34.

85. Tuman KJ, McCarthy RJ, March RJ, et al. Effects of epidural anesthesia and analgesia on coagulation and outcome after major vascular surgery [see comments]. Anesth Analg 1991; 73: 696–704.

86. Bode RH Jr, Lewis KP, Zarich SW, et al. Cardiac outcome after peripheral vascular surgery. Comparison of general and regional anesthesia. Anesthesiology 1996; 84: 3–13.

87. Baron JF, Bertrand M, Barre E, et al. Combined epidural and general anesthesia versus general anesthesia for abdominal aortic surgery. Anesthesiology 1991; 75: 611–18.

88. Norris EJ, Beattie C, Perler BA, et al. Double-masked randomized trial comparing alternate combinations of intraoperative anesthesia and postoperative analgesia in abdominal aortic surgery. Anesthesiology 2001; 95: 1054–67.

89. Shah MR, Hasselblad V, Stevenson LW, et al. Impact of the pulmonary artery catheter in critically ill patients: meta-analysis of randomized clinical trials. JAMA 2005; 294: 1664–70.
90. Nelson AH, Fleisher LA, Rosenbaum SH. Relationship between postoperative anemia and cardiac morbidity in high-risk vascular patients in the intensive care unit. Crit Care Med 1993; 21: 860–6.
91. Hogue CW Jr, Goodnough LT, Monk TG. Perioperative myocardial ischemic episodes are related to hematocrit level in patients undergoing radical prostatectomy. Transfusion 1998; 38: 924–31.
92. Carson JL, Terrin ML, Noveck H, et al. Liberal or restrictive transfusion in high-risk patients after hip surgery. N Engl J Med 2011; 365: 2453–62.
93. Frank SM, Fleisher LA, Breslow MJ, et al. Perioperative maintenance of normothermia reduces the incidence of morbid cardiac events. A randomized clinical trial. JAMA 1997; 277: 1127–34.
94. Adams JE, Sicard GA, Allen BT, et al. Diagnosis of perioperative myocardial infarction with measurement of cardiac troponin I. N Engl J Med 1994; 330: 670–4.
95. Hake U, Schmid FX, Iversen S, et al. Troponin T–a reliable marker of perioperative myocardial infarction? Eur J Cardiothorac Surg 1993; 7: 628–33.
96. Landesberg G, Shatz V, Akopnik I, et al. Association of cardiac troponin, CK-MB, and postoperative myocardial ischemia with long-term survival after major vascular surgery. J Am Coll Cardiol 2003; 42: 1547–54.
97. Lee TH, Thomas EJ, Ludwig LE, et al. Troponin T as a marker for myocardial ischemia in patients undergoing major noncardiac surgery. Am J Cardiol 1996; 77: 1031–6.
98. Lopez-Jimenez F, Goldman L, Sacks DB, et al. Prognostic value of cardiac troponin T after noncardiac surgery: 6-month follow-up data. J Am Coll Cardiol 1997; 29: 1241–5.
99. Kim LJ, Martinez EA, Faraday N, et al. Cardiac troponin I predicts short-term mortality in vascular surgery patients. Circulation 2002; 106: 2366–71.
100. Le Manach Y, Perel A, Coriat P, et al. Early and delayed myocardial infarction after abdominal aortic surgery. Anesthesiology 2005; 102: 885–91.
101. Vascular Events In Noncardiac Surgery Patients Cohort Evaluation Study Investigators. Devereaux PJ, Chan MT, Alonso-Coello P, et al. Association between postoperative troponin levels and 30-day mortality among patients undergoing noncardiac surgery. JAMA 2012; 307: 2295–304.
102. Rosenfeld BA, Beattie C, Christopherson R, et al. The effects of different anesthetic regimens on fibrinolysis and the development of postoperative arterial thrombosis. Perioperative Ischemia Randomized Anesthesia Trial Study Group. Anesthesiology 1993; 79: 435–43.

30

Disability and frailty in older patients with cardiovascular disease

John E. Morley and Michael W. Rich

SUMMARY

Cardiovascular disease, functional impairments, disability, diminished quality of life, and frailty are inextricably linked in older adults. This chapter reviews the pathophysiology of frailty and the interactions between cardiovascular disorders, especially coronary artery disease and heart failure, and functional decline. Often, the functional limitations imposed by cardiovascular disease in older adults contribute to progressive disability culminating in frailty or cardiac cachexia. Mechanisms underlying these interactions include alterations in protein metabolism and function, inflammation related in part to cytokine excess, neurohormonal changes, and inadequate intake of calories and other nutrients (i.e., malnutrition). Although limited data are available concerning the prevention and treatment of frailty in older patients with cardiovascular disease, aggressive control of symptoms (angina, heart failure) to limit functional decline, regular physical activity (including aerobic, resistance, and flexibility exercises), and a balanced diet with adequate caloric intake are recommended.

INTRODUCTION

Functional status plays an important role in maintenance of quality of life as people age. When an older person is admitted to the hospital, the best predictor of hospital mortality is the ability to perform routine activities of daily living (ADLs) (1). Loss of independence in even one ADL dramatically increases the chances of an older person either dying or requiring nursing-home placement within 6 months following hospital admission (1,2). Moreover, loss of ADLs is a better predictor of outcome than the Charlson comorbidity index or the New York Heart Association functional class.

Nagi has created a simple model of the pathway to disability (3,4). In this model, active pathology (e.g., heart failure) leads to impairment in bodily functions (e.g., dyspnea), which leads to functional limitations (e.g., walking, stair climbing, poor memory), and finally to disability (Fig. 30.1). In this model, disability is defined as a limitation in the performance of work or in the tasks essential to allow a person to live independently.

The disablement process plays an important role in the determination of health-related quality of life, often assessed with the short form (SF)-36 questionnaire. The more cardiovascular-related diseases a person has (i.e., hypertension, diabetes, angina pectoris, heart failure, myocardial infarction), the lower the SF-36 score (5). This assessment is true

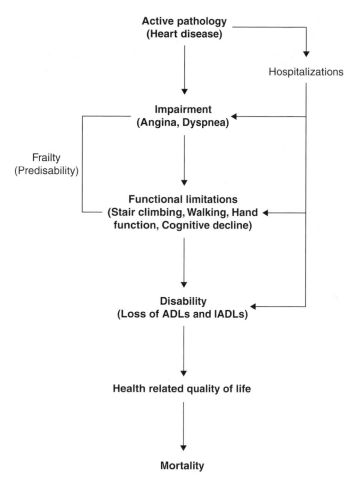

Figure 30.1 The pathway to disability in heart disease. *Abbreviations*: ADLs, activities of daily living; IADLs, instrumental activities of daily living.

for all eight domains of health-related quality of life (physical function, role-physical, bodily pain, general health, vitality, social function, role-emotional, and mental health). In addition, each cardiovascular disorder is individually related to the different domains, with the strongest associations being for angina and heart failure.

Similarly, as the number of comorbid diseases increases, so too does the likelihood of disability. The conditions most associated with the development of disability are hip fracture, stroke, arthritis, and heart disease (6). The number of hospitalizations (i.e., acute events) is also a strong predictor of disability (7). In an analysis combining data from the 2001 Mexican Health and Aging Study ($n = 4872$) and the Hispanic Established Population for Epidemiologic Studies of the Elderly ($n = 3050$), the likelihood of disability due to comorbid diseases was most closely linked to diabetes, stroke, and heart attack (8). In the Framingham study, angina pectoris was the best cardiovascular predictor of disability, while heart failure only predicted disability in women (9).

These studies clearly implicate cardiovascular disease and related hospitalizations as important factors contributing to disability and impaired quality of life in older adults. This chapter focuses on the role of heart disease in the pathophysiology of frailty. Frailty represents a form of predisability associated with both impairments and limitations.

FRAILTY—DEFINITION

Frailty is a condition in which a person has subclinical impairment of routine activities that exceeds normal age-related physiological deterioration. A frail person is at increased risk of developing disability when exposed to stressful conditions such as hospitalization for an acute medical illness.

Fried et al. (10,11) have objectively defined frailty as the presence of three or more of the following:

- Weight loss (10 lbs in 1 year)
- Exhaustion (self-report)
- Weakness (grip strength; lowest 20% for age and gender)
- Walking speed (15 ft; slowest 20% for age and gender)
- Low physical activity (kcal/wk; lowest 20% for age and gender)

Individuals with one or two of these factors are considered prefrail. Using this definition, the prevalence of frailty in a community-dwelling population of individuals aged 65 years or older was 6.9%, and the 4-year incidence of frailty was 7.2% (11).

Another objective definition of frailty utilizes the FRAIL mnemonic:

- Fatigue (self report)
- Resistance/power (inability to climb one flight of stairs)
- Activity (inability to walk one block without stopping)
- Illness (more than three illnesses diagnosed)
- Loss of weight (5% in 6 months)

A positive score for frailty is three out of five (12,13). Alternatively, Rockwood (14) considers frailty merely to be a reflection of the number of underlying diseases in a person.

FRAILTY AND HEART DISEASE

Cacciatore et al. (15) studied 1259 older subjects with a 9-year follow-up. In this population, frailty was more predictive of mortality in persons with chronic heart failure than in the general population.

Chronic heart failure is a classical condition that predisposes to frailty. It is associated with a decline in VO_2max leading to reduced mobility and strength. It can also be associated with anorexia and declines in both lean and fat mass (cardiac cachexia). Activation of the renin–angiotensin system, and of angiotensin II in particular, leads to an increased rate of cleavage of actinomysin, with resulting clearance of muscle protein by the ubiquitin–proteasome system, resulting in accelerated loss of muscle mass (sarcopenia).

Coronary artery disease (CAD) results in decreased mobility because of angina pectoris and dyspnea. In addition, persons with CAD often have peripheral arterial disease that may lead to decreased walking time and a loss of lower limb muscle. This combination provides "fertile soil" for frailty to develop.

In the Cardiovascular Health Study, subclinical cardiovascular disease (i.e., asymptomatic carotid intima-media thickening, abnormal ankle-arm blood pressure index, or decreased left ventricular ejection fraction) was present in 37% of older adults and was a strong independent predictor of frailty (16). Thus, the presence of clinical or subclinical cardiovascular disease is a potent risk factor for the development of frailty in older adults.

PATHOPHYSIOLOGY OF FRAILTY

Frailty occurs as an interaction between aging physiology, environment, and disease. The major lifestyle factor is physical activity, including formal exercise, for example, endurance, resistance, and balance exercises, as well as spontaneous physical activity, for example, the distance walked each day or the time spent gardening. Food intake leading to either obesity or under-nutrition represents a second lifestyle factor involved in the pathogenesis of frailty.

Factors contributing to frailty include sarcopenia and decline in executive function. Syndromes that can interact with heart failure to foster frailty include chronic pain, anemia, and cachexia. Anemia is an independent predictor of physical disability in older heart failure patients (17).

As noted above, sarcopenia refers to the loss of muscle mass that occurs with aging (18). Sarcopenia is considered pathological when the muscle mass is 2 SD below that of a young person. It is best measured using DEXA and dividing the appendicular muscle (lean) mass by height squared. Using this approach, approximately 18% of 70-year-old persons and 50% of 80-year-old persons are sarcopenic (19). Importantly, with aging, loss of strength and power is greater than loss of muscle mass. Many older persons also develop fatty infiltration of the muscles, that is, myosteatosis, which further decreases muscle function (20). Men with moderate sarcopenia have an adjusted odds ratio for physical disability of 3.65 relative to men without sarcopenia, while the adjusted odds ratio is 4.71 in men with more marked sarcopenia; corresponding odds ratios in women are 1.41 and 2.96 (21). While persons with moderate obesity and no sarcopenia have good outcomes, obesity associated with sarcopenia, that is, sarcopenic obesity or "fat frail", is a strong independent predictor of future disability and mortality (22).

The causes of sarcopenia are summarized in Table 30.1. Genetic factors and low birth weight have been associated with poor grip strength at age 70 years (23). In accordance with the adage "use it or lose it", lack of physical exercise, in particular resistance exercise is a major cause of loss of muscle mass. A daily energy intake of less than 21 kcal/kg leads to sarcopenia and frailty (24). To maintain muscle mass, most older persons require between 1.2 and 1.5 g/kg/day of protein, as opposed to the recommended 0.8 g/kg/day (25). Besides acting as building blocks for muscle, branched chain amino acids (leucine, isoleucine, valine) promote protein synthesis and inhibit proteolysis (26). Creatine intake has been shown to enhance lean mass and power in older persons performing resistance exercise (27). Insulin resistance leads to triglyceride accumulation in muscle and decreased strength (20).

Anabolic steroids play a key role in maintaining muscle mass and strength (28). Anabolic steroids increase protein synthesis and promote the conversion of stem cells to muscle satellite cells (cells responsible for skeletal muscle repair). Testosterone increases muscle

Table 30.1 Causes of Sarcopenia

- Genetic factors
- Low muscle mass at birth
- Physical inactivity
- Low calorie intake
- Low protein intake
- Insulin resistance
- Hypogonadism (male)
- Low growth hormone
- Low mechanogrowth factor
- Low vitamin D
- Myostatin
- Cytokine excess
- Loss of motor units
- Peripheral arterial disease

mass, strength, and function in older persons (29,30), and it has been shown to increase functional capacity and reduce symptoms in older men (31–33) and women (34) with moderate heart failure. Nandrolone, another anabolic steroid, increases muscle mass and strength in older women (35). Selective androgen receptor molecules (SARMs) increase muscle strength and prevent bone loss while having no adverse effects on the prostate gland. Ostarine is a SARM that has been shown to increase lean mass and power in men and women older than 60 years. In contrast, dehydroepiandrosterone at a dose of 50 mg daily for 1 year failed to increase muscle mass or strength (36).

Growth hormone increases nitrogen retention and muscle mass but fails to increase strength. Ghrelin, a peptide hormone secreted primarily from the fundus of the stomach, stimulates release of growth hormone and increases food intake and muscle mass. In addition, preliminary data indicate that ghrelin improves left ventricular function and exercise capacity in older persons with heart failure (37). Growth hormone acts by increasing insulin growth factor-1 (IGF-1), which increases muscle protein synthesis. Mechanogrowth factor is a splicing variant of IGF-1. It is increased by resistance exercise and enhances muscle strength by increasing satellite cell recruitment. Stem cells with mechanogrowth factor have been shown to reverse sarcopenia in older rats (38).

Vitamin D levels decline throughout life (39), and levels less than 30 ng/mL are associated with sarcopenia, falls, hip fracture, and disability (40). Vitamin D replacement reduces the risk of these conditions.

Myostatin is a protein that inhibits satellite cell proliferation. Inhibition of myostatin results in muscle regeneration. Early studies with myostatin antibodies in humans show promise for restoring skeletal muscle mass. At present, there are no data on the effects of myostatin antibodies on cardiac muscle.

Cytokines, such as tumor necrosis factor α and interleukin-6, are associated with loss of muscle mass, decreased strength, and poor physical function (41). Cytokine elevation is also associated with anemia, hypoalbuminemia, low cholesterol, and loss of bone mineral. Moreover, it has been suggested that cytokines may play a fundamental role in the aging process (41).

Motor units play a key role in the maintenance of muscle mass, but motor unit firing rates decrease with aging (42). In addition, there is a decline in the ciliary neurotrophic factor (CNTF) that correlates with a decline in muscle mass and strength. Conversely, CNTF administration has been shown to increase soleus muscle mass twofold (43). Peripheral arterial disease leads to decreased physical activity and muscle apoptosis, resulting in sarcopenia and diminished muscle strength.

In summary, the pathophysiology of frailty and sarcopenia are complex and multifactorial. In addition, interactions between these conditions and cardiovascular disease are bidirectional, such that cardiovascular disease contributes to the development and progression of frailty and sarcopenia, while the latter conditions accelerate the functional decline and disability associated with cardiovascular disorders in older people.

CARDIAC CACHEXIA

Cachexia or wasting disease, a condition in which anorexia and systemic inflammation lead to marked weight loss (both muscle and fat), occurs in 10–35% of patients with heart failure (44) and is a major cause of disability in such patients. Non-intentional weight loss of greater than or equal to 7.5% of body weight is associated with a marked increase in mortality (45), independent of VO_2max, left ventricular ejection fraction, New York Heart Association class, serum sodium, or age. Similarly, low cholesterol is highly predictive of mortality in heart failure (46). Moreover, heart failure patients with body adipose tissue content in the highest quartile have improved survival compared with those in the lowest quartile (47). Thus, obesity and overweight are "reverse" risk factors for mortality in patients with chronic heart failure, while weight loss and cachexia are strongly associated with functional decline and death (48). In addition, these associations are in part related to the presence of elevated cytokines (49).

The causes of cachexia in older persons with heart failure are multifactorial and include:

- Anorexia
- Early satiation
- Dyspepsia
- Protein enteropathy
- Abnormal catecholamine kinetics
- Malabsorption
- Increased metabolic rate
- Cytokine excess
- Medications
- Depression

Discussion of each of these factors is beyond the scope of this chapter, but it is becoming increasingly recognized that prevention of disability in older persons with heart failure requires prevention of weight loss.

PREVENTION AND TREATMENT OF FRAILTY

The key component of prevention and treatment of frailty is exercise (both resistance and aerobic) (50,51). In addition, a high protein diet (1.2 g/kg) with a protein supplement consisting of leucine-enriched essential amino acids is recommended (52,53). Potentially reversible causes of dry weight loss need to be sought and treated (54). Weight loss is associated with poor outcomes in frail persons with heart failure (55). The available data on testosterone suggest that it may be reasonable to consider testosterone treatment in hypogonadal males, recognizing that this will likely lead to fluid retention (56–58).

CONCLUSION

Disability is a common outcome of heart disease in older persons, and there is a growing body of evidence linking cardiovascular disease with sarcopenia, frailty, and progressive functional decline. Minimizing disability in older cardiac patients requires aggressive treatment of symptoms, especially angina and dyspnea, to enable such patients to engage in optimal levels of physical activity. In addition, regular aerobic and resistance exercise is, at present, the most effective means for preventing disability and maintaining functional capacity, independence, and quality of life in older cardiac patients (59,60). Proper nutrition, emphasizing prevention of weight loss, is also crucial for limiting the adverse impact of cardiovascular disease on functional outcomes. The role of other interventions, such as treatment of anemia and the use of anabolic hormones, for the prevention and management of disability in older cardiac patients requires further investigation.

REFERENCES

1. Thomas DR, Kamel H, Azharrudin M, et al. The relationship of functional status, nutritional assessment, and severity of illness to in-hospital mortality. J Nutr Health Aging 2005; 9: 169–75.
2. Narain P, Rubenstein LZ, Wieland GD, et al. Predictors of immediate and 6-month outcomes in hospitalized elderly patients. The importance of functional status. J Am Geriatr Soc 1988; 36: 775–83.
3. Nagi SZ. Some conceptual issues in disability and rehabilitation. In: Sussman MB, ed. Sociology and Rehabilitation. Washington, DC: American Sociological Association, 1963: 100–13.

4. Nagi SZ. An epidemiology of disability among adults in the United States. Milbank Mem Fund Q Health Soc 1976; 54: 439–67.

5. Wolinsky FD. Function assessment scales. In: Pathy MSJ, Sinclair AJ, Morley JE, eds. Principles and Practice of Geriatric Medicine, 4th edn. West Sussex, England: John Wiley & Sons, 2006: 132.

6. Fried LP, Guralnik JM. Disability in older adults: evidence regarding significance, etiology, and risk. J Am Geriatr Soc 1997; 45: 92–100.

7. Boyd CM, Xue QL, Guralnik JM, et al. Hospitalization and development of dependence in activities of daily living in a cohort of disabled older women: the Women's Health and Aging Study I. J Gerontol A Biol Sci Med Sci 2005; 60: 888–93.

8. Patel KV, Peek MK, Wong R, et al. Comorbidity and disability in elderly Mexican and Mexican American adults: findings from Mexico and the southwestern United States. J Aging Health 2006; 18: 315–29.

9. Pinsky JL, Jette AM, Branch LG, et al. The Framingham Disability Study: relationship of various coronary heart disease manifestations to disability in older persons living in the community. Am J Public Health 1990; 80: 1363–7.

10. Fried LP, Ferrucci L, Darer J, et al. Untangling the concepts of disability, frailty, and comorbidity: implications for improved targeting and care. J Gerontol A Biol Sci Med Sci 2004; 59: 255–63.

11. Fried LP, Tangen CM, Walston J, et al. Frailty in older adults: evidence for a phenotype. J Gerontol A Biol Sci Med Sci 2001; 56: M146–56.

12. Woo J, Leung J, Morley JE. Comparison of frailty indicators based on clinical phenotype and the multiple deficit approach in predicting mortality and physical limitation. J Am Geriatr Soc 2012; 60: 1478–86.

13. Abellan van Kan G, Rolland YM, Morley JE, Vellas B. Frailty: toward a clinical definition. J Am Med Dir Assoc 2008; 9: 71–2.

14. Rockwood K. Frailty and its definition: a worthy challenge. J Am Geriatr Soc 2005; 53: 1069–70.

15. Cacciatore F, Abete P, Mazzella F, et al. Frailty predicts long-term mortality in elderly subjects with chronic heart failure. Eur J Clin Invest 2005; 35: 723–30.

16. Chaves PH, Kuller LH, o'Leary DH, et al. Subclinical cardiovascular disease in older adults: insights from the Cardiovascular Health Study. Am J Geriatr Cardiol 2004; 13: 137–51.

17. Maraldi C, Volpato S, Cesari M, et al. Investigators of the Gruppo Italiano di Farmacoepidemiologia nell'Anziano Study. Anemia, physical disability, and survival in older patients with heart failure. J Card Fail 2006; 12: 533–9.

18. Morley JE. Anorexia, sarcopenia, and aging. Nutrition 2001; 17: 660–3.

19. Morley JE, Baumgartner RN, Roubenoff R, et al. Sarcopenia. J Lab Clin Med 2001; 137: 231–43.

20. Mazza AD, Morley JE. Metabolic syndrome and the older male population. Aging Male 2007; 10: 3–8.

21. Janssen I, Shepard DS, Katzmarzyk PT, et al. The healthcare costs of sarcopenia in the United States. J Am Geriatr Soc 2004; 52: 80–5.

22. Baumgartner RN, Wayne SJ, Waters DL, et al. Sarcopenic obesity predicts instrumental activities of daily living disability in the elderly. Obes Res 2004; 12: 1995–2004.

23. Yliharsila H, Kajantie E, osmond C, et al. Birth size, adult body composition and muscle strength in later life. Int J Obes (Lond) 2007; 31: 1392–9.

24. Bartali B, Frongillo EA, Bandinelli S, et al. Low nutrient intake is an essential component of frailty in older persons. J Gerontol A Biol Sci Med Sci 2006; 61: 589–93.

25. Wilson MM, Morley JE. Invited review: aging and energy balance. J Appl Physiol 2003; 95: 1728–36.

26. Volpi E, Kobayashi H, Sheffield-Moore M, et al. Essential amino acids are primarily responsible for the amino acid stimulation of muscle protein anabolism in healthy elderly adults. Am J Clin Nutr 2003; 78: 250–8.

27. Brose A, Parise G, Tarnopolsky MA. Creatine supplementation enhances isometric strength and body composition improvements following strength exercise training in older adults. J Gerontol A Biol Sci Med Sci 2003; 58: 11–19.

28. Horani MH, Morley JE. Hormonal fountains of youth. Clin Geriatr Med 2004; 20: 275–92.

29. Wittert GA, Chapman IM, Haren MT, et al. Oral testosterone supplementation increases muscle and decreases fat mass in healthy elderly males with low-normal gonadal status. J Gerontol A Biol Sci Med Sci 2003; 58: 618–25.

30. Sih R, Morley JE, Kaiser FE, et al. Testosterone replacement in older hypogonadal men: a 12-month randomized controlled trial. J Clin Endocrinol Metab 1997; 82: 1661–7.

31. Stout M, Tew GA, Doll H, et al. Testosterone therapy during exercise rehabilitation in male patients with chronic heart failure who have low testosterone status: a double-blind randomized controlled feasibility study. Am Heart J 2012; 164: 893–901.

32. Caminiti G, Volterrani M, Iellamo F, et al. Effect of long-acting testosterone treatment on functional exercise capacity, skeletal muscle performance, insulin resistance, and baroreflex sensitivity in elderly patients with chronic heart failure a double-blind, placebo-controlled, randomized study. J Am Coll Cardiol 2009; 54: 919–27.

33. Toma M, McAlister FA, Coglianese EE, et al. Testosterone supplementation in heart failure: a meta-analysis. Circ Heart Fail 2012; 5: 315–21.

34. Iellamo F, Volterrani M, Caminiti G, et al. Testosterone therapy in women with chronic heart failure: a pilot double-blind, randomized, placebo-controlled study. J Am Coll Cardiol 2010; 56: 1310–16.

35. Frisoli A, Chaves PH, Pinheiro MM, et al. The effect of nandrolone decanoate on bone mineral density, muscle mass, and hemoglobin levels in elderly women with osteoporosis: a double-blind, randomized, placebo-controlled clinical trial. J Gerontol A Biol Sci Med Sci 2005; 60: 648–53.

36. Percheron G, Hogrel JY, Denot-Ledunois S, et al. Effect of 1-year oral administration of dehydroepi-androsterone to 60- to 80-year-old individuals on muscle function and cross-sectional area: a double-blind placebo-controlled trial. Arch Intern Med 2003; 163: 720–7.

37. Nagaya N, Moriya J, Yasumura Y, et al. Effects of ghrelin administration on left ventricular function, exercise capacity, and muscle wasting in patients with chronic heart failure. Circulation 2004; 110: 3674–9.

38. Musaro A, McCullagh K, Paul A, et al. Localized Igf-1 transgene expression sustains hypertrophy and regeneration in senescent skeletal muscle. Nat Genet 2001; 27: 195–200.

39. Perry HM, Horowitz M, Morley JE, et al. Longitudinal changes in serum 25-hydroxyvitamin D in older people. Metabolism 1999; 48: 1028–32.

40. Morley JE. Should all long-term residents receive vitamin D? J Am Med Dir Assoc 2007; 8: 69–70.

41. Morley JE, Baumgartner RN. Cytokine-related aging process. J Gerontol A Biol Sci Med Sci 2004; 59: M924–9.

42. Knight CA, Kamen G. Modulation of motor unit firing rates during a complex sinusoidal force task in young and older adults. J Appl Physiol 2007; 102: 122–9.

43. Mizisin AP, Vu Y, Calcutt NA, et al. Ciliary neurotrophic factor improves nerve conduction and ame-liorates degeneration deficits in diabetic rats. Diabetes 2004; 53: 1807–12.

44. Morley JE, Thomas DR, Wilson MM. Cachexia: pathophysiology and clinical relevance. Am J Clin Nutr 2006; 83: 735–43.

45. Anker SD, Ponikowski P, Varney S, et al. Wasting as independent risk factor for mortality in chronic heart failure. Lancet 1997; 349: 1050–3.

46. Rauchhaus M, Clark AL, Doehner W, et al. Relationship between cholesterol and survival in patients with chronic heart failure. J Am Coll Cardiol 2003; 42: 1933–40.

47. Fonarow GC, Srikanthan P, Costanzo MR, et al. An obesity paradox in acute heart failure: analysis of body mass index and in-hospital mortality for 108,927 patients in the Acute Decompensated Heart Failure Registry. Am Heart J 2007; 153: 74–81.

48. Kalantar-Zadeh K, Block G, Horwich T, et al. Reverse epidemiology of conventional cardiovascular risk factors in patients with chronic heart failure. J Am Coll Cardiol 2004; 43: 1439–44.

49. Filippatos GS, Anker SD, Kremastinos DT. Pathophysiology of peripheral muscle wasting in cardiac cachexia. Curr Opin Clin Nutr Metab Care 2005; 8: 249–54.

50. Chou CH, Hwang CL, Wu YT. Effect of exercise on physical function, daily living activities, and qual-ity of life in the frail older adults: a meta-analysis. Arch Phys Med Rehabil 2012; 93: 237–44.

51. Theou O, Stathokostas L, Roland KP, et al. The effectiveness of exercise interventions for the management of frailty: a systematic review. J Aging Res 2011; 2011: 569194. Doi: 10.4061/2011/569194.

52. Dominguez LJ, Barbagallo M. Perspective: Protein supplementation in frail older persons: often nec-essary but not always sufficient. J Am Med Dir Assoc 2013; 14: 72–3. doi:pii:S1525-8610(12)00352-0. 10.1016/j.jamda.2012.09.029; Epub ahead of print.

53. Cesari M. Perspective: protein supplementation against sarcopenia and frailty: future perspectives from novel data. J Am Med Dir Assoc 2013; 14: 62–3.doi: 10.1016/j.jamda.2012.08.017; Epub 2012 Sep 30.

54. Morley JE. Weight loss in older persons: new therapeutic approaches. Curr Pharm Des 2007; 13: 3637–47.

55. Anker SD, von Haehling S. The obesity paradox in heart therapy: accepting reality and making rational decisions. Clin Pharmacol Ther 2011; 90: 188–90.

56. Chahla EJ, Hayek ME, Morley JE. Testosterone replacement therapy and cardiovascular risk factors modification. Aging Male 2011; 14: 83–90.

57. Morley JE. Frailty: Diagnosis and management. J Nutr Health Aging 2011; 15: 667–70.

58. Morley JE. Should frailty be treated with testosterone? Aging Male 2011; 14: 1–3. doi: 10.3109/13685538.2010.502271; Epub 2010 Jul 29.
59. Guerra-Garcia H, Taffet G, Protas EJ. Considerations related to disability and exercise in elderly women with congestive heart failure. J Cardiovasc Nurs 1997; 11: 60–74.
60. Ades PA, Waldmann ML, Meyer WL, et al. Skeletal muscle and cardiovascular adaptations to exercise conditioning in older coronary patients. Circulation 1996; 94: 323–30.

31

Ethical decisions and end-of-life care in older patients with cardiovascular disease

Craig Tanner and Sarah Goodlin

SUMMARY

Cardiovascular disease disproportionately affects older adults. Treatment of older patients with cardiovascular disease requires addressing many ethical and end-of-life issues. The ethical issues include assessment of decision-making capacity, surrogacy and advance directives, decisions related to cardiopulmonary resuscitation, and effective communication with patients. Palliative and end-of-life issues are common in the management of heart failure, acute stroke, and in caring for stroke survivors. Advanced surgical interventions and implantable devices have changed the course of coronary artery disease, advanced heart failure, and valvular disease. Such interventions are increasingly applied to older and more medically complicated patients. As the population ages and technology advances, issues of distributive justice and access to care will challenge health systems worldwide.

INTRODUCTION

Cardiovascular disease (CVD) has an enormous impact on patients, their families, and healthcare systems worldwide. Advancing technologies and an aging population have increased the number and complexity of ethical issues involved in caring for patients living and dying with CVD. Though survival has increased, so has the percentage of patients living with chronic illness and the cost of caring for them. Cardiovascular disease disproportionately affects the elderly, and older patients have a higher risk of complications and disability associated with CVD. Comorbidities particular to older patients (cognitive dysfunction, frailty, pre-existing functional impairment, etc.) and other chronic illnesses further complicate management of CVD in the elderly.

Deaths from CVD may be sudden and unexpected in the case of acute myocardial infarction, sudden cardiac death or acute stroke, or may follow years or decades of chronic illness such as heart failure or chronic disability from stroke or peripheral vascular disease. This chapter will discuss ethical issues commonly encountered in caring for older patients with CVD, including impaired decision-making capacity, issues of surrogate decision-making and advance directives, and ethical issues surrounding cardiopulmonary resuscitation (CPR). Disease-specific issues related to heart failure and stroke will then be discussed. We will also address end-of-life issues in patients with CVD including palliative care, end-of-life decision-making and hospice care. Finally, there will be a brief discussion of advanced surgical treatments for CVD in elderly patients.

DECISION-MAKING CAPACITY

The ability of patients to understand and consent to treatments is usually assumed and is fundamental to patient autonomy. In many clinical scenarios such as dementia or delirium, the patient's ability to make decisions may be unclear. The understanding of decision-making capacity and the ability to assess this capacity are essential skills for any clinician involved in obtaining informed consent for treatments or procedures, or in educating patients about their illness and treatment options. Older adults have a higher incidence of conditions which may impair decision-making capacity. These include dementia, mild cognitive impairment, and impairments in communicative ability (hearing, speech, and cognition).

This section will discuss assessment of the capacity to make treatment decisions and consent to treatment. This is only one domain of capacity (1) but is the most relevant to ethical decision making in patient care.

Determination of Decision-Making Capacity

Applebaum et al. (2) have described the fundamental components of capacity to make treatment decisions as the abilities to communicate a choice, to understand the relevant information, to appreciate the medical consequences of the situation, and to reason about treatment choices. These are further outlined in Table 31.1 with questions clinicians might use to assess each component. Contrary to common belief (3), psychiatric consultation is not routinely necessary to make an assessment of capacity. Decision-making capacity can be assessed by any provider caring for a particular patient. However, there are certain instances in which it is advisable to have capacity assessed by someone separate from the treatment providers or team. Such is the case when there is conflict between treatment providers or between the treatment team and the patient or family. In this instance, either a psychiatric consultant or an ethics committee may be best able to assess decision-making capacity. Another instance in which psychiatric consultation is advisable is when the presence of an active psychiatric illness contributes to the question of the patient's ability to make competent decisions. Another common misconception about decision-making capacity is that it is only necessary to undertake an assessment when a patient is going against medical advice (3). Informed consent for any treatment requires that the patient meet the criteria of ability to communicate and understand the choice, appreciate options and consequences, and demonstrate reasoning regardless of whether they are complying with medical recommendations. Furthermore, patients may have capacity to make certain decisions (such as designation of a surrogate) but not to make more complex medical decisions.

Formal Assessment Tools

Several tools have been developed to formally assess decision-making capacity (4). The most widely used and validated among these is the MacArthur Competence Assessment Tool for Treatment. This instrument involves a 15–20 minute semistructured interview which generates quantitative scores for each of the four criteria of decision-making capacity. Though this instrument can be a helpful guide (and can provide standardized data in the case of legal proceedings), the scores must be integrated with other available data to make an ultimate decision about the decision-making capacity of the patient.

SURROGACY AND ADVANCE DIRECTIVES
When the Patient Lacks Capacity

When it is determined that an individual lacks the ability to make his or her own medical decisions, medical providers must turn to others for assistance with such decisions.

Table 31.1   Criteria for Decision-Making Capacity and Questions for Assessment

Criterion	Questions for Assessment	Comments
Ability to communicate a choice	Have you decided whether to follow the treatment recommendation? Can you tell me what your decision is?	Frequent reversals of choice due to neurologic or psychiatric illness may be indicative of lack of capacity
Ability to understand relevant information	What have you been told about: The current problem with your health? What treatment has been recommended? The possible risks or benefits of the treatment? The alternatives to this treatment? What would happen if you got no treatment?	Ask patient to answer these questions in his/her own words. Patient need not use medical terminology to demonstrate understanding
Ability to appreciate the situation and its consequences	What do you know about your health? Tell me about the illness and the treatments you could choose. What is this treatment likely to do for you? What do you believe will happen if you do not get treatment?	Patients who do not acknowledge their illness cannot make valid treatment decisions Choosing no treatment is acceptable as long as the explanation of the decision process is rational.
Ability to reason about treatment options	How did you make your decision? Why is the option you chose better than the alternative option?	This is to assess the *process* not content of decision. Patients have the right to make poor choices

Source: Adapted from Ref. 2.

Ideally, the patient would have left specific instructions for medical providers and appointed surrogates to follow in the event of the loss of capacity, and such instructions would be clearly applicable to the patient's current condition. However, this ideal set of circumstances is rarely present. At a minimum, it is important to identify a surrogate who can act in the patient's best interest, even if they lack knowledge of the patient's wishes in specific circumstances. Most often a close family member (spouse, child, sibling, etc.) is the surrogate to whom medical providers turn in such situations. In the USA, all states have specific laws governing hierarchy of surrogates for medical decision making (in the absence of an advance directive designating a surrogate). Several European countries have similar laws, though there is more variability throughout Europe than within the USA (5).

Traditional Advance Directives

Traditional advance directives (AD), usually consisting of surrogate appointments and living wills, were developed with the hope of allowing patients to maintain control over their medical care when they were no longer able to speak for themselves. Despite this hope, evidence suggests that few patients complete AD and that, even when completed, AD have limited impact on treatment decisions near the end of life (6). The reasons for the failure of traditional AD have been outlined by Hickman et al. (7). These reasons include instructions that are too vague or too specific to apply to unanticipated and complex future health decisions, lack of integration of AD into clinical care, and the overvaluation of autonomy as a mode of decision-making. Furthermore, surrogates appointed by AD are frequently unfamiliar with the patient's wishes and many patients prefer that their surrogate's decisions respond dynamically to the clinical situation rather than adhere strictly to previously stated treatment preferences.

Newer Models for AD

Fortunately, there are emerging models of advance care planning which may overcome some of the failings of traditional AD. "Respecting Choices" is a community-wide advance planning system originally developed in La Crosse, Wisconsin. This program, described in detail elsewhere, involves community-wide education of healthcare providers and patients, training of advance care planning facilitators, integration of advance care planning into clinical care and written protocols allowing emergency personnel access to physician orders which reflect patient preferences (8). This program has been shown to increase the use of AD and the adherence to treatment preferences in AD; in addition, participants are less likely to die in the hospital. The "Respecting Choices" program is being implemented in greater than 50 communities and organizations in the USA, Canada, and Australia. Another effective system of advance planning and documentation is the "Physician Orders for Life-Sustaining Treatment" (POLST) paradigm. This model, originally developed in Oregon, is designed to be used with individuals who are frail or suffering from advanced illnesses. The main feature of this paradigm is a brightly colored physician order form that is completed following discussion between the physician and the patient and/or surrogates. This form orders the level of aggressiveness in medical care and serves to direct nurses in community based settings and emergency personnel. The document accompanies the patient across care settings to ensure knowledge of patient preferences throughout the healthcare system. The POLST form has been shown to represent patient treatment preferences and to match actual treatment at the end of life (9). Additionally, use of the form reduces unwanted cardiopulmonary resuscitation, intensive care, and ventilator support (10). A national task force for implementation of the POLST paradigm was established in 2004. Rather than a stand-alone system, the POLST paradigm is complementary to other AD systems and its use is strongly encouraged within the "Respecting Choices" program (11). Another model, the Five Wishes paradigm [agingwithdignity.org], is a legal advance directive in 23 states, and can be used to guide decisions by surrogates even where it is not a formal advance directive (7). Five Wishes walks people through decision-making and documentation of "1. The person I want to make care decisions for me when I can't; 2. The kind of medical treatment I want or don't want; 3. How comfortable I want to be; 4. How I want people to treat me; 5. What I want my loved ones to know."

CARDIOPULMONARY RESUSCITATION
History and Outcomes of CPR

In the 1960s, multiple advanced life support techniques were combined to form a new life-saving intervention known as cardiopulmonary resuscitation (CPR). In its infancy CPR was restricted to intraoperative use and cardiac arrest due to ventricular arrhythmias. Before long, however, CPR began to be applied more broadly both in and outside of healthcare facilities. In 1974, the American Medical Association recommended that "code status" be documented in the medial record. Hospital policies regarding do-not-resuscitate (DNR) orders first appeared in 1976, ushering in an era, extending to the present day, in which CPR became the default medical treatment after cardiopulmonary arrest in the absence of

a DNR order (12). Patients undergoing in-hospital CPR have a rate of return of spontaneous circulation of 30–45% but only between 10% and 18% will survive to hospital discharge
(13). Though older adults as a group have a lower rate of survival to discharge following
CPR, there are conflicting data as to whether age predicts poorer outcome independent of
illness burden (14). Cardiopulmonary arrest from cardiac disease may be more responsive
to CPR than other disease states, especially in the case of cardioversion for witnessed
ventricular fibrillation (15).

The Ethics of CPR and DNR Orders

Given the poor outcomes of CPR described above and even poorer outcomes in those with
advanced illnesses, there has been vigorous debate over the ethics of offering or withholding CPR. In the past, it was routine for physicians to unilaterally decide whether or not to
attempt resuscitation on a given patient. In recent decades, however, the rising prominence
of autonomy as a driving force in medical care and medical ethics has appropriately challenged this view (16). Multiple professional societies now recommend routine discussions
of resuscitation preferences with all patients suffering from chronic or advanced illness.
There is evidence that physicians do not conduct these discussions as frequently as recommended (17). Discussing resuscitation preferences can be seen as an informed consent
discussion. A conversation should begin by asking what the patient has told other clinicians
or their families that they would prefer when the time comes that the person's breathing or
heart stops. If the patient desires, or if needed to correct misimpressions, the clinician
should be prepared to share available data and estimates of outcomes of CPR in the context
of the patient's medical problems. Additionally, the physician should provide support for a
patient's choice to allow natural death versus attempting resuscitation and be prepared to
make a recommendation based on the patient's goals, values, and medical condition. Most
patients want their physician to initiate discussions of resuscitation preferences and to provide a recommendation. This is true even in patients who find the topic upsetting (18).
Table 31.2 describes the recommended contents of resuscitation discussions as well as
sample statement and questions that can be used in such discussions. To respect patient
autonomy fully, these discussions should be ongoing rather than a single event. There is
evidence that the resuscitation preferences of older adults and those with advanced illness
are not static and frequently change with changes in medical condition or other life circumstances. (19). Additionally, many patients may not want to make their own healthcare decisions, and these patients should be asked to identify someone who will make decisions for
them (20).

It is generally agreed that the wishes of the patient or his or her surrogate with regard
to resuscitation preferences should be followed. It is also generally agreed, however, that
physicians are not required to provide interventions that are "futile" or will have no benefit.
Ethicists disagree on how such futility should be defined and even whether it should ever
be used as a reason not to initiate CPR outside of extreme circumstances (e.g., decapitation,
rigor mortis, decomposition) (21,22). The clinician should lead an empathetic exploration
of patient goals, values, and preferences as well as educate the patient about his or her illness and expected outcome of potential resuscitation attempts. If a patient and/or surrogate
continue to insist on resuscitation in a case in which it is believed to be medically futile all
attempts should be made to obtain consensus. In the absence of such consensus, involvement of an institutional ethics board may be appropriate.

One concerning finding from multiple studies which may complicate discussion of
resuscitation preferences is that the presence of a DNR order affects physician decision-
making and aggressiveness of care separate from resuscitation (23,24). It has been stated
by some authors that a "Do Not Resuscitate" order is frequently interpreted as a "Do Not

Table 31.2   Discussing Resuscitation Preferences

General Guidelines:
–Eliminate distractions, sit at patient level, and be ready to listen
–Ask if the patient would like any family/loved ones present
–Name and validate emotions that arise
–Validate difficulty of discussing these issues
–Stress importance of discussion in order to provide care that is consistent with patient goals/values

Step	Example of Language to Use
Setting context/normalizing discussion	"I talk with all of my patients about what to do when the time comes that their heart or breathing stops" "Given the change in your condition, we need to review what to do when the time comes that your heart or breathing stops"
Describe alternatives and use "when" rather than "if"	"When the time comes when your heart stops or you stop breathing, do you want us to try to revive you or allow you to die naturally?"
Probing for understanding of patient's reasoning	"Help me understand how you think about this issue" "Have you or your family had experiences with being revived or resuscitated?"
Identify undesired states, describe broadly	"Are there states of health that you would never want to be kept alive in?" "Unable to communicate with family/friends" "Unable to make decisions for yourself" "Unable to live independently"
Discuss preferences for level/location of care	"How would you feel about being cared for in the hospital, an intensive care unit or a nursing home if your condition worsened?"
Closing the conversation Provide a professional recommendation	"Given what you describe (restate details) I recommend that we enter a do-not-resuscitate order"
Clarify the difference between DNR/ongoing treatment, state commitment to continue care	"We will continue to treat your illnesses and try to improve your length and quality of life"
Set expectation for ongoing discussions	"We will revisit these issues with you and/or your family if your condition changes or if you want to discuss this again"

Source: Adapted from Refs. 25,28.

Treat" order. It is not ethically justifiable to restrict nonresuscitation treatments based on the presence of a DNR order. It may be possible to avoid this problem by using explicit language in DNR orders clarifying that all other treatments should be continued or through educational initiatives targeted at medical and nursing staff.

ETHICAL DECISIONS IN THE MANAGEMENT OF HEART FAILURE

Among all CVDs, heart failure (HF) presents the greatest number and most complex ethical issues (25). HF is a chronic, often debilitating illness which slowly robs sufferers of functional capability and ultimately shortens their lives. The epidemiology, impact, and treatment of heart failure in the elderly are discussed in chapter 20. Advances in the management of heart failure have improved both length and quality of life. These advances include pharmaceutical approaches, chronic disease management, and therapy with devices to prolong life and improve functional capacity. This section will address advance care or preparedness planning in heart failure, both in general and in the setting of treatment with implanted devices.

Preparedness Planning in Heart Failure

The prolonged and highly variable trajectory of HF makes it difficult for clinicians to predict outcomes for individual patients and complicates discussions of advance care planning (26). Such discussions, however, are critical to supporting patient autonomy and allowing patients to avoid undue harm and any unwanted interventions. Unfortunately, such planning is often initiated in the last stages of heart failure and may be actively avoided by both clinicians and patients (27). While it is true that some patients may decline participation in such discussions, all patients should be given the opportunity to discuss expected disease trajectory, prognosis, and the uncertainties associated with a HF diagnosis. Ideally, discussions of preparedness planning would be initiated at or near the time of the heart failure diagnosis. These discussions should be focused around the patient's beliefs, values, and wishes and should openly acknowledge both the life-limiting nature of heart failure and the uncertainty in prognostication. We described an approach to communication in heart failure care that utilizes shared decision-making and empathetic responses to patient emotions and emphasizes the importance of discussing prognosis and patient wishes to whatever extent the patient desires (28).

Treatment with Implantable Devices in Heart Failure

Implantable devices such as automated defibrillators (ICDs), left ventricular assist devices (LVADs), and cardiac resynchronization therapy (CRT) pacemakers have revolutionized the care of patients with heart failure. These devices prevent sudden cardiac death (ICDs) (29), improve functional status and quality of life (LVADs and CRT) (30,31) and improve survival in heart failure (LVADs, ICDs, and CRT) (29–31). Informed consent for such devices must include not only the indications for the device and its potential risks and benefits, but also any reasonable alternatives to device implantation. Furthermore, the patient and his or her family should be aware of the role and management of the implanted device throughout the course of the illness, including its management at the end of life. Prior to device implantation, the possibility of future deactivation of the device and the circumstances under which this may be desired should be discussed with the patient and family (32).

ICD and CRT Devices

As with any procedure or intervention, the implantation of an ICD requires that the patient and/or their surrogate understand the risks, benefits and alternatives to the procedure. There is evidence, however, that patients frequently do not understand the purpose of an ICD, the reason for its implantation or the alternatives to implantation (33). Additionally, patients and providers report that they rarely discuss the possibility of future deactivation of an ICD prior to proceeding with implantation (34,35). By correcting ventricular arrhythmias and preventing sudden death, ICDs can prolong survival in patients for whom they are indicated. Rarely is it considered or explicitly discussed, however, that this makes a more prolonged death with diminished quality of life from deterioration of the failing heart more likely. The manner or mode of death may be a more important consideration for some patients than length of life (36). Because of this, it is critical that the purpose and expected effects of an ICD be clarified by the provider and understood by the patient prior to implantation. Additionally, the potential for future deactivation of the device should be discussed prior to implantation. Patients must understand that the device can easily be deactivated in the future if the benefits of the device no longer outweigh its burdens. This could be due to advancing heart failure, other non-heart failure illness, or a change in the patient's goals or priorities. Failure to address this issue may subject patients to unwanted painful and futile shocks near the end of life (37).

Most of the issues discussed above with ICDs also pertain to implantation of CRT devices. Informed consent for CRT implantation must include not only the risk, benefits, and alternatives but also the possibility that the device will not improve symptoms. The discussion of deactivation of CRT therapy is somewhat more complicated than that with ICDs, as patients may experience a rapid deterioration and worsening of symptoms when a CRT device is deactivated. Patients and their families must understand this prior to CRT device deactivation. In the USA combination CRT/ICD devices are frequently implanted. Informed consent discussions for such a device should address the possibility of future deactivation of the ICD alone if the patient's condition warrants. Guidelines have been published which discuss these issues in greater detail (38,39).

LVADs

Few other devices have carried both the promise and the ethical complexity associated with LVADs. Originally developed as bridging devices for patients awaiting cardiac transplant, LVADs have now become "destination" therapy for many patients with end-stage heart failure. For select patients, these devices have demonstrated the ability to both prolong life and dramatically improve quality of life. This promise is tempered by the significant risk of neurologic complications, sepsis, and repeated and prolonged hospitalization (31). With such powerful potential burdens and benefits, informed consent for LVAD implantation must carefully consider potential complications and clarify patient understanding of risk. It is also recommended that patients identify a desired surrogate prior to LVAD implantation, and specify their wishes in the event of certain complications (stroke, multiorgan system failure). Models of partnering with palliative medicine teams both in the preimplantation evaluation and on an ongoing basis after implantation have been described in centers offering LVADs (40–42). Such teams can assist in clarifying patient and family understanding, elucidating patient goals and values and in supporting patients and families during the course of the patient's illness. This is particularly important with LVAD placement, as there is evidence that families and caregivers of patients with these devices suffer high levels of anxiety, caregiver burden, and negative effects on their own health (43). Collaboration with palliative medicine teams can also promote ongoing discussion of patient goals and wishes, and ease the transition to end-of-life care when the time is appropriate.

Palliative and End-of-Life Care in Heart Failure

Among the population with heart failure, at least 60% will ultimately die of a cardiovascular cause. The majority of these will die from progressive pump failure with a steadily declining minority dying from sudden death (44). With the aging of the population and increasing incidence and prevalence of heart failure, more clinicians will be involved in end-of-life care for patients with advanced, progressive heart failure. The systems of end-of-life and hospice care in both the USA and Europe were largely developed to manage patients dying from malignant disease. Studies in the USA suggest that some hospice organizations may lack competence in management of heart failure at the end of life (45). Furthermore, specialists in CVD may lack confidence in providing end-of-life care for their patients with HF (46). The solution to this dilemma likely resides in collaboration between cardiovascular specialists, hospice and palliative medicine specialists and primary care providers in provision of end-of-life care to this population.

Prognostication in Advanced HF

Due to the variable disease trajectory and frequent exacerbations and stabilizations in heart failure, determination of prognosis and appropriateness for hospice care can be quite difficult. In the USA, hospice care is usually funded through Medicare, which requires an expected survival of 6 months or less. This model may be difficult to apply to many patients with HF. This is demonstrated by the fact that patients with heart failure are among those most often discharged alive from hospice programs in the USA (47). Nonetheless, clinicians must use available resources and tools to determine prognosis as accurately as possible. Among other tools, the Seattle Heart Failure Model may be helpful in this regard (48). An approach for communication around prognosis, uncertainty and death in HF involves acknowledging the uncertainty involved with a heart failure diagnosis and framing prognosis as average length of life associated with the current HF stage while allowing for exceptions in either direction (28). The clinician can then frame the approach as "hoping for the best while preparing for the worst" and assist the patient in elucidating his or her wishes as the disease progresses.

Symptom Management Versus Life Prolongation

Patients with HF have a burden of symptoms similar to that of patients with advanced malignancy (49). In contrast to malignant disease, where management of symptoms and prolongation of life usually require divergent therapeutic approaches, symptom management in HF initially consists of treatment with medications that also prolong life such as angiotensin-converting enzyme inhibitors, beta-adrenergic antagonists, and aldosterone antagonists (50). Symptom management in HF, therefore, usually begins at the time of diagnosis. As the disease progresses and the goals of the patient and family change, there may be a shift in focus from quantity to quality of life. This shift, however, should not automatically result in discontinuation of HF-directed medications, as would be the case in many other terminal illnesses. It is important that hospice providers, primary care providers, and cardiovascular specialists collaborate to determine the benefit and burden of each treatment prior to discontinuation. The most common symptoms in advanced heart failure are dyspnea, fatigue, pain, lack of energy, and depression. These symptoms cause a great deal of distress and significantly impact quality of life (51). The primary treatment for dyspnea in HF is maximal medical management of the heart failure. Opioids may be indicated if maximal HF management does not control dyspnea, but should not be considered first line treatment of dyspnea in HF. Depression, pain and spiritual suffering may be underrecognized and undertreated in HF (52,53). As with other chronic illnesses, adequate symptom assessment and management often require the involvement of professionals from multiple disciplines. All providers caring for patients with advanced HF should learn at least basic symptom assessment. Such assessment should, at the very minimum, include evaluation for fatigue, dyspnea, pain, and depression. Symptom assessment instruments such as the Edmonton Symptom Assessment Scale (ESAS) and the Memorial Symptom Assessment Scale Modified for HF (MSAS-HF) are appropriate for a more comprehensive evaluation in patients with HF (54,55).

Care at the End of Life in HF

As HF progresses and patient's lifespan is more limited, the goals of care may shift entirely to comfort and quality of life. As mentioned above, in HF this does not obviate the need for maximal disease management, as this can be important for managing distressing symptoms. However, the burdens of even simple oral therapies may become overwhelming near the end of life. Recognition of this important transition point requires ongoing assessment of patient's goals and wishes and discussion with not only the patient but also their family and other providers. Utilization of specialized palliative and hospice care can not only aid families in such transitions but also ease the burden of end-of-life care on both primary care and other specialty providers. Assessment for spiritual and existential distress is appropriate at any point in the management of chronic illness. As the end of life approaches such issues may predominate. Though data are limited on spiritual assessment specific to HF patients, instruments such as the Faith-Importance-Community-Address (FICA) tool are appropriate for use in such circumstances (56). Involvement of the multidisciplinary team, including social work and chaplaincy should also be considered. As discussed earlier in this chapter, many patients who die with HF are undergoing treatment with device therapy for symptoms and/or life prolongation. As the end of life approaches the use of such devices should be re-addressed. All hospice agencies should develop policies for the ongoing evaluation and deactivation of such devices when appropriate. This may require collaboration with cardiovascular specialists to ensure maximum patient benefit and comfort without undue burden.

ETHICAL DECISIONS IN STROKE/CVA

CVAs affect those older than 65 three times as frequently as those under 65 and older patients have a substantially higher risk of dying after a stroke (57). As many as 15–20% of patients will die in the acute post-CVA period with another 10% dying in the 6–12 months following the acute CVA. However, even among those initially requiring mechanical ventilation, as many as 25% may recover all or nearly all of their pre-CVA functional capacity (58). This section discusses the ethical issues relating to artificial nutrition in the post-CVA period as well as palliative and end-of-life care after CVA.

Artificial Nutrition in the Post-CVA Period

Nearly 80% of patients may have difficulty safely swallowing food and fluids after an acute CVA (59). For those who are expected to survive long term, or for those who wish to pursue aggressive interventions, artificial nutrition by feeding tube (FT) may be necessary. Though tube feeding in general does not prevent aspiration or prolong life in most patients with dysphagia, it may have a limited role in the acute post-CVA recovery period. Some patients (or family members/surrogates) may choose not to have a FT. The reasons for such a decision are varied and may include, among others, cognitive impairment or mood disorder caused by the stroke, misunderstanding of the role of artificial nutrition in recovery or a well-informed desire not to prolong a life that is seen as unacceptable to the patient (60). Careful evaluation of the patient's understanding of the situation, cognitive ability and motivations for refusing FT are important to act with beneficence while avoiding harm and preserving autonomy. A formal capacity evaluation may be necessary in such a situation. If it is determined that the patient has decision-making capacity, understands the risks and benefits of tube feeding and wishes to forgo this intervention to avoid life-prolongation, clinicians should respect the patient's autonomy and honor his or her wishes. Furthermore, many patients may wish to continue oral nutrition despite the risk of aspiration, pneumonia and death. This decision should be supported in the competent patient who is able to give informed consent. In the unfortunate case of an incompetent patient with no available surrogate, healthcare professionals face a difficult dilemma. If a patient's previously expressed wishes are known, this should guide the treatment—this may be true even if such wishes are not legally binding. In the absence of such expressed wishes, the healthcare professionals themselves (often with the assistance of an ethics committee or consult team) must be responsible for acting in the patient's best interest. If there is conflict or uncertainty among the healthcare team, legal counsel should be sought (61).

Symptom Prevalence and End-of-Life Care After Acute Stroke

The overall 30-day mortality rate after CVA ranges from 12–20%. The death rate is highest for hemorrhagic stroke and lowest for lacunar infarct and increases with increasing age across all stroke types (57). Families of patients dying after stroke frequently report inadequate symptom control, poor communication and failure to address psychological morbidity (62). Commonly reported symptoms in the acute post-CVA period include pain, fatigue, dyspnea, confusion, anxiety, depression, and emotional lability. A prospective study of 191 acute CVA patients admitted to a UK hospital assessed patients for palliative care needs using a screening tool developed to assess distress in advanced illness. In this cohort more than half of patients reported moderate or significant fatigue, while approximately 50% reported distress from physical or psychological symptoms (63). One quarter of this group expressed concerns about death and dying while two thirds had concerns about dependence and disability. Among patients dying in the hospital after acute CVA, Mazzocato et al. found that 81% had dyspnea and 69% had pain (64). Ninety-three percent of these patients had difficulties with communication. This study, which included patients referred to a palliative care consult service, found that 81% of patients were free of pain and 48% free of dyspnea during the final 48 hours of life. Treatments included opioid medications (for pain and dyspnea) and anticholinergic medications (for dyspnea and respiratory secretions).

Very few organized programs or protocols for end-of-life care in stroke have been described. The Liverpool Care Pathway, initially developed for dying cancer patients, was successfully applied to a small group of stroke patients in a UK study (65). This pathway focused on discontinuation of inappropriate interventions, appropriate use of subcutaneous medications, addressing spiritual needs and communication with family members. A separate study examined the implementation of locally developed palliative care guidelines in an acute stroke unit in Canada (66). These guidelines addressed discontinuation of inappropriate interventions as well as use of appropriate medications for symptom management in 104 dying stroke patients. Ninety percent of these patients were appropriately palliated based on a retrospective chart review. Although small, these studies demonstrate that standard palliative care interventions can be reasonably applied to stroke patients at the end of life. To this end, National Health Service Quality Improvement Scotland recently developed a detailed best practices statement defining quality end-of-life care after stroke (67). Further research is required to determine what, if any, stroke-specific end-of-life interventions may be beneficial. As with other terminal illness, the use of hospice services can be of great benefit to patients dying of stroke and to their families. A 2010 study of US Medicare Beneficiaries found that among patients dying within 30 days of an acute stroke, 23% utilized hospice services, which is on par with both malignant and other nonmalignant diseases (68).

Palliative Care for CVA Survivors

In the USA alone there are at least 4.5 million stroke survivors, with the large majority being over the age of 65 (57). The Framingham study found that in patients over age 65 surviving a stroke, the following were present at 6 months (% affected): hemiparesis (50%), inability to walk without assistance (30%), depressive symptoms (35%), aphasia (19%), and dependence in activities of daily living (25%) (69). One-quarter of elderly stroke survivors were institutionalized in a nursing home 6 months after a stroke. Though a great deal has been written about secondary prevention of stroke and poststroke rehabilitation, supportive or palliative treatments after CVA are rarely discussed. This section will discuss the symptom management and palliative care needs of stroke survivors.

Pain Syndromes in Stroke Survivors

Several pain syndromes specific to CVA survivors have been described, including central poststroke pain (CPSP), hemiplegic shoulder pain (HSP), tension-type headache and painful spasticity. CPSP is a neuropathic pain syndrome affecting as many as 12% of stroke survivors, arising in the weeks to months after the CVA (70). CPSP is most common when pain perception or processing areas are affected by the cerebral infarction. CPSP can be spontaneous or evoked and may be either intermittent or continuous. Similar to other neuropathic pain syndromes, CPSP may involve sensory abnormalities including hyperalgesia, allodynia, or dysthesthesia. Several pharmaceutical treatments have shown benefit in CPSP including tricyclic antidepressants, selective noradrenergic uptake inhibitors and anticonvulsants including lamotrigine and gabapentin. Opioids are not beneficial in CPSP (71). HSP arises in the weeks to months following stroke and is directly related to the degree of motor impairment. Physical therapy is generally recommended as are topical treatments (ice, heat, massage) and oral analgesics. Intra-articular steroid injections, botulinum toxin injections, and electrical stimulation are developments with potential promise in treatment of HSP (72). Fortunately, most patients with HSP have improvement or complete resolution by 6 months after CVA. Painful spasticity is common after CVA and is best addressed with physical therapy, positioning and range of motion exercises. Antispasmodic agents should be reserved for extreme cases, which do not respond to nonpharmacological interventions (71).

Psychiatric Symptoms in Stroke Survivors

Poststroke depression is common, affecting as many as one third of stroke survivors. Depression after CVA is associated with increased dependency, delayed rehabilitation, poor functional outcome and increased mortality (73). Treatments that have shown benefit in poststroke depression include tricyclic antidepressants (TCAs) and serotonin selective reuptake inhibitors (SSRIs). Psychotherapy, though a theoretically attractive option, has thus far not shown benefit in this setting. Anxiety is also common in both the acute and chronic poststroke period. A presentation consistent with generalized anxiety disorder is most common, but panic attacks may also be seen (74). Treatment with SSRI antidepressants is most appropriate, though benzodiazepines may be used in extreme cases and/or when the expected life span is short. Some patients will display mood lability and frequent crying or laughing after stroke. Treatment of emotional lability consists primarily of reassuring and educating the patient and family members.

Fatigue in Stroke Survivors

Fatigue affects more than half of patients surviving an acute CVA. Initially, a comprehensive assessment to rule out underlying metabolic or hematologic causes should be undertaken (75). Sleep disordered breathing, which affects more than half of stroke survivors, may also be an important cause of fatigue in this population. In the absence of an underlying cause, exercise and diet modification are recommended for fatigue in stroke survivors. Stimulant drugs may have a role (modafinil has shown benefit in a small study of brainstem stroke survivors) but should be used with caution due to common adverse effects (76).

Incontinence in Stroke Survivors

Six months after acute CVA as many as 20% of patients will have urinary incontinence and as many as 10% will suffer from fecal incontinence. These symptoms may be due to the effects of the stroke itself, but they are often related to immobility and impaired communication (77). Bladder training as well as scheduled voiding and bowel movements are generally recommended in the management of incontinence. Avoidance of indwelling urinary catheters and appropriate management of constipation may also be helpful. A 2008 Cochrane systematic review found insufficient evidence to guide treatment of poststroke urinary incontinence (78).

Care Giving in Stroke Survivors

At least one-quarter of stroke survivors will be dependent in activities of daily living 6 months after their CVA. At least this many will require some degree of assistance and care giving. While many poststroke patients reside in nursing homes or other care facilities, many receive care from family members or other caregivers. In contrast to conditions such as dementia or chronic heart disease, caregivers for stroke patients often have an abrupt transition from their previous routine to their new role in caring for their loved one. Stress and burnout are common in these caregivers and many report lack of support and poor quality of life (79). The degree of functional impairment of the stroke survivor is associated with decreasing quality of life in caregivers. Caregiver training has been shown to reduce depression and anxiety as well as improve quality of life in both caregivers and stroke survivors. Trained caregivers also experience less caregiver burden. Referral to a social worker familiar with resources in the community as well as connection with patient or caregiver advocacy groups may be beneficial (80).

AGE AND ETHICAL ISSUES IN ADVANCED CARDIOVASCULAR INTERVENTIONS

As described above in reference to LVADs, advanced cardiac interventions have the potential to lengthen life and improve quality of life. As with other invasive technologies, the application of advanced surgical interventions to the elderly population raises ethical and resource concerns. The following section examines the use of advanced cardiac surgical procedures in elderly patients.

Coronary Artery Bypass Grafting and Valve Replacement

Coronary artery bypass grafting (CABG) was first performed in 1960 and has since become a standard treatment for severe coronary artery disease (81). As techniques and outcomes have improved, CABG has been offered to increasingly complicated, medically ill and older patients. It is now routine for centers in the USA, Canada, and Europe to perform CABG on patients greater than 65 and even patients in their 70s or 80s. The outcomes and complications of CABG in octogenarians have been examined by several groups (see chap. 11). Multiple investigators have reported that, though the rate of perioperative complications and mortality is higher than for younger individuals, patients over age 80 have good long-term survival, improved quality of life and an acceptable operative risk for CABG (82–84). These results come, however, with higher resource utilization in the postoperative period (85). Similar results have been demonstrated for elderly patients undergoing valve replacement surgery, particularly with replacement of the aortic valve (86). Newer less invasive valve replacement procedures also show promise in reducing complications and mortality in older patients.

Cardiac Transplantation

The first cardiac transplant was performed in South Africa in 1967 (81). There are at least 3500 cardiac transplants performed worldwide each year. Less than 5% of cardiac transplant recipients are over the age of 70, but as many as one-quarter are between the age of 60 and 70 (87). When selected based on comorbidities and overall health it appears that patients over age 60 or even over age 70 have short- and long-term survival comparable to younger patients after cardiac transplantation (88). Many centers, however, still use age as an absolute contraindication to heart transplantation (89). In light of the available evidence it does not appear ethically justifiable to deny patients cardiac transplantation solely on the basis of age (90).

Though use of these advanced surgical interventions in elderly CVD patients appears ethically justifiable from a medical perspective, it does raise questions of distributive justice in health care systems already overtaxed in providing care for entire populations. Such overarching ethical dilemmas, which will only increase with aging of the population and development of more advanced interventions, will ultimately need to be addressed at societal and public policy levels.

CONCLUSION

As the worldwide population ages the burden of CVD will continue to rise. Technological advances and increasing survival challenge healthcare professionals and systems to address the ethical issues that arise, and professionals caring for chronically ill patients will increasingly encounter ethical decisions as well as care for patients at the end of life. Education is needed to improve the knowledge and skills of healthcare professionals to navigate complex ethical issues, communicate effectively with patients and their families and provide care that is centered on patient goals and values using models of shared decision-making. As the care of chronic illness becomes more complex and costly, policymakers will be challenged to address issues of distributive justice and access to care. By partnering with patients and advocacy groups these tasks can be approached with the values of individuals and societies as guiding principles.

REFERENCES

1. Moye J, Marson DC. Assessment of decision-making capacity in older adults: an emerging area of practice and research. J Gerontol B Psychol Sci Soc Sci 2007; 62: P3–P11.
2. Appelbaum PS. Clinical practice. Assessment of patients' competence to consent to treatment. N Engl J Med 2007; 357: 1834–40.
3. Ganzini L, Volicer L, Nelson WA, Fox E, Derse AR. Ten myths about decision-making capacity. J Am Med Dir Assoc 2004; 5: 263–7.
4. Dunn LB, Nowrangi MA, Palmer BW, Jeste DV, Saks ER. Assessing decisional capacity for clinical research or treatment: a review of instruments. Am J Psychiatry 2006; 163: 1323–34.
5. Lautrette A, Peigne V, Watts J, Souweine B, Azoulay E. Surrogate decision makers for incompetent ICU patients: a European perspective. Curr Opin Crit Care 2008; 14: 714–19.
6. Fagerlin A, Schneider CE. Enough. The failure of the living will. Hastings Cent Rep 2004; 34: 30–42.
7. Hickman SE, Hammes BJ, Moss AH, Tolle SW. Hope for the future: achieving the original intent of advance directives. Hastings Cent Rep 2005; Spec No: S26–30.
8. Hammes BJ, Rooney BL. Death and end-of-life planning in one midwestern community. Arch Intern Med 1998; 158: 383–90.
9. Hickman SE, Nelson CA, Moss AH, et al. The consistency between treatments provided to nursing facility residents and orders on the physician orders for life-sustaining treatment form. J Am Geriatr Soc 2011; 59: 2091–9.
10. Tolle SW, Tilden VP, Nelson CA, Dunn PM. A prospective study of the efficacy of the physician order form for life-sustaining treatment. J Am Geriatr Soc 1998; 46: 1097–102.
11. Hammes BJ, Rooney BL, Gundrum JD, Hickman SE, Hager N. The POLST program: a retrospective review of the demographics of use and outcomes in one community where advance directives are prevalent. J Palliat Med 2012; 15: 77–85.
12. Loertscher L, Reed DA, Bannon MP, Mueller PS. Cardiopulmonary resuscitation and do-not-resuscitate orders: a guide for clinicians. Am J Med 2010; 123: 4–9.
13. Ehlenbach WJ, Barnato AE, Curtis JR, et al. Epidemiologic study of in-hospital cardiopulmonary resuscitation in the elderly. N Engl J Med 2009; 361: 22–31.
14. Lannon R, O'Keeffe ST. Cardiopulmonary resuscitation in older people – a review. Rev Clin Gerontol 2010; 20: 20.
15. de Vos R, Koster RW, De Haan RJ, et al. In-hospital cardiopulmonary resuscitation: prearrest morbidity and outcome. Arch Intern Med 1999; 159: 845–50.

16. Burns JP, Edwards J, Johnson J, Cassem NH, Truog RD. Do-not-resuscitate order after 25 years. Crit Care Med 2003; 31: 1543–50.

17. Anderson WG, Chase R, Pantilat SZ, Tulsky JA, Auerbach AD. Code status discussions between attending hospitalist physicians and medical patients at hospital admission. J Gen Intern Med 2010; 26: 359–66.

18. Gorton AJ, Jayanthi NVG, Lepping P, Scriven MW. Patients' attitudes towards "do not attempt resuscitation" status. J Med Ethics 2008; 34: 624–6.

19. Fried TR, O'Leary J, Van Ness P, Fraenkel L. Inconsistency over time in the preferences of older persons with advanced illness for life-sustaining treatment. J Am Geriatr Soc 2007; 55: 1007–14.

20. Puchalski CM, Zhong Z, Jacobs MM, et al. Patients who want their family and physician to make resuscitation decisions for them: observations from SUPPORT and HELP. Study to Understand Prognoses and Preferences for Outcomes and Risks of Treatment. Hospitalized Elderly Longitudinal Project. J Am Geriatr Soc 2000; 48: S84–90.

21. Ardagh M. Futility has no utility in resuscitation medicine. J Med Ethics 2000; 26: 396–9.

22. Hilberman M, Kutner J, Parsons D, Murphy DJ. Marginally effective medical care: ethical analysis of issues in cardiopulmonary resuscitation (CPR). J Med Ethics 1997; 23: 361–7.

23. Beach MC, Morrison RS. The effect of do-not-resuscitate orders on physician decision-making. J Am Geriatr Soc 2002; 50: 2057–61.

24. Chen JLT, Sosnov J, Lessard D, Goldberg RJ. Impact of do-not-resuscitation orders on quality of care performance measures in patients hospitalized with acute heart failure. Am Heart J 2008; 156: 78–84.

25. Tanner CE, Fromme EK, Goodlin SJ. Ethics in the treatment of advanced heart failure: palliative care and end-of-life issues. Congest Heart Fail 2011; 17: 235–40.

26. Harding R, Selman L, Beynon T, et al. Meeting the communication and information needs of chronic heart failure patients. J Pain Symptom Manage 2008; 36: 149–56.

27. The AM, Hak T, Koeter G, van Der Wal G. Collusion in doctor-patient communication about imminent death: an ethnographic study. BMJ 2000; 321: 1376–81.

28. Goodlin SJ, Quill TE, Arnold RM. Communication and decision-making about prognosis in heart failure care. J Card Fail 2008; 14: 106–13.

29. Moss AJ, Zareba W, Hall WJ, et al. Prophylactic implantation of a defibrillator in patients with myocardial infarction and reduced ejection fraction. N Engl J Med 2002; 346: 877–83.

30. Cleland JG, Daubert JC, Erdmann E, et al. The effect of cardiac resynchronization on morbidity and mortality in heart failure. N Engl J Med 2005; 352: 1539–49.

31. Long JW, Kfoury AG, Slaughter MS, et al. Long-term destination therapy with the HeartMate XVE left ventricular assist device: improved outcomes since the REMATCH study. Congest Heart Fail 2005; 11: 133–8.

32. Berger JT, Gorski M, Cohen T. Advance health planning and treatment preferences among recipients of implantable cardioverter defibrillators: an exploratory study. J Clin Ethics 2006; 17: 72–8.

33. Goldstein NE, Mehta D, Siddiqui S, et al. "That's like an act of suicide" patients' attitudes toward deactivation of implantable defibrillators. J Gen Intern Med 2008; 23: 7–12.

34. Goldstein NE, Lampert R, Bradley E, Lynn J, Krumholz HM. Management of implantable cardioverter defibrillators in end-of-life care. Ann Intern Med 2004; 141: 835–8.

35. Goldstein NE, Mehta D, Teitelbaum E, Bradley EH, Morrison RS. "It's like crossing a bridge" complexities preventing physicians from discussing deactivation of implantable defibrillators at the end of life. J Gen Intern Med 2008; 23: 2–6.

36. MacIver J, Rao V, Delgado DH, et al. Choices: a study of preferences for end-of-life treatments in patients with advanced heart failure. J Heart Lung Transplant 2008; 27: 1002–7.

37. Fromme EK, Stewart TL, Jeppesen M, Tolle SW. Adverse experiences with implantable defibrillators in Oregon hospices. Am J Hosp Palliat Care 2011; 28: 304–9.

38. Epstein AE, DiMarco JP, Ellenbogen KA, et al. ACC/AHA/HRS 2008 Guidelines for Device-Based Therapy of Cardiac Rhythm Abnormalities: a report of the American College of Cardiology/American Heart Association Task Force on Practice Guidelines (Writing Committee to Revise the ACC/AHA/NASPE 2002 Guideline Update for Implantation of Cardiac Pacemakers and Antiarrhythmia Devices): developed in collaboration with the American Association for Thoracic Surgery and Society of Thoracic Surgeons. Circulation 2008; 117: e350–408.

39. Lampert R, Hayes DL, Annas GJ, et al. HRS Expert Consensus Document on the Management of Cardiac Implantable Devices (CIEDs) in patients nearing end of life or requesting withdrawal of therapy. Heart Rhythm 2010; 7: 1008–26.

40. Brush S, Budge D, Alharethi R, et al. End-of-life decision making and implementation in recipients of a destination left ventricular assist device. J Heart Lung Transplant 2010; 29: 1337–41.

41. Swetz KM, Freeman MR, AbouEzzeddine OF, et al. Palliative medicine consultation for preparedness planning in patients receiving left ventricular assist devices as destination therapy. Mayo Clin Proc 2011; 86: 493–500.

42. Swetz KM, Ottenberg AL, Freeman MR, Mueller PS. Palliative care and end-of-life issues in patients treated with left ventricular assist devices as destination therapy. Curr Heart Fail Rep 2011; 8: 212–18.

43. Bunzel B, Laederach-Hofmann K, Wieselthaler G, Roethy W, Wolner E. Mechanical circulatory support as a bridge to heart transplantation: what remains? Long-term emotional sequelae in patients and spouses. J Heart Lung Transplant 2007; 26: 384–9.

44. Cubbon RM, Gale CP, Kearney LC, et al. Changing characteristics and mode of death associated with chronic heart failure caused by left ventricular systolic dysfunction: a study across therapeutic eras. Circ Heart Fail 2011; 4: 396–403.

45. Goodlin SJ, Kutner JS, Connor SR, et al. Hospice care for heart failure patients. J Pain Symptom Manage 2005; 29: 525–8.

46. Goodlin SJ, Trupp R, Bernhardt P, Grady KL, Dracup K. Development and evaluation of the "Advanced Heart Failure Clinical Competence Survey": a tool to assess knowledge of heart failure care and self-assessed competence. Patient Educ Couns 2007; 67: 3–10.

47. Bain KT, Maxwell TL, Strassels SA, Whellan DJ. Hospice use among patients with heart failure. Am Heart J 2009; 158: 118–25.

48. Levy WC, Mozaffarian D, Linker DT, et al. The Seattle Heart Failure Model: prediction of survival in heart failure. Circulation 2006; 113: 1424–33.

49. Bekelman DB, Rumsfeld JS, Havranek EP, et al. Symptom burden, depression, and spiritual well-being: a comparison of heart failure and advanced cancer patients. J Gen Intern Med 2009; 24: 592–8.

50. Goodlin SJ. Palliative care in congestive heart failure. J Am Coll Cardiol 2009; 54: 386–96.

51. Blinderman CD, Homel P, Billings JA, Portenoy RK, Tennstedt SL. Symptom distress and quality of life in patients with advanced congestive heart failure. J Pain Symptom Manage 2008; 35: 594–603.

52. Goebel JR, Doering LV, Shugarman LR, et al. Heart failure: the hidden problem of pain. J Pain Symptom Manage 2009; 38: 698–707.

53. Cully JA, Johnson M, Moffett ML, Khan M, Deswal A. Depression and anxiety in ambulatory patients with heart failure. Psychosomatics 2009; 50: 592–8.

54. Zambroski CH, Moser DK, Bhat G, Ziegler C. Impact of symptom prevalence and symptom burden on quality of life in patients with heart failure. Eur J Cardiovasc Nurs 2005; 4: 198–206.

55. Chang VT, Hwang SS, Feuerman M. Validation of the Edmonton symptom assessment scale. Cancer 2000; 88: 2164–71.

56. Puchalski CM. Spirituality and end-of-life care: a time for listening and caring. J Palliat Med 2002; 5: 289–94.

57. Roger VL, Go AS, Lloyd-Jones DM, et al. Heart disease and stroke statistics–2012 update: a report from the American Heart Association. Circulation 2012; 125: e2–e220.

58. Steiner T, Mendoza G, De Georgia M, et al. Prognosis of stroke patients requiring mechanical ventilation in a neurological critical care unit. Stroke 1997; 28: 711–15.

59. Martino R, Foley N, Bhogal S, et al. Dysphagia after stroke: incidence, diagnosis, and pulmonary complications. Stroke 2005; 36: 2756–63.

60. Sandman L, Agren Bolmsjo I, Westergren A. Ethical considerations of refusing nutrition after stroke. Nurs Ethics 2008; 15: 147–59.

61. Blackmer J. Tube feeding in stroke patients: a medical and ethical perspective. Can J Neurol Sci 2001; 28: 101–6.

62. Stevens T, Payne S, Burton C, Addington-Hall J, Jones A. Palliative care in stroke: a critical review of the literature. Palliat Med 2007; 21: 323–31.

63. Burton CR, Payne S, Addington-Hall J, Jones A. The palliative care needs of acute stroke patients: a prospective study of hospital admissions. Age Ageing 2010; 39: 554–9.

64. Mazzocato C, Michel-Nemitz J, Anwar D, Michel P. The last days of dying stroke patients referred to a palliative care consult team in an acute hospital. Eur J Neurol 2010; 17: 73–7.

65. Jack C. Towards a good death: the impact of the care of the dying pathway in an acute stroke unit. Age Ageing 2004; 33: 625–6.

66. e BlacquierDP, Gubitz GJ, et al. Evaluating an organized palliative care approach in patients with severe stroke. Can J Neurol Sci 2009; 36: 731–4.

67. Cowey E. End of life care for patients following acute stroke. Nurs Stand 2012; 26: 42–6.

68. duPreez AE, Smith MA, Liou J-I, et al. Predictors of hospice utilization among acute stroke patients who died within thirty days. J Palliat Med 2008; 11: 1249–57.

69. Kelly-Hayes M, Beiser A, Kase CS, et al. The influence of gender and age on disability following ischemic stroke: the Framingham study. J Stroke Cerebrovasc Dis 2003; 12: 119–26.

70. Klit H, Finnerup NB, Jensen TS. Central post-stroke pain: clinical characteristics, pathophysiology, and management. Lancet Neurol 2009; 8: 857–68.

71. Creutzfeldt CJ, Holloway RG, Walker M. Symptomatic and palliative care for stroke survivors. J Gen Intern Med 2012; 27: 853–60.

72. Koog YH, Jin SS, Yoon K, Min BI. Interventions for hemiplegic shoulder pain: systematic review of randomised controlled trials. Disabil Rehabil 2010; 32: 282–91.

73. Hackett ML, Anderson CS, House A, Xia J. Interventions for treating depression after stroke. Cochrane Database Syst Rev 2008: CD003437.

74. Castillo CS, Starkstein SE, Fedoroff JP, Price TR, Robinson RG. Generalized anxiety disorder after stroke. J Nerv Ment Dis 1993; 181: 100–6.

75. Mead GE, Graham C, Dorman P, et al. Fatigue after stroke: baseline predictors and influence on survival. Analysis of data from UK patients recruited in the International Stroke Trial. PLoS One 2011; 6: e16988.

76. Brioschi A, Gramigna S, Werth E, et al. Effect of modafinil on subjective fatigue in multiple sclerosis and stroke patients. Eur Neurol 2009; 62: 243–9.

77. Nakayama H, Jorgensen HS, Pedersen PM, Raaschou HO, Olsen TS. Prevalence and risk factors of incontinence after stroke. The Copenhagen Stroke Study. Stroke 1997; 28: 58–62.

78. Thomas LH, Cross S, Barrett J, et al. Treatment of urinary incontinence after stroke in adults. Cochrane Database Syst Rev 2008: CD004462.

79. Han B, Haley WE. Family caregiving for patients with stroke. Review and analysis. Stroke 1999; 30: 1478–85.

80. Kalra L, Evans A, Perez I, et al. Training carers of stroke patients: randomised controlled trial. BMJ 2004; 328: 1099.

81. Weisse AB. Cardiac surgery: a century of progress. Tex Heart Inst J 2011; 38: 486–90.

82. Baskett R, Buth K, Ghali W, et al. Outcomes in octogenarians undergoing coronary artery bypass grafting. CMAJ 2005; 172: 1183–6.

83. Conaway DG, House J, Bandt K, et al. The elderly: health status benefits and recovery of function one year after coronary artery bypass surgery. J Am Coll Cardiol 2003; 42: 1421–6.

84. Stoica SC, Cafferty F, Kitcat J, et al. Octogenarians undergoing cardiac surgery outlive their peers: a case for early referral. Heart 2006; 92: 503–6.

85. Scott BH, Seifert FC, Grimson R, Glass PSA. Octogenarians undergoing coronary artery bypass graft surgery: resource utilization, postoperative mortality, and morbidity. J Cardiothorac Vasc Anesth 2005; 19: 583–8.

86. Ashikhmina EA, Schaff HV, Dearani JA, et al. Aortic valve replacement in the elderly: determinants of late outcome. Circulation 2011; 124: 1070–8.

87. Longo DL. Harrison's Principles of Internal Medicine, 18th edn. New York: McGraw-Hill, 2012.

88. Daneshvar DA, Czer LS, Phan A, Trento A, Schwarz ER. Heart transplantation in the elderly: why cardiac transplantation does not need to be limited to younger patients but can be safely performed in patients above 65 years of age. Ann Transplant 2010; 15: 110–19.

89. Mancini D, Lietz K. Selection of cardiac transplantation candidates in 2010. Circulation 2010; 122: 173–83.

90. Robbins RC. Ethical implications of heart transplantation in elderly patients. J Thorac Cardiovasc Surg 2001; 121: 0434–5.

Index